THE GUIDE TO CARDIOLOGY
THIRD EDITION

Edited by

Robert A. Kloner, MD, PhD
Professor of Medicine
Section of Cardiology
University of Southern California
Director of Research
Heart Institute
Good Samaritan Hospital
Los Angeles, California

Le Jacq Communications, Inc.
777 West Putnam Avenue
Greenwich, Connecticut 06830

Preface

Cardiology remains one of the most rapidly evolving fields of internal medicine in terms of diagnostic techniques, pharmacologic therapy, catheter intervention techniques, and surgical therapeutic options. Since 1990, when the second edition of *The Guide to Cardiology* was published, there have been tremendous advances in the field. Transesophageal echocardiography and intravascular ultrasound have given us new ways to assess cardiac and vascular structure. Electrophysiologic testing has become standard in many medical centers for aiding in the diagnosis and treatment of arrhythmias. The use of thrombolytic therapy for myocardial infarction continues to grow and new adjunctive therapies such as hirudin and hirulog are under investigation. Left ventricular remodeling has emerged as a major post-infarct complication that is amenable to therapy. Powerful lipid-lowering agents are on the market and atherosclerotic regression is becoming a reality. Interventional cardiology has continued to grow not only with the use of coronary angioplasty, but stents, atherectomy, and percutaneous balloon valvuloplasty devices. The automatic implantable cardioverter-defibrillator has been shown to prevent sudden death, while the wide use of antiarrhythmic pharmacologic therapy has come under question. The practice of medicine is rapidly changing as managed care sweeps across the United States; with it, changes in the practice of cardiology are inevitable.

A number of large and comprehensive cardiology texts offer detailed information about the ever-broadening knowledge base of cardiology. Realizing that many clinicians do not have the time to read these texts thoroughly, I've undertaken *The Guide to Cardiology* to provide a selective, concise, current, and practical handbook on the fundamentals of the specialty. As in the previous editions, the first half of the book reviews diagnostic techniques and procedures. Along with updating the existing chapters, we have completely rewritten sections on electrocardiography, exercise testing, electrophysiology, and advanced cardiac imaging.

The second half of the book presents chapters on specific problems in cardiology that the clinician is likely to encounter, such as hyperlipidemia, myocardial infarction, angina pectoris, cardiac arrhythmias, conduction abnormalities, valvular heart disease, cardiomyopathy and myocarditis, heart failure, hypertension, and congenital heart disease. These chapters have been revised. There is a thorough review of newer thrombolytic trials, updates on interventional cardiology, and therapy for heart failure. The section on congenital heart disease has been substantially expanded since the last edition. The chapters on pulmonary hypertension and pregnancy in heart disease have been totally rewritten. New additions include chapters on the implantable cardioverter defibrillator, left ventricular remodeling after myocardial infarction, and how managed care will impact the practice of cardiology. There are chapters that deal with the approach to patients with cardiac and non-cardiac surgery that the cardiology consultant may find especially useful. Also included are chapters on areas such as the effect of exercise on the heart, cardiopulmonary resuscitation, diseases of the aorta, and cardiac problems in systemic diseases, including AIDS.

My hope is that physicians will find the text a useful guide for clinical practice. It may also be a useful review text for physicians such as cardiology fellows, residents preparing for board examinations, and for trainees who are participating in rotations on cardiology services.

The drugs, indications for drugs, and drug dosages referred to throughout this book are commonly used by practicing cardiologists and suggested by the authors. However, not all drugs, doses, and indications mentioned are Food and Drug Administration approved. Therefore, it is suggested that the package inserts or Physicians' Desk Reference be consulted as well for drug indications, contraindications, side effects, and dosages as recommended by the Food and Drug Administration. While the procedures and treatments in this text are based upon current standard practices, they should serve as a guide and not as the sole reference or sole determinant for practice and therapy of individual patients.

I wish to acknowledge the excellent help and advice of Suzanne Del Gallo. I would also like to thank Cathy Davisson for her help with typing portions of this manuscript.

Robert A. Kloner, MD, PhD
Los Angeles, CA
October 1994

Contributors

Anil K. Bhandari, MD
Clinical Associate Professor of Medicine
Los Angeles County USC Medical School
Director, Electrophysiology Laboratory
Heart Institute
Good Samaritan Hospital
Los Angeles, CA

Edward J. Brown, MD
Director, Cardiology Division
Bronx-Lebanon Hospital Center
Bronx, NY

Bruce H. Brundage, MD
Professor of Medicine and Radiological Sciences
UCLA School of Medicine
Chief of Cardiology
Harbor-UCLA Medical Center
Scientific Director,
St. John's Cardiovascular Research Center
Torrance, CA

David S. Cannom, MD
Clinical Professor of Medicine
UCLA School of Medicine
Medical Director
Division of Cardiology
Good Samaritan Hospital
Los Angeles, CA

Richard Caso, MD
Medical Director
Orange County Heart Center
Aliso Viejo, CA

Maria F. De Guzman, MD
Assistant Professor of Medicine
University of Southern California
School of Medicine
Director, Electrocardiography
Los Angeles County USC Medical School
Los Angeles, CA

Victor Dzau, MD
Arthur L. Bloomfield, Professor of Medicine
Chairman, Department of Medicine
Stanford University School of Medicine
Stanford, CA

Andrew C. Eisenhauer, MD
Clinical Instructor in Medicine
Harvard Medical School
Boston, MA
Director, Cardiac Catheterization Laboratory
and Interventional Cardiovascular Medicine
Lahey Clinic
Burlington, MA

Michael B. Fowler, MB, MRCP
Associate Professor of Medicine
Division of Cardiovascular Medicine
Stanford School of Medicine
Stanford, CA

Peter L. Friedman, MD, PhD
Associate Professor of Medicine
Harvard Medical School
Co-Director, Cardiac Arrhythmia Service and
Clinical Electrophysiology Laboratory
Brigham and Women's Hospital
Boston, MA

Demetrios Georgiou, MD
Assistant Professor of Medicine
UCLA School of Medicine
Director of the Ultrafast CT Scanner
Saint John's Cardiovascular Research Center
Director of the Cardiology Clinic
Harbor-UCLA Medical Center
Torrance, CA

Samuel Z. Goldhaber, MD
Associate Professor of Medicine
Harvard Medical School
Physician, Brigham and Women's Hospital
Boston, MA

Lee Goldman, MD
Professor of Medicine
Chairman, Department of Medicine
Associate Dean for Clinical Affairs
University of California San Francisco
San Francisco, CA

Thomas B. Graboys, MD
Associate Clinical Professor of Medicine
Harvard Medical School
Director, Lown Cardiovascular Center
Physician, Brigham and Women's Hospital
Boston, MA

Brian P. Griffin, MD
Staff Cardiologist
Section of Cardiovascular Imaging
Department of Cardiology
The Cleveland Clinic Foundation
Cleveland, OH

James M. Hagar, MD
Associate Professor of Medicine
University of California at Irvine
Department of Veterans Affairs
Long Beach, CA

Haim Hammerman, MD
Director, Intensive Coronary Care Unit
Cardiology Department
Rambam Medical Center
Haifa, Israel

Joshua M. Hare, MD
Instructor in Medicine
Harvard Medical School
Junior Associate in Medicine,
Cardiovascular Division
Brigham and Women's Hospital
Boston, MA

Donald P. Harrington, MD
Professor and Chairman,
Department of Radiology
Stony Brook Health Sciences Center
State University of New York at Stony Brook
School of Medicine
Stony Brook, NY

L. David Hillis, MD
Professor of Medicine
James M. Wooten Chair in Cardiology
Associate Director, Cardiovascular Division
University of Texas
Southwestern Medical Center
Dallas, TX

Robert A. Kloner, MD, PhD
Professor of Medicine
Section of Cardiology
University of Southern California
Director of Research
Heart Institute
Good Samaritan Hospital
Los Angeles, CA

Dusan Z. Kocovic, MD
Assistant Professor of Medicine
University of Pennsylvania School of Medicine
Director, Electrophysiology Laboratory
Cardiovascular Division
Hospital of the University of Pennsylvania,
Philadelphia
Philadelphia, PA

Richard A. Lange, MD
Associate Professor of Medicine
University of Texas
Southwestern Medical Center
Director, Cardiac Catheterization Laboratory
Parkland Memorial Hospital
Dallas, TX

Thomas H. Lee, MD, ScM
Assistant Professor of Medicine
Harvard Medical School
Chief, Section for Clinical Epidemiology
Brigham and Women's Hospital
Boston, MA

Marlo F. Leonen, MD
Cardiology Fellow
Harper Hospital and Wayne State University
School of Medicine
Detroit, MI

Jonathan Leor, MD
Cardiology Fellow
University of Southern California
Heart Institute
Good Samaritan Hospital
Los Angeles, CA

Richard R. Liberthson, MD
Associate Professor of Pediatrics
Associate Physician in Medicine
Harvard Medical School
Pediatrician at Massachusetts General Hospital
Boston, MA

Leonard S. Lilly, MD
Associate Professor of Medicine
Harvard Medical School
Physician, Brigham and Women's Hospital
Boston, MA

Sylvia A. Mamby, MD
Assistant Professor of Medicine
Mayo Medical School
Consultant, Cardiovascular Diseases
Mayo Clinic Scottsdale
Scottsdale, AZ

James D. Marsh, MD
Professor of Medicine
Director of Cardiology Research
Harper Hospital and Wayne State University
School of Medicine
Detroit, MI

David T. Martin, MBBS
Instructor in Medicine
Harvard Medical School
Director, Cardiac Electrophysiology
Laboratory
Lahey Clinic
Burlington, MA

John H. McAnulty, MD
Professor of Medicine
Division of Cardiology
Oregon Health Sciences University
Portland, OR

Gary F. Mitchell, MD
Instructor in Medicine
Harvard Medical School
Cardiovascular Division
Brigham and Women's Hospital
Boston, MA

Gilbert H. Mudge, Jr, MD
Associate Professor of Medicine
Harvard Medical School
Director, Clinical Cardiology Service
Medical Director
Cardiac Transplantation Program
Cardiovascular Division,
Brigham and Women's Hospital
Boston, MA

Allen J. Naftilan, MD, PhD
Assistant Professor of Medicine
and Pharmacology
Division of Cardiology
Vanderbilt University School of Medicine
Nashville, TN

Stephen N. Oesterle, MD
Associate Professor of Medicine (Cardiovascular)
Director, Cardiac Catheterization and Coronary
Interventional Laboratories
Stanford University Medical Center
Stanford, CA

Harold G. Olson, MD
Associate Professor of Medicine
University of California at Irvine
Department of Veterans Affairs
Long Beach, CA

Natesa G. Pandian, MD
Associate Professor of Medicine and Radiology
Tufts University School of Medicine
Director, Cardiovascular Imaging and
Hemodynamic Laboratory
New England Medical Center
Boston, MA

Priscilla J. Peters, BA, RDCS
Division of Cardiology
Harper Hospital
Wayne State University
Detroit, MI

Marc A. Pfeffer, MD, PhD
Associate Professor of Medicine
Harvard Medical School
Cardiovascular Division
Brigham and Women's Hospital
Boston, MA

Joseph F. Polak, MD, MPH
Associate Professor of Radiology
Harvard Medical School
Department of Radiology
Brigham and Women's Hospital
Boston, MA

Charles Pollick, MB, CHB
Clinical Associate Professor of Medicine
UCLA School of Medicine
Medical Director Noninvasive Cardiology
Good Samaritan Hospital
Los Angeles, CA

Shereif Rezkalla, MD
Clinical Assistant Professor
University of Wisconsin, Madison, MI
Director of Cardiovascular Research
Department of Cardiology
Marshfield Clinic
Marshfield, WI

Steven L. Schwartz, MD
Assistant Professor of Medicine
Tufts University School of Medicine
Associate Director, Cardiovascular Imaging and
Hemodynamic Laboratory
New England Medical Center
Boston, MA

Thomas L. Shook, MD
Director, Coronary Care Unit
Director, Acute Myocardial Interventional Program
Heart Institute
Good Samaritan Hospital
Los Angeles, CA

Neil J. Stone, MD
Associate Professor of Medicine
Section of Cardiology
Northwestern University
School of Medicine
Chicago, IL

Peter H. Stone, MD
Associate Professor of Medicine
Harvard Medical School
Brigham and Women's Hospital
Co-Director, Samuel A. Levine Cardiac Unit
Director, Clinical Trials
Cardiovascular Division
Department of Medicine
Boston, MA

James D. Thomas, MD
Professor of Medicine
Ohio State University
Director of Cardiovascular Imaging
Department of Cardiology
The Cleveland Clinic Foundation
Cleveland, OH

Richard D. White, MD
Head, Section of Cardiovascular Imaging
Diagnostic Radiology
The Cleveland Clinic Foundation
Cleveland, OH

John E. Willard, MD
Assistant Professor of Medicine
University of Texas Southwestern
Medical Center
Dallas, TX

Richard F. Wright, MD
Assistant Professor of Medicine
UCLA School of Medicine
Los Angeles, CA
Director of Research
Pacific Heart Institute
Santa Monica, CA

Joshua Wynne, MD
Professor and Chief, Division of Cardiology
Wayne State University
Harper Hospital
Detroit, MI

Dedicated to Shirley and Philip Kloner

Contents

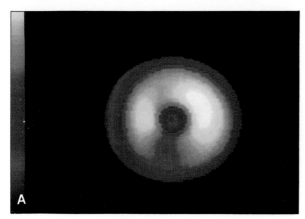 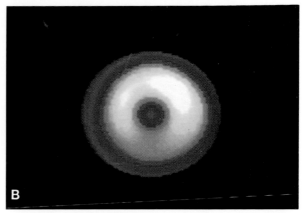

Figure 4. Thallium-201 Bullseye Plot. These short-axis SPECT images are a superposition of the quantitative information contained on multiple short axis views. The maximal uptake of thallium-201 for each point in the short axis is obtained as shown in Figures 2 and 3. The data are then displayed as a series of concentric color-encoded circles. The more central circle corresponds to the apex while the larger one represents the left ventricular base. The presence of a significant stenotic lesion in the inferior wall shows up nicely as a region of decreased thallium uptake (blue) (4A). This is then compared with resting (redistribution) view on the same patient. This confirms that the defect corresponds to ischemic yet viable myocardium (4B). **From Chapter 5.**

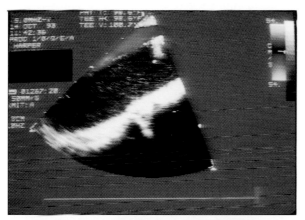 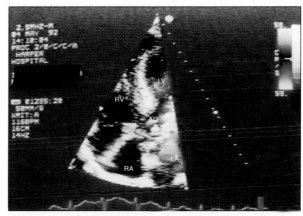

Figure 10B. From Chapter 7. Aortic dissection.

Figure 18D. From Chapter 7. Perforation into RA.

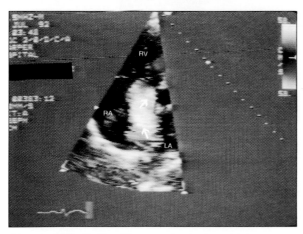 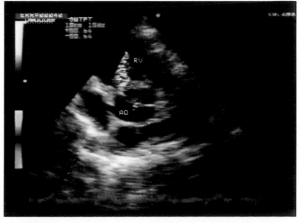

Figure 19B. From Chapter 7. Left-to-Right Shunt through ASD.

Figure 20. Short-axis view at the level of the aortic valve, demonstrating color flow across a perimembranous ventricular septal defect in a 21-year-old patient. Ao=Aorta; RV=Right ventricle. **From Chapter 7.**

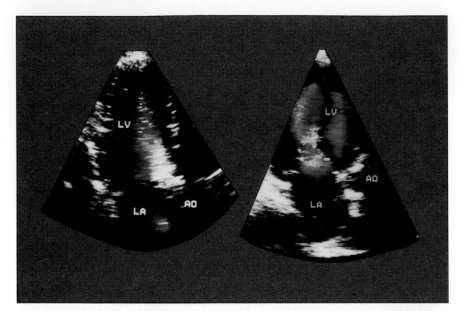

Figure 2. *Color-flow mapping of normal left ventricular flows as recorded from the apical long axis view. The systolic frame (left) illustrates left ventricular outflow. The flow is going away from the transducer and is encoded with a bright blue color. In the diastolic frame (right), flow is seen going from the left atrium (LA) to the left ventricle (LV). The blood is traveling toward the transducer and is depicted as red. The center of the flow jet, which is near the mitral annulus, contains flow velocity exceeding the Nyquist limit, and frequency aliasing is noted. There are progressively brighter shades of red with color reversal to blue in the central core. Also seen is vortex flow, or blood that has hit the apex and is turning toward the outflow tract. This is seen as faint blue. Ao=Aorta.* **From Chapter 8.**

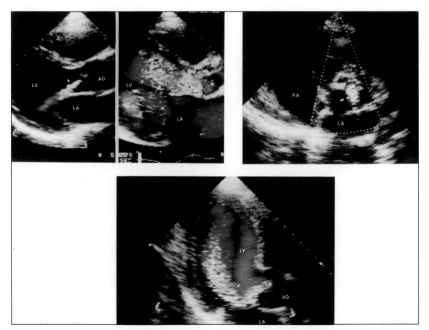

Figure 7. *Color Doppler images of aortic insufficiency from the parasternal long-axis (top left and center), short-axis (top right), and apical (bottom) views. In the parasternal long-axis view, the regurgitant flow is seen as a blue jet going from the left ventricular outflow tract toward the mitral valve and posterior wall (arrow). The recording on the top left is from a patient with mild AR; the jet in the center panel occupies the entire LV outflow and is from a patient with severe AR. The jet is seen as a bright area of turbulence within the outflow tract in the short-axis view. In the apical long-axis view (bottom), the predominantly red jet is seen first deflecting off the anterior mitral leaflet, then heading toward the center of the LV. Ao=Aorta; LA=Left atrium; LV=Left ventricle; RA=Right atrium.* **From Chapter 8.**

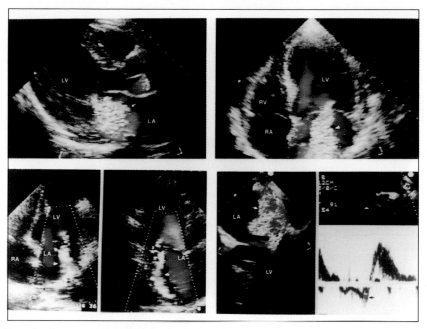

Figure 9A. *Color Doppler images recorded in the apical long axis view from 2 patients with mitral regurgitation (MR). The top left is from the parasternal long axis, top right is from the apical chambers. The mitral regurgitation jets (arrow) are seen as bright mosaic patterns in the left atrium due to high velocity turbulent flow. The jets occupy a large portion of the left atrium (LA) and signify severe MR. The frames on the bottom left are from a patient with mitral valve prolapse and severe MR. The jets are eccentric, hugging the wall of the LA. The frames on the right are recorded using TEE. The color jet in the LA is red, as it is traveling toward the transducer. The pulmonary venous tracing exhibits retrograde systolic flow (black arrow), denoting severe MR. LV=Left ventricle; RA=Right atrium; RV=Right ventricle.* **From Chapter 8.**

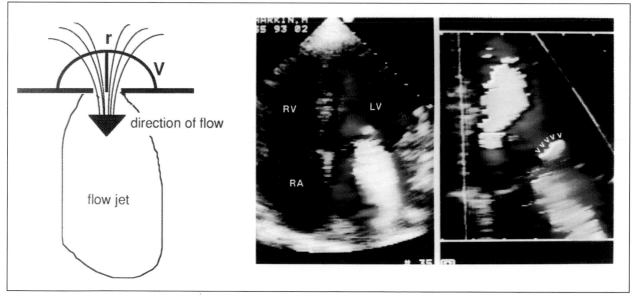

Figure 9B. *An illustration of the PISA method. The schematic on the left demonstrates the proximal flow convergence on the ventricular side of the mitral valve, through which isovelocity lines can be drawn. The surface area of the resultant hemiellipse can be calculated using the distance between the mitral valve and isovelocity line as the radius (r). Multiplying this surface area by the velocity at the line (V) provides the instantaneous volumetric flow. The center panel is an apical 4-chamber view from a patient with severe MR. By magnifying the region of the regurgitant orifice and altering the color bar so that the Nyquist limit is set low, the region of proximal flow convergence can be more accurately measured (right). The outline of the isovelocity line at which red-blue aliasing occurs is demarcated by the arrowheads. The distance from the valve to this point is the radius of the hemiellipse. LV=Left ventricle; RA=Right atrium; RV=Right ventricle.* **From Chapter 8.**

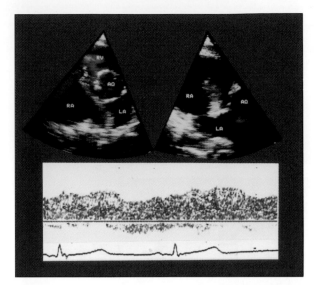

Figure 11. *Color Doppler and CW Doppler recordings from a patient with an atrial septal defect. The image in the top left is from a parasternal short axis view. The frame on the top right was recorded from a low right parasternal position. The interatrial septum lies almost perpendicular to the ultrasound beam in this orientation. In both images, the shunt flow is visualized as an orange jet traveling from the left atrium (LA) to the right atrium(RA). Ao=Aorta; RV=Right ventricle. The CW tracing (bottom) illustrates the typical continuous low velocity flow profile of an interatrial shunt.* **From Chapter 8.**

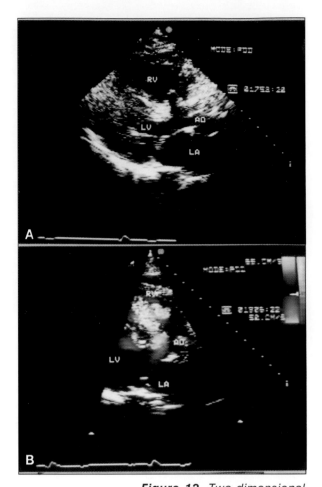

Figure 12. *Two-dimensional echocardiographic (A) and color Doppler images (B) from a patient with a congenital membranous ventricular septal defect and an aneurysm of the membranous septum as recorded from the parasternal long axis view. The 2-dimensional echo image in A is for orientation. The color Doppler image in B shows a bright red mosaic jet traveling from the left ventricle (LV) to the right ventricle (RV) through the defect. LA=Left atrium; Ao=Aorta.* **From Chapter 8.**

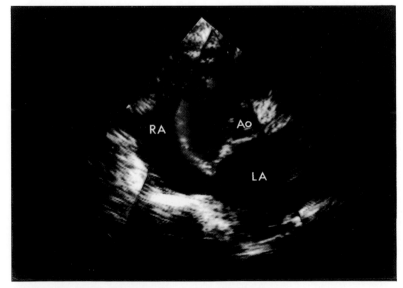

Figure 3C. From Chapter 25. *Left-to-Right shunt through an iatrogenic atrial septal defect.*

1

The Cardiac History

Robert A. Kloner, MD, PhD

Despite the recent surge in cardiac diagnostic technology, the history and physical examination remain the cornerstones of the patient work-up.[1-3] This chapter discusses the cardiac history and reviews the major symptoms directly related to the heart: chest pain, shortness of breath (dyspnea), syncope, edema, palpitations, cough, hemoptysis, cyanosis, and fatigue.

CHEST PAIN

In most cases the cause of chest pain can be derived from an adequate history. The patient should be questioned as to the quality, duration, radiation, exacerbating and ameliorating factors, and frequency of the pain. Chest pain due to angina pectoris is typically a dull, substernal pain or pressure that radiates down the arms and up into the jaw; typically lasts a few to 15 minutes; is exacerbated by exertion, anxiety, and cold; and is relieved by rest and nitroglycerin. Patients often will not refer to angina as pain but will describe it as an uncomfortable sensation or discomfort. Other descriptions include a "burning," "squeezing," or "tight" sensation. When angina is suspected, the patient should be questioned regarding the presence of cardiac risk factors such as smoking, hypertension, hyperlipidemia, and diabetes.

The chest pain of myocardial infarction may be similar to that of angina but is usually more severe, is not relieved by rest or nitroglycerin, and lasts longer. A careful history of drug use should be obtained, given recent data implicating cocaine as a cause of myocardial infarction.[4] Pericardial chest pain tends to be sharper than angina, positional (worse when the patient is lying down and often relieved by sitting up), and exacerbated by inspiration.

Several cardiac conditions cause chest pain that may mimic the pain of angina, such as hypertrophic cardiomyopathy, mitral valve prolapse, pulmonary hypertension, and myocarditis. The pain of mitral valve prolapse is often of shorter duration and may not be related to exertion.

Many noncardiac causes of chest pain may be confused with cardiac chest pain. Noncardiac causes of chest pain and their differentiating features are listed in the Table.

DYSPNEA

Dyspnea is defined as an uncomfortable awareness of breathing, with a need for increased ventilation. When dyspnea is due to chronic organic heart disease, it is typically exacerbated by exertion and develops gradually over weeks to months.[1-3,7]

Dyspnea at rest is more common in lung disease but is also exacerbated by exertion, making the distinction between cardiac and pulmonary dyspnea difficult. The dyspnea of bronchospasm may be relieved by bronchodilators and steroids; that of heart failure by diuretics, vasodilators, and digitalis. Further differentiating features between these 2 types of dyspnea will be discussed in later chapters. Both cardiac and pulmonary dyspnea should be differentiated from functional dyspnea, which occurs at rest, may not be exacerbated by exertion, and is often accompanied by anxiety. This form of dyspnea may be associated with atypical chest pain and actually relieved by exertion. Normal persons may experience dyspnea upon exercise depending upon their degree of training. Sudden onset of dyspnea at rest may be due to a variety of causes, including pneumothorax, pulmonary embolism, and pulmonary edema. End-stage heart disease is

---

Table 1. Noncardiac Causes of Chest Pain that May Mimic Cardiac Pain

DISEASE ENTITY	DIFFERENTIATING FEATURES
Musculoskeletal	Pain tends to be exacerbated by motion of certain extremities and certain postures; often follows a nerve route distribution; point tenderness may be present in costochondritis.
Herpes zoster	Chest wall pain occurs several days before development of typical rash; pain follows dermatome distribution.
Pleuritis, pneumonitis Pulmonary embolism	Pain is sharp, worse with inspiration, associated with fever, cough. pleuritic when there is an associated infarction; shortness of breath is typically present; massive pulmonary embolus associated with cardiovascular collapse, may be confused with myocardial infarction.
Esophageal	Esophagitis and esophageal spasm often mimic angina; esophageal spasm may be relieved by nitroglycerin; patient may complain of regurgitation of food and have relief with antacids; pain may radiate to back.[5]
Gastric and duodenal (gastritis, ulcers)	Epigastric discomfort typically is exacerbated by aspirin, alcohol, and relieved by food, antacids.
Gall bladder (cholecystitis)	Right upper quadrant cramping; pain exacerbated by fatty foods, occurs after eating; there may be associated ECG abnormalities.
Pancreatitis	Mid- and epigastric abdominal pain; possible history of associated alcohol ingestion; exacerbated by ingestion of food.
Functional	Nonexertional chest tightness often associated with anxiety, hyperventilation and perioral paresthesia; "panic attack."[6]
Aortic dissection	Pain typically is sharp, tearing in nature, may radiate to the back; onset of pain is often as severe as pain ever becomes, in contrast to myocardial infarction, in which the pain has a crescendo-like onset.

---

associated with chronic dyspnea at rest. A history suggesting cardiac dyspnea should lead the interviewer to question the patient about a history of rheumatic fever, a history of a heart murmur, a history of chest pain, and family history of heart disease.

Orthopnea is dyspnea that occurs while the patient is recumbent. It is due to redistribution of fluid from dependent parts of the circulation to the thorax. It occurs in patients with heart failure and is relieved by standing or sitting. Paroxysmal nocturnal dyspnea is an extreme form of orthopnea in which the patient wakes from sleep with a sense of severe breathlessness and suffocation. This symptom is due to interstitial pulmonary edema. In some patients with coronary artery disease, transient ischemic episodes may be experienced as dyspnea upon exertion, so called anginal equivalents. Such dyspnea may be an early marker of coronary artery disease.[8]

SYNCOPE

Syncope is a temporary loss of consciousness associated with muscle weakness and inability to stand. Common cardiac causes include arrhythmias (both tachyarrhythmias and bradyarrhythmias, including atrioventricular block and sick sinus syndrome). Stokes-Adams attacks are episodes of loss of consciousness due to asystole or ventricular fibrillation in the setting of high degrees of atrioventricular block. One form of cardiac syncope results from episodic ventricular fibrillation associated with prolonged QT interval, and may be familial. In this condition, ventricular fibrillation may spontaneously revert to sinus rhythm.

Other causes of cardiac syncope include valvular heart disease (especially aortic stenosis), hypertrophic obstructive cardiomyopathy, congenital heart disease (especially tetralogy of Fallot), atrial myxoma, cardiac tamponade, acute myocardial infarction, mitral valve prolapse, vasovagal attacks, and orthostatic hypotension, which is often associated with administration of certain antihypertensive medicines.

Cerebrovascular disease and subclavian steal syndrome may also result in syncope. A rare cause of syncope is excessive sensitivity of the carotid baroreceptor to pressure. In this condition — carotid sinus syncope — slight pressure to the neck (tight collar, rapid turning of the head) causes extreme bradycardia coupled with peripheral vasodilatation and hypotension.

Another rare cause is associated with excessive coughing, resulting in increases in intrathoracic pressure large enough to reduce systemic venous return. Other causes of syncope are hypoglycemia, hyperventilation, migraine headache, and micturition. Loss of consciousness may also occur with seizures and should be differentiated from syncope of cardiac origin.

The history may be extremely useful in differentiating the causes of syncope, especially if a witness observed the patient during the event. For example, if the patient was observed to develop loss of consciousness associated with typical epileptiform movements and incontinence, then seizure is more likely to be the diagnosis. However, Stokes-Adams attacks may be associated with a few clonic jerks due to reduced perfusion to the brain. Patients should be questioned about the presence of an aura before the loss of consciousness, which suggests seizures as a diagnosis. Also, recovery of consciousness tends to occur more slowly in patients with seizure disorders than with syncope due to cardiac disease. Abrupt loss of consciousness suggests Stokes-Adams attacks, other cardiac arrhythmias, or seizures as a cause. Gradual onset of syncope is more suggestive of a vasodepressor reaction or syncope due to a metabolic cause, such as

hypoglycemia or hyperventilation. The patient should be questioned about the presence of palpitations before syncope, which may suggest arrhythmias as a cause.

A history of syncope associated with a change in body position from lying to standing suggests orthostatic hypotension. Syncope associated with a change in body position, such as bending over or leaning forward, is suggestive of left atrial myxoma or ball-valve thrombus of the left atrium. Syncope independent of changes in body position occurs with arrhythmias, asystole, and hyperventilation; seizures also occur independent of body position. Syncope occurring after exertion of the upper extremities may suggest subclavian "steal" syndrome as a cause. The patient should be questioned in detail about antihypertensive drug use, which may contribute to orthostatic hypotension as a cause of syncope.

Vasodepressor syncope—the common faint—typically occurs in persons undergoing emotional or physical stress (such as pain). These patients often have a chronic history of such episodes. The episodes are accompanied by peripheral vasodilatation and bradycardia, and can be terminated by having the patient lie down.

The syncope of hypertrophic obstructive cardiomyopathy typically occurs after cessation of exercise, while the patient is in an upright position or maintaining an erect posture for a long period, when standing suddenly, or after coughing. A family history of syncope is not uncommon.

The patient should be questioned as to history of known valvular or congenital heart disease; history of transient ischemic attacks, which might suggest a cerebrovascular cause for syncope; epilepsy; migraine headaches; anxiety; and use of insulin, which might suggest a hypoglycemic episode.

Many of the same conditions that can cause syncope may cause dizziness, light-headedness, or faintness (sense of impending loss of consciousness, sometimes referred to as presyncope). Vertigo due to disturbances of the inner ear is associated with a sense of "the room spinning" but rarely is associated with loss of consciousness.

PALPITATIONS

The term palpitation refers to an uncomfortable awareness of the heart beat, usually associated with an arrhythmia. The patient may complain of a forceful pulsation of the heart, often with an increase in frequency of heart beats, with or without irregular rhythm. If patients describe a skipped beat or the heart stopping for an instant, they may be sensing the compensatory pause after a premature beat; it is not uncommon for patients to sense the post-extra-systolic beat as a forceful contraction. After strenuous exercise, palpitations due to rapid sinus tachycardia are common and normal.

Palpitations with sinus tachycardia at rest or with mild exertion may indicate a disease state, such as high cardiac output states due to thyrotoxicosis, AV fistulas, anemia, beriberi, and heart failure. Palpitations that come on suddenly and end abruptly may indicate paroxysmal supraventricular tachycardia, atrial fibrillation, or atrial flutter, whereas a gradual onset and end is more likely to reflect sinus tachycardia. The patient should be asked whether the palpitations feel like a regular fast rhythm or irregular rhythm, as the latter is more suggestive of atrial fibrillation. Palpitations may also be felt with very slow rates, as in AV block.

Patients should be questioned about concomitant symptoms. With very rapid heart rates of supraventricular tachycardias, patients may describe light-headedness or presyncope. Syncopal episodes after palpitations suggest asystole or severe bradycardia after a tachycardia (as in sick sinus syndrome) or may be due to a Stokes-Adams attack. If the patient has angina with rapid palpitations, the chest pain is probably ischemic in origin and due to an increase in oxygen demand greater than oxygen supply to the heart.

EDEMA

Edema is a perceptible accumulation of fluid in the tissues.[9] Questioning the patient on the location of the edema may be important in determining whether the edema is due to a cardiac or noncardiac cause. Common cardiac causes of edema include right- or left-sided heart failure, biventricular failure, constrictive pericarditis, restrictive cardiomyopathy, and tricuspid valvular disease. Peripheral edema due to a cardiac cause is usually distributed from the ankles upward; but in patients who are bedridden, the edema is more prominent in the presacral area. In patients who are upright during the day, edema of the lower extremities typically becomes more severe in the evening, a feature also common to peripheral edema due to venous insufficiency. Edema of the lower extremities associated with a history of prominent neck veins is suggestive of a cardiac cause rather than venous insufficiency alone.

In adults, edema of the face and upper extremities without edema of the lower extremities is more suggestive of a noncardiac cause, such as superior vena caval syndrome (obstruction of this vessel due to carcinoma of the lung, lymphoma, or aortic aneurysm) or angioneurotic edema. Periorbital edema with edema of the face often accompanies acute glomerulonephritis, the nephrotic syndrome, and myxedema; it is not uncommon in children with cardiac edema. When edema of one extremity occurs, local problems, such as thrombophlebitis, lymphatic obstruction, or varicose veins, are probably the cause. Patients should be questioned about accompanying symptoms, such as dyspnea, ascites, and jaundice. Cardiac edema associated with dyspnea may result from mitral stenosis, left ventricular failure, and cor pulmonale due to chronic obstructive lung disease. Cardiac edema without a history of dyspnea is more suggestive of constrictive pericarditis, tricuspid stenosis or regurgitation, or right heart failure. The patient will describe ascites as an increase in abdominal girth or a swelling of the abdomen. When ascites is of cardiac origin, the patient often has a history of peripheral edema before the development of ascites. Conversely, if the history of ascites occurs before peripheral edema, and especially if jaundice is present, the diagnosis is more likely hepatic dysfunction.

COUGH AND HEMOPTYSIS

Cough is defined as a sudden explosive expiration, initiated by an effort to expel mucus or foreign material from the tracheobronchial tree, while hemoptysis is defined as coughing up blood. Causes of cough due to cardiac disorders include pulmonary edema, pulmonary hypertension, pulmonary emboli leading to infarction, and aortic aneurysms compressing the tracheobronchial tree. Cough associated with dyspnea may be due to cardiac or pulmonary disease. Determining which of these is the cause may be difficult. A long history of productive cough in a patient who is a heavy smoker or a history of cough associated with wheezing in a patient with known allergic (extrinsic) asthma suggests a pulmonary cause. A cough that produces pink, frothy sputum is likely associated with acute pulmonary edema; a cough that produces thick yellow sputum is more likely of an infectious nature.

Hemoptysis may be due to a number of noncardiac causes, including pulmonary tuberculosis, pneumonia, bronchiectasis, carcinoma of the lung, and chronic obstructive lung disease. Cardiovascular causes include mitral stenosis, pulmonary emboli leading to infarction, Eisenmenger's physiology, pulmonary arteriovenous fistulas, and rupture of an aortic aneurysm into the tracheobronchial tree. Large amounts of blood (more than 1/2 cup) due to brisk bleeding are more likely to be due to focal ulceration, as in bronchogenic carcinoma, bronchiectasis, presence of a foreign body, and rupture of an arteriovenous aneurysm; less often, it may occur in mitral stenosis and pulmonary infarction. Exsanguinating hemoptysis suggests rupture of an aortic aneurysm into the bronchi.

Associated symptoms may clarify the cause. Hemoptysis associated with pleuritic chest pain suggests pulmonary infarction; hemoptysis associated with chronic cough and gray sputum in a patient who smokes suggests chronic bronchitis; hemoptysis associated with purulent sputum suggests pulmonary infection, including abscess; hemoptysis associated with dyspnea on exertion or during pregnancy may be associated with mitral stenosis; episodes of hemoptysis in an otherwise healthy young woman may be due to pulmonary adenoma.

OTHER SYMPTOMS OF CARDIAC DISEASE

Although fatigue and weakness are not specific symptoms of cardiac disease, they do occur with decreased forward cardiac output, as in heart failure. These symptoms may occur after massive diuresis with orthostatic hypotension and hypokalemia. In addition, fatigue and weakness are side effects of some antihypertensive medications, such as alpha methyldopa and, occasionally, beta blockers.

Either the patient or the patient's family may note cyanosis, but cyanosis often goes unnoticed. Cyanosis indicates that 4 gm/dl or more of reduced hemoglobin is present. Cyanosis occurs in certain forms of congenital heart disease with right to left shunts, pulmonary embolism, peripheral vascular disease, and low output states.

Gastrointestinal symptoms such as anorexia, nausea, and vomiting may occur in right-sided heart failure and may be secondary to digitalis toxicity. Epigastric distress is not uncommonly associated with left ventricular inferior wall infarction or ischemia. Indigestion may occur as the sole symptom of angina pectoris or myocardial infarction. Hiccups may occur in patients with myocardial infarction or after cardiac surgery.

REFERENCES

1. Braunwald E. The history. In: Braunwald E (ed). *Heart Disease: A textbook of Cardiovascular Medicine.* 4th Ed. Philadelphia: Saunders; 1992:1-12.
2. Hurst JW, Morris DC, Crawley IS, et al. The history: Symptom and past events related to cardiovascular disease. In: Hurst JW, Schlant RC, Rackley CE, Sonnenblick EH, Wenger NK (eds). *The Heart, Arteries, and Veins.* 7th Ed. New York: McGraw-Hill; 1990:122-134.
3. Chatterjee K. The History (Chapter 30). In: Parmley WW, Chatterjee K (eds). *Cardiology.* Philadelphia: JP Lippincott; 1988:1-12.
4. Kloner RA, Hale S, Alker K, et al. The effects of acute and chronic cocaine on the heart. *Circulation.* 1992;85:407-419.
5. Schofield PM, Whorwell PJ, Jones PE, et al. Differentiation of "esophageal" and "cardiac" chest pain. *Am J Cardiol.* 1986;13:315-316.

6. Beitman BD, Basha I, Flaker G, et al. Atypical or nonanginal chest pain and panic disorder or coronary artery disease? *Arch Intern Med.* 1987;147:1548-1552.

7. Wasserman K. Dyspnea on exertion. Is it the heart or the lungs? *JAMA.* 1982;248:2039-2043.

8. Cook DG, Shaper AG. Breathlessness, angina pectoris, and coronary artery disease. *Am J Cardiol.* 1989:67:921-924.

9. Braunwald E. Edema. In: Wilson J, Braunwald E, et al (eds). *Harrison's Principles of Internal Medicine.* 12th Ed. New York: McGraw Hill; 1991:228-232.

CHAPTER **2**

The Physical Examination

Robert A. Kloner, MD, PhD

GENERAL APPEARANCE AND VITAL SIGNS

A useful approach to the cardiovascular physical examination is to begin by recording the general appearance and vital signs, followed by examination of the patient from the head downward.

The general appearance of the patient may provide helpful clues as to the nature and severity of cardiac illness.[1] For example, cachexia is not uncommon in end-stage heart disease. If the patient appears short of breath at rest or when walking from one end of the examining room to another, significant disease is suggested. Body habitus should be noted; long extremities and an arm span exceeding height, kyphoscoliosis, and pectus excavatum or pectus carinatum suggest Marfan's syndrome. Extreme obesity, somnolence, and cyanosis suggest Pickwickian syndrome.

Vital signs (pulse rate, respiratory rate, blood pressure, and temperature) are crucial parts of the cardiovascular physical examination. Pulse rate should be determined by palpating the radial pulse for a full minute, noting the strength of the pulse and irregularities in rhythm. The apical rate should be determined by cardiac auscultation.

Blood pressure is recorded with a sphygmomanometer and a stethoscope over the brachial artery. The standard-size blood pressure cuff is designed for the average adult arm. In patients with large or obese arms, a standard cuff will overestimate arterial pressure; therefore, a leg cuff should be used to measure pressure in their upper extremities. As the cuff is deflated, the first appearance of clear tapping sounds (phase I of Korotkoff sounds) is the systolic pressure. Most physicians record the disappearance of sounds (phase V of Korotkoff

sounds) as the diastolic pressure, but if phase IV (a sudden muffling of sounds before their disappearance) is heard and is more than 10 mm Hg from phase V, then it should be recorded as well. An auscultatory gap is a period of silence occurring after phase I and before phase II of Korotkoff sounds. (Phase II is the period in which the clear tapping sounds of phase I are replaced by soft murmurs.) If the reappearance of sound is read mistakenly as systolic pressure, then this pressure is underestimated. The auscultatory gap occurs where there is reduced velocity of blood flow through the arms (i.e., aortic stenosis) or venous distention of the arms.

To determine blood pressure in the basal state, multiple readings must be obtained. Blood pressure should be measured in both arms, as differences between extremities greater than 10 mm Hg may signify obstructive lesions in the arterial tree. It is useful to measure both supine and standing blood pressures, especially in patients who have symptoms suggesting orthostatic hypotension and who are taking antihypertensive medicines. Normally, there is a small, transient decrease in systolic arterial pressure of 5-15 mm Hg and a rise in diastolic pressure when a person assumes upright posture. Systolic blood pressure in the legs may be up to 20 mm Hg higher than in the arms, but diastolic pressure should be the same. In patients with hypertension, pressures in the legs should be recorded to rule out coarctation of the aorta, in which case pressures are lower than in the arms.

Pulsus paradoxus is a fall in arterial pressure greater than 10 mm Hg during inspiration. It is associated with pericardial tamponade, but may also occur in chronic lung disease, asthma, pleural effusions, and pneumothorax. It may be appreciated by feeling the radial pulse diminish or disappear during inspiration. Pulsus alternans occurs during a regular rhythm when every other heart beat has a higher systolic pressure. This phenomenon is associated with end-stage left ventricular failure and can occur for several beats after a premature contraction.

EXAMINATION OF THE HEAD AND FACE

Facial edema may occur in myxedema, constrictive pericarditis, tricuspid valve disease, and superior vena caval syndrome. Several structural facial abnormalities are associated with various congenital cardiac diseases, as in Down's, Turner's, Hurler's, and Noonan's syndromes. In Down's syndrome, which is usually associated with endocardial cushion defect and ventricular septal defect, there is a prominent medial epicanthus and large protruding tongue. Turner's syndrome is associated with coarctation of the aorta, bicuspid aortic valve, and other congenital cardiac abnormalities; these patients characteristically have webbing of the neck and widely set eyes (hypertelorism). In Hurler's syndrome, in which aortic and mitral regurgitation, cardiomyopathy, and coronary artery disease may be present, the facies exhibit coarse features and there is corneal clouding. Patients with Noonan's syndrome, in which a characteristic cardiovascular abnormality is pulmonic stenosis, have hypertelorism, webbing of the neck, small chin, low-set ears, epicanthal folds, and ptosis. Patients with a nonfamilial form of supravalvular aortic stenosis may have a so-called "elfin facies," with a prominent, high forehead, low-set ears, hypertelorism, a small, pointed chin, epicanthal folds, overhanging upper lip, upturned nose, and dental abnormalities.

Examination of the eyes should include assessment for exophthalmos and stare, which occur in both hyperthyroidism and advanced right-sided heart failure. Arcus is a light-colored ring around the iris associated with hypercholesterolemia in young adults; this may be a normal finding in the elderly. Xanthelasma are lipid-filled plaques that surround the eyes and also are associated with hypercholesterolemia. Blue sclera can be seen in Marfan's syndrome, osteogenesis imperfecta, and Ehlers-Danlos syndrome; they are associated with aortic dilatation and dissection. Cataracts occur in a number of diseases associated with cardiovascular disorders, including Marfan's syndrome, myotonic dystrophy, homocystinuria, and rubella. Argyll Robertson pupils (small, unequal pupils that do not react to light but do react to accommodation) are classic for central nervous system syphilis and may be associated with luetic aortitis.

Fundi should be examined for the presence of hypertensive and atherosclerotic arterial changes. Roth's spots are hemorrhages with a white center, which are observed on funduscopic examination; they are usually due to infective endocarditis. Conjunctival hemorrhages also may be seen in endocarditis.

A deep vertical crease in the earlobe in young patients is associated with premature atherosclerosis, but this is a nonspecific finding.

EXAMINATION OF THE NECK

Examination of the neck includes assessing the jugular venous pressure and pulse, carotid pulse, and thyroid gland.

JUGULAR VENOUS PULSE

The internal jugular vein should be examined for determination of jugular venous pressure and is more reliable for this purpose than the external jugular vein. The pulsations caused by this vein are best visualized with a flashlight shining tangentially across the neck. Jugular venous pulses are effectively examined with the patient lying at a 45° angle, but if venous pressure is high, a greater inclination is desirable (60-90°). If it is low, the patient should be positioned at a 30° angle. To estimate central venous pressure, the patient is placed at 45° and the height of the oscillating meniscus of the jugular pulse is determined. Normally the height of the pulse wave is less than 4 cm above the sternal angle. Since the sternal angle is approximately 5 cm above the right atrium, central venous pressure is normally less than 9 cm H_2O (4 cm above the sternal angle plus 5 cm above the right atrium). Thus, to determine central venous pressure (in cm H_2O), one adds (in cm) the height of the jugular pulse above the sternal angle to 5.

The wave form of the jugular venous pulse yields important information. (Details of the components of the pulses are described in Chapter 7.) With the unaided eye, 2 waves per heart beat are visible: the A and V waves. The A wave reflects atrial contraction and occurs before the carotid pulse. After the A wave, pressure drops; this is called the X descent, due to atrial relaxation, and occurs just before the second heart sound. The V wave follows and results from a rise in right atrial pressure as blood flows into the right atrium while the tricuspid valve is closed. The V wave occurs just after the carotid pulse. After the V wave, there is a smaller fall in pressure, the Y descent, which is due to the fall in right atrial pressure as the tricuspid valve opens; it ends just after the second heart sound.

When the jugular venous pressure is elevated, the V wave becomes higher and the Y descent more prominent. Conditions in which jugular venous pressure increases reflect an increase in right atrial pressure, as occurs in right heart failure, pericardial disease (cardiac tamponade and constrictive pericarditis), and restrictive cardiomyopathies. The jugular venous pressure is also elevated in superior vena caval obstructions.

With cardiac tamponade, the X descent is prominent and the Y descent is small; with constrictive pericarditis the Y descent is prominent and deep. Large A waves are observed in pulmonary stenosis, tricuspid stenosis, right ventricular hypertrophy, pulmonary hypertension, and ventricular septal hypertrophy. In conditions of atrioventricular (AV) dissociation, when the atrium contracts against a closed tricuspid valve, giant or cannon A waves are observed. A prominent regurgitant V wave and absence of an X descent suggest tricuspid regurgitation. In tricuspid stenosis, the Y descent is typically gradual.

THE CAROTID PULSE

Normally, the carotid pulse has a rapid rise to a rounded peak followed by a less rapid decline, which is interrupted in its early phase by an incisura or dicrotic notch (a sharp downward deflection representing closure of the aortic valve). As the pulse wave is transmitted from the ascending aorta to the peripheral vessels, the systolic upstroke becomes steeper and its amplitude higher; the incisura or dicrotic notch becomes smoother in configuration.

The carotid pulse contour is abnormal in a number of disease states. A delayed systolic peak (pulsus tardus) is typical of aortic stenosis, in which there may also be an accentuated anacrotic notch (a pause on the ascending limb of the pulse). A bisferiens pulse occurs when there are 2 systolic peaks; it is associated with aortic regurgitation, a combination of aortic regurgitation and aortic stenosis, and hypertrophic obstructive cardiomyopathy (formerly called idiopathic hypertrophic subaortic stenosis). Pulsus paradoxus and pulsus alternans, described earlier, are appreciated by palpation of the pulse. Pulsus alternans, which occurs with a regular rhythm, should be distinguished from pulsus bigeminus, which occurs with ectopic bigeminal rhythm, usually ventricular. In this latter condition, the weaker beat follows a shorter interval. Pulsus parvus refers to a weak pulse and can be encountered in any condition in which left ventricular stroke volume is reduced. The arterial pulse may be accentuated or bounding in patients with high cardiac output states (e.g., hyperthyroidism and arteriovenous fistulas), aortic regurgitation, or rigid, sclerotic arteries. Excessive carotid pressure during the physical examination should be avoided in elderly patients, who may have atherosclerosis.

All peripheral pulses should be examined. Reduced, unequal pulses or bruits may indicate significant obstructive disease due to atherosclerosis or other causes (dissection, aneurysm, aortitis, embolism). Further discussion of carotid pulses appears in Chapter 7.

EXAMINATION OF THE LUNGS

Bilateral rales that are fine and crackling (like crackling cellophane) and that are often more prominent at the bases of the lungs occur in congestive heart failure. Rales, however, may be due to noncardiac causes (e.g., pneumonia), in which case the rales have a coarser sound and are unilateral. Auscultation of the lungs after

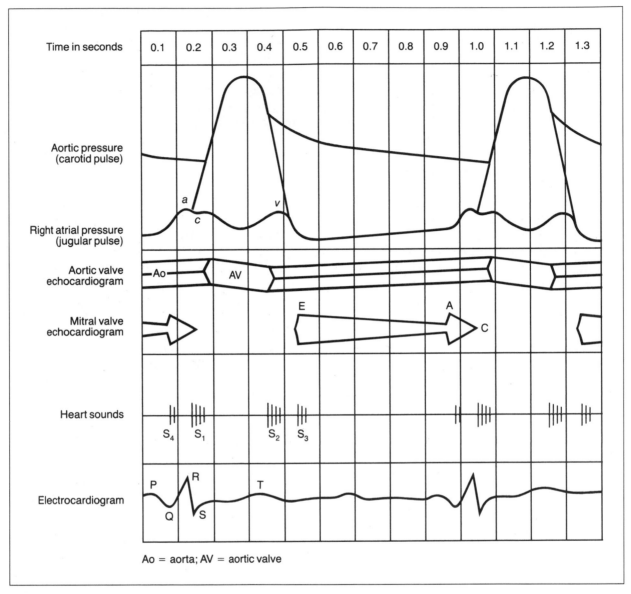

| Time in seconds | 0.1 | 0.2 | 0.3 | 0.4 | 0.5 | 0.6 | 0.7 | 0.8 | 0.9 | 1.0 | 1.1 | 1.2 | 1.3 |

Ao = aorta; AV = aortic valve

Figure 1. *Timing in the cardiac cycle. Most sounds are either systolic or diastolic (rarely both). Accurate timing is impossible by listening alone, for systole and diastole "sound" the same. The upstroke of the carotid arterial pulse marks the onset of systole. The first heart sound immediately precedes the carotid upstroke, whereas the second sound immediately follows the downstroke. Ao=Aorta; AV=Aortic valve. Reprinted with permission from Myers DG. Review of cardiac auscultation (Part 1). Hospital Medicine. October 1993;25-45.*

deep breathing and coughing decreases false-positive findings. Pleural effusions secondary to heart failure are usually bilateral; when they are unilateral, they tend to occur on the right side. The physical findings of pleural effusion include dullness to percussion and reduced or absent vocal fremitus.

EXAMINATION OF THE HEART

Inspection and palpation of the precordium provides information concerning the location and quality of the left ventricular impulse. The examiner should palpate the precordial movements of the heart with the patient both in

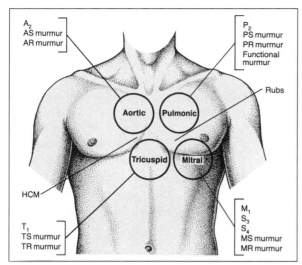

Figure 2. *Cardiac listening sites. Cardiac sounds and murmurs have maximal intensity at the chest wall sites closest to their origins. M1=Mitral component of S_1; T_1=Tricuspid component of S_1; A_2=Aortic component of S_2; P_2=Pulmonic component of S_2; S_3=Third heart sound; S_4=Fourth heart sound; AS=Aortic stenosis; AR=Aortic regurgirtation; PS=Pulmonic stenosis; PR=Pulmonic regurgitation; TS=Tricuspid stenosis; TR=Tricuspid regurgitation; MS=Mitral stenosis; MR=Mitral regurgitation; HCM=Hypertrophic cardiomyopathy. Reprinted with permission from Myers DG. Review of cardiac auscultation (Part 1). Hospital Medicine. October 1993;25-45.*

the supine and the left lateral decubitus position. This latter maneuver increases the ability to palpate the left ventricle. The apex beat is the lowest and most lateral point on the chest at which the cardiac impulse can be felt. Normally, it is superior to the fifth left intercostal space and within the left mid-clavicular line. It is often, but not always, the point of maximal impulse, since pulsations arising from other structures may be more forceful.

The normal precordial pulse is an outward systolic motion felt during isovolumetric contraction as the left ventricle rotates and strikes the anterior chest wall, followed by retraction of the left ventricle as blood is ejected from the cavity. With left ventricular hypertrophy, the outward systolic motion is exaggerated and sustained. Displacement of the left ventricular impulse downward and to the left suggests left ventricular dilatation, as occurs in

chronic aortic regurgitation or chronic congestive heart failure.

Aneurysms of the left ventricle result in a large systolic bulge, which is felt above and often medial to the apex beat. Left ventricular dyskinesia may be appreciated as 2 impulses separated by several centimeters. A presystolic impulse is felt when the atrial contribution to left ventricular filling is increased (in myocardial ischemia, left ventricular hypertrophy due to hypertension, aortic stenosis, or myocardial fibrosis) and is associated with a fourth heart sound.

Double systolic impulses plus a presystolic impulse typically are felt in hypertrophic obstructive cardiomyopathy. Parasternal lifts usually are due to right ventricular or left atrial enlargement in the setting of mitral regurgitation. Systolic retraction of the chest is associated with constrictive pericarditis. Prominent systolic pulsations in the left second intercostal space represent pulmonary hypertension or increased pulmonary blood flow. Finally, thrills may be palpated in association with loud murmurs (such as those resulting for aortic stenosis, ventricular septal defect, and pulmonary stenosis).

AUSCULTATION

Timing of heart sounds in relationship to other cardiac events and location for auscultation are shown in Figures 1 and 2.

FIRST HEART SOUND

The classic theory holds that the origin of the first heart sound (S_1) is due to closure of the mitral and tricuspid valves. The S_1 is often split with the first component representing mitral and the second component representing tricuspid valve closure.[2,3] The two components are separated by a narrow interval of 0.02-0.03 sec. The S_1 is heard best in the mitral area.

Conditions that increase the intensity of the S_1 include mitral stenosis (in cases where the valve is not extensively calcified and is still pliable), exercise, thyrotoxicosis, systemic hypertension, a short PR interval, and fast heart rates which result in the AV valves being widely separated at the beginning of ventricular contraction. Conditions that decrease the intensity of the S_1 include a prolonged (>0.20 sec) PR interval (AV valves have partially closed before a later onset of ventricular contraction), aortic insufficiency (also due to premature mitral valve closure), mitral insufficiency not due to mitral prolapse, cases of mitral stenosis in which the valve is severely calcified and rigid, and left ventricular failure. The intensity of the S_1 varies in complete heart block and in atrial fibrillation. Abnormally wide splitting of the S_1 is unusual, but may occur in Ebstein's anomaly when associated with right bundle branch block, occasionally in right bundle branch block alone, and in tricuspid stenosis.

SECOND HEART SOUND

The second heart sound (S_2) consists of 2 components: A_2, representing closure of the aortic valve, and P_2, representing closure of the pulmonic valve (Fig. 3A). A_2 is best heard in the second right intercostal space and P_2 is best heard in the second left intercostal space. The 2 components normally fuse with expiration and are separated (by 0.02-0.06 sec) with inspiration. Wide splitting of S_2 with preservation of respiratory variation occurs when P_2 is delayed relative to A_2. This situation occurs with complete right bundle branch block, occasionally in Wolff-Parkinson-White syndrome, with ventricular premature beats arising from the left ventricle, with pacing from the left ventricle, in pulmonic stenosis, in pulmonary hypertension with right ventricular failure, with massive pulmonary embolism, in severe mitral regurgitation and ventricular septal defect in which the left ventricular ejection time is shortened. Broad fixed splitting of S_2 occurs in atrial septal defect, with an average splitting interval of 0.05 sec (range, 0.03-0.08 sec). Fixed splitting may also occur in right ventricular failure due to any cause, although the splitting interval is not usually wide in this situation.

Reversed or Paradoxical Splitting of the S_2

When aortic valve closure is delayed, the A_2 and P_2 are separated during expiration and come together during inspiration. Thus, the splitting

is said to be reversed (Fig. 3A). The 2 most common causes of reversed splitting of the S_2 are left bundle branch block and aortic stenosis. Other causes include right ventricular paced and ectopic beats, hypertrophic obstructive cardiomyopathy, patent ductus arteriosus, and, less often, systemic hypertension and ischemic heart disease. The S_2 is single in tetralogy of Fallot, pulmonary atresia, severe pulmonary stenosis, complete transposition of the great vessels, hypoplastic left heart syndrome, and truncus arteriosus. The S_2 may appear single when the P_2 is very faint due to obesity and emphysema.

Intensity of the S_2

In adults, the A_2 is normally louder than the P_2. Hypertension within the aorta or pulmonary artery results in a loud A_2 or P_2 respectively. Dilatation of these vessels may also cause the S_2 to be accentuated. In thin-chested persons the S_2 may be loud. The A_2 is also accentuated in coarctation of the aorta and corrected transposition of the great arteries.

The A_2 is reduced in intensity in aortic stenosis, when the valve is rigid secondary to calcification; it may also be reduced in intensity in aortic regurgitation. The P_2 is reduced in both valvular and infundibular stenosis. In patients with a greater distance between the origin of the S_2 and chest wall, due to either a thoracic deformity or lung disease, especially emphysema, the intensity of the S_2 is reduced.

THIRD HEART SOUND

The third heart sound (S_3) is a low pitched sound occurring approximately 0.15 sec (range, 0.1-0.2 sec) after the S_2. It is probably due to rapid expansion and filling of the left or right ventricle in early diastole (Fig. 3B). One recent phonocardiographic, echocardiographic and Doppler study found that S_3s were associated with an "abnormally rapid deceleration of early diastolic left ventricular inflow."[4] An S_3 may be a normal finding in young persons; but when it is associated with a pathologic condition, it is also termed a protodiastolic gallop or an S_3 gallop. Left-sided S_3s are heard best at the apical area

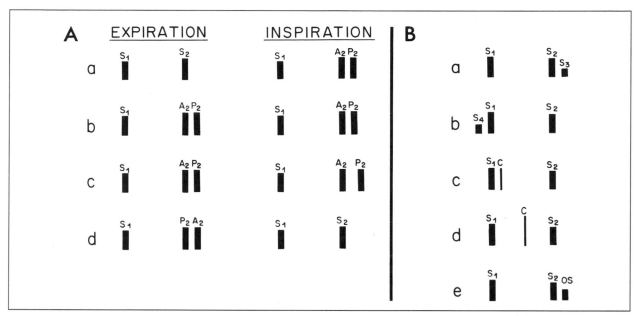

Figure 3. A: Respiratory variation of the second heart sound. S_1=First heart sound; S_2=Second heart sound; A_2=Aortic component of S_2; P_2=Pulmonic component of S_2. (a) Normal splitting of S_2 in inspiration. (b) Fixed splitting of S_2, as in atrial septal defect. (c) Splitting in expiration enhanced with inspiration, as in right bundle branch block. (d) Paradoxical splitting. Splitting in expiration but not in inspiration, as in left bundle branch block and aortic stenosis. B: Timing of the extra heart sounds in relationship to S_1 and S_2. S_3=Third heart sound; S_4=Fourth heart sound; C=Click; OS=Opening snap. (a) S_3 (b) S_4, (c) Early systolic ejection click (or sound). (d) Midsystolic ejection click. (e) Opening snap.

with the bell of the stethoscope. Right-sided S_3s are heard best along the left sternal border and are accentuated by inspiration.

Frequent causes of an S_3 gallop are high cardiac output states, as in anemia or thyrotoxicosis; mitral insufficiency, in which there is increased ventricular filling in early diastole; and congestive heart failure with a dilated ventricle. S_3s are commonly associated with reduced ventricular ejection fraction plus impaired diastolic filling rates.[5] When S_3s are present in the setting of mitral regurgitation they do not necessarily reflect left ventricular systolic dysfunction.[6] Other causes include atrial septal defect, ventricular septal defect, patent ductus arteriosus, and aortic insufficiency. An S_3 should be differentiated from an opening snap of mitral stenosis, which tends to be a higher frequency sound and occurs 0.03-0.12 sec — that is, earlier — after the S_2. An S_3 also may be confused with the pericardial knock of constrictive pericarditis, which tends to have a somewhat higher frequency, occurs earlier than

an S_3 (0.09-0.12 sec after A_2) and radiates more widely over the precordium.

FOURTH HEART SOUND

The fourth heart sound (S_4) or presystolic gallop, is a low-frequency vibration that occurs when the atrium contracts into a ventricle (left or right) with reduced compliance (Fig. 3B). An S_4 occurs when the ventricular walls are stiff due to hypertrophy, fibrosis, ischemia, or infarction. Thus, an S_4 is a common feature of systemic hypertension and aortic stenosis with left ventricular hypertrophy, hypertrophic obstructive cardiomyopathy, and coronary artery disease. A left-sided S_4 is best heard with the bell of the stethoscope at the apex; placing the patient in a left lateral decubitus position accentuates it. An S_4 originating from the right ventricle occurs with pulmonary hypertension and pulmonary stenosis.

When heart rates are very rapid, an S_3 and S_4 may merge to produce a "summation gallop." In general, S_4s are not present with atrial fibrillation due to loss of synchronized atrial contraction.

EJECTION SOUNDS AND CLICKS

Ejection sounds and clicks are high-frequency sounds that arise from the aortic or pulmonic valve areas and occur in early systole (Fig. 3B). Aortic ejection sounds occur in association with congenital aortic stenosis, bicuspid aortic valve, and acquired aortic stenosis; they imply that the valve is mobile and not heavily calcified. When due to an abnormal aortic valve, the sounds may radiate over the entire precordium. Ejection sounds also occur when the aortic root is dilated, as in systemic hypertension. Pulmonic ejection sounds are heard in cases of valvular pulmonic stenosis, pulmonary hypertension, and, occasionally, idiopathic dilatation of the pulmonary artery. In cases of pulmonary stenosis, the earlier in systole the ejection sound is heard, the more severe the stenosis. Pulmonary ejection sounds are absent in subvalvular pulmonic stenosis or when valvular stenosis is caused by severely immobilized valves. The pulmonic ejection sound is typically louder during expiration, unlike most other right-sided cardiac sounds. It tends to be localized to the left upper sternal border, in contrast to aortic ejection sounds, which are heard more widely over the precordium. Pulmonic ejection sounds also tend to occur slightly earlier than aortic ejection sounds, and, as noted earlier, vary with respiration, while aortic ejection sounds do not.

MIDSYSTOLIC CLICKS

A midsystolic click or multiple clicks that may be accompanied by a late systolic murmur occur in patients with mitral valve prolapse (Fig. 3B). Simultaneous echocardiographic and phonocardiographic studies show that the click or clicks correspond to the point of maximal prolapse of the valve.

OPENING SNAP

The opening snap (OS) is a high-frequency sound heard in early diastole in patients with mitral or tricuspid stenosis and results from the stiff valve snapping into its respective ventricle during the early filling phase (Fig. 3B). The S_2-OS interval is important, in that severe stenosis is associated with a shorter S_2-OS interval. The OS due to mitral stenosis is heard best between the mid-left sternal border and apex. Those due to tricuspid stenosis are heard at the lower left sternal border.

MURMURS

Murmurs are a series of vibrations due to turbulence of blood flow (Fig. 4). The intensity of a murmur depends upon blood velocity and volume of blood flowing across the sound-producing area and the distance from the sound-producing area to the stethoscope. The intensity of murmurs is graded on a scale of 1 to 6. Grade 1 is the faintest murmur that can be heard; grade 2 is faint but slightly louder; grade 3 is moderately loud; grade 4 is a loud murmur associated with a palpable thrill; grade 5 is a very loud murmur but still requires a stethoscope to be heard; a grade 6 murmur is so loud that it can be heard without the use of a stethoscope. Radiation of murmurs depends on the direction of blood flow responsible for the murmur, site of origin, and intensity of the murmur. Duration depends on the duration of the pressure gradient that causes the murmur. Timing of murmurs during systole or diastole is aided by simultaneous palpation of the carotid pulse.[7]

SYSTOLIC MURMURS

Systolic murmurs are classified as midsystolic ejection murmurs or as pansystolic regurgitant murmurs (Fig. 4). Midsystolic, diamond-shaped, crescendo-decrescendo ejection murmurs occur as a result of the forward ejection of blood into the root of the aorta or pulmonary arteries. They begin after the S_1 and end before the S_2. Pansystolic (or holosystolic) regurgitant murmurs occur due to backward flow of blood through the mitral or tricuspid valve or through a ventricular septal defect and have a more even intensity. They begin with the first heart sound and proceed to the second sound on their side of origin.

Midsystolic Murmurs

Causes of midsystolic murmurs associated with systolic ejection of blood include physiologic or functional ejection murmurs (not associated with any cardiac abnormality), aortic stenosis, aortic sclerosis (without significant stenosis) pulmonic stenosis, hypertrophic obstructive cardio-myopathy, ejection of blood through a normal valve into a dilated aorta or pulmonary artery, and increased rate of ejection of blood in otherwise normal persons due to anemia, fever, thyrotoxicosis, and exercise. An ejection murmur originating from 1 side of the heart always stops before closure of the semilunar valve on that side, but may continue through closure of the semilunar valve on the other side of the heart. Thus, the murmur of pulmonic stenosis continues through A_2 but stops before P_2. The murmur of aortic stenosis is best heard in the right second intercostal space and radiates into the neck. In elderly patients with aortic stenosis due to fibrosclerotic degeneration of the valve, the murmur of aortic stenosis tends to be harsh and noisy in the aortic area while radiation of the murmur to the left ventricular apex is musical in quality (Gallavardin dissociation[2]). It is now believed that most functional murmurs in adults are probably aortic in origin. They tend to peak in early systole (<0.20 sec after the QRS complex). Murmurs caused by high grades of aortic stenosis or pulmonic stenosis tend to be prolonged and peak in mid-to-late systole (>0.24 sec after the QRS complex). In Tetralogy of Fallot, the systolic ejection murmur becomes shorter with increased severity of the pulmonic stenosis, as less blood crosses the pulmonary valve and more is ejected through the ventricular septal defect. In some cases, mitral regurgitation may be associated with a midsystolic murmur. The murmur of aortic stenosis or sclerosis increases in loudness during the beat following an extrasystolic contraction; while the murmur of mitral regurgitation usually does not change its intensity in this setting.

Pansystolic Murmurs

Causes of pansystolic regurgitant murmurs include blood flowing retrogradely through the mitral and tricuspid valves and ventricular septal defect. The even intensity and long duration of these murmurs correspond to the duration of the pressure difference across the orifice producing the murmurs. These murmurs tend to have a higher frequency and a "blowing" quality compared with systolic ejection murmurs, which in general tend to be harsher. The murmur of tricuspid regurgitation increases with inspiration (Carvallo's sign), whereas that of mitral regurgitation does not.

Early Systolic Murmurs

Early systolic murmurs may be heard in acute mitral regurgitation due to rupture of a chordae tendineae or papillary muscle or in infective endocarditis. The murmurs may be confined to early and midsystole and taper off in late systole. Since a large volume of blood enters a small, previously normal left atrium during systole, the ventricular and atrial pressures equalize during the second half of systole, suppressing the murmur. Tricuspid regurgitation due to disease of the valve itself rather than related to pulmonary hypertension can cause an early systolic murmur. Early systolic murmurs are heard in very small ventricular septal defects or ventricular septal defects once Eisenmenger's complex (pulmonary hypertension) develops. The murmur of patent ductus arteriosus becomes confined to early systole once pulmonary hypertension develops.

Late Systolic Murmurs

Late systolic murmurs are most frequently due to mitral valve prolapse and often begin with a midsystolic click or clicks. These murmurs begin in mid-to-late systole, continue to the S_2, and tend to be of relatively high frequency. Sometimes, late systolic murmurs are musical in nature and sound like a honk or a whoop. Late systolic murmurs are rarely due to ventricular septal defect or coarctation of the aorta.

DIASTOLIC MURMURS

Diastolic murmurs occur due to regurgitation of blood across the aortic or pulmonic valves or to forward flow across the mitral or tricuspid valves (Fig. 4). When the cause is regurgitation across the semilunar valves, the murmurs begin in very early diastole, just after S_2; when the cause is flow across the AV valves, they tend to occur in mid-diastole.

Diastolic Murmurs Due to Insufficiency of the Semilunar Valves

These murmurs begin with an S_2; they are high frequency, blowing, and decrescendo. When the aortic cusps are torn or perforated, the murmur of aortic regurgitation may have a musical or cooing quality. These murmurs are heard best with the diaphragm of the stethoscope in the third or fourth intercostal space at the sternal edge, while the patient is sitting upright and leaning forward. Aortic insufficiency due to disease of the valve leaflets typically radiates to the left sternal border, while that due to aortic root dilatation radiates to the right sternal border. It may be difficult to differentiate the murmurs of aortic from those of pulmonary regurgitation; however, inspiratory augmentation favors the latter. The pulmonary regurgitant murmur due to pulmonary hypertension (Graham Steell murmur) has a higher pitch and may be heard earlier in diastole than the murmur of pulmonary regurgitation due to primary valvular disease.

An Austin Flint murmur is an apical diastolic rumbling murmur heard in aortic insufficiency. The mechanism of this murmur remains controversial. Rahka[8] performed a doppler and echocardiographic study in patients with this murmur and concluded that it was due to the aortic insufficiency jet causing shuddering of the anterior leaflet of the mitral valve. He could not confirm previous suggestions that the murmur was due to functional mitral stenosis. Another study, using similar results plus cine nuclear magnetic resonance imaging concluded that the Austin Flint murmur occurred when the aortic regurgitation jet abutted the left ventricular endocardium, causing the low pitched diastolic rumbling murmur.[9] Emi and colleagues[10] showed that the Austin Flint murmur did not depend on rapid mitral inflow.

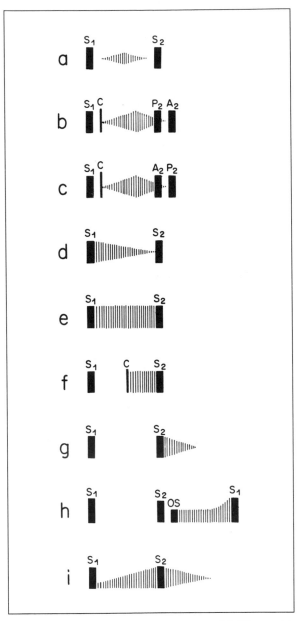

Figure 4. Principal cardiac murmurs. (a) Short mid-systolic murmur as in innocent murmur. (b) Aortic stenosis. Aortic ejection click, mid-to-late peaking systolic murmur, delayed A_2 (c) Pulmonic stenosis. Pulmonic ejection click, systolic ejection murmur stops before P_2 but extends through A_2. (d) Holosystolic murmur decreases in late systole as in acute mitral regurgitation. (e) Pansystolic regurgitant murmur as in mitral regurgitation. (f) Midsystolic murmur due to mitral valve prolapse. (g) Diastolic decrescendo murmur due to semilunar valve insufficiency. (h) Diastolic murmur of mitral stenosis. (i) Continuous murmur as in patent ductus arteriosus.

Diastolic Murmurs Due to Forward Flow Through the Mitral and Tricuspid Valves

Diastolic murmurs originating from the AV valves occur when forward flow through these valves is increased or when these valves become stenotic. These murmurs begin in early to mid-diastole, when ventricular pressure has fallen below atrial pressure and the valve opens, which may be associated with an opening snap. The murmur is low-pitched and rumbling and may intensify during atrial contraction just before the S_1 of the next beat.[11] This presystolic accentuation typically is absent in atrial fibrillation. Occasionally, however, mild accentuation of a mitral diastolic rumble occurs in the absence of atrial systole due to closer coaptation of the diseased mitral leaflets toward end-diastole.

The murmur of mild mitral stenosis is relatively short and may disappear in mid-diastole and reappear with atrial contraction in late diastole, while the murmur of severe mitral stenosis tends to be longer in duration and more even in intensity. Mitral stenosis murmurs are best heard at the apex with the bell of the stethoscope and with the patient in the left lateral decubitus position. The murmur of tricuspid stenosis has similarities to that of mitral stenosis, but is augmented with inspiration, is higher in frequency, is best heard at the left lower sternal border, and occurs slightly earlier in diastole. Murmurs due to left atrial myxoma often mimic those due to mitral stenosis but tend to change in quality and intensity with alterations in body position.

Diastolic murmurs that occur with increased blood flow across the mitral valve have a number of causes: mitral regurgitation, ventricular septal defect, and patent ductus arteriosus. Increased flow across the tricuspid valve may result in a diastolic murmur as in tricuspid regurgitation and atrial septal defect.

CONTINUOUS MURMURS

Continuous murmurs begin in systole and extend through the S_2 into all or part of diastole. They occur when there is a continuous pressure difference between areas. Abnormal connections between the systemic arterial and systemic venous systems or between the systemic and pulmonary systems may cause such murmurs. Continuous murmurs may be caused by patent ductus arteriosus, rupture of a sinus of Valsalva into the right side of the heart, systemic or pulmonary AV fistulas, and man-made fistulas (Blalock, Potts procedure, shunts for hemodialysis). Abnormalities in arteries may cause such murmurs, as occur in constriction of a peripheral systemic artery, constriction of a pulmonary artery, and coarctation of the aorta. The venous hum is a continuous murmur originating over the great veins of the lower part of the neck; it is a normal finding. It can be obliterated by recumbency, pressure over the veins of the neck, and by Valsalva maneuver.

MANEUVERS TO DIFFERENTIATE TYPES OF HEART SOUNDS AND MURMURS

Various physiologic and pharmacologic maneuvers may be useful in differentiating murmurs and sounds with similar characteristics. Table 1 summarizes the effect of these maneuvers on intensity of murmurs.

RESPIRATION

Inspiration results in increased right ventricular filling and stroke volume and decreased left ventricular filling and stroke volume. In general, the intensity of murmurs arising from the right side of the heart increases during inspiration, while the intensity of murmurs originating from the left side either does not change or decreases. In mitral valve prolapse, however, inspiratory decrease of left ventricular cavity size increases the redundancy of the valve, and the click occurs earlier and the murmur may become accentuated. An S_3 and S_4 originating from the right side are increased during inspiration.

VALSALVA MANEUVER

This maneuver involves forced expiration against a closed glottis. During phase I of the Valsalva maneuver, intrathoracic pressure rises and there is an increase in left ventricular output and blood pressure. During the strain phase (II), venous return is impaired with a reduction in right ventricular filling followed by a reduction in left ventricular filling, and there is a fall in stroke volume and blood pressure. During this strain phase, almost all murmurs and heart sounds diminish in intensity except the murmur of hypertrophic obstructive cardiomyopathy, which increases in intensity due to the reduction in left ventricular volume. The murmur of mitral prolapse occurs earlier due to more severe prolapse. During phase III (release of respiratory pressure), flow to the right side of the heart increases first, followed by increased flow to the left side. Thus, murmurs originating from the right side of the heart return to normal (or may actually temporarily increase) 1-2 cardiac cycles after release of the maneuver, while murmurs from the left side require 4-11 cardiac cycles to recover their intensity. Therefore, the Valsalva maneuver may aid in differentiating right-sided from left-sided murmurs.

When the cardiac cycle length varies, as in atrial fibrillation or with compensatory pauses after a premature contraction, systolic ejection murmurs after the pause are increased in intensity, whereas there is no change in left-sided pansystolic regurgitant murmurs or systolic murmurs due to ventricular septal defect. Therefore, this sign may be helpful in differentiating aortic stenosis from mitral regurgitation. There is, however, increased intensity after longer cycles in the murmur of tricuspid regurgitation.

ISOMETRIC EXERCISE

Isometric exercise consisting of hand grip for 30-40 sec causes an increase in systemic blood pressure and heart rate, cardiac output, and left ventricular filling pressure. This maneuver should be avoided in patients with myocardial ischemia and ventricular arrhythmias. Isometric exercise helps differentiate systolic murmurs due to valvular aortic stenosis and hypertrophic obstructive cardiomyopathy, which decrease during hand grip, from those due to mitral insufficiency and ventricular septal defect, which increase with this maneuver. The diastolic

murmur of aortic insufficiency increases with hand grip. The murmur of mitral stenosis increases with hand grip due to increased cardiac output. The systolic murmur and click of mitral prolapse are delayed by hand grip.

SQUATTING

Squatting increases systemic venous return; at the same time, it increases arterial blood pressure. The systolic murmur of hypertrophic obstructive cardiomyopathy characteristically is reduced by squatting; the murmur of aortic insufficiency is accentuated. Third and fourth heart sounds are augmented during squatting.

CHANGES IN POSTURE

Rapid changes in posture alter venous return; lying down from a standing position and elevation of the legs increase right ventricular filling and, hence, right ventricular stroke volume, followed by an increase in left ventricular stroke volume. Murmurs of aortic and pulmonic stenosis, functional systolic murmurs, mitral and tricuspid regurgitation, and ventricular septal defect are increased by maneuvers that increase venous return, while the murmur of hypertrophic obstructive cardiomyopathy is diminished and that of mitral prolapse is delayed or reduced. Gallop sounds are increased and splitting of the S_2 is widened with increased venous return.

Venous return is decreased by sudden standing, which has the opposite effect on murmurs. Specifically, the murmur of hypertrophic obstructive cardiomyopathy is increased by sudden standing.

PHARMACOLOGIC MANEUVERS

When amyl nitrite is inhaled, there is marked systemic vasodilatation with a fall in blood pressure and reflex tachycardia. This is followed by an increase in venous return and cardiac output. Because of the increase in forward flow, systolic murmurs of hypertrophic obstructive cardiomyopathy, aortic stenosis, pulmonic stenosis, functional flow murmurs, and the diastolic murmurs of tricuspid and mitral stenosis are increased. The systolic murmur of tetralogy of Fallot, however, is reduced in intensity. Blood flowing through the pulmonary outflow tract decreases in favor of increased flow through the right to left shunt, due to reduced systemic arterial pressure. The fall in systemic arterial pressure results in diminution of the systolic murmur of mitral insufficiency, ventricular septal defect (less left-to-right shunting), patent ductus arteriosus, and the diastolic murmur of aortic insufficiency. Increased pressures on the right side of the heart and a slight increase in pulmonary artery pressure cause the murmur of tricuspid and pulmonic insufficiency to increase. The murmur of mitral valve prolapse occurs earlier, and is thus longer; however, the intensity of the murmur may have a variable response to amyl nitrite.

Amyl nitrite is especially useful in differentiating the murmur of mitral insufficiency (decrease) from aortic stenosis (increase); differentiating the murmur of rheumatic mitral stenosis (increase) from an Austin Flint murmur due to aortic insufficiency (decrease); differentiating right-sided regurgitant murmurs (increase) from left-sided regurgitant murmurs (decrease); and differentiating small ventricular septal defects (decrease) from pulmonary stenosis (increase).

Vasopressors may be used to assess murmurs including phenylephrine (0.5 mg IV) and methoxamine (3-5 mg IV). These drugs increase systemic and vascular resistance, increase systolic and diastolic arterial pressure and increase systolic pressures within the ventricles. Phenylephrine is preferred because it elevates pressure for only 3-5 minutes; methoxamine has a duration of action of up to 15-20 minutes. The increased systemic pressure causes an increase in regurgitant flows, thus increasing the diastolic murmur of aortic insufficiency and the systolic murmur of mitral regurgitation. The systolic murmurs due to left-to-right shunts through ventricular septal defects and patent ductus arteriosus also are increased. Because these agents cause an increase in left ventricular size, they reduce the systolic murmur of hypertrophic obstructive cardiomyopathy and delay the onset of the click and murmur of mitral prolapse.

OTHER HEART SOUNDS AND RUBS

Artificial cardiac valves are associated with various heart sounds not normally heard. The caged-ball or disc valve has opening and closing sounds. Early evidence of valve dysfunction may result in a change in intensity or timing of these sounds. Pacemakers may produce a presystolic extra sound due to skeletal muscle contraction; and occasionally, the pacemaker wire causes a late systolic musical murmur due to its position across the tricuspid valve.

Pericardial friction rubs are described as scratching, grating, or squeaking sounds heard between the left sternal border and apex of the heart. The quality of the sound has been likened to the noise produced when 2 pieces of leather are rubbed together. These sounds may be inconstant, appearing or disappearing depending on the patient's position. They are easiest to hear with the diaphragm of the stethoscope pressed tightly against the chest while the patient is sitting up and leaning forward. Since the sound occurs as the heart moves within an inflamed pericardium, the rubs often have 3 components, reflecting movement of the heart during atrial systole, ventricular systole, and ventricular diastole. Three-component rubs are diagnostic of pericarditis; however, pericardial rubs may only have 1 or 2 components, in which case they may be confused with systolic or to-and-fro murmurs, respectively.

THE ABDOMINAL EXAMINATION

Valuable clues to the cardiac status may be derived from the abdominal exam. The liver may be enlarged and tender to palpation, due to venous congestion in cases of right heart failure or constrictive pericarditis. Pulsation of the liver occurs in severe tricuspid regurgitation, but can also be due to transmitted pulsations, as occurs in aortic aneurysms. Palpation of the spleen may reveal enlargement when there is concomitant hepatomegaly. The abdomen should be palpated for the presence of aortic aneurysms; if these are found, their width should be estimated. Auscultation should be performed to assess for bruits, which can be heard in cases of renovascular hypertension.

Table 1. Intensity Responses of Cardiac Murmurs to Hemodynamic Changes

CARDIAC LESION	INSPIRATION	SUPINE LEG ELEVATION	VALSALVA MANEUVER	POST-PVC	AMYL NITRITE	SQUATTING	HAND GRIP	EXPIRATION
Valvular aortic stenosis	—	↑	↓	↑	↑	↑	↓—	↑—
Obstructive hypertrophic cardiomyopathy	↓	↓	↑	↑	↑	↓	↓	—
Aortic regurgitation	—	—	↓	—	↓	↑	↑	—
Mitral stenosis	↓	↑	↓	—	↑	↑	↑	↑
Mitral regurgitation	—	—	↓	—	↓	↑	↑	—
Mitral valve prolapse	—	↓ and delayed click	↑ and early click	↓ and delayed click	↑ and early click	↓ and delayed click	↓ and delayed click	—
Pulmonic stenosis	↑	↑	↓	↑	↑	↑	—	—
Tricuspid stenosis	↑	↑	↓	—	↑ and early OS	↑	↑	↓
Tricuspid regurgitation	↑	↑	↓	↑	↑	—	—	—
VSD	—	—	—	—	↓	↑ (L—R) shunt)	↑	—
Functional murmur	—	↑	↓	↑	↑	↑	—	—

Reprinted with permission from Myers DG. Review of cardiac auscultation (Part 1). *Hospital Medicine.* October 1993:25-45.

EXAMINATION OF THE SKIN AND EXTREMITIES

Reduction of blood flow may result in cool, cyanotic extremities. Cyanosis is particularly marked in the nailbeds. The term peripheral cyanosis refers to cyanosis in this setting of reduced flow secondary to peripheral vascular disease or heart failure. Central cyanosis refers to that which occurs with intracardiac or intrapulmonary right-to-left shunting and is more prominent in the conjunctiva and mucous membranes. Differential cyanosis is cyanosis in the lower but not the upper extremities and is associated with patent ductus arteriosus with right-to-left shunting.

Raynaud's phenomenon is recognized as the presence of cold-induced pallor of the fingers or toes, followed by intense cyanosis and pain. During the recovery period, there may be a hyperemic phase, in which case the digits appear bright red. Raynaud's phenomenon is associated with certain collagen vascular diseases, atherosclerosis, and primary pulmonary hypertension.

With long-standing arterial vascular insufficiency, atrophic skin changes include a thin, shiny appearance to the skin, loss of hair on the backs of the hands and feet, and dry, brittle nails containing transverse ridges. Small round scars, ulcers, and, in severe cases, gangrene of the skin develops. Venous insufficiency is associated with varicose veins, edema, brownish pigmentation and induration of the skin, and stasis ulcers. Stasis ulcers due to chronic venous insufficiency of the lower extremity typically occur in the area of the internal malleolus.

The skin should be examined for the presence of petechiae and the nailbeds for splinter hemorrhages, both of which are signs associated with bacterial endocarditis. Xanthomas are cholesterol-filled nodules located subcutaneously or along extensor surfaces of tendons and occur in certain types of hyperlipidemias. Clubbing of the fingers and toes is seen with right-to-left shunts, pulmonary disease, and endocarditis as well as a number of noncardiac conditions.

A number of congenital heart diseases are associated with bony abnormalities. Patients with Holt-Oram syndrome have a thumb with an extra phalynx and atrial septal defect. Ellis-van Creveld syndrome includes polydactyly, hypoplastic fingernails, and atrial or ventricular septal defects. Long, thin, spiderlike fingers — arachnodactyly — are seen in Marfan's syndrome. Turner's syndrome includes short stature, cubitus vulgus and can be associated with coarctation of the aorta and bicuspid aortic valve.

REFERENCES

1. Braunwald E. The Physical Examination. In: Braunwald E (ed). *Heart Disease: A Textbook of Cardiovascular Medicine.* Philadelphia: W.B. Saunders; 1992:13-42.
2. Perloff JD. Heart sounds and murmurs: Physiological Mechanisms. In: Braunwald E (ed). *Heart Disease: A Textbook of Cardiovascular Medicine.* Philadelphia: W.B. Saunders; 1992:43-63.
3. Perloff WP. *Physical examination of the Heart and Circulation.* Philadelphia: W.B. Saunders; 1982.
4. Downes TR, Dunson W, Stewart K, et al. Mechanism of physiologic and pathologic S3 gallop sounds. *J Am Soc Echocardiography.* 1992;5:211-218.
5. Patel R, Bushnell DL, Sobotka PA. Implications of an audible third heart sound in evaluating cardiac function. *Western J Med.* 1993;158:606-609.
6. Folland ED, Kriegel BI, Henderson WG, et al. Implications of third heart sounds in patients with valvular heart disease. The Veterans Affairs Cooperative Study on Valvular Heart Disease. *N Engl J Med.* 1992;327:458-462.
7. Meyers DG. Review of cardiac auscultation (Part 1). *Hospital Medicine.* 1993;29(October):25-45.
8. Rahko PS. Doppler and echocardiographic characteristics of patients having an Austin Flint murmur. *Circulation.* 1991;83:1940-1950.
9. Landzberg JS, Pflugfelder PW, Cassidy MM, et al. Etiology of the Austin Flint murmur. *J Am Coll Cardiol.* 1992;20:408-413.
10. Emi S, Fukuda N, Oki T, et al. Genesis of the Austin Flint murmur: relation to mitral inflow and aortic regurgitant flow dynamics. *J Am Coll Cardiol.* 1993;21:1399-1405.
11. Meyers DG. Auscultatory findings in the heart (Part 2). *Hospital Medicine.* 1993;29(November):23-38.

Electrocardiography

CHAPTER **3**

Maria F. DeGuzman, MD

THE NORMAL ELECTROCARDIOGRAM

The normal electrocardiogram (ECG) consists of the P wave, QRS complex, ST segment, T wave and U wave (Fig. 1).

The P wave represents atrial depolarization which originates from the sinoatrial (SA) node and spreads to both atria.[1,2] The early portion of the P wave represents electrical forces from the right atrium, the late portion from the left atrium and the middle portion from both atria and the interatrial septum.

In normal adults, the P duration varies from 0.08 to 0.11 sec, and the amplitude seldom exceeds 2.5 mm in the limb leads and 1.5 mm in the pre-cordial leads. The negative deflection in the right precordial leads is usually less than 1 mm.

The normal P vector is directed to the left and inferiorly; initially it is anterior and terminally is posterior. The P axis in the frontal plane varies from 0° to +75°, and is usually between +45° and +60°. Thus, the P wave is always upright in leads I and II and inverted in AVR. When the mean P axis is directed more inferiorly, for example, in tall, thin individuals, then the P waves in leads II, III and AVF are larger than the P wave in lead I. When the P axis is more leftward, for example, in short, stocky individuals, the P wave is larger in lead I than in the inferior leads. In the horizontal plane, the P

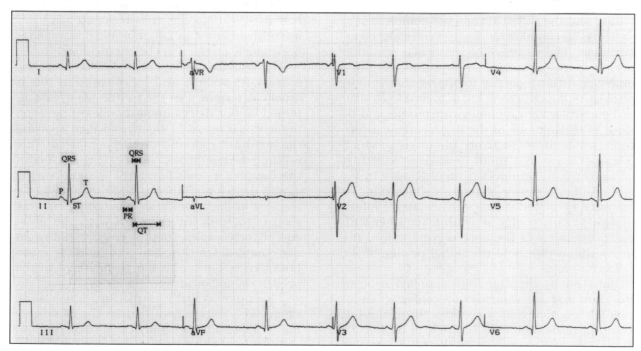

Figure 1. The normal ECG. PR=0.14 sec; QRS=0.08 sec; QTc=0.40 sec. Septal activation rightward (Q in lead I), anteriorly (R in V₁) and superiorly (Q in AVF).

23

waves in leads V_1 and V_2 are usually diphasic with a positive-negative morphology, corresponding to the initial anterior right atrial forces and the terminal posterior left atrial forces. The P wave is always upright in the remaining precordial leads because of the right-to-left atrial activation sequence.

Atrial repolarization (Ta) has the same direction as atrial depolarization, unlike that of the ventricles, because the atria are thin-walled and at low-pressure. The Ta wave produces a negative deflection after the P wave, but is usually not seen in the normal ECG because it is buried in the QRS complex. The Ta, however, may deform the ST segment especially with rapid heart rates or the PR segment when it is prolonged.

The PR interval, measured from the beginning of the P wave to the beginning of the QRS complex, represents the conduction time from the upper right atrium through the atrioventricular (AV) node, bundle of His, left and right bundle branches and the Purkinje fibers until the beginning of ventricular activation. The normal PR interval in the adult is 0.12 to 0.20 sec[3] and varies with the heart rate; the slower the heart rate the longer the PR interval. It is most accurately measured in the lead with the largest P wave and the widest P and QRS complexes.

The QRS complex represents ventricular depolarization. The sequence of ventricular activation occurs in an organized fashion and one must understand this sequence to appreciate the morphology of the QRS complex in every ECG lead.

Ventricular activation begins from the middle third of the left side of the interventricular septum and is directed from left to right which inscribes a normal small Q wave in lead I, is anterior which produces a small R wave in V_1, and is either superior or inferior which explains an initial Q or R wave, respectively, in the inferior leads. This septal activation together with early activation of the anteroseptal wall of the myocardium represent the initial portion of the QRS complex.

Subsequent simultaneous depolarization of the right and left ventricles follows in an endocardial-to-epicardial direction. Since the left ventricle is the dominant ventricle in the normal adult, the major portion of the QRS complex will reflect this and produce mean forces directed to the left and posteriorly, and usually inferiorly. Electrocardiographically, there will be large R waves in leads I, AVL, V_5 and V_6 (left-

ward forces), and a large S wave in V_1 and V_2 (posterior forces).

The terminal portion of the QRS complex represents the last areas of the ventricles to be depolarized, the basal portion of the septum and the posterobasal portion of the free wall of the left ventricle. This results in a mean vector oriented posteriorly to produce an S wave in V_1, and often to the right producing a small s wave in leads I, V_5 and V_6. In 5% of normal adults, however, the terminal vector may be oriented anteriorly, inscribing a small r' in leads V_1 and V_2.

In normal adults the QRS duration varies from 0.06 to 0.10 sec. This represents the total ventricular depolarization time and should be measured from the QRS complex that is widest in either the frontal or horizontal plane. Some leads may show narrower-looking QRS complexes because the initial or terminal forces may be perpendicular to the particular lead and are thus inscribed on the isoelectric line.

The normal mean QRS axis in the frontal plane is between –30° to +105°,[4,5] and in most individuals is between +30° to +75°. In individuals under 40 years of age the axis is 0° to +105°. The axis shifts leftward with age and at 40 years and older, the axis is –30° to +90°. The body habitus also affects the axis which becomes more inferiorly oriented in tall, thin individuals and is horizontally oriented in obese individuals.

The QRS axis represents the direction of the mean QRS vectors and by convention this is usually determined in the frontal plane. A simplified way of determining the axis is by using the hexaxial reference figure and then applying the quadrant rule and the perpendicular rule utilizing the equiphasic complex (Fig. 2). A positive complex in leads I and AVF would place the axis to the left and inferior and therefore locate the axis in the left-inferior quadrant. The next step is to look for the lead with the most equiphasic complex (sum of positive and negative complexes is closest to zero) and the mean QRS axis is perpendicular to this lead in the predetermined quadrant (Fig. 3).

The normal QRS amplitude has a wide range. The voltage recorded on the ECG tracing is dependent not only on cardiac but also extracardiac factors such as chest-wall thickness, emphysema, etc. In general, the QRS voltage is considered to be abnormally low if the amplitude of the entire QRS complex is equal to or less than 5 mm in all the limb leads or equal to

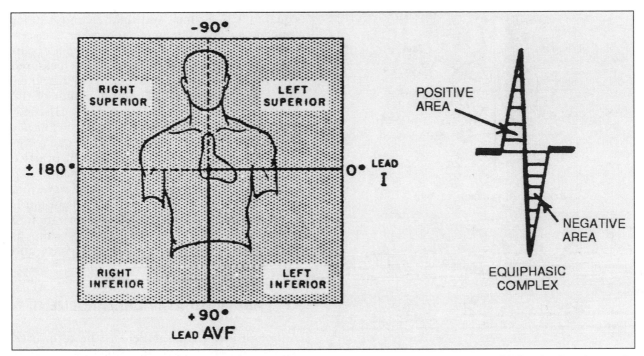

Figure 2. *Use of the quadrant and perpendicular rules in determining the mean frontal QRS axis. Quadrant rule localizes the mean QRS vector to 1 of the 4 quadrants by utilizing the 2 best leads representing left-right axis (lead I) and superior-inferior axis (lead AVF). Perpendicular rule states that the mean QRS axis is perpendicular to the lead with the most equiphasic complex and in the predetermined quadrant.*

or less than 7 mm in all the precordial leads. Lepeschkin[3] has data tabulating the normal ranges of the amplitudes of the Q, R, S, and T waves in men and women of different age groups. In practice, it is difficult to determine upper limits of QRS voltage although the generally accepted maximum in a precordial lead is 25 to 30 mm.

The QRS morphology in the frontal plane depends on the direction of the mean QRS vectors. Since the normal QRS axis is usually in the left inferior quadrant and in most adults is between +30° to +75°, leads I and II will usually inscribe a prominent R wave and AVR will record a negative deflection. The QRS complex in lead III is variable. An axis of +30° will be perpendicular to lead III and a shift in either direction will change the QRS morphology in this lead. The R wave increases and the S wave decreases in amplitude from V_1 to V_5 and/or V_6. A QS complex may be present in V_1 and rarely in V_2. The tallest R wave is usually recorded in V_4 or V_5, and V_6 usually has a lower R wave than V_5. The S wave is usually deepest in V_2 and is

usually absent in V_5 and V_6.

The ST segment is the portion between the end of the QRS complex and the beginning of the T wave. It represents the state when the end of depolarization and the beginning of repolarization are superimposed and neutralize each other. In 75% of healthy adults, the ST segment is isoelectric in the frontal plane,[4] and an elevation or depression of up to 1 mm is within normal.[6] In the precordial leads, however, 90% of healthy adults have some ST elevation[4] most commonly in leads V_2 and V_3. This elevation may reach 3 mm. Since the ST segment vector, if present, is directed to the left, inferiorly and anteriorly, ST depressions are usually abnormal if present in leads I, II, AVF and in any precordial lead.

The T wave represents ventricular repolarization in an epicardial-to-endocardial direction.[7] In healthy individuals, the T vector is directed to the left and inferiorly. In most adults it is anterior or may be slightly posterior, and this is especially true in children and young adults. The T wave is therefore normally upright in

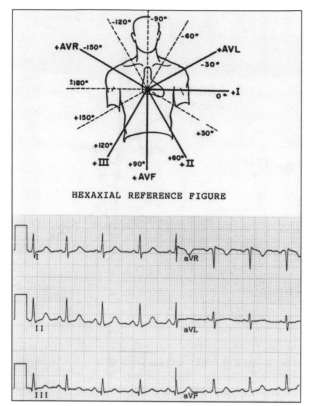

HEXAXIAL REFERENCE FIGURE

Figure 3. Determining mean frontal QRS axis. Positive deflection in lead I (left), positive deflection in AVF (inferior), axis left-inferior quadrant; equiphasic complex in AVL, axis perpendicular to AVL (either +60° or −120°) in the preselected quadrant (+60°).

leads I and II and V_3 to V_6, inverted in AVR, and is variable in leads III, AVL, AVF, V_1 and V_2. The normal T wave is asymmetric with an initial gradual upward slope and when diphasic has a positive-negative direction. The T waves normally are not more than 5 mm high in the limb leads, and 10 mm in the precordial leads although occasionally they may reach up to 12 mm or more in healthy individuals.

The QT interval represents the total duration of ventricular systole and is measured from the beginning of the QRS complex to the end of T wave. Often it is technically difficult to accurately measure the QT interval. It should be obtained from the lead with a large T wave and a distinct end point, and this is usually in either leads V_2 or V_3. The normal limits are 0.30 to 0.46 sec. The most commonly used formula to calculate the QT interval is the Bazett formula:[8] Normal QT interval = K $\sqrt{RR}$, where K is a constant

equal to 0.37 for men and children and 0.40 for women, and RR is the interval between 2 successive R waves. The QT interval corrected for heart rate, QTc, is obtained by dividing the measured QT interval by the square root of the RR interval: QTc = QT/ $\sqrt{RR}$. The upper limit of the QTc interval is 0.39 sec for men and 0.41 sec for women.[3] Minor deviations may not be clinically significant especially since accurate measurements are not always possible and in practice QTc up to 0.44 sec is accepted as normal.

The U wave is a small, low-voltage wave that often follows the T wave. Although its origin is controversial, it may represent repolarization of the Purkinje fibers.[9] Its polarity is the same as the T wave, that is to the left, inferiorly and anteriorly.

LEFT AND RIGHT ATRIAL ENLARGEMENT

Although atrial enlargement is the term used when there are P wave abnormalities, the ECG does not distinguish between atrial hypertrophy, dilatation or intraatrial conduction delay or any combination of these. Perhaps "atrial abnormality" would be a better term to use.

The left atrium is activated after the right atrium and is located posterior and to left of the right atrium. With left atrial enlargement (LAE) the P wave duration is prolonged, the P axis in the frontal plane will be more horizontally oriented, and the posterior component of the P wave in V_1 and V_2 will be larger.

DIAGNOSTIC CRITERIA FOR LAE (FIG. 4)

P wave duration is >0.11 sec.

There seems to be a significant correlation between P wave duration and left atrial dilatation.[10,11] Two-thirds of patients with documented LAE have prolonged P wave duration.

The terminal P vector is posterior in V_1 and is ≥ 0.04 mm-sec.

This measurement is obtained by getting the product of the depth of the terminal negative portion of the P wave in mm and its duration in seconds. This correlates more closely with the left atrial volume than the left atrial pressure.

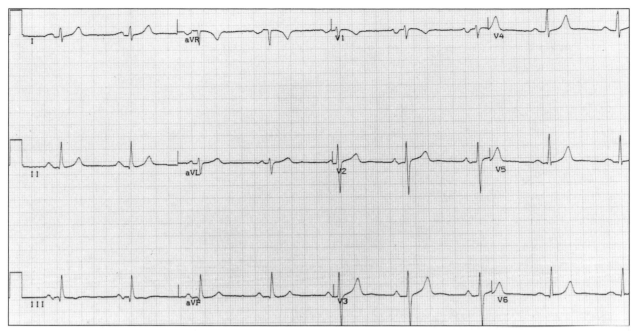

Figure 4. LAE. P duration=0.14 sec in lead II, P terminal posterior vector=0.10 mm-sec in V₁.

Leftward shift of the P axis in the frontal plane to +15° or more (from the normal +45° to +60°).

Atrial activation begins in the SA node which is located in the posterior-superior portion of the right atrium. Therefore, the initial portion of the P wave is the result of right atrial depolarization which is directed inferiorly and anteriorly.

Right atrial enlargement (RAE) causes the frontal plane P axis to shift vertically, with tall peaked P waves in the inferior leads, and in V_1 and V_2 the anterior component will be larger. Since the right atrial forces are responsible only for the initial part of the P wave, the total P wave duration is not prolonged in RAE.

DIAGNOSTIC CRITERIA FOR RAE (FIG. 5)

P wave is ≥ 2.5 mm tall in leads II, III, AVF.

Diagnosis is more specific if a 3 mm criterion is used. Tall peaked P waves may be seen in normal subjects with asthma or long, thin body habitus and is due to the vertical position of the heart.

P wave axis is +75° or greater in the frontal plane.

An axis of greater than +90° is uncommon and therefore almost never is there a negative P wave in lead I even in severe RAE.

P wave is ≥ 1.5 mm tall in V₁ or V2.

Biatrial enlargement is diagnosed when criteria for LAE and RAE are present (Fig. 6).

LEFT VENTRICULAR HYPERTROPHY (LVH)

The increased left ventricular mass results in an exaggeration of the normal dominance of the left ventricle. Therefore, an increased QRS voltage is directed to the left and posteriorly; a prolongation of ventricular activation time, prolongs the QRS duration; and the onset of the intrinsicoid deflection (ID) may be delayed. Because there is a delay in the endocardial-to-epicardial ventricular depolarization, a reversal of the repolarization process occurs from endocardium to epicardium. This results in secondary repolarization abnormality of the ST

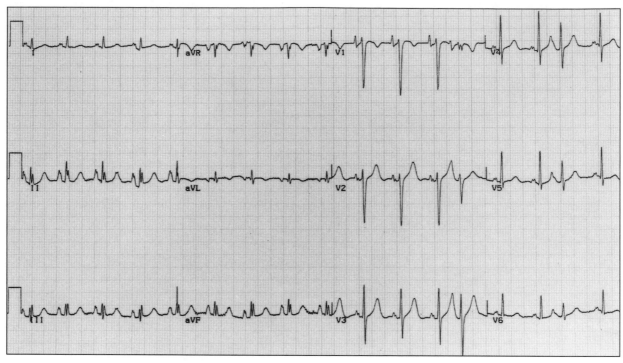

Figure 5. RAE. P amplitude=4 mm in lead II and 3 mm in V_1, P axis +75°.

segment and the T wave and is directed opposite to the left ventricle; that is, to the right and anteriorly.

DIAGNOSTIC CRITERIA FOR LVH (FIG. 7)

Increased QRS voltage.

The electrocardiographic diagnosis of LVH is difficult to establish because it is predominantly dependent on an increase of the QRS voltage, which can be altered by many noncardiac and cardiac factors. These include proximity factors, such as body habitus, large breasts, cardiac position, pneumonectomy, etc.; conduction factors, such as obesity, pericardial fluid, pleural fluid, emphysema, etc.; and impulse formation factors, such as chamber enlargement, age, etc. There are numerous voltage criteria proposed but those suggested by Sokolow and Lyon[12] are commonly used:

R in AVL >11 mm (horizontal heart)
R in AVF >20 mm (vertical heart)
R in V_5 or V_6 >26 mm
R in V_5 or V_6 + S in V_1 >35 mm.

Criteria proposed by other authors[13–15] are:

Largest R+largest S in precordial leads >45 mm
R in lead I + S in lead III >25 mm
S in AVR >14 mm.

Sensitivity of the combined criteria is reported as 60% to 85%[16,17] and specificity is 85% to 89%.[17,18]

In general, increased voltage in the precordial leads was the most sensitive criterion (up to 56%) but gave up to a 15% false-positive diagnosis. On the other hand, high voltage in the limb leads is less sensitive (up to 11%) but very specific, with no false-positive diagnosis.[19]

Secondary ST-T abnormality directed opposite to the left ventricle.

ST segment is depressed and T wave inverted in the left precordial leads, V_5 and V_6. In the limb leads, similar changes occur in leads I and AVL with a horizontal QRS axis, and in leads II, III and AVF if the axis is vertical. These are secondary repolarization abnormalities and are directed rightward.

In the right precordial leads, V_1 and V_2, the ST segment may be elevated and the T wave upright. These are secondary repolarization abnormalities

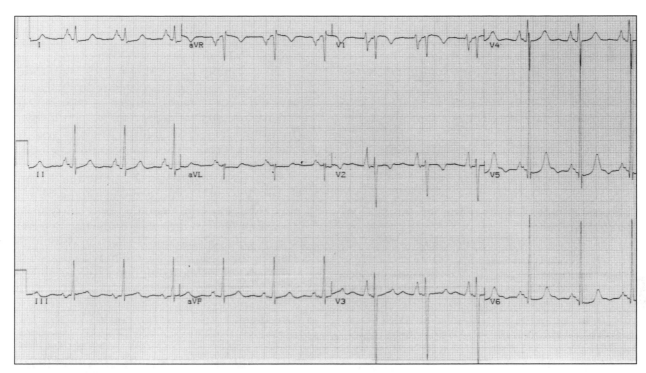

Figure 6. *Biatrial enlargement. P duration=0.12 sec and P amplitude=4 mm in lead II; P terminal posterior vector=0.32 mm sec and P amplitude=5.5 mm in V$_{1-2}$.*

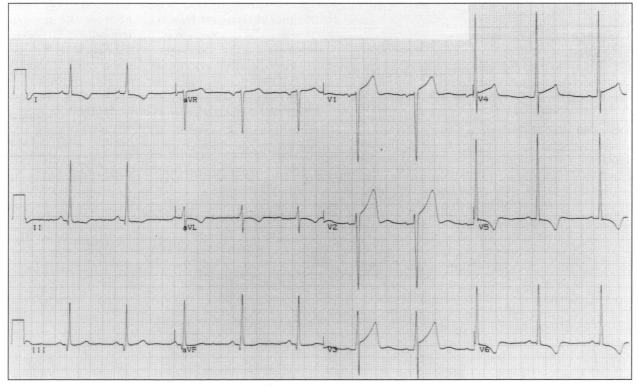

Figure 7. *LVH. Increased QRS voltage left and posterior: R-AVF=21 mm, R-V$_5$=35 mm, R-V$_5$ + S-V$_1$=63 mm; repolarization abnormality right and anterior: depressed ST and inverted T in leads I, AVL, V$_{5-6}$ and elevated ST and upright T in V$_{1-2}$.*

and are directed anteriorly. Although these ST-T changes are secondary abnormalities, primary T wave changes, if present, will also rotate the T vector away from the left ventricle and create the same abnormally wide QRS-T angle; thus, the term "strain" is used. However, it is preferable to view these as secondary changes and not use the word, "strain."

When voltage criteria and the classical ST-T changes are present, a false-positive diagnosis of LVH is seldom made.[17]

Delayed onset of ID over the left ventricle of up to ≥ 0.05 sec.

The onset of intrinsicoid deflection (ID) represents the time period for the impulse to pass through the ventricles from endocardium to epicardium underlying the exploring electrode and is measured from the onset of the QRS to the peak of the R wave. The upper limit of normal for the left ventricle measured in V_5 or V_6 is 0.045 sec and for the right ventricle measured in V_1 or V_2 is 0.035 sec.

This criterion is highly insensitive but quite specific especially if other criteria are also present.

Prolonged QRS duration.

An increase in left ventricular mass results in a longer depolarization time and therefore an increased duration of the QRS but not up to 0.12 sec.

Left axis deviation.

LVH shifts the mean QRS axis leftward although it is unusual for the axis to shift to more than –30°.

Romhilt and Estes[20] developed a point score system to diagnose LVH as follows:

QRS Voltage — 3 points for presence of any 1 criterion:
  R or S in limb lead ≥ 20 mm
  S in V_1 or V_2 ≥ 30 mm
  R in V_5 or V_6 ≥ 30 mm.
Typical ST-T repolarization abnormality
  Without digitalis — 3 points
  With digitalis — 1 point
LAD –30° or more — 2 points
QRS duration ≥ 0.09 sec — 1 point
ID V_{5-6} ≥ 0.05 sec — 1 point
LAE (terminal negative P wave
  in V_1 ≥ 0. 04 mm-sec)— 3 points
A score of 5 or more points is diagnostic of

LVH, and of 4 points suggests probable LVH.

Some physiologic factors can affect the diagnosis of LVH such as age — children and young adults normally have higher QRS amplitude; body habitus — thin, emaciated individuals may have tall QRS voltages; gender — men in general have higher voltages than women in both the frontal and horizontal planes; and race — blacks are reported to have higher voltages than whites.

Some pathologic states also affect the diagnosis of LVH such as lung disease, pleural and pericardial effusion, pneumothorax, myocardial disease and intraventricular conduction defects.

It is generally accepted that the commonly used electrocardiographic criteria are less sensitive than the echocardiogram (20% to 50% vs 88%) in the diagnosis of LVH. Both are equally highly specific but the echocardiogram also detects concentric versus eccentric LVH.

RIGHT VENTRICULAR HYPERTROPHY (RVH)

An increase in right ventricular mass results in an increase of QRS vectors directed to the right and anteriorly. However, because the normal electrical dominance of the left ventricular forces is several times stronger than the right ventricular forces, RVH has to be severe to abolish or modify left ventricular forces that are oriented to the left and posteriorly. The changes in RVH are best seen in the right precordial leads, V_1 and V_2 which are directly over the right ventricle.

DIAGNOSTIC CRITERIA FOR RVH (FIG. 8)

QRS voltage and R/S ratios

Proposed by Sokolow and Lyon.[21]
$RV_1 + SV_5$ or V_6 ≥ 10.5 mm
RV_1 > 7 mm
R/S ratio in V_5 or V_6 < 1
SV_1 < 2 mm
RAVR ≥ 5 mm
RV_5 or V_6 < 5 mm
SV_5 or V_6 ≥ 7 mm
$$\frac{\text{R/S ratio in } V_5}{\text{R/S ratio in } V_1} \leq 0.4$$

The first 4 are the more frequently used criteria. Other criteria that are proposed:

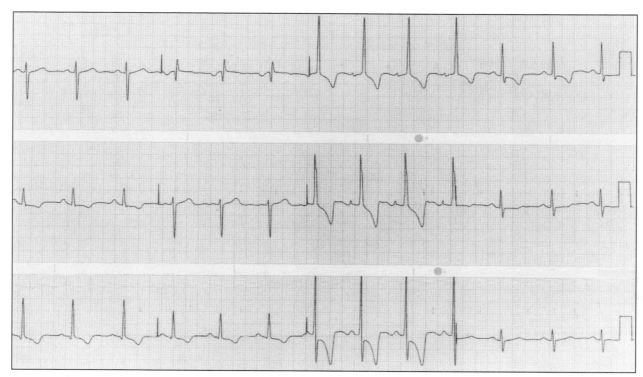

Figure 8. *RVH. Increased QRS voltage right and anterior: R-V$_1$=23 mm, R-V$_1$ + S-V$_6$=27 mm, no S in V$_1$; RAD=+135°; repolarization abnormality left and posterior: upright T in lead I and depressed ST and inverted T in V$_1$.*

R/S ratio V$_1$ >1
qR in V$_1$
RAD +110° or more
Onset of ID in V$_1$ 0.035–0.055 sec
R ≥ 10 mm if rSR' pattern in V$_1$

In general the R/S ratio decreases in the precordial leads from right to left.

Secondary ST-T abnormality directed opposite to the right ventricle.

There is ST-segment depression and T-wave inversion in the right precordial leads (V$_1$ and V$_2$). The presence of repolarization abnormality often suggests severe RVH.

Delayed onset of ID over the right ventricle >0.035 sec.

The onset of ID in V$_1$ is prolonged to >0.035 sec, whereas that in the left precordial leads is within normal limits.

Normal QRS duration.

The thickness of the hypertrophied right ventricle does not exceed that of the left ventricle and

therefore the QRS duration is seldom prolonged in RVH. In some congenital heart diseases where the right ventricle may be thicker than the left ventricle, the QRS may be prolonged to 0.10 sec or more.

A Q wave in V$_1$ may be present in RVH. This is because of the marked clockwise rotation of the heart so that septal activation may be directed posteriorly, or because of the presence of lower right septal forces being greater than the left, resulting in the septal vector being directed to the left and posteriorly. When present, a Q wave in V$_1$ is one of the most specific signs of RVH.

Right axis deviation (RAD) between +90° and +150°.

Right axis deviation may be absent when RVH is not severe. On the other hand, it is also seen in healthy infants and children, tall, thin subjects, chronic obstructive lung disease, lateral wall infarct and left inferior posterior hemiblock.

The sensitivity of the electrocardiographic criteria for RVH varies tremendously from 23% to 66%[22,23] and depends on the patient population. If the patient population has a large num-

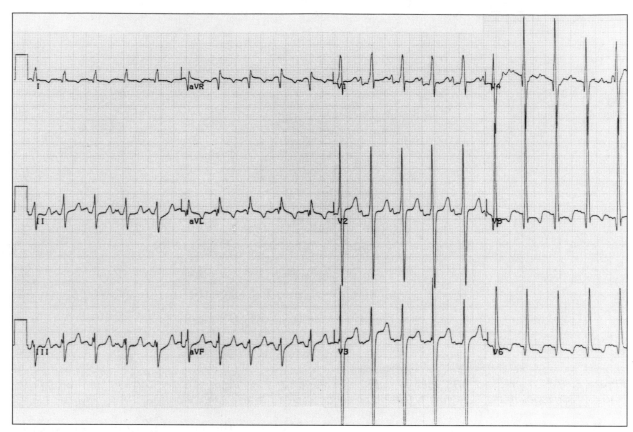

Figure 9. *Combined ventricular hypertrophy. R-V$_1$=10.5 mm (RVH), R-V$_5$= 42 mm (LVH) and repolarization abnormality of LVH.*

ber of congenital heart diseases and, therefore, severe RVH, the sensitivity is increased. The sensitivity of individual criterion is low and is generally less than 20%.

COMBINED VENTRICULAR HYPERTROPHY

Biventricular hypertrophy is often difficult to recognize, especially when the left or right ventricular forces counterbalance each other, which causes the usual voltage criteria to be absent.

DIAGNOSTIC CRITERIA FOR COMBINED VENTRICULAR HYPERTROPHY (FIG. 9)

Tall R in V$_1$ and V$_2$ (RVH) and tall R in V$_5$ and V$_6$ (LVH)
Delayed onset of ID over both ventricles
Repolarization abnormalities over the involved ventricle

Rs in V$_1$ to V$_5$ in the presence of LVH
LAD in limb leads and RVH in precordial leads
RAD in limb leads and LVH in precordial leads
Katz-Wachtel sign — very high voltage in V$_2$, V$_3$, and V$_4$ with combined R and S voltage >60 mm

RIGHT BUNDLE BRANCH BLOCK (RBBB)

The right bundle branch is a long, slender stalk that does not give off branches until it reaches the base of the anterior papillary muscle of the right ventricle near the interventricular septum. In the presence of RBBB, activation of the right septum and the right ventricle is delayed. The initial septal activation from the middle of the left septum proceeds normally to the right and anteriorly. Then, instead of simultaneous depolarization of both ventricles, the left and right ventricles are

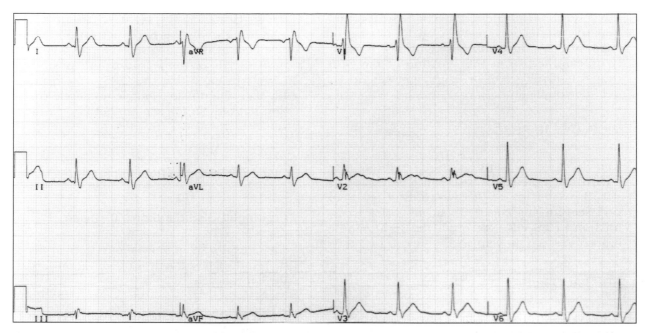

Figure 10. *RBBB. QRS duration=0.14 sec, normal septal activation: Q-lead I and R-V₁, delayed onset of ID in V₁=0.08 sec, delayed right ventricular forces right and anterior: wide slurred S-lead I and R'-V₁, and repolarization abnormality left and posterior: upright T-lead I and inverted T-V₁.*

depolarized sequentially, the left ventricle first via the intact left bundle branch, resulting in vectors directed to the left and posteriorly. Up to this point the QRS complex looks normal. The terminal QRS portion represents the delayed abnormal activation of the right ventricular septum and free wall. These terminal forces, unopposed by potentials from the left ventricle which has already completed its activation, are directed to the right (S in leads I, V_5 and V_6) and anteriorly (R' or r' in leads V_1 and V_2), and are wide and slurred due to the slow muscle-to-muscle conduction.

Secondary repolarization abnormality occurs so that the ST segment and T wave are directed to the left and posteriorly opposite to the terminal QRS vectors directed to the right and anteriorly (right ventricular forces).

DIAGNOSTIC CRITERIA FOR RBBB (FIG. 10)

Prolonged QRS duration ≥ 0.12 sec.

This is due to delayed muscle-to-muscle activation of the right ventricular septum and free wall.

Delayed onset of ID in the right precordial lead V_1 >0.05 sec.

This is also due to delayed activation of the

right ventricle and must be present to make the diagnosis.

Increased amplitude of the R' in the right precordial leads V_1 and V_2.

The R' has a higher amplitude than the initial septal R wave (rsR' or rSR') because these terminal anterior forces are unopposed by the left ventricular posterior forces. The S wave (in V_1) which represents left ventricular activation may be absent or not as deep as usual because the left ventricular forces are being opposed by the septal forces.

Wide, slurred S wave in leads I, V_5 and V_6.

This is due to delayed abnormal right ventricular forces directed rightward.

Secondary ST-T abnormality directed to the left and posteriorly.

The right precordial leads V_1 and V_2 may show depressed ST segment and inverted T wave; the left precordial leads, V_5 and V_6, and lead I may show elevated ST segment and upright T wave.

Other common electrocardiographic findings

are a terminal positive deflection in AVR and negative deflection in AVL, and a normal or rightward axis deviation. The QRS axis is usually determined from that portion of the QRS (initial 0.06–0.08 sec) prior to right ventricular delayed conduction.

INCOMPLETE RBBB

The electrocardiographic findings in incomplete RBBB are essentially the same as complete RBBB except for a QRS duration of less than 0.12 sec. Incomplete RBBB suggests slow transmission of impulses through the right bundle branch to the right ventricle.

RBBB AND RVH

Some criteria proposed to diagnose RVH in the presence of complete RBBB are an R in V_1 >15 mm[24] and an abnormal RAD of the unblocked portion of the QRS complex. However, these have been found to have a low sensitivity and specificity.

RBBB AND LVH

Voltage criteria for LVH are often counterbalanced by the presence of complete RBBB. However, when present, they are highly specific.

LEFT BUNDLE BRANCH BLOCK (LBBB)

In LBBB ventricular activation is abnormal from the start and the main delay is in the septum. Instead of normally originating from the mid-left septal surface, septal activation starts from the right midseptal and lower septal mass and is directed from the right to left (absence of normal septal q wave in lead I), anteriorly and inferiorly toward the apex. Muscle-to-muscle activation of the septum continues from apex to base and this delayed septal activation is believed to cause the QRS prolongation.[25,26] Once the activation front reaches the base of the septum, it reenters the normal Purkinje system below the block and proceeds to depolarize the left ventricle in a normal fashion. As in RBBB the ventricles are depolarized successively rather than simultaneously, but in LBBB the left ventricle is depolarized after the right ventricle. However, the right ventricular forces which occur during early activation are canceled out by the strong septal forces going in an opposite direction leftward and posteriorly. Others propose that the QRS prolongation in LBBB is due to slow muscle-to-muscle conduction not only in the septum but also in the left ventricular wall.

DIAGNOSTIC CRITERIA FOR LBBB (FIG. 11)

Prolonged QRS duration ≥ 0.12 sec.

This results from slow septal activation and therefore delayed arrival of activation forces to the left ventricle.

Delayed onset of ID in leads over the left ventricle, V_5 and V_6.

This is a fundamental criterion to make the diagnosis of LBBB and signifies delayed activation of the left ventricle. The onset of ID in V_5 and V_6 is abnormally prolonged up to 0.10 sec (normal = 0.035–0.055 sec).

Absence of Q wave in leads I, V_5 and V_6.

Septal activation starts from mid- and low-right septal surface and goes leftward, resulting in the absence of the normal septal Q wave in leads over the left ventricle.

Increased amplitude of the R' in the left precordial leads.

Following the initial septal force, activation of the lower septum occurs and is directed to the left and posteriorly, giving rise to the upstroke and peak of the R wave in leads I, V_5 and V_6, and the downstroke of the S wave in leads V_1 and V_2. Continued activation of the upper two-thirds of the left side of the septum is very slow and produces the slurring and notching of the R wave in V_5 and V_6. and the slurring and notching of the S wave in V_1 and V_2. Delayed onset of left ventricular activation, unopposed by right ventricular forces, produces an R of greater than normal amplitude in the left precordial leads. Left ventricular activation pro-

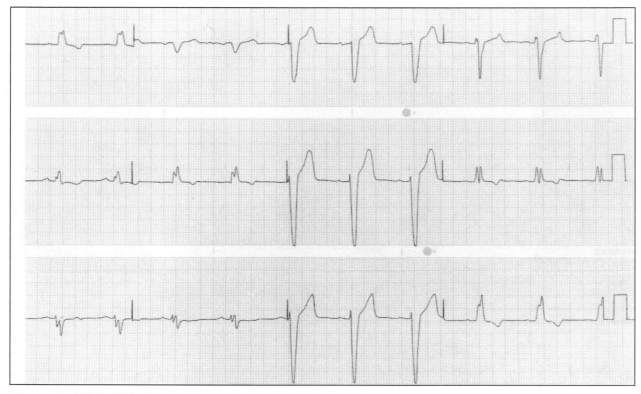

Figure 11. *LBBB. QRS duration=0.16 sec, abnormal septal activation leftward (absent Q-lead I), delayed onset of ID in V_{5-6}=0.10 sec, slurring and notching of R-V_{5-6} and S-V_{1-2}, and repolarization abnormality right and anterior: inverted T-lead I, elevated ST and upright T-V_1.*

ceeds rapidly as the activation wave reenters the Purkinje system.

Secondary ST-T abnormality directed to the right and anteriorly.

Leads I, V_5 and V_6 may show depressed ST segment and inverted T wave; V_1 and V_2 may show ST-segment elevation and upright T wave.

There is controversy whether or not uncomplicated complete LBBB produces an abnormal left axis deviation (LAD). In LBBB the leftward shift in axis is not significant[27] and in the presence of an abnormal LAD some investigators propose additionally the presence of left anterior superior hemiblock (LASH) as its cause.[28] If after septal activation is completed the excitation wave reenters the Purkinje network below the block and LASH coexists, then there will be an abnormal LAD. Other investigators, however, have shown that LBBB alone is responsible for marked LAD.[29,30]

INCOMPLETE LBBB (a controversial subject)

Most patients with incomplete LBBB have LVH and it may not be clinically important to make the differentiation. Some of the diagnostic criteria are:
  Diminished or absent Q wave in V_5 and V_6
  Initial slurring of R wave in V_5 and V_6
  QRS duration usually not more than 0.11 sec
  Delayed onset of intrinsicoid deflection in V_5 and $V_6 \geq 0.06$ sec
  Small or absent R wave in V_1 and V_2

LBBB AND LVH

Although patients with LBBB may have LVH, the usual voltage criteria for LVH are not applicable. One study[31] reported an 86% sensitivity and a 100% specificity using the criterion of SV_2 + RV_6 >45 mm to diagnose LVH. A markedly prolonged QRS duration up to 0.18–0.20 sec may support the diagnosis of LVH.

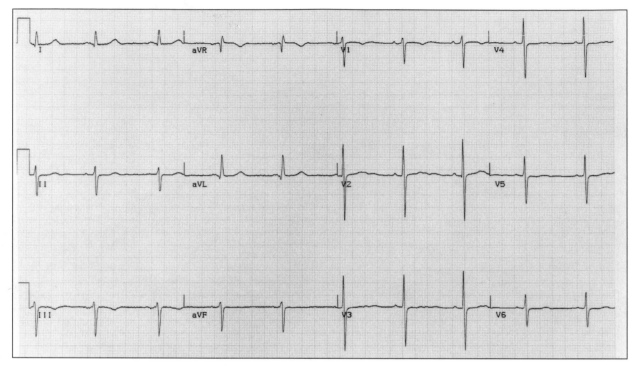

Figure 12. LASH. LAD $-60°$, qR-lead I, rS-AVF, and persistent S-V_{5-6}.

LBBB AND RVH

It is not possible to diagnose RVH in the presence of LBBB. A few case reports propose that if the frontal plane axis shows an abnormal right axis deviation (RAD) in the presence of typical LBBB changes in the precordial leads, this is suggestive of RVH.

HEMIBLOCKS

The left bundle branch divides into 2 major divisions of clinical import, the anterior-superior division which supplies the anterior and lateral walls of the left ventricle, and the posterior-inferior division which supplies the inferior and posterior portion of the left ventricle. A branching network of Purkinje fibers interconnect these major fascicles.

Conduction through the anterior fascicle results in a vector oriented to the left and superiorly; conduction through the posterior fascicle results in a vector oriented to the right and inferiorly. Normally, conduction through these fascicles occurs simultaneously. A delay or inter-ruption of conduction through either one of the fascicles produces a hemiblock.

In left anterior superior hemiblock (LASH), the impulse initially travels to the right and inferiorly, and terminally to the left and superiorly. Because these late forces are unopposed, they are prominent and also shift the axis to the left and superiorly.

In left posterior inferior hemiblock (LPIH) the opposite occurs. Initial vectors will go left and superiorly, and terminally to the right and inferiorly. Again, these terminal forces are mostly unopposed and result in right axis deviation.

DIAGNOSTIC CRITERIA FOR LASH (FIG. 12)

Abnormal LAD ($-30°$ to $-90°$).

This is a major criterion. There are differences in opinion as to how much LAD results from LASH. Rosenbaum,[29] who has probably given the most significant contribution regarding the electrocardiographic changes in hemiblocks, suggests an axis of at least $-45°$.

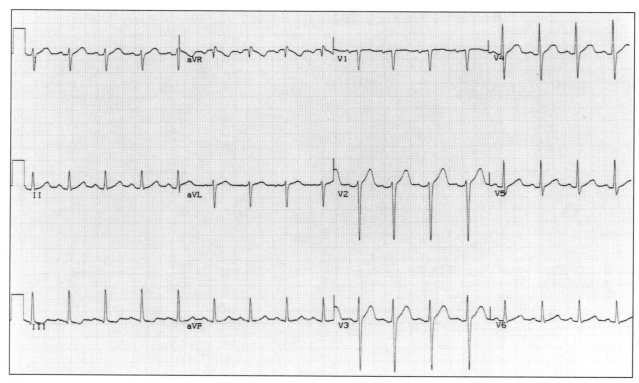

Figure 13. *LPIH. RAD=+105°, rS-lead I, qR-AVF, and no RVH.*

A qR in leads I and AVL and an rS in leads II, III and AVF.

This results from initial vectors to the right and inferiorly and terminal vectors to the left and superiorly. Because of the prominent forces leftward, large R waves may be present in leads I and AVL and may mimic LVH. The S wave in lead III is usually larger than the S wave in lead II because the axis shift in the left superior quadrant is more parallel to lead III than to lead II.

Normal or slightly prolonged QRS duration.

The QRS prolongs by 0.02 sec with the development of the hemiblock.

Other electrocardiographic findings include poor R wave progression across the precordial leads with persistent S waves in leads V_5 and V_6 due to the left superior axis deviation; the persistent S waves in leads V_5 and V_6 will disappear if the electrodes are placed 1 or 2 interspaces higher; and the peak of the R wave in AVR occurs after the peak of the R wave in AVL.

DIAGNOSTIC CRITERIA FOR LPIH (FIG. 13)

Abnormal RAD (+90° to +180°).

Other causes of RAD must be excluded before making a diagnosis of LPIH.

An rS in leads I and AVL and qR in leads II, III and AVF.

This results from initial vectors to the left and superiorly and terminal vectors to the right and inferiorly.

Normal or slightly prolonged QRS duration.

Absence of RVH.

A large R wave in V_1 with secondary repolarization changes favors RVH.

BIFASCICULAR, BILATERAL AND TRIFASCICULAR BLOCKS

The right bundle branch and the 2 divisions of the left bundle branch comprise a trifascicular

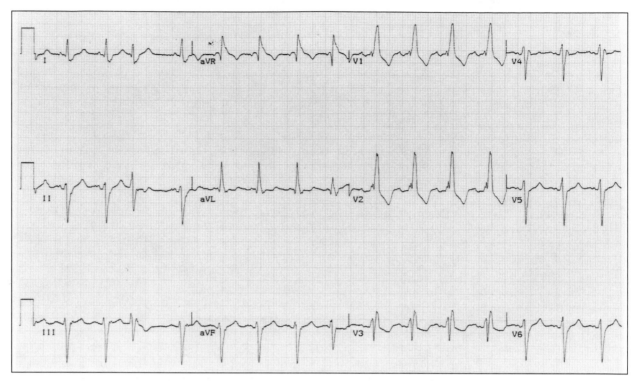

Figure 14. *RBBB + LASH (bifascicular block).*

system. RBBB with either LASH or LPIH is called a bifascicular block. RBBB plus LASH is the more common type of bifascicular block (Fig. 14). Involvement of both the right bundle branch and the main left bundle branch or its fascicles is also called bilateral bundle branch block. When all 3 fascicles are blocked, completely or incompletely, it is called trifascicular block. The ECG features of trifascicular block are varied and only His bundle electrocardiography can locate the exact site of the block.

MYOCARDIAL INFARCTION, INJURY, AND ISCHEMIA

The ECG is an excellent tool for the diagnosis and localization of myocardial necrosis (QRS changes), injury (ST-segment changes) and ischemia (T-wave changes). The electrocardiographic diagnostic hallmarks for acute myocardial infarction are abnormal Q waves, ST-segment elevation and T-wave inversion. Since many other clinical conditions can produce these ECG changes, the diagnosis of myocardial infarction must be based on the total clinical picture, including the history and the laboratory data, and serial ECG changes.

Myocardial necrosis produces an electrically dead zone. The resultant vectors which become dominant as they are unopposed, will be directed away from this area. An electrode facing the infarcted myocardium will thus inscribe an abnormal Q wave if the unopposed potentials are large.

Myocardial injury is represented by ST-segment changes. Injured muscle, when stimulated, becomes less negatively charged than the stimulated uninjured muscle at the end of depolarization. The injury vector is always directed toward the area of injury. If the injury is subepicardial, leads overlying the injured muscle will show ST-segment elevation and the opposite leads will show ST-segment depression (reciprocal changes). If the injury is subendocardial, the injury vector will be directed from the uninjured epicardial muscle toward the injury and leads overlying the area will show ST-segment depression.

Myocardial ischemia, represented by changes in the T wave, delays the repolarization process and prolongs the QT interval. Normally, repo-

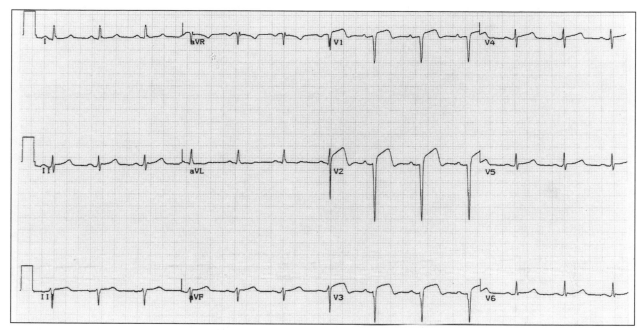

Figure 15. *Anteroseptal MI. Q wave, ST-elevation, and T-wave inversion in V$_{1-3}$.*

larization is delayed in the endocardium and therefore proceeds from epicardium to endocardium. Since the repolarization wave has a negative front, the T waves are normally upright over the epicardium.

In subepicardial myocardial ischemia, repolarization is reversed and proceeds in an endocardial-to-epicardial direction. The ischemic vector is therefore directed away from the area of ischemia and produces inverted T waves. In subendocardial ischemia the normal subendocardial delay is exaggerated but the repolarization sequence is not altered from epicardium to endocardium. The T wave then remains upright in the leads overlying the ischemia and is tall, peaked and increased in duration.

It is important to recognize clinically that numerous nonischemic conditions can produce T-wave abnormalities. Primary T-wave changes are characterized by being symmetrically inverted, or the T waves may be peaked with either isoelectric or slightly elevated J-junction.

When abnormal Q, ST-segment and T-wave changes are present in an acute myocardial infarction, it is called a Q-wave infarct; when only the ST-T changes occur, it is called a non-Q-wave infarct. The terms transmural and nontransmural myocardial infarction are not used because the ECG changes correlate poorly with the pathological findings. Non-Q and Q-wave myocardial infarction imply a different clinical course and thus this classification seems more meaningful.

DIAGNOSTIC CRITERIA FOR Q-WAVE MYOCARDIAL INFARCTION

Anteroseptal (Fig. 15).

QS deflection in leads V$_1$, V$_2$, and V$_3$ and absence of septal q wave in leads V$_5$, V$_6$.

Strictly anterior.

rS in lead V$_1$ and QS in leads V$_2$, V$_3$, V$_4$. Initial septal forces are preserved.

Anterolateral (Fig. 16).

Abnormal Q wave in leads V$_4$, V$_5$, V$_6$, I, AVL. The Q wave should be at least 0.04 sec.

Extensive anterior.

This is a combination of anteroseptal, strictly anterior, and anterolateral. QS in all precordial

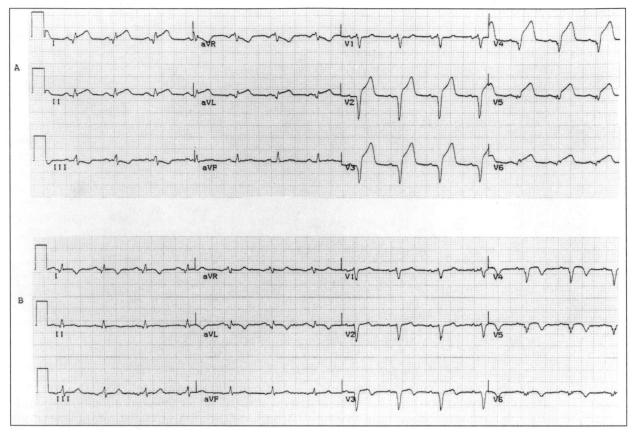

Figures 16A and B. *Evolution of acute anterolateral MI. ECG B: 1 day after ECG A.*

leads with or without Q wave in leads I and AVL.

High lateral.

Abnormal Q wave in leads I and AVL.

Inferior.

Abnormal Q wave ($\geq$ 0.04 sec) in leads II, III and AVF. A Q wave in lead III alone is not diagnostic.

Infero-lateral.

Abnormal Q wave in leads II, III, AVF, V_5, V_6 and sometimes in leads I and AVL.

True posterior.

Loss of posterior forces exaggerates the normal initial anterior vectors giving rise to an R wave in leads V_1 and V_2 $\geq$ 0.04 sec and with an R/S ratio $\geq$ 1. In the acute phase, leads V_1/V_2 will show ST-segment depression (ST vector toward

injury) and upright T wave (ischemic vector away from ischemia). Isolated posterior myocardial infarction is rare.

Inferior-posterior (Fig. 17).

Combination of inferior and posterior.

Posterolateral.

Tall, wide R wave in leads V_1 and V_2 with an R/S ratio of $\geq$ 1 and abnormal Q wave in leads V_5, V_6 and sometimes in leads I and AVL.

Right ventricular infarction.

Acute inferior or infero-posterior changes, plus ST-segment elevation of $\geq$ 1 mm in 1 or more of the right precordial leads, especially in lead V_4R.

Accompanying laboratory data and ST-segment and T-wave changes and their evolution seen in serial ECGs confirm the diagnosis and determine the acuteness of the infarction.

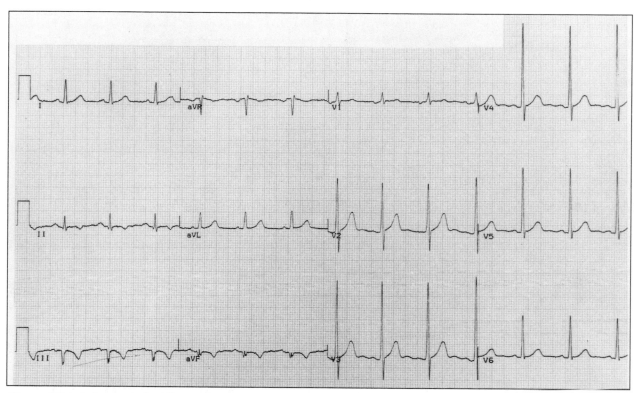

Figure 17. *Inferior-posterior MI.*

In the acute phase, the first ECG change that is usually seen is ST-segment elevation in the lead facing the infarct and ST-segment depression in the opposite leads (Figs. 18A, 18B). ST-segment elevation varies from 1 mm to several mm. It lasts for hours or days and in the majority resolve within 2 weeks. When the ST-segment elevation persists for at least 4 weeks, the possibility of a left ventricular aneurysm is considered.

Abnormal Q waves usually develop within a few hours of the infarction and they usually appear while the ST segment is still elevated. They may persist for years or indefinitely; in some patients they disappear.

During the hyperacute stage of the infarction, tall, peaked T waves may actually be the very first ECG change but are quite transient, and accompany the marked ST elevation (Fig. 19). The T waves then become symmetrically inverted while the ST segment is still elevated but is returning to baseline. These T-wave inversions become prominent as evolution continues and may persist for days, weeks, months, or even years.

The major effects of reperfusion on the electrocardiogram are a rapid evolution of the infarct pattern and arrhythmias. The ST-segment elevation starts decreasing rapidly, maybe within 30 minutes of the reperfusion therapy and continues to do so for many hours thereafter. Q waves also develop earlier, and may decrease in size, or are seen in fewer leads in the succeeding hours. The most common rhythm disturbance is an accelerated idioventricular rhythm.

MYOCARDIAL INFARCTION AND RBBB (FIGS. 20–22)

As was previously discussed, in RBBB only the terminal QRS vectors are altered. And since most myocardial infarctions result in abnormalities of the initial QRS vectors, the usual diagnostic criteria for both RBBB and MI are not affected. A true posterior infarct may be an exception wherein an exaggeration of the anterior forces (R in V_1) may be difficult to differentiate from that of RBBB. However, the ischemic T wave vector in posterior infarct is directed anteriorly (upright T wave in lead V_1) and in RBBB is posterior (inverted T wave in lead V_1).

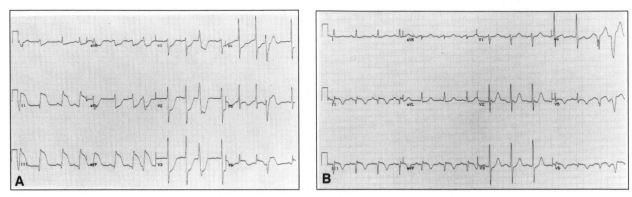

Figures 18A and B. *Evolution of acute inferior-posterior-lateral MI and PVCs. ECG B: 1 day after ECG A.*

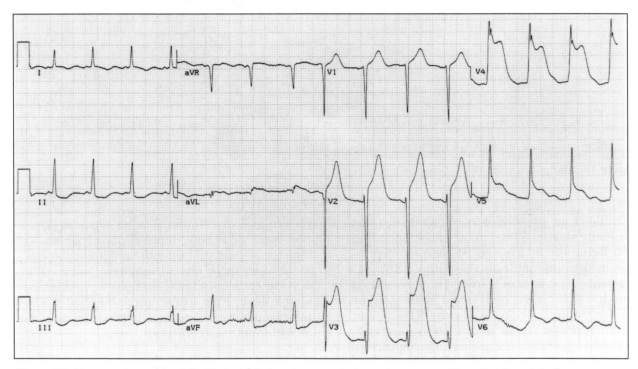

Figure 19. *Hyperacute anterior MI. Marked ST elevation anteriorly, up to 16 mm in V₃, with tall upright T waves.*

MYOCARDIAL INFARCTION AND COMPLETE LBBB

Myocardial infarction is difficult to diagnose because complete LBBB alters the ventricular activation sequence from the start. Again, since most of the infarcts result in abnormalities of the initial vectors, the standard criteria are not applicable. The following changes may suggest the presence of infarction:

Presence of Q wave in leads I, V_5 and V_6:

With septal infarct, the septal forces leftward disappear and the right ventricular potentials directed rightward produce a Q wave in leads I, V_5 and V_6.

ST-T vectors directed opposite the secondary repolarization changes: For example, in acute lateral MI the depressed ST segment seen in V_5 and V_6 in LBBB will become elevated. This is further confirmed by evolutionary changes.

Thus, LBBB can mimic or mask MI, whereas RBBB neither mimics nor masks MI.

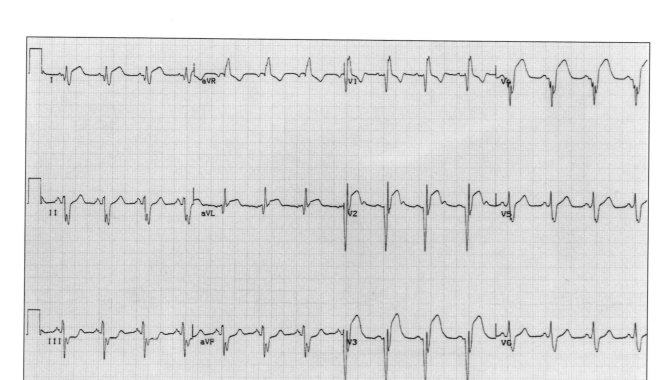

Figure 20. *RBBB + LASH (bifascicular block) + anterolateral MI.*

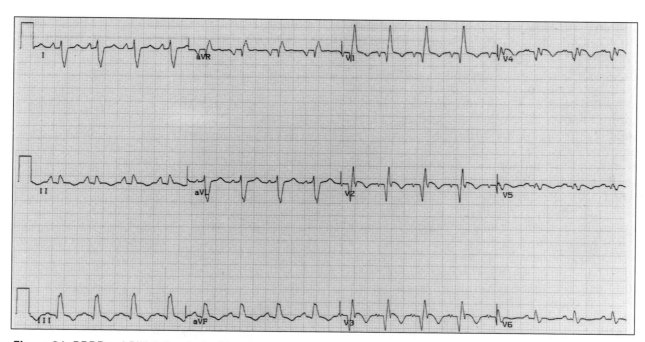

Figure 21. *RBBB + LPIH (bifascicular block) + anteroseptal and inferior MI; probable biatrial enlargement.*

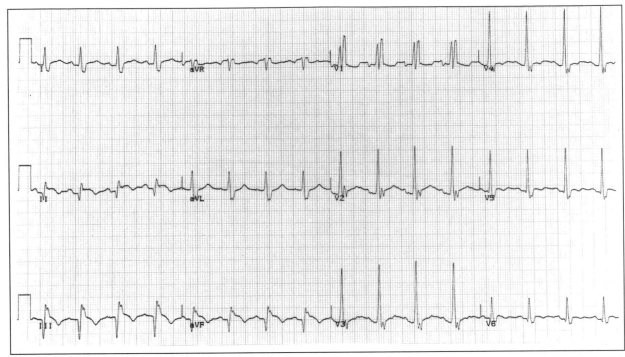

Figure 22. *RBBB + inferior-posterior MI. Initial tall, broad R wave in V_{1-2} suggests posterior MI along with the inferior MI.*

SIGNAL-AVERAGED ELECTROCARDIOGRAPHY

The signal-averaged electrocardiogram (SA ECG) has its greatest use in identifying late ventricular potentials. They serve as a marker for a substrate with slow and inhomogeneous activation from which reentrant tachyarrhythmias originate. The application of an abnormal SAECG has been studied best following an MI.

The presence of late ventricular potentials after an MI has an important prognostic implication although the timing of these recordings can affect the prevalence and its significance. An abnormal SAECG a few hours or a few days after the infarction may not be meaningful and is usually transient. The best time to record the SAECG is 7–10 days after the infarct during which period the incidence of late ventricular potentials, as well as the clinically significant arrhythmic events, is highest.

In 5 large studies[32–36] 325 of 1,069 patients (30%) had late ventricular potentials, and 744 (70%) had normal SAECGS. During a follow-up period of from 12–20 months, 19% of patients with an abnormal SAECG had arrhythmic events (sudden death and sustained ventricular tachycardia) and only 3% of those with normal SAECGS

had such events. Thus, the absence of an abnormal SAECG following an infarction makes it unlikely that an arrhythmic event will occur.

The electrocardiographic patterns of arrhythmias are presented in the arrhythmia and electrophysiologic sections of this book.

REFERENCES

1. Boineau JP, Canavan TE, Schuessler RB, et al. Demonstration of a widely distributed atrial pacemaker complex in the human heart. *Circulation.* 1988; 77:1221-1237.
2. Durrer D, Vandam RT, Freud GE, et al. Total excitation of the isolated human heart. *Circulation.* 1970;41:899-912.
3. Lepeschkin E. Duration of electrocardiographic deflections and intervals: Man. In: Altman BE, Dittmer DS (eds). *Respiration and Circulation.* Bethesda: Federation of American Societies for Experimental Biology; 1971:277.
4. Hiss RG, Lamb LE, Allen MF. Electrocardiographic findings in 67,375 asymptomatic subjects. *Am J Cardiol.* 1960;6:200-231.
5. Simonson E. The effect of age on the electrocardiogram. *Am J Cardiol.* 1972;29:64-73.
6. Kossman CE. The normal electrocardiogram. *Circulation.* 1953;8:920-936.
7. Franz MR, Bargheer K, Rafflebeul W, et al. Monophasic action potential mapping in human subjects with normal electrocardiograms: Direct evidence for the gene-

sis of the T wave. *Circulation.* 1987;75:379-386.

8. Bazett HC. An analysis of the time-relations of electrocardiograms. *Heart.* 1920;7:353-370.

9. Watanabe Y. Purkinje repolarization as a possible cause of the U wave in the electrocardiogram. *Circulation.* 1975;51:1030-1037.

10. de Oliveira JM, Zimmerman HA. Auricular overloading: Electrocardiographic analysis of 193 cases. *Am J Cardiol.* 1959;3:453-471.

11. Reynolds G. The atrial electrogram in mitral stenosis. *Br Heart J.* 1953;15:250-258.

12. Sokolow M, Lyon TP. The ventricular complex in ventricular hypertrophy as obtained by unipolar precordial and limb leads. *Am Heart J.* 1949;37:161-186.

13. Gubner R, Ungerleider HE. Electrocardiographic criteria of left ventricular hypertrophy. *Arch Intern Med.* 1943;72:196-209.

14. Schack JA, Rosenman RH, Katz LN. The aV limb leads in the diagnosis of ventricular strain. *Am Heart J.* 1950;40:696-705.

15. Noth PH, Myers GB, Klein HA. The precordial electrocardiogram in left ventricular hypertrophy: A study of autopsied cases. *J Lab Clin Med.* 1947;32:1517.

16. Rosenfeld I, Goodrich C, Kassebaum G, et al. The electrocardiographic recognition of left ventricular hypertrophy. *Am Heart J.* 1962;63:731-742.

17. Selzer A, Ebnother CL, Packard P, et al. Reliability of electrocardiographic diagnosis of left ventricular hypertrophy. *Circulation.* 1958;17:255-265.

18. Chou TC, Scott RC, Booth RW, et al. Specificity of the current electrocardiographic criteria in the diagnosis of left ventricular hypertrophy. *Am Heart J.* 1960;60:371-377.

19. Mazzoleni A, Wolff R, Wolff L, et al. Correlation between component cardiac weights and electrocardiographic patterns in 185 cases. *Circulation.* 1964;30:808-829.

20. Romhilt DS, Estes EH Jr. A point-score system for the ECG diagnosis of left ventricular hypertrophy. *Am Heart J.* 1968;75:752-758.

21. Sokolow M, Lyon TP. The ventricular complex in right ventricular hypertrophy as obtained by unipolar precordial and limb leads. *Am Heart J.* 1949;38:273-294.

22. Pruitt RD, Robinson JG. The electrocardiographic findings in patients undergoing surgical exploration of the mitral valve. *Am Heart J.* 1956;52:880-886.

23. Chou TC, Masangkay MP, Young R, et al. Simple quantitative vectorcardiographic criteria for the diagnosis of right ventricular hypertrophy. *Circulation.* 1973;48:1262-1267.

24. Barker JM, Valencia F. The precordial electrocardiogram in incomplete right bundle branch block. *Am Heart J.* 1949;38:376-406.

25. Wyndham CRC, Smith T, Meran MK, et al. Epicardial activations in patients with left bundle branch block. *Circulation.* 1980;61:696-703.

26. Kennamer R, Prinzmetal MM. Depolarization of the ventricle with bundle-branch block. *Am Heart J.* 1954;47:769-779.

27. Jones AN, Feil H. On axis deviation in human bundle branch block. *Am Heart J.* 1948;36:98-111.

28. Lichstein E, Mahapatra R, Gupta PK, et al. Significance of complete left bundle branch block with left axis deviation. *Am J Cardiol.* 1979;44:239-242.

29. Rosenbaum MB, Elizari MV, Lazzari JO. *The Hemiblocks.* Oldsmar, Florida: Tampa Tracings; 1970:71-96.

30. Swiryn S, Abben R, Denes P, et al. Electrocardiographic determinations of axis during left bundle branch block: Study in patients with intermittent left bundle branch block. *Am J Cardiol.* 1980;46:53-58.

31. Klein RC, Vera Z, DeMaria JA, et al. Electrocardiographic diagnosis of left ventricular hypertrophy in the presence of left bundle branch block. *Am Heart J.* 1984;108:502-507.

32. Kuchar DL, Thorburn CW, Sammel NL. Prediction of serious arrhythmic events after myocardial infarction. Signal-averaged electrocardiogram, Holter monitoring and radionuclide ventriculography. *J Am Coll Cardiol.* 1987;9:531-538.

33. Gomes JA, Winters SL, Martinson M, et al. The prognostic significance of quantitative signal-averaged variables relative to clinical variables, site of myocardial infarction, ejection fraction and ventricular premature beats: A prospective study. *J Am Coll Cardiol.* 1989;13:377-384.

34. El-Sherif N, Ursell SN, Bekhett S, et al. Prognostic significance of the signal-averaged ECG depends on the time of recording in the postinfarction period. *Am Heart J.* 1989;118:256-264.

35. Steinberg JS, Regan A, Sciacca R, et al. Predicting arrhythmic events after acute myocardial infarction using the signal-averaged electrocardiogram. *Am J Cardiol.* 1992;69:13-21.

36. Farrell TG, Bashir Y, Cripps T, et al. Risk stratification for arrhythmic events in postinfarction patients based on heart rate variability, ambulatory electrocardiographic variables and the signal-averaged electrocardiogram. *J Am Coll Cardiol.* 1991;18:687-697.

CHAPTER 4

Chest Radiograph in the Evaluation of Acquired Cardiac Disease

Donald P. Harrington, MD

After the discovery of x-rays by Konrad Roentgen in 1895, the chest radiograph was rapidly incorporated into evaluation of cardiac disease and became an essential component of that evaluation. For many years, all diagnostic efforts in cardiac disease were based on the triad of clinical examination, electrocardiogram, and chest radiograph. Beginning with the era of cardiac catheterization and followed by the widespread use of echocardiography, the usefulness of the plain film has been questioned, but chest radiography survives despite technologic advances. This chapter reviews the basic principles of plain chest film examination in cardiac disease and looks at this safe, inexpensive, and reproducible screening procedure in the context of other tests that are more sophisticated but often more invasive.

PLAIN FILM EXAMINATIONS

Plain films may be separated into 3 categories. The first is the posteroanterior (PA) and lateral chest radiograph, which represents the most basic and useful examination of the heart by plain radiographic means; in both positions the patient is upright with deep inspiration (Fig. 1). The second examination, 4 views of the heart with barium, is an extension of the first; the presence of barium within the esophagus provides a posterior cardiac marker, and the right and left oblique views of the heart (Figs. 2, 3) provide a greater appreciation of cardiac structures. This examination is also made with the patient in the upright position during deep inspiration. The third examination is the supine chest radiograph, which is sometimes confused with the portable film. The term *portable* refers to the x-ray equipment that is used to perform the study. In fact, the

portability of this equipment limits the power and flexibility of the system, and portable film examinations may not be as useful as the standard PA chest radiograph, particularly if the patient is very obese. The term *supine* refers only to the position of the patient when the radiograph is taken. The limitation of this study is the heightened position of the diaphragm because of the lessened ability of the patient to take a deep breath. By necessity, the view is anteroposterior (AP) in direction, which also tends to widen the mediastinal and cardiac outline as compared to the PA upright chest. In a portable x-ray examination the PA position cannot be achieved, but the patient can be seated upright for an AP radiograph. The position in which the examination is performed should always be clearly identified on the film itself.[1-4]

CARDIAC CONTOURS AND OVERALL SIZE

For the most part, the heart itself appears totally homogeneous on the film; muscle and blood are indistinguishable. Calcium deposits within the heart shadow can be distinguished from soft tissue, as can concentrations of normal fat around the heart; both may be significant clues to pathology.[2,5] The contours of the heart are seen most readily in relationship to the air-filled lungs that surround it on 2 sides. We are easily able to distinguish the heart from aerated lung. This, in turn, allows a preliminary judgment about heart size, as a first step in the evaluation of the heart.

The simplest method for assessing overall heart size involves the use of the *cardiothoracic ratio* (Fig. 1).[6-8] The cardiothoracic ratio is generally expressed as a percent, with any value below 50% considered to be within normal

47

limits; some authors suggest that 55% is a better limit of normal. The result is that while the number of true positives increases with a higher cardiothoracic ratio, so does the rate of false negatives. This value should be increased to 60% for children and infants.

Care must be taken in the use of the cardiothoracic ratio in several common situations. The heart appears larger in both the supine and the AP positions in comparison with the standard upright PA positioning. There may also be a 1.0- to 1.5-cm difference in heart size between systole and diastole in the same patient. Abnormalities of the spine, such as kyphosis and scoliosis, and of the sternum, as in pectus excavatum, preclude the use of the cardiothoracic ratio as a measure of cardiac size. Finally, the established norms for the cardiothoracic ratio assume a deep inspiration on the part of the patient, so that an expiration film will tend to overestimate heart size (Fig. 1B). This fact affects the supine radiograph as well because of the difficulty with a standardized deep inspiration in this position.

Several other methods of evaluating cardiac size have been developed, but those that provide the most precise measurements of heart volume also require complex analyses of both PA and lateral projections. With increasing availability and ease of use, computer methods may come in to more clinical favor than in the past.[6] At present, no method has received the same wide acceptance as the cardiothoracic ratio.

Lesions associated with moderate to severe cardiomegaly include the volume overload lesions of mitral, aortic, and tricuspid regurgitation, as well as congestive cardiomyopathy and pericardial effusion. Those acquired cardiac diseases in which the patient is not in heart

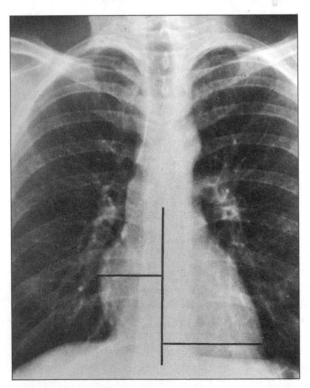 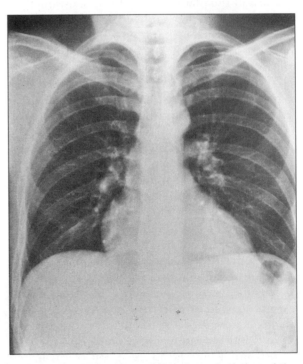

Figure 1. *Normal posteroanterior (PA) chest radiographs. (A) Inspiration film with markings for calculation of the cardiothoracic ratio. The vertical reference line is established using the spinous processes. The numerator of the cardiothoracic ratio is established by adding the longest distance to the right and left heart borders from the reference line. The denominator is the longest length between the inner aspects of the rib cage. Note also the normal distribution of the pulmonary vacularity, with pulmonary venous vessels seen in the lower lung fields but none in the upper lung fields. (B) Normal expiration film for comparison with A. The normal value of 50% cardiothoracic ratio is not valid with an expiration film.*

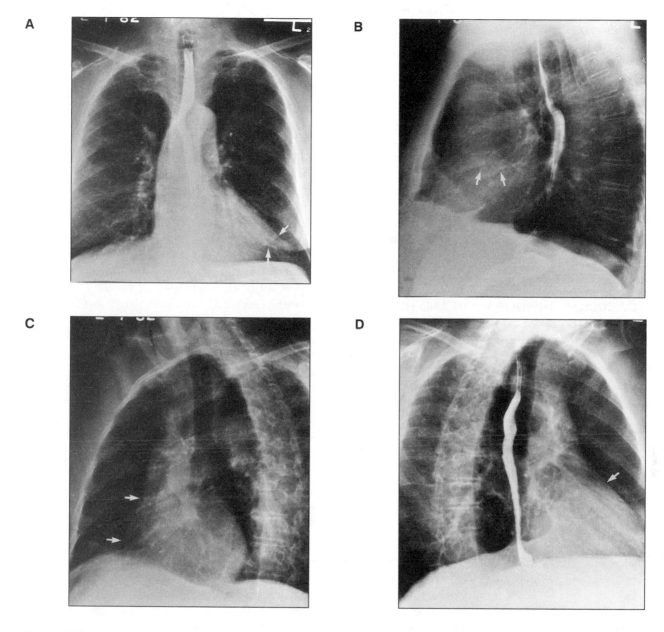

Figure 2. *Four views of the heart with barium from a patient with mild aortic stenosis. (A) PA radiograph. The heart size is normal. A fat pad is present at the cardiac apex, accentuated by the density of the overlying left breast (arrows). Some rounding of the left ventricular contour is present, consistent with left ventricular hypertrophy. The ascending arch and descending portions are dilated and ectatic due to a combination of aortic stenosis and aging. If post-stenotic dilatation were the only factor, the arch and descending portion of the aorta would be normal. (B) Lateral radiograph. Minimal aortic calcification is seen (arrows). This calcification was better seen fluoroscopically at the time of cardiac catheterization but was identified first by plain film examination. The ascending aorta is prominent above the aortic valve. The retrosternal space is clear. The left ventricle does not extend beyond the inferior vena cava, and the esophagus is not significantly displaced posteriorly. (C) Left anterior oblique (LAO) radiograph. Aortic calcification is obscured by overlying lung markings. The right atrial and right ventricular margin has a normal straight line configuration (arrows). The normal clear space is present between the right atrium and the left mainstem bronchus. (D) Right anterior oblique (RAO) radiograph. No deviation of the esophagus is present, and the right ventricular outflow tract is normal (arrow).*

failure and which show normal or only slight enlargement of the heart include all pressure overload lesions, such as mitral and aortic stenosis and systemic hypertension. Other disease processes in this group include acute myocardial infarction, hypertrophic cardiomyopathy, and constrictive pericarditis. Left ventricular failure from any of these or other causes results in cardiomegaly with left ventricular enlargement, left atrial enlargement, and pulmonary venous changes. An exception is if left ventricular failure is acute, as in acute myocardial infarction; then, hours are needed for ventricular and atrial dilatation, whereas the pulmonary vasculature changes can be seen acutely.[3,9–11]

CARDIAC CONFIGURATION AND HEART BORDERS

Our next step in assessment of the heart is related to cardiac configuration and individual chamber enlargement.[2,3] As previously stated, it is important to look at changes at the interface between the heart and the lung. These can be seen more readily at the points where the right and the left borders are outlined by the lungs. The PA radiographs in Figures 1 and 2 will serve as the visual reference for evaluation of the normal heart contours, since the first is normal and the second is an example of mild aortic stenosis, which only slightly alters cardiac configuration. Beginning at the left cardiophrenic angle, the apex of the heart is gently rounded and sharply delineated. Fat, a normal finding, can be seen in this area because fat is less dense than the heart and more dense than the lung (Fig. 2A). The presence of fat at the cardiophrenic angle may blunt the distinction between these organs and falsely increase the cardiothoracic ratio. An extension of the cardiac contour outward and downward suggests left ventricular enlargement; when enlargement is severe, the air bubble within the stomach will be indented by the heart, since an enlarged left ventricle will press through the diaphragm. This can be best evaluated in the lateral projection. When the right ventricular chamber is enlarged, there may also be leftward extension of the ventricular contour, but the apex

tends to be deviated upward rather than downward, giving the appearance of a boot-shaped heart.

Localized bulging of the cardiac contour on the left lateral and posterior aspects of the cardiac border is seen frequently in aneurysms of the left ventricle. Ascending toward the pulmonary hilum, the left heart border rises diagonally as a line which either remains straight or becomes slightly concave in the region of the left atrial appendage before reaching the main pulmonary artery segment. A bulging of the segment is noted when the left atrium and its appendage are dilated (Figs. 3, 4).

In assessing the right heart border, we begin at the cardiophrenic angle on the right. A small portion of the right side of the heart is usually seen beyond the vertebral bodies; this represents the right atrium. Enlargement of either the right atrium or the right ventricle causes extension of the right border further to the right of the spine so that it appears more prominent than normal (Fig. 5). Advancing further up the right side of the heart, the junction between the right atrium and the superior vena cava may be noted as a change in direction of these structures as they form a small niche. The superior vena cava is the only border-forming element above this level. Just above the mainstem bronchus and right hilum lies the azygos vein, which is seen as a small mass density in supine radiographs (or in the upright radiograph when there is systemic venous distention). There are no absolute normal values for the extensions of these structures to the right or the left of the heart shadow; experience teaches how to differentiate normal from abnormal.

PULMONARY VASCULARITY

The functional significance of the radiographic evaluation of the pulmonary vascularity has only come about since the widespread use of cardiac catheterization. Thus, a more invasive, more sophisticated procedure has actually enhanced the plain film examination rather than replacing it.[7,12–16]

The main pulmonary artery segments should be evaluated first, followed by the right and left

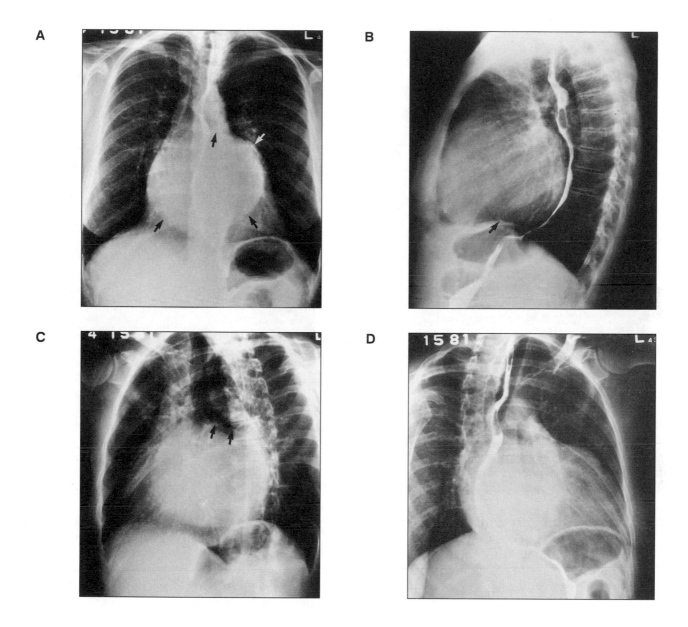

Figure 3. *Four views of the heart with barium from a patient with severe mitral stenosis. (A) PA radiograph. Cardiothoracic ratio is just above 50%. The left atrium is massively enlarged, causing a double density with the cardiac contour (lower black arrows). The left atrial appendage is dilated (white arrow). The left mainstem bronchus is markedly elevated by the left atrial enlargement (upper black arrow). Upper lobe vascularity on the right is easier to visualize than on the left because it is not obscured by the heart. In this case, the heart contour is displaced to the right by the left atrial enlargement and not right ventricular or right atrial dilatation. (B) Lateral radiograph. There is marked posterior deviation of the esophagus by the enlarged left atrium. The retrosternal clear space is still present despite the distortion caused by the enlarged left atrium, suggesting that right-sided enlargement is not present. Calcification (black arrow) is noted in the wall of the left atrium, (C) LAO radiograph. The left mainstem bronchus (arrows) is in contact with the enlarged left atrium and elevated. No vascular calcification is seen. (D) RAO radiograph. Further illustration of the size of the left atrium and deviation of the trachea. This series of films illustrates how the cardiothoracic ratio may underestimate the extent of cardiac enlargement, particularly when the dilatation is in the posterior direction with the left atrial enlargement.*

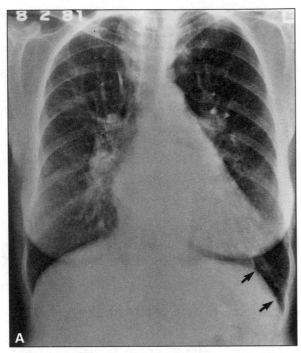
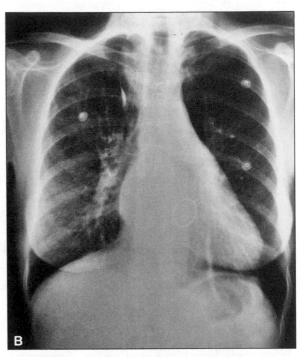

Figure 4. Radiographs before and after replacement of the mitral valve in a patient with mitral stenosis. (A) PA radiograph preoperatively shows mild cardiomegaly, double density of enlarged left atrium, and prominent left atrial appendage. The left mainstem bronchus is only minimally elevated. The pulmonary vascular changes also demonstrate the classic changes of this disease process. Pulmonary vascularity is shifted to the upper lung fields, with diminution of the venous pattern in the lower lungs. There is diffuse blurring of the pulmonary hila. Kerley B lines (arrows) are noted at the left costophrenic angle. Increased density throughout both lung fields indicates early pulmonary edema. (B) Postoperative PA chest radiograph after replacement of the mitral valve. The previously noted pulmonary changes have been reversed. Overall heart size and slight prominence of the left atrial appendage remain.

pulmonary arteries and hilum, continuing into the smaller, more peripheral veins and arteries, and ending with the pulmonary parenchyma and pleural space. Enlargement of the main pulmonary artery segment is generally caused either by increased flow through the pulmonary artery, as in a left-to-right shunt, or by pulmonary hypertension. A third and uncommon cause of arterial prominence is post-stenotic dilatation of this segment due to pulmonary stenosis. Idiopathic dilatation of the pulmonary artery without pulmonary stenosis may occasionally be seen in women younger than 30 years of age. Increased blood flow or increased pressure can also cause enlargement of the right and left pulmonary artery segments. The vascularity in the more peripheral portions of the pulmonary arteries is helpful in differentiating between these 2 causes. This vascularity is best evaluated by covering over the

hilum and proximal pulmonary arteries and viewing only the vessels in the outer two-thirds to one-half of the lung. Normal pulmonary vascularity is defined by experience; but except in the base of the lungs, only small, well-delineated vessels are seen. Increased vascularity or larger peripheral vessels are seen in high-flow shunt lesions (Fig. 6), whereas no vessels are seen in pulmonary hypertension because of pruning of the peripheral pulmonary vessels.

Differentiation between arterial and venous vascularity is difficult at first. In the normal patient in the upright projection, an increased number of vessels may be seen in the lower lung fields. These are both arterial and venous, and the difference will become apparent on close inspection. The arterial vessels tend to be vertical, while the venous tend to be horizontal in their passage into the left atrium. The normal upper lobe has less arterial and venous vascularity than the lower lobe (Fig. 1). As pulmonary venous pressure rises (15-20 mm Hg), no matter what the cause, the visible vascularity in the upper and lower lungs tends to equalize (Fig. 7). As pressure rises further in the venous system (20-25 mm Hg), the lower lobe veins tend to disappear while upper lobe veins become more prominent (Figs. 3, 4A). This change occurs entirely on the venous side of the pulmonary circulation. Differentiation between arterial and venous vascularity is somewhat more difficult in the upper lung than in the lower; but here, too, the arteries tend to have a more vertical orientation than the veins, as in the lower lung fields. *Warning*: pulmonary vascular changes are accurately interpreted only if recorded in the upright position.[7,12–16]

As pressure rises within the pulmonary venous bed, the capillary oncotic pressure is exceeded and pulmonary edema occurs above 25 mm Hg. The first manifestation of this is generally a bilateral haziness and confluence of structures within the pulmonary hila. Normally, the structures in the hila are distinct. A second sign is the appearance of short, horizontal lines at the costophrenic angles, representing interstitial edema; these are the classic Kerley B lines (Fig. 4). The next step in the process is haziness throughout the lung fields with frank pulmonary edema, also indicated by the so-called alveolar pattern and pleural effusion. Pulmonary edema of cardiac origin is usually associated with an increase in the cardiothoracic ratio, caused by left ventricular dilatation. This is not true when edema is rapid in onset, such as in an acute myocardial infarction, or when it is noncardiac in origin, as in the case of drowning or overhydration.

CARDIAC CALCIFICATION

Calcification within the left ventricular muscle is associated with injury and repair after myocardial infarction (Fig. 8). In general, this calcification is more localized than pericardial calcification and

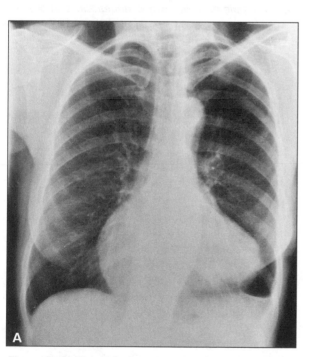
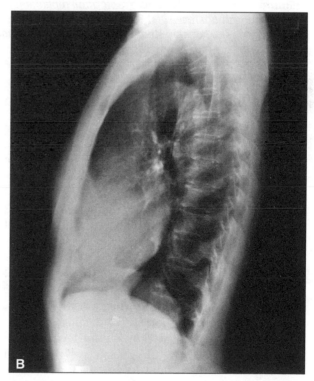

Figure 5. Radiographs from a patient with combined mitral and tricuspid valvular disease, in whom tricuspid disease is the major component. (A) PA radiograph. Cardiomegaly is present with prominence of the right heart border. No double density of left atrial enlargement is present. Pulmonary vascularity is normal. (B) Lateral radiograph. Filling in of the retrosternal clear space, with no abnormal posterior displacement of the left ventricle or left atrium. The findings are specific for right-sided enlargement due to the patient's predominant tricuspid valvular disease.

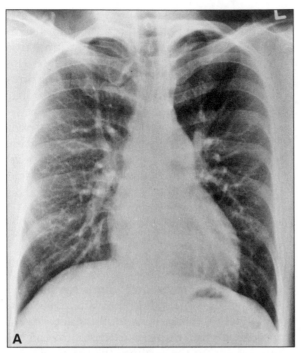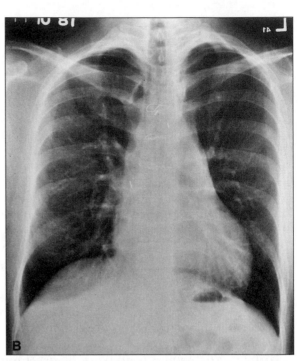

Figure 6. *PA and lateral chest radiographs from a patient with an atrial septal defect (ASD). (A) Normal heart size in a patient with a large ASD. The increased pulmonary arterial vascularity is evident in both lungs, as is prominence of the main pulmonary artery segment. Note the vertical orientation of the vessels. (B) PA radiograph after surgical closure of the ASD. The sternal sutures and slightly larger heart size are consistent with the preceding surgical procedure. The pulmonary vascularity is now normal and in striking contrast to that seen in panel A.*

can be associated with a bulging of the ventricular contour in aneurysm formation.

Cardiac calcification is useful in delineating specific pathologic processes within the heart.[2,3,5] Calcification occurring within the pericardium, as shown in Figure 9, is indicative of pericarditis. In this example, calcification involves the entire pericardial space, whereas the calcification is usually seen in only parts of the pericardium. Calcification is a good indication of old pericarditis; only half the patients with constrictive pericarditis have evidence of calcification. Tuberculous pericarditis is the most common cause of pericardial calcification.

Calcification of the aortic and mitral valves is another common pathologic and radiologic phenomenon. Frequently, these valves are not seen clearly in the PA projection because they overlap the spine and tend to be superimposed on one another. The lateral and oblique projections are more useful in delineating valvular calcifications. In the lateral projection, the calcified aortic valve tends to be horizontally located in the middle third of the cardiac shadow, whereas the calcified mitral valve is in the posterior third and obliquely oriented. C-shaped calcification is frequently seen in the mitral annulus, and while the mitral valve is not directly calcified, mitral insufficiency is associated with this phenomenon. Valvular calcification itself is usually irregular and spiculated and is more extensive in the aortic as opposed to the mitral valve. Calcification of any cardiac structure is better appreciated using fluoroscopy rather than films because the motion of the calcified structure enhances visualization. Pathologic calcification of cardiac valves is far more frequent than radiologically evident calcification.

Calcification of the coronary arteries is frequently associated with atherosclerotic coronary artery disease. However, the calcium deposits are usually too small to be seen on the plain chest radiograph. When calcification is seen, its linear arrangement and railroad-track configuration are good indications of its origin.

OTHER CARDIAC DENSITIES

Fat densities within the heart are normal findings; for example, in the lateral film, a radiolucent stripe of epicardial fat can frequently be seen in the retrosternal area, or the slight radiolucent density of a cardiac fat pad may be found at the left cardiophrenic angle. The retrosternal fat stripe is indicative of pericardial effusion if it lies well within the cardiac shadow in the lateral projection and away from the normal retrosternal location. As the pericardial fluid accumulates, it does so outside the epicardium, thus displacing the fat into a more central location in the overall cardiac shadow.

SPECIFIC CHAMBER ENLARGEMENT

The pathophysiologic response of the heart to a volume overload, such as aortic insufficiency, is chamber dilatation; the response to a pressure overload, such as aortic stenosis, is myocardial hypertrophy.[2,3] Dilatation of the ventricles will result in cardiomegaly and an abnormal cardiothoracic ratio, whereas ventricular hypertrophy generally only rounds out the left ventricular contour. Isolated dilatation of the left atrium does not result in cardiomegaly. Right atrial enlargement is difficult to distinguish from right ventricular enlargement; the 2 phenomena are usually considered together as right-sided dilatation. Ventricular hypertrophy subtly changes the cardiac contour but does not increase the size of the heart or of the cardiothoracic ratio (Figs. 2, 10).

Differentiation between right and left ventricular enlargement is somewhat difficult. One must first establish whether or not the right ventricle is enlarged (Fig. 5). If it is, it is seen as abnormal displacement of the cardiac shadow to the right of the ventral bodies and as a filling in of the retrosternal clear space in the lateral projection. There is also extension of the heart upward and to the left into the shape of a boot.

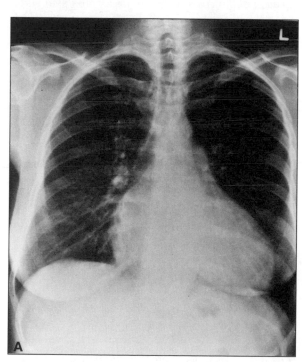
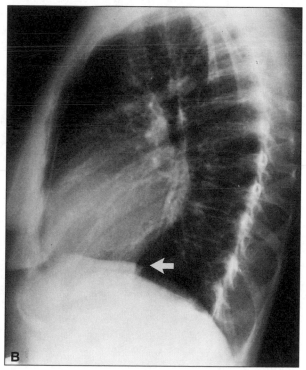

Figure 7. *Chest radiographs from a patient with hypertrophic cardiomyopathy and clinical evidence of intermittent congestive heart failure. (A) PA radiograph. Cardiomegaly with left ventricular and left atrial dilatation. The pulmonary vasculature has normal to slightly increased upper lobe vascularity. (B) Lateral radiograph. The retrosternal clear space is present. The enlarged left ventricle is displaced posteriorly to the inferior vena cava (arrow).*

The left anterior oblique (LAO) projection can also be used to evaluate the right ventricle. In this projection, the right border is seen as a relatively vertical line as it rises to meet the superior vena cava (Fig. 2). If there is a step formed between the right side of the heart and the superior vena cava, right-sided enlargement is present. Right ventricular enlargement can mimic all the signs of left ventricular enlargement, so the latter cannot be adequately determined. If right ventricular enlargement is *not* clearly shown, evaluation of the left ventricle can proceed. Extension of the ventricle downward and outward to the left is one indication of enlargement. Another radiographic sign involves extracardiac organ relationships. In the lateral projection, one normally sees the posterior wall of the inferior vena cava as it rises from the abdomen. This is seen as a vertical structure arising from the diaphragm into the heart, and normally no cardiac shadow will be seen posteriorly. However, left ventricular enlargement will cause a portion of the left ventricle to extend beyond this vertical

line (Fig. 7). The outward and downward expansion of left ventricular dilatation will also encroach on the left diaphragm and, in extreme cases, indent the gastric air bubble.

Of all radiographic signs of chamber enlargement, those involving the left atrium are the most reliable. Left atrial enlargement is indicated in the PA projection by formation of a double density as the left atrium expands posteriorly and by prominence of the left atrial appendage on the left heart border (Figs. 3, 4). As the left atrium enlarges, it tends to encroach upon and elevate the left mainstem bronchus. This encroachment is especially clear in the LAO projection, where there is normally a clear space between the upper portion of the cardiac shadow and left mainstem bronchus (Fig. 2C). As the left atrium increases in size, this space is encroached upon by the cardiac silhouette until finally the left mainstem bronchus is displaced upward by the cardiac mass (Fig. 3C). The LAO

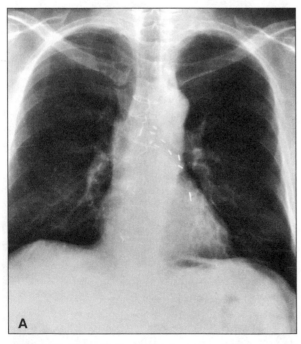

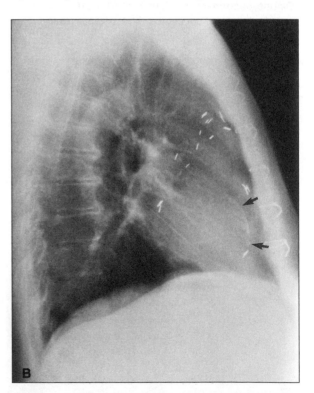

Figure 8. Chest radiographs from a patient who had a previous myocardial infarction and coronary artery bypass graft. (A) PA radiograph. Postoperative changes and normal heart size are present. No calcification or abnormalities of the left heart border are present (B) Lateral radiograph. An area of left ventricular infarction (arrows) shows calcification. At the time of cardiac catheterization, a contrast left ventriculogram demonstrated an aneurysm in the region of calcification. This calcification is more centrally located than in patients with pericardial calcification.

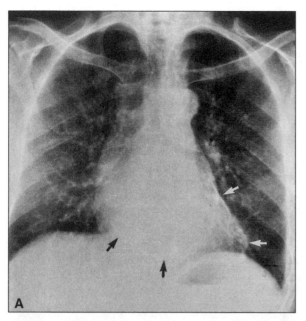 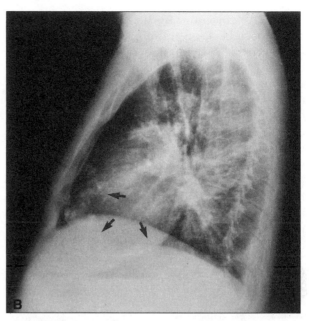

Figure 9. *Chest radiographs from a patient suspected of having constrictive pericarditis. (A) PA radiograph. Marked calcification of the entire pericardium (arrows). The overall heart size is normal, as is the pulmonary vascularity. Diffuse pulmonary parenchymal disease is noted. (B) The lateral film confirms the previous findings of extensive pericardial calcification, cardiac catheterization did not demonstrate evidence of pericardial constriction, and no other cardiac abnormalities were noted. The calcification is unequivocal evidence of previous pericarditis, but it is not specific for the present activity of the disease process or its cause, although most cases of calcific pericarditis are tubercular in nature.*

projection is also useful for separating the calcified mitral and aortic valves.

SPECIFIC PATHOLOGIC PROCESSES

A number of specific diseases may be identified on chest radiograph. Aortic valvular disease can present as aortic stenosis, as aortic insufficiency, or as a combination of these. When aortic stenosis is the predominant lesion, the overall cardiac size is not increased. The result is a pressure overload of the left ventricle, which leads to myocardial hypertrophy. Myocardial hypertrophy can cause subtle changes in cardiac contour, but it does not lead to an increased cardiothoracic ratio. Calcification of the aortic valve frequently accompanies aortic stenosis, whether the underlying process is rheumatic heart disease or a congenital bicuspid aortic valve. Isolated dilatation of the ascending aorta, which results in an apparent increased density of the retrosternal space above the heart and a deviation of the superior vena cava to the right,

is a further indication of aortic stenosis. This post-stenotic dilatation is caused by turbulent blood flow through the stenotic valve (Fig. 2).

Dilatation of the ascending arch and descending portion of the aorta may result from the normal aging process or from sustained systemic hypertension.

When aortic regurgitation is the predominant lesion, there is volume rather than pressure overload of the left ventricle. This results in dilatation of the left ventricle and an increase in the cardiothoracic ratio.

Mitral valve disease is another example of a process that is usually a combination of stenosis and insufficiency. When stenosis predominates, the left atrium dilates because of pressure overload, while the left ventricle tends to remain normal-sized. Left atrial enlargement is indicated by prominence of the left atrial appendage along the left heart border density in the PA projection with posterior extension of the left atrial chamber, and—in the most severe cases—elevation of the left mainstem bronchus in the PA projection. In the LAO projection, the clear space between the cardiac shadow and the left mainstem bronchus is obliterated, with ultimate elevation of the mainstem bronchus. Also in the most severe enlargement, the left atrium can extend beyond the right heart border and give the impression of right-sided enlargement (Fig. 3). With left atrial hypertension, the pressure is transmitted into the pulmonary venous bed, and there is a shift of pulmonary venous vascularity, from the lower lung fields to an equal balance between upper and lower vessels, finally giving marked prominence to those in the upper lobe (Figs. 3, 4). In the presence of mitral regurgitation, left

ventricular enlargement is added to these findings, reflecting the volume overload of the left ventricle by the regurgitation.

Tricuspid valve disease, regardless of its etiology, is usually not associated with radiographically identifiable calcification, as is mitral or aortic valve disease; rather, it is indicated by enlargement of the right side of the heart without evidence of pulmonary arterial or venous hypertension (Fig. 5).

When any valvular disease is combined with ventricular failure, or when multiple valves are involved, the previously noted distinctions are blurred and generally unreliable. The greatest

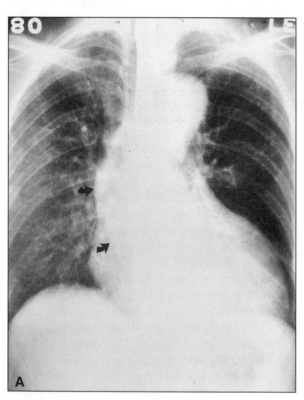 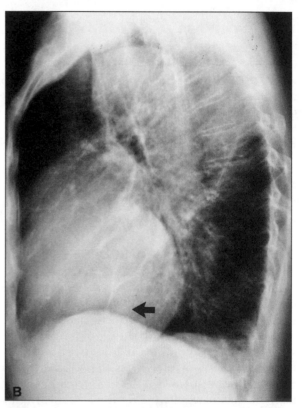

Figure 10. Chest radiographs from a patient with signs and symptoms of aortic insufficiency. (A) PA radiograph. The heart is enlarged, with outward and downward displacement of the left heart border. The right heart border appears normal. The aortic knob is prominent, which may relate to patient age or preexisting chronic hypertension, but the dilatation of the ascending aorta (arrows) suggests aortic valve disease (although an aneurysm involving the ascending aorta is a possibility). Equalization of the upper and lower pulmonary vascularity is present. (B) Lateral radiograph. The retrosternal clear space is maintained, with marked enlargement of the heart posteriorly beyond the inferior vena cava, where it passes through the diaphragm (arrow). No calcification of valves or of the ascending aorta is noted. Blunting of the posterior angle of the left diaphragm is incidentally noted. The overall cardiac enlargement and configuration of the ventricles indicate left ventricular dilatation. Prominence of the ascending aorta suggests aortic valve disease. Together these observations suggest that aortic regurgitation is the predominant element. Increased pulmonary venous pressure is indicated by the shift of venous vascularity.

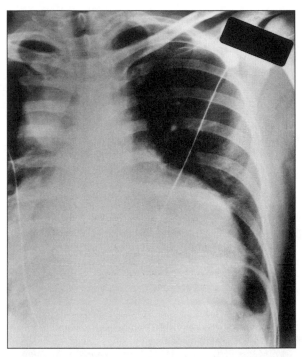

Figure 11. *Portable AP chest radiograph from a patient with pericardial effusion and mediastinal mass lesion. Obvious cardiomegaly is present, with uniform distribution that has been termed the water bottle heart. The pulmonary vascularity is normal in distribution, but the hila of the lung are obscured by the enlarging pericardial space. Cardiomegaly, other than from pericardial effusion, will not obscure the pulmonary vessels and hila. The mediastinal mass lesion is just above the right mainstem bronchus. This mass was a mediastinal tumor with pericardial metastasis, which led to the pericardial effusion.*

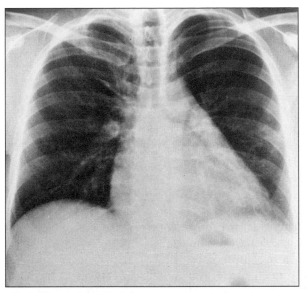

Figure 12. *PA chest radiograph from a patient with idiopathic pericardial effusion. The overall heart size is only slightly larger than normal, but the left hila and pulmonary vessels are totally obscured and the right hila is partially obscured. The pulmonary artery and pulmonary vascularity are normal.*

value of the chest x-ray in these cases is its ability to delineate the progressive physiologic and pathologic changes that accompany ventricular failure.

In patients with coronary artery disease, the chest radiograph is usually normal. This is true for other acute and chronic myocardial ischemia. Cardiomegaly, left ventricular and left atrial enlargement, and the accompanying signs of increased pulmonary venous hypertension are evident when ventricular failure results from myocardial ischemia. All of these findings are associated with a poorer prognosis than with a normal chest film.[3,9,10] Infarction may lead to aneurysm formation, which may be identifiable on chest radiographs as a localized bulging of the left ventricle, and may calcify. Other complications of infarction, such as papillary muscle infarction and acute mitral regurgitation or septal infarction with ventricular septal defect formation, are evident radiographically, although congestive heart failure is often the most obvious finding in these complications.

Myocarditis can only be identified as the myocardium fails with resultant left ventricular dilatation. This is a late sign, and such a limitation in radiographic identification also holds for cardiomyopathy, whether restrictive or hypertrophic (Fig. 7).

Pericardial disease processes may be identified if calcification is present in pericarditis (Fig. 9) or, in the case of pericardial effusion, when the effusion is large enough to give identifiable cardiomegaly, and to displace the retroperitoneal fat stripe (Figs. 11, 12). Echocardiography has superseded all other diagnostic methods for identifying pericardial effusion, especially if the effusion is small. Once pericardial effusion has been established, the chest radiograph can be used to follow resolution of this process by changes in cardiac size.

SUPINE AND PORTABLE FILMS

The supine chest film is used to evaluate patients in the intensive care area and recovery room, when standard radiographic views cannot be obtained. As noted earlier, a limitation of this technique is that the standard cardiothoracic ratio cannot be used. Despite this, the serial nature of the film provides much diagnostic information. First, it shows increasing or decreasing cardiac size on a day-to-day basis; second, it shows change in the pulmonary venous vascularity, which can indicate cardiac function and/or pulmonary venous pressure. Portable chest films taken in the intensive care unit are limited by the variations in technique, patient positioning, and the respirator, from 1 film to the next. However, when this draw-back is taken into account, the chest film can provide a good anatomic and physiologic study.

REFERENCES

1. Milne ENC, Pistolesi M. Intensive care unit radiology. In: Milne ENC, Pistolesi M (eds). *Reading the Chest Radiograph—A Physiologic Approach*. St. Louis, MO: Mosby; 1993:311-342.
2. Steiner RM, Levin DC. Radiology of the heart. In: Braunwald E (ed). *Heart Disease—A Textbook of Cardiovascular Medicine*. 4th Ed. Philadelphia: W.B. Saunders; 1992:204-234.
3. Higgins CB. Radiography of acquired heart disease. In: Higgins CB (ed). *Essentials of Cardiac Radiology and Imaging*. Philadelphia: J.B. Lippincott;1992:1-48.
4. Klein JS. Intensive and coronary care radiology. In: Higgins CB (ed). *Essentials of Cardiac Radiology and Imaging*. Philadelphia: J.B. Lippincott;1992:1-48.
5. Chen JTT. The significance of cardiac calcifications. *Applied Radiology*. 1992;11-18.
6. Nakamori H, Doi K, MacMahon H, et al. Effect of heart-size parameters computed from digital chest radiographs on detection of cardiomegaly. *Invest Radiol*. 1991;26:546-550.
7. Manninen H, Remes J, Partanen K, et al. Evaluation of heart size and pulmonary vasculature. *Acta Radiologica*. 1991;32(3)226-231.
8. Murphy ML, Blue LR, Thenabadu PN, et al. The reliability of the routine chest roentgenogram for determination of heart size based on specific ventricular chamber evaluation at postmortem. *Invest Radiol*. 1985;20:21-25.
9. Battler A, Karliner JS, Higgins CB, et al. The initial chest x-ray in acute myocardial infarction: Prediction of early and late mortality and survival. *Circulation*. 1980;61:1004-1009.
10. Higgins CB, Lipton MJ. Radiography of acute myocardial infarction. *Radiol Clin North Am*. 1980;18:359-368.
11. Newell JD, Higgins CD, Kelley MJ. Radiographic-echocardiographic approach to acquired heart disease: Diagnosis and assessment of severity. *Radiol Clin North Am*. 1980;18:387-409.
12. Milne ENC, Pistolesi M. Reading the chest radiograph—the value of adding the physiologic approach. In: Milne ENC, Pistolesi M (eds). *Reading the Chest Radiograph—A Physiologic Approach*. St. Louis, MO: Mosby; 1993:1-8.
13. Milne ENC, Pistolesi M. Radiologic appearances of pulmonary edema, anatomic and physiologic basis. In: Milne ENC, Pistolesi M (eds). *Reading the Chest Radiograph—A Physiologic Approach*. St. Louis, MO: Mosby; 1993:9-50.
14. Milne ENC, Pistolesi M. Quantification of pulmonary blood volume, flow, and pressure: Practice. In: Milne ENC, Pistolesi M (eds). *Reading the Chest Radiograph—A Physiologic Approach*. St. Louis, MO: Mosby; 1993:202-241.
15. Ravin CE. Pulmonary vascularity: Radiographic considerations. *J Thorac Imag*. 1988;3:1.
16. Balbarini A, Limbruno U, Bertoli D, et al. Evaluation of pulmonary vascular pressures in cardiac patients: The role of the chest roentgenogram. *J Thorac Imag*. 1991;6:62-68.

Nuclear Cardiology

CHAPTER **5**

Joseph F. Polak, MD

INTRODUCTION

Nuclear medicine procedures directed to the evaluation of the heart require specialized instrumentation and use specific radiopharmaceuticals. Selecting the most useful diagnostic procedure is difficult even to the nuclear medicine specialist. Since local experience with a test and its availability vary, clinicians should confer with their nuclear cardiology consultants before ordering the tests described in this chapter.

In the following pages, examinations that are noninvasive, require the intravenous administration of radiopharmaceuticals, and use standard imaging and processing instrumentation will be discussed in detail.

MYOCARDIAL IMAGING OVERVIEW

INSTRUMENTATION

The basic instrument used in nuclear medicine imaging is the Anger gamma camera. This device encodes information on the spatial distribution of a radioisotope onto a new dimensional image. It is capable of resolving objects separated by 1 to 2 cm. Combined with a computer interface, it can be used to acquire blood pool images that are gated to the electrocardiogram (ECG). Depending on the type of study acquired, computer analysis software can then determine right and left ventricular function or measure myocardial perfusion. This approach has helped to standardize the way that nuclear cardiology examinations are done and has improved their sensitivity and specificity.

Rotating gamma cameras capable for performing single-photon emission computed tomography (SPECT) are now a common feature of most nuclear medicine departments. This imaging approach works best in combination with myocardial perfusion tracers, improving sensitivity and specificity for the diagnosis of coronary artery disease. It also improves spatial localization and helps to delineate the size of infarcted myocardium with infarct-specific tracers. Finally, although time intensive, these acquisitions can be gated to depict regional myocardial function. The recently introduced 2- and 3-headed rotating gamma cameras now facilitate more rapid image acquisition and further improve on image quality and reliability. It may also help decrease the amount of radiopharmaceuticals needed for the examination and thereby reduce financial costs.

Although the use of positron emission tomography (PET) is spreading, it remains available in only a few centers throughout the country. Reimbursement is either lacking or does not meet expenses. Cyclotrons and specialized radiochemistry are needed to image O^{15}, C^{11}, or N^{13} labeled compounds. The availability of inexpensive on site ^{82}Rb generators makes it possible to perform perfusion imaging without purchasing a cyclotron. This technology has not yet been proven cost effective.

RADIOPHARMACEUTICALS

The radiopharmaceuticals available to aid in the assessment of both the functional and metabolic integrity of the heart can be categorized as follows: 1) myocardial perfusion and viability with thallium-201 (^{201}Tl) and the technetium-99m (^{99m}Tc) complexes (sestamibi, teboroxime, tetrofosmin), 2) cardiac function studies with gated or first-pass ventriculography, 3) detection and sizing of myocardial infarction using ^{99m}Tc pyrophosphate or ^{111}In and now ^{99m}Tc antimyosin antibody complexes, and 4) evaluation of myocardial metabolism with fatty acid analogs (labeled with ^{123}I or positron emitters) or glucose analogs.

Perfusion/Viability Imaging (Table I)

Thallium-201 is a potassium analog. Its administration results in a lower radiation dose and improved spatial resolution when compared with other potassium analogs such as rubidium and cesium. It is used clinically for the assessment of regional myocardial perfusion.

Immediately after an intravenous injection of thallium, the pattern of myocardial uptake reflects regional blood flow. Cardiac muscle has an extraction efficiency of 80% to 90% for this cation. Approximately 4% of the administered dose is captured by the myocardium.

In a healthy subject at rest, local myocardial uptake of this isotope depends on blood flow and is therefore homogeneously distributed throughout the left ventricle. With exercise, increased myocardial perfusion causes increased uniform myocardial uptake of the tracer. In patients with coronary artery disease (CAD), thallium uptake is unchanged if regional blood flow is normal. Areas of exercise-induced ischemia show a decrease in thallium uptake since regional delivery of the isotope is compromised.

Soon after the intravenous administration of this radiopharmaceutical, a "redistribution" occurs. This is a transition between early thallium distribution, proportional to blood flow, and later steady state during which thallium uptake reflects the size of the local potassium pool, i.e., viable cardiac muscle. Clinically, this transition begins soon after the injection. If the tracer is injected at the time of exercise, the myocardial segments supplied by

Table 1. Perfusion Imaging Agents

ISOTOPE	PHYSICAL HALF-LIFE	COMPLEX	PRINCIPLE	USE
^{201}Tl	73 hr	Ion Thallous chloride	Potassium analog; extraction	Perfusion imaging; intravenous injection
^{99m}Tc MIBI	6 hr	Hexakis nitrile	Myocyte uptake and trapping	Perfusion imaging; intravenous injection
^{99m}Tc Teboroxime	6 hr	Boronic acid adduct of technetium dioxime	Extraction and then rapid washout	Perfusion imaging; intravenous injection
^{82}Rb	75 sec	Dissolved in saline	Potassium analog; extraction	Perfusion imaging; intravenous injection positron emitter, on-site generator
^{13}N	10 min	Ammonia	Extraction but retention affected by local metabolism	Perfusion imaging; intravenous injection positron emitter, cyclotron needed

stenosed coronary arteries have decreased thallium uptake. After the patient stops exercising, the redistribution phase begins and is usually completed in 3 to 5 hours (Fig. 1). Areas with persistent thallium defects are thought to represent irreversibly damaged myocardium or scar. In some patients, local perfusion is so reduced that a repeat resting study must be performed if the size of resting metabolically active myocardium is to be assessed. This can be done either at the time of a separate visit or with reinjection immediately after the 4-hour rest-redistribution image. [1]

The procedure is conducted with the use of an Anger type gamma camera with either medium sensitivity or high resolution collimators. Images of the heart are obtained from the anterior and at least 2 other left anterior oblique (LAO) projections (40° and 70°) so that all the cardiac segments are well visualized. Single photon emission computed tomography (SPECT) image acquisition performed with an anterior 180° rotation of the gamma camera is preferred over 360° acquisitions. Correction for attenuation can

be done although it probably does not improve the accuracy of the test. Following reconstruction of the images, analysis is normally performed with images reformatted to give long axis and short axis views.

When this test is performed during stress or exercise, the patient should reach a maximal exercise point (most commonly 85% of the maximum predicted heart rate of the Bruce protocol) before being injected with a dose of approximately 3 mCi. He or she should also continue to exercise for 1 or 2 minutes or until the tracer has cleared the blood. For best results, imaging should start 5 minutes after injection. Redistribution images are also obtained at 3 to 5 hours after the injection. If necessary, a repeat resting study can be ordered over the next week or reinjection done immediately.

Two alternate means of actively assessing coronary perfusion reserve is the use of vasodilators such as dipyridamole and adenosine.[2] Dipyridamole is given either intravenously or orally in patients who are unable to exercise, i.e., patients with peripheral arterial disease. It

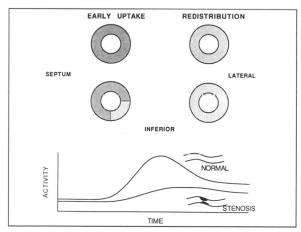

Figure 1A. *Diagram showing myocardial kinetics for thallium-201 uptake in normal (top) and ischemic myocardium (bottom). The bottom section to the left shows a relative decrease in uptake in the inferolateral segment due to a circumflex stenosis, in these idealized short-axis images of the left ventricle. This is also shown on the time-activity graph of myocardial uptake drawn below. With redistribution (section at bottom right), uptake will later become more homogeneous so that the ischemic segment will be indistinguishable from the normal segments.*

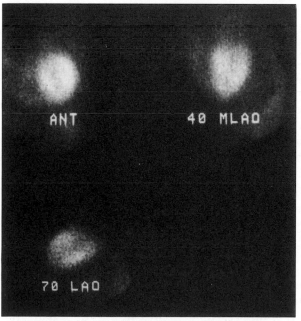

Figure 1B. *Myocardial perfusion scintigraphy showing normal thallium distribution. See color plate (Fig. 4, front of book) for ischemic thallium image.*

is normally given intravenously over a 4-minute interval (0.56 mg/kg). A second dose of 0.28 mg/kg is optional if heart rate and blood pressure remain unchanged. Thallium is injected 5 minutes later and imaging begins after another 5 minute delay. A moderate increase in heart rate is normally seen. Arrhythmia or chest pain caused by the coronary steal induced by this agent can be reversed with aminophylline (typical dose, 75–100 mg). The oral administration of dipyridamole requires larger doses (300–400 mg) but is less likely to cause arrhythmias compared to the intravenous route. Thallium is injected 45 minutes after administration. Adenosine is normally given intravenously at a rate of 140 µgm/kg/min for 6 minutes. Injection of the radioisotope is made half-way through the infusion. Imaging can start 5 minutes after the injection is finished. Infusion of dobutamine (≤ 40 µg/kg/min, by increments of 10 µg/kg/min every 3 min) has also been proposed as another way of increasing myocardial demand and thereby unmasking CAD. This is a viable option in patients with asthma or chronic pulmonary obstructive disease.[3]

A consistent scoring system is used to describe the results of a thallium scan. A normal study either shows a homogeneous distribution of the isotope in the left ventricular walls or a small apical defect best seen in the anterior and 30° LAO views. This apparent apical thinning is attributable both to ventricular geometry and motion during the cardiac cycle. Localized areas of decreased uptake can be related to the territories supplied by diseased coronary arteries. Multiple focal defects that fail to conform to those distributions may represent involvement by other processes such as sarcoidosis. Diffuse decreases in uptake suggest the presence of a cardiomyopathy. Myocardial dysfunction induced during exercise can cause ventricular dilation or increased thallium uptake in the lung.

Accuracy is increased if proper contrast enhancing schemes are used: decreases in uptake of 10% that affect 20% to 30% of the circumference of the heart are usually considered abnormal. Most computer-assisted methods of analysis rely on measurements of

isotope uptake along the circumference of the heart (Fig. 2). These techniques can be used on planar as well as on tomographic (SPECT) images. They have improved both sensitivity and specificity of the test for detecting coronary artery disease (Figs. 3, 4 [see color plate in front of book for Fig. 4]).

Technetium-99m complexes are used as alternatives to ^{201}Tl perfusion imaging. They offer better imaging characteristics and lower radiation dose to the patient. These complexes do not necessary share the same kinetics as ^{201}Tl. The major differences are in the myocardial extraction efficiency and clearance (redistribution) of the complexes.

Technetium-99m sestamibi (MIBI) is extracted slightly less efficiently by the myocardium than ^{201}Tl. There is, however, almost no redistribution of this isonitrile complex. Rest imaging requires that a second dose of isotope be injected. Conversely, there is no urgency to start imaging since the myocardial distribution of MIBI does not change significantly over 30 to 60 minutes. A delay of

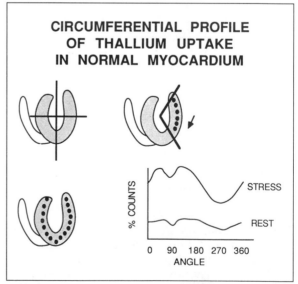

Figure 2. *The principle of quantitative thallium-201 scintigraphy is shown here. As a computer searches the left ventricular contour, points of maximal uptake are plotted as percent counts versus the angular location. Profiles are acquired for stress and rest studies. Interpretation is made by comparing uptake curves for the patient's study to a library of normal values.*

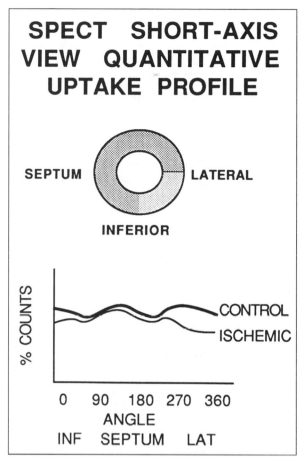

SPECT SHORT-AXIS VIEW QUANTITATIVE UPTAKE PROFILE

SEPTUM — LATERAL

INFERIOR

% COUNTS

CONTROL
ISCHEMIC

ANGLE
0   90   180   270   360
INF   SEPTUM   LAT

Figure 3. A similar quantitative approach can be used to quantify uptake on single-photon emission computed tomographic (SPECT) short-axis slices of the ventricle. Here, uptake of the isotope is decreased in the inferolateral segment when compared with a library of controls. This technique can be used for thallium-201 as well as technetium-99m sestamibi or any other analogue that maintains a relatively constant myocardial concentration over 20 to 30 minutes. The range of normal values must however be adjusted for the compound in use.

30 to 60 minutes is in fact used to permit clearance of the metabolized compound by the hepatobiliary system. Typically, a dose of up to 20 mCi is given at the point of maximal exercise or pharmacologic stress. Imaging starts later than for ^{201}Tl (30–60 min vs 5 min). The imaging protocol and the interpretation of the final images are similar to those in use for ^{201}Tl. Rest imaging can be done following a new injection of the compound on a separate day or 4 hours after stress imaging.

A much newer complex, Tetrofosmin—a lipophilic cation diphosphin—behaves similarly to the MIBI complex although clearance of background activity is somewhat more rapid.

The myocardium shows higher extraction efficiency for ^{99m}Tc teboroxime, a boronic acid adduct, than for ^{201}Tl. Clearance is, however, very rapid. Typically, the half-life of the complex is 10 to 12 minutes. Imaging must therefore be finished within 10 minutes. In general, planar imaging is achieved within this time interval. If SPECT imaging is done, it is with a series of 180 rotations lasting approximately 1 to 2 minutes each rather than with a single 10- to 20-minute acquisition. A dose of 10 to 15 mCi is normally injected.

Nitrogen-13 ammonia and rubidium-82 are used to assess myocardial perfusion in conjunction with a positron camera. They both have short half-lives and are more useful for determining perfusion than myocardial mass. Uptake of ^{13}N ammonium and ^{82}Rb is proportional to blood flow. Rubidium-82 is not metabolized whereas uptake of ^{13}N ammonium is modified if local metabolic changes affect the glutamine synthetase pathway. Imaging requires a positron camera. With ^{13}N ammonium, a cyclotron is needed. With ^{82}Rb, a ^{82m}Sr generator is used. Concurrent dipyridamole injection offers the best opportunity for stress imaging.

Myocardial Contractility (Table 2)

Left and right ventricular function can be assessed with first-pass, gated blood-pool radionuclide angiocardiography, while gated wall-motion analysis can be used to evaluate left ventricular function. This assumes the use of a computer package for data acquisition and processing. Whereas gated blood-pool imaging with labeled ^{99m}Tc red blood cells is considered the standard approach, other strategies may be more cost effective. Compounds such as ^{99m}Tc MIBI and teboroxime are injected in sufficient amounts to permit first-pass blood pool angiocardiography in addition to being useful for perfusion imaging. Uptake of ^{99m}Tc MIBI is sufficient to permit gated SPECT acquisitions and subsequent analysis of contractile motion in those areas of the ventricle that are still viable.[4]

Table 2. Myocardial Contractility Agents

ISOTOPE	HALF-LIFE	COMPLEX	PRINCIPLE	USE
^{99m}Tc	6 hr	Labeled red cells	Blood volume change synchronized to ECG	RV and LV ejection fraction; regional function; filling rates; volumes
^{99m}Tc	6 hr	Varied: DTPA, pertechnetate,	First-pass transit	RV and LV ejection fraction; regional function; filling rates; volumes and shunt lesions
^{99m}Tc		MIBI, teboroxime	First-pass transit	RV and LV ejection fraction; regional function; filling rates; volumes
^{99m}Tc	6 hr	MIBI	Wall motion synchronized to ECG	RV and LV ejection fraction; regional function; filling rates; volumes
^{81m}Kr	13 sec	Dissolved in saline from generator	First-pass transit	Mostly RV function
^{191m}Ir	4.7 sec	Dissolved in saline from generator	First-pass transit	Mostly RV function
^{195m}Au	30.5 sec	Dissolved in saline from generator	First-pass transit	Mostly RV function Shunt lesions

DTPA= Diethylenetriaminepentaacetic acid; MIBI=Technetium-99m sestamibi; ECG=Electrocardiogram; RV=Right ventricular; LV=Left ventricular.

Radionuclide angiography can be used to measure a number of useful indices of ventricular performance. The ejection fraction is a sensitive index of the contractile state of the left ventricle. Detection and quantification of regional changes in contractility correlate well with contrast ventriculography and with the absence of contracting myocardium, either when it is replaced by scar or when ischemia is present.

With exercise, patients with hemodynamically significant coronary artery stenoses will usually have changes suggesting decompensation of normal myocardial contractility, global decreases of left ventricular ejection fraction, or the appearance of new wall-motion abnormalities.[5]

Resting studies are more often performed with the patient supine (Fig. 5). In the first-pass study, a rapid bolus is injected so that the bolus remains compact when it reaches the left ventricle. The multicrystal camera is the instrument of choice for such a study, since it possesses a high count rate capability and permits the extraction of statistically significant information during the short transit time of the injected bolus. Since most of the isotope is in the ventricular cavity during the critical imaging period, there is minimal interference from the small amount distributed to adjacent anatomic structures such as the lungs. The patient can therefore be positioned in the anterior, left anterior oblique, or right anterior oblique position.

The blood-pool radionuclide angiocardio-

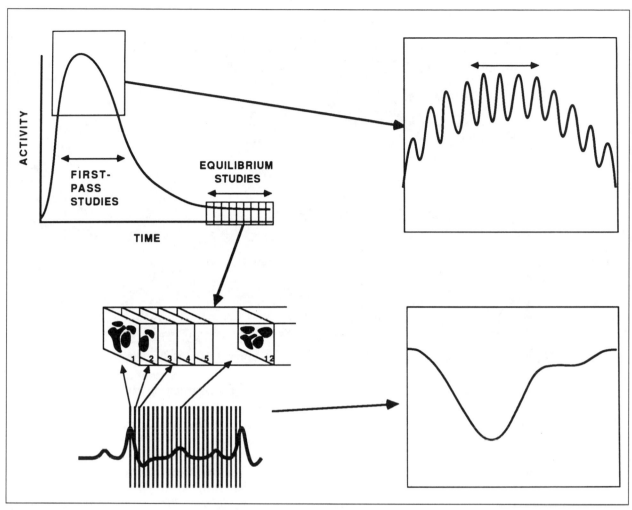

Figure 5A. *The difference between first-pass and gated radionuclide angiocardiography is summarized in this diagram. The first-pass angiocardiogram can be done without gating. The amount of activity over either the right or left ventricles is measured. Ejection fraction is normally calculated for the 3 to 5 cardiac cycles, located near the point of maximal activity in the ventricular region of interest. The gated blood-pool ventriculogram is the summation of activities detected during 100 to 300 cardiac cycles. The acquisition is synchronized to the electrocardiogram and is made when the activity in the blood pool is in a quasi-steady state.*

gram requires a greater degree of sophistication. First, the contents of the heart chambers must be labeled and remain so for the duration of the study. Technetium-99m-labeled red blood cells are the agent of choice. Second, patient radiation exposure must be kept to a minimum while collecting images with satisfactory statistics. This is achieved by the synchronization of individual cardiac beats to the R wave of the ECG and by the summation of many individual cycles into a representative cardiac cycle. This is easily done if the cardiac

rhythm is regular and without serious ectopy. Quantitative assessments of ejection fraction are more reproducible when a left anterior oblique projection is used. There is minimal overlap of the left ventricle with other cardiac chambers. Supplementary projections are used for additional qualitative interpretations (anterior, right anterior oblique, left lateral, or left posterior oblique positions).

The first-pass study can be performed with the patient doing exercise in either the supine or upright position with either the right anterior

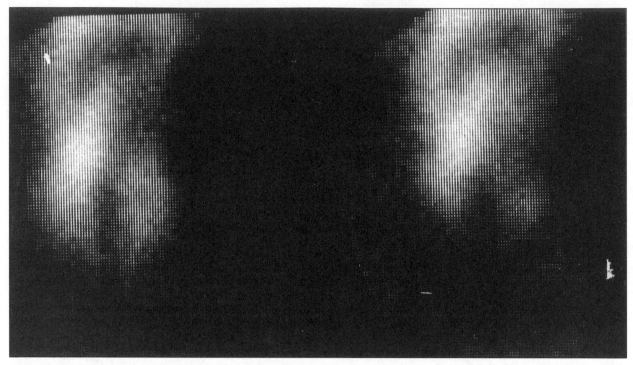

Figure 5B. *This is a gated blood-pool radionuclide angiocardiogram in the left anterior oblique position. Left diastolic image showing ventricles maximally dilated. Right-systolic image shows emptying of ventricles.*

oblique, anterior, or left anterior oblique projections. When the predefined exercise level is attained, a repeat injection of radionuclide is given and a study acquired. This approach is difficult to use for graded levels of exercise, since more than two injections are necessary. This type of angiocardiogram can be done with a compound that does not show too much myocardial uptake or persistent blood pool activity. With gated blood-pool imaging, a commonly used protocol increases the exercise stage every 3 minutes. Imaging is conducted in the last 2 minutes of each stage.

With both modalities, regional wall-motion abnormalities are assessed qualitatively during the dynamic display of a reconstructed representative cardiac cycle or with computer processed images of ejection fraction or paradox. Global ejection fraction is determined using a validated analysis package. There is some gain in accuracy if ventricular volumes are measured at rest with SPECT. However, the time available for the acquisition of an exercise ventriculogram is too short to permit quality SPECT imaging. Analysis of wall motion can

also be done with gated SPECT acquisition of a compound that binds to myocardium, 99mTc MIBI, for example.

The lower limits of ejection fraction for the left ventricle range from 45% to 55% and for the right ventricle from 40% to 50%, depending on the laboratory. Similarly, the criteria for an abnormal exercise response vary from laboratory to laboratory. Frequently cited criteria include either a fall of global ejection fraction, a failure to increase by 5%, or the development or worsening of regional wall-motion abnormalities. A depressed global left ventricular resting early diastole peak-filling rate is a more-sensitive criterion of ventricular dysfunction than any other parameter measured at rest. Early diastolic dysfunction has been measured in patients with CAD, with hypertrophic cardiomyopathy, and with hypertension.

Myocardial Necrosis (Table 3)

Technetium-99m pyrophosphate, a bone scanning agent, is one of the first radio-

Table 3. Myocardial Necrosis

ISOTOPE	HALF-LIFE	COMPLEX	PRINCIPLE	USE
^{111}In	67 hr	DTPA complex bound to antimyosin antibody	Binding to exposed myosin	Confirming infarct and measuring extent
^{201}Tl	73 hr	Thallous chloride injected at rest	Lack of uptake in nonviable myocardium	Extent of myocardial infarct
^{99m}Tc	6 hr	MIBI	Lack of uptake in nonviable myocardium	Extent of myocardial infarct
^{99m}Tc	6 hr	Pyrophosphate	Uptake by necrotic myocytes	Confirming infarct (measuring extent)

DTPA=Diethylenetriaminepentaacetic acid; MIBI=Technetium-99m sestamibi.

pharmaceuticals used to image the site of recent myocardial necrosis.

The distribution of pyrophosphate uptake parallels the amount of calcium present in the region of recently damaged myocardium. Absorption onto crystalline hydroxyapatite, amorphous calcium phosphate and to calcium linked to myofibrils accounts for most of the uptake of the pharmaceutical. Highest myocardial concentration of the tracer occurs in zones with 20% to 50% of normal resting blood flow. Optimal imaging time is 36 to 72 hours after transmural infarction whereas increased myocardial uptake can be seen as early as 4 hours after infarction.

A standard gamma camera is used. Anterior, LAO, and lateral projections are taken. Single-photon emission computed tomography imaging has shown higher sensitivity for nontransmural infarcts. Imaging should start at least 3 hours after the intravenous injection of this pharmaceutical.

Focal accumulations or diffuse massive uptake are unequivocal using ^{99m}Tc pyrophosphate for myocardial infarction. Diffuse patterns of uptake, if they are as intense as the bones of the sternum, are suspicious for an infarct. Diffuse uptake over the myocardium less than the ribs is less likely to be the result of an infarct.

When myocardial uptake is focal, it can be localized to 1 or more segments of the myocardial wall from an analysis of the scintigrams obtained in multiple projections. Frequently, contiguous segments are involved, especially with inferior infarcts extending into the right ventricle. Imaging by SPECT alleviates uncertainties in localization of the infarct and has in fact been shown to be superior to planar imaging.

Labeled antibodies to myosin localize at the site of recent myocardial infarcts. Although iodine ^{131}I can be labeled to the antibody, Indium-111 chelates are more readily available.[6] Fab fragments are chosen in order to improve the quality of the images, mainly by more rapid clearance of the background activity.

The myosin protein is exposed after disruption of the cell membrane in the zone of an infarct or of ongoing damage to the cell membrane. Labeled antimyosin antibodies, normally excluded by the intact membrane, can now reach the protein and bind to it.

Accumulation is best in zones of lowest flow. Image quality is improved when the time interval between injection is long. Typically, 24 hours are needed to build up the concentration in the infarct and to clear the nonspecific uptake in the surrounding tissues.

Although planar scintigraphy can be used, SPECT imaging is preferred. Imaging is performed at 24 and 48 hours after an injection of 1.2 to 2.0 mCi of DTPA coupled Fab fragments.

As with pyrophosphate imaging, zones of infarction can be clearly shown. False positives are less likely, since many of the causes of pyrophosphate uptake (bones, fractures) do not affect labeled antimyosin. Persistent uptake can also be seen long after the myocardial infarct.[6]

Myocardial Metabolism (Table 4)

Two categories of agents can be used to estimate myocardial metabolism. The first are single photon emitters such as ^{123}I bound to fatty acids (heptadecanoic acid). The second are compounds labeled to positron emitters.

Myocardial cells can extract and use glucose, fatty acids, or lactate as energy substrates. Nonesterified fatty acids are the preferred substrate of well-perfused myocardium. Carbon-11 palmitate extraction and clearance are decreased in ischemic myocardium due to impaired free fatty acid oxidation. Labeled heptadecanoic acid (methyl-^{11}C or ^{123}I) extraction is decreased in ischemia.

Glucose uptake and mainly anaerobic metabolism predominate during ischemia. Uptake of an analogue such as ^{18}F fluoro-deoxyglucose will therefore reflect ischemic but viable myocardium.

Carbon-11 acetate uptake parallels the level of oxidative metabolism in the myocytes.

These approaches are expensive because of the cost of the radiocompounds and the devices required for acquisition and analysis of the images.

DETECTION OF CORONARY ARTERY DISEASE

With the proliferation of noninvasive diagnostic tests aimed at evaluating CAD, it is critically important that the clinician keep very clearly in mind the questions he or she wishes answered and the population on which the pertinent test have been validated. The application of decision-making theory and, more importantly of Bayes' theorem gives us insight into the limitations of these screening procedures. Consider, for example, the patient with a finite pretest likelihood of disease (determined by integrating all of the available clinical data). After a positive or negative test, the likelihood of disease depends not only on the sensitivity and specificity of the procedure but also on the pretest likelihood of disease. If the patient has a high pretest likelihood of disease, it becomes almost impossible to rule out disease with a negative test, whereas a low pretest likelihood of diseases makes it very difficult to rule in diseases with a positive test.

If we apply the same logic to standard exercise ECG testing, there is no doubt that the test will do well in a group of symptomatic patients. In asymptomatic patients, the test is a poor discriminator between the presence or absence of disease.

THE ROLE OF STRESS PERFUSION IMAGING

The following arguments assume that ^{201}Tl is considered as a gold standard for perfusion imaging and that the ^{99m}Tc complexes have similar diagnostic accuracy.[7–9] For the detection of CAD, a set of "sensitive" criteria can be used, in the same way that the presence of resting Q waves on an ECG adds to the detection sensitivity of an ECG stress or exercise treadmill test. When the presence of either a stress-induced or a resting decrease in thallium uptake is used, the sensitivity of an abnormal test is 84%, whereas the specificity is 87%.[10] For similar population groups, the exercise test is 68% sensitive and 77% specific.[11]

More specific criteria can be introduced if the clinical question is the assessment of ongoing ischemia in patients suspected of having significant CAD. A fair proportion of these patients have resting Q waves on ECG or resting defects on thallium testing. The appearance of a new defect or the worsening of a previously present thallium defect on exercise is 73% sensitive and 90% specific for the presence of significant CAD.[12,13] The appearance of ST-segment changes is 77% sensitive and 86% specific in the sample populations when acceptable ECG exercise tolerance tests are reviewed.

Table 4. Myocardial Metabolism

ISOTOPE	HALF-LIFE	COMPLEX	PRINCIPLE	USE
[18]F	108 min	FDG; glucose analog	Uptake in viable myocytes, more so in ischemic ones	Detection of viable myocytes
[11]C	20 min	Fatty acid (palmitate)	Oxidative metabolism	Decreased oxidation; retention in ischemia
[11]C	20 min	Acetate	Uptake in metabolically active cells	Viability
[123]I	3.3 hr	Fatty acid analog (heptadecanoic acid)	Uptake in metabolically active, non-ischemic cells	Nonischemic cells
[13]N	10 min	Ammonia	Perfusion; uptake in viable cells	In combination with ^{11}C palmitate, ^{18}F FDG

FDG=Fluorodeoxyglucose.

Thallium studies play an important role in the assessment of patients with an unsatisfactory ECG stress test. Resting ECG abnormalities (left bundle branch block, ST-segment depression secondary to digitalis effect) or the inability to reach established exercise endpoints occur in 5% to 20% of the population groups commonly screened. Under these circumstances, the stress thallium test can be 73% sensitive and 72% specific for the detection of coronary artery disease.[12,13]

The sensitivity and specificity of ^{201}Tl imaging are improved when computer assisted analysis is applied to planar images.[14] With the introduction and dissemination of SPECT imaging, sensitivity has increased and specificity may have decreased slightly.[15–18]

Slow redistribution of ^{201}Tl can be circumvented by the use of a second injection of isotope. This improves the sensitivity for detecting severely ischemic and viable—possibly hibernating—myocardium.[1] The cost effectiveness of this approach needs to be evaluated further. Hybrid

techniques that evaluate combined injections of ^{201}Tl and MIBI can lead to very efficacious patient management. For example, resting injection of ^{201}Tl imaging and then MIBI exercise imaging can be done sequentially rather than requiring delayed imaging.

In general, stress perfusion imaging protocols that rely on any of the pharmacological agents mentioned above perform with accuracies similar to those of exercise stress testing.[3,19–21]

THE ROLE OF EXERCISE VENTRICULOGRAPHY

For the detection of CAD, sensitive criteria include the presence of a reduced resting ejection fraction, with or without regional wall motion abnormalities; and, with exercise, either the appearance of new or the worsening of old regional wall motion abnormalities and/or failure of the ejection fraction to rise by 0.05 resting ejection fraction units or 4% of the resting ejection fraction. Sensitivity is over 90%

and specificity is 58% when this method is used to attempt to differentiate those patients with CAD from those presenting with chest pain not due to CAD.[22] An abnormal response is, however, rarely seen in normal asymptomatic subjects. In fact, it is not the change in ejection fraction with exercise that helps predict outcome in symptomatic patients or patients after myocardial infarction (MI) but rather the actual ejection fraction at exercise.[23,24]

This test has lost favor as a screening test for the detection of CAD because of the poor specificity of the test and the wide availability of stress echocardiography.

LIMITATIONS OF RADIONUCLIDE METHODS

Right ventricular (RV) involvement secondary to CAD cannot be reliably assessed by perfusion scintigraphy—[201]Tl or Tc analogs—since the RV walls cannot be visualized under normal circumstances. By inference, resting or exercise defects seen in the inferior wall of the left ventricle may suggest right coronary disease. The sensitivity of perfusion deficits for identifying involvement of specific coronary artery territories is worse for the circumflex artery. Performance is slightly better when the right coronary artery is affected, and sensitivity is best when the left anterior descending artery is involved. Detection accuracy has improved slightly with SPECT.

Although the overall detection efficiency is quite good, planar thallium imaging does not offer much specificity in assessing the extent of significant CAD. For example, a perfusion defect in the territory of the left anterior descending artery (anterolateral left ventricular wall) is seen in 80% of cases with solitary involvement of this vessel but in only 50% of cases with concomitant involvement of the other coronaries. This is improved with SPECT imaging. High-risk perfusion scans are characterized by: 1) acute dilatation of the left ventricle, 2) increased lung uptake and, 3) multiple defects in 2 or more coronary artery perfusion regions. Patients with left main disease or extensive CAD are likely to have these findings.[25]

The value of thallium uptake as a predictor of operative response to saphenous aortocoronary bypass surgery is twofold. Preoperatively, it confirms the physiologic significance of a coronary artery lesion. Postoperatively, it offers a noninvasive means of assessing graft patency and surgical effectiveness.[26] For example, those areas where preoperative perfusion defects show redistribution at rest or delayed redistribution typically show improved ventricular function after revascularization.[1,27]

In combination with dipyridamole, the test can be used for risk stratification of patients undergoing noncardiovascular surgery. Normal ^{201}Tl dipyridamole scanning is predictive of an intra- and postoperative period free of cardiac events, whereas the extent of transient perfusion defects is positively correlated to the likelihood of perioperative cardiac events.[28]

Radionuclide ventriculography has poor specificity when used to screen patients presenting with chest pain. Global and regional left ventricular function can also be abnormal in patients with false-positive test results who have valvular disease, cardio-myopathies, left bundle branch block, or therapy requiring a concomitant assessment by another imaging modality, such as echo-cardiography. It is also of limited utility when arrhythmias are present.

The interpretation of exercise ventriculography should take into consideration the distinction between the screening for the presence of CAD and assessing its physiological importance. The resting study should serve as a first step. A low ejection fraction and/or regional wall-motion abnormalities are suggestive of ischemic heart disease. The results of the exercise test will more sensitively reflect the physiologic state of the ventricle. For example, patients with previously abnormal ventriculographic responses to exercise often demonstrate a return to normal exercise ejection fraction response in the early post–aortocoronary bypass surgery period.

Ideally propranolol therapy should be withdrawn 48 hours before exercise stress thallium imaging and stress radionuclide ventriculography since it may blunt the heart rate response. Nitroglycerin may also reverse areas of decreased thallium uptake or areas of ventricular dysfunction.

ACUTE MYOCARDIAL INFARCTION

PYROPHOSPHATE 99MTC/111IN ANTIMYOSIN ANTIBODY IMAGING

The overall sensitivity of pyrophosphate for the detection of acute myocardial infarction varies between 51% and 100% and is best for large transmural myocardial infarctions.[29] This is surpassed by the antimyosin antibody.[30] False-positive test results are often attributable to uptake in a zone of previous myocardial infarction. False-negative results occur in 6% to 7% of cases (75% of which are inferior infarcts). The sensitivity for detecting nontransmural infarcts is 43%. SPECT imaging can further increase the sensitivity of pyrophosphate infarct imaging.

Abnormal pyrophosphate uptake is seen in patients presenting with unstable angina yet without acute infarcts. Pathological correlations suggest that subclinical ongoing myocardial necrosis probably accounts for a large proportion of these cases.[31] Technetium-99m pyrophosphate imaging can delineate any extension of inferior infarcts into the right ventricle, a phenomenon seen in more than one-third of the cases of inferior infarction.

Infarct avid scintigraphy is also a sensitive and specific means of establishing whether myocardial infarction occurred in the perioperative period. It can assist in the clinical problem of documenting recent myocardial damage in a patient presenting with an unreliable ECG (as in the case of left bundle branch block) or presenting too late in the clinical course for serial elevation of the cardiospecific enzymes. The pattern and intensity of pyrophosphate uptake also holds prognostic significance. The greater the amount of radiopharmaceutical taken up by the infarcted myocardium, the higher the mortality and morbidity in the early period after discharge. There are no similar data available for antimyosin antibodies.

PERFUSION IMAGING WITH 201TL OR 99MTC ANALOGS

This imaging procedure detects both infarction and regions of peri-infarct ischemia. The overall sensitivity in acute (<6 hr) events is 100%; for events occurring between 6 and 24 hours before the imaging period, the sensitivity decreases to 88%. When imaging is performed more than 24 hours after the onset of symptoms, the sensitivity decreases to 72%.[32] The overall detection rate for transmural events is 88%; for nontransmural infarctions, the sensitivity is 63%. The test is not specific enough to be of use in screening patients with acute chest pain (i.e., infarct vs noninfarct). There has, however, been increased use of the test for documenting the value of acute interventions aimed at preserving myocardium at risk. Technetium-99m sestamibi may be better suited than 201Tl for monitoring the efficiency of thrombolysis. The distribution of isotope remains stable over hours, making the subsequent images an accurate depiction of the extent of myocardium at risk, as it was before therapy started. Subsequent administration of either 201Tl or 99mTc MIBI can be used to monitor improvement in perfusion.[33] Successful thrombolysis is associated with a normalization of 201Tl uptake in the reopened coronary artery, even if regional wall-motion abnormalities persist as a result of stunned myocardium. Persistently depressed 201Tl uptake after percutaneous transluminal coronary angioplasty (PTCA) may indicate delayed recovery of coronary reserve or may indicate a higher likelihood of recurrent stenosis.[34]

Submaximal exercise or pharmacologic 201Tl stress testing can be done after MI—possibly subsequent to therapies such as thrombolysis or angioplasty—to document the presence of persistent ischemia. This may suggest a still-active culprit stenosis or a second significant stenosis in a different coronary branch. Transient perfusion defects increase the likelihood of cardiac events in the subsequent days.[35,36] The presence of a reversible perfusion defect is less than 50% accurate for determining the presence of a second significant lesion if it is located in a coronary branch distant from the infarct related artery.[37]

Stress thallium imaging can be used in patients after aortocoronary bypass surgery when graft patency is questioned. Exercise and redistribution thallium images are obtained pre- and postoperatively. The graft patency rate is over 80% if new defects are not seen on rest-redistribution images or if transient defects are present on the postoperative study. A persistent defect suggests graft occlusion (73%) and, by inference, myocardial damage. Bypass surgery seems to normalize thallium uptake in those regions showing either complete or partial redistribution on preoperative scans.[38] Surprisingly, up to 50% of fixed defects seem also to improve, presumably because they represent areas of hibernating myocardium.[1]

Right ventricular infarction cannot be appreciated on thallium images unless abnormally increased uptake is present in this wall. This is possible only in patients with hypertrophied right ventricular walls, a finding common in patients with chronic elevations of pulmonary artery pressures.[39]

The technetium complexes—sestamibi, teroboxime, tetrofosmin—are believed to give similar information, although the imaging protocols can vary markedly.

RADIONUCLIDE ANGIOGRAPHY

This imaging modality is used to identify alterations in regional and/or global ventricular function seen during and after ischemic damage. Left ventricular ejection fraction may be depressed coincident with an anterior transmural infarction, while it is often not affected during inferior myocardial infarctions. Serial evaluations of both global left ventricular ejection fraction and regional wall-motion abnormalities in the postinfarction period have shown that regional and global asynergy improve slowly, with little change at 2 weeks after infarction and more dramatic results at 2 to 4 months.[40]

A depressed global left ventricular ejection fraction identifies patients with increased mortality in the postinfarction period; the presence of both low left and right ventricular ejection fractions can further define a group of high-risk patients.[41] Inferior wall infarction, associated with depressed resting right ventricular (RV) ejection fraction, is an especially important indicator of poor prognosis.[42]

PREVIOUS MYOCARDIAL INFARCTION

Evidence of previous myocardial infarction can be seen with perfusion agents (^{201}Tl, ^{99m}Tc sestamibi, ^{99m}Tc teboroxime, ^{99m}Tc tetrofosmin) or radionuclide ventriculographic (first-pass or gated) studies. Abnormal myocardial uptake of pyrophosphate and antimyosin antibody[6] decreases in intensity in the first 2 to 3 weeks after infarction in most patients, whereas defects on ^{201}Tl scintigraphy shrink with time after infarction and, by 7 months, have disappeared entirely in 25% of patients with previous infarction. The wall-motion abnormalities measured by radionuclide angiocardiography do not change significantly in the first 4 to 6 weeks postinfarction.

The amount of "stunned" myocardium can be detected by combining the information from different studies. Loss of myocardial function as detected by gated blood pool, first-pass ventriculography, gated MIBI images can be correlated against preserved perfusion and uptake in myocardium as indicated by ^{201}Tl, ^{99m}Tc MIBI. The presence of metabolically active cells is, however, unequivocally proved by showing ^{18}F FDG or ^{11}C acetate uptake. "Hibernating" myocardium shows markedly decreased perfusion and loss of contractile function. These zones may show uptake after rest-reinjection of ^{201}Tl when a defect is seen on stress-redistribution imaging.[1] The diagnosis is certain if active glucose metabolism (uptake of ^{18}F FDG) is shown in the same area of the myocardium.[43,44]

ASSESSMENT OF MISCELLANEOUS DISORDERS

THALLIUM-201

Areas of absent or decreased myocardial uptake may result from an invasive process that replaces cardiac muscle with fibrous tissue, granulomas, or tumor. Thus, focal areas of decreased thallium uptake may be seen in patients with myocardial sarcoidosis, amyloidosis, or other infiltrative processes.[45]

In patients with asymmetrical hypertrophic cardiomyopathy, the relative asymmetry of uptake between septum and left ventricular free wall can confirm the presence of this entity. Patients with symmetrical hypertrophy secondary to pressure overload show relatively normal ratios of left ventricular and septal wall uptake. The amount of RV wall uptake also appears to correlate with pulmonary artery pressure elevation and increased pulmonary vascular resistance.

Patients with congestive cardiomyopathy can be expected to have large areas of decreased left ventricular uptake (>40% circumference) when an underlying ischemic etiology is responsible (sensitivity, 100%). Idiopathic cardiomyopathies more often present with an inhomogeneous diffuse pattern of decreased uptake; large focal areas are less common (incidence, 25%).[46]

VENTRICULOGRAPHY

The feasibility of using gated ventriculography to detect large atrial myxomas and left ventricular aneurysms is overshadowed by the performance of other noninvasive tests such as magnetic resonance imaging and echocardiography. Postoperative success or ventricular aneurysmectomy can be predicted based on residual ejection fraction of the left ventricular walls not involved by the aneurysm.

Although the therapeutic effects of calcium-channel blockers or inotropic agents can be monitored using either exercise or resting indices of ventricular function, there are no outcome data to suggest that this needs to be done in a routine fashion.

Congestive cardiomyopathy is likely when the ejection fraction is decreased at rest (<40%) and the left ventricular cavity is enlarged. Coronary artery disease is likely to be the etiology if: 1) contraction of the basal portions of the left ventricle is the last to be compromised, 2) regional asynergy involves a large contiguous portion of the ventricular contour (>40%), and 3) if the right ventricle is spared. Generalized hypokinesia, with focal areas of dyskinesia, is more common in idiopathic cardiomyopathy. Depression of right and left ventricular ejection fraction holds prognostic information in those patients with severe left ventricular dysfunction.[41]

Diastolic dysfunction of the left ventricle has been observed in patients with CAD, hypertrophic cardiomyopathy, and hypertension, despite normal systolic function. Of the 2 parameters commonly measured, peak-early diastolic filling rate and time to peak-diastolic filling rate, the former more accurately predicts early ventricular dysfunction.[47] Improvement in this parameter of ventricular function has been shown after coronary bypass surgery in patients with CAD and after calcium-channel blocker therapy in patients with hypertrophic cardiomyopathy.[48]

Left-sided valvular regurgitation and left ventricular volume overload in the absence of concomitant right-sided valvular regurgitation can be documented in cases of significant (regurgitant fraction >0.20) valvular incompetence.[49] The method most frequently used relies on good geometric separation of both ventricles and atria and considers the ratio of left-to-right ventricular stroke volume counts: (LV stroke volume – RV stroke volume)/LV stroke volume = Regurgitant fraction).

Abnormal blood pool increase in the liver during systole can also be used to document tricuspid regurgitation.

[111]I ANTIMYOSIN ANTIBODY

Uptake of [111]I antimyosin antibody is seen in patients with acute myocarditis,[50] following cardiac transplantation,[51] and doxorubicin toxicity.[52] Uptake in acute myocarditis seems to correlate with a positive prognosis, whereas it has negative connotations in cases of transplantation—possible rejection—and during the administration of doxorubicin—developing toxicity.

CENTRAL CIRCULATION

The transit of an intravenously injected bolus of a radiopharmaceutical can be followed and recorded providing qualitative information about the anatomy of the heart chambers and the major vessels. This yields gross anatomic and functional information in patients—mostly pediatric—with suspected congenital anomalies (Fig. 6).

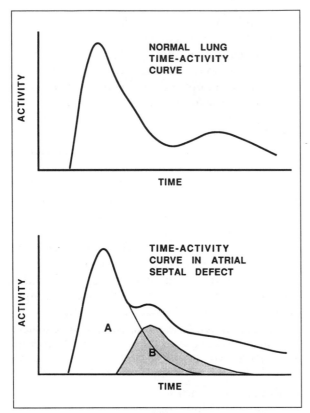

Figure 6. *Measurement of the time-activity curve over the lung normally shows an initial, high-amplitude peak as a bolus or intravenously administered radioisotope passes through the lung. A second, smaller peak, is caused by systemic recirculation. In the case of a left to right shunt, such as in an arterial septal defect, an early recirculation peak is detected. The area corresponding to this second peak is representative of the shunt lesion while A–B represents systemic flow.*

Tricuspid atresia and Ebstein's anomaly have right-to-left shunts through atrial septal defects. In pulmonary atresia without a right-to-left shunt, the bolus persists in the right atrium. The bolus persists in either the right atrium or right ventricle if either tricuspid stenosis or pulmonic stenosis is present. On the left side of the heart, the left atrium is enlarged in the presence of mitral stenosis. Transit into the left ventricle and aorta is also delayed. In severe aortic stenosis at birth or in patients with a hypoplastic left heart, a right-to-left shunt via a patent ductus arteriosus may be detected. In transposition of the great vessels, cardiac activity

disappears quickly, with only the right heart and aorta being identified.

Right-to-left shunts are measured using either of 2 techniques. Radioactive particles, such as ^{99}Tc-labeled macroaggregated albumin (20–50 μ diameter), are injected intravenously. The number of particles transiting the pulmonary, renal and cerebral circulations is then measured. Since a small number of particles (20,000–100,000) is injected, no side effects have been reported. The calculation is made as follows:

$$\% \text{ right-to-left-shunt} = \frac{\text{Counts (total body – lung)}}{\text{Counts (total body)}} \times 100\%$$

Alternatively, the time-activity curve (the relationship between time and the quantity of a radioactive tracer in an organ or region of an organ as measured by an external detector) can be analyzed as the bolus passes over the left ventricle. For left-to-right shunts, time-activity information is generated over the lung field and is mathematically processed to obtain a curve representing the pulmonary circulation and a second curve representing pulmonary recirculation. The difference between these 2 curves is proportional to systemic flow. The shunt is then calculated as a pulmonary to systemic (QP:QS) flow ratio; ratios greater than 1.2:1 are abnormal.

In conclusion, nuclear cardiology remains an important aspect in the diagnosis and characterization of a host of cardiac diseases.

REFERENCES

1. Dilsizian V, Rocco TP, Freedman NMT, et al. Enhanced detection of ischemic but viable myocardium by the reinjection of thallium after stress-redistribution imaging. *N Engl J Med.* 1990;323:141-146.
2. Iskandrian AS. Single-photon emission computed tomography thallium imaging with adenosisne, dipyridamole, and exercise. *Eur Heart J.* 1991;122:279-284.
3. Hays JT, Mahmarian JJ, Cochran AJ, et al. Dobutamine thallium-201 tomography for evaluating patients with suspected coronary artery disease unable to undergo exercise or vasodilatory pharmacologic testing. *J Am Coll Cardiol.* 1993;21:1583-1590.

4. Chua T, Kiat H, Germano G, et al. Gated technetium-99m sestamibi for simultaneous assessment of stress myocardial perfusion, post-exercise regional ventricular function and myocardial viability: Correlation with echocardiography and rest thallium-201 scintigraphy. *J Am Coll Cardiol*. 1994;23:1104-1111.

5. Borer JS, Bacharach SL, Green MV, et al. Real time radionuclide cineangiography in the noninvasive evaluation of global and regional left ventricular function at rest and during exercise in patients with coronary artery disease. *N Engl J Med*. 1977;296:839-844.

6. Bhattacharya S, Liu XJ, Senior R, et al. [111]In antimyosin antibody uptake is related to the age of myocardial infarction. *Am Heart J*. 1991;122:1583-1587.

7. Labonte C, Taillefer R, Lambert R, et al. Comparison between technetium-99m-teboroxime and thallium-201 dipyridamole planar myocardial perfusion imaging in detection of coronary artery disease. *Am J Cardiol*. 1992;69:90-96.

8. Pozzoli MM, Fioretti PM, Salustri A, et al. Exercise echocardiography and technetium-99m MIBI single-photon emission computed tomography in the detection of coronary artery disease. *Am J Cardiol*. 1991; 67:350-355.

9. Sridhara BS, Braat S, Rigo P, et al. Comparison of myocardial perfusion imaging with technetium-99m tetrofosmin versus thallium-201 in coronary artery disease. *Am J Cardiol*. 1993;72:1015-1019.

10. Kotler TS, Diamond GA. Exercise thallium-201 scintigraphy in the diagnosis and prognosis of coronary artery disease. *Ann Intern Med*. 1990;113:684-702.

11. Gianrossi R, Detrano R, Mulvihill D, et al. Exercise-induced ST depression in the diagnosis of coronary artery disease. A meta-analysis. *Circulation*. 1990;80:87-98.

12. Ritchie JL, Zaret BL, Stauss HW, et al. Myocardial imaging with thallium-201: A multicenter study in patients with angina pectoris or acute myocardial infarction. *Am J Cardiol*. 1978;42:345-350.

13. McCarthy DM, Blood DK, Sciacca RR, et al. Single dose myocardial perfusion imaging with thallium-201: Application in patients with nondiagnostic electrocardiographic stress tests. *Am J Cardiol*. 1979;43:899-906.

14. Beller GA. Current status of nuclear cardiology techniques. *Curr Probl Cardiol*. 1991;16:449-535.

15. DePasquale EE, Nody AC, DePuey EG, et al. Quantitative rotational thallium-201 tomography for identifying and localizing coronary artery disease. *Circulation*. 1988;77:316-327.

16. Maddahi J, Van Train K, Prigent F, et al. Quantitative single photon computed thallium-201 tomography for detection and localization of coronary artery disease by planar and tomographic methods. *J Am Coll Cardiol*. 1989;14:1689-1699.

17. Mahmarian JJ, Boyce TM, Goldberg RK, et al. Quantitative exercise thallium-201 single photon emission computed tomography for the enhanced diagnosis of ischemic disease. *J Am Coll Cardiol*. 1990;15:318-329.

18. Fintel DJ, Links JM, Brinker JA, et al. Improved diagnostic performance of exercise thallium-201 single photon emission computed tomography over planar imaging in the diagnosis of coronary artery disease: A receiver operating characteristics analysis. *J Am Coll Cardiol*. 1989;13:600-612.

19. Leppo JA. Dipyridamole-thallium imaging: The lazy man's test. *J Nucl Med*. 1989;30:281-287.

20. Gupta N, Esterbrooks DJ, Hilleman DE, et al. Comparison of adenosine and exercise thallium-201 single-photon emssion computed tomography (SPECT) myocardial perfusion imaging. *J Am Coll Cardiol*. 1992;19:248-257.

21. Nishimura S, Mahmarian JJ, Boyce TM, et al. Equivalence between adenosine and exercise thallium-201 myocardial tomography: A multicenter, prospective, crossover trial. *J Am Coll Cardiol*. 1992;20:265-275.

22. Rozanski A, Diamond GA, Berman D, et al. The declining specificity of exercise radionuclide ventriculography. *N Engl J Med*. 1983;309:518-522.

23. Pryor DB, Harrell FE, Lee KL, et al. Prognostic indicators from radionuclide angiocardiography in medically treated patients with coronary artery disease. *Am J Cardiol*. 1984;53:18-22.

24. Lee KL, Pryor DB, Pieper KS, et al. Prognostic value of radionuclide angiography in medically treated patients with coronary artery disease: A comparison with clinical and catheterization variables. *Circulation*. 1990;82:1705-1717.

25. Nygaard TW, Gibson RS, Ryan JM, et al. Prevalence of high-risk thallium-201 scintigraphic findings in left main coronary artery stenosis: Comparison with patients with multiple- and single-vessel coronary artery disease. *Am J Cardiol*. 1984;53:462-469.

26. Kolibash AJ, Call TD, Bush CA, et al. Myocardial perfusion as an indicator of graft patency after coronary bypass surgery. *Circulation*. 1980;61:882-887.

27. Ragosta M, Beller GA, Watson DD, et al. Quantitative planar rest-redistribution Tl-201 imaging in detection of myocardial viability and prediction of improvement in left ventricular function after coronary bypass in patients with severely depressed left ventricular function. *Circulation*. 1993;86:1630-1641.

28. Eagle KA, Coley CM, Newell JB, et al. Combining clinical and thallium data optimizes preoperative assessment of cardiac risk before surgery. *Ann Intern Med*. 1989;110:859-866.

29. Holman BL, Lesch M, Alpert JS. Myocardial scintigraphy with technetium-99m pyrophosphate during the early phase of acute infarction. *Am J Cardiol*. 1978;41:39-42.

30. Johnson LL, Seldin DW, Becker LC, et al. Antimyosin imaging in acute transmural myocardial infarctions: Results of a multicenter clinical trial. *J Am Coll Cardiol*. 1989;13:27-35.

31. Buja LM, Tofe AJ, Kulkarni PV, et al. Sites and mechanisms of localization of technetium-99m phosphorous radiopharmaceuticals in acute myocardial infarcts and other tissues. *J Clin Invest*. 1977;60:724-740.

32. Wackers FJT, Lie KI, Lien KL, et al. Potential value of thallium-201 scintigraphy as a means of selecting patients for the coronary care unit. *Br Heart J*. 1979;41:111-117.

33. Wackers FJT, Gibbons RJ, Verani MS, et al. Serial quantitative planar technetium-99m isonitrile imaging in acute myocardial infarction: Efficacy for noninvasive assessment of thrombolytic therapy. *J Am Coll Cardiol*. 1989;14:861-873.

34. Hecht HS, Shaw RE, Chin HL, et al. Silent ischemia after coronary angioplasty: evaluation of restenosis and extent of ischemia in asymptomatic patients by tomographic thallium-201 exercise imaging and comparison with symptomatic patients. *J Am Coll Cardiol*. 1991;17:670-677.

35. Leppo JA, O'Brien J, Rothendler JA, et al. Dipyridamole-thallium-201 scintigraphy in the prediction of future cardiac events after acute myocardial infarction. *N Engl J Med*. 1984;310:1014-1018.

36. Brown KA, O'Meara J, Chambers CE, et al. Ability of dipyridamole-thallium-201 imaging one to four days after acute myocardial infarction to predict in-hospital and late recurrent myocardial ischemic events. *Am J Cardiol*. 1990;65:160-167.

37. Haber HL, Beller GA, Watson DD, et al. Exercise thallium-210 scintigraphy after thrombolytic therapy with or without angioplasty for acute myocardial infarction. *Am J Cardiol*. 1993;71:1257-1261.

38. Gibson RS, Watson DD, Taylor GJ, et al. Prospective assessmant of regional myocardial perfusion before and after coronary revascularization surgery by quantitative thallium-201 scintigraphy. *J Am Coll Cardiol*. 1983;1:804-815.

39. Kaaja F, Alah M, Goldstein S, et al. Diagnostic value of visualization of the right ventricle using thallium-201 myocardial imaging. *Circulation*. 1979;59:182-188.

40. Reduto LA, Berger HJ, Cohen LS, et al. Sequential radionuclide assessment of left and right ventricular performance after actue transmural myocardial infarction. *Ann Intern Med*. 1978;89:441-447.

41. Shah PK, Maddahi J, Staniloff HM, et al. Variable spectrum and prognostic implications of left and right ventricular ejection fractions in patients with and without clinical heart failure after acute myocardial infarction. *J Am Coll Cardiol*. 1986;5:387-393.

42. Zehender M, Kasper W, Kavder E, et al. Right ventricular infarction as an independent predictor of prognosis after acute inferior myocardial infarction. *N Engl J Med*. 1993;328:981-988.

43. Brunken R, Schwaiger M, Grover-McKay M, et al. Positron emission tomography detects tissue metabolic activity in myocardial segments with persistent thallium perfusion defects. *J Am Coll Cardiol*. 1987;10:557-567.

44. Bonow RO, Dilsizian V, Cuocolo A, et al. Identification of viable myocardium in patients with chronic coronary artery disease and left ventricular dysfunction: Comparison of thallium scintigraphy with reinjection and PET imaging with ^{18}F-Fluorodeoxyglucose. *Circulation*. 1991;83:26-37.

45. Strauss HW, McKusick KA, Boucher CA, et al. Of linens and laces: The eighth anniversary of the gated blood pool scan. *Semin Nucl Med*. 1979;9:296-309.

46. Bulkley BH, Hutchins GM, Bailey I, et al. Thallium-201 imaging and gated cardiac blood pool scans in patients with ischemic and idiopathic congestive cardiomyopathy: A clinical and pathologic study. *Circulation*. 1977;55:753-760.

47. Inouye I, Massie B, Loge D, et al. Abnormal left ventricular filling: An early finding in mild to moderate systemic hypertension. *Am J Cardiol*. 1984;53:120-126.

48. Bonow RO, Rosing DR, Bacharach SC, et al. Effects of verapamil on left ventricular systolic function and diastolic filling in patients with hypertrophic cardiomyopathy. *Circulation*. 1981;64:787-796.

49. Bough EW, Gandsman EJ, North DL, et al. Gated radionuclide angiographic evaluation of valve regurgitation. *Am J Cardiol*. 1980;46:423-428.

50. Dec GW, Palacios I, Yasuda T, et al. Antimyosin antibody cardiac imaging: its role in the diagnosis of myocarditis. *J Am Coll Cardiol*. 1990;16:97-104.

51. Ballester M, Obrador M, Carrio I, et al. Indium-111-monoclonal antimyosin antibody studies after the first year of heart transplantation: Identification of risk groups for developing rejection during long-term follow-up and clinical implications. *Circulation*. 1990;82:2100-2107.

52. Carrio I, Estorch M, Berna L, et al. Assessment of anthracycline-induced myocardial damage by quantitative indium-111 myosin-specific monoclonal antibody studies. *Eur J Nucl Med*. 1991;18:806-812.

CHAPTER 6

Exercise Testing and Noninvasive Assessment of Coronary Artery Disease

Charles Pollick, MB ChB

The predictable association between activity and angina provides the basis for the exercise testing of patients with chest pain of unknown etiology. Many studies, performed in the early part of this century, contributed to the framework for our current approach.[1,2] The realization that ST-segment depression occurs in angina, together with the accessibility of an electrocardiogaph (ECG) machine and treadmill apparatus has made the treadmill test the most common method of assessing patients for coronary disease.

The main initial thrust of ECG exercise testing was to diagnose patients with chest pain. Later studies demonstrated that ECG responses could be gauged to assess the extent and prognosis of coronary disease. Recently, therefore, exercise testing is performed increasingly on patients with known coronary disease.

Two major developments in the latter quarter of this century are likely to produce a major impact on ECG exercise testing. First, is the development of other non-invasive markers of exercise induced ischemia, e.g., stress echocardiography,[3] and nuclear myocardial perfusion studies.[4] Both have been demonstrated to have superior accuracy to ECG assessment alone, and have thereby questioned the time-honored role of ECG testing in patients with suspected or known coronary artery disease. Second, is the introduction of non-exercise noninvasive techniques for the assessment of coronary disease, e.g. ultrafast CT scanning[5] which questions the initial "exercise centered" approach developed in the first quarter of the century.

Despite these caveats, the ECG, as a marker of ischemia, has a continued pivotal place in cardiology as it is relatively inexpensive, and relatively "operator independent," unlike nuclear or echocardiography techniques. The place of exercise also seems secure in the assessment of patients as the "fitness generation" equates exercise with good health.

In this chapter, I shall discuss the relationship between exercise and myocardial ischemia, the indications for noninvasive exercise assessment of coronary artery disease, methods of exercise testing, and interpretation of test results.

EXERCISE PATHOPHYSIOLOGY AND MYOCARDIAL ISCHEMIA

Myocardial ischemia occurs when myocardial oxygen demand exceeds supply. The 3 major determinants of demand are heart rate, myocardial contractility, and afterload. Exercise induces an increase in sympathetic activity which produces an increase in heart rate and contractility. Parasympathetic withdrawal also enhances heart rate. The normal left ventricular end-diastolic dimension diminishes, as does end-systolic dimension to a greater extent, producing an increase in stroke volume. Increased stroke volume increases blood pressure and thereby afterload, or left ventricular wall stress; the increase in blood pressure is lessened by the decrease in peripheral vascular resistance that accompanies exercise, and mean increases in arterial pressure are modest. Systolic blood pressure should increase with exercise, and diastolic pressure usually stays the same. Large studies have shown that a "normal" rise in systolic blood pressure up to 210 mm Hg may occur. Levels beyond this and diastolic pressures greater than 100 mm Hg likely reflect a hypertensive response. While stroke volume increases by a maximum of 50%, cardiac output increases up to 5 times. These findings underscore the importance of heart rate increase as the major determinant of myocardial ischemia in patients with coronary artery disease undergoing exercise testing. This fact also emphasizes the importance of achieving an adequate heart rate response (usually defined as 85% of the maximum) in ensuring an interpretable test.

Several factors affect an individual's maximum exercise induced heart rate. Age accounts for most of the variability, with gender and fitness the other major determinants. Various algorithms exist for predicting an individual's maximum response. A failure to achieve this maximum is usually due to reduced exercise capacity, although chronotropic incompetence from sinus node disease is another possibility.

In patients with coronary artery disease, various deviations from the normal physiologic response may be seen. Myocardial ischemia can induce an increase in end-diastolic volume, and to a greater extent, end-systolic volume which may also increase producing a fall in blood pressure or a failure of the blood pressure to increase. Exercise-induced hypotension (fall in systolic blood pressure below resting levels) may also be seen in dilated cardiomyopathy and in patients with aortic stenosis and hypertrophic obstructive cardiomyopathy.

INDICATIONS FOR EXERCISE TESTING

The major indication for stress testing is to determine if myocardial ischemia is the etiology of a patient's atypical chest pain.[6] Stress testing is also used to screen individuals with risk factors for developing coronary disease (e.g., high cholesterol, smoker, family history, hypertension, diabetes). Among patients with known coronary disease (or male patients with typical chest pain in whom the pre-test likelihood of coronary disease is 90%), stress testing is used to help determine the severity of coronary disease, assess efficacy of anti-anginal therapy, to look for restenosis following percutaneous coronary angioplasty, to determine effectiveness of coronary artery bypass surgery, and to "risk stratify" patients following myocardial infarction.

Stress testing is also used to determine exercise capacity and myocardial reserve in patients with valvular heart disease, especially aortic and mitral regurgitation. Cardiac arrhythmias in patients may also be usefully studied during exercise to determine their onset and response to antiarrhythmic drugs.

CONTRAINDICATIONS TO EXERCISE TESTING

Recent studies have demonstrated that exercise is sometimes associated with myocardial infarction, probably through the mechanism of coronary artery plaque rupture. It is common practice, therefore, to wait at least 48 hours following myocardial infarction and to limit the degree of stress testing to a submaximal test up to 75% of maximum predicted heart rate. Patients with congestive heart failure, rest angina, pericarditis, severe hypertension (e.g., blood pressure greater than 200 mm Hg systolic or 100 mm Hg diastolic) and second- or third-degree heart block are some examples of situations where exercise testing poses a significant risk and should be avoided. The risk of death with exercise testing clearly depends on the individual being tested. Normal healthy individuals are usually quoted a risk of death of 1 in 50,000. To put this in perspective, the annual risk of an average motorist dying from a motor vehicle accident is 1 in 4,500.

EXERCISE END-POINTS

In general, the severity of coronary artery disease correlates well with the degree of myocardial ischemia induced by exercise. Patients with single vessel disease need to be exercised much further (e.g., to maximum heart rate) to produce ischemia than patients with triple vessel and proximal disease who can develop ischemia with small increases in heart rate. Therefore exercise duration must be tailored to the individual. Ideally, all asymptomatic patients who are being screened should be exercised to exhaustion (i.e., to 100% or more of their maximum predicted heart rate) (Table 1). Sedentary patients are often reluctant to exercise and should be coaxed to achieve at

Table 1. Age-Related Heart Rate

AGE	75%	85%	100%
20	150	170	200
25	146	166	195
30	142	162	190
35	139	157	185
40	135	153	180
45	131	149	175
50	127	145	170
55	124	140	165
60	120	136	160
65	116	132	155
70	112	128	150
75	109	123	145
80	105	119	140
85	101	115	135
90	98	111	130

least 85% of their predicted heart rate, otherwise the test loses its accuracy as insufficient myocardial oxygen demand is achieved and significant coronary disease may not manifest as ischemia. Patients with chest pain should be exercised to the point of significant chest pain (subjective scale of >5/10) where the patient wishes to stop. Fall in systolic blood pressure below resting levels, increase in systolic levels above 260 mm Hg or diastolic above 115 mm Hg, multifocal premature ventricular beats, ventricular tachycardia, rapid atrial fibrillation, second or third degree heart block, or pronounced ST depression (e.g., 3 mm) are all further indications to stop exercise.

EXERCISE PROTOCOLS

Maximal exercise testing is best achieved by use of the treadmill. Various protocols have been introduced, all of which gradually increase the speed and degree of incline of the treadmill at regular time periods. The Bruce protocol uses 2-3 metabolic equivalent (MET) increments every 3 minutes. The Bruce protocol, however, has been criticized as taking too long to achieve maximum heart rate, and other tests, e.g. the Ellestad[1] test, have been proposed that produce maximum heart rate response in approximately

75% of the time required for the Bruce protocol. Froelicher[2] advocates the "ramp test" in which the speed and incline of the treadmill gradually and continually increases, avoiding the sudden increases seen with the Bruce protocol, which tends to overestimate exercise capacity. Despite these caveats, the Bruce protocol remains the most widely used test in North America, and exercise capacity is often referred to as "4 minutes on the Bruce protocol" etc.

Exercise capacity, however, is more properly measured in METs. Metabolic equivalents are a unit of basal oxygen consumption equal to approximately 3.5 ml of O_2/kg/min. One MET is the oxygen requirement to maintain life in the resting state. Some examples of MET demands for common activities may clarify the understanding of this unit which is often used as a way of classifying a patient's exercise capacity. Typing calls for about 1.5 METs; playing the violin—2 METs; walking at 3 mph—3 METs; golf—5 METs: dancing—6 METs; jogging a 10 minute mile—10 METs etc. The patient's maximal exercise capacity can be compared for age and sedentary versus active lifestyle, to provide an objective indication of ability.

TECHNICAL CONSIDERATIONS

The test must be fully explained to the patient and, if necessary, through an interpreter if there is a language barrier. Although controversial, a consent form should be signed by the patient.

TREADMILL ELECTROCARDIOGRAPHIC TESTING

Good ECG electrode contact must be made with the skin and this may require shaving, removing oil with acetone, and the use of devices to produce a mild abrasion. Better sensitivity and specificity is achieved with 12 leads which are placed on the chest in the Mason-Likar method. A blood pressure cuff, with separate or built-in stethoscope is wrapped around the arm and secured with a tape or elastic strapping to ensure its stability during exercise. Electrocardiograph and blood pressure should be recorded supine, standing, and at each stage of the exercise protocol. Various computerized exercise ECG machines are available which smooth the raw ECG signal and may be of help in certain patients. It should be explained to the patient how to use the treadmill, in particular, to take slow long strides, hold on to the hand rail, and to stay near the front of the treadmill. When the test is finished, the patient is helped back to bed; ECG and blood pressure are recorded every 1 to 3 minutes for a further 10 minutes or until the ECG returns to normal.

STRESS ECHOCARDIOGRAPHY

Stress echocardiography involves the acquisition of resting images of left ventricular function before exercise and then immediately after terminating exercise (preferably within 1 minute of the end of the test so that transient ischemia and left ventricular wall motion abnormalities will not be missed). Special computerized equipment is used in conjunction with the echocardiographic machine to perform this test properly.[3] The images are best gated to the R wave—8 images are collected every 50 msec at rest, and every 33 msec with exercise. The images are digitized and played back in a cine loop format. Only those cardiac cycles that are clear and not obscured by respiratory artefact are chosen for analysis. Four views are routinely assessed: parasternal long, parasternal short, apical 4-chamber, apical 2-chamber. To enhance interpretation, the same views at rest and exercise are positioned side by side. A fixed point superimposed in the left ventricular cavity on the video screen facilitates the assessment of wall motion.

NUCLEAR PERFUSION TEST

Two isotopes are used to assess myocardial perfusion.[4] The most widely used is Thallium-201 (^{201}Tl), a potassium analogue, which is avidly extracted in proportion to myocardial blood flow. The physical properties of ^{201}Tl limits its usefulness because it produces images of various and sometimes suboptimal quality. Technetium-99m sestamibi (^{99m}Tc) can be injected in higher amounts than ^{201}Tl improving image quality. Unlike ^{201}Tl, which redistributes into areas of ischemia necessitating image acquisition soon after injection, ^{99m}Tc does not exhibit significant redistribution permitting imaging several hours after injection. One- and 2-day acquisition protocols are used. Two-day: exercise, inject ^{201}Tl, image within 1 hour, image for redistribution after 24 hours. One-day: ^{201}Tl injection, image after 10 minutes, exercise, inject ^{99m}Tc sestamibi, continue 1 more minute of exercise, image 15 minutes following injection. Single-photon emission computed tomography (SPECT) has proved superior to planar imaging and involves the acquisition of multiple planar images of the myocardium over 180°.

NON-EXERCISE STRESS TESTING

Approximately 35% of patients being evaluated for coronary artery disease are unable to perform sufficient exercise to produce an adequate heart rate pressure product that would produce myocardial ischemia. Reasons include arthritis, peripheral vascular disease, chronic lung disease, recent surgery, infirmity, etc. These patients can be adequately assessed by pharmacological stress testing.

Dobutamine is rapidly becoming the agent of choice as its inotropic and chronotropic effects mimic the effects of exercise.[7] Dobutamine produces myocardial ischemia in patients with coronary artery disease mainly by increasing heart rate: the increase in heart rate with the usually recommended doses is generally less than with exercise—often the maximum achieved is 85% of the maximum predicted heart rate for any patient. The effects on blood pressure are variable because of its peripheral vasodilating capabilities. A fall in blood pressure below resting levels occurs in approximately 25% of patients and does not represent an adverse ischemic response. Dobutamine has been widely used without significant morbidity and to date no mortality. About 10% of patients experience shaking or tremor associated with its catecholamine effects; other side-effects include atrial arrhythmias (atrial premature beats, atrial tachycardia, and less commonly atrial fibrillation), and ventricular arrhythmias (ventricular premature beats and non-sustained ventricular tachycardia).

Dobutamine is given through a peripheral arm vein in graduated doses starting at 5 or 10 mcg/kg/min and increasing by 10 mcg/kg/min increments every 3-5 minutes to a maximum of 40 mcg/kg/min. An increase of heart rate to 85% of maximum predicted heart rate is the usual goal and intravenous atropine (.25 mg/min to a total of 1 mg) may be needed to augment the heart rate response, particularly in patients taking ß-blocking medications. Esmolol can be given intravenously (.25-.5 mg/kg) to abort atrial tachycardia or bring the tachycardia under control more quickly than waiting for the dobutamine-induced tachycardia to dissipate. Reasons to terminate the test include significant arrhythmias, systolic blood pressure below 90 mm Hg, and significant chest pain. Undue hypotension can be treated by raising the legs, and giving volume (e.g., 100 ml 5% dextrose or normal saline).

When dobutamine is given as part of an *echocardiographic stress test*, left ventricular function is assessed at rest, during low-dose (5 or 10 mcg/kg/min), at peak dose, and in recovery. During a *nuclear perfusion* dobutamine protocol, the isotope is injected approximately 1 minute before the anticipated end of the test.

Dipyridamole is the other widely used pharmacologic stress agent. This exerts its effect to produce myocardial ischemia by a "coronary steal," diverting blood flow away from myocardium supplied by stenosed coronary arteries, to myocardium supplied by normal or less stenosed arteries. Dipyridamole generally causes more discomfort to the patient than dobutamine, with headache, nausea, and chest pain being common. Arrhythmias and heart block may also be precipitated, and bronchospasm in susceptible patients (patients with obstructive airways disease should not receive dipyridamole). Aminophylline (1.5 mg/kg IV) usually terminates most side effects. Dipyridamole is given at 0.14 mg/kg/min for 4 minutes. When administered as part of a *nuclear perfusion study*, the isotope is given approximately 4 minutes after the end of the infusion. When administered as part of a *stress echocardiographic study*,[8] left ventricular function is assessed during the infusion and for 5-10 minutes afterward. If no wall motion abnormalities are

seen, then some authors advocate an additional 0.14 mg/kg/min over 2 minutes and echocardiographic examination continued for a further 5-10 minutes.

INTERPRETATION OF EXERCISE ELECTROCARDIOGRAPHIC CHANGES

ST CHANGES

The "classic" ECG response to myocardial ischemia is ST-segment depression (Fig. 1). It has been speculated that myocardial ischemia invokes a leak of potassium from the ischemic subendocardial cells, causing a current flow from endo to epicardium and toward the overlying ECG electrode which in diastole will produce an upward deviation of the ECG baseline. With the onset of the QRS complex, however, ventricular depolarization terminates the current flow and the elevated ECG baseline returns to zero—giving the impression of ST depression as the major abnormality (when, in fact, the major perturbation is elevation of the TQ segment in the rest of the cardiac cycle). ST depression may also occur, in the absence of myocardial ischemia, as a result of prominent atrial depolarization (the atrial T wave) which can superimpose on the ST segment to cause a net deflection of the ST segment.[9] ST-segment elevation may occur with transmural ischemia with coronary spasm. ST-segment elevation, however, usually is associated with worsening of a preexisting wall motion abnormality and does not usually indicate ischemia, per se.

Initial enthusiasm for ST depression as a marker of ischemia has been markedly dampened. There are clearly many reasons other than myocardial ischemia that can produce ST depression, and there are also many patients with myocardial ischemia who do not develop ST depression. A whole body of statistical jargon has developed largely due to the conflicting ST responses in patients with and without coronary artery disease (Table 2). As ST depression often occurs in healthy patients, various empirical criteria for "significant" ST depression have been developed to be able to separate normal from abnormal responses. The criteria most accepted is greater than or equal to

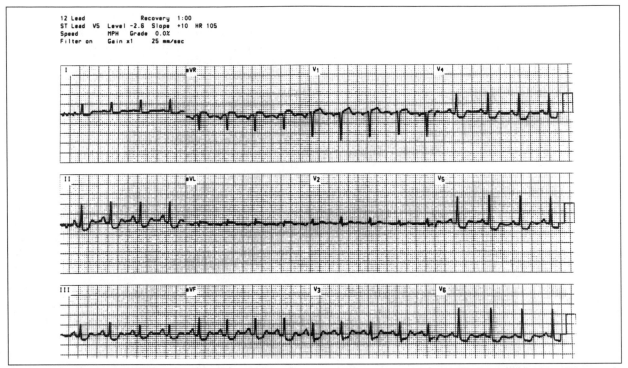

```
12 Lead              Recovery  1:00
ST Lead  V5  Level -2.6  Slope  +10  HR 105
Speed       MPH   Grade   0.0%
Filter on    Gain x1    25 mm/sec
```

Figure 1. *An example of classic ST-segment depression showing 2 mm horizontal ST depression 80 milliseconds from the J point.*

1 mm horizontal or greater than or equal to 1.5 mm upsloping ST depression measured 80 msec from the J point occurring at peak exercise. In a usual group of patients being tested in a large hospital setting, the recommended criteria will lead to 65% sensitivity and 75% specificity.[10] Criteria of ST depression of 0.5 mm horizontal will lead to more false-positives (lower specificity of 60%) and less false-negatives (higher sensitivity of 75%); using criteria of 2 mm horizontal for a "positive test" will lead to more false-negatives (higher specificity of 95%) and few false-positives (lower sensitivity of 35%) (Fig. 2). For the detection of multivessel disease ST depression criteria have higher sensitivities (0.5 mm, 85%; 1 mm, 75%; 2 mm, 45%). ST depression occurring only in recovery may also

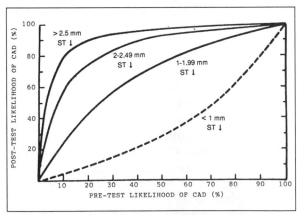

Figure 2. *Family of ST-segment depression curves and the likelihood of coronary artery disease depending on the pretest probability of disease. From Epstein SE. Implications of probability analysis on the strategy used for non-invasive detection of coronary artery disease. Am J Cardiol. 1980;46:491. With permission.*

Table 2. Definitions

Sensitivity = $\dfrac{\text{True Positive}}{\text{True Positive + False Negative}}$

Specificity = $\dfrac{\text{True Negative}}{\text{False Positive + True Negative}}$

Predictive Value of Positive Test = $\dfrac{\text{True Positive}}{\text{True Positive + False Positive}}$

represent myocardial ischemia and appears to have similar accuracy as ST depression judged at peak exercise, although this is controversial.

Exercise-induced ST depression is less likely to indicate myocardial ischemia in the following circumstances: otherwise normal young healthy individuals without risk factors for coronary artery disease, concurrent digoxin administration, left ventricular hypertrophy, bundle branch block, resting ST depression, and late onset e.g., ST depression of 1 mm occurring at 12 minutes of the Bruce protocol. Exercise induced ST depression is more likely to indicate coronary disease in the following circumstances: typical chest pain and 2 or more risk factors, and prolonged (3 minutes or more) ST depression in recovery. Early positivity (significant ST depression in the first 3 minutes of the Bruce protocol) and profound ST depression (greater than or equal to 3 mm) are both associated with a higher incidence of left-main and 3 vessel disease and subsequent cardiac events than later onset and less pronounced ST depression.

Using new computerized equipment, the raw ECG signal can be smoothed and the ST changes can be more accurately quantified. Various indexes have been derived and correlated with coronary angiography. Heart rate adjusted ST depression (maximal ST depression/exercise-resting heart rate), which can be easily determined by computer (but can

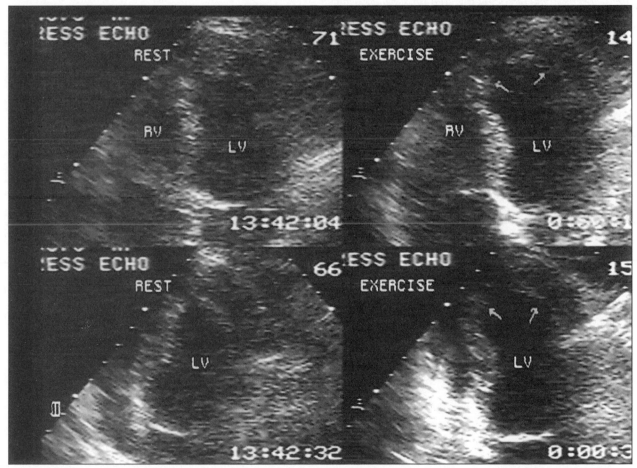

Figure 3. *Stress echo study in a 74-year-old man with mild angina, apical 4-chamber view (upper panel), 2-chamber view (lower panel); end-systolic image at rest (left panel) is normal. Ejection fraction is 60%. After exercise, the distal septum, anterior wall and apex become akinetic (right panel—arrows) Ejection fraction is 35%. Subsequent coronary angiogram revealed a single 90% mid left anterior descending stenosis (LAD) lesion—*

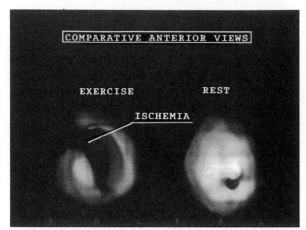

Figure 4. *Stress Technetium-99m sestamibi (MIBI) study in a 65-year-old man with mild angina. The tomographic images show a perfusion defect following exercise associated with a proximal 90% left anterior descending coronary artery lesion. Courtesy of Gerald J. Kavanagh, Nuclear Medicine Department, Good Samaritan Hospital, Los Angeles, CA.*

also be determined manually) has been shown by some authors[10] to have an approximately 10% higher sensitivity (for the same specificity). Other authors,[11] however, contend that simple ST depression as analyzed from the raw uncomputerized tracing is as good as computerized data.

R-WAVE CHANGES

R-wave amplitude usually decreases in normal subjects at peak exercise, possibly due to decreased left ventricular diastolic size. With myocardial ischemia, left ventricular size and R-wave amplitude increase. The sensitivity of R-wave increase for significant coronary artery disease is approximately 50% with 60% specificity.

INVERTED T AND U WAVES

T-wave inversion during exercise is often seen in patients with left ventricular hypertrophy and does not indicate ischemia. Inverted T waves that develop in recovery may reflect ischemia, but it is still considered a non-specific finding. Normalization of flat or inverted T waves is also most often not due to ischemia. U-wave

inversion with exercise is also most commonly associated with left ventricular hypertrophy (80%) and with myocardial ischemia in the minority (20%).

PREMATURE VENTRICULAR CONTRACTIONS

Approximately 35% of asymptomatic men develop PVCs and this is more common with advancing age. Neither frequent (>10% of beats in any 1 minute) PVCs nor non-sustained ventricular tachycardia, in the absence of ST depression, are associated with coronary disease or with an adverse prognosis as determined in several studies. Suppression of PVCs by exercise does not rule out coronary disease, although most often this is a clue to a benign arrhythmia.

INTERPRETATION OF STRESS ECHOCARDIOGRAPHIC CHANGES

The generally accepted criteria for a positive stress (exercise or pharmacologic) echo test is the development of new wall motion abnormality (Fig. 3) or significant worsening of an existing wall motion abnormality, which suggests exercise induced myocardial ischemia. The presence of a resting wall motion abnormality gives the diagnosis of coronary disease even before the test has begun. Overall sensitivity is approximately 80% and specificity 80%. For multivessel disease these numbers are higher at approximately 90%. Unlike ECG changes which poorly correlate between lead and vessel stenosed, there is good correlation between the abnormal wall segment and vessel e.g., inferior wall changes reflect right coronary, and septal abnormalities reflect left anterior disease. Wall motion abnormalities, in the absence of obstructive coronary disease may be due to technical factors, e.g. motion of the heart with respiration causing an apparent wall motion abnormality, or noncoronary causes like cardiomyopathy. The degree of mitral regurgitation, pulmonary artery pressure, and aortic velocity (as a marker of stroke volume, and in patients with aortic stenosis) can also be assessed at the time of stress echocardiography and may be of value in selected patients.

INTERPRETATION OF NUCLEAR PERFUSION STUDIES

The presence of a reversible defect is evidence of myocardial ischemia (Fig. 4). Fixed defects represent previous myocardial infarction. Exercise and pharmacologic stress produce virtually equal sensitivities for both nuclear perfusion and stress echocardiography studies for the detection of coronary artery disease and myocardial ischemia.[12] False positive studies may be seen in patients with bundle branch block, cardiomyopathy, and particularly in women, sometimes associated with breast artefact.

REFERENCES

1. Ellestad MH. Stress testing. *Principles and Practice,* 3rd Ed. Philadelphia: FA Davis; 1986.
2. Froelicher VF, Myers J, Follansbee WP, et al. *Exercise and the Heart,* 3rd Ed. St. Louis: Mosby; 1993.
3. Marwick TH, Nemec JJ, Pashkow FJ, et al. Accuracy and limitations of exercise echocardiography in a routine clinical setting. *J Am Coll Cardiol.* 1992;19:74-81.
4. Berman DS, Kiat H, Friedman J. Separate acquisition rest thallium-201/Stress technetium-99, sestamibi dual isotope myocardial perfusion SPECT: a clinical validation study. *J Am Coll Cardiol.* 1993;22:1455-1466.
5. Wong ND, Kouwabunpat D, Vo AN, et al. Coronary calcium and atherosclerosis by ultrafast computed tomography in asymptomatic men and women: Relation to age and risk factors. *Am Heart J.* 1994;127:422-430.
6. Schlant RC, Friesinger GC, Leonard JJ. ACP/ACC/AHA task force statement. Clinical competence in exercise testing. *J Am Coll Cardiol.* 1990;16:1061-1065.
7. Sawada SG, Segar DS, Ryan T, et al. Echocardiographic detection of coronary artery disease during dobutamine infusion. *Circulation.* 1991;83:1605-1614.
8. Picano E, Lattanzi F, Masini M, et al. High dose dipyridamole echocardiography test in effort angina pectoris. *J Am Coll Cardiol.* 1986;8:848-854.
9. Gettes LS, Sapin P. Concerning falsely negative and falsely positive electrocardiographic responses to exercise. *Br Heart J.* 1993;70:205-207.
10. Detrano R, Salcedo E, Passalacqua M, et al. Exercise electrocardiographic variables: A critical appraisal. *J Am Coll Cardiol.* 1986;8:836-847.
11. Morise AP, Duval RD. Accuracy of ST/heart rate index in the diagnosis of coronary artery disease. *Am J Cardiol.* 1992;69:603-606.
12. Quinones MA, Verani MS, Haichin RM, et al. Exercise echocardiography versus Tl single-photon emission computed tomography in evaluation of coronary artery disease. Analysis of 292 patients. *Circulation.* 1992;85:1026-1031.

7 Echocardiography and Pulse Recordings

CHAPTER

Joshua Wynne, MD
Priscilla Peters, BA, RDCS

Echocardiography is the most widely used noninvasive cardiac diagnostic method available (aside from the chest x-ray and electrocardiogram), and it may provide definitive information in a wide variety of valvular, pericardial, myocardial, and congenital diseases. It uses short pulses (1–2 μsec duration) of high-frequency (1.9–5 million cycles/sec or MHz) sound waves, repeated many times each second (typically, 1,000 Hz). Because of the short duration of the ultrasound pulses, no deleterious effects occur with echocardiography. The sound waves are generated by a piezoelectric crystal, which has the unique property of transforming electrical energy into mechanical energy (i.e., sound) and vice versa. A transducer containing the crystal is placed on the chest wall and acts as both a transmitter and receiver of the short pulses of ultrasound that reflect off surfaces of the heart and return to the crystal. Ultrasound waves are reflected when they strike an interface composed of 2 tissues of differing acoustic impedance, which is related to tissue density.

All current echocardiographic machines provide a cross-sectional or 2-dimensional (2D) view by steering the echocardiographic beam through an arc of up to 90°, producing a tomographic image of excellent spatial resolution (Fig. 1). If many such images are obtained each second (typically, 30–60 images/sec), the motion of the heart can be viewed in real time.

The transesophageal (TEE) technique is now well established as a useful adjunct to the standard precordial examination; in the evaluation of pathology of the aorta, especially dissection, it is the preferred technique. The esophageal approach frequently provides more specific morphologic and anatomic information with better resolution of intracardiac structures than the precordial technique allows.[1,2]

When TEE is employed in the conscious patient, some form of sedation generally is used. Topical anesthesia, such as Xylocaine® (lidocaine hydrochloride) spray, is administered to the oropharynx to suppress the gag reflex, and a bite guard typically is used to prevent damage to the probe. During probe insertion, the patient may be in the left lateral decubitus position, which aids in the elimination of salivary secretions, or in a sitting position, depending on imaging needs and physician and patient interaction. The probe is lubricated with surgical jelly and introduced in the same fashion as a standard gastroscope. In addition to the physician performing the procedure, at least 1 assistant should be present to monitor vital signs, suction the patient as needed, and adjust machine controls to ensure adequate image quality. A routine examination is completed in approximately 20 minutes.

The TEE technique is particularly useful in the evaluation of the thoracic aorta, prosthetic valves, mitral regurgitation, intracardiac and paracardiac masses, and congenital heart disease, especially when the precordial images are inadequate and/or additional detailed information is required. In the operating room, TEE is used to evaluate the success of valve repair and the repair of congenital heart disease, especially intracardiac shunts, and to monitor left ventricular function.

CLINICAL APPLICATIONS OF ECHOCARDIOGRAPHY

Echocardiography is probably the best method currently available, invasive or noninvasive, for evaluating structural cardiac abnormalities larger than 1–2 mm. Because air within the lungs disperses echocardiographic signals, adequate images occasionally may be difficult or impossible to obtain in patients in whom an optimal transducer position cannot be found, particularly those with obstructive lung disease. All 4 cardiac valves

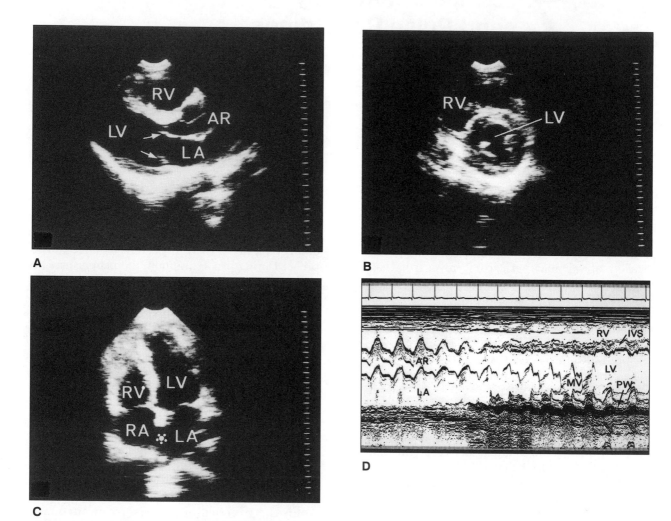

Figure 1. *Two-dimensional echocardiographic views from a normal subject. (A) Long-axis parasternal view, demonstrating the coaptation in diastole of 2 of the aortic valve leaflets in the center of the aorta. (B) Short-axis parasternal view at the level of the papillary muscles, which are the indentations within the LV at 3 and 8 o'clock. (C) Apical 4-chamber view, showing the normal dropout of echo signal from the region of the fossa ovalis (*). (D) M-mode echocardiographic sweep of a normal subject. AR=Aortic root; LA=Left atrium; LV=Left ventricle; RA=Right atrium; RV=Right ventricle; IVS=Interventricular septum; MV=Mitral valve; PW=Posterior wall. The arrows indicate the anterior and posterior mitral valve leaflets.*

and chambers usually can be seen, as well as the interventricular and interatrial septum. The main pulmonary artery, the base of the aorta and proximal aortic root, and the inferior vena cava can be imaged easily. Direct visualization of the ostia of both the right and left coronary arteries is also possible. However, because the ultrasound beam can typically evaluate only the proximal portions of the vessels, consistently reliable and reproducible assessment of coronary artery stenosis is not yet practical. The left ventricular (LV) wall motion abnormalities seen with myocardial infarction or myopathy can be readily imaged and are valuable for initial assessment and follow-up.

VALVULAR HEART DISEASE

Echocardiography provides reliable evaluation of the site, cause, and severity of a variety of forms of valvular heart disease. Differentiation of subvalvular, valvular, and supravalvular involvement is usually easily determined. Although in adult patients obstruction at sites other than the valve is usually a consideration only with the LVOT, muscular obstruction in the subpulmonary area and membranous obstruction above the mitral valve occasionally are found in adults as well as children.[3,4] The causes of valvular disease can frequently be delineated, since current transthoracic (TTE) and TEE techniques can evaluate thickening and calcification of the valve and supporting apparatus (as in rheumatic deformity or mitral annular calcification); abnormal motion of the valve (doming from congenital or rheumatic commissural fusion, mitral valve prolapse with or without myxomatous changes, or frank disruption of chordal apparatus); and secondary disease processes, such as valvular tumors, vegetations, aneurysms, or abscesses. In addition to the assessment of valvular anatomy, morphology, and motion, the extent of disease can be assessed from changes in chamber size, thickness, and function. Left ventricular and left atrial volume overload and enlargement may result from left-sided regurgitant lesions, and LV hypertrophy will be seen with aortic stenosis. Current Doppler techniques, including color-flow mapping, provide substantial additional information regarding the severity of valvular disease.

Mitral Valve

The normal mitral valve appears as 2 thin mobile leaflets with the anterior leaflet demonstrating the larger excursion. The motion of the posterior leaflet is a mirror image of the anterior leaflet, although its excursion is substantially less. The pattern of motion of the leaflets is one of rapid opening in diastole (during the period of rapid ventricular filling), with anterior and posterior leaflets moving in opposite directions. At the end of the rapid filling phase and the start of the slow filling phase, the leaflets float toward each other, assuming a more neutral position. With left atrial systole, transmitral flow again increases, and the leaflets are driven farther apart, only to coapt completely during ventricular systole.

Mitral Stenosis. Mitral stenosis, almost always a consequence of rheumatic involvement, is characterized echocardiographically by doming of the anterior leaflet in diastole, which occurs as a result of fusion of the commissures (Fig. 2). In addition, leaflet mobility typically is diminished, and there is fusion and diminished separation of the leaflet tips. The morphologic appearance of the valve typically is one of thickened, fibrotic leaflets supported by a shortened, thickened, and fused chordal apparatus. Deformity of the valve ranges from mild (rheumatic deformity without significant stenosis) to severe (densely thickened, immobile leaflets with calcium throughout the leaflet body, extending into and

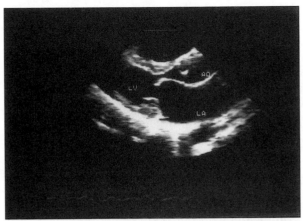

Figure 2. *Parasternal long axis view of mitral stenosis, demonstrating thickening and doming of the anterior leaflet. LA=Left atrium; LV=Left ventricle; Ao=Aorta.*

fusing the supporting apparatus). The changes in the supporting apparatus can significantly contribute to the overall degree of inflow obstruction. While the most common etiology of LV inflow obstruction is rheumatic mitral stenosis, an occasional adult will present with parachute deformity of the valve, in which all chordal structures are congenitally fused into a single papillary muscle. The hemodynamic consequences of parachute deformity typically are obstructive, but these valves may be regurgitant as well.[5-7]

The noninvasive evaluation of mitral stenosis is crucial to the selection of appropriate patients for balloon valvuloplasty. A morphologic scoring system has been devised, based on TTE images, that assesses valve thickness, valve mobility, the presence and extent of calcium, and the appearance of the subvalvular apparatus.[8,9] Each variable is assigned a score of 0 to 4; a totally normal valve would score 0. A higher morphologic score (>12) typically is associated with a suboptimal valvuloplasty result, while a lower score (<8) generally is associated with a good result. The scoring system includes only morphologic characteristics of the valve; it does not include assessment of mitral regurgitation.

Mitral Regurgitation. Structural abnormalities of the mitral valve that cause mitral regurgitation include diseases of the leaflets (including rheumatic deformity and myxomatous degeneration with prolapse) and disruption or deformity of the valvular supporting apparatus. Functional abnormalities of the valve apparatus and papillary muscles typically are associated with normal-appearing leaflets (although annular calcium may extend into the base of the leaflets). When there is significant papillary muscle dysfunction, LV regional wall motion abnormalities frequently are identified. Additional information that can aid in the indirect assessment of mitral regurgitation, including LV size and function and left atrial dilatation, is also easily obtained with echocardiography.

Doppler color-flow mapping is invaluable in the assessment of mitral regurgitation. In this technique, the Doppler signal is superimposed on the echocardiographic image, resulting in a graphic depiction of regurgitant blood flow. It is particularly useful in the evaluation of the direction of the regurgitant jet (anterior, posterior, or central)[10] and the origin of the jet (between the leaflets or through a leaflet perforation) and can effectively evaluate the severity of the regurgitation via jet width, number, and extent.

Pathologic causes of mitral regurgitation include rheumatic disease, chordal rupture, trauma, papillary muscle rupture following myocardial infarction, endocarditis, hypertrophic cardiomyopathy, annular calcification, and prolapse. Rheumatic disease directly affects the valve and supporting apparatus, while annular calcification usually appears behind the posterior leaflet. Extensive annular calcification can involve the base of both leaflets (although leaflet tips are free, there can be significant obstruction to flow) and can extend into the base of the aorta. When chordal rupture occurs, hypermobile and flail segments can be identified. Transesophageal imaging is especially valuable in characterizing leaflet motion when chordal or papillary muscle rupture occurs (Fig. 3).

Valve repair for mitral regurgitation offers substantial advantages over valve replacement. Recent work has shown that intraoperative echocardiography, either TEE or epicardial, provides a consistently reliable assessment of the mechanisms (not the same as etiology) of mitral regurgitation.[11] These mechanisms include flail leaflets, papillary muscle infarction, restricted leaflets, annular dilatation, and leaflet perforation. Reliably identifying the mechanism of mitral regurgitation enables the surgeon to apply appropriate repair techniques. In addition to preoperative evaluation, intraoperative TEE imaging immediately after valve repair can reliably detect persistent mitral regurgitation

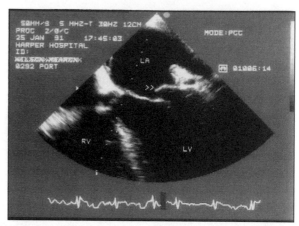

Figure 3. *Transesophageal 4-chamber view demonstrating a flail posterior mitral leaflet (arrow). LA=Left atrium; LV=Left ventricle; RV=Right ventricle.*

(and thus a failed repair) and can allow for immediate additional surgical treatment, such as valve replacement.

Aortic Valve

The anatomically normal aortic valve is composed of 3 thin, mobile, generally symmetric leaflets. In diastole, the leaflets meet in the center of the aorta; during systole, the normal valve opens until the leaflets are adjacent to the aortic wall. Anomalies of the number of leaflets range from total congenital absence of the valve to the very rare hexacuspid valve.[12]

The bicuspid aortic valve is the most common congenital malformation of the heart, occurring in up to 2% of the population.[13] Bicuspid valves may be associated with critical aortic stenosis in children or may lead to surgical aortic stenosis in adults. In addition, bicuspid valves may be purely incompetent and are prone to infective endocarditis. They may also be found in association with other congenital malformations, especially aortic coarctation and ventricular septal defects (VSDs). Interestingly, the mechanism by which a bicuspid valve becomes incompetent or stenotic is not known, nor is it understood why some bicuspid valves remain functionally normal.[13]

The echocardiographic diagnosis of a bicuspid valve is best made from the short axis views of the valve (Fig. 4). Anatomically, these valves have 2 principal orientations. In 50% of cases, the commissures may be oriented right-left with leaflets that open anterior-posterior; in the remaining 50%, the commissures insert anteri-

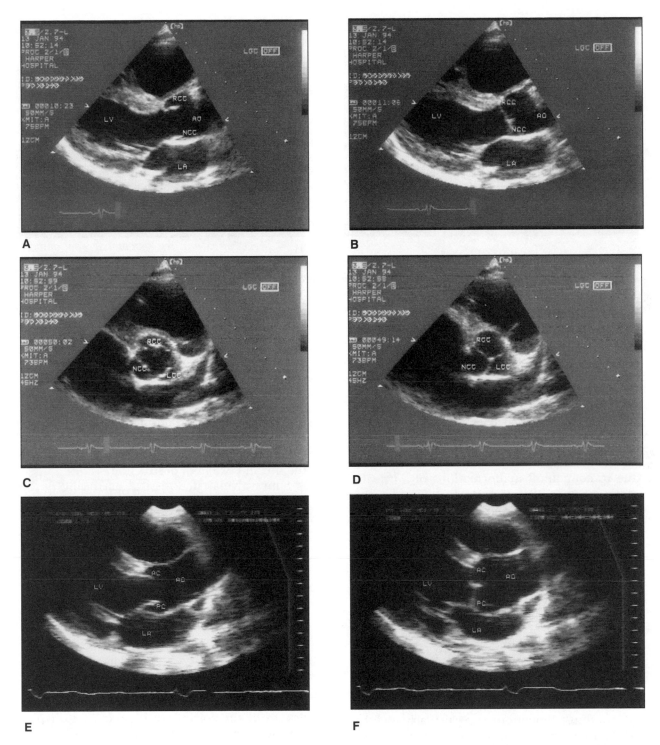

Figure 4. *(A) Parasternal long axis view of a normal aortic valve in systole. (B) Diastolic frame of a normal aortic valve in the parasternal long axis plane.C) Parasternal short axis view of the normal aortic valve in systole. (D) The same valve at end-diastole from the parasternal short axis view. (E) A bicuspid aortic valve as seen from the parasternal long axis plane. The cusps dome in systole. (F) The same valve from the long axis plane at end-diastole. Note the central closure line of this bicuspid valve. Ao=Aorta; LA=Left atrium; LV=Left ventricle; AC=Anterior cusp; PC=Posterior cusp; RCC=Right coronary cusp; LCC=Left coronary cusp; NCC=Noncoronary cusp.*

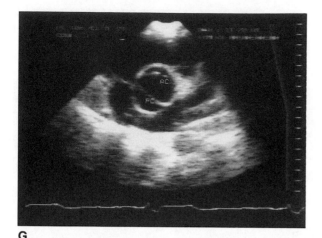 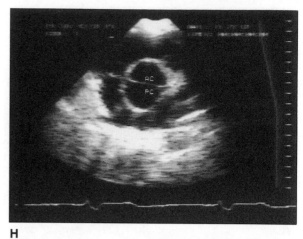

G   H

Figure 4 continued. (G) Short axis view of a bicuspid aortic valve in systole. The commissures are oriented right-left, and the leaflets open anterior-posterior. (H) The same valve at end-diastole. No raphe is seen.

or-posterior, and the leaflets open right-left. Raphes are present in approximately half of all bicuspid valves, and most typically are on the anterior cusp or the right cusp.[13] The long axis views of the valve may demonstrate eccentric closure or doming in systole when there is commissural fusion. Once a bicuspid valve is heavily calcified, however, echocardiographic differentiation from a calcified trileaflet valve is neither necessary nor reliable.

Aortic Stenosis. Valvular aortic stenosis may be due to congenital malformations of a trileaflet valve, rheumatic commissural fusion, or acquired senile calcific changes. The typical echocardiographic features of the stenotic valve include thick deformed cusps, usually with some degree of calcium, demonstrating diminished leaflet mobility and decrease in orifice size (Fig. 5). It is important to note that LV dysfunction and reduced cardiac output can alter leaflet mobility, and it is possible to overestimate the severity of stenosis based on imaging alone. Valve leaflet separation may also vary depending on the segment interrogated by the ultrasound beam. Evaluation of Doppler flow across the valve (using either the modified Bernoulli equation or the continuity equation) is particularly useful in determining the severity of aortic stenosis.[14–17]

While valvular aortic stenosis is the most common cause of LVOT obstruction, echocardiography can identify other sites of obstruction. Discrete subvalvular obstruction accounts for approximately 10% of all LVOT obstruction in children and may be caused by a thin fibrous membrane located just below the valve or a thicker, muscular ring that tends to extend well below the aortic valve.[18–20] With discrete membranous subaortic disease, the remainder of the outflow tract is generally normal, although associated disease of the aortic valve is common (Fig. 6). With the more diffuse fibromuscular obstruction, a more extensive area of obstruction is present and involvement of the base of the anterior mitral leaflet is common. Doppler techniques are adjunctive in the localization of the site and extent of obstruction.

Supravalvular stenosis is a narrowing of the ascending aorta that may be localized or diffuse, originating distal to the insertion of the coronary arteries at the superior margins of the sinuses of Valsalva. This lesion is not common in adults. Patients with supravalvular obstruction are often mentally retarded, with abnormal facial appearance ("elfin facies") and a history of infantile hypercalcemia. Echocardiography can identify the site of aortic narrowing, and Doppler techniques can define its severity.

Aortic Regurgitation. Aortic regurgitation typically results from disease of the cusps (due to rheumatic or calcific disease or endocarditis) or disease of the aortic root (secondary to hypertension or aneurysmal dilatation). Echocardiography usually can distinguish between these 2 etiologies. Acute severe aortic regurgitation with markedly elevated LV end-diastolic pressure, usually seen in the context of leaflet disruption from endocarditis, may result in premature closure of the mitral valve or premature opening of

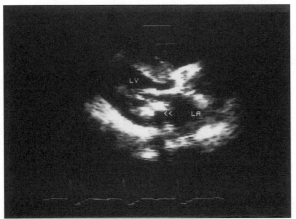

A

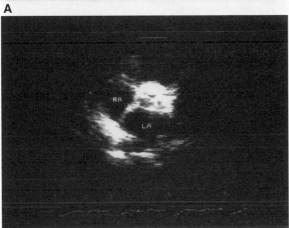

B

Figure 5. (A) Parasternal long axis view of calcific aortic stenosis. Calcification of the mitral annulus is also noted (arrow). (B) Parasternal short axis view of the same valve. LV=Left ventricle; LA=Left atrium; RA=Right atrium.

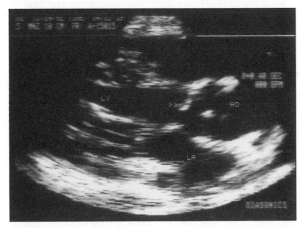

Figure 6. Parasternal long axis view of a subaortic membrane (arrow). There is some thickening of the aortic valve as well. LA=Left atrium; LV=Left ventricle; Ao=Aorta.

the aortic valve. Patients with these findings are often in severe heart failure and in need of urgent surgical intervention.

While reliable in distinguishing causes of aortic regurgitation, echocardiography is less useful in estimating its severity, although the degree of LV enlargement in chronic isolated aortic regurgitation is an indirect parameter of severity. Doppler color-flow mapping is a useful adjunct for estimating the severity of regurgitation by demonstrating the width of the jet; more severe regurgitation is associated with a wider jet.

Tricuspid Valve

The tricuspid valve is anatomically more complex than the mitral valve and is composed of 3 leaflets of unequal size: the anterior, posterior, and septal leaflets. It can be evaluated from the parasternal long axis right ventricular (RV) inflow view (anterior and posterior leaflets); the short axis at the base of the heart (septal and anterior leaflets); and the apical 4-chamber view (anterior and septal leaflets).

The important structural causes of tricuspid valve dysfunction include rheumatic deformity (the most common cause of tricuspid stenosis), carcinoid, and fibroelastosis; endocarditis (most commonly seen in intravenous drug abusers but also associated with central venous catheters); tricuspid valve prolapse; trauma; and congenital malformations, especially Ebstein's anomaly. In rheumatic tricuspid stenosis, the commissures fuse and the thickened leaflets dome in diastole. With carcinoid involvement, fibrous thickening on the surfaces of the valve leaflets markedly restricts motion and typically causes some obstruction to flow but also renders the valve grossly incompetent.

Vegetations on the tricuspid valve are seen most commonly in drug abusers and appear as distinct, shaggy, amorphous masses usually attached to the valve leaflets. Trauma to the valve can result from either blunt or penetrating injury, and both frank chordal rupture and leaflet perforation can occur.[21] Ebstein's anomaly is a congenital deformity of the valve that results in a highly variable appearance of the valve, typically characterized by inferior displacement of all or part of the valve.[22] Right heart chambers usually are dilated (a portion of the right ventricle is "atrialized" by the displacement of the valve), and there is some degree of RV dysfunction, dependent on the degree of valve displacement.

The most common cause of tricuspid regurgitation, in general, is right ventricular enlargement with annular dilatation, typically due to left heart problems, such as mitral valve disease or LV dysfunction. The leaflets usually are intrinsically normal. Doppler techniques, especially color flow, are particularly useful in evaluating the presence and severity of the regurgitation; continuous wave peak velocities provide a reliable assessment of RV (and hence pulmonary artery) systolic pressure.

Pulmonary Valve

The pulmonary valve is the most anterior of the cardiac valves and consists of 3 semilunar leaflets. It is the least likely of all cardiac valves to be structurally abnormal in the adult patient. The typical 2-dimensional exam allows for visualization of the anterior and posterior leaflets of the valve as they open and close in the pulmonary artery.

Structural deformity of the pulmonary valve is unusual except for mild thickening with congenital pulmonic stenosis. Rarely, it may occur from a vegetation involving the cusps or with the carcinoid syndrome. Abnormalities of motion of the valve are more common. Doming of the valve may indicate the presence of congenital pulmonic stenosis. Enhanced imaging of the valve, with systolic fluttering of the valve cusps and ablation of the movement of the valve after right atrial systole, often indicate pulmonary hypertension.

While the echocardiogram can determine the presence and location of RV outflow tract obstruction, the echocardiographic estimation of the severity of valvular pulmonic stenosis is only a rough semiquantitative guide. The addition of the Doppler technique can provide further information about the site and degree of obstruction. Cardiac catheterization may be required in the adult patient in order to be confident about the degree of obstruction and to look for associated lesions.

Prosthetic Valves

Two principal forms of prosthetic valves are used: an entirely mechanical one, with a rigid ball or disc occluder; and a bioprosthetic type, with a rigid or semirigid prosthetic base and cusps composed of human or animal tissue (most commonly the aortic valve of the pig). Regular assessment of prosthetic valves is important, as echocardiography may detect evidence of preclinical dysfunction. Current noninvasive techniques can provide baseline (early postoperative) functional status and can follow valve and myocardial performance over time.[23]

Artificial valves create special problems for standard imaging because of the different acoustic properties of the prosthetic material. Reverberations behind the prosthesis can create artifact that may obscure normal anatomy and can mimic pathology. Attenuation of sound creates acoustic shadowing that can also distort normal anatomy and obscure important Doppler signals. Alteration in gain control settings on the standard TTE examination, as well as the use of multiple imaging planes, helps to avoid confusion due to this distortion. Transesophageal imaging is particularly useful in the evaluation of prosthetic valves, especially of the mechanical type. In general, leaflet or occluder motion can be reliably evaluated, as well as the integrity of the sewing ring. Doppler techniques are important to assess flow across the prosthesis, although velocities are dependent on valve type and surgical orientation. It is important to obtain and compare serial studies.

Prosthetic Dysfunction. Stenosis and/or regurgitation may be seen with each type of valve. Partial dehiscence of the sewing ring of either valve type from its annulus leads to paraprosthetic regurgitation, which is easy to detect with TEE color evaluation. If the valve prosthesis is sufficiently detached, abnormal rocking of the valve will be seen.

Dysfunction of a mechanical prosthesis may be caused by thrombosis, ingrowth of fibrous tissue, or vegetations. If the motion of the occluder is disturbed as a result, echocardiography will identify such abnormalities of motion, especially sticking. Mobile vegetations or pedunculated clots typically are easier to identify than laminated thrombus or fibrous ingrowth.

Acquired bioprosthetic dysfunction usually is heralded by thickening and, at times, visible calcification of the cusps. Diminished or abnormal motion of the leaflets may be identified when stenosis is present. Spontaneous tearing of a leaflet (or dysfunction as a consequence of endocarditis) usually results in a dramatic and virtually diagnostic echocardiographic appearance, with the flail portion of the valve vibrating violently and chaotically in the associated regurgitant jet of blood.

THE LEFT VENTRICLE

Echocardiography has demonstrated great clinical utility in the evaluation of LV function. Cavity size, contour, orientation, and thickness are evaluated easily. Echocardiography plays an important role in the evaluation of ventricular function following myocardial infarction, allowing for early identification of the location and extent of wall motion abnormalities.[24] The ready availability of echocardiography in the coronary care unit makes it an ideal method for the rapid assessment and diagnosis of the mechanical complications of myocardial infarction.

In addition to the ablation of thickening of the interventricular septal myocardium with ischemia and infarction, other types of abnormal septal motion can be observed. These include paradoxical (anterior in systole or posterior in diastole) septal motion of the RV volume overload type, such as that seen with atrial septal defects; delayed or abnormal electrical activation, such as that seen with left bundle branch block; or the abnormal paradoxical septal motion commonly seen after open heart surgery. The factors that contribute to this postoperative abnormality are complex and poorly understood. [25,26]

Left Ventricle in Valvular Disease

Left ventricular pressure or volume overload is an important consequence of aortic stenosis, aortic regurgitation, and mitral regurgitation. Echocardiography reliably evaluates the attendant changes in wall thickness, chamber size, and chamber contractility. In chronic aortic regurgitation, the end-systolic dimension (>5.5 cm) appears to be an important predictive parameter; higher values are associated with persistence of symptoms postoperatively, heart failure, and a higher mortality.[27,28] Aortic stenosis increases pressure and leads to increased LV mass and wall thickness, while systolic function usually remains normal. In patients with end-stage aortic stenosis, systolic function may decrease. After aortic valve replacement, those patients may experience an improvement in systolic function.

Chronic mitral regurgitation causes a volume loading of both left-sided chambers. The most frequent cause of death following mitral valve replacement is postoperative LV dysfunction; hence, there is substantial interest in which parameters of preoperative myocardial function are most important in predicting outcome. A recent study of 176 patients found that LV systolic function, as defined by the ratio of LV free wall thickness to LV end-systolic dimension, was a powerful predictor of postoperative outcome: a lower ratio, indicating increased systolic dimension and diminished wall thickness, was always found in patients who died a cardiac death.[29] In addition, the patients who died had larger left atrial dimensions than those who survived.

Coronary Artery Disease

It has long been known that a severe reduction in coronary perfusion results in cessation of systolic motion of ischemic myocardium. However, many patients with coronary artery disease have near normal coronary blood flow at rest, and these patients demonstrate normal LV wall motion. With stress such as exercise, the limited coronary reserve cannot keep pace with the increased demand, and ischemia results. Echocardiographic studies performed during exercise can identify these ischemic segments, because they become hypokinetic or akinetic when compared with normal LV regions. These wall motion abnormalities can be induced by either dynamic or pharmacologic stress.

Dynamic exercise can be accomplished on either a bicycle or a treadmill. Using the treadmill, echocardiographic images are obtained before and immediately after exercise, when the patient resumes the supine position. The 2D images obtained usually include the parasternal short and long axis views and the apical 2- and 4-chamber views. The same views are obtained post-exercise and may be stored and analyzed on-line or with the use of an off-line analysis system. Post-exercise data acquired within 60 seconds of cessation of exercise are most useful. Typically, the response of the various wall segments identified is termed normal only if the segment becomes hypercontractile post exercise, regardless of resting function. The overall "normal" response to stress includes generalized hyperkinesis, increase in myocardial systolic thickening in all segments, and increase in ejection fraction. An abnormal response is the appearance of a new regional wall motion abnormality or the failure of any myocardial wall segment to become hyperkinetic.[30] When doing bicycle exercise, in addition to the images taken post-exercise when the patient is returned to the table, the 2 apical images are recorded while the patient is still on the bicycle; occasionally subcostal imaging during exercise is obtained.

Pharmacologic agents infused to increase heart rate and blood pressure include isoproterenol and dobutamine. Vasodilatory agents, used to alter coronary blood flow, include dipyridamole and adenosine. The obvious advantage of pharmacologic agents is that the response is not dependent on patient effort; in addition, it is much easier to maintain an adequate imaging portal without patient movement and respiratory interference. Dobutamine typically is infused with an initial dose of 5 μg/kg/min, increasing the dose (10, 20, 30 μg/kg/min) every 3 minutes, usually to a maximal 3 minute infusion of 40 μg/kg/min. Echocardiographic images and an electrocardiogram are acquired with every stage of infusion and approximately 5 minutes after cessation of infusion (depending, obviously, on results during each stage). Reasons for terminating dobutamine include angina, significant dysrhythmia, ST-segment depression of greater than 2 mm, severe hypertension, decrease in systolic pressure of greater than 20 mm Hg (although some drop in systolic pressure from baseline is not uncommon), achievement of 85% of maximum heart rate, or a new wall motion abnormality on echocardiography.[31] In general, stress echocardiography appears to be reliable for the identification of wall motion abnormalities and associated coronary artery disease and can provide useful management and prognostic information.[32]

In addition to the identification of wall motion abnormalities, echocardiography is useful in the evaluation of the chronic and acute complications of myocardial infarction.[33] True and false LV aneurysms, papillary muscle rupture, and ventricular septal rupture can be readily evaluated in the post-infarction patient, especially via the TEE approach (Fig. 7). The chronic complications that can be followed include papillary muscle dysfunction, with varying degrees of mitral regurgitation, and LV thrombi.

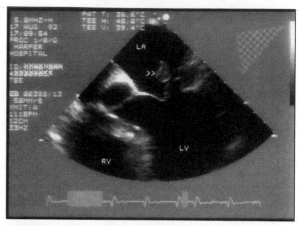

Figure 7. *Transesophageal image of a ruptured papillary muscle (arrow) prolapsing into the left atrium, following acute myocardial infarction. LA=Left atrium; LV=Left ventricle; RV=Right ventricle.*

Table 1. Echocardiographic Features of the Cardiomyopathies

	DILATED	RESTRICTIVE	HYPERTROPHIC
LV size	↑	N	N or ↓
LV systolic function	↓	N (or ↓)	N or ↑
LV wall thickness	N	↑	↑
Other features		PE	ASH
			SAM

LV=Left ventricular; N=Normal; PE=Pericardial effusion; SAM=Systolic anterior motion of the mitral valve; ASH=Asymmetric septal hypertrophy; ↑=Increased; ↓=Decreased.

Cardiomyopathy

It is often useful to divide the cardiomyopathies into groups with similar echocardiographic, hemodynamic, and clinical findings, rather than grouping them by cause (Table 1). Echocardiography permits definitive evaluation of some of these cases, although the precise causal factor rarely is apparent from the echocardiogram.

The 3 principal functional groups are dilated (formerly called congestive), restrictive, and hypertrophic.[34] The primary feature of the dilated form is LV dilatation and dysfunction; of the restrictive type, increased wall stiffness producing elevated filling pressures; and of the hypertrophic form, inappropriate myocardial hypertrophy. The distinctions are not absolute, and a given disease may have features from 2 of the functional groups.

Dilated Cardiomyopathy. Although caused by a variety of toxic substances (alcohol, drugs such as Adriamycin® [doxorubicin hydrochloride], etc.), this cardiomyopathy is most frequently of unknown cause. Although four-chamber cardiac enlargement is the rule, the left ventricle typically is most involved, demonstrating enlargement and hypokinesis. The asynergy commonly is diffuse and involves all LV segments, which in many cases distinguishes dilated cardiomyopathy from coronary artery disease. However, end-stage LV damage due to multiple infarctions also may appear diffusely hypokinetic, and conversely, dilated cardiomyopathy may demonstrate regional dysfunction on occasion. Wall thickness typically is normal, and left ventricular thrombi may be found. No intrinsic valvular pathology is seen.

Restrictive Cardiomyopathy. Grouped in this category are primary restrictive processes and secondary diseases, most frequently infiltrative diseases of the myocardium (e.g., amyloid, sarcoid, and iron overload). The typical echocardiographic feature is a normal-sized left ventricle with increased wall thickness. While the rigorous classification of the restrictive cardiomyopathies excludes secondary types (i.e., infiltrative diseases), these in fact constitute the most commonly encountered form of restrictive disease in clinical practice. Although systolic function is normal in idiopathic restrictive cardiomyopathy, it often is depressed in the infiltrative diseases. One characteristic echocardiographic feature of amyloidosis is a granular, speckled appearance of the myocardium. Doppler techniques are valuable in the assessment of the diastolic abnormalities that typically dominate the clinical picture.[35]

Hypertrophic Cardiomyopathy. The characteristic feature in this category is inappropriate LV hypertrophy.[36,37] In many cases, there is asymmetric involvement of the septum (asymmetric septal hypertrophy), with the septum at least 1.5 times

the thickness of the posterior wall. In occasional cases, other LV locations are preferentially involved, including the anterolateral wall and apex. In a minority of cases, symmetric hypertrophy is noted. Wall motion typically is normal or increased, and the LV cavity size is small.

When dynamic LVOT obstruction is present, systolic anterior motion of the anterior leaflet of the mitral valve is found. The subaortic pressure gradient produces turbulent blood flow, which causes the aortic valve to vibrate violently. Cardiac Doppler studies, with the sample volume placed in the LV outflow tract below the aortic valve, provide useful information about the presence and degree of pressure gradient.

PERICARDIUM

The posterior pericardium generates a strong echocardiographic signal and usually is easily identified. A minimal separation may normally be found between the epicardial and pericardial surfaces and probably represents less than 15 ml of pericardial fluid.

Pericardial Effusion

More than a minimal separation of epicardium and pericardium identifies a pericardial effusion. Free-flowing fluid will move to dependent locations within the pericardial space, so the apparent size of an effusion depends on the position of the patient during imaging. Precise estimation of the size of a pericardial effusion is probably both unnecessary and unreliable, but semiquantitative distinctions (trivial, small, moderate, and large) are clinically meaningful; these estimates are based on the degree of epicardial/pericardial separation. Pericardial thickening is suggested by an unusually broad and prominent pericardial signal and is often associated with concordant movement of the epicardium and pericardium, suggesting symphysis of these structures as a consequence of fibrosis. In large pericardial effusions, fibrous strands occasionally can be imaged within the pericardial fluid, as can tumor masses with neoplastic involvement of the pericardium.

Echocardiography is highly reliable in detecting pericardial effusions (Fig. 8), and specific echocardiographic signs, such as gross cardiac oscillation and respirophasic right atrial and RV

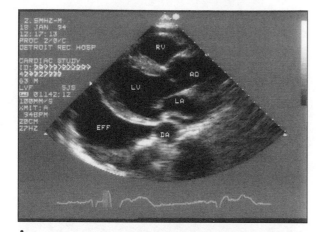

A

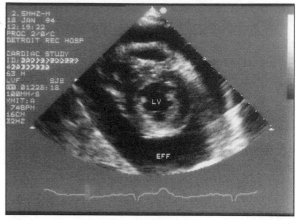

B

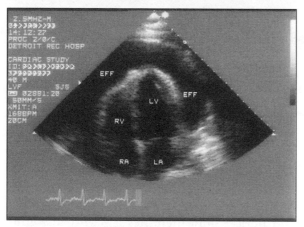

C

Figure 8. *(A) Long axis view of a large circumferential pericardial effusion. (B) The same effusion as seen in the short axis. (C) The large effusion seen from the apex. DA=Descending aorta; LA=Left atrium; LV=Left ventricle; RA=Right atrium; RV=Right ventricle; Eff=Effusion; AO=Aorta.*

diastolic collapse, suggest hemodynamic compromise.[38] Recent Doppler studies have assessed respiratory variation in diastolic filling velocities in pericardial tamponade. These studies have demonstrated marked respiratory change in LV and RV inflow velocities and isovolumic relaxation times in patients with pericardial tamponade, compared with patients with or without effusion, but without tamponade.[39,40] These changes were most evident on the first beat after inspiration and the first beat after expiration. In addition, hepatic vein flow demonstrated a decrease in diastolic forward flow and an increase in reverse flow with tamponade. After pericardiocentesis, in most patients respiratory variations in flow velocities significantly decreased. In some patients in whom flow velocities do not normalize, effusive-constrictive physiology may be operant. It is important to emphasize that these Doppler findings must be

interpreted in the context of the clinical and echocardiographic findings.

AORTA

Echocardiography, especially the TEE approach, is particularly useful in the evaluation of the aorta. Transthoracic imaging can interrogate the aortic root and several centimeters of the proximal ascending aorta. Color Doppler studies can identify aortic regurgitation associated with any root abnormalities.

Aneurysms of the sinuses of Valsalva can also be detected by echocardiography. Most are congenital and originate in the right coronary sinus or the right portion of the noncoronary sinus; involvement of the left coronary sinus is uncommon.[41] Unruptured aneurysms can be asymptomatic and incidental findings or may actually

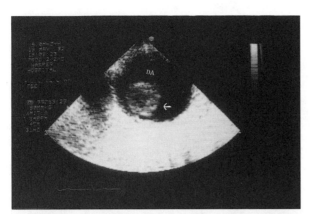

Figure 9. *Transesophageal short axis image of the descending aorta demonstrating a pedunculated mass (arrow), found to be thrombus at surgery. DA=Descending aorta.*

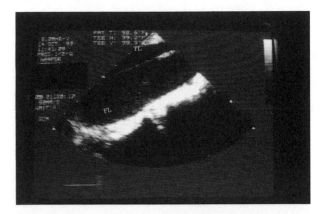

A

Figure 10. *(A) Long axis transesophageal image demonstrating aortic dissection and intimal flap. (B) Color flow demonstration of site of communication between true and false lumen. (see color plate in front of book.) TL=True lumen; FL=False lumen.*

protrude into the RV outflow tract and cause outflow obstruction.[42] With abrupt rupture, chest pain and dyspnea often initiate the onset of heart failure in association with a continuous murmur. Rupture can be catastrophic and quickly fatal if untreated, but the physiologic and hemodynamic consequences of rupture ultimately depend on the size of the shunt, the rapidity with which it develops, and the recipient chamber.[41] Small perforations in otherwise normal hearts can progress slowly with hemodynamic compensation; asymptomatic rupture has been reported.[43] Two-dimensional echocardiography can localize the abnormal sinus; color Doppler studies are invaluable in visualizing the origin and pathway of shunt flow.

Echocardiography has long been used to evaluate for intracardiac source of embolus. While the yield of transthoracic imaging is low, TEE has been found to have a significantly higher yield in the diagnosis and detection of cardiac source of embolism.[44] One potential source is atheroma of the aorta (Fig. 9). Intra-aortic debris can be readily identified and characterized by TEE.[45] Identification of atheromatous plaques is also important to the surgeon who will be cross-clamping the aorta during cardiac surgical procedures.

The role of TEE imaging in diagnosing aortic dissection is well established.[46] Transesophageal imaging is as good as, if not superior to, other diagnostic imaging technology.[47] Easily identified are the true and false lumen, as well as the extent of the dissection and presence of

stasis or luminal thrombus (Fig. 10). It is also possible to identify the entry site and to determine dissection into the coronary arteries. The technique is readily available, expeditiously accomplished, and arguably the procedure of choice to diagnose or exclude aortic dissection.

INTRACARDIAC MASSES

Echocardiography is the procedure of choice for the evaluation of suspected intracardiac masses, including intracavitary tumors, atrial and ventricular thrombi, and valvular vegetations.

Tumors

The most common primary cardiac tumor by far is the myxoma (Fig. 11).[48] Myxomas most commonly are found in the left atrium, but they may be seen in any cardiac chamber or directly attached to valves; a myxoma originating from the inferior vena cava has been described. Typically, myxomas are pedunculated and attached to the left atrium at the level of the fossa ovalis. They are often heterogeneous in appearance, with frond-like protuberances and cavitations not uncommon. Myxomas usually move with the cardiac cycle and often prolapse through the mitral valve in diastole; the erroneous clinical diagnosis of mitral stenosis is not uncommon. Transesophageal techniques confirm the presence, point of attachment,

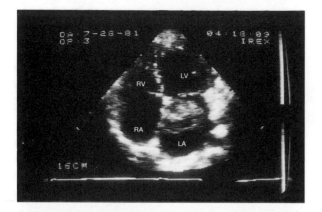

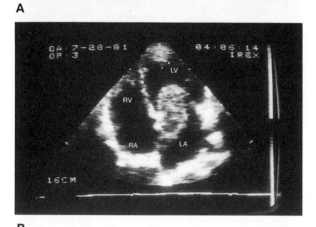

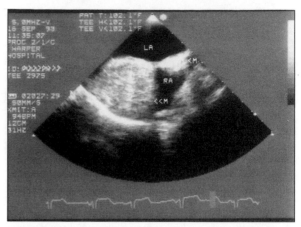

Figure 12. *Transesophageal image of large fatty infiltrate ("lipomatous hypertrophy") of the atrial septum. Note the dumbbell shape and sparing of the fossa ovalis. LA=Left atrium; RA=Right atrium; M=Mass.*

Figure 11. *Apical 4-chamber transthoracic image demonstrating an atrial myxoma attached to the interatrial septum. (A) Systole (B) Diastole, during which the myxoma prolapses through the mitral orifice into the left ventricle. LV=Left ventricle; LA=Left atrium; RV=Right ventricle; RA=Right atrium.*

and size of the mass and preclude any further diagnostic studies. As these tumors frequently embolize, surgery is indicated.

Other primary benign tumors of the heart include lipomas (intracavitary and intrapericardial), fibroelastomas, rhabdomyomas, and fibromas. Rhabdomyomas are most commonly found in children, often in association with tuberous sclerosis. There is evidence now that these tumors may resolve completely, so surgery is not always necessary and some period of "watchful waiting" is appropriate in asymptomatic patients.[48] Fibromas are the second most common cardiac tumor of childhood, and, while rare, are usually found infiltrating and displacing ventricular

myocardium. These tumors may be associated with lethal ventricular arrhythmias, so surgical resection, if feasible, is indicated. Complete resection of these tumors is difficult. While reliable localization of these tumors is possible, echocardiography cannot characterize tissue, and magnetic resonance imaging may be indicated. Primary malignant tumors of the heart are rare, and, as with most other tumors, cannot be characterized histologically by ultrasound.

Fatty infiltration of the atrial septum ("lipomatous hypertrophy") is an occasional echocardiographic finding and is characterized by its typical "dumbbell" shape (Fig. 12).[49] The fossa ovalis typically is spared fatty infiltration. Fat may extend into both atria, and infiltrates up to 8 cm have been described.[50] Because this is typically an incidental autopsy finding, when discovered premortem no treatment is necessary, except perhaps when associated with atrial dysrhythmias.

Metastatic tumors of the heart are up to 40 times more common than primary tumors. (Fig. 13).[51] Those malignancies that frequently metastasize to the heart include lung, breast, and esophageal by direct extension; renal cell (hypernephroma) and hepatoma by venous extension; and melanoma, leukemia, and lymphoma via lymphangitic spread. As is the case with primary cardiac neoplasms, ultrasound cannot histologically characterize these masses, but their presence, extent, and origin can reliably be determined, especially with the TEE technique.

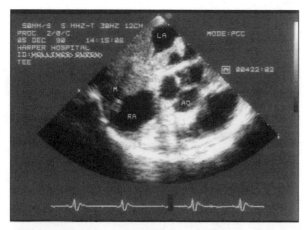

Figure 13. *Transesophageal short axis view of metastatic lung cancer invading both atria. LA=Left atrium; RA=Right atrium; Ao=Aorta; M=Mass.*

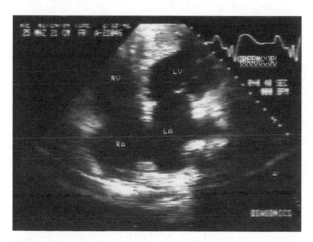

Figure 14. *Apical 4-chamber view demonstrating large laminar thrombus in the apex (arrow). LV=Left ventricle; LA=Left atrium; RV=Right ventricle; RA=Right atrium.*

Thrombi

Thrombi are readily identified with echocardiography. Left ventricular thrombi post-myocardial infarction, especially those involving the anteroseptal apex, are commonly detected in those regions of significant hypokinesia or akinesia (Fig. 14).[52] While thrombus in the left ventricle typically occurs in areas of marked reduction in wall motion, in patients with hypercoagulable states, such as those associated with malignancies or inflammatory bowel diseases, thrombus has been identified in normally contracting ventricles.[53] Left atrial thrombus and "smoke"

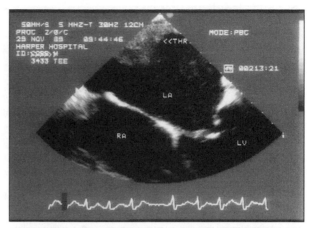

Figure 15. *Four-chamber transesophageal view demonstrating mitral stenosis, with thrombus and smoke (stasis) in the left atrium. LV=Left ventricle; LA=Left atrium; RA=Right atrium; Thr=Thrombus.*

(indistinct swirling intracavitary reflections as a consequence of low flow) can be identified with TTE imaging, but they are best evaluated with the TEE approach (Fig. 15).[54] Thrombus in the left atrium is most commonly seen in patients in atrial fibrillation with mitral stenosis.

A common type of thrombus now regularly identified in the right heart is the so-called pulmonary embolus in transit (Fig. 16).[55] These lesions originate from leg veins and are identified as they pass through the heart in transit to the lungs. They are striking in appearance: unattached, coiling, serpiginous, with a striking mobility independent of the cardiac cycle. Occasionally, these thrombi will traverse the fossa ovalis, become entrapped, and bobble about in the left atrium as well as the right. Because these lesions are notoriously unstable, urgent treatment is necessary and thus appropriate expeditious diagnosis is imperative.

Vegetations

Echocardiography is invaluable in the diagnosis of infective endocarditis and should be considered in all patients in whom the diagnosis is suspected. While there is no question that the technology is still operator/interpreter dependent, the high detection rate of vegetations makes it an extremely useful diagnostic tool. Transesophageal images are more sensitive than TTE images for detecting vegetations,[56,57] and, even when TTE provides the diagnosis, should

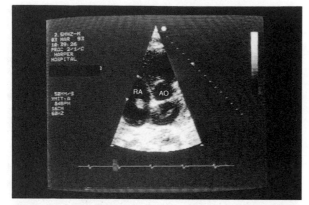

A

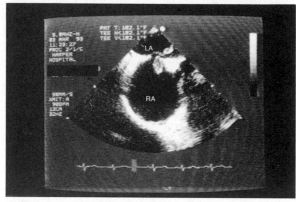

B

Figure 16. *(A) Short axis transthoracic view of the base of the heart, demonstrating thrombus (arrow) traversing the interatrial septum (pulmonary embolus-in-transit). (B) Transesophageal view of the atrial septum demonstrating the embolus crossing the fossa ovalis. LA=Left atrium; RA=Right atrium; Ao=Aorta.*

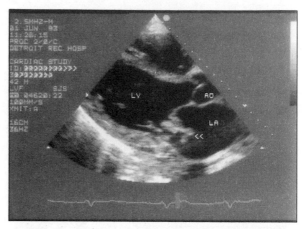

Figure 17. *Parasternal long axis view demonstrating a large prolapsing vegetation of the mitral valve (arrow). LV=Left ventricle; LA=Left atrium; Ao=Aorta.*

still be performed to evaluate the heart for the common and important complications of endocarditis, especially abscesses, leaflet perforations, and perforation of the tissue surrounding the vegetation.[58,59] Transesophageal imaging is also indicated when TTE is negative, but the index of suspicion is high for the diagnosis or when prosthetic valves are in place.

Active vegetations typically appear as oscillating masses attached to either valve leaflets or supporting apparatus (Figs. 17,18). They usually do not interfere with valve mobility, although large vegetations can obstruct a valve orifice. Vegetations can also seed in the path of a septic regurgitant jet, such as that of the left atrial wall jet of mitral regurgitation. Old healed vegeta-

tions in general appear smaller and more dense ("echo reflective"), consistent with the pathologic evolution of the lesion. The distinction between new and old vegetations is not always easy or reliable, however, especially in patients with old right-sided lesions and new febrile illnesses.

There is considerable debate regarding any correlation between the size, shape, and location of vegetations and eventual clinical outcome. In one study mitral valve vegetations were associated with a higher incidence of embolic events than were vegetations on aortic valves; risk factors for embolization were vegetation size of greater than 10 mm and mitral valve location.[60] Interestingly, except for the rate of embolic events, mitral endocarditis had a lower risk of death and surgical intervention than aortic endocarditis. Patients without visualized vegetations less frequently developed complications, required surgery, or died. Other studies suggest that while larger vegetations have a higher incidence of embolization, size was not significantly different in patients with and without severe heart failure or in patients surviving or dying during acute endocarditis.[61] There is no consensus as to whether the type of organism involved is a specific independent risk factor for complications. Nonetheless, careful echocardiographic characterization of vegetation location, size, and mobility forms an important component of the baseline evaluation of any patient with endocarditis. The TEE approach is superior to TTE both in determining the presence of vegetations

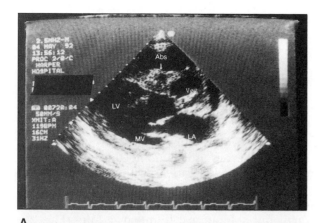

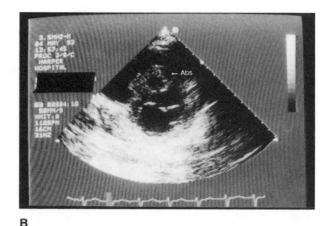

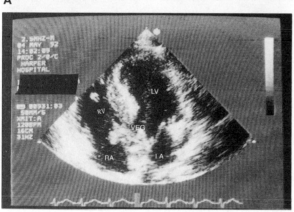

Figure 18. *(A) Parasternal long axis view of extensive endocarditis involving the base of the heart. There is a large vegetation of the aortic valve and an abscess that extends into the base of the interventricular septum. (B) Short axis of the left ventricular outflow tract demonstrating the abscess cavity. (C) Apical 4-chamber view demonstrating prolapsing aortic vegetation and extension of the infectious process into the right atrium (arrow). (D) Color flow image demonstrating flow (blue) through the perforation into the right atrium (see color plate in front of book). MV=Mitral valve; Veg=Vegetation; Abs=Abscess; LV=Left ventricle; RV=Right ventricle; LA=Left atrium; RA=Right atrium; Ao=Aorta.*

and in the assessment of associated complications, information which may alter the clinical and therapeutic course.

CONGENITAL HEART DISEASE

The development of 2-dimensional echocardiography had its earliest and perhaps its most profound influence in the evaluation of congenital cardiac anomalies. Because of its wide field of view, 2-dimensional echocardiography permits analysis of often complex spatial relationships and orientations. Atrial, ventricular, and great vessel anatomy, orientation, and connections can be evaluated with a high degree of accuracy

and reliability. Cardiac catheterizations have become more stylized since the introduction of 2-dimensional echocardiography, because now the anatomical features often are known prior to catheterization and only specific questions (such as pressures, flows, and resistances) remain to be determined. In selected patients with certain lesions, such as secundum-type atrial septal defect (ASD) and coarctation of the aorta, catheterization is no longer required or routine before surgery but rather is performed only when there are unresolved issues following echocardiography.

Since a review of all congenital cardiac anomalies is beyond the scope of this chapter, the discussion will be limited to several of the most com-

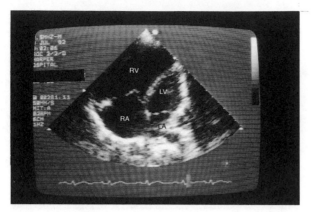

A

Figure 19. *(A) Apical 4-chamber view of a patient with an atrial septal defect, demonstrating marked prominence of the right heart chambers. (B) Color flow recording of left-to-right shunt flow (see color plate in front of book). LV=Left ventricle; LA=Left atrium; RV=Right ventricle; RA=Right atrium.*

mon nonvalvular congenital defects found in the adult. Coarctation of the aorta may not cause symptoms until after 20 years of age. Most patients who survive infancy with this defect reach adulthood, although on average death occurs in the mid-30s. The most common associated lesion is a bicuspid aortic valve. The echocardiographic images are obtained from the suprasternal notch, and the lesion is characterized by a localized decrease in the diameter of the aortic lumen, usually with the area of maximal narrowing just distal to the left subclavian. In the absence of other lesions that can affect flow velocity, Doppler studies are accurate in determining the pressure gradient across the lesion.

Secundum ASD is among the more common congenital lesions seen in adults (Fig. 19). Symptoms may be absent for decades. The findings of dilated right heart chambers and "paradoxical" septal motion (the RV volume overload pattern) are the typical echocardiographic findings. Occasionally, direct visualization of the defect is possible. One must be cautious about assessment of normal echo "drop out" in the region of the fossa ovalis. The subcostal view is probably the most reliable in assessing the integrity of the interatrial septum, as in this plane the atrial septum is perpendicular to the ultrasound beam. Doppler color flow is very sensitive for detecting flow across the atrial septum, and the abnormal color flow crossing the atrial septum can frequently be seen even when the anatomic defect itself cannot be visualized.[62] Mitral valve prolapse, with or without mitral regurgitation, is commonly found with ASDs. Transesophageal imaging is particularly reliable in imaging atrial septal defects and should always be performed when TTE imaging is inconclusive and there is unexplained dilatation of the right heart.[63] There is usually no need for catheterization in young adult patients with this lesion.

Ventricular septal defects are among the most common congenital cardiac malformations at birth but seldom are found in adults (Fig. 20 color plate). Many close spontaneously or significantly shrink in size. Ventricular septal defects are often clinically apparent, so the echocardiographic examination is directed toward evaluating the site and size of the defect, as well as associated lesions and the hemodynamic consequences of the shunt. The parasternal long and short axis planes and the apical 4-chamber and subcostal 4-chamber views are most useful in detecting VSDs. In defects with left-to-right shunts, an abnormal Doppler flow signal is recorded in the right ventricle; Doppler studies are occasionally diagnostic even when the defect cannot be directly visualized. Using the Bernoulli equation, the pressure difference between the left and right ventricles can be calculated from the maximal Doppler jet velocity. Right ventricular systolic pressure may be estimated by subtracting the gradient from the LV(systemic) systolic blood pressure. Color flow is extremely valuable in localizing the site and direction of flow, especially when the defects are quite small and cannot be directly imaged.

Tetralogy of Fallot is the most common cyanotic cardiac lesion that allows uncorrected survival to adulthood. It is characterized by 4 anomalies: a subaortic VSD (malalignment type); hypertrophy of the right ventricle; infundibular narrowing; and overriding of the aorta. Echocardiography is used to identify the VSD and the degree of truncal override. Normally, the anterior mitral leaflet is contiguous with the base of the aorta, and the interventricular septum is contiguous with the anterior wall of the aorta. With aortic override, the septal-aortic continuity is distorted. Doppler techniques provide important information concerning the degree and location of RV outflow tract obstruction. Occasionally, patients with only mild outflow obstruction and left-to-right shunt flow may be acyanotic.

PULSE RECORDINGS

By placing an ultrasound transducer over the carotid artery, internal jugular vein, and cardiac apex impulse, a tracing may be obtained that displays in graphic form the pressure and volume fluxes of the underlying structures. Although the resulting external recordings are not direct measurements of intraluminal pressure, the morphology of the carotid, jugular, and apical pulse tracings closely mirrors the intracavitary pressure tracings obtained from within the aorta, right atrium, and left ventricle, respectively. In specific pathologic conditions, tracings may be obtained from other locations, such as recording the RV impulse with pressure overload of the right ventricle or the hepatic pulse with tricuspid regurgitation. The use of pulse recordings as clinical tools has been replaced by the echocardiographic and Doppler techniques, but pulse recordings remain invaluable as teaching aids.

CAROTID PULSE

The normal carotid pulse tracing is composed of a rapid upstroke (anacrotic limb), terminating in an initial peak or percussion wave (Fig. 21). The percussion wave is followed by a less prominent, somewhat more rounded tidal wave. The percussion wave appears to be primarily related to the peak aortic flow rate, while the tidal wave is related to peak aortic pressure. Thus, the tidal wave often becomes more prominent with systemic hypertension, following the infusion of a vasoconstrictor, and in elderly patients. The descending limb of the carotid pulse tracing, which normally is less steep than the ascending limb, is interrupted by the incisura or dicrotic notch. The notch is due to aortic valve closure. Although the morphology of the carotid pulse tracing resembles that of an intra-aortic pressure recording, it is delayed by approximately 20–50 msec, which is the time it takes the pulse wave to travel from the chest to the neck. Systolic time intervals (STI)—measurements derived from the simultaneous recording of the electrocardiogram, the indirect carotid pulse,

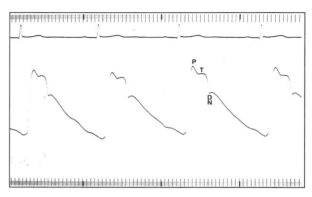

Figure 21. *Normal carotid pulse tracing. The percussion wave (P) is more prominent than the subsequent tidal wave (T). DN=Dicrotic notch.*

and the phonocardiogram—include total systole, the pre-ejection period, and the LV ejection time. Used in the past to aid in the evaluation of valvular heart disease and ventricular performance, STIs have been supplanted by echocardiographic and Doppler techniques.

Carotid Pulse Abnormalities

Atherosclerosis of the carotid artery may produce abnormalities of the carotid pulse tracing. In the absence of local carotid disease, abnormalities of the pulse may be generally categorized as hyperkinetic or hypokinetic (Table 2). In a variety of disease states, specific abnormalities of the carotid pulse often can be identified. Aortic stenosis typically shows a small hypokinetic pulse with a delayed systolic peak (Fig. 22). An anacrotic shoulder, occurring in the early to mid-portion of the ascending limb of the carotid pulse tracing, reflects decreased aortic flow secondary to obstruction to LV emptying, as well as turbulent flow. A "shudder" is often noted, also as a consequence of turbulent blood flow.

In contrast to the findings in fixed-orifice LV outflow obstruction, in the dynamic obstruction seen with hypertrophic cardiomyopathy there is a hyperkinetic pulse of large amplitude with a rapid upstroke (Fig. 23). As LV volume decreases during systole, the anterior leaflet of the mitral valve moves toward the septum and narrows the outflow tract. Consequently, there is a sudden decrease in the carotid pulse amplitude, reflecting a sudden fall in ejection rate. A secondary wave is generated until the end of systole, resulting in the characteristic "spike and dome" pulse curve configuration.

Table 2. General Causes of Abnormalities of the Carotid Pulse Tracing

HYPERKINETIC PULSE
  Increased cardiac output states, such as anxiety, fever, exercise, pregnancy, and anemia
  Widened pulse pressure, as with aortic regurgitation, persistent ductus arteriosus, and Paget's diesease of the bone
  Decreased arterial distensibility

HYPOKINETIC PULSE
  Fixed left ventricular outflow tract obstruction, as with aortic stenosis and discrete subaortic stenosis
  Reduced forward stroke volume, as with myocardial infarction, cardiomyopathy, and severe mitral regurgitation
  Narrow pulse pressure, as with cardiac tamponade and constrictive pericarditis

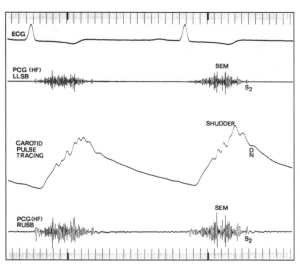

Figure 22. *Carotid pulse tracing from a patient with severe valvular aortic stenosis, showing a low anacrotic shoulder and systolic shudder. The phonocardiogram (PCG) demonstrates a mid-to-late peaking systolic ejection murmur (SEM) with soft aortic component of the second heart sound (S2). ECG=Electrocardiogram; DN=Dicrotic notch; HF=High frequency; LLSB=Left lower sternal border; RUSB=Right upper sternal border. From Borow KM, Wynne J. External pulse recordings, systolic time intervals, apexcardiography, and phonocardiography. In: Cohn PF, Wynne J (eds). Diagnostic Methods in Clinical Cardiology. Boston: Little Brown; 1982:144. With permission.*

JUGULAR VENOUS PULSE

The normal jugular venous pulse recording consists of 2 major peaks (A and v) and 2 major descents (x and y) (Fig. 24). The A wave is the result of displacement of blood into the jugular vein by right atrial systole; it is the most prominent positive wave and is absent when effective atrial systole is lacking. Atrial relaxation is associated with the x descent, which continues to the x trough, the most negative wave of the normal jugular venous pulse recording. The x descent usually is interrupted by the c wave, a small wave resulting from closure of the tricuspid valve. Further accumulation of blood behind the still-closed tricuspid valve results in the v wave, due to passive filling of the right atrium. The y descent is generated by the open tricuspid valve and flow of blood from the right atrium into the right ventricle.

Jugular Venous Pulse Abnormalities

A prominent A wave is found when right atrial systole is unusually forceful as a consequence of an impediment to right atrial emptying. This is

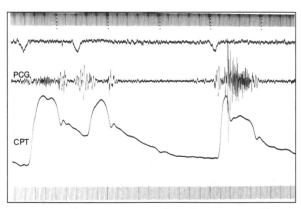

Figure 23. *Carotid pulse tracing (CPT) and phonocardiogram (PCG), recorded at the left lower sternal border, and electrocardiogram in a patient with provocable dynamic subaortic obstruction due to hypertrophic cardiomyopathy. Recordings made after an atrial premature beat demonstrate precipitation of a spike and dome configuration on CPT and accentuation of the systolic murmur, indicating that dynamic obstruction was provoked. From Borow KM, Wynne J. External pulse recordings, systolic time intervals, apexcardiography, and phonocardiography. In: Cohn PF, Wynne J, (eds). Diagnostic Methods in Clinical Cardiology. Boston: Little Brown: 1982:148. With permission.*

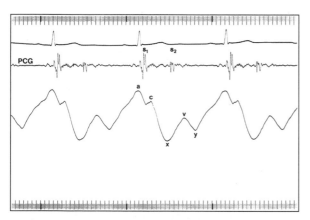

Figure 24. *Jugular venous pulse recording from a normal subject. The A wave is the largest positive wave, while the X-trough is the more prominent negative wave. The phonocardiogram (PCG) is a low frequency recording at the lower left sternal border, showing first (S₁) and second (S₂) heart sounds.*

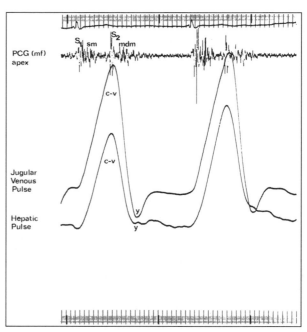

Figure 25. *Jugular venous and hepatic pulse tracings from a patient with Ebstein's anomaly and tricuspid regurgitation. A giant C-V systolic wave is noted, with an abrupt Y-descent. The hepatic pulse recording is similar to the jugular pulse tracing. PCG=Phonocardiogram; SM=Systolic murmur; MF=Mid-frequency; MDM=Mid-diastolic murmur. From Borow KM, Wynne J. External pulse recordings, systolic time intervals, apexcardiography, and phonocardiography. In: Cohn PF, Wynne J, (eds). Diagnostic Methods in Clinical Cardiology. Boston: Little Brown; 1982:131. With permission.*

usually the result of increased stiffness (diminished compliance) of the right ventricle as a consequence of RV hypertrophy of any etiology. The x descent is reduced in atrial fibrillation, since atrial relaxation is absent. It is shallow or obliterated in tricuspid insufficiency, since there is active regurgitation of blood into the right atrium. A positive systolic wave (or c-v wave) replaces the x trough in severe tricuspid regurgitation. With severe tricuspid regurgitation, a similar systolic pulsation may often be recorded over the liver (Fig. 25). In cardiac tamponade, a prominent x descent is noted. Conversely, the x descent is reduced with constrictive pericarditis; a prominent x descent in this setting strongly suggests effusive-constrictive disease.

The v wave is more prominent with enhanced passive filling of the atrium, as seen in an atrial septal defect. As noted above, an early and large systolic regurgitant wave is seen in tricuspid regurgitation. Although by common usage regurgitant waves have been referred to as v waves, strictly speaking, a v wave is solely the result of passive atrial filling, while the systolic wave is due to active systolic filling of the atrium.

The y descent is unusually rapid and brief in constrictive pericarditis and ends with an early diastolic plateau. This reflects the small RV end-diastolic volume and restriction to filling, resulting in the so-called square-root sign. A deep and sharp y descent may also be found with RV failure.

THE APEXCARDIOGRAM

The movement of the heart against the chest wall throughout the cardiac cycle results in motion against the left precordial surface, which can be recorded on the apexcardiogram. This closely resembles the LV pressure pulse in morphology (Fig. 26).

The rapid upstroke of the apexcardiogram begins with LV isovolumic systole (c point). The upstroke terminates at the e point, which coincides with the onset of LV ejection. During the second half of LV systole, the curve usually undergoes a gentle decline. At approximately the time of aortic valve closure, the curve begins a sharp decline, correlating with the onset of the ventricular isovolumic relaxation period. This

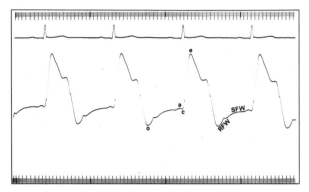

Figure 26. *Normal apexcardiogram. RFW=Rapid filling wave; SFW=Slow filling wave.*

downward deflection terminates near the end of the mitral valve opening (end of isovolumic relaxation period), an event that is approximated by the 0 point of the apexcardiogram. Vigorous ventricular filling in early diastole produces the rapid filling wave, which is followed by the less vigorous slow filling wave. The A wave is the final diastolic wave and corresponds to the distension of the left ventricle as a consequence of atrial contraction.

Apexcardiographic Abnormalities

The A wave is absent in patients with atrial fibrillation and is increased in cases of diminished LV compliance (Fig. 27). The systolic bulge of the apexcardiogram may be unusually forceful, although typically not sustained, in volume overload of a compensated left ventricle (increased stroke volume). This may be found in mitral or aortic regurgitation, anemia, anxiety, thyrotoxicosis, etc. A sustained apical impulse, on the other hand, is found with LV pressure overload (aortic stenosis or systemic hypertension), and with LV dysfunction (Fig. 27).

An unusual double or bifid apical impulse may be seen with hypertrophic cardiomyopathy with LVOT obstruction. Since diminished LV compliance also is found, the A wave may be quite prominent as well, resulting in a characteristic triple apical impulse.

A prominent rapid filling wave is found in patients with augmented early diastolic filling, often as a result of LV volume overload. The rapid filling wave is reduced with diminished LV compliance, since the increased stiffness of the ventricle limits its ability to expand in early dias-

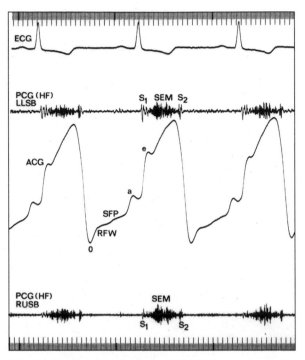

Figure 27. *Apexcardiogram (ACG) in a patient with severe valvular aortic stenosis. The systolic wave is sustained, with a continuous rise throughout ventricular ejection. The A wave is exaggerated. ECG=Electrocardiogram; HF=High frequency; LLSB=Left lower sternal border; PCG=Phonocardiogram; RFW=Rapid filling wave; RUSB=Right upper sternal border; SEM=Systolic ejection murmur; SFP=Slow filling period. From Borow KM, Wynne J. External pulse recordings, systolic time intervals, apexcardiography, and phonocardiography. In: Cohn PF, Wynne J, (eds). Diagnostic Methods in Clinical Cardiology. Boston: Little Brown, 1982:145. With permission.*

tole. The rapid filling wave is blunted and shortened in mitral stenosis.

The apexcardiogram is particularly useful in clarifying the timing of auscultatory events. An ejection sound occurs in relationship to the e point. A mitral opening snap is found near the 0 point, while a third heart sound is found later, at the peak of the rapid filling wave. The fourth heart sound is found at the time of the A wave.

REFERENCES

1. Seward JB, Khandheria BK, Oh JK, et al. Transesophageal echocardiography: Technique, anatomic

correlations, implementation, and clinical applications. *Mayo Clin Proc.* 1988;63:649-680.

2. Seward JB, Khandheria BK, Edwards WD, et al. Biplanar transesophageal echocardiography: Anatomic correlations, image orientation, and clinical applications. *Mayo Clin Proc.* 1990;65:1193-1213.

3. Swan JW, Chambers JB, Monaghan MJ, et al. Echocardiographic appearance of pulmonary artery stenosis. *Br Heart J.* 1990;63:175-177.

4. Fagan LF, Penick DR, Williams GA, et al. Two dimensional, spectral Doppler, and color flow imaging in adults with acquired and congenital cor triatriatum. *J Am Soc Echocardiogr.* 1991;4:177-184.

5. Vitarelli A, Landolina G, Gentile R, et al. Echocardiographic assessment of congenital mitral stenosis. *Am Heart J.* 1984;108:523-531.

6. Pan GVS, Fripp RR, Whitman V, et al. Anomalous mitral arcade: Echocardiographic and angiographic recognition. *Ped Cardiol.* 1983;4:163-165.

7. Davachi F, Moller J, Edwards JE. Diseases of the mitral valve in infancy. An anatomic analysis of 55 cases. *Circulation.* 1971;43:565-579.

8. Wilkins QT, Weyman AE, Abascal VM, et al. Percutaneous balloon dilatation of the mitral valve: An analysis of echocardiographic variables related to outcome and the mechanism of dilatation. *Br Heart J.* 1988;60:299-308.

9. Marwick TH, Torelli J, Obarski T, et al. Assessment of the mitral valve splittability score by transthoracic and transesophageal echocardiography. *Am J Cardiol.* 1991;68:1106-1107.

10. Pearson AC, St. Vrain J, Mrosek D, et al. Color Doppler echocardiographic evaluation of patients with a flail mitral leaflet. *J Am Coll Cardiol.* 1990;16:232-239.

11. Stewart WJ, Currie PJ, Salcedo EE, et al. Evaluation of mitral leaflet motion by echocardiography and jet direction by Doppler color flow mapping to determine the mechanism of mitral regurgitation. *J Am Coll Cardiol.* 1992;20:1353-1361.

12. Roberts WC. Valvular, subvalvular, and supravalvular aortic stenosis. *Cardiovasc Clin.* 1973;5:97-126.

13. Roberts WC. The congenitally bicuspid aortic valve. A study of 85 autopsy cases. *Am J Cardiol.* 1970;26:72-83.

14. Requarth JA, Goldberg S, Vasko SD, et al. In vitro verification of Doppler prediction of transvalve pressure gradient and orifice area in stenosis. *Am J Cardiol.* 1984;53:1369-1373.

15. Ohlsson J, Wranne B. Noninvasive assessment of valve area in patients with aortic stenosis. *J Am Coll Cardiol.* 1986;7:501-508.

16. Otto CM, Pearlman AS, Comess KA, et al. Determination of the stenotic aortic valve area in adults using Doppler echocardiography. *J Am Coll Cardiol.* 1986;7:509-517.

17. Nishimura RA, Tajik AJ. Quantitative hemodynamics by Doppler echocardiography: A noninvasive alternative to cardiac catheterization. *Prog Cardiovasc Dis.* 1994;36:309-342.

18. Choi JY, Sullivan I. Fixed subaortic stenosis: Anatomical spectrum and nature of progression. *Br Heart J.* 1991;65:280-286.

19. Frommelt MA, Snider AR, Bove EL, et al. Echocardiographic assessment of subvalvular aortic stenosis before and after operation. *J Am Coll Cardiol.* 1992;19:1018-1023.

20. Friedman W. Aortic stenosis. In: Adams FH, Emmanouilides GC, Riemenschneider TA (eds). *Heart Disease in Infants, Children, and Adolescents.* Baltimore: Williams and Wilkins; 1989:224-243.

21. Berkery W, Hare C, Warner RA, et al. Nonpenetrating traumatic rupture of the tricuspid valve. *Chest.* 1987;91:778-780.

22. Guiliani ER, Fuster V, Brandenburg RO, et al. Ebstein's anomaly. The clinical features and natural history of Ebstein's anomaly of the tricuspid valve. *Mayo Clin Proc.* 1979;54:163-173.

23. Zabalgoitia M. Echocardiographic assessment of prosthetic heart valves. *Curr Probl Cardiol.* 1992;17:271-325.

24. Feigenbaum H. Role of echocardiography in acute myocardial infarction. *Am J Cardiol.* 1990;66:17H-22H.

25. Wranne B, Pinto F, Siegel LC, et al. Abnormal postoperative interventricular motion: New intraoperative transesophageal echocardiographic evidence supports a novel hypothesis. *Am Heart J.* 1993;126:161-167.

26. Lehmann KG, Lee FA, McKenzie WB, et al. Onset of altered interventricular septal motion during cardiac surgery. Assessment by continuous intraoperative transesophageal echocardiography. *Circulation.* 1990;82:1325-1334.

27. Gaasch WH, Carroll JD, Levine H, et al. Chronic aortic regurgitation: Prognostic value of left ventricular end-systolic dimension and end-diastolic radius/thickness ratio. *J Am Coll Cardiol.* 1983;13:775-782.

28. Henry WL, Bonow RO, Borer J, et al. Observation on the optimum time for operative intervention for aortic regurgitation. I. Evaluation of the results of aortic valve replacement in symptomatic patients. *Circulation.* 1980;61:471-483.

29. Reed D, Abbott RD, Smucker ML, et al. Prediction of outcome after mitral valve replacement in patients with symptomatic chronic mitral regurgitation. The importance of left atrial size. *Circulation.* 1991;84:23-34.

30. Ryan T, Vasey CG, Presti CF, et al. Exercise echocardiography: Detection of coronary artery disease in patients with normal left ventricular wall motion at rest. *J Am Coll Cardiol.* 1988;11:993-999.

31. Rosamond TL, Vocek JL, Hurwitz A, et al. Hypotension during dobutamine stress echocardiography: Initial description and clinical relevance. *Am Heart J.* 1992;123:403-407.

32. Armstrong WF. Stress echocardiography for detection of coronary artery disease. *Circulation.* 1991;84(suppl I):I-43–I-49.

33. Buda AJ. Role of echocardiography in the evaluation of mechanical complications of acute myocardial infarction. *Circulation.* 1991;84(suppl I):I-109–I-121.

34. Wynne J, Braunwald E. The cardiomyopathies and myocardities: Toxic, chemical and physical damage to the heart. In: Braunwald E (ed). *Heart Disease. A Textbook of Cardiovascular Medicine,* 4th Ed. Philadelphia: WB Saunders; 1992:1394-1450.

35. Klein AL, Cohen GI. Doppler echocardiographic

assessment of constrictive pericarditis, cardiac amyloidosis, and cardiac tamponade. *Clev Clin J Med.* 1992;59:278-290.

36. Maron BJ. Hypertrophic cardiomyopathy. *Curr Probl Cardiol.* 1993;18:637-704.

37. Louie EK, Edwards LC. Hypertrophic cardiomyopathy. *Prog Cardiovasc Dis.* 1994;36:275-308.

38. Chandraratna PAN. Echocardiography and Doppler ultrasound in the evaluation of pericardial disease. *Circulation.* 1991:84(suppl I):I-303–I-310.

39. Burstow DJ, Oh JK, Bailey K, et al. Cardiac tamponade: Characteristic Doppler observations. *Mayo Clin Proc.* 1989;64:312-324.

40. Appleton CP, Hatle LK, Popp RL. Cardiac tamponade and pericardial effusion: Respiratory variation in transvalvular flow velocities studied by Doppler echocardiography. *J Am Coll Cardiol.* 1988;11:1020-1030.

41. Sakakibara S, Konno S. Congenital aneurysms of the sinus of valsalva. Anatomy and classification. *Am Heart J* 1962; 63:405-423.

42. Desai AG, Sharma S, Kumar A, et al. Echocardiographic diagnosis of unruptured aneurysm of right sinus of valsalva: An unusual case of right ventricular outflow obstruction. *Am Heart J.* 1985;109:363-364.

43. Peters P, Juziuk E, Gunther S. Doppler color flow mapping detection of ruptured sinus of valsalva aneurysm. *J Am Soc Echocardiogr.* 1989;2:195-197.

44. Kronzon I, Tunick P. Transesophageal echocardiography as a tool in the evaluation of patients with embolic disorders. *Prog in Cardiovasc Dis.* 1993;36:39-60.

45. Karalis DG, Chandrasekaran K, Victor MF, et al. Recognition and embolic potential of intraaortic atherosclerotic debris. *J Am Coll Cardiol.* 1991;17:73-78.

46. Ballal RS, Nanda NC, Gatewood R, et al. Usefulness of transesophageal echocardiography in assessment of aortic dissection. *Circulation.* 1991;84:1903-1914.

47. Erbel R, Daniel W, Visser C, et al. Echocardiography in diagnosis of aortic dissection. *Lancet.* 1989;1:457-460.

48. Salcedo EE, Cohen GI, White RD, et al. Cardiac tumors: Diagnosis and management. *Curr Probl Cardiol.* 1992;17:73-137.

49. Applegate PM, Tajik AJ, Ehman RL, et al. Two dimensional echocardiographic and magnetic resonance imaging observations in massive lipomatous hypertrophy of the atrial septum. *Am J Cardiol.* 1987;59:489-491.

50. Shirani J, Roberts WC. Clinical, electrocardiographic and morphologic features of massive fatty deposits ("lipomatous hypertrophy") in the atrial septum. *J Am Coll Cardiol.* 1993;22:226-238.

51. McAllister HA. Primary tumors of the heart and pericardium. *Curr Probl Cardiol.* 1979;4:1-51.

52. Funkekupper AJ, Verheugt FWA, Peels CH, et al. Left ventricular thrombus incidence and behavior studied by serial two-dimensional echocardiography in acute anterior myocardial infarction: Left ventricular wall motion, systemic embolism, and oral anticoagulation. *J Am Coll Cardiol.* 1989;13:1514-1520.

53. Chin WW, Van Tosh A, Hecht SR, et al. Left ventricular thrombus with normal left ventricular function in ulcerative colitis. *Am Heart J.* 1988;116:562-563.

54. Black IW, Hopkins AP, Lee LCL, et al. Left atrial spontaneous echo contrast: A clinical and echocardiographic analysis. *J Am Coll Cardiol.* 1991;18:398-404.

55. Farfel Z, Shechter M, Vered Z, et al. Review of echocardiographically diagnosed right heart entrapment of pulmonary emboli in transit with emphasis on management. *Am Heart J.* 1987;113:171-178.

56. Sochowski RA, Chan K-L. Implication of negative results on a monoplane transesophageal echocardiographic study in patients with suspected infective endocarditis. *J Am Coll Cardiol.* 1993;21:216-221.

57. Khandheria BK. Suspected bacterial endocarditis: To TEE or not to TEE. *J Am Coll Cardiol.* 1993;21:222-224.

58. Karalis DG, Bansal RC, Hauck AJ, et al. Transesophageal echocardiographic recognition of subaortic complications in aortic valve endocarditis. *Circulation.* 1992;86:353-362.

59. Daniel WG, Mugge A, Martin R, et al. Improvement in the diagnosis of abscesses associated with endocarditis by transesophageal echocardiography. *N Engl J Med.* 1991;324:795-800.

60. Rohmann S, Erbel R, Gorge J, et al. Clinical relevance of vegetation localization by transesophageal echocardiography in infective endocarditis. *Eur Heart J.* 1992;13:446-452.

61. Sanfilippo AJ, Picard MH, Newell J, et al. Echocardiographic assessment of patients with infectious endocarditis: Prediction of risk for complications. *J Am Coll Cardiol.* 1991;18:1191-1199.

62. Faletra F, Scarpini S, Moreo A, et al. Color Doppler echocardiographic assessment of atrial septal defect size: Correlation with surgical measurements. *J Am Soc Echocardiogr.* 1991;4:429-434.

63. Kronzon I, Tunick PA, Freedburg RS, et al. Transesophageal echocardiography is superior to transthoracic echocardiography in the diagnosis of sinus venosus atrial septal defect. *J Am Coll Cardiol.* 1991;17:537-542.

8 Doppler Echocardiography

Steven L. Schwartz, MD
Natesa G. Pandian, MD

Echocardiography is the most useful diagnostic technique for evaluation of most cardiac disorders. Two-dimensional echocardiography provides detailed information on the morphology of the valves, myocardium and pericardium, function of the valves, and size of the cardiac chambers. The last decade has established Doppler echocardiography as an important tool for studying cardiac flow dynamics. Based on the capability of Doppler to determine the direction and velocity of blood flow, an enormous amount of hemodynamic information can be deduced in a noninvasive manner. In obstructive valvular lesions, transvalvular pressure gradients and estimation of the valve areas can be obtained. Regurgitant and shunt flows are readily detected and evaluated. The technique is also very useful in the assessment of ischemic heart disease, constrictive and restrictive disorders, and cardiac tamponade. The combination of hemodynamic information gained from the various Doppler modalities with the anatomic information provided by 2-dimensional echocardiographic imaging makes the ultrasound technique a powerful diagnostic tool.

PRINCIPLES AND TECHNICAL ASPECTS

The fundamental basis of ultrasound Doppler is relatively simple. A high frequency sound signal, ultrasound, is generated by a crystal within a transducer, and aimed at various regions within the cardiovascular system where red blood cells reflect the ultrasound signals back to the transducer.[1-3] The frequency of the reflected ultrasound waves is altered according to the relative motion of the reflective surface encountered. The difference between the emitted and the reflected frequency is termed the Doppler shift. If the reflected surface is stationary, then the emitted and reflected signals will have identical frequencies and no Doppler shift is observed. If the reflective surface is moving toward or away from the ultrasound source, then the reflected signal will be "shifted" to a higher or lower frequency, respectively. A higher frequency shift will be displayed as a positive deflection on the spectral display screen and a lower frequency shift as a negative deflection. The magnitude of the frequency shift is proportional to the velocity with which the reflective surface is moving toward or receding away from the ultrasound source. Thus the application of these Doppler principles allow for the determination of flow direction and flow velocity.

The precise mathematical relationship between flow velocity and the Doppler shift is illustrated by the Doppler equation:

$$F(d) = \frac{2f}{c} V \cos \theta$$

where F(d)=the frequency or Doppler shift, f=the frequency of the ultrasound generated by the transducer, c=the velocity of ultrasound in tissues (1,540 m/s), V=the velocity of the blood column that is being interrogated and θ, or the Doppler angle=the angle between the ultrasound beam and the long axis of the column of blood. Inspection of the Doppler equation reveals that the shift in frequency is not only related to blood flow velocity but also to the Doppler angle. The larger the angle, the less the magnitude of the frequency shift detected. Only the velocity of the vector component in the direction of the ultrasound beam will be measured. A large Doppler angle will underestimate the blood velocity. It is therefore desirable for the ultrasound beam to be as parallel as possible to the column of blood being interrogated. Generally, when the

Doppler angle is 20° or less, the under-estimation of true velocity is negligible.

Two forms of Doppler modalities are commonly used: continuous-wave (CW) Doppler and pulsed-wave (PW) Doppler. Both are used in a complementary fashion. The differences between the 2 are illustrated in Figure 1. In CW Doppler, the transducer is continuously emitting and receiving ultrasound data and the CW display depicts Doppler shift information reflected from every red blood cell along the path of the ultrasound beam. The advantage of such a system is that high velocity flows can be accurately measured.

In PW Doppler, the transducer alternates between transmission and reception of ultrasound waves. By so doing, depth dis-

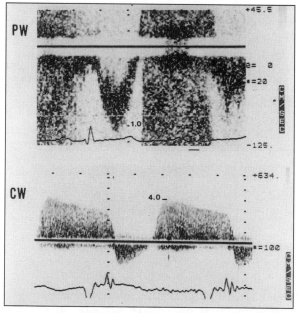

Figure 1. *Pulsed- and continuous-wave Doppler. The tranducer is placed at the apex. The top tracing is a PW recording where the sample volume is placed in the left ventricular outflow tract. The negative deflection which follows the QRS complex represents systolic ejection. Note the normal laminar appearance (hollow center). The curtain-like signals seen in diastole represent turbulent flow of aortic regurgitation which aliases, making it difficult to determine its true direction and velocity. The CW Doppler tracing seen at the bottom clearly characterizes the aortic regurgitation flow as having a direction toward the transducer (positive deflection and a peak velocity of 4 m/s).*

crimination becomes possible. The pulsing of the ultrasound waves allows the selective sampling of an operator-defined region along the path of the ultrasound beam known as the "sample volume." The PW Doppler examination is frequently performed with the guidance of 2-dimensional echocardiography[4] or color-flow Doppler where the sample volume is moved to varying depths and positioned in the regions of interest by the examiner. The number of transmitted pulses per second, or the sampling rate, is limited by their round-trip travel time to and from the target distance (depth of the sample volume). When high velocity flows are encountered, the sampling rate in the pulsed Doppler mode is too slow to accurately measure their velocity and an artifact phenomenon known as "aliasing" occurs. Aliasing on the spectral display is depicted as a cut off of a given flow velocity envelope and the placement of the cut portion on the other side of the reference (zero velocity) baseline. When the blood velocity is high enough, signals on both sides of the baseline merge and a curtain-like pattern is seen as shown in Figure 1. In this situation, it becomes difficult to discern the direction and velocity of blood flow with certainty. The maximum velocity which can be recorded without aliasing (generally 1.5-2 msec) is termed the Nyquist limit, which varies according to the transducer frequency, depth of the sample volume, and the position of the reference baseline.

Color-flow Doppler imaging allows direct, 2-dimensional real-time visualization of flow velocity as a color-coded pattern superimposed on a 2-dimensional echo image (Fig.2, see color plates for all color Doppler figures in this chapter).[5-7]It is essentially a form of PW Doppler where hundreds of sampling sites within a given sector are simultaneously analyzed and assigned a color according to blood flow direction and velocity relative to the transducer. The most commonly used algorithm assigns a red or blue color to blood flow that is moving toward or away from the transducer, respectively. High velocities are represented by brighter hues of these colors. Since color Doppler is a form of PW Doppler, it is subject to the same aliasing phenomenon. If the Nyquist limit is exceeded, color reversal will occur. Thus, high velocity flows travelling toward the transducer may have a central mosaic core containing blue, and those travelling away from the trandsucer may exhibit regions of bright red. This occurs at a lower velocity than pulsed Doppler because of a lower pulse repetition frequency. A third color, usually green, can be added to the map to denote variance. Turbulent flows exhibit a wide range of velocities, or variance. Use of a variance map will add a green color to the mosaic of aliased flow velocities.

INSTRUMENTATION AND EXAMINATION

The frequency of Doppler transducers used today commonly vary between 1.8 and 2.5 MHz. Modern 2-dimensional echocardiographic imaging transducers contain PW, CW, and color Doppler transducers as well, so that placement of the PW sample volume or CW beam is guided by the 2-dimensional image and can be steered electrically to the desired location with a track ball on the imaging console. Although these combined transducers provide high-quality spectral recordings, we still recommend use of the dedicated or "blind" transducer when accurate measurements are required, such as in patients with aortic stenosis. These dedicated transducers, with improved signal-to-noise ratio, smaller transducer heads, and lighter weight are easier to manipulate in the intercostal and suprasternal spaces and thus, can more accurately detect higher velocities.

Controls that must be optimized on the spectral Doppler examination include gain or signal amplitude, compression, and low velocity filter. The gain is adjusted so that the wave form is of appropriate strength; if too low then signals will appear weak or may go undetected, if set too high then noise may interfere with wave-form analysis. The filter is adjusted to eliminate low velocity signals produced by the motion of cardiac walls. In general, when one is examining high-velocity flows, turning up the filter will improve signal quality. Angle correction is also available on most imaging systems but its use is not recommended for cardiac Doppler as over correction may result in

falsely elevated velocity recordings.

Important color-flow controls include gain setting and sector size and location. Their proper adjustment is essential for obtaining optimum results. When the gain is set too high for example, there are excessive bright color signals which obscure the image. If set too low, signals will appear weak, flow jets will appear small, and the severity of regurgitant flows will be underestimated. The gain setting should be carefully set in as standardized a manner as possible. This may be achieved by initially turning the color gain up to saturate the image with artifact, then slowly decreasing the gain to the point were this artifact is virtually gone. Sector size and location can also be selected. In general, the smallest sector size that allows visualization of the desired flow should be chosen, as sector size varies inversely with frame rate. Therefore large sector sizes result in a slower sampling rate compromising the spatial and temporal resolution.

The Doppler examination should be performed as part of the routine 2-dimensional echocardiogram. The path and course of abnormal flow jets are unpredictable and usually do not travel parallel to normal flows. Therefore, to improve detection and assessment of abnormalities, we perform PW, CW, and color-flow Doppler in every view. Using the image guided transducer, the PW sample volume or CW beam is directed to the desired location. Although color-flow imaging has predominantly replaced PW in the assessment of regurgitant jet size, the latter is still useful to define antegrade flows such as aortic and transmitral flow, and also for improved definition and timing of flow jets that may be ambiguous or those jets whose etiology are difficult to define by the color appearance alone.

DOPPLER CHARACTERISTICS OF NORMAL AND ABNORMAL FLOW

When a normally functioning valve opens, full communication between the two chambers (or chamber and great vessel) separated by this valve is established. Only a minimal pressure difference exists (1-2 mm Hg) providing the driving force for forward blood flow, therefore, normal blood flow across the cardiac valves is low in velocity. Normal, physiologic flows contain red blood cells that are moving at approximately the same velocity and are said to be laminar. Because the blood is advancing at uniform velocity, when the PW sample volume is placed within a laminar jet, the resultant tracing exhibits a dark outline and a clear envelope.

The direction of the flow velocity envelope on the spectral display depends on the location of the transducer relative to the direction of blood flow. Flows coming toward the transducer are displayed as positive, and those going away from the transducer are negative. When the transducer is placed at the cardiac apex and the sample volume is placed in the left ventricular outflow tract (Fig. 3) or in the aorta just beyond the aortic valve, blood ejected by the left ventricle into the aorta is moving away from the transducer and is therefore depicted as a negative or downward deflection which follows the QRS complex. The same flow will have a positive deflection when interrogated from the suprasternal notch. Normal aortic flow is also characterized by a rapid rise in velocity reaching its peak value of up to 1.5 m/s usually during the first third of systole.

From the apex, the sample volume may be placed in the left ventricle beneath the mitral valve where the direction of mitral flow is oriented toward the transducer and will therefore be depicted by a positive or an upward deflection. Normal mitral flow, as depicted in Figure 3A, is also laminar and low in velocity, usually under 1 m/s and is biphasic in an individual with an intact sinus mechanism. Most of left ventricular filling takes place in early diastole (E-wave) followed by diastasis and then by a smaller A-wave representing late diastolic filling which occurs as a result of atrial contraction.

Flows within the right-sided chambers and vessels are interrogated in a similar manner to left-sided flows by placing the sample volume of the PW Doppler or directing the CW beam to intercept the flow in question. Generally when comparing right- and left-sided flows across their respective atrioventricular and semilunar valves, right-sided flow profiles tend to have similar morphology to, but lower velocity than their counterpart left-sided flow (Fig. 3A).

Doppler can also be used to interrogate venous flows. Pulmonary venous flow is best depicted using transesophageal echocardiography but can be recorded from the apical transthoracic views. Color guidance of sample volume placement may be useful when the latter is being performed. The normal pattern consists of a systolic and diastolic wave, with the systolic wave being slightly higher (Fig. 3B). At the end of diastole, a retrograde component due to atrial contraction (or atrial reversal) is noted. Systemic venous flow is best recorded from the hepatic vein in the subcostal view of the superior vena cava in the suprasternal view. Systemic venous flow is similar to pulmonary venous flow but exhibits a greater variation with respiration.

Several features characterize abnormal flows. They have increased velocity reflecting the pressure gradient driving the flow, as will be discussed later. When blood passes through a narrowed or deformed orifice, a turbulent jet is created, consisting of red blood cells which have varying direction and velocity, depicted on the PW spectral display as a broad spectral pattern. The resultant jet will have a higher velocity, and because of the turbulence, the envelope recorded will appear "filled in" as opposed to a clear envelope seen with laminar jets. In the case of regurgitant lesions, the abnormal flow will travel in a retrograde direction in relation to the valve.

HEMODYNAMICS

Traditionally, hemodynamic assessment of cardiovascular disorders has been done primarily in the catheterization laboratory. The advent of flow-directed, balloon-tipped catheters has brought hemodynamic monitoring to the bedside in the intensive care unit. These methods require invasive techniques. Doppler echocardiography allows one to assess intracardiac hemodynamics noninvasively. The key to the noninvasive hemodynamic assessment is the Bernoulli equation, which describes the relationship between the pressure gradient and flow velocity across a restrictive orifice. In most clinical situations, pressure gradients can be determined using the modified Bernoulli equation: $P_2 - P_1 = 4 (V_2^2 - V_1^2)$, where $P_2 - P_1 =$ the

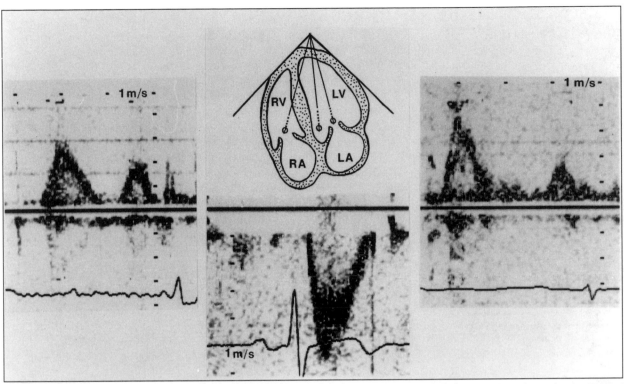

Figure 3A. *PW recording of normal flow patterns obtained from the cardiac apex. The sample volume is positioned within the flow of interest. The tracing on the left represents diastolic tricuspid flow. In the center tracing, the left ventricular outflow tract flow is seen during systole. In the right tracing, diastolic mitral flow is recorded. Note the biphasic appearance of flow across the atrioventricular valves.*

pressure gradient, V_1=the flow velocity proximal to the stenosis, and V_2=the maximum velocity of the stenotic jet. Usually V_1^2 is much less than V_2^2 and is therefore assumed to equal zero. The modified Bernoulli equation is even further simplified: $P_2 - P_1 = 4 V^2$, where V=the maximum post-stenotic flow velocity. This technique has been applied to jets across stenotic valves[8] as well as regurgitant valves.[9-11]

By knowing the maximal velocity across a stenotic valve, one can calculate the gradient across that valve, as in aortic stenosis. Likewise, with knowledge of maximal velocity of a regurgitant jet, we may then be able to determine the pressure on 1 side of the regurgitant valve if the pressure on the other side is known. This can be applied to examination of right ventricular systolic pressures in patients with tricuspid regurgitation. As will be discussed later, the changes in velocity, time intervals, and slopes of spectral tracings can give important hemodynamic information as well.

When using this method to calculate pressure gradients, the following factors must be adhered to in order to insure accuracy: the Doppler beam must be as parallel as possible to the jet in order to record maximal velocity, and the proximal velocity (V_1) should be much less than V_2.

Another hemodynamic variable that can be assessed noninvasively is cardiac output. Flow across an orifice can be determined by the following equation: Q=A x V, where Q=flow, A=orifice area, and V=the integral of velocity curve over time, or time-velocity integral. Using this equation, stroke volume can be determined by measuring the area of any valve orifice and obtaining the velocity across that valve. Cardiac output can be calculated by simply multiplying the stroke volume by the heart rate. Usually, aortic flows and dimensions are used in such calculations because the velocity across a normal aortic valve is easily obtainable, the aortic orifice is relatively circular so the area can be calculated from its diameter, and the

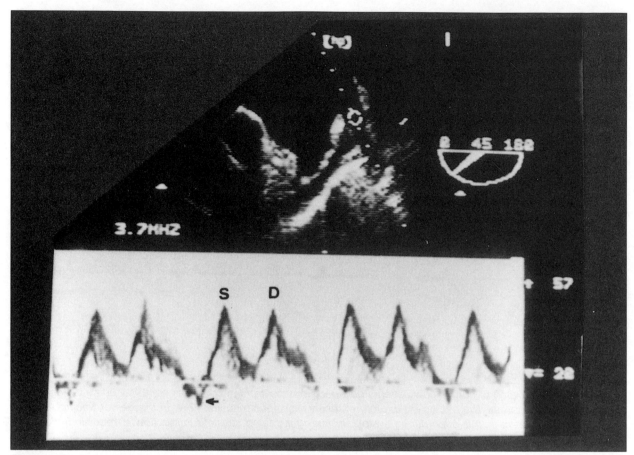

Figure 3B. *Pulsed-wave recording from the left upper pulmonary vein using multiplane transesophageal echocardiography. Antegrade flow into the left atrium is noted in systole (S) and early diastole (D). Late in diastole, there is a small retrograde component (arrow) corresponding to atrial systole.*

orifice size remains relatively constant throughout systole.

Determination of stroke volume in this manner can be applied to other situations as well. Comparing flow across the pulmonic valve to that across the aortic valve in patients with an intracardiac shunt gives the shunt ratio, or Qp:Qs. The continuity equation is another application of stroke volume measurement. This equation states that flow on 1 side of an orifice must equal that on the other side of that orifice, and is expressed in the following manner: $A_1 \times V_1 = A_2 \times V_2$, where V_1 and V_2 are flow velocities proximal and distal to the orifice, and A_1 and A_2 are the areas at the site where velocity is measured. By rearranging this equation, one can solve for a stenotic valve area by knowing the area and velocity proximal to the valve and the maximal flow velocity through the valve.

This equation has proven to be very useful for noninvasive assessment of aortic stenosis.

VALVULAR HEART DISEASE

STENOTIC LESIONS

Doppler echocardiography provides several ways to assess valvular stenoses, as alluded to above. Maximal and mean gradients can be calculated with the Bernoulli equation; and valve areas can be calculated as well.

AORTIC STENOSIS

The 2-dimensional echocardiographic study is useful in delineating the aortic valve morphology. While the presence of valvular thickening and limitation of aortic cusp separation readily identifies patients with abnormal aortic valves, it is unreliable in determining the degree of aortic valvular narrowing.[12,13] It is not uncommon to note valvular restriction on the 2-dimensional examination and ultimately find no trans-valvular pressure gradient. The use of Doppler provides the necessary information to assess the hemodynamic significance of the stenotic valve. Significant aortic valvular obstruction creates turbulent flow, the pressure drop across the valve during systole results in increased flow velocity (Fig. 4), and peak velocity is reached later in systole. Although PW Doppler may be used for the detection and localization of such turbulent flows, it has little value in estimating severity because of its inability to measure high-flow velocities. Such flows are accurately measured with CW Doppler and when applied to the modified Bernoulli equation, the pressure gradient across the aortic valve can be readily derived.[8,14,15] When the maximum velocity is used in the calculation, the maximum instantaneous gradient or "peak gradient" is obtained reflecting the largest systolic pressure difference between the left ventricle and aorta. Although there is a strong correlation between the 2, the maximum instantaneous gradient is somewhat higher than the customary "peak-to-peak" gradient obtained in the catheterization laboratory. One may also average the instantaneous gradient over time to obtain a mean gradient.

Accurate estimation of pressure gradients depends on the precise measurement of blood flow velocity through the stenotic orifice. In order to record the true maximum velocity, it is imperative that the ultrasound beam is aligned as parallel as possible to the long axis of the stenotic jet flow, otherwise the flow velocity and the calculated pressure gradient may be significantly underestimated. Since the direction of stenotic jets is often eccentric and un-predictable in a given patient, the examiner must utilize multiple sampling sites for CW Doppler interrogation of the ascending aorta and use the highest value obtained in the calculation of pressure gradients. Doppler sampling sites in patients with aortic stenosis should include the apical, subcostal, right parasternal and suprasternal views. The

acquisition of the highest possible flow velocity requires a compulsive, systematic examination by an experienced operator.

It is important to note that pressure gradients, whether obtained by Doppler or catheterization, are related not only to valve area but cardiac output as well. Therefore, in states of abnormal cardiac output, the use of velocity and pressure gradients alone to assess the severity of valvular stenosis may lead to erroneous conclusions. Flow velocity is increased in high cardiac output states such as encountered with a hyperdynamic left ventricle or in aortic regurgitation and will therefore overestimate the severity of aortic stenosis. Conversely, velocity is decreased in low output states such as ischemic cardiomyopathy or end-stage aortic stenosis and will therefore underestimate true severity. However, Doppler validation studies with cardiac catheterization show that peak aortic velocity flow of greater than 3 m/s or the ratio of left ventricular outflow velocity to aortic velocity of less than 0.25 are highly sensitive indicators for detecting critical aortic stenosis (AS), and therefore their absence can be used reliably to exclude the condition.[15] Flow velocity greater than 4.5 m/s is highly specific for critical aortic stenosis but not sensitive.[15,16] Values in between have less diagnostic value. A velocity of only 3.5 m/s for example, may represent the maximum velocity obtained in patients with critical AS with co-existing depressed left ventricular function. In such settings of abnormal cardiac output, the noninvasive calculation of aortic valve area using the continuity equation, rather than the use of pressure gradients alone, more accurately reflects aortic stenosis severity. The previously discussed continuity equation is based on the principal that flow volume proximal to, distal to, and at the site of obstruction are identical. The equation may be rearranged in the following manner to solve for the stenotic aortic valve area:

$$A_2 = \frac{A_1 \times V_1}{V_2}$$

The diameter of the left ventricular outflow tract is measured in the parasternal long axis view and its cross sectional area (A_1), which is assumed to have a circular configuration is

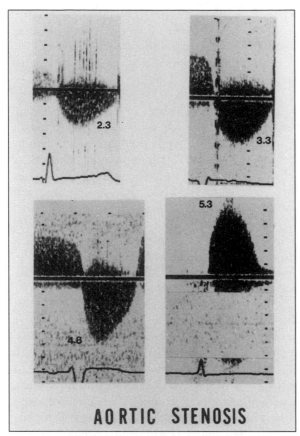

AORTIC STENOSIS

Figure 4. Continuous-wave Doppler recordings from 4 patients with aortic stenosis of varying severity. The peak velocity of the tracing on top left is 2.3 m/s which corresponds to a maximal instantaneous gradient (MIG) of 21 mm Hg which is consistent with mild aortic stenosis. The tracing on top right is from a patient with moderate aortic stenosis, MIG is 44 mm Hg. The recording on bottom left, taken from a patient with critical aortic stenosis, as a peak velocity of 4.8 m/s which translates to a MIG of 92 mm Hg. The tracing on bottom right was recorded from the suprasternal position in a patient with critical aortic stenosis, the flow is toward the transducer and recorded as positive. MIG is 110 mm Hg.

calculated with the simple algebraic formula: Area $= \Pi r^2$, substituting one-half the diameter for r. Flow velocity in the left ventricular outflow tract (V_1) is obtained by PW Doppler from the apical views where the sample volume is positioned immediately beneath the aortic valve. V_2 is the maximum flow velocity obtained at or beyond the valve by CW Doppler examination from multiple transducer orientations. In using

the continuity equation, V_1 and V_2 may be expressed as peak velocities, mean velocities, or time velocity integrals. In the presence of atrial fibrillation, the average of multiple consecutive beats is used in the calculation. Because velocity information from the left ventricular outflow tract proximal to the obstruction, which is directly influenced by cardiac output, is incorporated into the continuity equation, this method is especially useful in estimating aortic stenosis severity in the setting of abnormal cardiac output and is theoretically valid even in the setting of severe aortic insufficiency.

Some cautions should be expressed in the use of the continuity equation method to derive aortic valve area. Derivation of the left ventricular outflow tract area (A_1) assumes a circular configuration. The left ventricular outflow tract, bounded by the interventricular septum and the anterior mitral leaflet is dynamic throughout the cardiac cycle and may not have a perfectly circular cross-section. Furthermore the diameter of the left ventricular outflow tract may be difficult to accurately measure in patients with stenotic valves which are occasionally surrounded by echo bright calcifications. This measurement has been identified as the greatest source of interobserver variability.[17] Flow velocity in the left ventricular outflow tract (V_1) may vary with minor alterations in the position of the sample volume, especially in the region where prestenotic acceleration of flow occurs. The sample volume should be withdrawn to a region just proximal to this acceleration. Finally, obtaining the maximum velocity across the stenotic valve (V_2) via proper alignment of the CW beam with the stenotic jet is time consuming and requires a considerable amount of operator expertise. Despite these difficulties however, the non-invasive calculation of aortic valve area has been validated with values obtained at cardiac catheterization in numerous centers with excellent correlations.[15–20]

RIGHT VENTRICULAR OUTFLOW OBSTRUCTION

Obstruction to right ventricular outflow can be at the valvular level (pulmonic stenosis), subvalvular level (infundibular stenosis), or peripheral level (pulmonary artery stenosis). Interrogation of the infundibulum, pulmonic valve, pulmonary trunk, and proximal right and left pulmonary arteries can be accomplished from either parasternal or subcostal windows. Flow profiles seen in valvular pulmonic stenosis and main pulmonary artery stenosis are similar to those seen in aortic stenosis, while infundibular stenosis gives a similar profile to subaortic obstruction. As with other valvular lesions, gradients calculated from CW Doppler recordings correlate well with hemodynamic data.[21] Increased flow across the pulmonic valve, seen in patients with right ventricular volume overload, can lead to mildly elevated flow velocities recorded across the pulmonic valve. These patients can be differentiated from those with stenotic lesions by noting increased flow in the right ventricle as well as the pulmonary artery, without a localized increase in flow velocity.[22]

MITRAL STENOSIS

Two-dimensional echocardiography plays an important role in the evaluation of mitral stenosis (MS). It is used to survey the various cardiac chambers sizes and to provide detailed morphological information pertaining to the mitral valve and submitral structures. Estimation of mitral valve area is possible by direct planimetry of the valve orifice in those with technically satisfactory parasternal short axis images. Doppler is used to provide important hemodynamic information to supplement and confirm the 2-dimensional echocardiographic findings.[23-25] When a normally functioning mitral valve opens, early diastolic filling occurs and the left atrium and left ventricular diastolic pressures rapidly equalize as depicted by the normal swift diastolic descent of the Doppler flow velocity profile. In MS, the transmitral pressure gradient is initially elevated and persists longer into diastole, resulting in a high-peak velocity at the onset of left ventricular filling and a slow decline of the diastolic velocity profile. The rate of decline corresponds to the degree of obstruction and is used to gauge its severity (Fig. 5). The best mitral flow velocity profile is obtained when the transducer is placed at the cardiac apex. Since the Doppler flow velocity does not usually exceed the Nyquist limit even in severe MS, either PW or CW Doppler may be utilized. Color Doppler may serve as a guide to orient the Doppler ultrasound beam as parallel to the stenotic jet as possible. The mean transmitral pressure gradient is derived by measuring multiple instantaneous velocities at small time intervals throughout diastole and employing the modified Bernoulli equation. Doppler may also be used for the noninvasive estimation of mitral valve area using the principle of pressure half-time. This is especially pertinent in situations where factors other than the degree of valvular stenosis may influence the mean gradient such as increased flow across the mitral valve from significant co-existent mitral regurgitation or in changes in diastolic filling times from variations in heart rate. Pressure half-time ($t_{1/2}$), is defined as the time in milliseconds that it takes for the transvalvular diastolic gradient to decay to half its initial peak value. Since the spectral display reflects velocity measurements and the relationship between pressure and velocity is quadratic ($\Delta P = 4 \times V^2$), $t_{1/2}$ may be expressed in terms of velocity rather than pressure, (i.e., the time required for the velocity to fall to a value corresponding to the initial velocity divided by $\sqrt{2}$ [or simply multiplied by 0.7]). The $t_{1/2}$ in normal individuals ranges from 20-60 msec. The narrower the mitral orifice, the flatter the diastolic slope of the velocity profile and the more prolonged the $t_{1/2}$ will be. Hatle and coworkers have shown that a mitral valve area of 1 cm^2 corresponds to a $t_{1/2}$ of 220 msec. Accordingly, mitral valve area may be estimated by dividing 220 by the $t_{1/2}$:

$$\text{MVA} = \frac{220 \text{ msec}}{t_{(1/2)}}$$

The pressure half-time derivation of mitral valve area is independent of heart rate, stroke volume, mitral regurgitation, and the presence of atrial fibrillation. Pressure half-time, because it relates the rate of decline of the gradient between the left atrium and left ventricle, may be affected by ventricular abnormalities such as severe aortic regurgitation, left ventricular hypertrophy, or coronary artery disease.[26,27] Altered left atrial compliance, observed immediately following balloon valvuloplasty, also effects pressure half-time and one should use caution in its use in the acute period following balloon valvuloplasty.[28]

In these circumstances, the continuity equation described above has been advocated to assess mitral valve area.[29] The time velocity integral of the aortic flow multiplied by the area of the LV outflow tract, divided by the time velocity integral of the mitral flow will provide the mitral valve area. This method is not valid when there is more than trivial regurgitation across either the mitral or aortic valve, as the presence of such regurgitation will alter the forward flow. In our laboratory, we reserve use of the continuity equation to those circumstances when the pressure half-time does not apply and 2-dimensional planimetry of the valve is not feasible because of poor image quality, heavily calcified mitral leaflets, or inability to obtain adequate short axis views of the mitral valve.

To ensure diagnostic accuracy, both Doppler derived $t_{1/2}$ and planimetry of the mitral orifice in the 2-dimensional echocardiographic examination should be utilized whenever possible and their results compared in each patient with MS.

TRICUSPID STENOSIS

Tricuspid stenosis (TS) should be carefully searched for in all patients with rheumatic heart disease. Like MS, the hallmark of TS is the demonstration of valve thickening and diastolic doming on the 2-dimensional echocardiographic study. The direct planimetry of the tricuspid orifice however, is not possible. Doppler evaluation of tricuspid flow in TS is similar to that of mitral flow in MS but because of the relatively uncommon nature of TS, it is less well-studied. With increasing severity of TS, the peak tricuspid flow is increased and the diastolic descent of the flow velocity is prolonged.[30] The mean diastolic gradient and pressure half-time are calculated in the same manner as in MS but the latter is less useful as

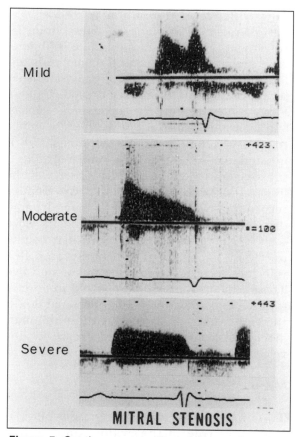

Figure 5. *Continuous-wave Doppler recordings from the apex in mitral stenosis. The top tracing is from a patient with mild mitral stenosis, valve area was calculated to be 2.2 cm2. The middle tracing is from a patient with moderate mitral stenosis. The tracing on the bottom was recorded from a patient with critical mitral stenosis, mitral valve area was 0.5 cm2. Notice the deceleration slope becomes more flat as mitral stenosis becomes more severe.*

the mathematical relationship required to estimate tricuspid valve area has not yet been fully elucidated.

REGURGITANT LESIONS

Assessment of valvular regurgitation requires integration of all modes of Doppler echocardiography. PW Doppler can be used to systematically "map" the jet by carefully moving the sample volume to various locations proximal to the valve orifice. This method is tedious and time consuming and has largely been abandoned as color-flow mapping provides the same information but requires less time to perform and interpret. The size of the turbulent regurgitant jet as displayed by color Doppler correlates with the severity of the regurgitation and is discussed in greater detail below. When performing and interpreting color Doppler examinations, one must keep in mind that the color-flow display is merely a velocity map of moving blood cells and is not a volumetric representation of regurgitant flow, nor is it analogous to angiography (which is also an imperfect technique). Factors such as gain setting, pulse repetition frequency, and even imaging system may have vast effects on the appearance of a given flow jet.[31] Furthermore, there is no true gold standard by which to measure any method of assessment of regurgitation.

Quantification of the regurgitant volume and fraction can be calculated for both aortic and mitral regurgitation using 2-dimensional echocardiography in conjunction with PW Doppler by measuring volumetric forward flow across the valves.[32-34] As mentioned earlier in this chapter, volumetric flow equals the time velocity integral multiplied by the area of the orifice. Thus, forward flow through the aortic valve, or aortic stroke volume, can be calculated by multiplying the area of the LV outflow tract by the time velocity integral of aortic flow. Likewise, mitral flow or stroke volume is the product of the area of the mitral annulus (derived from the diameter of the annulus, assuming a circular shape and employing the formula Πr^2) and the time velocity integral of the mitral flow with the PW sample volume placed at the level of the mitral annulus. The following formulae can be used to calculate regurgitant volume and fraction.

For MR: RV = Mitral stroke volume- aortic stroke volume
RF = RV/mitral stroke volume
For AR: RV = Aortic stroke volume- mitral stroke volume
RF = RV/aortic stroke volume

RV is regurgitant volume and RF is regurgitant fraction. These methods are quantitative as opposed to the semiquantitative techniques of color-flow analysis and angiography. Another index, the regurgitant orifice area, can be calculated by dividing the regurgitant volume by the time velocity integral of the regurgitant flow from the CW tracing.[35] Unfortunately, these methods can only be used when one valve is regurgitant; if more than trivial regurgitation is present across both valves, these equations are invalid. In these cases, pulmonic flow may be substituted as the reference for forward stroke volume, however care must be taken to accurately measure the diameter of the pulmonic annulus as the anterior surface is often poorly defined in adults. Other applications of PW, CW, and color-flow Doppler specific to the various types of regurgitation are discussed below.

AORTIC REGURGITATION

Doppler echocardiography has proven to be a highly sensitive method for the diagnosis of aortic insufficiency. The presence of aortic regurgitation detected by Doppler echocardiography, even if very mild, indicates at least a minor abnormality of the aortic valve.[36] Both pulsed and continuous-wave Doppler recordings of aortic regurgitation are seen as a high velocity, holodiastolic flow, as shown in Figure 1. The appearance of aortic insufficiency on PW tracings is that of a curtain-like holodiastolic flow pattern due to aliasing. Continuous-wave Doppler recorded from the apex, as illustrated in Figures 1 and 6, reveals a characteristic profile with a decrescendo pattern in which the peak velocity, at least 3 m/s, occurs immediately after aortic valve closure. The timing of onset of flow is an important point in differentiation from mitral flow, which commences after the isovolumic relaxation phase. Spectral recordings of the flow in the proximal descending aorta with the transducer in the suprasternal position may exhibit a retrograde diastolic flow signal. In the presence of severe regurgitation, these tracings may resemble a "sine wave" pattern (Fig. 6). Color Doppler is useful for the identification of aortic insufficiency. As shown in Figure 7, a bright, mosaic, retrograde jet emanating from the aortic valve that persists throughout diastole is seen in the left ventricular outflow tract in the parasternal long axis, short axis, or apical views.

The color of the jet depends upon transducer location and jet orientation. From the apical views, the jet is predominantly red, however from the parasternal views the color is variable. If the jet is directed toward the anterior mitral leaflet, as in the majority of cases, it will be a shade of blue. However, if the jet is directed toward the septum, a reddish hue will be seen.

Pulsed Doppler, CW, and color-flow imaging can be used to grade the severity of aortic insufficiency. Pulsed Doppler sampling of the left ventricular outflow tract may be employed to "map" the jet. The further from the aortic valve the jet is detected, the more severe the regurgitation. Grading systems have employed intracardiac landmarks for determination of severity, just beneath the valve is grade I, up to the tip of the anterior mitral leaflet is grade II, up to the papillary muscles is grade III, and beyond the papillary muscle level is grade IV. The problems with this method are that the technique may be time consuming and tedious to accurately perform, the depth at which regurgitant flow is detected can vary with different sized ventricles; additionally, antegrade mitral flow, especially in the presence of mitral stenosis or prosthesis, may contaminate the aortic regurgitation flow signal. For these reasons, other Doppler methods are preferable.

The ability to measure instantaneous gradients with CW Doppler has proven useful in assessing the severity of aortic insufficiency. Severe regurgitation tends to result in rapid equalization of diastolic aortic and ventricular pressures. This relationship forms the basis for analysis of CW tracings. Steeper deceleration slope and shorter pressure half-time, both indicative of a more rapidly diminishing gradient between the aortic and left ventricle, are observed with increasing severity of aortic insufficiency (Fig. 6).[37–39] In general, a slope of greater than 2 m/s^2 and a pressure half-time of less than 400 msec are indicative of at least moderate aortic insufficiency, and a slope of greater than 4 m/s^2 represents severe regurgitation. Acute, severe aortic regurgitation is associated with a steep slope and rapid pressure half-time (<180 msec); flow may stop before the end of diastole. Drawbacks to quantification of aortic regurgitation in this manner include the overlap between groups and the properties of the ventricle may also effect the aortic-ventricular gradient and the flow velocity profile. Patients with elevated ventricular diastolic pressures for reasons other than aortic insufficiency (i.e., aortic stenosis) may have relatively steeper deceleration slopes and shorter pressure half-times, therefore this method may overestimate the severity of regurgitation in these patients.[40]

Color-flow mapping, with the ability to visualize regurgitant jets, is an attractive method to rate severity of valvular insufficiency. Attempts to use the length and area of the jet in the ventricle as recorded from the apical views have proven to be less than satisfactory.[41,42] Examination of the regurgitant jets in the parasternal views is useful. By comparing the height of the jet in the left ventricular outflow tract as seen in the parasternal long axis view to the height of the outflow tract, one can accurately assess the severity of aortic insufficiency.[41] Likewise, the ratio between the area of the jet as visualized on the parasternal short axis view and the area of the outflow tract also correlates well with the severity of regurgitation.[41,43] Though the grading system has yet to be precisely defined, data from 1 report supports the following scheme: for parasternal long axis, a jet height/outflow tract height ratio of less than 25% would signify grade I; 25% to 46%, grade II; 47% to 64%, grade III; and >65%, grade IV.[44] These cutoff points, while useful, have yet to be validated by independent investigators. There are some potential problems that must be kept in mind with this type of analysis. The regurgitant jet can spread out and disperse very quickly after entering the left ventricular outflow tract; care must be taken to evaluate the jet as close as possible to the valve itself. Aortic valve morphology can also affect the appearance of the jet.[44] Patients with bicuspid valves frequently have very eccentric jets that travel anteriorly directly toward the interventricular septum or posteriorly directly at the anterior mitral leaflet. The appearance of the jet by color Doppler as it emanates from the aortic valve is almost vertical and is therefore not amenable to the type of analysis mentioned above.

PULMONIC REGURGITATION

Mild regurgitation across the pulmonic valve is a common finding in healthy adults. It can be detected by pulsed and CW Doppler, and as with aortic insufficiency a holodiastolic flow is recorded. The flow profile recorded using CW Doppler is similar to that of aortic insufficiency, except that an accentuated decrease in velocity following atrial contraction is seen in patients in normal sinus rhythm. The peak velocities are lower than those recorded with aortic regurgitation, which is an expected finding as the

gradient between the pulmonary artery and right ventricle in diastole is lower than that between the aorta and left ventricle. In normal individuals, the peak diastolic velocity is less than 2.0 m/s, though it is higher in patients with pulmonary hypertension. Pulmonic regurgitation is seen on color Doppler display as a red, flame-shaped jet emanating from the valve cusps. It can be visualized in the right ven-

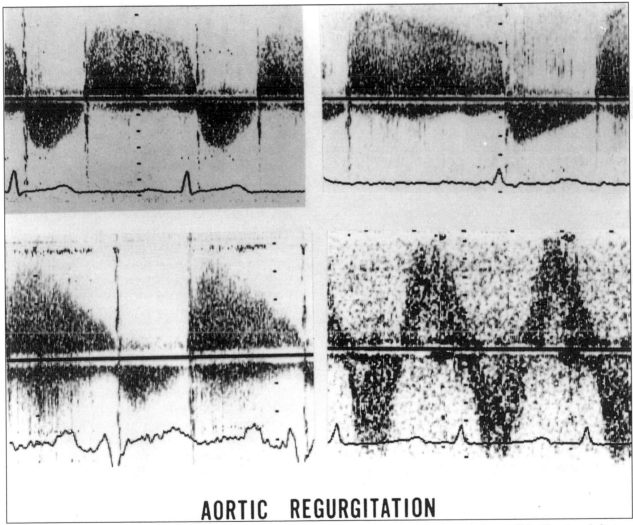

AORTIC REGURGITATION

Figure 6. Doppler recordings from four patients with varying degrees of aortic insufficiency (AI). The top left, top right, and bottom left tracings are CW Doppler recordings from the apex. The tracing in the top left was recorded from a patient with mild AI. The deceleration slope is 1.8 m/s². The deceleration slope seen on the top right is 3.2 m/s², which corresponds with moderate AI. The bottom left recording was obtained from a patient with severe AI who required valve replacement. The downslope of the tracing in this patient is quite steep at 6.9 m/s². The tracing on bottom right is a PW Doppler recording with the transducer at the suprasternal postion and the sample volume in the descending aorta. The retrograde flow seen in diastole is almost equal to the forward flow in systole, consistent with severe AI.

tricular outflow view and the parasternal short axis view.

No system has been devised yet for grading pulmonic insufficiency, though regurgitant jets seen by PW Doppler or color Doppler that are restricted to 1 or 2 cm proximal to the pulmonic valve are considered within normal limits, and can be detected in the majority of healthy individuals.[45,46] In patients with pathologic pulmonic regurgitation, the jets are wider and extend deeper into the right ventricle.

Analysis of the pulmonary insufficiency profile also gives hemodynamic information. Peak diastolic velocity correlates well with mean pulmonary artery pressure; values over 2 m/s indicate pulmonary hypertension. End-diastolic velocity measured by Doppler correlates well with hemodynamic measurements of end-diastolic gradient between the pulmonary artery and right ventricle as well as the right ventricular end-diastolic pressure. Though the correlation is excellent, predicted values are consistently underestimated by this technique.[47] Nevertheless, a pulmonary regurgitant profile that exhibits a steep deceleration slope or premature cessation of flow is a reliable sign of elevated right ventricular end-diastolic pressure.

MITRAL REGURGITATION

All Doppler modalities, PW, CW, and color-flow Doppler have demonstrated excellent sensitivity and specificity for detecting mitral regurgitation (MR). With PW Doppler, when the sample volume is placed in the left atrium just above a normally functioning mitral valve, only diastolic mitral flow is recorded. There is no systolic flow. In the presence of MR, a retrograde turbulent signal which aliases will be detected during systole. The full flow profile maybe obtained with CW Doppler. As shown in Figure 8, it is characterized by a high peak velocity reaching 4-6 m/s reflecting the systolic pressure gradient across the mitral valve. The flow profile also appears symmetric and broad-based spanning both isovolumic contraction and relaxation phases of the cardiac cycle. This serves as a useful feature to distinguish MR flow from aortic flow. With color-flow Doppler, MR is readily identified as a bright systolic jet (because of its high velocity)

spurting out from the mitral valve orifice and receding to fill a portion of the left atrial cavity. When the transducer is placed at the cardiac apex, the jet is blue in color (flow is oriented away from the transducer), and usually displays a mosaic pattern reflecting the velocity spectrum variance within turbulent flow (Fig. 9A).

There are several possible approaches for gauging MR severity. As mentioned previously, quantitation of regurgitant volume is possible by subtracting forward systolic aortic flow from total mitral diastolic flow. The signal intensity and the deceleration rate of the CW derived flow profile may also yield useful information. The most widely used approach however, is a semiquantitative grading system using PW or color-flow Doppler. With PW Doppler, the sample volume is systematically moved to explore various regions within the left atrial cavity to map out the size of the flow disturbance.[48] Grading is based on the maximum depth where the flow disturbance is detected within the left atrium. Although this approach has shown acceptable correlation with angiographic grading of MR, the technique requires the point by point mapping of the entire left atrium in multiple views, which can be time consuming and may underestimate severity, especially when the jet is eccentric, clinging to an atrial wall, or over-estimate severity when a narrow jet extends far onto the left atrium.

Although PW mapping of the regurgitant jet is being outmoded in favor of color-flow mapping, recording pulmonary venous flow velocities with PW is useful in the assessment of mitral regurgitation. Normally, the systolic component of pulmonary venous flow is slightly greater than the diastolic component. With increasing severity of mitral regurgitation, the systolic component becomes less prominent (Fig. 9A). In patients with 3+ mitral regurgitation, the systolic component is markedly blunted. Systolic reversal is noted in severe (4+) mitral regurgitation.[49] While such analysis is most easily performed using transesophageal echocardiography, careful interrogation of the pulmonary veins from the transthoracic apical windows can provide this information as well. When assessing pulmonary venous flow, it is imperative that both left and right pulmonary veins are assessed, as

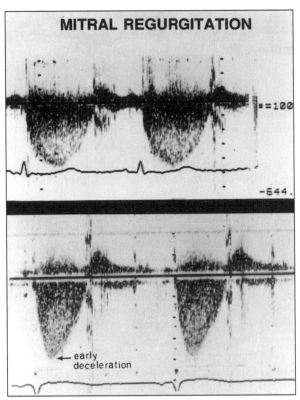

Figure 8. *These tracings were obtained from 2 different patients with mitral regurgitation. Note the symetric contour of the top tracing. In contrast, the bottom tracing shows early deceleration signifying a rapid decline in pressure gradient between the left ventricle and left atrium during systole that results from the precipitous rise in left atrial pressure. This is the correlate of the hemodynamic presence of a V-wave.*

patients with eccentric jets can exhibit different patterns in the right or left pulmonary vein, depending on the direction of the flow jet. Although we have found this method useful in our laboratory, we have noted some patients with severe mitral insufficiency who exhibit antegrade systolic pulmonary venous flow. These patients have large left atria that are presumably very compliant. One must also realize that other factors, such as left atrial pressure effect the pulmonary venous tracing. This will be discussed in more detail later in this chapter.

Color-flow Doppler allows direct observation of the dynamic features and orientation of a regurgitant jet and thus permits rapid and more precise evaluation of MR severity (Fig. 9A).[50–52] From multiple orthogonal views, the 3-dimen-

sional characteristics of the jet may be mentally reconstructed. It has been shown that the best correlation with angiographic grading of MR is achieved when jet area, rather than length, as considered from multiple views or when the ratio of jet area to cross sectional left atrial area were utilized. A maximum jet area from multiple views measuring 8 cm² or more, or a jet area to left atrium area ratio of 40% or more indicates severe MR, whereas a jet area measuring 4 cm² or less or a jet area to left atrium area ratio of 20% or less indicates mild MR.[51,52]

Several points should be considered when using the color Doppler approach to gauge MR severity. Factors other than regurgitation volume may influence jet area. Jets visualized with color Doppler are composed not only of regurgitant flows but also atrial blood displaced by the regurgitant flow making it difficult to define the precise boundaries of the jet. When using transesophageal echocardiography, the appearance of the regurgitant jet is larger than on transthoracic echocardiography in the same patient.[53,54] Eccentric jets, those that track along a valve leaflet and the atrial wall, also pose a problem when using jet area to grade severity (Fig. 9A). These jets are usually seen in patients with severe mitral valve prolapse and chordal rupture (i.e., flail leaflet), endocarditis with leaflet perforation or flail, paraprosthetic leaks, or systolic anterior motion. The disparity between jet size and degree of regurgitation is not merely because such jets are of markedly different sizes in different echocardiographic views. For eccentric jets, the area of turbulence displayed by color-flow mapping markedly underestimates the regurgitant volume. Additionally, the correlation between regurgitant volume and area of eccentric jets is poor.[55,56] When such eccentric jets are present, we rely on a combination of factors in grading jet severity. These include proximal jet width, pulmonary venous flow, density of the CW jet, and early systolic velocity, and the 2-dimensional appearance of the valve. Severe regurgitation is present if the actual regurgitant orifice can be seen, the CW tracing of the jet is intense, the regurgitant jet is wide at the mitral orifice, and/or the "E" wave velocity is elevated.

Other factors, such as the effect of the

interaction between incoming pulmonary venous flow and the regurgitant jet's velocity is not well known. Jet areas may also vary from one machine to another depending on their respective converter algorithm and resolution.[31,57] Also, since the area of flow disturbance represents velocity data, it is subject to underestimation when the Doppler angle is large. This is not likely to represent a significant confounding factor however, because multiple views are used and MR flow velocity is high, the precise measurement of which is less relevant than its mere detection in a given area. Despite these potential influences the technique yields good correlations with angiography and serves as a very useful noninvasive means of detecting MR, gauging its severity, and serially following progression over time.

Newer Methods

Although analysis of color-flow mapping in the assessment of regurgitant lesions is predominantly semiquantitative, quantitative techniques are being investigated. These involve measuring the proximal flow convergence region or the proximal isovelocity surface area (PISA). This analysis is based on the principles that flow accelerates proximal to a restrictive orifice (a regurgitant orifice is restrictive) with increasing velocity closer to the orifice. The pattern of flow acceleration is such that a series of isovelocity lines can be drawn around the orifice, approximating a hemielliptical shape. As discussed earlier in this chapter, volumetric flow is the product of area and velocity. Thus, the instantaneous flow volume at any of these isovelocity lines can be calculated by multiplying the velocity and the surface area of the hemielliptical shell created by the isovelocity line. Expressed in another way:

$$Q = A \times V$$
$$A = 2\Pi r^2$$
$$Q = 2\Pi r^2 \times V$$

where Q=instantaneous regurgitant flow, A=area of the hemiellipse, r=the radius of the hemiellipse, and V=instantaneous flow velocity.

When color Doppler is applied to patients with mitral regurgitation (or any lesion with a restrictive orifice), the proximal acceleration or flow convergence region can be identified by a mosaic pattern on the ventricular side of the mitral valve. An isovelocity line can be identified as the point of red-blue aliasing (Fig. 9B). The velocity along this line of aliasing, the Nyquist limit, is known. The radius is measured as the distance from the orifice to the aliasing line. By multiplying the square of this radius by the Nyquist velocity and 2Π, the instantaneous regurgitant volume can be calculated.[58,59] The color map is set for a low Nyquist number, which will increase the radius of the aliased isovelocity line, making this measurement more accurate. Using this method, the instantaneous regurgitant volumes calculated have demonstrated excellent agreement with in vitro models of regurgitation, as well as angiographic grade of mitral regurgitation, and regurgitant volume in clinical use.[58] Total regurgitant volume has been derived by multiplying the instantaneous volume by the ratio of the time velocity integral and the peak velocity of the regurgitant jet, both measured from the CW tracing.[60] Regurgitant orifice area has also been calculated by dividing the instantaneous regurgitant flow volume by the maximal flow velocity.[61]

Advantages to the flow convergence method include that it is quantitative, independent of orifice shape in vitro,[62] and independent of technical factors such as gain and pulse repetition frequency.[62] It has also been applied to the assessment of shunt flows[63] and stenotic lesions.[64] However, the clinical use of flow convergence remains limited; measurements are made from 1 frame in 1 view which may not apply to the entire period of regurgitation, orifice shape may have an effect in clinical use, and cardiac motion has been shown to alter radius measurements.[65] Additionally, analysis of flow convergence may not be feasible in most patients with aortic regurgitation. While the flow convergence or PISA method is a promising quantitative tool, further work needs to be done before employing it clinically.

TRICUSPID REGURGITATION

Tricuspid regurgitation may be diagnosed by the presence of a retrograde holosystolic flow disturbance proximal to the tricuspid valve. The spectral tracings observed are similar to those seen in the presence of mitral regurgitation, except that the peak velocity recorded from tricuspid regurgitation is lower due to the lower pressure gradient between the right atrium and right ventricle in systole. Color-flow images of tricuspid regurgitant jets also appear similar to mitral regurgitant jets, though the lower flow velocity of tricuspid insufficiency leads to less frequency aliasing. Many views can be employed to detect tricuspid regurgitation, including the right ventricular inflow view, the parasternal short axis view at the aortic valve level, apical 4 and 5 chamber views, subcostally via the four chamber or the short axis view, and the right parasternal view. Flow is away from the transducer and is therefore depicted as "negative" on spectral tracings and blue on color imaging, though when imaged subcostally or from the right thorax, this is not always the case.

When assessing the severity of tricuspid regurgitation, one should keep in mind that depending on age, 15% to 80% of otherwise healthy individuals have tricuspid regurgitation detectable by Doppler.[45,66] In general, tricuspid regurgitant flows detectable only in the vicinity of the tricuspid valve and with flow velocities in the range of 2.0-2.6 m/s in the presence of a normal-sized right atrium are considered "physiologic." Patients with more severe tricuspid regurgitation are identified by a regurgitant jet that can be detected in a larger portion of the right atrium or by retrograde systolic flow in the hepatic vein (Fig. 10). A regurgitant jet seen by color Doppler occupying greater than one-third of the area of the right atrium is seen in patients judged to warrant tricuspid annuloplasty at surgery.[67] As illustrated in Figure 10, in the presence of severe valvular pathology such as Ebstein's anomaly, carcinoid, or endocarditis, the profile of the regurgitant jet may be of relatively low velocity (<3m/s) and may appear laminar in PW tracings. This signifies a very large regurgitant orifice that blood can flow through without turbulence, which, in extreme cases, represents a functionally common right-sided chamber.[68]

PROSTHETIC VALVES

The basic principles described for Doppler assessment of normal valves apply to prosthetic valves as well. The normally functioning prosthetic valve differs from the native valve in that higher flow velocities are recorded across prosthetic valves in the absence of pathology. Transvalvular flow velocities of up to 4.0 m/s have been recorded across normal prosthetic valves in the aortic position.[69-75] Despite high flow velocities, Doppler recordings of prosthetic valves differ from stenotic native valves in that the peak velocity occurs earlier and the acceleration slope is steeper. There is a weak inverse correlation between peak velocity and valve size. In general, velocities and gradients are higher and observed valve areas lower for ball-in-cage valves, followed by bioprosthetic valves and disc valves. Doppler echocardiography can be used to assess prosthetic valve function in a manner similar to native valves, however there are some caveats. Gradients calculated by the Bernoulli equation and valve areas calculated by the pressure half-time method correlate well with those obtained by catheterization in some studies.[72,73,76-79] Other studies point out overestimation of gradient and underestimation of valve area when echocardiographic methods are used, often despite good correlation.[77,80-82] These differences appear to be dependent upon valve type, and are most notable in St. Jude and Starr-Edwards valves. Pressure recovery distal to the valve and localized gradients produced by the geometry of the valve itself have been the proposed reasons for the discrepancies.[80,81] Evaluation of a patient with possible prosthetic valve obstruction should not depend only on the velocity observed during a given echocardiographic evaluation, but on the clinical status of the patient and on the results of prior echocardiographic studies. In many laboratories, including our own, patients undergo an echocardiographic examination prior to discharge following prosthetic valve implantation to determine the baseline hemodynamics of that particular valve.

Regurgitation across prosthetic valves is common, detectable by Doppler across virtually all normally functioning valves. This however, is usually trivial or mild, and limited to the vicinity of the prosthesis. Each valve type has its own distinct pattern of regurgitation. In general, bioprosthetic valves demonstrate small central

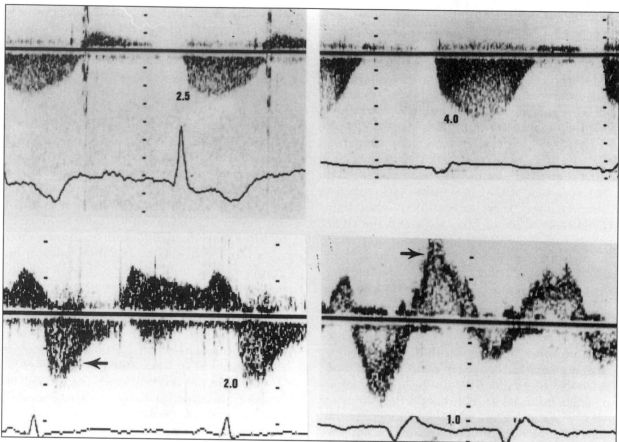

Figure 10. *Doppler recordings of tricuspid regurgitation. The tracing on top left was recorded from a patient with mild tricuspid regurgitation and normal right ventricular pressures. Peak velocity is 2.5 m/s. The recording on top right is from a patient with tricuspid regurgitation. Peak velocity is 4.0 m/s and corresponds to a 64 mm Hg systolic pressure gradient between the right ventricle and right atrium indicating the presence of pulmonary hypertension. The bottom 2 tracings are recorded from a patient with severe tricuspid regurgitation secondary to carcinoid heart disease. The regurgitant orifice is large, the right atrial pressure is markedly elevated, but right ventricular systolic pressure is only mildly elevated so the peak velocity recorded is only 2.0 m/s. Right atrial pressure rises rapidly causing the flow velocity to decelerate rapidly (arrow). The bottom right tracing is a pulsed Doppler recording from the hepatic vein in the same patient. The severe tricuspid regurgitation causes retrograde systolic flow in the systemic veins (arrow).*

regurgitant jets; the jets in mechanical valves arise from the interfaces between the disc and the sewing ring.[83-85] Using transesophageal echocardiography, the appearance of the jet changes as the imaging plane changes from the horizontal to vertical planes. Color Doppler has proven useful in the detection of pathologic prosthetic valve insufficiency, being able to differentiate between transvalvular and paravalvular regurgitation. However, assessment of regurgitation by the transthoracic echocardiography is often difficult due to reverberation artifact. While precordial Doppler examination can be useful in patients with suspected valvular regurgitation,[74,75,86] transesophagal echocardiography is superior and should be performed in all patients in whom prosthetic valve regurgitation is suspected but not adequately defined by transthoracic examination.[87-89] Not only is the diagnosis and assessment of the severity of regurgitation more precise using transesophegeal echocardiography, but the differentiation between transvalvular and paravalvular regurgitation is also more accurately made, especially when the prosthesis is in the mitral position.

INTRACARDIAC SHUNTS

Doppler plays a major role in the evaluation of acquired and congenital shunt flows.[90] The detection of such flows has been greatly facilitated by the advent of color-flow Doppler. Figures 11 and 12 are examples of intracardiac shunt flows, which are visualized as jets originating on 1 side of the interatrial or interventricular septum (where prestenotic acceleration of flow begins), crossing it to reach the receiving chamber. The width of the color-flow jet loosely correlates with the size of the defect noted at surgery.[91] Although interatrial shunting may be seen in several views, the subcostal and modified right parasternal views, which allow parallel alignment of the ultrasound beam with shunt flow, are particularly useful (Fig. 11). A PW Doppler recording of interatrial shunt flow may be obtained with or without the guidance of color-flow Doppler by placing the sample volume within the shunt flow. Because the pressure difference between the right and left atria is relatively small, the interatrial shunt flow is low in velocity and thus must be differentiated from physiologic venous flows. The inferior vena cava, superior vena cava, and coronary sinus flow dynamics within the right atrium may often make the diagnosis of atrial septal defect flows difficult. The latter flow, depicted in Figure 11, is characterized by being continuous throughout the cardiac cycle and showing only minor variation with respiration when compared with caval flows. Shunt flows across ventricular septal defects are evaluated in a similar manner. Membranous ventricular septal defects are easily seen in the parasternal long and short axis views (Fig. 12). These lesions are characterized by systolic flow jets with a high velocity commensurate with the systolic pressure gradient across the interventricular septum. Shunt flow which occurs between the aortic right sinus of Valsalva and the right ventricle is also high in velocity but occurs during both systole and diastole.[92] Shunt flow across a patent ductus arteriosus is best evaluated from the parasternal view, though visualization from the suprasternal window is also possible. This is a high velocity flow occurring during systole and diastole. All flows described thus far occur initially in a left-to-right direction. With progression over time, the elevation of right-sided pressures result in the reversal of shunt flow direction.

The quantitative assessment of shunt size is based on the comparison of pulmonary and systemic flow rates (Qp:Qs). Noninvasive right ventricular and left ventricular stroke volumes can be estimated by calculating the product of the flow velocity integral obtained by PW Doppler and the cross sectional area of the right ventricular and left ventricular outflow tracts, respectively.[93,94] Shunt volume can be measured by subtracting the Qs from the Qp, or by applying the continuity equation. The mean velocity of the shunt flow, determined by spectral Doppler, multiplied by the diameter of the jet and the duration of the flow provides the volumetric flow for one beat. Shunt flow/min is the product of the flow/beat times the heart rate.[91]

Doppler derived shunt flow ratio correlates well with other modalities but is subject to limitations that result primarily from defining the precise borders of the right ventricular and left ventricular outflow tracts and to a lesser extent, the recording of their flow measurements. It is important to note that the pulmonary to systemic ratio as calculated by any technique, whether invasive or noninvasive, is not reliable in the presence of significant valvular regurgitation.

The Doppler technique is useful not only for the detection of shunt flows and estimation of pulmonary to systemic flow ratio but also for the detection and evaluation of concomitant congenital lesions, and the estimation of pulmonary artery systolic pressure using TR flow velocity as previously discussed. The hemodynamic information gained by the Doppler examination, along with the anatomic information gathered by the 2-dimensional echocardiographic examination, are complementary and provide comprehensive evaluation in most patients with abnormal shunt flows.

ASSESSMENT OF VENTRICULAR FUNCTION

SYSTOLIC FUNCTION

The aortic flow velocity curve can be used to assess left ventricular systolic function as well as stroke volume and cardiac output. In patients with left heart failure, decreases in peak velocity and acceleration have been described. The aortic tracing exhibits a more rounded form, with the peak velocity occurring later in systole.[95] A normal flow pattern, however, does not exclude the presence of a myopathic ventricle and overlap between groups has been noted.[96,97] Continuous-wave tracings from mitral regurgitant jets can also supply information about left ventricular performance. The rate of rise in a systolic pressure, or dp/dt, is reflected in the upslope of the mitral regurgitation tracing. Those patients with impaired systolic function, therefore, would have a more gradual upslope.[98] Analysis of this tracing in combination with the Bernoulli equation allows for the noninvasive calculation of dp/dt.[99,100]

DIASTOLIC FUNCTION

With increasing realization that left ventricular diastolic dysfunction can lead to symptoms of congestive heart failure (CHF), recent work has focused on mitral flow patterns to gain insight into this phenomenon. Several abnormalities in mitral flow patterns have been described, including alterations in the early filling velocity (E wave), atrial filling velocity (A wave), and the ratio of the former to the latter (E/A ratio). Other useful parameters are the isovolumic relaxation time, the period between aortic closure and mitral opening, and the deceleration time, or the interval between peak early velocity and cessation of flow (if the A wave commences prior to cessation of flow, the deceleration slope is extrapolated to baseline). Figure 13 depicts the 2 basic patterns which have been described. The first pattern is seen in patients with ischemic heart disease, left ventricular hypertrophy, hypertrophic cardiomyopathy, and aortic stenosis, and is characterized by a lower peak E velocity, increased atrial filling velocity, E/A ratio <1, prolonged deceleration slope, and a prolonged isovolumic relaxation time.[101] These changes have been attributed to impaired relaxation of the left ventricle, as patients with coronary disease who exhibit this pattern also have prolonged time constants of relaxation.[102] The other pattern

described is caused by restriction to filling, and consists of an elevated early velocity, decreased atrial filling velocity, high E/A ratio, and shortened isovolumic relaxation and deceleration times.[101] This pattern is usually seen in patients with restrictive cardiomyopathy and constrictive pericarditis.

Assessment of diastolic properties in this manner is confounded by a variety of factors. The mitral flow velocity profile has been shown to change with age,[103,104] heart rate, and most importantly, loading conditions.[105,106] The magnitude of the E velocity is dependent upon the difference between the left atrial pressure and left ventricular diastolic pressure in early diastole.[107] Progressive increases in left atrial pressure in patients with ischemic or dilated cardiomyopathy cause the mitral valve to open earlier, and the resultant higher early diastolic gradient leads to a higher E velocity. Therefore, despite prolonged relaxation as determined by hemodynamic recordings, the isovolumic relaxation time shortens, and the E/A ratio increases. The mitral flow tracing observed in this situation may change from the abnormal relaxation pattern to the restrictive pattern.[108] In patients with dilated cardiomyopathy, elevated E velocities and E/A ratio signify higher pulmonary capillary wedge pressure, greater functional impairment, and portend a worse prognosis.[109] However, in patients with modest elevation in filling pressure an intermediate stage in this process has been described during which the mitral flow profile may appear normal. This finding has been described in patients with chronic ischemic disease and those with aortic stenosis and elevated end-diastolic pressures.[108,110] In attempts to clarify problems produced by this "pseudonormalization" of the mitral flow pattern and better assess left ventricular diastolic pressure, pulmonary venous flow patterns have been investigated. In general, systolic flow velocity decreases and the retrograde flow at atrial contraction increases as left atrial pressure rises.[111–113] Not only is the magnitude of the atrial reversal velocity useful, but its duration is as well. Elevated left ventricular end-diastolic pressure can be diagnosed with relatively high sensitivity and specificity if the duration of the atrial reversal wave exceeds that of the transmitral A wave.[112,113] Unfortunately, such analysis requires careful interrogation of the pulmonary venous flow in patients with good quality ultrasound windows or transesophageal echocardiography.

ESTIMATION OF RIGHT VENTRICULAR AND PULMONARY ARTERIAL PRESSURE

Hemodynamic analysis of the right heart has become one of the important uses of Doppler. One way this can be done is by evaluating the characteristics of flow velocity in the pulmonary artery. There is an inverse correlation between acceleration time, defined as the interval between onset of flow and peak velocity, and pulmonary artery pressure. Patients with pulmonary hypertension, defined as mean pulmonary artery pressure greater than 22 mm Hg, have acceleration times of less than 100 msec. The downslope of the velocity profile is also altered, with a small period of reacceleration sometimes evident.[114] Other Doppler indices that have been shown to correlate well with pulmonary artery pressure are the interval between pulmonic valve closure and tricuspid valve opening and the ratio of the pre-ejection period to ejection time.[115]

The most widely used method for estimation of right ventricular or pulmonary artery systolic pressure is analysis of the tricuspid regurgitation flow profile. As demonstrated in Figure 10, by measuring the peak velocity, pressure gradient can be determined using the Bernoulli equation.[10,11] Pulmonary artery systolic pressure can then be determined by adding an estimate of the right atrial pressure to the pressure gradient. The advantage to this method is the ease in which pulmonary arterial systolic pressure can be estimated from a spectral tracing. The tricuspid regurgitant profile can be enhanced by intravenous injection of agitated saline.[116] Estimation of right atrial pressure can lead to some error, but several methods have been proposed to minimize this limitation.[10,11,117] In our laboratory, we estimate right atrial pressures as follows: if right atrial size is normal, right atrial pressure is estimated to be 5 mm Hg; if the right atrium is enlarged, 10 mm Hg; if the inferior vena cava is dilated as well, 15

mm Hg; and if inspiratory collapse is not evident in a dilated inferior vena cava, 20 mm Hg. Using the peak velocity of the tricuspid regurgitation profile to estimate pulmonary artery pressure allows for the acquisition of accurate, clinically relevant information without the need for invasive monitoring.

ISCHEMIC HEART DISEASE

DETECTION

As previously mentioned, measurements of global left ventricular systolic function such as cardiac output and stroke volume can be measured by Doppler echocardiography. Exercise induced changes in the aortic flow velocity profile have been examined with the hope that changes in global left ventricular function resulting from ischemia could be detected. While initial work suggested that aortic flow velocity falls during exercise in patients with coronary disease,[118] later reports have shown that though aortic flow velocity may not decrease with exercise in those with ischemia; the increases in peak velocity and peak acceleration in patients with coronary disease are often less than those seen in normal individuals.[96,119] Aortic flow velocity is influenced by a number of factors such as changes in loading conditions and heart rate, and thus, is not a useful parameter to detect ischemia.

The effects of ischemia on diastolic function have been previously described (Fig. 13). Diminution of the E/A ratio occurs frequently during ischemia and is often noted in patients with myocardial infarction. Changes in the mitral flow pattern however, can not be used to reliably detect ischemic heart disease.

COMPLICATIONS OF ACUTE MYOCARDIAL INFARCTION

A major area where Doppler is extremely useful in patients with ischemic disease is in the diagnosis of complications of myocardial infarction, namely ventricular septal defect and acute mitral regurgitation. Prompt, accurate diagnosis is important as they are both life-threatening conditions. The details of Doppler

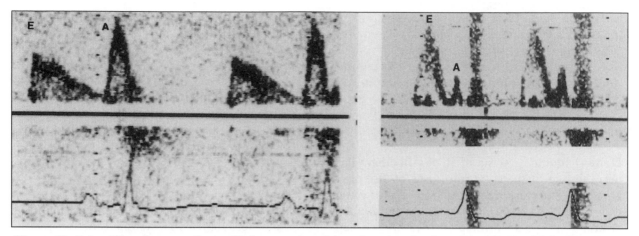

Figure 13. *Pulsed Doppler recordings with the sample volume placed at the tips of the mitral valve leaflets from 2 patients. The tracing on the left, taken from a patient with coronary disease, represents the abnormal relaxation pattern, with a slow deceleration time of the E wave and an E/A ratio of <1. The recording on the right is from a patient with restrictive cardiomyopathy. Note the rapid downslope of the E wave and an E/A ratio of approximately 2:1.*

flow patterns in ventricular septal defect and mitral regurgitation are discussed elsewhere in this text, though some differences may be present in the patient in whom these conditions complicate an acute myocardial infarction. Both are heralded by new murmurs. Early deceleration of the mitral regurgitant jet profile, indicative of a noncompliant left atrium, is highly suggestive of an acute increase in left atrial pressures (and a prominent "v" wave) and may give a clue about the acuity of the regurgitation.[120] Patients with acute, acquired ventricular septal defects may have a low velocity diastolic flow across the septum due to elevated left ventricular diastolic pressure, though the predominant flow is systolic.[121] Triphasic flow, consisting of a low velocity mid-diastolic flow, a presystolic wave, and high velocity systolic flow, has also been described.[122–124] Patients with elevated right ventricular diastolic pressure exhibit a transient reversal of flow in diastole.[125] This finding is an indicator of poor prognosis. Color-flow imaging adds to the detection and localization of acquired ventricular septal defects and is especially useful in patients with serpiginous tracts through the interventricular septum.[123,124] The width of the color jet correlates with the size of the rupture and pulmonary-to-systemic flow ratio.[125]

HYPERTROPHIC OBSTRUCTIVE CARDIOMYOPATHY

The presence of a subaortic obstruction can be detected by a high velocity systolic jet directed away from the apex. This jet can be differentiated from that seen with aortic stenosis by the contour and relative time of the peak velocity. The typical tracing, seen in Figure 14, has been described as "dagger-shaped," with a gradual early systolic upslope and a late systolic peak. The maximal instantaneous gradient derived from the peak systolic velocity is indicative of the severity of the intraventricular obstruction.[126–128] The peak velocity also occurs simultaneously with maximal septal contact of the anterior mitral leaflet in patients with systolic anterior motion of the mitral valve.[129] Using CW Doppler, the outflow jet may overlap with the MR jet, making the peak velocity difficult to discern. If this problem is not appropriately detected, erroneously elevated pressure gradients may result. Diligent interrogation with the Doppler transducer, especially from the right parasternal location, may help avoid this problem.

The site of obstruction can be localized using pulsed Doppler by moving the sample volume within the left ventricle and noting the location of flow acceleration. Cessation of flow can be

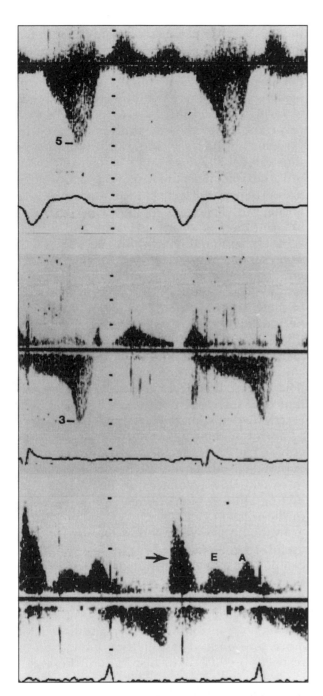

Figure 14. *Continuous-wave recordings from the apex illustrating altered flows in patients with hypertrophic or hyperdynamic ventricles. The top recording is from a patient with hypertrophic obstructive cardiomyopathy. The recording with the Doppler beam aimed at the left ventricular outflow tract exhibits the typical dagger-shaped appearance. Peak flow velocity is 5 m/s. The patient from whom the middle tracing was recorded had a hyperdynamic ventricle without obstruction or hypertrophy. The increased flow velocity late in systole is presumably caused by obliteration of the outflow tract due to markedly increased systolic function. Note that the peak velocity is relatively later in systole than the example above. The bottom tracing illustrates exaggerated flow velocity during the isovolumic relaxation period (arrow). This can be observed in patients with hypertrophic cardiomyopathy or in the setting of a hyperdynamic ventricle with cavity obliteration.*

Diastolic flow abnormalities are also seen in the majority of patients with hypertrophic cardiomyopathy. The mitral flow pattern typically resembles the abnormal relaxation pattern, with an E/A ratio less than 1 and a prolonged deceleration time. An additional flow during the isovolumic relaxation period can be recorded. As shown in Figure 14, this flow is typically directed toward the apex, and is thought to be due to an interventricular gradient caused by asynchronous relaxation.[130] Flow from apex to base during isovolumic relaxation has been described in patients with mid-cavity obstruction, felt to be secondary to a residual postsystolic gradient between the apex and the basal portion of the ventricle.[131] It should be noted that the systolic and diastolic flow abnormalities described are not specific, and may be observed in the presence of a hyperdynamic ventricle or left ventricular hypertrophy with partial cavity obliteration in systole (Fig. 14). Hypertrophic cardiomyopathy can be nonobstructive, so the absence of a systolic gradient does not exclude the diagnoses.

RESTRICTIVE CARDIOMYOPATHY

The hallmark of restrictive cardiomyopathy is abnormal ventricular diastolic function, elevation of ventricular and atrial pressures, and

observed during mid-systole in patients with mid-ventricular obstruction when the pulse sample is placed at the point of cavity obliteration. Color-flow mapping can locate the site by noting a narrow, mosaic flow pattern that is seen at the site of obstruction. These methods can be employed to determine if the obstruction is subaortic, mid-ventricular, or apical.

a "dip and plateau" appearance to the ventricular pressure tracings. These findings are reflected in mitral and tricuspid recordings as a shortened isovolumic relaxation time, increased E velocity and E/A ratio, and decreased deceleration time (Fig. 13). Inspiration is associated with an exaggeration of these abnormalities for tricuspid flows, but mitral flows are essentially unchanged throughout the respiratory cycle.[132,133] Diastolic mitral and tricuspid regurgitation, due to markedly elevated ventricular pressures, can be present. Marked elevations in right ventricular end-diastolic pressure can be demonstrated by the presence of antegrade flow across the pulmonic valve at end-diastole.

Examination of venous flow patterns may also be useful. Normally, the flow pattern recorded from systemic veins consists of a systolic and diastolic phase, with the systolic velocity slightly higher. In the presence of restrictive cardiomyopathy, systemic and pulmonary venous flow patterns exhibit higher flow velocities in diastole. Diastolic velocities in systemic veins increase with inspiration, but are relatively constant in the pulmonary veins.[132,134] Systolic flow reversal is seen in the presence of severe tricuspid regurgitation. Additionally, atrial systole is accompanied by an exaggerated flow reversal in the pulmonary veins.[134] It should be noted that the above-mentioned signs are seen in patients with symptomatic restrictive cardiomyopathy or those with advanced disease; early in the course of amyloidosis the mitral flow pattern may show an abnormal relaxation pattern.[134] Also, other disorders, namely constrictive pericarditis, may be accompanied by similar Doppler findings. Thus, when evaluating for the presence of restrictive cardiomyopathy, clinical, 2-dimensional echocardiographic, and other findings play an important role.

CONSTRICTIVE PERICARDITIS

Constrictive pericarditis is associated with preserved systolic function and impairment of ventricular filling. Clinical, hemodynamic and Doppler findings of constrictive pericarditis and restrictive pericarditis may be similar, but differentiation is possible. Normally, intra-

thoracic and intracardiac pressures are altered to a similar degree throughout the respiratory cycle. In constrictive pericarditis, the abnormal pericardium acts as a "buffer" to changes in pressure, hence there is a dissociation between intrathoracic and intracardiac pressures with respiration. This dissociation is detected by variations in flow velocities with respiration as illustrated in Figure 15.[133] With inspiration, intrathoracic and pulmonary capillary wedge pressures decrease, yet ventricular pressures are unchanged. This leads to a decreased gradient between the pulmonary circulation and the left ventricle, so mitral flow velocity decreases. The reverse happens with expiration. A 25% difference between inspiratory and expiratory E velocity (compared to <10% in healthy patients or those with restriction) is noted in constrictive pericarditis.[135] Right-sided flow velocities vary in the opposite direction; tricuspid flow increases with inspiration and decreases with expiration. While the typical atrioventricular flow pattern, high E velocity, rapid deceleration time, and increased E/A ratio, are seen in both restrictive cardiomyopathy and constrictive pericarditis, these respiratory variations, seen only in the latter, are useful in differentiating the two.[133] Additionally, the respiratory changes in mitral flow velocities are useful in predicting clinical improvement following pericardiectomy.[135]

Evaluation of venous flow patterns is also useful. In constrictive pericarditis, the systolic component of systemic venous flow is greater than the diastolic component. An early, rapid deceleration with late systolic retrograde flow may be seen in this condition.[136] Pulmonary venous flows in constrictive pericarditis exhibit more pronounced systolic flow compared to restriction.[137,138] With inspiration, there is a modest decrease in systolic flow and a marked reduction in diastolic flow, whereas there is little respiratory change in the pulmonary venous flow patterns in patients with restriction. Other abnormalities, such as diastolic mitral and tricuspid regurgitation and end-diastolic antegrade flow across the pulmonic valve, can be seen in constrictive pericarditis, though they are more common in patients with restrictive cardiomyopathy. Thus, the hemodynamic and physiologic differences between restrictive cardiomyopathy and constrictive pericarditis can be used to help differentiate the 2.

CARDIAC TAMPONADE

The hemodynamic alterations seen in tamponade are caused by the pericardium exerting positive pressure on the cardiac chambers, with resultant impairment to ventricular filling. As with constrictive pericarditis, there is dissociation between alterations in pericardial pressures and pulmonary pressures with respiration. The gradient between the pulmonary circulation and the left heart decreases with inspiration, so the mitral flow velocity decreases as well. Respiratory changes in flow velocities, or "flow velocity paradoxus" has been shown across all four valves (Fig. 15). Flow velocity decreases with inspiration

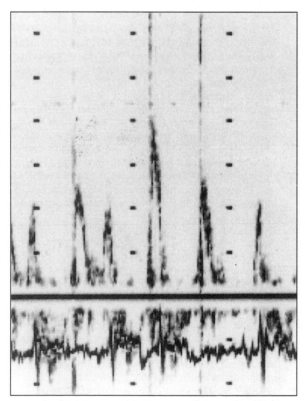

Figure 15. Pulsed Doppler recording of mitral inflow in a patient with calcific constrictive pericarditis. The flow velocity during inspiration (Insp) is at least 35% lower than that during expiration (Exp). Similar changes with respiration, often to a greater degree, are seen in patients with tamponade.

and increases with expiration across the mitral and aortic valves. Changes in the opposite direction are observed across the tricuspid and pulmonic valves.[139-144] The magnitude, as well as the presence of these respiratory variations in flow velocities is of diagnostic importance. Percent change in mitral flow velocity with respiration varies with the degree of hemodynamic compromise.[143,144] Patients who have effusion without tamponade have lesser degrees of respiratory changes in flow velocity;[140,144] these modest respiratory changes are noted prior to the onset of right ventricular collapse.[142-144] These findings support the notion that tamponade is a continuum and not an all-or-none phenomenon. The presence of these Doppler findings, in association with right ventricular diastolic collapse and right atrial collapse seen on 2-dimensional echocardiography, strongly indicates the presence of cardiac tamponade.

CLINICAL IMPACT

The ability of Doppler echocardiography to describe both flow dynamics and hemodynamics make it a valuable noninvasive tool. When combined with 2-dimensional echocardiography, the full range of cardiac pathologic conditions can be described, with the lone exception being the coronary anatomy. This comprehensive noninvasive evaluation has made hemodynamic assessment using cardiac catheterization obsolete in many circumstances. Many centers are no longer performing right-heart catheterization in patients with cardiac tamponade, constrictive pericarditis, and simple congenital abnormalities such as atrial and ventricular septal defects. When evaluated prospectively in a blinded manner, echocardiography has provided clinicians with the ability to make accurate management decisions in patients with valvular heart disease without catheterization.[145-148] The greatest discrepancy was in patients with mitral regurgitation.[147] However, one should keep in mind that the "gold standard" for assessment of regurgitation, contrast ventriculography and angiography, are fraught with errors,[149-151] and improved, quantitative echocardiographic methods are being evaluated. In the future, clinical evaluation in combination with echocardiography (and perhaps coronary angiography) may be all that is performed prior to surgical intervention for patients with valvular heart disease.

REFERENCES

1. Kremkau FW. Transducers and sound beams. In: *Diagnostic Ultrasound—Physical Principles and Exercises.* New York: Grune & Stratton; 1980:54-78.
2. McDicken WN. Detection of motion by the Doppler effect. In: *Diagnostic Ultrasonics—Principles and Use of Instruments.* New York: Wiley; 1976:219-235.
3. Wells PNT. Fundamental physics. In: *Physical Principles of Ultrasonic Diagnosis.* London: Academic Press; 1969:1-27.
4. Griffith JM, Henry WL. An ultrasound system for combined cardiac imaging and Doppler blood flow measurement in man. *Circulation.* 1978;57:925-930.
5. Miyatake K, Okamoto M, Kinoshita N, et al. Clinical application of a new type of real-time 2-dimensional Doppler flow imaging system. *Am J Cardiol.* 1984;54:857-868.
6. Pandian NG, Thanikachalam S, Elangovan D, et al. Color Doppler flow imaging in valvular stenosis. *Echocardiography.* 1987;4:515-526.
7. Pandian NG, Kusay BS, Caldeira M, et al. Color Doppler flow imaging in cardiac diagnosis. *Echocardiography.* 1989;6:99-117.
8. Stamm RB, Martin RP. Quantification of pressure gradients across stenotic valves by Doppler ultrasound. *J Am Coll Cardiol.* 1983;2:707-718.
9. Nishimura RA, Tajik AJ. Determination of left-sided pressure gradients by utilizing Doppler aortic and mitral regurgitant signals: Validation by simultaneous dual catheter and Doppler studies. *J Am Coll Cardiol.* 1988;11:317-321.
10. Yock PG, Popp RL. Noninvasive estimation of right ventricular systolic pressure by Doppler ultrasound in patients with tricuspid regurgitation. *Circulation.* 1984;70:657-662.
11. Currie PJ, Seward JB, Chan KL, et al. Continuous wave Doppler determination of right ventricular pressure: A simultaneous Doppler-catheterization study in 127 patients. *J Am Coll Cardiol.* 1985;6:750-756.
12. DeMaria AN, Bommer W, Joye J, et al. Value and limitations of cross-sectional echocardiography of the aortic valve in the diagnosis and quantification of valvular aortic stenosis. *Circulation.* 1980;62:304-312.
13. Godley RW, Green D, Dillon JC, et al. Reliability of 2-dimensional echocardiography in assessing the severity of valvular aortic stenosis. *Chest.* 1981;79:657-662.
14. Berger M, Berdoff RL, Gallerstein PE, et al. Evaluation of aortic stenosis by continuous wave ultrasound. *J Am Coll Cardiol.* 1984;3:150-156.
15. Oh JK, Taliercia CP, Holmes DR Jr, et al. Prediction of the severity of aortic stenosis by Doppler aortic valve area determination: Prospective Doppler-catheterization correlation in 100 patients. *J Am Coll Cardiol.* 1988;11:1227-1234.
16. Harrison MR, Gurley JC, Smith ME, et al. A practical application of Doppler echocardiography for the assessment of severity of aortic stenosis. *Am Heart J.* 1988:115:622-628.
17. Geibel A, Gornandt L, Kasper W, et al. Reproducibility of Doppler echocardiographic quantification of aortic and mitral valve stenoses: Comparison between two echocardiography centers. *Am J Cardiol.* 1991; 67:1013-1021.
18. Otto CM, Pearlman AS, Comess KA, et al. Determination of stenotic aortic valve area in adults using Doppler echocardiography. *J Am Coll Cardiol.* 1986;7:509-517.
19. Skjaerpe T, Hegrenaes L, Hatle L. Noninvasive estimation of valve area in patients with aortic stenosis by Doppler ultrasound and 2-dimensional echocardiography. *Circulation.* 1985;72:810-818.
20. Zoghbi WA, Farmer KL, Soto JG, et al. Accurate non-invasive quantification of stenotic aortic valve area by Doppler echocardiography. *Circulation.* 1986;73:452-459.
21. Hatle L, Angelsen B. *Doppler Ultrasound in Cardiology: Physical Principles and Clinical Applications.* Philadelphia: Lea & Febiger; 1985:149.
22. Hatle L, Angelsen B. *Doppler Ultrasound in Cardiology: Physical Principles and Clinical Applications.* Philadelphia: Lea & Febiger; 1985:145.
23. Hatle L, Brubakk A, Tromsdal A, et al. Noninvasive assessment of pressure drop in mitral stenosis by Doppler ultrasound. *Br Heart J.* 1978;40:131-140.
24. Hatle L, Angelsen B, Tromsdal A. Noninvasive assessment of atrioventricular pressure half-time by Doppler ultrasound. *Circulation.* 1979;60:1096-1104.
25. Holen J, Aaslid R, Landmark K, et al. Determination of pressure gradient in mitral stenosis with a noninvasive ultrasound Doppler technique. *Acta Med Scand.* 1976;199:455-460.
26. Thomas JD, Weyman AE. Doppler mitral pressure half-time: a clinical tool in search of theoretical justification. *J Am Coll Cardiol.* 1987;10:923-929.
27. Flachskampf FA, Weyman AE, Gillam L, et al. Aortic regurgitation shortens Doppler pressure half-time in mitral stenosis: clinical evidence, in vitro simulation and theoretic analysis. *J Am Coll Cardiol.* 1990;16:396-404.
28. Thomas JD, Wilkins GT, Choong CYP, et al. Inaccuracy of mitral pressure half-time immediately after percutaneous mitral valvotomy: dependence on transmitral gradient and left atrial and ventricular compliance. *Circulation.* 1990;78:980-993.
29. Nakatani S, Masuyama T, Kodama K, et al. Value and limitations of Doppler echocardiography in the quantification of stenotic mitral valve area: comparison of the pressure half-time and the continuity equation methods. *Circulation.* 1988;77:78-85.
30. Parris TM, Pandidis IP, Ross J, et al. Doppler echocardiographic findings in rheumatic tricuspid stenosis. *Am J Cardiol.* 1987;60:1414-1416.

31. Stevenson JG. Two-dimensional color Doppler estimation of the severity of atrioventricualr valve regurgitation: Important effects of instrument gain setting, pulse repetition frequency, and carrier frequency. *J Am Soc Echo.* 1989;2:1-10.

32. Karen G, Katz S, Strom J, et al. Non-invasive quantification of mitral regurgitation in dilated cardiomyopathy: Correlation of two Doppler echocardiographic methods. *Am Heart J.* 1988;116:758-764.

33. Rokey R, Sterling LL, Zoghbi WA, et al. Determination of regurgitant fraction in isolated mitral or aortic regurgitation by pulsed Doppler 2-dimensional echocardiography. *J Am Coll Cardiol.* 1986;7:1273-1278.

34. Enriquez-Sarano M, Bailey KR, Seward JB, et al. Quantitative Doppler assessment of valvular regurgitation. *Circulation.* 1993;87:841-848.

35. Enriquez-Sarano M, Seward JB, Bailey KR, et al. Effective regurgitant orifice area: A noninvasive Doppler development of an old hemodynamic concept. *J Am Coll Cardiol.* 1994;23:443-451.

36. Berger M, Hecht SR, Van Tosh A, et al. Pulsed and continuous wave Doppler echocardiographic assessment of valvular regurgitation in normal subjects. *J Am Coll Cardiol.* 1989;13:1540-1545.

37. Masuyama T, Kodama K, Kitabatake A, et al. Non-invasive evaluation of aortic regurgitation by continuous-wave Doppler echocardiography. *Circulation.* 1986;73:460-466.

38. Teague SM, Heinsimer JA, Anderson JL, et al. Quantification of aortic regurgitation utilizing continuous wave Doppler ultrasound. *J Am Coll Cardiol.* 1986;8:592-599.

39. Labovitz AJ, Ferrara RP, Kern MJ, et al. Quantitative evaluation of aortic insufficiency by continuous wave Doppler echocardiography. *J Am Coll Cardiol.* 1986;8:1341-1347.

40. Beyer RW, Ramirez M, Josephson MA, et al. Correlation of continuous-wave Doppler assessment of chronic aortic regurgitation with hemodynamics and angiography. *Am J Cardiol.* 1987;60:852-856.

41. Perry GJ, Helmcke F, Nanda NC, et al. Evaluation of aortic insufficiency by Doppler color flow mapping. *J Am Coll Cardiol.* 1987;9:952-959.

42. Smith MD, Grayburn PA, Spain MG, et al. Observer variability in the quantitation of Doppler color flow jet areas for mitral and aortic regurgitation. *J Am Coll Cardiol.* 1988;11:579-584.

43. Baumgartner H, Kratzer H, Helmreich G, et al. Quantitation of aortic regurgitation by colour coded cross-sectional Doppler echocardiography. *Eur Heart J.* 1988;9:380-387.

44. Taylor AL, Eichhorn EJ, Brickner ME, et al. Aortic valve morphology: An important in vitro determinant of proximal regurgitant jet width by Doppler color flow mapping. *J Am Coll Cardiol.* 1990;16:405-412.

45. Yoshida K, Yoshikawa J, Shakudo M, et al. Color Doppler evaluation of valvular regurgitation in normal subjects. *Circulation.* 1988;78:840-847.

46. Takao S, Miyatake K, Izumi S, et al. Clinical implications of pulmonary regurgitation in healthy individuals detection by cross sectional pulsed Doppler echo-cardiography. *Br Heart J.* 1988;59:542-550.

47. Masuyama T, Kodama K, Kitabatake A, et al. Continuous-wave Doppler echocardiographic detection of pulmonary regurgitation and its application to non-invasive estimation of pulmonary artery pressure. *Circulation.* 1986;74:484-492.

48. Quinones MA, Young JB, Waggoner Ad, et al. Assessment of pulsed Doppler echocardiography in detection and quantification of aortic and mitral regurgitation. *Br Heart J.* 1980;44:612-620.

49. Klein AL, Obarski TP, Steward WJ, et al. Transesophageal Doppler echocardiography of pulmonary venous flow: A new marker of mitral regurgitation severity. *J Am Coll Cardiol.* 1991;18:518-526.

50. Miyatake K, Izumi S, Okamoto M, et al. Semiquantitative grading of severity of mitral regurgitation by real-time 2-dimensional Doppler flow imaging technique. *J Am Coll Cardiol.* 1986;7:82-88.

51. Helmke F, Nanda NC, Hsiung MC, et al. Color Doppler assessment of mitral regurgitation with orthogonal planes. *Circulation.* 1987;75:175-183.

52. Spain MG, Smith MD, Grayburn PA, et al. Quantitative assessment of mitral regurgitation by Doppler color flow imaging: Angiographic and hemodynamic correlations. *J Am Coll Cardiol.* 1989;13:585-590.

53. Smith MD, Harrison MR, Pinton R, et al. Regurgitant jet size by transesophageal compared with transthoracic Doppler color flow imaging. *Circulation.* 1991;83:79-86.

54. Castello R, Lenzen P, Aguirre F, et al. Variability in the quantitation of mitral regurgitation by Doppler color flow mapping: Comparison of transthoracic and transesophageal studies. *J Am Coll Cardiol.* 1992;20:433-438.

55. Chen C, Thomas JD, Anconina J, et al. Impact of impinging wall jet on color Doppler quantification of mitral regurgitation. *Circulation.* 1991;84:712-720.

56. Enriquez-Sarano M, Tajik AJ, Bailey KR, et al. Color flow imaging compared with quantitative Doppler assessment of severity of mitral regurgitation: Influence of eccentricity of jet and mechanism of regurgitation. *J Am Coll Cardiol.* 1993;21:1211-1219.

57. Bolger A, Eigler N, Pfaff JM, et al. Computer analysis of Doppler color flow mapping images for quantitative assessment of in vitro fluid jets. *J Am Coll Cardiol.* 1988;12:450-457.

58. Bargiggia GS, Tronconi L, Sahn DJ, et al. A new method for quantitation of mitral regurgitation based on color flow Doppler imaging of flow convergence proximal to regurgitant orifice. *Circulation.* 1991; 84:1481-1489.

59. Utsunomiya T, Ogawa T, Tang HA, et al. Doppler color flow mapping of the proximal isovelocity surface area: A new method for measuring volume flow rate across a narrowed orifice. *J Am Soc Echo.* 1991;4:338-348.

60. Utsunomiya T, Doshi R, Patel D, et al. Regurgitant volume estimation in patients with mitral regurgitation: Initial studies using the color Doppler "proximal isovelocity surface area" method. *Echocardiography.* 1992;9:63-70.

61. Vandervoort PM, Rivera JM, Mele D, et al. Application of color Doppler flow mapping to calculate effective regurgitant orifice area: An in vitro study and initial clinical observations. *Circulation.* 1993;88:1150-1156.

62. Utsunomiya T, Ogawa T, Doshi R, et al. Doppler color flow "proximal isovelocity surface area" method for estimating volume flow rate: Effects of orifice shape an machine factors. *J Am Coll Cardiol.* 1991;17:1103-1111.

63. Rittoo D, Sutherland GR, Shaw TRD. Quantification of left-to-right atrial shunting and defect size after balloon mitral commissurotomy using biplane transesophageal echocardiography, color flow Doppler mapping, and the principle of proximal flow convergence. *Circulation.* 1993;87:1591-1603.

64. Rodriguez L, Thomas JD, Monterroso V, et al. Validation of the proximal flow convergence method: Calculation of orifice area in patients with mitral stenosis. *Circulation.* 1993;88:1157-1165.

65. Cape EG, Kim YH, Heinrich RS, et al. Cardiac motion can alter proximal isovelocity surface area calculations of regurgitant flow. *J Am Coll Cardiol.* 1993;22:1730-1737.

66. Akasaka T, Yoshikawa J, Yoshida K, et al. Age-related valvular regurgitation: A study by pulsed Doppler echocardiography. *Circulation.* 1987;76:262-265.

67. Chopra HK, Fan PH, Daruwala D, et al. Can color Doppler/2-dimensional echocardiography identify the need for tricuspid valve repair? *J Am Coll Cardiol.* 1987;13:24A. Abstract.

68. Hatle L, Angelsen B. *Doppler Ultrasound in Cardiology: Physical Principles and Clinical Applications.* Philadelphia: Lea & Febiger; 1985:174.

69. Ramirez ML, Wong M, Sadler N, et al. Doppler evaluation of bioprosthetic and mechanical aortic valves: Data from four models in 107 stable, ambulatory patients. *Am Heart J.* 1988;115:418-425.

70. Bhatia S, Moten M, Werner M, et al. Frequency of unusually high transvalvular Doppler velocities in patients with normal prosthetic valves. *J Am Coll Cardiol.* 1987;9:238A. Abstract.

71. Sagar KB, Wann LS, Paulsen WHJ, et al. Doppler echocardiographic evaluation of Hancock and Bjork-Shiley prosthetic valves. *J Am Coll Cardiol.* 1986;7:681-687.

72. Cooper DM, Stewart WJ, Schiavone WA, et al. Evaluation of normal prosthetic valve function by Doppler echocardiography. *Am Heart J.* 1987;114:576-582.

73. Alam M, Rosman HS, Lakier JB, et al. Doppler and echocardiographic features of normal and dysunctioning bioprosthetic valves. *J Am Coll Cardiol.* 1987;10:851-858.

74. Panidis IP, Ross J, Mintz GS. Normal and abnormal prosthetic valve function as assessed by Doppler echocardiography. *J Am Coll Cardiol.* 1986;8:317-326.

75. Williams GA, Labovitz AJ. Doppler hemodynamic evaluation of prosthetic (Starr-Edwards and Bjork-Shiley) and bioprosthetic (Hancock and Carpentier-Edwards) cardiac valves. *Am J Cardiol.* 1985;56:325-332.

76. Burstow DJ, Nishimura RA, Bailey KR, et al. Continuous wave Doppler echocardiographic measurement of prosthetic valve gradients: A simultaneous Doppler-catheter correlative study. *Circulation.* 1989;80:504-514.

77. Chafizadeh ER, Zoghbi WA. Doppler echocardiographic assessment of the St. Jude medical prosthetic valve in the aortic position using the continuity equation. *Circulation.* 1991;83:213-223.

78. Rothbart RM, Castriz JL, Harding LV, et al. Determination of aortic valve area by 2-dimensional and Doppler echocardiography in patients with normal and stenotic bioprosthetic valves. *J Am Coll Cardiol.* 1990;15:817-824.

79. Dumesnil JG, Honos GN, Lemieux M, et al. Validation and applications of indexed aortic prosthetic valve areas calculated by Doppler echocardiography. *J Am Coll Cardiol.* 1994;16:637-643.

80. Baumgartner H, Khan SS, DeRobertis M, et al. Doppler assessment of prosthetic valve orifice area: An in vitro study. *Circulation.* 1992;85:2275-2283.

81. Stewart SFC, Nast EP, Arabia FA, et al. Errors in pressure gradient measurement by continuous wave Doppler ultrasound: Type, size and age effects in bioprosthetic aortic valves. *J Am Coll Cardiol.* 1991;18:769-779.

82. Baumgartner H, Khan S, DeRobertis M, et al. Effect of prosthetic aortic valve design on the Doppler-catheter gradient correlation: An in vitro study of normal St. Jude, Medtronic-Hall, Starr-Edwards and Hancock valves. *J Am Coll Cardiol.* 1992;19:324-332.

83. Flachskampf FA, O'Shea JP, Griffin BP, et al. Patterns of normal transvalvular regurgitation in mechanical valve prosthesis. *J Am Coll Cardiol.* 1991;18:1493-1498.

84. Vandenberg BF, Dellsperger KC, Chandran KB, et al. Detection, localization, and quantitation of bioprosthetec mitral valve regurgitation. An in vitro 2-dimensional color-Doppler flow mapping study. *Circulation.* 1988;78:529-538.

85. Mohr-Kahaly S, Kupferwasser I, Erbel R, et al. Regurgitant flow in apparently normal valve prostheses: improved detection and semiquantitative analysis by transesophageaal 2-dimensional color coded Doppler echocardiography. *J Am Soc Echo.* 1990;3:187-195.

86. Dittrich H, Nicod P, Hoit B, et al. Evaluation of Bjork-Shiley prosthetic valves by real-time 2-dimensional Doppler echocardiographic flow mapping. *Am Heart J.* 1988;115:133-138.

87. Nellessen U, Schnittger I, Appleton CP, et al. Transesophageal 2-dimensional echocardiography and color Doppler flow velocity mapping in the evaluation of cardiac valve prostheses. *Circulation.* 1988;78:848-855.

88. Taams MA, Gussenhoven EJ, Cahalan MK, et al. Transesophageal Doppler color flow imaging in the detection of native and Bjork-Shiley mitral valve regurgitation. *J Am Coll Cardiol.* 1989;13:95-99.

89. Currie PJ, Calafiore P, Stewart WJ, et al. Transesophageal echo in mitral prosthetic dysfunction: Echo-surgical correlation. *J Am Coll Cardiol.* 1989;13:69A. Abstract.

90. Stevenson JG. Echo Doppler analysis of septal defects. In: Peronneau P, Diebold B (eds). *Cardiovascular Application of Doppler Echocardiography.* Paris: Inserm; 1983;515-540.

91. Mehta RH, Helmcke F, Nanda N, et al. Transesophageal Doppler color flow mapping assessment of atrial septal defect. *J Am Coll Cardiol.* 1990;16:1010-1016.

92. Yokoi K, Kambe T, Ichimiya S, et al. Ruptured aneurysm of the right sinus of Valsalva: Two pulsed Doppler echocardiographic studies. *J Clin Ultrasound.* 1981;9:505-510.

93. Goldberg SJ, Sahn DJ, Allen HD, et al. Evaluation of pulmonary and systemic blood flow by 2-dimensional Doppler echocardiography using fast Fourier transform spectral analysis. *Am J Cardiol.* 1982;50:1394-1400.

94. Sanders SP, Yeager S, Williams R. Measurement of systemic and pulmonary blood flow and QP:QS ratio using Doppler and 2-dimensional echocardiography. *Am J Cardiol.* 1983;51:952-956.

95. Hatle L, Angelsen B. Doppler *Ultrasound in Cardiology: Physical Principles and Clinical Applications.* Philadelphia: Lea & Febiger; 1985:265.

96. Pandian NG, Wang SS, Thanikachalam S. Role of Doppler echocardiography in ischemic heart disease. In: Kerber RE (ed). *Echocardiography in Coronary Artery Disease.* Mount Kisko: Futura; 1988:259-280.

97. Gardin JM, Iseri LT, Elkayam U, et al. Evaluation of dilated cardiomyopathy by pulsed Doppler echocardiography. *Am Heart J.* 1983;106:1057-1065.

98. Hatle L, Angelsen B. Doppler *Ultrasound in Cardiology: Physical Principles and Clinical Applications.* Philadelphia: Lea & Febiger; 1985:188.

99. Bargiggia GS, Bertucci C, Recusani F, et al. A new method for estimating left ventricular dP/dt by continuous wave Doppler-echocardiography. *Circulation.* 1989;80:1287-1292.

100. Chen C, Rodriguez L, Guerrero JL, et al. Noninvasive estimation of the instantaneous first derivative of left ventricular pressure using continuous-wave Doppler echocardiography. *Circulation.* 1991;83:2101-2110.

101. Nishimura RA, Abel MD, Hatle LK, et al. Assessment of diastolic function of the heart: Background and current applications of Doppler echocardiography. Part II. Clinical studies. *Mayo Clin Prac.* 1989;64:181-204.

102. Stoddard MF, Pearson AC, Kern MJ, et al. Left ventricular diastolic function: Comparison of pulsed Doppler echocardiographic and hemodynamic indexes in subjects with and without coronary artery disease. *J Am Coll Cardiol.* 1989;13:327-336.

103. Gardin JM, Rohan MK, Davidson DM, et al. Doppler transmitral flow velocity parameters: relationship between age, body surface area, blood pressure and gender in normal subjects. *Am J Noninvasive Cardiol.* 1987;1:3-10.

104. Kitzman DW, Sheikh KH, Beere PA, et al. Age-related alterations of Doppler left ventricular filling indexes in normal subjects are independent of left ventricular mass, heart rate, contractility and loading conditions. *J Am Coll Cardiol.* 1991;18:1243-1250.

105. Choong CY Herrmann HC, Weyman AE, et al. Preload dependence of Doppler-derived indexes of left ventricular diastolic function in humans. *J Am Coll Cardiol.* 1987:10:800-808.

106. Courtois M, Vered Z, Barzilai B, et al. The transmitral pressure-flow velocity relation: effect of abrupt preload reduction. *Circulaton.* 1988;78:672-683.

107. Masuyama T, St. Goar FG, Alderman EL, et al. Effects of nitroprusside on transmitral flow velocity patterns in extreme heart failure: A combined hemodynamic and Doppler echocardiographic study of varying loading conditions. *J Am Coll Cardiol.* 1990;16:1175-1185.

108. Appleton CP, Hatle LK, Popp RL. Relation of transmitral flow velocity patterns to left ventricular diastolic function: New insights from a combined hemodynamic and Doppler echocardiographic study. *J Am Coll Cardiol.* 1988;12:426-440.

109. Vanoverschelde JLJ, Raphael DA, Robert AR, et al. Left ventricular filling in dilated cardiomyopathy: Relation to functional class and hemodynamics. *J Am Coll Cardiol.* 1990;15:1288-1295.

110. Gallino RA, Milner MR, Goldstein SA, et al. Left ventricular filling patterns in aortic stenosis in patients older than 65 years of age. *Am J Cardiol.* 1989; 63:1103-1106.

111. Nishimura RA, Abel MD, Hatle LK, et al. Relation of pulmonary vein to mitral flow velocities by transesophageal Doppler echocardiography. Effect of different loading conditions. *Circulation.* 1990;81:1488-1497.

112. Rossvoll O, Hatle LK. Pulmonary venous flow velocities recorded by transthoracic Doppler ultrasound: relation to left ventricular diastolic pressures. *J Am Coll Cardiol.* 1993;21:1687-1696.

113. Appleton CP, Galloway J, Gonzalez MS, et al. Estimation of left ventricular filling pressures using 2-dimensional and Doppler echocardiography in adult patients with cardiac disease. *J Am Coll Cardiol.* 1993;1972-1982.

114. Kitabatake A, Inoue M, Masao M, et al. Noninvasive evaluation of pulmonary hypertension by a pulsed Doppler technique. *Circulation.* 1983;68:302-309.

115. Hatle L, Angelsen B. Doppler Ultrasound in Cardiology: *Physical Principles and Clinical Applications.* Philadelphia: Lea & Febiger; 1985:252-264.

116. Himelman RB, Stulbarg M, Kircher B, et al. Noninvasive evaluation of pulmonary artery pressure during exercise by saline-enhanced Doppler echocardiography in chronic pulmonary disease. *Circulation.* 1989;79:863-871.

117. Simonson JS, Schiller NB. Sonospirometry: A new method for noninvasive estimation of mean right atrial pressure based on 2-dimensional echographic measurements of the inferior vena cava during measured inspiration. *J Am Coll Cardiol.* 1988;11:557-564.

118. Bryg RJ, Labovitz AJ, Mehdirad AA, et al. Effect of coronary artery disease on Doppler-derived parameters of aortic flow during upright exercise. *Am J Cardiol.* 1986;58:14-19.

119. Harrison MR, Smith MD, Friedman BJ, et al. Uses and limitations of exercise Doppler echocardiography in the diagnosis of ischemic heart disease. *J Am Coll Cardiol.* 1987;10:809-817.

120. Hatle L, Angelsen B. *Doppler Ultrasound in Cardiology: Physical Principles and Clinical Applications.* Philadelphia: Lea & Febiger; 1985:180.

121. Hatle L, Angelsen B. *Doppler Ultrasound in Cardiology: Physical Principles and Clinical Applications.* Philadelphia: Lea & Febiger; 1985:238.

122. Bhatia SJS, Plappert T, Theard MA, et al. Transseptal Doppler flow velocity profile in acquired ventricular septal defect in acute myocardial infarction. *Am J Cardiol.* 1987;60:372-373.

123. Amico A, Iliceto S, Rizzo A, et al. Color Doppler findings in ventricular septal dissection following myocardial infarction. *Am Heart J.* 1989;117:195-198.

124. Smyllie JH, Sutherland GR, Geuskens R, et al. Doppler color flow mapping in the diagnosis of ventricular septal rupture and acute mitral regurgitation after myocardial infarction. *J Am Coll Cardiol.* 1990;15:1449-1455.

125. Helmcke F, Mahan EF, Nanda NC, et al. Two-dimensional echocardiography and Doppler color flow mapping in the diagnosis and prognosis of ventricular septal rupture. *Circulation.* 1990;81:1775-1783.

126. Sasson Z, Yock PG, Hatle LK, et al. Doppler echocardiographic determination of the pressure gradient in hypertrophic cardiomyopathy. *J Am Coll Cardiol.* 1988;11:752-756.

127. Panza JA, Petrone RK, Fananapazir L, et al. Use of continuous wave Doppler echocardiography in the noninvasive assessment of left ventricular outflow tract pressure gradient in patients with hypertrophic cardiomyopathy. *J Am Coll Cardiol.* 1992;19:91-99.

128. Schwammenthal E, Block M, Schwartzkopff B, et al. Prediction of the site and severity of obstruction in hypertrophic cardiomyopathy by color flow mapping and continuous wave Doppler echocardiography. *J Am Coll Cardiol.* 1992;20:964-972.

129. Yock PG, Hatle L, Popp RL. Patterns and timing of Doppler-detected intracavitary and aortic flow in hypertrophic cardiomyopathy. *J Am Coll Cardiol.* 1986;8:1047-1058.

130. Sasson Z, Hatle L, Appleton CP, et al. Intraventricular flow during isovolumic relaxation: Description and characterization by Doppler echocardiography. *J Am Coll Cardiol.* 1987;10:539-546.

131. Zoghbi WA, Haichin RN, Quinones MA. Mid-cavity obstruction in apical hypertrophy: Doppler evidence of diastolic intraventricular gradient with higher apical pressure. *Am Heart J.* 1988;116:1469-1474.

132. Appleton CP, Hatle LK, Popp RL. Demonstration of restrictive ventricular physiology by Doppler echocardiography. *J Am Coll Cardiol.* 1988;11:757-768.

133. Hatle LK, Appleton CP, Popp RL. Differentiation of constrictive pericarditis and restrictive cardiomyopathy by Doppler echocardiography. *Circulation.* 1989;79:357-370.

134. Klein AL, Hatle LK, Burstow DJ, et al. Doppler characterization of left ventricular diastolic function in cardiac amyloidosis. *J Am Coll Cardiol.* 1989;13:1017-1026.

135. Oh JK, Hatle LK, Seward JB, et al. Diagnostic role of Doppler echocardiography in constrictive pericarditis. *J Am Coll Cardiol.* 1994;23:154-162.

136. von Bibra H, Schober K, Jenni R, et al. Diagnosis of constrictive pericarditis by pulsed Doppler echocardiography of the hepatic vein. *Am J Cardiol.* 1989;63:483-488.

137. Schiavone WA, Calafiore PA, Salcedo EE. Transesophageal Doppler echocardiographic demonstration of pulmonary venous flow velocity in restrictive cardiomyopathy and constrictive pericarditis. *Am J Cardiol.* 1989;63:1286-1288.

138. Klein AL, Cone GI, Pietrolungo JF, et al. Differentiation of constrictive pericarditis from restrictive cardiomyopathy by Doppler transesophageal echocardiographic measurements of respiratory variations in pulmonary venous flow. *J Am Coll Cardiol.* 1993;22:1935-1943.

139. Leeman DE, Levine MJ, Come PC. Doppler echocardiography in cardiac tamponade: Exaggerated respiratory variation in transvalvular blood flow velocity integrals. *J Am Coll Cardiol.* 1988;11:572-578.

140. Appleton CP, Hatle LK, Popp RL. Cardiac tamponade and pericardial effusion: Respiratory variation in transvalvular flow velocities studied by Doppler echocardiography. *J Am Coll Cardiol.* 1988;11:1020-1030.

141. King SW, Pandian NG, Gardin JM. Doppler echocardiographic findings in pericardial tamponade and constriction. *Echocardiography.* 1988;5:361-372.

142. Gonzalez MS, Basnight MA, Appleton CP, et al. Experimental pericardial effusion: Relation of abnormal respiratory variation in mitral flow velocity to hemodynamics and diastolic right heart collapse. *J Am Coll Cardiol.* 1991;17:239-248.

143. Picard MH, Sanfilippo AJ, Newell JB, et al. Quantitative relation between increased intrapericardial pressure and Doppler flow velocities during experimental cardiac tamponade. *J Am Coll Cardiol.* 1991;18:234-242.

144. Schutzman JJ, Obarski TP, Pearce GL, et al. Comparison of Doppler and 2-dimensional echocardiography for assessment of pericardial effusion. *Am J Cardiol.* 1992;70:1353-1357.

145. Jaffe WM, Roche AHG, Coverdale HA, et al. Clinical evaluation versus Doppler echocardiography in the quantitative assessment of valvular heart disease. *Circulation.* 1988;78:267-275.

146. van den Brink RBA, Verheul HA, Hoedemaker G, et al. The value of Doppler echocardiography in the management of patients with valvular heart disease: Analysis of one year of clinical practice. *J Am Soc Echo.* 1991;4:109-120.

147. Slater J, Gindea AJ, Freedberg RS, et al. Comparison of cardiac catheterization and Doppler echocardiography in the decision to operate in aortic and mitral valve disease. *J Am Coll Cardiol.* 1991;17:1026-1036.

148. Galan A, Zoghbi WA, Quinones MA. Determination of severity of valvular aortic stenosis by Doppler echocardiography and relation of findings to clinical outcome and agreement with hemodynamic measurements determined at cardiac catheterization. *Am J Cardiol.* 1991;67:1007-1012.

149. Mennel RG, Joyner CR, Thompson PD, et al. The preoperative and operative assessment of aortic regurgitation: Cineaortography vs. electromagnetic flowmeter. *Am J Cardiol.* 1972;29:360-366.

150. Croft CH, Lipscomb K, Mathis K, et al. Limitations of qualitative angiographic grading in aortic or mitral regurgitation. *Am J Cardiol.* 1984; 53:1593-1598.

151. Carabello BA. What exactly is 2+ to 3+ mitral regurgitation? *J Am Coll Cardiol.* 1992;19:339-340.

Cardiac Catheterization

CHAPTER **9**

John E. Willard, MD
Richard A. Lange, MD
L. David Hillis, MD

Since its inception in the 1940s, cardiac catheterization has played an important role in our understanding of cardiovascular physiology and pathophysiology. More recently, it has been used with increasing frequency as a therapeutic procedure in patients with valvular abnormalities and atherosclerotic coronary artery disease (CAD). During its early years, catheterization was performed sparingly and with substantial risk. Over time, however, it has become established throughout the world, and the associated morbidity and mortality rates have fallen drastically. Today, diagnostic cardiac catheterization is performed with minimal risk, and therapeutic catheterization (i.e., coronary angioplasty and valvuloplasty) is performed without incident in the vast majority of patients. Therefore, cardiac catheterization now plays a vital role in the *diagnostic* evaluation of the patient with suspected or known cardiac disease; in addition, it offers percutaneous *therapeutic* possibilities in these individuals.

INDICATIONS AND CONTRAINDICATIONS

Diagnostic cardiac catheterization is appropriate in several circumstances. First, it is indicated to confirm or exclude the presence of a condition already suspected from the history, physical examination, or noninvasive evaluation. In such a circumstance, it allows the establishment of the presence and the assessment of the severity of cardiac disease. Second, catheterization is indicated to clarify a confusing or obscure clinical problem, that is, to arrive at a diagnosis in a patient whose clinical presentation and noninvasive evaluation are inconclusive. Third, catheterization is performed in some patients for whom corrective cardiac surgery is contemplated to confirm the suspected abnormality and to

exclude associated abnormalities that might require the surgeon's attention. Fourth, catheterization is occasionally performed purely as a research procedure.

Therapeutic catheterization is appropriate in several circumstances. Percutaneous coronary revascularization (e.g., angioplasty, atherectomy, rotational ablation, or endovascular stenting) may be indicated in the patient with symptomatic atherosclerotic coronary artery disease whose coronary anatomy is suitable for the procedure. Valvuloplasty is indicated in the subject with symptomatic isolated pulmonic stenosis and is an acceptable alternative to surgery in the patient with aortic or mitral stenosis in whom surgery may offer an unfavorable risk:benefit ratio, due, for example, to advanced age or comorbid medical conditions (such as chronic pulmonary, hepatic, or renal disease or an underlying malignancy).

Catheterization is absolutely contraindicated if a mentally competent individual does not consent. It is relatively contraindicated if an intercurrent condition exists which, if corrected, would improve the safety of the procedure. Examples of such conditions include ventricular irritability, uncontrolled cardiac failure, digitalis toxicity, electrolyte imbalance, acute renal insufficiency, infection, severe anemia, hypovolemia, uncontrolled systemic arterial hypertension, and an uncorrected bleeding diathesis.

TECHNIQUES OF CARDIAC CATHETERIZATION

Catheterization of the right and left sides of the heart can be accomplished by the introduction of catheters (a) by direct vision (into the brachial vein and artery)[1] or (b) by percutaneous punc-

145

ture (of the femoral or brachial vein and artery).[2] In the brachial cutdown approach, local anesthetic is introduced into an area 3-4 cm in diameter about 1 cm above the flexor crease of the arm, after which a transverse cutdown is performed. If both right and left heart catheterization is planned, the incision should be wide (2-3 cm in length) and located over the brachial artery; if only right-heart catheterization is contemplated, a small incision can be made directly over a brachial vein. Once the skin incision is made, the subcutaneous tissues are separated by blunt dissection with a curved hemostat. The vein and artery are isolated with bands, separated from adjacent tissues, and cleaned. The catheters are introduced under direct vision and are advanced into the great vessels and heart.

Following catheterization by the brachial approach, the catheters are removed, and the vein used for right-heart catheterization is ligated. The artery used for left-heart catheterization is rendered free of thrombi, and the arteriotomy is repaired. After blood flow has been successfully restored to the distal arm, the wound is flushed with saline, the incision is sutured, and the site of the cutdown is appropriately dressed.

To use the percutaneous femoral approach, local anesthetic is introduced into an area 3-4 cm in diameter 3-4 cm below the inguinal ligament (the inguinal ligament extends from the anterior superior iliac spine to the symphysis pubis). The anticipated puncture site should overlie bone, thus allowing for adequate vessel compression when the sheaths are removed. A small incision (about .5 cm long) is made over the vessels to be used for catheter introduction and passage, after which a "tunnel" is constructed (using a straight hemostat) at a 30° to 45° angle to the surface of the skin and to the approximate depth of the desired femoral vessel. An 18-gauge needle is introduced through the skin incision and tunnel into the lumen of the femoral artery or vein. Once blood flows freely through the needle, a Teflon-coated guide wire is advanced into the lumen of the punctured vessel. The wire is held firmly in place as the needle is removed, and the wire is wiped to remove blood and thrombi. Then, a sheath is threaded over the wire into the vessel lumen, and the wire is removed.

Following catheterization, the vascular sheaths are removed, and hemostasis is achieved by applying pressure over the puncture site

(generally 1-1.5 cm cephalad to the skin incision) for sufficient time to insure the cessation of bleeding. Hemostasis is generally obtained by applying direct pressure to the puncture site on the femoral vein for 5-10 min and on the femoral artery for 25-30 min. Subsequently, the patient is required to remain in bed and to immobilize the involved limb for 8-24 hours, depending on the size of the sheaths. The percutaneous brachial technique is performed in a similar manner by creating a tunnel 1 cm above the flexor crease of the arm.

The choice of approach (brachial or femoral) for both venous and arterial catheterization is determined by the preference and experience of the operator as well as the anatomic and pathophysiologic abnormalities of the patient. In general, right-heart catheterization is easier via the brachial approach in the patient with right ventricular and right atrial dilatation. In contrast, in the patient with a secundum atrial septal defect, a right-heart catheter can be passed across the defect more easily from the femoral approach. Thus, in choosing the route for right-heart catheterization, it is necessary to know anatomic abnormalities and specific disease entities. In most patients, left-heart catheterization can be performed by the brachial or femoral approach. Certain conditions make it difficult to perform left-heart catheterization by the femoral approach, such as extensive peripheral vascular disease, severe obesity, severe systemic arterial hypertension, bleeding diatheses, and any disorder that causes a markedly augmented arterial pulse pressure (e.g., severe aortic regurgitation). In turn, the brachial approach for left-heart catheterization is relatively contraindicated if there is evidence of severe brachiocephalic arterial disease.

In most catheterization laboratories, the brachial or femoral approach is used in almost all procedures. Occasionally, catheterization of 1 or more cardiac chambers is necessary via another route. For example, patients with tilting-disc prosthetic aortic valves require a direct left ventricular puncture to measure left ventricular pressure and to perform a ventriculogram.

HEMODYNAMIC ASSESSMENTS

CARDIAC OUTPUT

The role of the heart is to deliver an adequate quantity of blood to the body. This flow of blood

Table 1. Normal Hemodynamic Values

Flows	
Cardiac index (l/min/m²)	2.6-4.2
Stroke volume index (ml/m²)	35-55
Pressures (mm Hg)	
Systemic arterial	
Peak systolic/end diastolic	100-140/60-90
Mean	70-105
Left ventricle	
Peak systolic/end diastolic	100-140/3-12
Left atrium (PCW)	
Mean	1-10
a-wave	3-15
v-wave	3-15
Pulmonary arterial	
Peak systolic/end diastolic	16-30/0-8
Mean	10-16
Right ventricle	
Peak systolic/end diastolic	16-30/0-8
Right atrium	
Mean	0-8
a-wave	2-10
v-wave	2-10
Resistances	
Systemic vascular resistance	
Dynes-sec-cm⁻⁵	770-1500
Resistance units	10-20
Pulmonary vascular resistance	
Dynes-sec-cm⁻⁵	20-120
Resistance units	0.25-1.5
Oxygen consumption (ml/min/m²)	110-150
AV O₂ difference (ml/dl)	3.0-4.5

PCW=Pulmonary capillary wedge;
AV=Arteriovenous.

is known as the cardiac output (CO) and is expressed in liters per minute. Since the magnitude of CO is proportional to body surface area, one person may be compared to another by means of the cardiac index (CI), that is, the CO adjusted for body surface area. The normal CI is 2.6 to 4.2 l/min/m² of body surface area (Table 1).

There are 2 major methods of measuring CO: the Fick method and the indicator dilution technique. The latter can be performed by thermodilution or the injection of indocyanine green.

Fick Method

The measurement of CO by the Fick method is based on the hypothesis that the uptake or release of a substance by an organ is the product of the blood flow to that organ and the regional arteriovenous (AV) concentration difference of the substance.[3] To measure CO in humans, this principle is applied to the lungs, and the substance measured is oxygen (O_2). By measuring the amount of O_2 extracted from inspired air by the lungs and the AV-O_2 difference across the lungs, pulmonary blood flow may be calculated. Since pulmonary blood flow equals systemic blood flow in most people, the Fick method allows one to measure systemic blood flow. The Fick formula for the calculation of CO is:

$$CO\ (l/min) = \frac{O_2\ consumption(ml/min)}{AV\ O_2\ difference\ across\ the\ lungs}$$

The O_2 consumption is determined directly by collecting a timed sample (usually 3-4 min) of expired air in a special receptacle called a Douglas bag. The volume of this collection is measured, and the difference in O_2 content between inspired and expired air is calculated. From these data, the person's O_2 consumption (in ml/min) is determined.

The normal O_2 consumption index (O_2 consumption/m² of body surface) is 110-150 ml/min/m² (Table 1).[4] In general, the O_2 consumption decreases gradually with age. It increases with hyperthyroidism, hyperthermia, and exercise, whereas it decreases with hypothyroidism and hypothermia.

Determining the AV-O_2 difference across the lungs requires that blood from the vessels entering and draining the lungs (i.e., the pulmonary artery and vein) be analyzed for O_2 content. Since the O_2 content of pulmonary venous blood is similar to that of systemic arterial blood (provided that a right-to-left shunt is not present), systemic and pulmonary arterial samples are usually obtained for the Fick determination of CO. The O_2 content of pulmonary and systemic arterial blood may be measured directly or calculated from the O_2 saturation of the blood: O_2 content = Hgb (in gm/100 ml) x 1.39 (ml O_2/gm Hgb) x saturation, where 1.39 is the maximum O_2-carrying capacity of 1 gm of Hgb. The normal AV-O_2 difference is 3.0-4.5 volumes percent (ml O_2/dl of blood). The following is an example of the Fick calculation of cardiac output: (a) O_2 consumption = 250 ml/min; (b) Hgb = 15 gm/dl; (c) systemic arterial O_2 saturation =

0.95 (95%); (d) pulmonary arterial O_2 saturation = 0.70 (70%); and (e) 10 = dl/l (conversion factor).

$$CO=\frac{250}{(15)(1.39)(10)(0.95)-(15)(1.39)(10)(0.70)}=4.80\ l/min$$

The Fick method has several potential sources of error.[5] First, an incomplete collection of expired air causes an underestimation of O_2 consumption, leading to the calculation of a falsely low value for CO. This is the most common source of error. Second, incorrect timing of the expired air collection leads to an inaccurate estimate of O_2 consumption. Third, analysis of the Douglas bag contents should be performed soon after its collection, since air diffuses in and out of the bag if there is a substantial delay. Fourth, the spectrophotometric determination of the O_2 saturations may be inaccurate if certain substances, such as indocyanine green, have been introduced into the blood. Finally, the mixed venous blood sample must, indeed, be mixed venous. It is generally obtained from the pulmonary artery; it must not be partially contaminated by pulmonary capillary wedge blood or left-to-right shunted blood.

The average error in determining O_2 consumption is about 6%, and that for AV-O_2 difference is 5%. When the AV-O_2 difference is small, errors in measurement are magnified. Therefore, the Fick method is most accurate in the patient with a low CO (i.e., one with a relatively wide AV-O_2 saturation difference) and least accurate in one with a high CO (i.e., one with a relatively narrow AV-O_2 saturation difference).

Indicator Dilution Technique

This technique is based on the principle that the volume of fluid within a container can be measured if one adds a known quantity of indicator to the fluid and then measures the concentration of the indicator after it has been completely mixed with the fluid. The indicator most often used to measure CO is cold saline or 5% dextrose-in-water. The catheter used for this measurement is a balloon-tipped, flow-directed, polyvinylchloride catheter with 2 openings, one at the tip and the other 25-30 cm proximal to the tip. In addition, a small thermistor is located 2-5 cm from the tip. This catheter is inserted into a vein and advanced to the pulmonary

artery. Thus, the distal opening is in a large pulmonary artery, and the proximal opening is in the right atrium. Iced fluid is injected into the right atrial opening, and the temporary change in temperature at the thermistor is recorded.[6,7]

Indocyanine green, an easily detectable, water-soluble, nontoxic substance, can also be used for the indicator dilution measurement of CO.[8] To do so, (a) a known concentration of indicator must be injected; (b) there must be complete mixing of the indocyanine green between the sites of injection and sampling; and (c) there must be no metabolism or disappearance of the indicator between the sites of injection and sampling. In most catheterization laboratories, CO is measured by injecting indocyanine green into the pulmonary artery as blood is withdrawn at a constant rate from a systemic artery through an optical densitometer. The lungs, left atrium, and left ventricle act as adequate mixing sites, and there is no degradation of indocyanine green between the pulmonary and systemic arteries.

The calculation of CO by the indicator dilution technique is usually done by a minicomputer, which establishes that the downslope of the inscribed curve is exponential and then computes the area inscribed by the curve, excluding the recirculation peak. These calculations can be done manually but require a clear separation of the initial circulation peak from that of normal recirculation.

With both indocyanine green and cold saline or dextrose, therefore, CO can be determined by assessing the concentration of an indicator after adequate mixing with blood has occurred. To insure an accurate assessment of CO, great care must be taken, first, to inject an exact amount of indicator; second, to inject the indicator as rapidly as possible (so that, in fact, it is delivered as a bolus); third, to calibrate the densitometer and recorder systems precisely; and fourth, to insure that the withdrawal of blood (in the case of indocyanine green) at the sampling site is uniform and not accompanied by air bubbles. If care is taken to eliminate these sources of error, the indicator dilution technique is a reliable method of measuring CO. This technique is most accurate for individuals with a high CO. It is least accurate in those with a low CO and in those with valvular regurgitation between the sites of indicator injection and sampling (i.e., tricuspid or pulmonic regurgitation

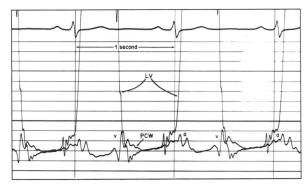

Figure 1. *Simultaneous recording of left ventricular (LV) and pulmonary capillary wedge (PCW) pressures in a patient without mitral valve disease. The distance between each horizontal line above the baseline represents 4 mm Hg, and the distance between each vertical line represents 1 sec. The PCW A wave occurs in conjunction with the A wave of the LV pressure trace, and the PCW V wave occurs with the down-slope of the LV trace. Note that during diastole the LV and PCW pressures are superimposed; that is, there is no pressure gradient between the PCW and LV.*

with thermodilution, aortic or mitral regurgitation with indocyanine green).

PRESSURE MEASUREMENTS

One of the most important functions of cardiac catheterization is the accurate measurement and recording of intracardiac pressures. Once a catheter has been positioned in the desired cardiac chamber, it is connected directly or through stiff, fluid-filled tubing to a pressure transducer, which transforms a pressure signal into an electrical signal (via a Wheatstone bridge). The accurate measurement of pressures requires close attention to the details of the catheter-transducer system, including proper transducer balancing as well as removing air bubbles and blood from the catheters and connections. Errors in pressure measurement may occur in several ways. An accurate zero reference is essential. All manometers must be referenced to the same zero level, which must be adjusted if the patient's position is altered. Pressure transducers must be calibrated frequently, preferably before each pressure recording. To allow for a meaningful interpretation of hemodynamic data, they should be collected (a) with the patient in a steady state, (b) in close temporal proximity to one another (all pressure

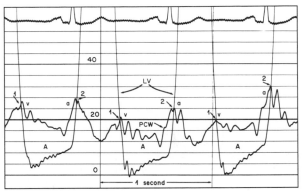

Figure 2. *Simultaneous recording of LV and PCW pressures in a patient with mitral stenosis. Throughout diastole, from points 1 to 2, there is a pressure gradient between the PCW and LV pressures. The patient, a 28-year-old woman, had a cardiac output of 3,740 ml/min, measured simultaneously with this pressure tracing. The heart rate was 68 beats/min, the mean diastolic filling period was 0.49 sec/beat, and the mean pressure gradient, derived by dividing A by the average gradient duration, was 12.7 mm Hg. Using the Gorlin formula, the mitral valve area was $\frac{3740/(68)(0.49)}{(38)(\sqrt{12.7})} = 0.8$ cm².*

measurements and assessments of CO should be completed within 10-15 min), and (c) before the introduction of contrast material or other agents known to alter hemodynamics.

During most catheterizations, pressures are measured directly from each of the cardiac chambers except the left atrium. A direct pressure measurement is obtained with a catheter in the right atrium, right ventricle, pulmonary artery, ascending aorta, and left ventricle. In contrast, the left atrium is seldom entered unless a transseptal catheterization is performed (passage of a catheter from the right atrium across the interatrial septum into the left atrium). The left atrial pressure is generally recorded "indirectly," that is, as the pulmonary capillary wedge pressure. To accomplish this, an end-hole catheter is placed in the pulmonary artery and advanced into the pulmonary arterial tree until it is effectively wedged. If the catheter is wedged adequately, the resultant pressure is left atrial, and the blood withdrawn from it is fully saturated. The demonstration that fully saturated blood can be withdrawn from the catheter confirms that the pressure is indeed left atrial.

In addition to the recording of pressures from each of the cardiac chambers, it is impor-

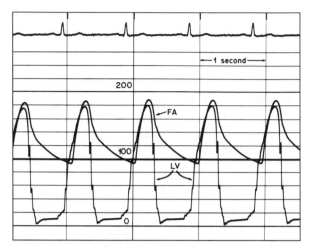

Figure 3. *Simultaneous recording of LV and femoral arterial (FA) pressures in a patient without LV outflow tract obstruction. Pressures are indicated in mm Hg on the vertical scale. Note that there is no pressure gradient during systole between LV and FA; in fact, the peak systolic FA pressure is about 5 mm Hg higher than LV. See Figure 4 for an explanation of this phenomenon.*

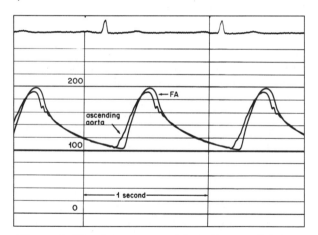

Figure 4. *Simultaneous recording of ascending aortic and FA pressures in a normal individual. The peak systolic FA pressure is slightly higher than the peak systolic ascending aortic pressure, due to peripheral amplification of pressure, a normal phenomenon.*

tant that the pressures from certain chambers be examined simultaneously to confirm or exclude the presence of valvular abnormalities. Thus, left ventricular and pulmonary capillary wedge pressures should be recorded simultaneously to

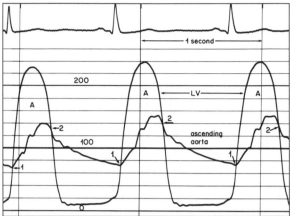

Figure 5. *Simultaneous recording of LV and ascending aortic pressures in a patient with severe aortic stenosis. Throughout systole, from points 1 to 2, there is a pressure gradient between LV and aorta. The patient, a 50-year-old man, had a cardiac output of 3,350 ml/min, a heart rate of 62 beats/min, a mean systolic ejection time of 0.36 sec/beat, and a mean pressure gradient throughout systole of 83 mm Hg, determined by dividing A by the average duration of the gradient. Thus, the aortic valve area equals*

$$\frac{3,350/(62)(0.36)}{(44.5)\,(\sqrt{83})} = 0.4 \text{ cm}^2$$

ascertain if mitral stenosis is present (Figs. 1, 2). Likewise, the left ventricular and systemic arterial pressures should be displayed concurrently to evaluate the presence or absence of left ventricular outflow tract obstruction (Figs. 3–5).

Recording intracardiac and peripheral vascular pressures can demonstrate hemodynamic evidence of valvular regurgitation. For instance, large regurgitant waves in the pulmonary capillary wedge tracing may indicate mitral regurgitation or other causes of pressure or volume overload of the left atrium (Fig. 6). Conversely, a wide peripheral arterial pulse pressure in conjunction with a greatly elevated left ventricular end-diastolic pressure suggests aortic regurgitation (Fig. 7). In short, both the absolute level and the qualitative configuration of the intracardiac and peripheral vascular pressures are important in the diagnosis and quantitation of valvular heart disease. The normal intracardiac and peripheral vascular flows, pressures, and resistances are listed in Table 1.

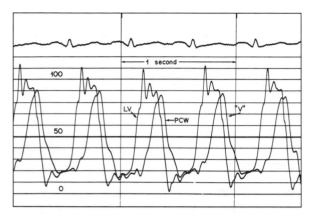

Figure 6. *Simultaneous recording of LV and PCW pressures from a patient with severe, acute mitral regurgitation due to an inferior myocardial infarction with resultant papillary muscle rupture. Note that there is no gradient between LV and PCW during diastole. However, the PCW tracing demonstrates large regurgitant V waves as high as 90 mm Hg.*

RESISTANCES

The resistance of a vascular bed can be calculated by dividing the pressure gradient across the bed by the flow through it. Thus, systemic vascular resistance =

$$\frac{\text{mean systemic arterial pressure} - \text{mean right atrial pressure}}{\text{systemic blood flow}}$$

and

pulmonary vascular resistance =

$$\frac{\text{mean pulmonary arterial presure} - \text{mean pulmonary venous pressure}}{\text{pulmonary blood flow}}$$

Resistances are expressed in resistance units (mm Hg/l/min), dynes-sec-cm^{-5} (resistance units x 80), or Wood units (resistance units x body surface area in m^2). The normal values for vascular resistances are displayed in Table 1.

An increased systemic vascular resistance is usually present in patients with systemic arterial hypertension. It may also be seen in the patient with a reduced forward CO and compensatory arteriolar vasoconstriction. In turn, a reduced systemic vascular resistance may be present in the patient with an inappropriately increased CO, the causes of which include AV fistula, severe anemia, high fever, sepsis, and thyrotoxicosis. An elevated pulmonary vascular resistance may be caused by primary lung disease,

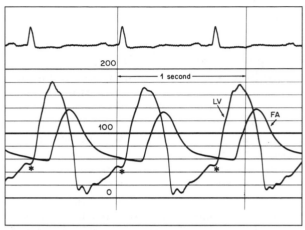

Figure 7. *Simultaneous recording of LV and FA pressures from a patient with mixed aortic stenosis and regurgitation. The FA upstroke occurs later than that of the LV, due to the time required for pulse wave transmission from the LV to the FA. There is a systolic gradient between LV and FA of about 40 mm Hg peak to peak. The FA pulse pressure is only minimally widened. During diastole, the LV pressure demonstrates a gradual and steady rise, so that the LV pressure at end-diastole (*) is about 50 mm Hg.*

Eisenmenger's syndrome (alterations in the pulmonary vasculature in response to increased pulmonary flow and pressure), and a greatly elevated pulmonary venous pressure due to left-sided myocardial and/or valvular dysfunction.

VALVE AREAS

Through the application of standard fluid dynamic principles, the resistance to blood flow through a stenosed valve can be expressed as an effective valve orifice area.[9] The data required for the calculation of a valve area may be obtained during cardiac catheterization. Specifically, the pressures on either side of a stenotic valve and the flow across it must be known. The Gorlin equation is then used to calculate the valve area:

$$\text{valve area} = \frac{\text{CO/(DFP or SEP) (heart rate)}}{\text{(constant) } (\sqrt{\text{mean pressure gradient}})}$$

where DFP = diastolic filling period, and SEP = systolic ejection period. If an atrioventricular valve (mitral or tricuspid) is being evaluated, the diastolic filling period is employed; if the aortic or pulmonic valve is involved, the systolic ejection period is used. The constant used is 38 for the mitral valve and 44.5 for the other valves. The mean pressure gradient is the average gradient throughout systole (for aortic and pulmonic valves) or diastole (for mitral or tricuspid valves).

The normal mitral valve orifice area is 4-6 cm². Substantial stenosis can develop before a pressure gradient appears. A mitral valve with an effective orifice area of ≤ 1.0 cm² is considered severely stenotic (Fig. 2); 1.1 to ≤ 1.5 cm², moderately stenotic; and 1.6 to ≤ 2.0 cm², mildly stenotic. A valve area >2.0 cm² is not necessarily normal but does not usually constitute a hemodynamically significant obstruction to flow. The normal aortic valve has a cross-sectional area of 3-4 cm², but hemodynamically important aortic stenosis does not develop until the valve orifice area falls below 1.1-1.3 cm². Specifically, an aortic valve with an effective orifice area of ≤ 0.7 cm² is severely stenotic (Fig. 5); 0.8 to ≤ 1.0 cm², moderately stenotic; and 1.1 to ≤ 1.3 cm², mildly stenotic. The normal pulmonic valve has a cross-sectional area similar to the aortic valve. Although the Gorlin equation can be applied to the pulmonic valve, by convention the severity of stenosis in adults is based on the peak right ventricular systolic pressure. Pulmonic stenosis with an RV peak systolic pressure of 25 to <50 mm Hg is termed mild; 50 to <100 mm Hg, moderate; and ≥ 100 mm Hg, severe. Finally, the tricuspid valve is very large, with a normal orifice area of 6-10 cm². The assessment of the severity of tricuspid stenosis is most accurate when simultaneous right atrial and right ventricular pressures are recorded. Patients with a tricuspid valve area of ≤ 3.0 cm² in the presence of medically refractory right-sided heart failure should be considered for appropriate mechanical interventions (i.e., balloon valvuloplasty, open commissurotomy, or valve replacement).

It is essential that all the variables used to calculate a valve area (CO, systolic ejection period or diastolic filling period, heart rate, and pressure gradient) are measured in close temporal proximity to one another and with the patient hemodynamically stable. Great care must be exercised in acquiring these data, since the decision for surgical intervention is based on the calculated valve area.

BALLOON-TIPPED, FLOW-DIRECTED (SWAN-GANZ) CATHETERS

In 1970, the balloon-tipped, flow-directed catheter was introduced for right-heart catheter-

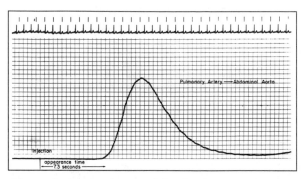

Figure 8. *A normal curve following the injection of 5 mg of indocyanine green into the pulmonary artery, with simultaneous withdrawal of blood from the abdominal aorta. The time between injection and first appearance of the indicator is 7.3 sec.*

ization at the bedside, without the need for fluoroscopy.[10] At present, it is widely used to monitor pulmonary arterial and pulmonary capillary wedge pressures in the critically ill patient in an intensive care unit. The catheter, which has an inflatable balloon at its tip, is made of polyvinylchloride and is extremely soft. The standard balloon-tipped catheter has 2 lumina — the smaller lumen allows inflation of the balloon and the larger lumen allows one to measure pressures and to obtain blood specimens.

Before using the balloon-tipped catheter, the balloon should be inflated in saline to exclude an air leak, and the catheter lumen should be flushed with saline. A temporary transvenous pacing catheter should be positioned in the right ventricle in patients with a preexisting left bundle branch block before passage of any catheter from the right atrium to the pulmonary artery, since such passage may induce a transient right bundle branch block, leading to complete heart block. The balloon-tipped catheter may be inserted at the bedside either percutaneously (via the femoral, internal jugular, subclavian, or basilic vein) or by direct exposure of the brachial vein. When it is introduced without the use of fluoroscopy, it should be passed into the vasculature for 10-30 cm (depending on the site of introduction) before the balloon is inflated. The catheter is marked at 10-cm intervals to facilitate this procedure. Before advancing the catheter, blood should be aspirated through it to insure that it is intravascular. The balloon is inflated gently with up to 1 ml of air to facilitate its flow-directed passage from the right atrium to the pulmonary artery. If there is resistance to bal-

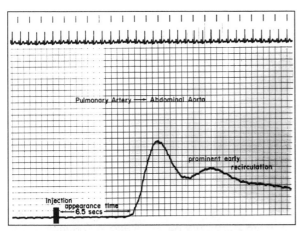

Figure 9. *A curve following the injection of 5 mg of indocyanine green into the pulmonary artery, with blood withdrawal from the abdominal aorta, in a patient with a large left-to-right intracardiac shunt (in this case, an atrial septal defect). In comparison to a normal curve (Fig. 8), there is a very prominent early recirculation peak. The appearance time is normal, thus excluding a right-to-left shunt distal to the site of injection.*

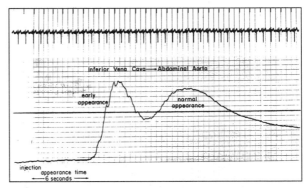

Figure 10. *A curve following the injection of 5 mg of indocyanine green into the inferior vena cava, with blood withdrawal from the abdominal aorta, in a patient with a large right-to-left intracardiac shunt (in this case, a large ventricular septal defect with pulmonary infundibular stenosis, or tetralogy of Fallot). The initial peak represents early appearance of indocyanine green in the abdominal aorta, reflecting the right-to-left through the VSD. The second peak represents normal appearance of indocyanine green.*

loon inflation, the catheter should be advanced or withdrawn carefully until the balloon can be inflated freely. The catheter is then connected to a pressure transducer to record right atrial pressure. It is also valuable to obtain a blood sample for oximetric analysis in each right-heart chamber or vessel where pressures are recorded to exclude left-to-right intracardiac shunting.

Once a blood sample and pressure have been obtained from the right atrium, the balloon is inflated and the catheter gently advanced while observing pressure and the electrocardiogram. If the catheter does not pass easily from the right ventricle to the pulmonary artery or significant ventricular ectopy occurs, it should be withdrawn to the right atrium and the procedure repeated. Once it has passed to the pulmonary artery and the pressure has been recorded (Fig. 11), it is advanced gently (with the balloon still inflated) until the wave-form changes to that of a pulmonary capillary wedge pressure (Fig. 12). A fully oxygenated blood specimen from this site confirms that the catheter is truly in a wedged position. When the balloon is deflated, the waveform should change to that of pulmonary arterial pressure.

It is occasionally impossible to pass the balloon-tipped catheter without the use of fluoroscopic guidance, particularly in the patient with a

large right atrium, ventricle, or pulmonary hypertension. It may be necessary to introduce a 0.025 in. J-tipped guide wire into the catheter to stiffen it, after which it is advanced under fluoroscopic visualization. Passage of the catheter without the use of fluoroscopy is easier when the site of vascular entry is central (i.e., internal jugular or subclavian vein) rather than peripheral.

The balloon-tipped, flow-directed catheter offers several advantages over the more traditional stiff catheter used for right-heart catheterization; at the same time, it has certain drawbacks. Since it is unusually soft, perforation of the major vessels and heart is virtually impossible, whereas such perforation occasionally occurs with a stiff catheter. As indicated, the flow-directed catheter can be inserted and advanced without fluoroscopic control, although catheter manipulation is easier with fluoroscopic assistance. Apart from its safety, the balloon-tipped, flow-directed catheter can be equipped with a distal thermistor and CO can be measured by the thermodilution technique.

The major disadvantages of the balloon-tipped, flow-directed catheter stem from the same features that are responsible for its advantages. First, because the catheter is unusually soft, the pressure recordings obtained through it contain a good deal of "catheter whip," that is, artifact introduced by the movement of the

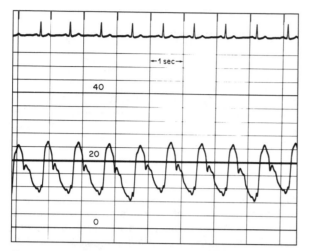

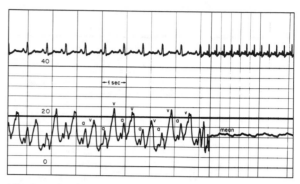

Figure 12. A recording of PCW pressure from the same patient as in Figure 11. For each QRS complex, there are 2 pressure waves: A and V. The mean PCW pressure is 13 mm Hg.

Figure 11. A recording of pulmonary arterial pressure with a Swan-Ganz catheter; the pressure averages about 25/10 mm Hg.

catheter itself within the heart. Second, since the catheter is no larger than 7 French in size yet contains 2 or more lumens, the distal lumen is small in size, making the aspiration of blood difficult. Third, since this catheter is advanced in the direction of blood flow, its placement in the pulmonary artery may be impossible if flow within the right-heart chambers is bidirectional. For example, advancing a balloon-tipped, flow-directed catheter to the pulmonary artery in a patient with severe tricuspid regurgitation may be technically difficult, since the regurgitation jet directs the catheter from the right ventricle back into the right atrium. Despite these limitations, this catheter almost always allows one to measure right- and left-sided filling pressures and to make appropriate therapeutic decisions regarding fluid and drug administration.

The risks and complications of the balloon-tipped, flow-directed catheter are similar to those of any catheter used for right-heart catheterization: ventricular irritability or transient right bundle branch block during passage through the right ventricle and local inflammation or infection at the site of entrance. In addition, because of its softness, the balloon-tipped catheter is easily knotted. Improper or prolonged inflation of the balloon can lead to rupture of a small pulmonary artery or to subsegmental pulmonary infarction, respectively. By and large, however, the balloon-tipped, flow-

directed catheter is extremely safe. Once it is positioned in the pulmonary artery, it may be left in place for 48-96 hours.

SHUNT DETECTION AND MEASUREMENT

The detection and quantitation of an intracardiac shunt can be accomplished by several techniques.[11] First, the measurement of O_2 content within the cardiac chambers and the great vessels allows one to locate the site of intracardiac shunting and to determine its magnitude. Once the site of shunting is determined, one can calculate the blood flow to the pulmonary and systemic circulations. The oximetric determination of intracardiac shunting is highly specific but relatively insensitive; that is, an oximetric assessment reliably demonstrates the presence of a moderate-to-large shunt but usually fails to detect a small one.[12,13]

Second, the presence and magnitude of an intracardiac shunt can be demonstrated and quantitated by indicator dilution injections.[14] By performing the injection of indocyanine green and the simultaneous withdrawal of blood from several sites within the heart and great vessels, one can determine the site and size of the intracardiac shunt (Figs. 8–10). Indocyanine green injections are more sensitive than oximetry for detecting and quantitating small intracardiac shunts.[15,16]

Third, the inhalation of hydrogen with simultaneous sensing with a platinum-tipped elec-

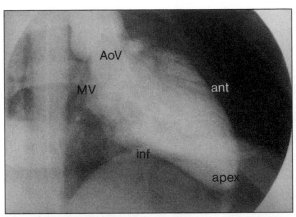

Figure 13. *The end-diastolic image from a right anterior oblique (RAO) left ventriculogram in a patient with normal wall motion. AoV=Aortic valve; MV=Mitral valve; inf=Inferior wall; ant=Anterior wall; apex=Apex of the left ventricle.*

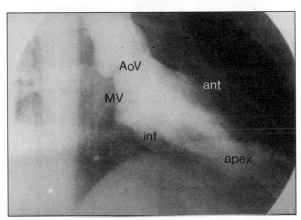

Figure 14. *The end-systolic image from a RAO left ventriculogram in the same patient as shown in Figure 13. Abbreviations are also similar. In comparison to Figure 13, all segments of the left ventricular wall have contracted normally.*

trode in the pulmonary artery can be used to detect very small left-to-right shunts.[17,18] This technique is the most sensitive method available for the detection of left-to-right shunts.[19]

Fourth, angiography may be used to demonstrate an intracardiac shunt, but this technique does not allow quantitation of the shunt. For example, a ventricular septal defect with shunting from the left to the right ventricle can be demonstrated with a left ventriculogram in a 30°-40° left anterior oblique projection. Alternatively, a patent ductus arteriosus with shunting from the aorta to the pulmonary artery can be detected via a proximal aortogram in the lateral projection.

ANGIOGRAPHY

LEFT VENTRICULOGRAPHY

Cineangiocardiography of the left ventricle allows one to assess global and segmental left ventricular function, left ventricular volumes and ejection fraction, and the presence and severity of mitral regurgitation. To achieve adequate opacification, a large bolus of radiographic contrast material must be delivered to the left ventricle over a short period of time. In the normal adult, 40-60 ml of contrast material is injected over 3-4 seconds; thus, 10-20 ml are injected per second. As the contrast material is injected into the left ventricle, cineangiography is performed. Ventriculography may be performed in 2 projections (biplane) or more commonly in 1 projection (single plane), which is usually performed in the 30° right anterior oblique projection (Figs. 13, 14). If biplane cineangiographic equipment is available, 2 projections, 90° apart in obliquity (60° left anterior oblique and 30° right anterior oblique) are performed.

A variety of catheters can be used for left ventriculography, but all have certain features in common. First, the catheter should be of sufficient size so that a high-pressure injection of contrast material does not cause it to recoil, with resultant ventricular ectopy. Second, the catheter should be designed so that the jet of injected contrast material exits through a series of side-holes rather than just an end-hole; the chance of a high-pressure jet of contrast material being injected into the endocardium (so-called endocardial staining) is minimized. Finally, although the angiographic catheter should have multiple side-holes for the injection of contrast material, these holes should be confined to the distal 2-3 cm of the catheter to avoid contrast injection into both the left ventricle and the proximal ascending aorta.

Left ventriculography allows for calculation of left ventricular volumes and ejection fraction using a standard area-length formula.[20–22] End-diastolic and end-systolic volumes are measured; from these, left ventricular stroke volume is derived (end-diastolic volume minus end-systolic volume), and ejection fraction is calculated (stroke volume divided by end-diastolic volume). The normal values for left ventricular volumes

Table 2. Normal Angiographic Values	
LV end-diastolic volume index	50-90 ml/m²
LV end-systolic volume index	15-35 ml/m²
LV stroke volume index	35-55 ml/m²
LV ejection fraction	0.55-0.70
LV=Left ventricular.	

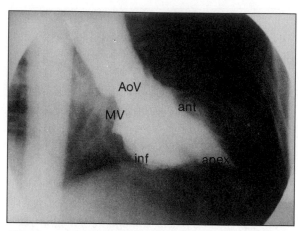

Figure 16. *The end-systolic image from a RAO left ventriculogram in the same patient as shown in Figure 15. Note that the anterior wall (ant) and apex move normally during systole but that the inferior wall (inf) is akinetic; that is, it does not move during systole. Ao=Aortic valve.*

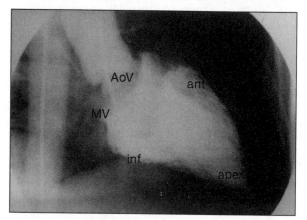

Figure 15. *The end-diastolic image from a RAO left ventriculogram in a patient with a previous inferior myocardial infarction. AoV=Aortic valve; MV=Mitral valve; inf=Inferior wall; ant=Anterior wall; apex=Apex of the left ventricle.*

and ejection fraction are displayed in Table 2. In addition to the calculation of left ventricular volumes, segmental wall motion can be assessed. A segment of the left ventricular wall with reduced systolic motion is said to be hypokinetic; a segment that does not move at all during ventricular contraction is akinetic; and one that moves paradoxically during ventricular systole is dyskinetic (Figs. 15, 16). Finally, the presence and severity of mitral regurgitation may be qualitatively evaluated during sinus beats as trivial (1+), mild (2+), moderate (3+), or severe (4+): (a) with 1+, contrast dye enters the left atrium during systole and clears with each beat; (b) with 2+, contrast opacification of the left atrium does not clear with each beat and is less dense than the left ventricle; (c) with 3+, opacification of the left atrium is equal to that of the left ventricle; and (d) with 4+, the presence of 1 of 3 findings is observed—opacification of the left atrium greater than that of the left ventricle, opacification of the left atrium in one systolic ejection period, or the presence of contrast material in a pulmonary vein (Fig. 17).[23]

RIGHT VENTRICULOGRAPHY

Cineangiography of the right ventricle allows one to assess global right ventricular function as well as the presence and severity of tricuspid regurgitation. Right ventriculography can be performed in single or biplane projections. Single plane right ventriculography is usually performed in a 30° right anterior oblique projection. If biplane angiography is available, a 60° left anterior oblique projection is also performed. To achieve adequate opacification, a bolus of 24-36 ml of radiographic contrast is injected over 2 seconds. As the contrast material is injected into the ventricle, cineangiography is performed. The presence and severity of tricuspid regurgitation can be qualitatively evaluated in a manner similar to mitral regurgitation: trivial (1+), mild (2+), moderate (3+), or severe (4+). There are no reliable methods for the quantitative assessment of right ventricular volumes or ejection fraction by ventriculography.

AORTOGRAPHY

Aortography is the rapid injection of a large amount of contrast material into the aorta. A proximal aortogram is performed to assess the competency of the aortic valve, to evaluate the anatomy of the proximal aorta and large vessels that supply the head and neck, and occasionally

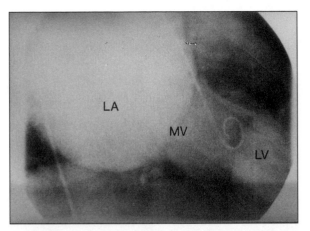

Figure 17. *A selected frame from a RAO left ventriculogram in a patient with severe, long-standing mitral regurgitation. Note that the left atrium (LA) is larger than the left ventricle (LV) and that it is more densely opacified with contrast material. MV=Mitral valve.*

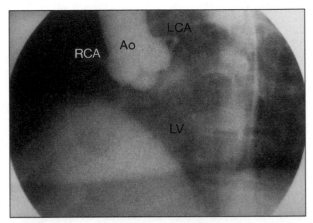

Figure 18. *A selected frame from a left anterior oblique (LAO) aortogram in a patient without aortic regurgitation. Ao=Proximal aorta; RCA=Proximal right coronary artery; LCA=Proximal left coronary artery; LV=Left ventricle. The three aortic valve cusps are easily discernible.*

to assess the presence of bypass graft anastomoses that have been difficult or impossible to cannulate selectively. In turn, a distal aortogram is performed to assess the presence of vascular abnormalities (e.g., aneurysm, dissection, intraluminal thrombus, coarctation). The catheters employed for aortography are similar to those used for left ventriculography. For proximal aortography, 50-60 ml of contrast material is injected over 2-2.5 seconds and filmed either by cineangiography or rapid cut-film angiography. The standard proximal aortogram is filmed in a 45°-60° left anterior oblique projection (Fig. 18). The severity of aortic regurgitation may be qualitatively evaluated during sinus beats as trivial (1+), mild (2+), moderate (3+), or severe (4+): (a) with 1+, contrast dye enters the left ventricle during diastole and clears with each beat; (b) with 2+, contrast opacification of the left ventricle does not clear with each beat and is less dense than the ascending aorta; (c) with 3+, opacification of the left ventricle is equal to that of the aorta; and (d) with 4+, opacification of the left ventricle is greater than that of the aorta, or the left ventricle is opacified in 1 diastolic filling period.[23]

PULMONARY ANGIOGRAPHY

Pulmonary angiography is performed primarily to confirm or exclude the presence of pulmonary emboli.[24,25] A large-bore angiographic

catheter is advanced from a systemic vein to the main pulmonary artery and is positioned so that it does not recoil into the right ventricle during the injection of contrast material, with resultant ventricular irritability. A large amount of contrast material (40-60 ml) is injected over 2-3 seconds. During the injection, cineangiography or rapid cut-film angiography is performed.

If injection into the main pulmonary artery does not provide a definitive diagnosis, subselective injections are made into those segments of lung where the suspicion of pulmonary emboli is highest. These injections can be made with either a small power injection through the same angiographic catheter or a hand injection through a balloon-tipped catheter.

Analysis of the films must be meticulous, as the radiographic findings associated with pulmonary embolism may be subtle. Radiographic signs diagnostic of pulmonary embolism include a large intraluminal filling defect or an abrupt pulmonary arterial cut-off. Other radiographic signs, such as localized oligemia and asymmetry of pulmonary blood flow, are suggestive but not strictly diagnostic of embolism.

SELECTIVE CORONARY ARTERIOGRAPHY

Selective coronary arteriography is usually performed to determine the presence and severity of fixed, atherosclerotic coronary artery disease.

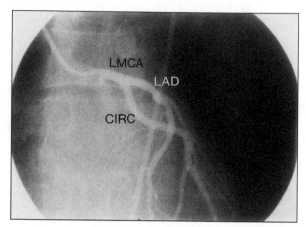

Figure 19. *An anteroposterior view of a normal left coronary artery. LMCA=Left main coronary artery; LAD=Left anterior descending artery; CIRC=Left circumflex artery.*

It is occasionally performed to evaluate the presence of dynamic alterations of coronary arterial tone, that is, coronary arterial spasm. Each coronary arterial ostium is selectively engaged with a catheter, after which injections of contrast material are made by hand.[1,2] The angiographer should design each coronary injection to evaluate the vessel segment of interest. To accomplish this, the vessel of interest should be positioned over a homogenous background; contrast material should be injected with sufficient force to opacify the coronary artery completely without injecting an excessive amount of contrast material in the aortic root; each vessel should be imaged in projections that display the area of interest in an unforeshortened and unoverlapped view; and injections of each of the coronary arteries should be performed and filmed in several obliquities, since atherosclerotic coronary artery disease is often eccentric (Figs. 19–24).

Several important features about selective coronary arteriography deserve emphasis. Systemic arterial pressure and heart rate should be observed closely during coronary arteriography, since it may induce transient hypotension and/or bradycardia. The latter can be treated with intravenous atropine and, if necessary, placement of a temporary transvenous ventricular pacemaker. Cineangiography of the coronary arteries should be performed with as much image magnification and, at the same time, as little distortion as possible. With very few exceptions, coronary arteriography should not be performed during an episode of angina. Rather, the patient should receive sublingual nitroglycerin, and sufficient time should be allowed for pain to

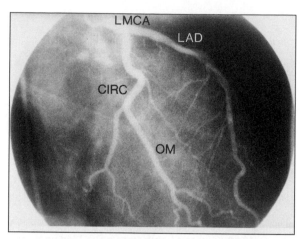

Figure 20. *A RAO projection of a normal left coronary artery. LMCA=Left main coronary artery; LAD=Left anterior descending artery; CIRC=Left circumflex artery; OM=Obtuse marginal branch of the circumflex artery.*

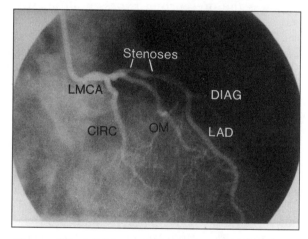

Figure 21. *A RAO projection of the left coronary artery in a patient with 2 stenoses of the proximal LAD. LMCA=Left main coronary artery; CIRC=Left circumflex coronary artery; OM=Obtuse marginal branch of circumflex coronary artery; LAD=Left anterior descending coronary artery; DIAG=Diagonal branch of the LAD.*

resolve. Then, coronary arteriography may proceed. Coronary angiography should be recorded on a permanent medium to allow for repeated review.

CORONARY ANGIOPLASTY

Percutaneous transluminal coronary angioplasty (PTCA) involves the inflation of a distensible balloon within a coronary stenosis, with subse-

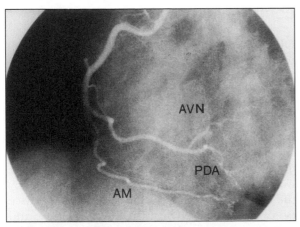

Figure 22. *A LAO projection of a normal right coronary artery. AM=Acute marginal branch of the right coronary artery; PDA=Posterior descending artery; AVN=Atrioventricular nodal artery.*

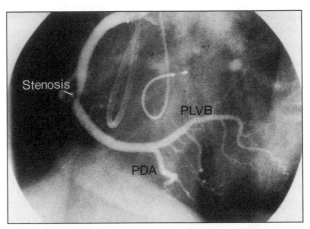

Figure 24. *A LAO projection of a right coronary artery with a severe stenosis in its midportion. PDA=Posterior descending artery; PLVB=Posterior left ventricular branch of the right coronary artery.*

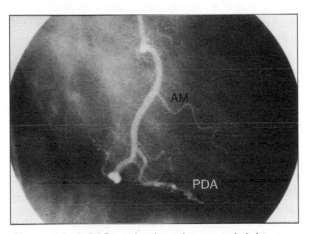

Figure 23. *A RAO projection of a normal right coronary artery. AM=Acute marginal branch of the right coronary artery; PDA=Posterior descending artery; AVN=Atrioventricular nodal artery.*

quent compression or disruption of the atheromatous stenosis. Successful angioplasty requires a skilled operator, well-trained support personnel, competent cardiothoracic surgical support, high-resolution fluoroscopic equipment to allow adequate visualization of the coronary arteries, a large lumen "guide" catheter, a flexible guide wire, and a balloon dilation catheter. Vascular access is usually attained through the femoral artery and vein. Generally, a prophylactic transvenous pacing catheter is advanced to the right ventricular apex when the stenosis to be dilated is located in the dominant vessel. The guide

catheter is stiffer, and it has a larger internal diameter than the catheters used for diagnostic angiography. These features provide for superior catheter support and angiographic visualization of the artery when the guide wire and balloon dilation catheter are within the guide catheter.

With the guide catheter positioned in the coronary ostium, angiography of the diseased artery is performed to visualize the stenosis and the artery proximal and distal to it. The flexible guide wire, 0.010-0.018 inches in diameter, is advanced through the guide catheter, navigated into the artery and across the stenosis, and positioned distally in the artery. The deflated balloon dilation catheter is advanced over the guide wire, and its position at the stenosis is confirmed by visualizing the artery as contrast material is injected through the guide catheter. Once positioned, the balloon is inflated for 1-2 min at 3-8 atmospheres of pressure with a mixture of saline and contrast material, so that balloon inflations can be visualized fluoroscopically. In an occasional patient, other inflation parameters are utilized. If an adequate result is achieved, the guide wire and balloon dilation catheter are removed. If the stenosis is not adequately dilated, the guide wire remains across the stenosis, and the initial balloon dilation catheter is replaced with a larger one. Once balloon inflations are completed, a final angiogram is obtained to confirm that the result is satisfactory and that other segments of the artery, including branches, have not been compromised.

Coronary angioplasty has been successfully in a variety of patients with ischemic heart disease. First, it has been widely employed in patients with stable angina of effort who have limiting symptoms despite appropriate medical therapy.[26,27] Second, angioplasty has been performed safely and effectively in patients with unstable angina pectoris.[28-30] In these individuals, the risk of myocardial infarction and need for emergent coronary artery bypass grafting is about twice that reported for patients with stable angina. Third, angioplasty has been used in patients with acute myocardial infarction, either alone or in close temporal proximity to thrombolytic therapy.[31-40] When used alone, the procedure is often successful in restoring antegrade flow in an occluded infarct artery. When used 2-48 hours after thrombolytic therapy, angioplasty allows the operator to dilate a high-grade residual coronary stenosis that presumably was the site of thrombus formation. In so doing, it is hoped that angioplasty might reduce the risk of reocclusion during the hours to days following the event.

Fourth, angioplasty has been employed with modest success in patients with stable angina and an occluded coronary artery not in the setting of acute myocardial infarction.[41-46] In these individuals, the chance of restoring antegrade flow is related to the elapsed time from occlusion to attempted angioplasty. If the procedure is performed within 12 weeks of occlusion, the chance of success is good (75%-90%); if it is performed later than 12 weeks after occlusion, the chance of success falls to below 50%. Finally, angioplasty has been used successfully in patients with saphenous vein or internal mammary grafts who have angina and angiographic evidence of a discrete graft stenosis.[47-55]

In experienced hands, PTCA is an effective therapeutic modality in patients with limiting angina who would otherwise require bypass surgery for symptomatic relief. Its overall success is dependent on patient selection, but in most series it averages 85%-90%.[26-27] Although complications are reported in 3%-7% of patients undergoing angioplasty, most are corrected with additional dilations or emergent bypass surgery, so that the mortality associated with the procedure is less than 1%.[56-59] During the 4-6 months after successful angioplasty, 25%-60% of stenoses recur, but these are usually amenable to repeat angioplasty.[60-64]

CORONARY ATHERECTOMY

Other than PTCA, directional coronary atherectomy (DCA) is the most widely used device for percutaneous coronary revascularization. With this device, a windowed cylindrical housing is pressed against the stenosis by an attached balloon. Once positioned appropriately, a rotating metal cutting blade is advanced through the housing, shaving plaque from the vessel wall, and depositing shaved debris in the catheter's flexible nosecone. Luminal enlargement is achieved by the dilating effect of positioning the bulky device (so-called "Dotter" effect), balloon inflation, and the removal of atherosclerotic material.[65-66] When used on non-calcified stenoses, the incidence of initial success, abrupt closure, and restenosis with DCA is similar to that of PTCA.[66-69] Further refinements in the device, additional operator experience, and analysis of the results of ongoing trials comparing DCA and PTCA may identify specific stenosis characteristics that are better approached with DCA.[64]

BALLOON VALVULOPLASTY

Percutaneous balloon valvuloplasty has been used with success in patients with aortic, mitral, and pulmonic stenosis as an alternative to surgical commissurotomy or valve replacement. The procedure is performed by positioning 1 or 2 large balloon catheters across the stenotic valve, followed by inflation of the balloons with 3-5 atmospheres of pressure for 15-30 seconds. Balloon inflations are usually repeated several times to achieve the desired result.

Several studies suggest that balloon valvuloplasty is modestly successful in many patients with aortic stenosis, but a recurrence of stenosis occurs in the majority within 6-12 months of dilatation.[70-73] As a result, aortic balloon valvuloplasty is recommended only for those with severe symptoms of aortic stenosis in whom valve replacement is thought to carry a prohibitive risk, another disease that requires urgent surgical intervention and in whom the presence of severe aortic stenosis substantially increases the risk of the planned procedure, or severe heart failure or cardiogenic shock due to aortic stenosis, thus making the risk of aortic valve replacement extraordinarily high.

Percutaneous mitral balloon valvuloplasty

(PMV) yields successful results in patients who are carefully selected based on echocardiographic evaluation of the mitral valve and subvalvular apparatus.[74-76] The presence of left atrial thrombus, a recent embolic event, extensive valvular or subvalvular calcification, severe valvular or subvalvular thickening and fibrosis, or concomitant significant mitral regurgitation are contraindications to PMV. Randomized trials of closed mitral commissurotomy (the most common treatment for mitral stenosis in geographic areas where rheumatic mitral stenosis is endemic) and PMV demonstrate similar results for mid-range (3-5 yr) follow-up.[77] The results of trials designed to compare open commissurotomy and PMV are not yet available.

Pulmonic balloon valvuloplasty, although originally described for pediatric patients, is successful in the treatment of adults with noncalcified valvular pulmonic stenosis.[78-79] Late follow-up data (4-8 yr) demonstrate that patients undergoing this procedure have a lower incidence of valve insufficiency and ventricular arrhythmias than those undergoing surgical valvulotomy.[80] Pulmonic balloon valvuloplasty is the procedure of choice for patients with isolated noncalcified valvular pulmonic stenosis.

RISKS AND COMPLICATIONS

As cardiac catheterization has been performed more frequently, the incidence of complications has diminished; however, even in the most skilled hands, the procedure is not without risk.[81-84] The overall incidence of a major complication—death, myocardial infarction, or cerebrovascular accident—during or within 24 hours of catheterization is 0.2% to 0.3%. Of these major complications, death during or within 24 hours of catheterization occurs in 0.1% to 0.2% of patients, the majority of whom have extensive cardiac disease. Such deaths may be caused by perforation of the heart or great vessels, cardiac arrhythmias, or acute myocardial infarction. Myocardial infarction during or immediately following catheterization occurs in 0.3% of patients, but most infarctions are small and uncomplicated. Importantly, patients with significant left main coronary artery (LMCA) stenosis have a substantially greater risk of periprocedural death (2.8%) compared to those without LMCA stenosis (0.1%).[85,86] Cerebrovascular accidents in the

pericatheterization period are either embolic (from the arterial catheter, guide wire, thrombus in the left ventricle or atrium, or dislodged atherosclerotic plaque) or thrombotic (i.e., existence of previous extensive cerebrovascular disease that, in association with the hemodynamic alterations induced by arteriography, leads to inadequate cerebral perfusion).

Numerous minor complications may cause morbidity but have no effect on mortality. Following arterial catheterization by the brachial approach, restoration of blood flow to the arm can be compromised, and the patient may require a thrombectomy after catheterization. Hemorrhage or hematoma formation may occur at the site of the femoral arterial puncture and, if severe, may require limited surgical exploration. Occasionally, a femoral arterial thrombectomy is required. Local infection may occur at the site of catheter entrance and manipulation, but this can usually be treated effectively with meticulous wound care and antibiotics. The injection of contrast material commonly causes nausea and vomiting as well as a transient fall in systemic arterial pressure. Occasionally such injections are associated with allergic reactions of varying severity, and a rare individual has anaphylaxis. In addition, the endocardial injection of contrast material during ventriculography may cause ventricular irritability. Finally, use of excessive quantities of contrast material may result in transient renal insufficiency. This is particularly important in patients with pre-existing renal dysfunction and diabetes mellitus.

POST CATHETERIZATION CONCERNS

During the 24 hours after catheterization, there are several important considerations. The patient should remain at complete bed rest after catheterization from the femoral artery, depending on the size of the arterial sheath inserted, for 8-24 hours. Close observation following catheterization is imperative, to insure that heart rate and blood pressure are stable and that the arterial and venous entrance sites do not show evidence of bleeding. Since radiographic contrast material is extremely hyperosmolar, it causes an osmotic diuresis during the 12-24 hours after catheterization. Therefore, sufficient oral and intravenous fluids should be administered to insure that such a diuresis does not induce intravascular volume depletion.

REFERENCES

1. Sones FM Jr, Shirey EK. Cine coronary arteriography. *Mod Concepts Cardiovasc Dis.* 1962;31:735-738.
2. Judkins MP. Percutaneous transfemoral selective coronary arteriography. *Radiol Clin N Amer.* 1968;6:467-492.
3. Fick A. Uber die Messung des Blutquantums in den Herzventriken'. *Phys-med Ges.* Wurzburg, July 9, 1870.
4. Dehmer GJ, Firth BG, Hillis LD. Oxygen consumption in adult patients during cardiac catheterization. *Clin Cardiol.* 1982;5:436-440.
5. Hillis LD, Firth BG, Winniford MD. Analysis of factors affecting the variability of Fick versus indicator dilution measurements of cardiac output. *Am J Cardiol.* 1985;56:764-768.
6. Branthwaite MA, Bradley RD. Measurement of cardiac output by thermal dilution in man. *J Appl Physiol.* 1968;24:434-438.
7. Forrester JS, Ganz W, Diamond G, et al. Thermodilution cardiac output determination with a single flow-directed catheter. *Am Heart J.* 1972;83:306-311.
8. Hamilton WF, Moore JW, Kinsman JM, et al. Studies on the circulation. IV. Further analysis of the injection method, and of changes in hemodynamics under physiological and pathological conditions. *Am J Physiol.* 1932;99:534-551.
9. Gorlin R, Gorlin SG. Hydraulic formula for calculation of the area of the stenotic mitral valve, other cardiac valves, and central circulatory shunts. I. *Am Heart J.* 1951;41:1-29.
10. Swan HJC, Ganz W, Forrester J, et al. Catheterization of the heart in man with use of a flow-directed balloon-tipped catheter. *N Engl J Med.* 1970;283:447-451.
11. Boehrer JD, Lange RA, Willard JE, et al. Advantages and limitations of methods to detect, localize, and quantitate intracardiac left-to-right shunting. *Am Heart J.* 1992;124:448-455.
12. Dexter L, Haynes FW, Burwell CS, et al. Studies of congenital heart disease. II. The pressure and oxygen content of blood in the right auricle, right ventricle, and pulmonary artery in control patients, with observations on the oxygen saturation and source of pulmonary "capillary" blood. *J Clin Invest.* 1947;26:554-560.
13. Hillis LD, Firth BG, Winniford MD. Variability of right-sided cardiac oxygen saturations in adults with and without left-to-right intracardiac shunting. *Am J Cardiol.* 1986;58:129-132.
14. Carter SA, Bajec DF, Yannicelli E, et al. Estimation of left-to-right shunt from arterial dilution curves. *J Lab Clin Med.* 1960;55:77-88.
15. Hillis LD, Winniford MD, Jackson JA, et al. Measurements of left-to-right intracardiac shunting in adults: oximetric versus indicator dilution techniques. *Cathet Cardiovasc Diagn.* 1985;11:467-472.
16. Niggemann EH, Ma PTS, Sunnergren KP, et al. Detection of intracardiac left-to-right shunting in adults: a prospective analysis of the variability of the standard indocyanine green technique in patients without shunting. *Am J Cardiol.* 1987;60:355-357.
17. Hugenholtz PG, Schwark T, Monroe RG, et al. The clinical usefulness of hydrogen gas as an indicator of left-to-right shunts. *Circulation.* 1963;28:542-551.
18. Glamann DB, Lange RA, Willard JE, et al. Hydrogen inhalation for detecting intracardiac left-to-right shunting in adults. *Am J Cardiol.* 1993;72:711-714.
19. Flores ED, Lange RA, Bedotto JB, et al. Assessment of the sensitivity of hydrogen inhalation in the detection of left-to-right shunting. *Cathet Cardiovasc Diagn.* 1990;20:94-98.
20. Dodge HT, Sandler H, Baxley WA, et al. Usefulness and limitations of radiographic methods for determining left ventricular volume. *Am J Cardiol.* 1966;18:10-24.
21. Kennedy JW, Trenholme SE, Kasser IS. Left ventricular volume and mass from single-plane cineangiocardiogram. A comparison of anteroposterior and right anterior oblique methods. *Am Heart J.* 1970;80:343-352.
22. Hillis LD, Winniford MD, Dehmer GJ, et al. Left ventricular volumes by single-plane cineangiography: in vivo validation of the Kennedy regression equation. *Am J Cardiol.* 1984;53:1159-1163.
23. Croft CH, Lipscomb K, Mathis K, et al. Limitations of qualitative angiographic grading in aortic or mitral regurgitation. *Am J Cardiol.* 1984;53:1593-1598.
24. Sasahara AA, Stein M, Simon M, et al. Pulmonary angiography in the diagnosis of thromboembolic disease. *N Engl J Med.* 1964;270:1075-1081.
25. Dalen JE, Brooks HL, Johnson LW, et al. Pulmonary angiography in acute pulmonary embolism: indications, techniques, and results in 367 patients. *Am Heart J.* 1971;81:175-185.
26. Gruentzig AR, King SB III, Schlumpf M, et al. Long-term follow-up after percutaneous transluminal coronary angioplasty. The early Zurich experience. *N Engl J Med.* 1987;316:1127-1132.
27. Parisi AF, Folland ED, Hartigan P, et al. A comparison of angioplasty with medical therapy in the treatment of single vessel coronary artery disease. *N Engl J Med.* 1992;326:10-16.
28. Myler RK, Shaw RE, Stertzer SH, et al. Unstable angina and coronary angioplasty. *Circulation.* 1990;82:II-88–II-95.
29. Bentivoglio LG, Holubkov R, Kelsey SF, et al. Short and long term outcome of percutaneous transluminal coronary angioplasty in unstable versus stable angina pectoris: A report of the 1985-1986 NHLBI PTCA Registry. *Cathet Cardiovasc Diagn.* 1991;23:227-238.
30. de Feyter PJ, Serruys PW, van den Brand M, et al. Percutaneous transluminal coronary angioplasty for unstable angina. *Am J Cardiol.* 1991;68:125B-135B.
31. Zijlstra F, Jan de Boer M, Hoorntje JCA, et al. A comparison of immediate coronary angioplasty with intravenous streptokinase in acute myocardial infarction. *N Engl J Med.* 1993;328:680-684.
32. Gibbons RJ, Holmes DR, Reeder GS, et al. Immediate angioplasty compared with the administration of a thrombolytic agent followed by conservative treatment for myocardial infarction. *N Engl J Med.* 1993;328:685-691.
33. Grines CL, Browne KF, Marco J, et al. A comparison of

immediate angioplasty with thrombolytic therapy for acute myocardial infarction. *N Engl J Med.* 1993; 328:673-679.

34. Topol EJ, Califf RM, George BS, et al. A randomized trial of immediate versus delayed elective angioplasty after intravenous tissue plasminogen activator in acute myocardial infarction. *N Engl J Med.* 1987;317:581-588.

35. The TIMI Research Group. Immediate vs delayed catheterization and angioplasty following thrombolytic therapy for acute myocardial infarction. TIMI II A results. *J Am Med Assn.* 1988;260:2849-2858.

36. Simoons ML, Arnold AER, Betriu A, et al. Thrombolysis with tissue plasminogen activator in acute myocardial infarction: No additional benefit from immediate percutaneous coronary angioplasty. *Lancet.* 1988;1:197-203.

37. Arnold AER, Simoons ML, Van de Werf F, et al. Recombinant tissue-type plasminogen activator and immediate angioplasty in acute myocardial infarction. One-year follow-up. *Circulation.* 1992;86:111-120.

38. SWIFT (Should We Intervene Following Thrombolysis?) Trial Study Group. SWIFT trial of delayed elective intervention v conservative treatment after thrombolysis with anistreplase in acute myocardial infarction. *Br Med J.* 1991;302:555-560.

39. The TIMI Study Group. Comparison of invasive and conservative strategies after treatment with intravenous tissue plasminogen activator in acute myocardial infarction. Results of the Thrombolysis in Myocardial Infarction (TIMI) phase II trial. *N Engl J Med.* 1989; 320:618-627.

40. Williams DO, Braunwald E, Knatterud G, et al. One-year results of the Thrombolysis in Myocardial Infarction Investigation (TIMI) phase II trial. *Circulation* 1992;85:533-542.

41. Meier B. Total coronary occlusion: A different animal? *J Am Coll Cardiol.* 1991;17:50B-57B.

42. Bell MR, Berger PB, Bresnahan JF, et al. Initial and long-term outcome of 354 patients after coronary balloon angioplasty of total coronary artery occlusions. *Circulation.* 1992;85:1003-1011.

43. Ivanhoe RJ, Weintraub WS, Douglas JS Jr, et al. Percutaneous transluminal coronary angioplasty of chronic total occlusions. Primary success, restenosis, and long-term clinical follow-up. *Circulation.* 1992;85:106-115.

44. Stone GW, Rutherford BD, McConahay DR, et al. Procedural outcome of angioplasty for total coronary occlusion: An analysis of 971 lesions in 905 patients. *J Am Coll Cardiol.* 1990;15:849-856.

45. Ruocco NA Jr, Ring ME, Holubkov R, et al. Results of coronary angioplasty of chronic total occlusions (the National Heart, Lung, and Blood Institute 1985-1986 Percutaneous Transluminal Angioplasty Registry). *Am J Cardiol.* 1992;69:69-76.

46. Kereiakes DJ, Selmon MR, McAuley BJ, et al. Angioplasty in total coronary artery occlusion: Experience in 76 consecutive patients. *J Am Coll Cardiol.* 1985;6:526-533.

47. Meester BJ, Samson M, Suryapranata H, et al. Long-term follow-up after attempted angioplasty of saphenous vein grafts: The Thoraxcenter experience 1981-1988. *Eur Heart J.* 1991;12:648-653.

48. Webb JG, Myler RK, Shaw RE, et al. Coronary angioplasty after coronary bypass surgery: Initial results and late outcome in 422 patients. *J Am Coll Cardiol.* 1990;16:812-820.

49. Platko WP, Hollman J, Whitlow PL, et al. Percutaneous transluminal angioplasty of saphenous vein graft stenosis: Long-term follow-up. *J Am Coll Cardiol.* 1989; 14:1645-1650.

50. Douglas JS, Gruentzig AR, King SB III, et al. Percutaneous transluminal coronary angioplasty in patients with prior coronary bypass surgery. *J Am Coll Cardiol.* 1983;2;745-754.

51. Plokker HWT, Meester BH, Serruys PW. The Dutch experience in percutaneous transluminal angioplasty of narrowed saphenous veins used for aortocoronary arterial bypass. *Am J Cardiol.* 1991;67:361-366.

52. de Feyter PJ, van Suylen R-J, de Jaegere PPT, et al. Balloon angioplasty for the treatment of lesions in saphenous vein bypass grafts. *J Am Coll Cardiol.* 1993;21:1539-1549.

53. Cote G, Myler RK, Stertzer SH, et al. Percutaneous transluminal angioplasty of stenotic coronary artery bypass grafts: 5 years' experience. *J Am Coll Cardiol.* 1987;9:8-17.

54. Pomerantz RM, Kuntz RE, Carrozza JP, et al. Acute and long-term outcome of narrowed saphenous venous grafts treated by endoluminal stenting and directional atherectomy. *Am J Cardiol.* 1992;70:161-167.

55. Urban P, Sigwart U, Golf S, et al. Intravascular stenting for stenosis of aortocoronary venous bypass grafts. *J Am Coll Cardiol.* 1989;13:1085-1091.

56. Cowley MJ, Dorros G, Kelsey SF, et al. Acute coronary events associated with percutaneous transluminal coronary angioplasty. *Am J Cardiol.* 1984;53:12C-16C.

57. Craver JM, Weintraub WS, Jones EL, et al. Emergency coronary artery bypass surgery for failed percutaneous angioplasty. A 10-year experience. *Ann Surg.* 1992; 215:425-434.

58. Talley JD, Weintraub WS, Roubin GS, et al. Failed elective percutaneous transluminal coronary angioplasty requiring coronary artery bypass surgery. In-hospital and late clinical outcome at 5 years. *Circulation.* 1990;82:1203-1213.

59. Holmes DR, Vlietstra RE, Smith HC, et al. Restenosis after percutaneous transluminal coronary angioplasty (PTCA): A report from the PTCA Registry of the National Heart, Lung, and Blood Institute. *Am J Cardiol.* 1984;53:77C-81C.

60. Leimgruber PP, Roubin GS, Hollman J, et al. Restenosis after successful coronary angioplasty in patients with single-vessel disease. *Circulation.* 1986;73:710-717.

61. Ernst SMPG, van der Feltz TA, Bal ET, et al. Long term angiographic follow up, cardiac events, and survival in patients undergoing percutaneous transluminal coronary angioplasty. *Br Heart J.* 1987;57:220-225.

62. Hirshfeld JW Jr, Schwartz JS, Jugo R, et al. Restenosis after coronary angioplasty: A multivariate statistical model to relate lesion and procedure variables to restenosis. *J Am Coll Cardiol.* 1991;18:647-656.

63. The Multicenter European Research Trial with Cilazapril after Angioplasty to Prevent Transluminal Coronary

Obstruction and Restenosis (MERCATOR) Study Group. Does the new angiotensin converting enzyme inhibitor cilazapril prevent restenosis after percutaneous transluminal coronary angioplasty? Results of the MERCATOR study: A multicenter, randomized, double-blind placebo-controlled trial. *Circulation.* 1992;86:100-110.

64. Topol EJ, Leya F, Pinkerton CA, et al. A comparison of directional atherectomy with coronary angioplasty in patients with coronary artery disease. *N Engl J Med.* 1993;329:221-227.

65. Tenaglia AN, Buller CE, Kisslo KB, et al. Mechanisms of balloon angioplasty and directional coronary atherectomy as assessed by intracoronary ultrasound. *J Am Coll Cardiol.* 1992;20:685-691.

66. Safian RD, Gelbfish JS, Erny RE, et al. Coronary atherectomy. Clinical, angiographic, and histological findings and observations regarding potential mechanisms. *Circulation.* 1990;82:69-79.

67. Hillis LD. Efficacy and safety of coronary balloon angioplasty and directional atherectomy. *Circulation.* 1990;82:305-307.

68. Hinohara T, Rowe MH, Robertson GC, et al. Effect of lesion characteristics on outcome of directional coronary atherectomy. *J Am Coll Cardiol.* 1991;17:1112-1120.

69. Popma JJ, Topol EJ, Hinohara T, et al. Abrupt vessel closure after directional coronary atherectomy. *J Am Coll Cardiol.* 1992;19:1372-1379.

70. Safian RD, Berman AD, Diver DJ, et al. Balloon aortic valvuloplasty in 170 consecutive patients. *N Engl J Med.* 1988;319:125-130.

71. Block PC. Aortic valvuloplasty—a valid alternative? *N Engl J Med.* 1988;319:169-171.

72. Bernard Y, Etievent J, Mourand J-L, et al. Long-term results of percutaneous aortic valvuloplasty compared with aortic valve replacement in patients more than 75 years old. *J Am Coll Cardiol.* 1992;20:796-801.

73. O'Neill WW, for The Mansfield Scientific Aortic Valvuloplasty Registry Investigators. Predictors of long-term survival after percutaneous aortic valvuloplasty: Report of the Mansfield Scientific Balloon Aortic Valvuloplasty Registry. *J Am Coll Cardiol.* 1991;17:193-198.

74. Wilkins GT, Weyman AE, Abascal VM, et al. Percutaneous balloon dilatation of the mitral valve: An analysis of echocardiographic variables related to outcome and the mechanism of dilatation. *Br Heart J.* 1988;60:299-308.

75. Palacios IF, Block PC, Wilkins GT, et al. Follow-up of patients undergoing percutaneous mitral balloon valvotomy. Analysis of factors determining restenosis. *Circulation.* 1989;79:573-579.

76. Cohen DJ, Kuntz RE, Gordon SPF, et al. Predictors of long-term outcome after percutaneous balloon mitral valvuloplasty. *N Engl J Med.* 1992;327:1329-1335.

77. Block PC, Palacios IF. Aortic and mitral balloon valvuloplasty: The United States Experience. In: Topol EJ (ed). *Textbook of Interventional Cardiology.* Philadelphia: W.B. Saunders; 1994:1189-1205.

78. al Kasab S, Ribeiro PA, al Zaibag M, et al. Percutaneous double balloon pulmonary valvotomy in adults: One- to two-year follow-up. *Am J Cardiol.* 1988;62:822-824.

79. Fawzy ME, Mercer EN, Dunn B. Late results of pulmonary balloon valvuloplasty in adults using double balloon technique. *J Interven Cardiol.* 1988;1:35-42.

80. O'Connor BK, Beekman RH, Lindauer A, et al. Intermediate-term outcome after pulmonary balloon valvuloplasty: Comparison with a matched surgical control group. *J Am Coll Cardiol.* 1992;20:169-173.

81. Adams DF, Fraser DB, Abrams HL. The complications of coronary arteriography. *Circulation.* 1973;48:609-618.

82. Davis K, Kennedy JW, Kemp HG Jr, et al. Complications of coronary arteriography from the Collaborative Study of Coronary Artery Surgery (CASS). *Circulation.* 1979;59:1105-1112.

83. Kennedy JW, the Registry Committee of the Society for Cardiac Angiography. Symposium on catheterization complications. Complications associated with cardiac catheterization and angiography. *Cathet Cardiovasc Diagn.* 1982;8:5-11.

84. Gersh BJ, Kronmal RA, Frye RL, et al. Coronary arteriography and coronary artery bypass surgery: Morbidity and mortality in patients ages 65 years or older. *Circulation.* 1983;67:483-491.

85. Gordon PR, Abrams C, Gash AK, et al. Pericatheterization risk factors in left main coronary artery stenosis. *Am J Cardiol.* 1987;59:1080-1083.

86. Boehrer JD, Lange RA, Willard JE, et al. Markedly increased periprocedure mortality of cardiac catheterization in patients with severe narrowing of the left main coronary artery. *Am J Cardiol.* 1992;70:1388-1390.

10 Electrophysiologic Testing: General Principles and Clinical Applications

Anil K. Bhandari, MD

The era of modern cardiac electrophysiology began in 1958 when Alanis et al[1] first recorded a His bundle potential in an isolated animal preparation. Ten years later, Scherlag and colleagues[2] reported on the use of an electrode catheter technique to record His bundle potentials in the intact dog. However, it was not until 1971 that Durrer et al[3] and Wellens[4] used the technique of programmed stimulation to reproducibly induce and terminate both supraventricular and ventricular tachycardias. In the ensuing decade, several investigators used electrophysiologic studies (EPS) to define the mechanisms of cardiac tachyarrhythmias and help in selecting optimum antiarrhythmic regimens.[5–32] In the 1980s, it became apparent that the available antiarrhythmic agents had limited efficacy in suppressing inducibility of ventricular arrhythmias. This provided an important incentive for the development of nonpharmacologic antiarrhythmic modalities e.g., implantable cardioverter defibrillators (ICD),[26] antiarrhythmic surgery and electrode catheter ablation.[33–38] Several prospective trials are in progress to compare the effectiveness of pharmacologic versus nonpharmacologic approaches in treating patients with life-threatening ventricular arrhythmias.[39] This chapter will attempt to provide a comprehensive understanding of the general principles involved in EPS, summarize the technical considerations, and evaluate the clinical utility and limitations of EPS.

GENERAL PRINCIPLES AND TECHNICAL CONSIDERATIONS

A comprehensive EPS involves recording of intracardiac signals and electrical stimulation of the heart at multiple sites. The baseline recordings provide information on the conduction properties of the cardiac tissue. The electric stimulation allows the inducibility and termination characteristics of the cardiac arrhythmias to be determined. Before performing EPS, one ought to critically appraise the indication for the procedure and make every attempt to obtain an electrocardiographic (ECG) documentation of the index cardiac arrhythmia.

PREOPERATIVE EVALUATION

The EPS is performed in a postabsorptive state. The preoperative use of sedative drugs has traditionally been considered undesirable, as it may adversely affect the conduction and refractoriness of the sinus node, atrioventricular (AV) node and His-Purkinje system. Another disadvantage in the use of sedative drugs may be a potential interference in suppressing the inducibility of supraventricular tachycardias. On the other hand, a judicious use of sedative drugs relieves apprehension on the part of the patient. It has been our practice to use intermittent boluses of intravenous midazolam or fentanyl to achieve adequate sedation. Another practice is to discontinue the use of all antiarrhythmic drugs for at least 5 half-lives before EPS. Other cardioactive drugs (e.g., diuretics, digoxin, vasodilators, ACE inhibitors) need not be discontinued. Before undertaking EPS, the serum electrolytes (including magnesium) and digoxin levels (whenever appropriate) must be routinely checked.

EPS LABORATORY AND EQUIPMENT

The performance of EPS requires a cardiac catheterization laboratory equipped with single-

or biplane fluoroscopy and an ability to record multiple electrocardiographic leads and intracardiac electrograms. At least 3 of the orthogonal electrocardiographic leads (leads I, AVF, and V1) and 5 intracardiac electrograms need to be recorded. Modern EPS laboratories have 16- or 32-channel recording systems with an ability to record all 12 ECG leads. For the surface ECG leads, the frequency settings are 0–1 Hz for the low-pass filter and 25–30 Hz for the high-pass filter; the corresponding values for the intracardiac electrograms are 30–40 Hz and 500 Hz, respectively. The notch filter (clamp) serves to apply a cutoff limit to the size of maximally or near maximally gained intracardiac signals. The notch function is especially valuable for the His bundle recordings where high-gain settings are often needed and may result in large atrial or ventricular deflections. In general, a reliance on excessive gain settings and notch filter ought to be avoided, and it is better to appropriately place the electrode catheters. Moreover, the high-gain settings can also unmask otherwise inconspicuous noise signals that may be related to the faulty techniques of grounding and isolation, improper shielding of the power lines, and loose recording cables.

The intracardiac electrograms may be recorded in unipolar or bipolar modes. The unipolar electrograms represent the electric activity between an index electrode catheter and a reference electrode that is extracardiac and remote. Unipolar recordings suffer from significant baseline drifts and contain low-frequency electric signals representing the far field activity. This may distort as well as mask an otherwise discrete local electric signal. In contrast, the bipolar electrograms represent the discrete electric activity between 2 closely (2–10 mm) spaced electrodes, do not have far field low frequency signals, and are the preferred mode of recording. The signals are displayed on a multichannel (8, 16, 24, or 32) physiologic oscilloscope, and may be simultaneously displayed and recorded in an analog or digital system. A digital system is preferred, as it allows for a better display of the intracardiac signals, provides an easier

storage system, and makes it possible to perform on-line (or off-line) electrophysiologic measurements.

EPS PROTOCOL

After the patient is brought into the EP laboratory, the right groin is prepared and draped under sterile conditions. Electrode catheters are introduced into the right femoral vein using Seldinger percutaneous technique and are advanced under fluoroscopic guidance through the inferior vena cava to the right sided cardiac chambers. For the baseline EPS, 2 or more quadripolar electrode catheters are used and placed at the high right atrium (near the sinus node), across the tricuspid valve to record the His bundle electrogram, and at the right ventricular apex. The distal electrode pair is used to stimulate the myocardium and the proximal electrode pair to record the bipolar electrogram. For patients with supraventricular tachycardia, another electrode catheter is advanced to the coronary sinus via the left subclavian or the internal jugular vein. We do not routinely place an arterial line (radial or femoral) unless left ventricular stimulation is contemplated.

After being placed at appropriate locations, the electrode catheters are connected via an isolation junction box to a multichannel oscilloscope and recording system. The electric signals may then be displayed and recorded simultaneously at various speeds (range, 10–400 mm/sec).

A comprehensive EPS involves the components listed in Table 1. A typical EPS may take 1 to 3 hours. The study steps and the protocols vary depending upon the patient needs and the clinical situation. The range of normal values for the electrophysiologic variables is given in Table 2. In addition to the clinical electrophysiologist, 2 other laboratory personnel who are fully trained in the use of EP and catheterization equipment should be present; one of them should preferably be a registered nurse. The EP laboratory should also be equipped with 1 or 2 functioning external cardioverter defibrillators, Ambu bag, laryngoscope, endotracheal intubation set and pericardiocentesis set.

Table 1. A Comprehensive EPS

1. Baseline intervals:
   sinus cycle length
   atrio-His (AH) interval
   His-ventricular (HV) interval
   ECG measurements (PR interval, QRS duration and interval)
2. Sinus node function:
   sinus node recovery time
   sinoatrial conduction time
   direct sinus node potential recording
3. Intra-atrial conduction time and atrial refractoriness
4. Conduction and refractoriness of the AV node and His–Purkinje system
5. Programmed atrial stimulation with up to triple extrastimuli
6. Right ventricular conduction and refractoriness
7. Programmed ventricular stimulation with up to triple extrastimuli
8. Evaluation of the mechanisms of inducible ventricular or supraventricular tachycardia
9. Effectiveness of antiarrhythmic drug in suppressing the inducibility of tachycardia
10. Evaluation and programming of implantable cardioverter defibrillator (ICD)
11. Radio frequency catheter ablative procedures
12. Tilt-table testing

COMPLICATIONS OF EPS

The risks associated with EPS are comparable with those reported with other cardiac catheterization procedures.[40,41] Death during EPS is rare, and the reported frequency is less than 0.1%. The vast majority of induced arrhythmias can be resolved by pace termination, cardioversion, or defibrillation; only rarely is there any need for closed chest cardiac compression or endotracheal intubation. The overall morbidity ranges between 2% and 5% and includes complications of pneumothorax (1%), pericardial tamponade (<1%), thrombophlebitis (1%–2%), pulmonary embolism (<1%), or cerebrovascular accident (<1%). Local hematomas may develop in 2%–3% of the patients.

CLINICAL UTILITY OF ELECTROPHYSIOLOGIC TESTING

In clinical practice, EPS is performed to: 1) establish the diagnosis of cardiac arrhythmia, 2)

Table 2. The Range of Normal Values for Electrophysiologic Variables

VARIABLE	RANGE OF VALUES
Sinus node recovery time:	
uncorrected	<1,400–1,600 ms
corrected	<354–680 ms
Sinoatrial conduction time	40–156 ms
Atrio-Hisian (AH) conduction time	60–140 ms
His–ventricular (HV) conduction time	30–55 ms
Atrial effective refractory period	170–300 ms
AV nodal effective refractory period	230–425 ms
AV nodal functional refractory period	320–525 ms
Ventricular effective refractory period	170–290 ms
AV nodal Wenckebach cycle length	350–500 ms

monitor antiarrhythmic therapy, and 3) cure certain forms of supraventricular and ventricular tachycardia.

SINUS NODE DISORDERS

This study is performed infrequently in patients with sinus node disorders. It is indicated in symptomatic patients with syncope or near syncope in whom sinus node dysfunction is suspected but not documented to be the cause of symptoms. Another indication may be to exclude the presence of other arrhythmic mechanisms in patients who have syncope and a known sinus node dysfunction. It is not indicated in asymptomatic patients with sinus pauses or sinus bradycardia.

During EPS, the sinus node function is evaluated by measuring the sinus node recovery time[8] (SNRT) and sinoatrial conduction time (SACT).[8,9] For SNRT, the high right atrium is paced at cycle lengths of 600, 500, 400, and 300 ms, respectively, for 30 seconds each; the interval between the last atrial paced beat and the first sinus escape beat represents the uncorrected SNRT (Fig. 1). The corrected SNRT is obtained by subtracting the sinus cycle length from the uncorrected SNRT. The normal values for both uncorrected and corrected SNRT are given in Table 2. SACT represents the time needed for a sinus impulse to exit from the sinus node and excite the adjoining atrial myocardium. It may be measured indirectly by

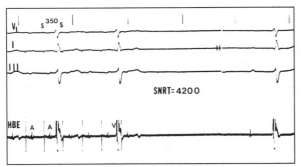

Figure 1. *Prolonged sinus node recovery time (SNRT) in a 60-year-old patient with a history of recurrent syncope and mild systemic hypertension. Three surface electrocardiographic leads (V₁, I, III) and intracardiac electrograms from the His-bundle region (His) are displayed. The high right atrium was paced at 350 ms. Paper speed 50 mm/s.*

atrial extrastimulus technique[8] (Strauss Method), or atrial pacing for 8 beats at a rate slightly faster than the sinus cycle length[9] (Narula Method), or directly by recording the sinus node potential.[10]

When interpreting the significance of abnormal SNRT and SACT, it is important to emphasize that the sensitivity ranges from 50% to 64% and the specificity from 80% to 88% in detecting the sinus node dysfunction. Mildly abnormal values are probably of no clinical significance.

AV CONDUCTION DISORDERS

First-degree AV block is characterized by a prolonged PR interval of greater than 0.20 seconds. The site of conduction delay may be within the AV node or the His bundle-Purkinje system. EPS is almost never needed in asymptomatic patients with first-degree AV block. At times, patients with first-degree AV block may present with recurrent syncope or syncope that may be suspected to be related to an intermittent occurrence of high-grade AV block. EPS may be needed in such patients.

Chronic second-degree or third-degree AV blocks are relatively uncommon disorders. The etiology may be congenital, rheumatic disease, sclerodegenerative, ischemic heart disease, valvular heart disease, or connective tissue disorders. At times, the etiology is not apparent. The prognostic significance depends upon both the type and severity of underlying heart disease and anatomic site of the AV block. A 12-lead ECG may be helpful but the findings are often not diagnostic. EPS allows for an accurate localization of the site of AV block (Fig. 2).[11] In general, the AV nodal blocks are considered to be benign as the junctional escape rhythm is predictable, stable in rate (40–50 beats/min), and hemodynamically well tolerated. In contrast, the Hisian- and infra-Hisian AV blocks are known to carry a poor prognosis as the idioventricular escape rhythm is unpredictable, slow in rate (20–40 beats/min), and hemodynamically poorly tolerated.[12]

In patients whose symptoms are documented to be due to second- or third-degree AV block, permanent cardiac pacing is indicated

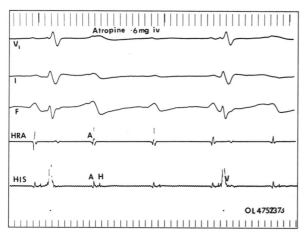

Figure 2. Infra-Hisian 3:1 atrioventricular (AV) block in a 40-year-old woman with recurrent dizziness. The display format is the same as in Figure 1. In the conducted beats, the AH interval is 60 ms and the HV interval 30 ms. The conducted QRS complexes are 100 ms in duration and show nonspecific IVCD. Note that atropine infusion increased the severity of the AV block from 2:1 to 3:1.

regardless of the site of AV block; EPS is not indicated. However, in patients whose symptoms are intermittent and, hence, not shown to be related to high-grade AV block, EPS is indicated to define the anatomic site and severity of the block.[13] EPS may also be indicated in asymptomatic patients with second- or third-degree AV block where the location of AV block is suspected to be infra-Hisian and a concern exists regarding its progression to high-grade AV block.

BUNDLE BRANCH AND FASCICULAR BLOCKS

Chronic bundle branch or fascicular blocks are common conduction disorders and may affect 1% to 2% of the population. The prevalence appears to increase with age. Syncope may occur in up to one-third of such patients, but the incidence of progression to complete AV block is relatively low at 2% to 3% per annum.[14,15] Thus, in the vast majority, the cause of syncope is unrelated to the AV block and needs to be investigated. Malignant ventricular tachyarrhythmias have been implicated to be the cause of syncope, especially when bundle branch block exists in the setting of structural heart disease

and left ventricular dysfunction.

In patients with bundle branch block, the utility of EPS lies in its ability to define the integrity of conduction over the remaining bundle branch and to exclude other arrhythmic mechanisms of syncope. The His-ventricular (HV) interval is a measure of conduction time over the contralateral bundle branch, and when greatly prolonged (HV >100 ms), identifies a high-risk subset with 20% to 25% incidence of progression to the complete AV block.[14,15] When the HV interval is moderately prolonged (75–100 ms), the risk of complete AV block is still high (5% to 10%) and the decision regarding permanent cardiac pacing should take into account the severity of clinical symptoms, and other known causes of syncope ought to be excluded in such patients. Another abnormality of clinical significance is the development of intra- or infra-Hisian AV block during incremental atrial pacing or programmed atrial stimulation. This abnormality may reflect the presence of severe hisian- or infra-Hisian disease and permanent cardiac pacing is recommended in such patients. EPS is not recommended in asymptomatic patients with bundle branch block or bifascicular block.

SUPRAVENTRICULAR TACHYCARDIA

Until recently, all forms of paroxysmal supraventricular tachycardias (PSVT) were lumped together under the term "paroxysmal atrial tachycardia." With the advent of EPS, it is now feasible to define the mechanisms of the PSVT, select antiarrhythmic therapy on a more judicious basis, and develop nonpharmacologic modalities in the treatment of patients with PSVT.

During EPS in patients with PSVT, clinical arrhythmia can be reproducibly initiated and terminated in up to 95% of the patients. Once induced, the SVT characteristics may be studied in detail, thus allowing for determining its anatomic-electrophysiological substrate. Moreover, the response of induced SVT to antiarrhythmic drugs can be systematically evaluated during serial electropharmacologic testing and the need for nonpharmacologic options may be better defined.

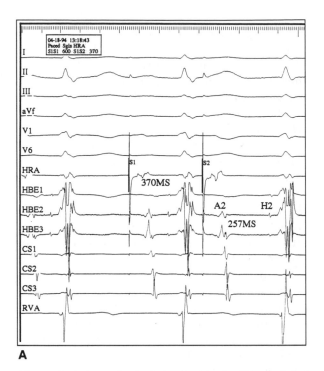

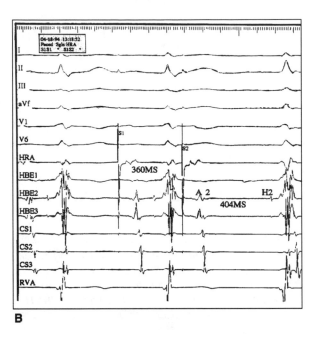

Figure 3. *Antegrade dual atrioventricular (AV) nodal physiology in a patient with recurrent PSVT. Six ECG leads and intracardiac electrograms from His-bundle position (HBE), proximal coronary sinus (CS₁), middle CS (CS₂), distal CS (CS₃), and right ventricular apex (RVA) are displayed at paper speed of 100 mm/s. (A): Following an 8-beat paced train of 600 ms at high right atrium (RA), an atrial extrastimulus (S₂) is delivered with coupling interval of 370 ms. The ensuing A₂H₂ interval is 257 ms. (B): The coupling interval of atrial extrastimulus was decreased to 360 ms. The ensuing A₂H₂ interval is 404 ms, which represents an increment of 147 ms from the previous A₂H₂ and is consistent with shift of conduction from the fast to the slow pathway.*

AV NODAL REENTRANT TACHYCARDIA

Dual AV nodal reentrant tachycardia is the commonest form of PSVT and accounts for 60% to 70% of the arrhythmias in patients without manifest preexcitation syndrome.[17] The vast majority of patients do not have underlying heart disease. The PSVT occurs with bimodal age distribution in those 20 to 30 years old and those older than 50 years. The reentrant substrate appears to result from the presence of 2 electrophysiologically distinct functional pathways within (or in the immediate vicinity) of the AV node. The fast pathway (ß-pathway) conducts rapidly and has a longer refractory period, whereas the slow pathway conducts slowly and has a shorter refractory period. The differing electrophysiologic properties may allow a premature ectopic beat to conduct in an antegrade fashion over 1 of the pathways and in

a retrograde manner over the other pathway, thus setting up the reentrant loop. In typical AV nodal reentry (the most common form of PSVT), the impulse follows an antegrade trail over the slow (α) pathway and a retrograde direction over the fast pathway. As the atrium and the ventricle are almost simultaneously activated, P waves are not evident during tachycardia, but the atrial activity may easily be recognized on the intracardiac electrograms (Figs. 3, 4).

In the atypical AV nodal reentry (rare form of PSVT), the reentrant loop is reversed with antegrade conduction over the fast pathway and the retrograde conduction over the slow pathway. This tachycardia may be frequently incessant, is characterized by the presence of the retrograde P waves with long RP' interval, and may not respond favorably to many anti-arrhythmic agents.

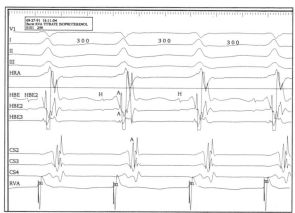

Figure 4. *Inducible dual atrioventricular (AV) nodal reentry supraventricular tachycardia (SVT). Four surface ECG leads and intracardiac electro-cardiograms with 3 His-bundle electrogram (HBE) channels, 3 coronary sinus channels, and right ventricular apex (RVA) channel displayed in the same format as in Figure 3. The tachycardia cycle length is 300 ms. Note that the atrial activation is almost simultaneous with the ventricular activation, thus explaining the lack of discernable P waves on the surface ECG leads.*

AV ORTHODROMIC RECIPROCATING TACHYCARDIA

This is the next most common mechanism of PSVT, accounting for 20% to 30% of the PSVT in patients who do not have manifest pre-excitation syndrome.[16] The reentrant loop requires participation of an accessory pathway that conducts in the retrograde direction. On a routine 12-lead ECG, delta waves are not seen; the pathway has no antegrade conduction—and hence the term "concealed" accessory pathway.

During tachycardia, antegrade conduction takes place over the AV nodal–His Purkinje axis and the retrograde conduction over the accessory pathway. The retrograde *P* waves are, therefore, inscribed immediately after the preceding QRS complex with AV intervals of 80 to 140 ms (Fig. 5). The retrograde atrial activation sequence is eccentric, depending upon the location of the accessory pathway. The pathways are left sided in 60% to 70% and right sided in 30% to 40%. During EPS, the AV orthodromic reciprocating SVT may be easily differentiated from the AV nodal reentrant SVT based on its longer VA conduction times (>80

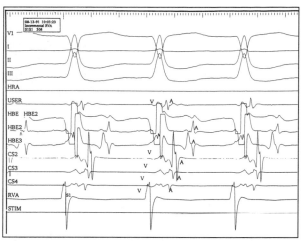

Figure 5. *Inducible atrioventricular (AV) orthodromic reciprocating tachycardia in a 40-year-old man with recurrent palpitations. The display format is the same as in previous figures. Paper speed is 200 mm/s. During tachycardia, the sequence of retrograde atrial activation is eccentric, with the earliest activation in the electrogram recorded at the distal coronary sinus. The findings indicate the presence of a left lateral accessory pathway participating in the tachycardia. The mapping probe (user) was placed at the left lateral mitral annulus, where the VA interval was shortest (68 ms). The delivery of radio frequency energy at this site terminated the supraventricular tachycardia (SVT) and abolished conduction over the accessory pathway.*

ms), eccentric sequence of retrograde atrial activation, and advancement of atrial depolarization by a ventricular stimulus delivered at the time of the His deflection.

INTRAATRIAL REENTRANT TACHYCARDIAS

In less than 10% of the patients with PSVT is the tachycardia circuit confined to the atrium. The atrial tachycardias originate in the right atrium in 60% to 80% and in the left atrium in 20% to 30% of the patients. The site of reentry may be in the low atrium when the P waves are inverted during tachycardia or in the high right atrium near the sinus node when the P waves are upright and may be indistinguishable, at times, from the sinus P waves. The tachycardia rate ranges between 100 and 250 beats/min, and the AV conduction may be 1:1, or there may be varying degrees of AV block (2:1, 3:2, 3:1). This is in contrast with the patients with AV nodal reentry or AV orthodromic reciprocating tachycardias where the presence of variable AV conduction ratio almost excludes the diagnosis of such arrhythmias. Infrequently, there may be an incessant form of atrial tachycardia when the affected patient may present with cardiomegaly and frank congestive heart failure. The electrophysiologic mechanisms are variable and may be related to abnormal automaticity, reentry or triggered activity.

INDICATIONS FOR EPS IN PSVT

EPS is indicated in symptomatic PSVT when the condition fails to respond to treatment with digoxin, ß-blockers or calcium-channel blockers. Before initiating treatment with class IA or IC drugs, EPS should probably be performed in such patients. EPS is indicated in patients whose PSVT results in hemodynamically compromising symptoms. It elucidates the mechanism of the PSVT, provides important data regarding the EP properties of the tachycardia substrate, and allows for more judicious selection of the treatment modalities. Finally, EPS is recommended in the symptomatic patients who desire not to take long-term antiarrhythmic drugs and in the patients who have high-risk professions. EPS is not recommended in the evaluation of asymptomatic or mildly symptomatic patients with PSVT.

PREEXCITATION SYNDROME

The preexcitation or the Wolff–Parkinson–White (WPW) syndrome results from the presence of an accessory pathway, a muscular strand(s) that connects the atrium to the ventricle across the mitral (left-sided) or the tricuspid (right-sided) annulus. As compared with the AV node, the conduction time over the accessory pathway is usually shorter and, hence, part of the ventricle is depolarized ahead of time via the accessory pathway. On the surface ECG, the early ventricular depolarization is manifested as a slurred upstroke (delta wave) on the initial part of the QRS complex. The preexcitation syndrome affects 0.1% to 0.3% of the population. It is not a hereditary abnormality but may rarely occur on a familial basis.

ARRHYTHMIAS IN WPW SYNDROME

Tachyarrhythmias occur in about two-thirds of the patients with WPW syndrome.[16,18-20] The most common arrhythmia is the AV orthodromic reciprocating tachycardia where antegrade conduction occurs over the AV node–His Purkinje axis and the retrograde conduction over the accessory pathway. During tachycardia, the QRS complexes are not preexcited, as the antegrade conduction is exclusively over the AV node. At times, there may be development of functional bundle branch block, resulting in widening of the QRS complexes. The retrograde P waves are inscribed immediately after the QRS complex with VA interval of 80 to 120 ms.

Atrial fibrillation is the second most common arrhythmia in WPW syndrome and may occur in 10% to 30% of the patients. It may arise as a *de novo* arrhythmia but results more often from degeneration of AV orthodromic reciprocating tachycardia to atrial fibrillation. During atrial fibrillation, atrial impulses may conduct to the ventricle over the AV node (narrow QRS complexes), over the AV accessory pathway (preexcited QRS complexes), or both resulting in varying degrees of fusion. Depending upon its refractoriness and conduction properties, the accessory pathway may allow for conduction of 300 or more atrial impulses to the ventricle per minute. This may lead to severe systolic hypotension and disorganization of cardiac rhythm to ventricular fibrillation.[19] Ventricular fibrillation is an infrequent complication of the WPW syndrome, with an estimated incidence of 1 per 1,000 patient-years of follow-up.

A less common form of tachyarrhythmia (<5%) is the AV antidromic reciprocating tachycardia variety, where the reentrant loop is reversed; the antegrade conduction occurs over the AV accessory pathway and the retrograde conduction over the AV nodal-His Purkinje axis. During tachycardia, the QRS complexes are completely preexcited and appear to be wide and bizarre, often mimicking ventricular tachycardia. The retrograde atrial activation is normal in sequence with His deflection appearing before the septal atrial depolarization. The AV antidromic reciprocating tachycardia needs to be differentiated from other PSVTs (e.g., atrial tachycardias, atrial flutter, and AV nodal reentry tachycardias) which involve AV accessory pathway as a bystander.

INDICATIONS FOR EPS

EPS provides information about the electrophysiologic properties of the accessory pathway, type and rates of inducible arrhythmias, location of 1 or more accessory pathways, and effects of the antiarrhythmic drugs on conduction and refractoriness of the accessory pathway. EPS is indicated in those with WPW syndrome who have symptomatic SVT or in those with a history of atrial fibrillation or syncope.[18,20] EPS is not indicated in patients with asymptomatic WPW syndrome unless they are in high-risk profession or have a family history of premature sudden death.

VENTRICULAR TACHYCARDIA AND SURVIVORS OF CARDIAC ARREST

The evaluation of patients with sustained VT or out-of-hospital cardiac arrest represents the most common indication for EPS. The vast majority of such patients have underlying structural heart disease. Coronary artery disease (with or without previous myocardial infarct) is present in 50% to 70% and dilated idiopathic cardiomyopathy in 10% to 20% of the patients. Less common etiologies include hypertensive or valvular heart disease, mitral valve prolapse, acute myocarditis, cardiac trauma, cardiac tumors, sarcoidosis, and the long QT syndromes. Rarely, no structural heart disease is evident despite an extensive workup (including myocardial biopsy). Many of the patients have concomitant congestive heart failure and LV wall motion abnormalities.

RATIONALE OF EPS

The utility of EPS in patients with sustained ventricular tachycardia (VT)/ventricular fibrillation (VF) is based on the following premises:[5,6,23,24] 1) EPS induces sustained VT/VF with high sensitivity in patients presenting with

this arrhythmia; 2) EPS does not induce sustained VT/VF in patients who did not experience such arrhythmias in the past and are not considered to be at high risk for development of such arrhythmias; 3) the inducible VT during EPS is similar in rate and morphology to the clinical VT; 4) the suppression of VT inducibility by an antiarrhythmic drug predicts its long-term clinical efficacy; and 5) conversely, the VT nonsuppressibility by an antiarrhythmic drug predicts a high rate of VT recurrence during treatment with the ineffective drug.

The validity of the above premises has been generally established. In the EP laboratory, sustained VT can be induced and terminated in 90% of the patients presenting with this arrhythmia (Figs. 6, 7). The yield of inducibility is high (>95%) in patients with coronary artery disease but falls to 70% to 80% for patients with other etiologies. In survivors of cardiac arrest, sustained VT/VF are inducible in 50% to 70% of the patients.[23] In addition to the type of the presenting arrhythmia and the underlying heart disease, the inducibility is also affected by aggressiveness of stimulation protocol.

Inducibility of sustained monomorphic VT is a specific finding regardless of its mode of induction. However, polymorphic VT or VF may be induced in up to 5% to 10% of the patients without a history of experiencing such arrhythmias. These are considered to be arrhythmias of low specificity. Serial electropharmacologic testing has been shown to be useful in finding an effective antiarrhythmic drug regimen. If the VT inducibility is suppressed in the EP laboratory, the antiarrhythmic drug is likely to be effective in suppressing clinical recurrences as well. Conversely, the use of an ineffective drug (with the notable exception of amiodarone) as predicted by EPS is associated with high recurrence rate during follow-up.

VT STIMULATION PROTOCOL

Before conducting EPS, all antiarrhythmic drugs should be stopped for at least 5 half-lives. No consensus exists on a standard stimulation protocol. In our laboratory, we use a stepwise and progressive introduction of 1, 2, and 3 extrastimuli linked to an 8-beat paced drive at

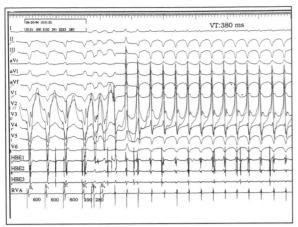

Figure 6. *Induction of sustained monomorphic ventricular tachycardia (VT) by 2 extrastimuli (S_2S_3) after an 8-beat paced train of 600 ms. The patient had a history of recurrent sustained VT, and the EPS was performed in a drug free state. Twelve surface ECG leads and intracardiac electrograms from the His bundle electrogram (HBE) channels and right ventricular apex (RVA) are displayed. Paper speed is 25 mm/s.*

cycle lengths of 600 ms and then 400 ms. Programmed stimulation is first performed at the RV apex using single and double ventricular extrastimuli and then at the RV outflow tract with the same protocol. Triple extrastimuli are used when the double extrastimuli fail to induce sustained VT/VF. Isoproterenol infusion may be needed when the VT is not inducible despite using triple extrastimuli at 2 RV sites. The isoproterenol is infused at 2–6 μg/min to increase the heart rate up to 120 beats/min or by 30% of the baseline value. Isoproterenol facilitates induction of the VT related to reentry or triggered activity mechanisms. It may also provoke the spontaneous development of automatic VT, which, as a rule, are not inducible by programmed ventricular stimulation. The LV programmed stimulation is only rarely needed when the above modalities fail.

INDICATIONS FOR EPS

The utility of EPS in patients with VT is severalfold. First, not all wide QRS complex tachycardias are ventricular in origin,[22] and the differential diagnosis may include 1) supra-ventricular tachycardia with functional or

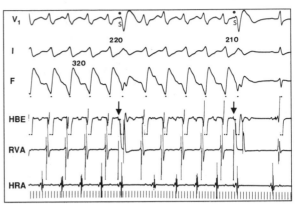

Figure 7. *Termination of inducible sustained ventricular tachycardia (VT) (cycle length, 320 ms) by synchronized ventricular extrastimulus(s). The VT was terminated abruptly by the ventricular extrastimulus with a coupling interval of 210 ms. The display format and abbreviations are as in previous figures. Paper speed is 100 mm/s.*

preexistent bundle branch block, 2) AV antidromic reciprocating tachycardia in patients with WPW syndrome, 3) atrial flutter or fibrillation with preexistent functional bundle branch block, and 4) atrial flutter/fibrillation with preexcited QRS complexes in patients with WPW syndrome. Frequently, the only available documentation of the clinical arrhythmia is an ECG rhythm strip which, by itself, is inadequate in the differential diagnosis of VT. Hemo-dynamic instability is an unreliable indicator for sustained VT, and its absence does not exclude the diagnosis of VT. A 12-lead ECG, when available, provides the most useful information and may allow for reaching a correct diagnosis in up to 80% to 90% of the patients. EPS is indicated when the diagnosis of VT remains in doubt despite clinical and ECG evaluation.

EPS is helpful in selection of optimum antiarrhythmic therapy for patients with sustained VT/VF.[6,23,24] Antiarrhythmic drugs are the first line of treatment. During EPS, the efficacy of a drug may be tested by determining its ability to suppress the VT inducibility. However, an effective drug, as predicted by EPS, can be identified in only 30% to 40% of the patients with sustained VT/VF. The drug efficacy is even less (which is as low as 10% to 20%) in those with impaired LV ejection fraction. In patients with nonsuppressible VT, the treatment options include amiodarone, implantable cardioverter defibrillator, or antiarrhythmic surgery. Amiodarone is the most effective antiarrhythmic agent but is associated with significant side effects, requiring discontinuation in up to 10% to 20%. Persistent VT inducibility in patients receiving amiodarone does not necessarily equate with poor prognosis, and some have used a significant slowing in the VT rate as an acceptable end point.[24] In such patients, the incidence of sudden death appears to be low, and the VT recurrences are likely to be nonlethal and hemodynamically well tolerated. Implantable cardioverter defibrillators can pace-terminate, cardiovert, or defibrillate the clinical arrhythmias, as and when they occur, and are the preferred mode of treatment when the antiarrhythmic drugs fail. The incidence of sudden death in patients with ICD is about 5% to 8% at 5 years of follow-up.[25] About half of the patients may require concomitant antiarrhythmic drugs to reduce the frequency of ICD discharges.

EPS is not indicated in evaluation of patients whose cardiac arrest occurred within the first 48 hours of acute myocardial infarction or in whom the cardiac arrest was related to drug toxicity or electrolyte abnormality. A routine use of EPS is also not recommended for patients with premature ventricular complexes. The role of EPS-guided antiarrhythmic treatment in patients with LV dysfunction and nonsustained VT needs to be investigated.[26]

UNEXPLAINED SYNCOPE

Syncope is a common medical problem. It accounts for about 1% of the hospital admissions, occurs at an incidence of 6% in the elderly patients, and has a recurrence rate of 30% to 40%. The etiology of syncope remains unexplained in up to half of the patients despite an extensive history, physical examination, neurologic study, and noninvasive diagnostic studies. The prognosis depends upon the mechanism of the syncope and the presence of heart disease. The mortality is high for patients with syncope of cardiac origin.[27] EPS is of great utility in these patients as it helps define the mechanisms of the syncope and helps to select an optimum antiarrhythmic therapy.

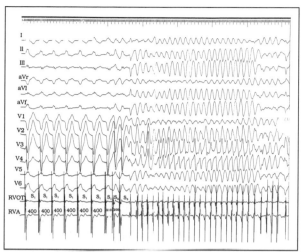

Figure 8. *Induction of sustained polymorphic ventricular tachycardia (VT) in a patient with recurrent syncope and coronary artery disease. The VT was reproducibly induced by double extrastimuli during pacing at right ventricular (RV) outflow tract. Administration of procainamide suppressed inducibility of the polymorphic VT.*

During EPS, the function of sinus node, AV node, and the His–Purkinje system is systematically evaluated, and an attempt is made to induce ventricular or supraventricular tachycardias. The diagnostic yield of EPS varies from 40% to 70% and depends upon the presence or absence of structural heart disease and the aggressiveness of the stimulation protocol employed. The findings of diagnostic importance include the inducibility of monomorphic VT, pacing-induced His–Purkinje block, and marked sinus node dysfunction.[28–30] Abnormal findings of less specificity include the inducibility of nonsustained monomorphic VT, VF induced with double extrastimuli (Fig. 8), or the presence of sluggish AV-nodal conduction despite atropine/isoproterenol administration. Induction of atrial fibrillation and polymorphic VT is probably a nonspecific response of little clinical significance.

In patients with syncope but no structural heart disease, the diagnostic yield of EPS is low and is thus not recommended. In the vast majority of these patients, neurocardiogenic syncope accounts for their symptoms. The syncope is provoked by an abnormally increased vagal tone (and a probable withdrawal of the

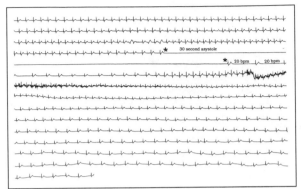

Figure 9. *A 30-second asystole after 12 minutes of head-up tilt (in drug-free state) in a 28-year-old school teacher with recurrent syncope. Thereafter, a slow junctional rhythm appeared at 20 beats/min. The patient required both ß-blockers and permanent dual chamber cardiac pacemakers for symptom relief.*

sympathetic tone), which leads to bradycardia and systolic hypotension. At times, the syncope may be triggered by stress, pain, fear, severe fatigue, hunger or thirst, overcrowded and humid environment, and prolonged standing. The syncope is typically preceded by symptoms of dizziness, nausea, abdominal discomfort, yawning, or diaphoresis, and the symptoms of urinary or bowel incontinence are conspicuously absent. The symptom complex may last several minutes to half an hour in duration, and an attempt to sit or stand up sooner results in recurrence of syncope.

Until recently, the diagnosis of neuro-cardiogenic syncope could only be based on the clinical findings. In recent studies, head-up tilt test has been used to provoke neurocardiogenic syncope with reported sensitivity of 42% to 80%.[28,31] The patient is tilted head up at 60°–70° angle for 20 to 30 minutes, during which time the heart rate and blood pressure are continuously monitored. An abnormal test is defined by provocation of severe presyncope or syncope associated with a sudden fall in the systolic blood pressure (<70 mm Hg), the heart rate (<60 beats/min), or both (Fig. 9). If the response to head up tilt is negative, iso-proterenol is infused to increase the heart rate by 50% or up to maximum of 120 beats/min, and the tilt test is repeated.

In patients with neurocardiogenic syncope, the recurrence of syncope may be prevented by the use of ß-adrenergic blocking agents,[32] anticholinergic drugs (disopyramide, scopolamine), or plasma volume expanding drugs (e.g., fludrocortisone). Rarely, dual chamber cardiac pacing is needed as well. The head-up tilt test may be repeated to test the efficacy of treatment. The prognosis is good in successfully treated patients and the syncope recurs in less than 10% of the patients.

RADIO FREQUENCY ELECTRODE CATHETER ABLATION

Until a decade ago the use of electrode catheter ablation was limited to patients with atrial fibrillation with an uncontrollable ventricular rate whose symptoms were refractory to drug treatment.[33] In these patients, direct current electric energy was used to interrupt the AV conduction, and the patients needed permanent cardiac pacing. Some attempted to use direct current electrode catheter ablation to cure both the AV nodal reentrant supraventricular tachycardia and atrial flutter, but the outcome was unpredictable and the complication of complete AV block occurred in up to 10% to 15%. Furthermore, direct-current electric shocks produced diffuse and nonhomogeneous myocardial lesions, were associated with significant barotrauma, and required administration of general anesthesia. Also, in some reports, a concern was raised regarding the development of sudden cardiac death in long-term follow-up as a complication of the procedure.[34] Thus, direct-current electrode catheter ablation never gained wide acceptance in the medical community.

The technique of radio frequency (RF) catheter ablation has revolutionized the approach to patients with symptomatic tachyarrhythmias. Unlike direct-current electric energy, RF energy produces a superficial and discrete lesion, is not associated with baro trauma, and does not require general anesthesia. Moreover, RF ablation has been associated with a high success rate and low incidence of both early and late complications.

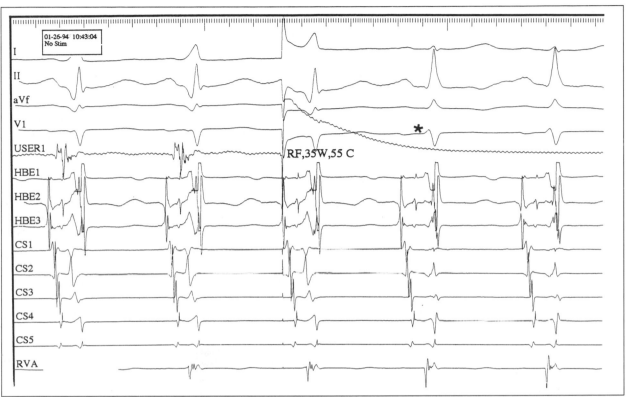

Figure 10. *Radio frequency (RF) catheter ablation of manifest right posteroseptal accessory pathway in a 16-year-old girl. The display format is the same as in previous figures. Paper speed is 100 mm/s. The mapping probe (user) was placed at the posteroseptal aspect of the tricuspid annulus but recorded atrial and ventricular signals superimposed upon each other and the ventricular electrogram preceded the onset of delta waves by 30 ms. Radio frequency application eliminated the delta-wave in less than a second, and the QRS complexes (marked by *) were normalized.*

AV NODAL REENTRANT TACHYCARDIA

In the initial reports, AV nodal reentrant tachycardia was cured by selectively ablating the fast pathway conduction.[35] This was achieved by targeting RF energy to a site just anterior and superior to the electrode catheter recording the His bundle potential during sinus rhythm. The endpoint for fast pathway ablation was a sudden and marked prolongation of the AH and PR intervals and noninducibility of the AV nodal reentry tachycardia. The procedure gained popularity because of its ease of performance and a high success rate (80% to 90%). However, complete AV block occurred in up to 3% to 19%,[16,35] and this complication limited the widespread use of the fast pathway ablative technique.

More recently, slow pathway ablation has become the procedure of choice to cure AV nodal reentrant tachycardia.[36] The slow pathway fibers appear to be located in the triangle of Koch at a site that is immediately posterior and inferior to the compact AV node. It may be successfully ablated by delivering RF energy to the posteroseptal or the mid-septal tricuspid annulus. Using this technique, the success rate has been 95% to 100% and the risk of AV block is less than 1%.[36]

PREEXCITATION SYNDROME

Radio frequency electrode catheter ablation has become the procedure of choice in symptomatic patients with concealed or manifest pre-excitation syndrome.[36] The success rate has ranged from

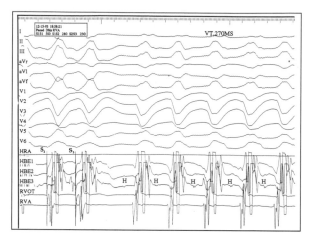

95% to 98% and the incidence of complications is low.[16,36] For right-sided accessory pathways, the tricuspid annulus is mapped by advancing a deflectable and steerable multielectrode catheter (4-mm tip electrode) through the right femoral, the subclavian, or the internal jugular vein. For

Figure 11. *Induction of bundle branch reentry ventricular tachycardia (VT) in a 55-year-old patient with idiopathic dilated cardiomyopathy. The display format is the same as in previous figures. Paper speed is 100 mm/s. The ventricular tachycardia (VT) was induced by 2 extrastimuli (S_2S_3) and had a cycle length of 270 ms. During VT, the QRS complexes were preceded by a His deflection, with HV interval of 80 ms. During sinus rhythm, the HV interval was 65 ms.*

the left-sided accessory pathways, the mitral annulus may be mapped by advancing the ablative catheter retrogradely across the aortic valve or by transseptal left atrial catheterization. The precise location of the accessory pathway can be mapped during sinus rhythm or atrial pacing in patients with manifest preexcitation (Fig. 10) or during induced AV orthodromic reciprocating tachycardia and ventricular pacing in patients with concealed accessory pathway (Fig. 11).

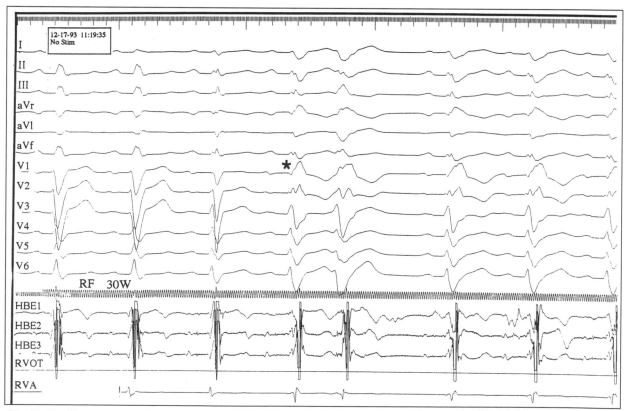

Figure 12. *The same patient as in Figure 11. The right bundle branch was successfully ablated by delivering radio frequency energy at the anteroseptal tricuspid annulus, where a large right bundle potential was recorded. The appearance of right bundle branch is indicated by *. Postablation, ventricular tachycardia could not be induced despite using triple extrastimuli. The HV interval lengthened to 80 ms after ablation of the right bundle branch.*

Table 3. Indications for Radio Frequency Catheter Ablative Procedures

ARRHYTHMIA	INDICATIONS IN PATIENTS WITH:
PSVT without WPW syndrome	Drug-refractory symptomatic PSVT Hemodynamically severe symptoms during PSVT PSVT in high risk professionals Intolerant to, or desire not to take drugs
WPW syndrome	Symptomatic PSVT (before initiating class Ia or class III antiarrhythmic agents) History of AF, presyncope, syncope, or cardiac arrest WPW with family history of sudden death WPW in high risk professionals
Atrial tachycardia and atrial flutter	Symptomatic and drug refractory tachycardias Hemodynamically severe symptoms during paroxysms of tachycardias Desire not to take drugs
VT	Idiopathic VT Fascicular VT VT due to bundle branch reentry Hemodynamically stable VT with frequent recurrences despite drugs

PSVT=Paroxysmal supraventricular tachycardia; VT=Ventricular tachycardia; CHF=Congestive heart failure; AF=Atrial fibrillation; WPW=Wolff–Parkinson–White.

ATRIAL TACHYCARDIA AND FLUTTER

The experience with RF ablation in patients with atrial tachycardias and atrial flutter is somewhat limited, but the results have been promising.[37] In up to 70% of the patients with atrial tachycardia, the reentrant substrate is located in the right atrium and is thus amenable to RF ablation. In others where the tachycardia focus is in the left atrium, a transseptal approach may be utilized to map and ablate the atrial tachycardia. Initial success is high (80%–90%) but the tachycardia has recurred in up to 20% of the patients who had successful ablation procedures. More recently, atrial flutter has also been successfully ablated by delivering RF energy to a narrow isthmus on the right atrial floor which is located between the low septal tricuspid annulus and the entry of the inferior vena cava.

VENTRICULAR TACHYCARDIA

Earlier investigators used direct-current electrode catheter ablation to ablate the focus of sustained VT in patients who had drug refractory arrhythmias and were considered to be too poor a surgical risk. The Percutaneous Cardiac Mapping and Ablation Registry[34] reported the experience of 164 patients with sustained VT. The procedure was successful in 18% (no inducible VT), partially successful in 42% (inducible but no recurrence on antiarrhythmic drugs) and unsuccessful in 40%. However, there was a 7% incidence of procedure related deaths and a 10% incidence of sudden death during mean follow-up of 12 months.

More recently, the RF electrode catheter ablation technique has been successfully used in patients who have sustained VT but no structural heart disease. In these patients, the

Table 4. Complications of Radio Frequency Ablative Procedures in 400 Patients	
COMPLICATIONS	NUMBER OF PATIENTS
Pneumothorax	4 (1%)
Pericardial tamponade	3 (0.77%)
Complete atrioventricular block:	
atrioventricular nodal reentrant	
supraventricular tachycardia (n=85)	4 (4.7%)
Wolff–Parkinson–White syndrome (n=245)	3 (1.2%)
Iliac artery dissection	1 (0.25%)
Venous thrombophlebitis	1 (0.25%)
Subclavian hematoma	1 (0.25%)

Notes: None had acute myocardial infarction, coronary artery dissection, acute cerebrovascular accident, aortic dissection, or pulmonary embolism. Early or late mortality were not observed. Atrioventricular block was not detected in the last 200 patients.

VT originates either in the RV outflow tract or the LV septum in its posteroinferior aspects. Such tachycardias may be successfully ablated in up to 90%, and the incidence of late recurrence has been less than 10%.[38] Another variety amenable to RF ablation includes the sustained VT related to bundle branch reentry. This macro-reentry circuit may be responsible for up to 30% of the sustained VTs originating in patients with idiopathic dilated cardiomyopathy. It can be successfully ablated by interrupting conduction through the right bundle branch (Figs. 11, 12). The results with RF ablation in

patients with sustained VT related to coronary artery disease have been disappointing but are likely to improve as catheter technology and mapping techniques are further refined.

CLINICAL UTILITY AND COMPLICATIONS OF RADIO FREQUENCY ELECTRODE CATHETER ABLATION

It should be emphasized that the performance of the RF ablative procedure requires a highly specialized EPS laboratory with fully trained and dedicated personnel. Typically, this procedure (both diagnostic and ablative components) may take 4 to 8 hours with a median fluoroscopic exposure of approximately 15 to 20 minutes. Data on the long-term efficacy and safety of RF ablative procedure are now available on large numbers of patients from multiple centers, and the findings have been encouraging. Table 3 lists the generally accepted indications for RF electrode catheter ablation. The experience with the first 400 patients at the Hospital of the Good Samaritan is displayed in Figure 13, and the complications are described in Table 4.

OVERVIEW

EPS has assumed an important role in the diagnosis and management of patients with cardiac arrhythmias. It is no longer merely considered a research tool and has matured into

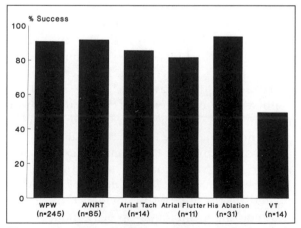

Figure 13. Radio frequency ablative experience in the first 400 patients at the Hospital of the Good Samaritan, Los Angeles. WPW=Wolfe-Parkinson-White; AVNRT=AV nodal reentrant tachycardia.

a separate subspecialty within the field of cardiology. Not every cardiologist finishing a cardiovascular training program is fully trained in clinical electrophysiology. Given the complexity of the cardiac arrhythmias and the rapidly evolving knowledge in this field, EPS should best be performed by those who have a special interest in cardiac electrophysiology, are well trained in this subspecialty, and are cognizant of the value and limitations of EPS.

REFERENCES

1. Alanis J, Gonzalez H, Lopez E. Electrical activity of the bundle of His. *J Physiol.* 1958;142:127-140.
2. Scherlag BJ, Lau SH, Helfant RA, et al. Catheter technique for recording His bundle activity in man. *Circulation.* 1969;39:13-18.
3. Durrer D, Shoo L, Schuilenburg RM, et al. The role of premature beats in the initiation and termination of supraventricular tachycardia in WPW syndrome. *Circulation.* 1967;36:644-662.
4. Wellens HJJ. Electrical stimulation of the heart in the study and treatment of tachycardias. *Circulation.* 1972;46:216-226.
5. Josephson ME, Horowitz LN, Farshidi A, et al. Recurrent sustained ventricular tachycardia: 1. Mechanisms. *Circulation.* 1978;57:431-440.
6. Horowitz LN, Josephson ME, Farshidi A, et al. Recurrent sustained ventricular tachycardia: 3. Role of the electrophysiologic study in the selection of antiarrhythmic regimens. *Circulation.* 1978;58:90-94.
7. Mirowski M, Reid PR, Mower MM, et al. Termination of malignant ventricular arrhythmias with an implanted automatic defibrillator in human beings. *N Engl J Med.* 1980;303:322-324.
8. Strauss HC, Bigger JT, Saroff AL, et al. Electrophysiologic evaluation of sinus node function in patients with sinus node dysfunction. *Circulation.* 1978;53:763-767.
9. Narula OS, Shanto N, Vasquez M, et al. A new method for measurement of sinoatrial conduction time. *Circulation.* 1978;58:706-714.
10. Hariman RJ, Krongrad E, Boxer RA, et al. Method of recording electrical activity of the sinoatrial node and automatic atrial foci during cardiac catheterization in human subjects. *Am J Cardiol.* 1980;45:775-781.
11. Damato AN, Lau SH, Helfant R, et al. A study of heart block in man using His bundle recordings. *Circulation.* 1969;39:297-305.
12. Strasberg B, Amat-Y-Leon F, Dhingra RC, et al. Natural history of chronic second degree atrioventricular nodal block. *Circulation.* 1981;63:1043-1049.
13. Bhandari AK, Rahimtoola SH. Intracardiac electrophysiologic studies in patients with atrioventricular and intraventricular conduction blocks not associated with acute myocardial infarction. *Circulation.* 1987;75(suppl III):107-109.
14. Dhingra RC, Palileo E, Stasberg P, et al. Significance of the HV intervals in 517 patients with chronic bifascicular block. *Circulation.* 1981;64:1265-1271.
15. Scheinman MM, Peters RW, Modin G, et al. Prognostic value of infranodal conduction time in patients with chronic bundle branch block. *Circulation.* 1977;55:240-244.
16. Sager PT, Bhandari AK. Narrow complex tachycardias: Differential diagnosis and management. In: Shah PK (ed). *Cardiology Clinics. Acute Cardiac Care.* Philadelphia: W.B. Saunders; 1991;9:619-641.
17. Akhtar M, Zazayeri MR, Sra JS. Atrioventricular nodal reentry. Clinical, electrophysiologic and therapeutic considerations. *Circulation.* 1993;388:282-295.
18. Morady F, Sledge C, Shen E, et al. Electrophysiologic testing in the management of patients with the WPW syndrome and atrial fibrillation. *Am J Cardiol.* 1983;51:1623-1628.
19. Klein GJ, Bashore TM, Sellers GD, et al. Ventricular fibrillation in Wolff-Parkinson-White syndrome. *N Engl J Med.* 1979;301:1080-1085.
20. Waldo AL, Akhtar M, Benditt DG, et al. Appropriate electrophysiologic study and treatment of patients with Wolff-Parkinson-White syndrome. *J Am Coll Cardiol.* 1988;11:1124-1129.
21. Wu D, Amat-Y-Leon F, Simpson RJ Jr, et al. EPS with multiple drugs in patients with atrioventricular reentrant tachycardias utilizing an extranodal pathway. *Circulation.* 1977;56:727-736.
22. Wellens HFF, Bar FW, Leik I. The value of the ECG in the differential diagnosis of a tachycardia with a widened QRS complex. *Am J Med.* 1978;64:27-33.
23. Wilber DJ, Garan M, Kelly E, et al. Out of hospital cardiac arrest: Role of electrophysiologic testing in prediction of long-term outcome. *N Engl J Med.* 1988;318:19-24.
24. Horowitz LN, Greenspan AM, Spielman SR, et al. Usefulness of electrophysiologic testing in evaluation of amiodarone therapy for sustained ventricular tachyarrhythmias associated with coronary heart disease. *Am J Cardiol.* 1985;55:367-371.
25. Marchlinski FE, Flores BT, Buxton AE, et al. The automatic implantable cardioverter defibrillator, efficacy, complications and device failures. *Ann Intern Med.* 1986;104:481-488.
26. Buxton AE, Marchlinski FE, Flores FT, et al. Nonsustained ventricular tachycardia in patients with coronary artery disease: role of electrophysiologic study. *Circulation.* 1987;75:1178-1185.
27. Kapoor WN, Karpf M, Wieand S, et al. A prospective evaluation and follow-up of patients with syncope. *N Engl J Med.* 1983;309:197-204.
28. Sra JS, Anderson AG, Sheikh SH, et al. Unexplained syncope evaluated by electrophysiologic studies and head-up tilt testing. *Ann Intern Med.* 1991;114:1013-1019.
29. Morady F, Shen E, Schwartz, A et al. Long-term follow-up of patients with recurrent unexplained syncope evaluated by electrophysiologic testing. *J Am Coll Cardiol.* 1983;2:1053-1059.

30. Glick RL, Gersh BJ, Sugiue DD, et al. Role of invasive electrophysiologic testing in patients with symptomatic bundle branch block. *Am J Cardiol.* 1987; 59:817-823.

31. Fitzpatrick AP, Theodorikis G, Valdes P, et al. Methodology of head-up tilt testing in patients with unexplained syncope. *J Am Coll Cardiol.* 1991;17:125-130.

32. Sra JS, Jazayeri MR, Avitall B, et al. Comparison of cardiac pacing with drug therapy in the treatment of neurocardiogenic (vasovagal syncope) with bradycardia or asystole. *N Engl J Med.* 1993;328:1080-1085.

33. Scheinman M, Morady F, Hess DS, et al. Catheter induced ablation of the atrioventricular junction to control refractory supraventricular arrhythmias. *JAMA.* 1982;.248:851.

34. Evans GT, Scheinman MM, Zipes DP, et al. The Percutaneous Cardiac Mapping Ablation Registry: Summary of results. *PACE.* 1986;9:923-926.

35. Jazayeri MR, Hemple SL, Sra JS, et al. Selective transcatheter ablation of the fast and slow pathways using radio frequency energy in patients with atrio-ventricular nodal reentrant tachycardia. *Circulation.* 1992;85:1318-1328.

36. Jackman WM, Wang X, Friday KJ, et al. Catheter ablation of accessory atrioventricular pathway (Wolff-Parkinson-White syndrome) by radio frequency current. *N Engl J Med.* 1991;324:1605-1611.

37. Kay GL, Chong F, Epstein AE, et al. Radio frequency ablation for treatment of primary atrial tachycardias. *J Am Coll Cardiol.* 1993;21:901-909.

38. Coggins DL, Lee RJ, Sweeney J, et al. Radio frequency catheter ablation as a cure for idiopathic tachycardia of both left and right ventricular origin. *J Am Coll Cardiol.* 1994;23:1333-1341.

39. Connolly SJ, Yusuf S. Evaluations of the implantable cardioverter defibrillators in survivors of cardiac arrest for randomized trials. *Am J Cardiol.* 1992;69:959-962.

40. DiMarco JP, Garan H, Ruskin JN. Complications in patients undergoing cardiac electrophysiologic procedures. *Ann Intern Med.* 1982;97:490-493.

41. Horowitz LM. Safety of electrophysiologic studies. *Circulation.* 1986;73:11-13.

CHAPTER **11** **Advanced Imaging Techniques**

Brian P. Griffin, MD
Richard D. White, MD
James D. Thomas, MD

Understanding the structure, function, and metabolism of the heart requires high-quality images. The delineation of anatomical detail requires high spatial resolution whereas the dynamic nature of cardiac function requires high temporal resolution. Images are acquired by the differential interaction of some form of energy with the heart. Four basic forms of energy are used to image the heart: 1) x-rays—radiography; 2) sound waves—echocardiography; 3) gamma rays—radionuclide imaging; 4) electromagnetic radiation—magnetic resonance imaging. Thus, radiography exploits the fact that x-rays are attenuated differently by various tissues and these differences can be increased by the injection of radioopaque contrast media. Echocardiography displays the reflection of ultrasonic energy from the border of 2 tissues with different acoustic impedance. Radionuclide techniques are different in that they deliver an energy source (the radionuclide compound) to the body where it is differentially concentrated in structures of interest and then localized by external detectors. Magnetic resonance imaging utilizes a powerful external magnet to define the differential distribution of weak magnetic characteristics within the body.

Current advances in imaging have been produced by manipulating the basic energy sources outlined above in order to obtain images of the heart with higher spatial and temporal resolution. These advances have involved the provision of more appropriate energy packets (such as the higher frequency ultrasound with transesophageal echocardiography), the process of getting the energy source to areas of the cardiovascular system previously not imaged (such as intravascular ultrasound) and the use of more sophisticated computerized technology whereby the energy scattered by the heart is reconstructed.

NEW ULTRASOUND TECHNIQUES

TRANSESOPHAGEAL ECHOCARDIOGRAPHY

Transesophageal echocardiography is a technique whereby imaging of the heart is performed from the esophagus using a modified gastroscope. High-quality images are acquired in most patients due to the higher frequency transducer used and the lack of acoustic interference. When first developed, transesophageal echocardiography utilized a single transducer mounted on the gastroscope. This limited the planes available for imaging to the transverse plane. Newer probes have been developed which allow biplane and multiple plane imaging. The biplane probe consists of two transducers mounted at the end of the gastroscope in series but which are aligned at right angles, allowing imaging in orthogonal planes. Biplane probes currently available do not allow simultaneous imaging in both planes but such probes are under development. The additional longitudinal imaging plane provided by the biplane probe is useful in imaging the aorta, the interatrial septum, and eccentric jets of mitral regurgitation and in imaging the long-axis of the left ventricle, thus facilitating quantitative volumetric measurements.[1]

Newer probes are capable of imaging in multiple planes (multiplane probes). Multiplane imaging is achieved by mechanically rotating the transducer at the tip of the probe. The transducer can rotate through 180°. The transverse plane is conventionally considered 0° and the longitudinal plane is at 90°. The multiple additional imaging planes are useful in obtaining images of complex pathologies such as eccentric mitral regurgitation, congenital heart

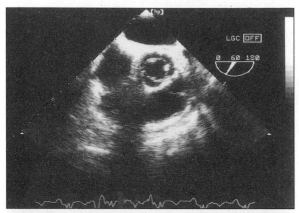

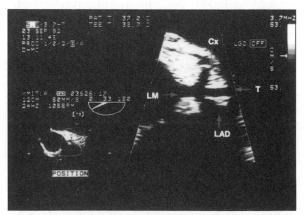

Figure 1. *True short-axis (A) and long-axis views (B) of the aortic root and valve acquired using a multiplane TEE probe. These images are acquired at 60° and 150°. These are planes not available with either a monoplane or biplane imaging transducer.*

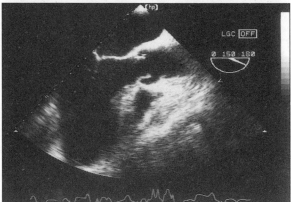

Figure 2. *Multiplane TEE image of the left main coronary artery (LM) as it branches into the left anterior descending (LAD), circumflex (Cx) and trification (T) arteries. The optimal display of the branches was possible in an imaging plane available only with the multiplane probe.*

disease, prosthetic valves, and in the assessment of the aortic valve (Fig. 1). The coronary ostia can be imaged (Fig. 2) and coronary flow may be sampled with Doppler. Furthermore, with multiplane imaging, three-dimensional reconstruction is feasible. The mitral annulus has been successfully reconstructed in this manner.

Current transesophageal probes are capable of imaging at multiple frequencies (3.5 MHz, 5 MHz, 7.5 MHz). The lower frequencies are useful in imaging far-field structures whereas the high frequency improves resolution of near-field structures. These probes have multiple Doppler capabilities also including continuous wave, color flow and pulsed Doppler. A complete hemodynamic examination of the heart valves is now possible with these transducers.

INTRAVASCULAR ULTRASOUND

Intravascular ultrasound is an exciting new technology in which the lumen and wall of a blood vessel are imaged by an ultrasound transducer mounted on a catheter within the lumen. Although this technology has been in development for many years, recent advances in the miniaturization of the transducer have led to its increasing clinical application. This technology is capable of determining the size of the lumen and the wall characteristics of both normal and abnormal blood vessels.[2,3]

The intravascular ultrasound imaging system consists of a transducer mounted on an angiographic catheter which is connected to an ultrasound machine. Images are acquired at 10–30 frames/sec and are recorded on videotape for storage. Catheters of 3.5 to 9F are available for different parts of the vascular system. The smallest catheters are used to examine the coronary tree. The smaller diameter catheters typically use a frequency of 20–40 MHz whereas the larger catheters use a frequency of 10–20 MHz. The higher frequencies allow resolution of the component structures of the vascular wall as they can resolve structures 150 μm apart. All of the imaging catheters have an area around the transducer where the image is degraded due to artifact (ring-down artifact). Two different types of imaging catheters are available. One catheter type uses a single-element transducer which is rotated at 1,000–2,000 rpm. The mechanical transducer is mounted on a drive shaft within the catheter

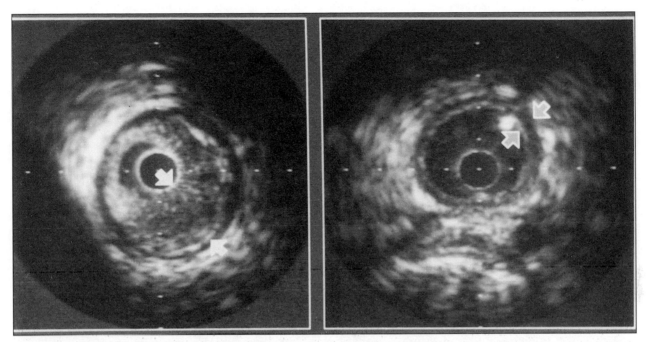

Figure 3. *Coronary artery plaque imaged using intravascular ultrasound. The image on the right illustrates a thin layer of plaque whereas that on the left shows a thicker area of plaque. The dark area in the center of the lumen is the signal void due to the imaging catheter.*

housing. In a modification of this type of transducer, a mirror is used to deflect the sound beam. In this modification, the mirror rather than the transducer is rotated. Another type of catheter uses a multiple-element array placed around the catheter. The elements are sequentially activated to produce an image. Advantages of the mechanical system are simplicity of design and greater power output and signal to noise ratio as compared to the multi-element system. Disadvantages of the mechanical system are 1) the need for a central drive-shaft precluding the use of a central guide-wire, 2) inflexibility of the tip which decreases the steerability of the catheter, 3) image distortion due to variable rotation of the drive-shaft (especially when the catheter is in contact with a wall), and 4) the need for an external guide-wire which lies beside the catheter, takes up space, and often appears in the image display. Advantages of the multi-element catheter are its flexibility and the ability to use a central lumen guide-wire. Disadvantages of this catheter type are decreased power and a larger area adjacent to the catheter in which images cannot be obtained due to ring-down artifact.

Intravascular ultrasound is used in the evaluation of all forms of vascular disease including coronary, pulmonary, and peripheral vascular disease. Intracardiac imaging has also been performed with intravascular ultrasound catheters. With the availability of smaller transducers, more distal segments of even diseased coronary vessels can be imaged. Intravascular ultrasound is now used clinically at the time of cardiac catheterization or coronary interventions in order to define the nature and extent of coronary disease and to monitor the effect of interventions on the vessel wall. Used in this way, intravascular ultrasound appears to be quite safe. Vasospasm is the most commonly reported complication.

Intravascular ultrasound gives rise to a 3-layered appearance of the arterial wall, although variations occur between arteries of the muscular and elastic type. The intima and internal elastic lamina give rise to a single circumferential echo, beneath which lies the hypoechoic area of the media. The adventitia is usually represented as dense echoes due to the presence of collagen. These observations were initially made in vitro but have now been extended to in vivo animal and human studies. Atherosclerotic plaque by its nature is echogenic and is represented as increased echodensities and irregular thickness of the intimal layer which extends into the lumen (Fig. 3). The presence of calcium within the plaque gives rise to focally dense echo

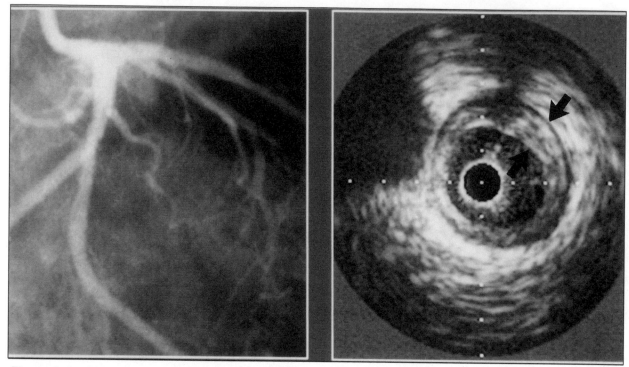

Figure 4. *Angiogram and intravascular ultrasound image of the left main coronary artery. No plaque is identified with angiography whereas the ultrasonic image demonstrates a concentric plaque (arrows).*

reflections and acoustic shadowing of underlying structures in the media and adventitia.

Excellent correlation has been recorded between measurements of lumen size by intravascular ultrasound and in vitro measurements.[4] In normal peripheral and coronary vessels excellent correlation between angiographic measurements of vessel diameter and intravascular ultrasound have been recorded in vivo.[5] In diseased vessels, the correlation between angiography and intravascular ultrasound is more variable.[6] Intravascular ultrasound frequently demonstrates abnormalities at sites which appear normal angiographically (Fig. 4). These abnormalities may be seen in excess of 75% of angiographically normal sites in patients with coronary artery disease (CAD). Luminal diameter of stenoses by angiography and intravascular ultrasound correlate closely if the stenosis is concentric. However, with eccentric plaque, the correlation between the two techniques is much poorer. Intravascular ultrasound is a tomographic technique and is therefore superior to angiography in imaging irregularly-shaped lumens. Intravascular ultrasound is also superior to angiography in defining a truly normal refer-

ence segment with which to derive stenosis severity. Intravascular ultrasound appears to be superior to angiography in defining the characteristics of plaques such as the presence of calcium. Thrombus is more difficult to reliably detect by intravascular ultrasound because it has acoustic qualities similar to both blood and soft plaque. However, thrombus has been correctly identified by this technique in vitro and in vivo, but the sensitivity and specificity of detection are unknown.

One major potential application of intravascular ultrasound is in the determination of the need for intervention in patients with coronary disease, the selection of the appropriate device with which to perform the intervention, and the assessment of the results and complications (Fig. 5).[7] Initial studies have indicated that the morphology of the plaque by intravascular ultrasound can help predict the likelihood of dissection or abrupt closure. The site and extent of dissections are more readily identified by intravascular ultrasound as compared to angiography. Intravascular ultrasound is increasingly used to guide atherectomy and to optimize the amount of debulking produced. Studies have

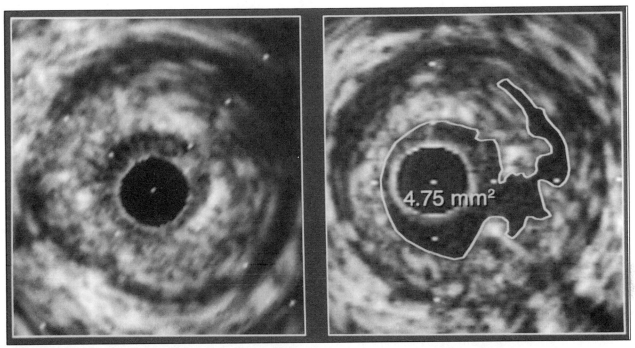

Figure 5. *Intravascular ultrasound images of a coronary plaque before (left) and after (right) percutaneous coronary angioplasty. The lumen increased by 4.75 mm².*

shown that following successful atherectomy, angiography underestimates the amount of residual plaque as compared to intravascular ultrasound.

Intravascular ultrasound has been used in peripheral arteries in a similar manner to that which it is used in coronary vessels. It has also been used to evaluate the aorta and pulmonary arteries.[8] Aortic dissection and coarctation and the site and extent of atherosclerotic disease have been reliably detected and characterized.[9] The aorta is imaged well with less invasive techniques such as transesophageal echocardiography and magnetic resonance imaging and intravascular ultrasound has not as yet been widely used for aortic imaging. Intravascular ultrasound has been used in the evaluation of pulmonary vascular disease. Abnormal structure of the distal vessels in pulmonary hypertension is identifiable with this technique as is abnormal vascular reactivity in response to vasodilators.

Intravascular ultrasound has great promise in both the research and clinical environment. In order to facilitate coronary interventions, angioplasty and atherectomy catheters are being developed which are also capable of intravascular imaging.[10] Intravascular ultrasound is also

being used to characterize atherosclerotic plaque using tissue characterization algorithms based on the reflected sound waves.[11] Similarly, three-dimensional reconstruction of the vessel wall has been performed in order to quantify the extent of the plaque and to gain insight into the mechanism of plaque rupture.[12] Intravascular ultrasound will be used increasingly to determine the extent of disease in patients with multiple risk factors for atherosclerosis and to follow the effects of risk-factor modification on the extent of disease.

INTRACARDIAC IMAGING

Intravascular ultrasound is also being used to image within the heart itself.[13] Catheters with 20 MHz transducers have been used to image intracardiac structures including the interatrial septum, the walls of the chambers and valvular structure but their field of view is extremely limited. More recently, catheters with 12.5 MHz transducers have become available which can image up to a 2-cm radius from the catheter. These catheters allow complete imaging of the semilunar valves and most of the mitral and tricuspid valve can be imaged at any one time. Ideally, an intravascular catheter which would allow complete imaging of both sides of the heart from the right side would be available. This is not yet possible as catheterization of the left side is necessary in order to achieve adequate images of left-sided structures. In the future, with modification of transducers, imaging of most intracardiac structures will be possible from a transducer within the right heart.[14] This technology is most likely to be beneficial in determining the severity of valvular lesions and the effect of balloon dilatation. Another potential use is in obtaining high-quality images of myocardial contrast perfusion studies in patients undergoing interventions.

MYOCARDIAL CONTRAST ECHOCARDIOGRAPHY

It has been known for many years that the presence of microbubbles within the blood stream produces increased echoreflectivity. This property has been used to detect intracardiac shunts and to improve the quality of Doppler signals. More recently, contrast enhancement of the myocardium has been produced by the injection of microbubbles into the aorta or directly into the coronary arteries themselves. This technique was initially developed in animals but is now used in humans.[15] Contrast is produced by mechanical sonication of a neutral medium such as radiographic dye or, more recently, a suspension of human albumen particles.[16] The latter has the advantage that the microbubbles persist longer in the circulation and that the size of the particles (4–5μ) is more physiological. Recent developments have concentrated on the production of a contrast agent which enhances the left heart following a venous injection.[17,18] Initial reports with a number of agents have been encouraging. At the simplest level, contrast enhancement of left-sided chambers and of the left ventricle improves endocardial border resolution and improves quantification of chamber volume and assessment of wall motion particularly with stress. However, this technique has proven potential in a number of other important areas.[19]

Myocardial contrast echocardiography (MCE) is capable of determining the area of perfusion of a coronary blood vessel injected following selective injection (Fig. 6).[20] This perfusion terri-

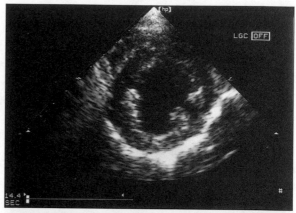

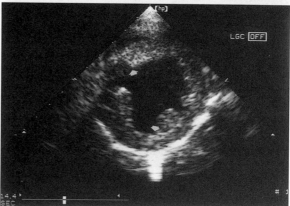

Figure 6. *Myocardial contrast echocardiography with sonicated albumen particles. The image on the top illustrates a cross-sectional view of the left ventricle before an intracoronary contrast injection. The image on the bottom illustrates the enhancement of the myocardium following injection of contrast. The area of contrast enhancement (area to the right of the arrows) represents the myocardium supplied by the left coronary artery.*

tory has been shown in animal studies to indicate the "area at risk" for infarction following coronary occlusion. Determining the "area at risk" is important in defining the value of interventional strategies in order to preserve the myocardium early after coronary occlusion. Myocardial contrast echocardiography can determine the likely size of infarction once reperfusion has taken place. A recent study has indicated that patients with large areas of no reflow by MCE early following thrombolysis are more likely to have severe left ventricular dysfunction or poor outcome.[21] Myocardial contrast echocardiography is more sensitive than angiography in the detection of collateral flow. Studies have indicated that post-infarct patients whose myocardium is well-collateralized as assessed by MCE are more likely to show improvement in regional left ventricular function following angioplasty as compared to those with poor collateral supply.[22] MCE can also determine coronary flow reserve.[23] This is determined by constructing a plot of the intensity of the contrast effect in a myocardial segment over time following the contrast injection. The time intensity curve can be characterized in a number of ways including the peak intensity, the area under the curve, and the time taken for the intensity to fall to one-half of its peak value (t1/2).[24] Following coronary vasodilatation, peak intensity and the area under the curve increase in normal vessels but not in vessels with a critical stenosis. The changes in the time intensity curve reflect those measured by a Doppler flow wire. Thus, MCE has the potential to assess the functional success of interventions such as coronary angioplasty. MCE has also been used at the time of surgical revascularization in order to determine the adequacy of protection with cardioplegia, to determine the sequence of graft placement and to assess the functional success of revascularization.[25,26]

Limitations to the use of MCE at present are the need for left heart catheterization in order to achieve optimal opacification of myocardium and the difficulty of obtaining high-quality echocardiographic images in patients lying supine in the catheterization laboratory. In the future, when left ventricular opacification is consistently possible from a venous injection, MCE is likely to be more widely applied particularly in acute infarction. Intracardiac imaging may, in the future, allow stable high-quality echocardiographic images to be obtained before and after interventions. Improved contrast agents with more physiological tracer profiles and stability within the circulation may allow estimation of regional myocardial blood flow.

ULTRASONIC TISSUE CHARACTERIZATION

Ultrasonic tissue characterization refers to the ability of ultrasound to determine the composition of cardiac tissue. At a simple level this is possible with the unaided eye, as certain tissues have acoustic properties which readily identify them from others. For example, calcification within the heart gives rise to brighter images than normal tissue because calcium is a better reflector of sound. A number of methods based on either qualitative or quantitative differences in the acoustic properties of tissues have been devised in order to detect abnormal myocardium.[27] These methods can be divided into those which manipulate the image or video data by color encoding or by statistical analysis of the image texture and those which exploit the acoustic properties of tissue contained in radiofrequency data such as integrated backscatter or tissue attenuation.

Alterations in tissue attenuation and backscatter following the onset of ischemia have been shown in many studies. The mechanism by which this occurs is multifactorial and involves alterations in tissue water content, blood flow and collagen content.[28] Cyclic variation in backscatter is a normal phenomenon which is sensitive to perturbations in myocardial function. Thus, cyclic variation is reduced in cardiomyopathy, acute ischemia, and infarction but normalizes following the onset of reperfusion.[29,30] Cyclic variability is potentially an important marker of reperfusion as the resumption of cyclic variability is independent of and antedates changes in regional contraction. Unfortunately, alterations in cyclic variability and in backscatter are non-specific in nature; many alterations in myocardial structure and function cause similar derangements in these parameters. Research is currently underway to uniquely characterize individual derangements by analysis of the frequency dependence of the backscatter.

Methods based on quantitative textural analysis of video images have also been shown to differentiate separate disease states such as amyloid cardiomyopathy or hypertrophic cardiomyopathy.[31] One of the significant limitations of these methodologies is their dependence on the settings of the ultrasound machine.[32] At present, quantitative tissue characterization is a research tool which has not been widely applied clinically due to the limited availability of the required technology and the absence of unique identifiers of specific abnormalities with the technology available.

THREE-DIMENSIONAL RECONSTRUCTION

Computerized reconstruction of three-dimensional (3-D) images has been used with comput-

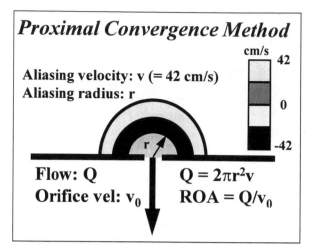

Proximal Convergence Method

Aliasing velocity: v (= 42 cm/s)
Aliasing radius: r

cm/s 42

0

-42

Flow: Q $Q = 2\pi r^2 v$
Orifice vel: v_0 $ROA = Q/v_0$

Figure 7. *Proximal isovelocity method of estimating regurgitant flow. See text for details. ROA= Regurgitant orifice area.*

ed tomography (CT) scanning and magnetic resonance imaging (MRI) for some time. Three-dimensional reconstruction is feasible with tomographic techniques and is easiest for static structures. Generation of 3-D cardiac images is more difficult because of the confounding effects of cardiac and respiratory motion. Three-dimensional reconstruction has been applied successfully to a number of different tomographic imaging modalities including MRI and echocardiography.[33] In echocardiography, 2 methods exist to obtain 3-D images. In 1 method, the transducer is fixed in space and moved incrementally to provide tomographic cuts. In the other method, the transducer is free to move but is localized in space by some form of locator. Both methods have produced computer-derived 3-D images of cardiac structures such as the mitral valve and the left ventricle.[34] Multiplane probes available with Transesophageal Echocardiography (TEE) have also been used to generate 3-dimensional images.[35] Three-dimensional reconstruction facilitates the representation of complex shapes such as the right ventricle, the abnormal left ventricle, and complex congenital lesions. It has also been shown to allow more accurate volumetric measurements. Difficulties in its routine clinical application relate to the time and difficulty in acquiring high-quality images and the time to reconstruct these images. The appropriate representation of images is also a problem, particularly of depth and texture. However, with the

increasing availability and sophistication of imaging technology, it is likely that 3-D reconstruction will be available routinely in the future.

ADVANCES IN DOPPLER ECHOCARDIOGRAPHY

Doppler echocardiography is increasingly used in the definitive evaluation of valvular heart disease, particularly stenotic lesions. Valvular regurgitation is readily detected by Doppler but accurate on-line quantitation has been difficult. Recent work suggests that valvular regurgitation may be quantified by color-flow mapping by analyzing the flow disturbance proximal to the regurgitant site (proximal isovelocity method).[36] In the region proximal to a regurgitant orifice, blood accelerates predictably to form a series of concentric shells of decreasing area and increasing velocity. For blood flow moving at velocity v and at a radius r from the regurgitant orifice, flow rate Q can be calculated as: $Q = 2\pi\ r^2\ v$ with simple correction factors used for distortion of the velocity field resulting from local and geometric factors (Fig. 7).[37] This process can be simplified by automated analysis of digital velocity maps available in echocardiographic machines.[38] In vitro, animal and initial clinical studies have indicated that this method can accurately determine mitral regurgitant flow and the flow across atrial septal defects.[39] One of the limitations in the application of this technique is the difficulty in validation posed by the lack of a true gold standard in the measurement of regurgitant flow, especially in the clinical setting. Once regurgitant flow rate (Q) and peak orifice velocity (v_0) are known, then the effective regurgitant orifice area can be calculated as Q/v_0. Regurgitant orifice area appears to be a fundamental measure of valvular regurgitation and may be an excellent parameter with which to follow regurgitant severity and the responses to pharmacologic intervention over time.[40]

The mitral regurgitant velocity spectrum has been used to reconstruct the ventriculo-atrial pressure difference throughout systole by means of the modified Bernoulli equation ($P=4v^2$). This permits estimation of the peak left ventricular dp/dt in early systole which is an index of contractile function (Fig. 8). Good correlation has been reported with this method of determining dp/dt when compared to simultaneous

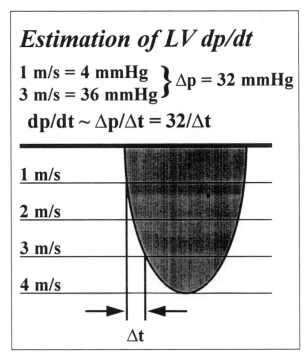

Estimation of LV dp/dt

$$1 \text{ m/s} = 4 \text{ mmHg}$$
$$3 \text{ m/s} = 36 \text{ mmHg}$$
$$\left.\right\} \Delta p = 32 \text{ mmHg}$$

$$dp/dt \sim \Delta p/\Delta t = 32/\Delta t$$

1 m/s

2 m/s

3 m/s

4 m/s

Δt

Figure 8. Method of estimating left ventricular dp/dt from the mitral regurgitant Doppler velocity trace. Velocity (v) is converted to pressure (P) using the modified Bernoulli equation where P = 4v².

invasive measurements.[41] LV dp/dt measured noninvasively can help predict outcome of surgery for mitral regurgitation and may be useful in the optimal timing of surgery for this condition. The time constant of ventricular relaxation (tau), an important measure of diastolic function, can also be determined from the mitral regurgitant velocity spectrum by derivation from negative dp/dt.[42]

ADVANCES IN NUCLEAR IMAGING

For many years thallium-201 has been the radionuclide of choice in the detection of myocardial ischemia and in the assessment of myocardial viability. Tomographic imaging has improved sensitivity as compared to planar imaging with some sacrifice in specificity as minor heterogeneity in uptake may be amplified by the tomographic display. Quantitation and graphic display of the regional uptake of the radionuclide agent help in the interpretation of

the findings. In patients who cannot exercise, pharmacologic agents now used include adenosine, dobutamine, and dipyridamole.

ASSESSMENT OF VIABILITY WITH THALLIUM

Thallium-201 scans have been used to assess myocardial viability.[43] Traditionally, absence of thallium uptake 3–4 hours following exercise was used to indicate scar. A number of studies have challenged this interpretation.[44] Following revascularization, up to 50% of fixed defects demonstrate improvement in thallium uptake.[45] Additionally, most defects which are fixed at 4 hours will show further improvement in uptake if scanned again at 24 hours.[46,47] Furthermore, reinjection of thallium prior to the resting images leads to improvement in uptake in up to half of the patients.[48] A second dose of thallium should, therefore, be injected prior to imaging at rest.

NEW AGENTS

Although thallium-201 is still widely used in myocardial perfusion studies, a number of new agents based on technetium 99m (99mTc) have become available.[49] Technetium has advantages over thallium as an imaging agent because it is eluted continuously from a generator in the nuclear medicine laboratory whereas thallium must be generated in a cyclotron. Additionally, the 140 keV technetium photon yields a higher quality image than the lower energy (69–83 keV) thallium photon. Furthermore, the shorter half-life of 99mTc allows up to 10 times the radioactive dose to be given safely. This leads to higher counts particularly in large patients and improved spatial resolution.

Two different compounds are approved for clinical use (sestamibi and teboroxime) and one is under investigation (tetrofosmin). 99mTc sestamibi is an isonitrile compound which is distributed in myocardium in proportion to blood flow. The mechanism of extraction is different to thallium in that it is independent of the Na-K ATPase pump. Sestamibi is bound within the mitochondria of the cell, and thus requires cell viability for binding. Once bound, washout occurs relatively slowly, allowing an image of myocardial perfusion at the time of the injection to be obtained for a number of hours. First-pass studies of ventricular function can also be obtained with ^{99m}Tc sestamibi. Teboroxime is a boronic acid derivative. Its short half-time (10–15 minutes) makes acquisition of tomographic images difficult with conventional systems.

^{99m}Tc sestamibi, unlike conventional thallium imaging, requires an exercise and rest injection. As hepatobiliary clearance of this agent is relatively slow even with exercise, imaging is usually begun 15–30 min following the exercise injection and 60–90 min following a resting injection. Completion of imaging in a single day is therefore more difficult than with thallium and the resting and exercise injections are often performed on separate days. Perfusion imaging with sestamibi is safe and is at least as sensitive as thallium in the detection of coronary disease in reported clinical studies.[50] Although sestamibi is capable of detecting scar, it is not clear whether it can detect chronically underperfused but viable (hibernating) myocardium because of its relative absence of redistribution. Ongoing investigation into this area is currently in progress. Clinical and animal studies have indicated that sestamibi imaging is highly sensitive for detecting perfusion defects in acute MI.[51] The stability of the perfusion distribution allows imaging to be performed a number of hours following injection once the patient has stabilized. The effects of interventions such as thrombolysis can be assessed and infarct size can be quantitated.[52,53] First-pass estimations of ejection fraction using ^{99m}Tc sestamibi correlate closely with standard first-pass determinations.[54] Imaging with this agent therefore allows an assessment of perfusion and function in the same imaging session. Other radionuclide agents are under investigation. Preliminary reports of tetrofosmin suggest that it is clinically valid, and may allow shorter imaging time than sestamibi due to its more rapid excretion through the hepatobiliary system.

OTHER NUCLEAR IMAGING TECHNIQUES

ANTIMYOSIN IMAGING

Antimyosin is a monoclonal antibody which binds to myosin in irreversibly-damaged myocytes. By labeling antimyosin within indium-111, its uptake in the myocardium can be imaged and necrotic areas are represented as brighter (hotter) than normal areas. Studies in myocardial infarction indicate that antimyosin imaging is sensitive and specific for myocardial damage.[55] One drawback of this imaging modality is that the area of increased uptake persists and limits its application in determining the acuity of the myocardial insult.[56] Antimyosin imaging has also been used to detect acute myocarditis[57] and acute rejection in transplant patients.[58]

IMAGING OF THROMBUS

Accurate detection and localization of intracardiac and intravascular thrombus is relatively difficult with all currently available noninvasive imaging techniques. Two nuclear techniques have been used: one in which platelets are labeled with indium;[59] the other uses radiolabeled monoclonal antibodies to platelet glycoproteins.[60] Clinical experience with these agents has been limited. A current limitation of these imaging modalities is that small thrombi are not as yet reliably imaged.

IMAGING OF SYMPATHETIC NERVES

Norepinephrine analogs such as metaiodobenzylguanidine (MIBG) labeled with iodine-123 are taken up in preganglionic sympathetic nerves. This imaging modality has been used to study the destruction of sympathetic nerve fibers in ischemia and infarction and their relationship to arrhythmogenesis.[61] MIBG imaging has also been used to study the depletion of catecholamines in patients with congestive heart failure.[62]

POSITRON EMISSION TOMOGRAPHY

Positron emission tomography (PET) uses positrons or positively charged electrons as a source of energy. These particles typically travel a very short distance following their generation before they collide with an electron. Combination of a positron with an electron causes annihilation of both particles with the release of 2 very high-energy (512 keV) photons. The photons are released at 180° from each other and are detected by an array of detectors. The simultaneous arrival of photons at detectors on opposite sides of the patient is used to register an

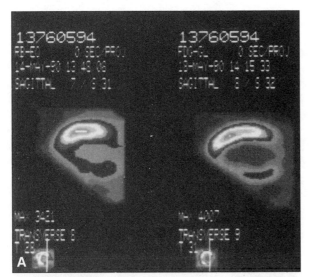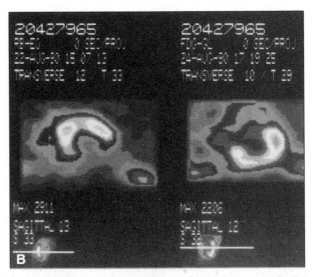

Figure 9. *Rubidium (on the left) and ¹⁸F deoxyglucose (on the right) images of the left ventricle. In A, no uptake is seen in the inferior wall by either technique indicating myocardial scar in this area. In B, a perfusion defect is seen in the inferior wall on the rubidium image but avid uptake is demonstrable by FDG in this area indicating the presence of viable myocardium.*

annihilation event. The annihilation events are filtered and transformed into images by back-projection. Advantages of PET scanning over conventional nuclear imaging are: 1) the 2 high-energy photons released give images of high-quality, and 2) the positron emitting substances used are biologically active or can be tagged onto biological substances. This allows evaluation of metabolic events within the heart in addition to blood flow.

A number of different tracer agents have been used in clinical PET imaging. Rubidium-82, nitrogen-13 ammonia, and oxygen-15 water have been used to assess myocardial perfusion in a manner similar to thallium. Rubidium has the advantage of being available continuously from a generator whereas the other agents require a cyclotron for their generation. Imaging protocols used are similar to those used with exercise or dipyridamole thallium. Quantification of regional flow is possible with N^{13} ammonia and O^{15} water. Other agents are used to trace cardiac metabolism. For example, ¹⁸F deoxyglucose is used to assess glucose utilization and ¹¹C palmitate is used to assess fatty acid metabolism. Other metabolic tracers are becoming available in which amino acid metabolism, adenosine concentration, and adrenergic neural activity can be monitored under normal conditions and in pathological states.

CLINICAL USE OF PET

Perfusion imaging with PET is sensitive and specific in the detection of coronary artery disease with reported sensitivities of 93% to 96% and specificities of 78% to 100%.[63,64] A number of comparative studies have reported improved sensitivity and specificity in the detection of coronary artery disease for PET as compared to conventional thallium imaging.[65] Flow tracers have also been used to detect myocardial infarction and scar.[66] The metabolic derangements resulting from ischemia have also been studied by PET scanning. Thus, in ischemia, fatty acid oxidation is impaired and the myocardium switches to glucose utilization as a major fuel source. Glucose utilization can be assessed with ¹⁸F deoxyglucose. A number of studies have indicated that avid glucose utilization may be present in myocardial segments which show no uptake of tracer on conventional nuclear imaging and which demonstrate severe wall motion abnormalities or perfusion abnormalities by other techniques.[67,68] Myocardial scar demonstrates a matched defect with perfusion and metabolic imaging with ¹⁸F deoxyglucose (Fig. 9). These findings of inadequate perfusion, mechanical dysfunction, and altered but preserved metabolism represent stunned or hibernating myocardium which is potentially functional upon restoration of an adequate blood flow (Fig. 9).[69] A number of studies have indicated that such myocardium does recover function following revascularization or thrombolytic reperfusion and that PET scanning is superior to other imaging modalities in predicting recovery of function in this setting. This is currently the largest indication for PET scanning.

Wider application of PET scanning has been limited by the availability of appropriate nuclear agents and machines and because third-party payers have been slow to allow reimbursement for its use. However, this is likely to change given the high sensitivity of this technology in the detection of coronary disease and its ability to detect hibernating myocardium. In the future, PET scanning will be used to elucidate the role of metabolic abnormalities in disease states other than coronary disease and to aid in the diagnosis and treatment of these diseases.

ULTRAFAST COMPUTED TOMOGRAPHY

Ultrafast CT allows rapid acquisition of images by using an electron beam rather than the rotating x-ray tube used in conventional CT imaging.[70] The electron beam is electromagnetically steered through an arc of 210° onto 4 tungsten targets thus generating x-rays. The x-rays pass through the body structure to be imaged onto detectors. X-ray attenuation is measured by the detector and stored in a digital format for subsequent computer aided reconstruction. A number of different imaging acquisition sequences are available in which the timing and the width of the slices acquired can be varied. Up to 8 imaging levels can be acquired in a single cardiac cycle as each image takes 50 msec with an obligatory 8 msec pause between images. Gating to different parts of the cardiac cycle is possible using the electrocardiograph. Radiographic contrast is generally required for all cardiovascular examinations.

Ultrafast CT provides accurate measurements of the mass and volume of individual cardiac chambers.[71,72] Thus, cardiac output, regurgitant volumes, and left and right ventricular mass have been reliably quantified in vivo with this technique.[73] Ultrafast CT has also been used in global and regional assessment of ventricular function both at rest and during exercise.[74] Ultrafast CT has also proved reliable in the eval-

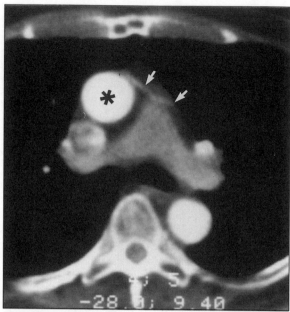

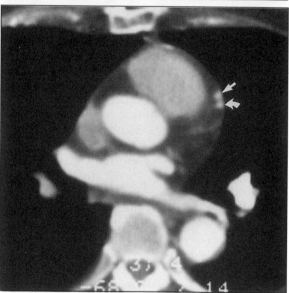

Figure 10. *Ultrafast CT images of patent aortocoronary grafts. Patent coronary grafts originating from the ascending aorta (*) are noted at several levels. They include a graft to the LAD (arrows) seen tangentially in the more cranial level (A) and another graft to a diagonal branch (curved arrow) seen at the more caudal level (B). (Images courtesy of William Stanford, MD, University of Iowa).*

uation of the patency of coronary artery bypass grafts (CABG) and is probably the most reliable noninvasive method of determining graft patency (Fig. 10). Ultrafast CT has also been used to detect the presence of coronary calcification as a marker of significant coronary artery disease. Coronary calcification is reliably detected and quantitated by this technique. However, coronary calcification appears sensitive but not very specific for the presence of significant obstructive disease.[75] Ultrafast CT also appears reliable in detecting the transmural extent of myocardial infarcts but may underestimate true infarct size. Similarly, ultrafast CT has reliably measured myocardial blood flow at low flow rates but is less reliable at higher flow rates probably due to the washout of contrast into the cardiac veins.[76] Peak blood flow and thus flow reserve have been accurately determined. Diastolic filling indices have also correlated well with measurements using other techniques in normal subjects.[77] Research has recently focused on the computation of 3-dimensional velocity flow fields by ultrafast CT which potentially may allow measurement of intracardiac velocities and pressures.[78]

Ultrafast CT is a technology capable of precise depiction of dynamic cardiac structure. Application of this technology has been limited to relatively few centers due to its expense and the more widespread application and familiarity of competing technologies such as magnetic resonance imaging and Doppler echocardiography. In the future, improved spatial and temporal resolution may allow noninvasive coronary arteriography as well as more precise measurements of myocardial function.

MAGNETIC RESONANCE IMAGING

Magnetic resonance imaging is increasingly applied in the demonstration of normal and abnormal anatomy and function of the heart and great vessels.[79] Recent advances in technology and processing whereby more rapid acquisition of images is possible have facilitated dynamic display.[80-82]

Magnetic resonance imaging is based on the existence of microscopic magnetic moments within atomic nuclei. The most important of these nuclei in medical imaging is the single proton of ^{1}H which is both abundant in tissues and very sensitive to external magnetic fields. When a proton is exposed to an external magnetic field it spins or *precesses* about the vector of the main magnetic field. A magnetic field which changes over time (such as a precessing proton) will radiate electromagnetic energy outward at

the precessional frequency, which can then be received by an antenna and amplified electronically. This radiated signal forms the basis for magnetic resonance imaging.

Normally, the proton moments are randomly oriented in space such that the energy radiated by their precession cancels out and their net magnetization vector is zero. Applying a strong external magnetic field causes protons to become aligned either with or against the field. Protons aligned with the field are in a lower energy state and more numerous than those aligned against the field. This generates a net magnetization vector. In order to detect this vector, it must be directed away from the direction of the external magnetic field by applying a pulse of electromagnetic radiation at the precessional frequency (RF pulse). This pulse of energy causes some of the protons to enter a higher energy state from which they return slowly (relax) toward equilibrium. The energy produced as the protons relax back to equilibrium is used to produce magnetic resonance images. The strength of this signal is dependent primarily on the density of the protons. Unfortunately, proton density does not vary sufficiently within the body to allow sufficient contrast in order to characterize different tissues. However, other magnetic properties of the signal can be used to produce additional contrast. The first of these is the rapidity with which the protons relax back toward equilibrium. This is the T1, the longitudinal relaxation time, or spin-lattice time, and which is typically 200 ms to 3 sec in duration. The second time constant, T2, refers to the speed with which the magnetic vector produced by the application of the external magnetic energy dissipates in the transverse plane. This is due to the interaction of adjacent magnetic vectors and is called the transverse or spin-spin relaxation time. Typically, T2 is shorter than T1 and lasts 20–400 ms. The differences in T1 or T2 between tissues can be highlighted by adjusting the timing of signal reception. The motion of the heart and the necessity for gating increases the complexity of cardiac imaging.

Magnetic resonance spectroscopy is capable of identifying the chemical composition of myocardium and has been used in both experimental and clinical studies.[83,84] The external magnetic field excites nuclei within the tissue of interest causing them to emit energy as they return to the unexcited state. The emitted energy

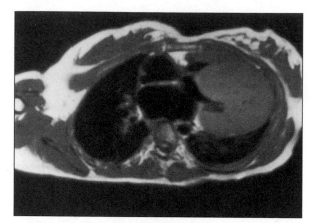

Figure 11. *Spin echo magnetic resonance image of the heart in a patient with hypertrophic cardiomyopathy.*

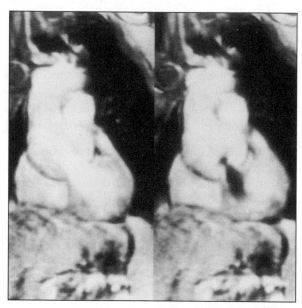

Figure 12. *Spin echo magnetic resonance image of the heart in a patient with Marfan's syndrome and aortic regurgitation. The image on the left is systolic in timing whereas that on the right is diastolic. Aortic regurgitation is demonstrated as the dark area of signal void.*

gives rise to a signal which is mathematically transformed using Fourier analysis into a spectrum of frequency shifts of different intensities. Identification and quantification of different molecules in the spectrum can be determined from their known pattern and the intensity of the signal. The phosphorus nucleus which is intimately involved in energy transfer within cells (ATP, ADP) is readily detected by magnetic resonance spectroscopy and has been studied most often. Other nuclei of interest such as hydrogen and carbon are also studied but are technically more difficult to utilize. Other limitations of this technology include the relatively large volume of tissue required to produce a signal which makes interrogation of regional pathology more difficult.

CLINICAL USE OF MRI

MRI provides high-quality tomographic images of the heart and great vessels. Application of these images is increasing particularly in the assessment of diseases of the aorta[85] (aneurysm, dissection, coarctation), pericardial disease,[86] tumors, hypertrophic cardiomyopathy (Fig. 11), and in complex congenital heart disease.[87] The high spatial resolution provided by magnetic resonance images allows precise determination of chamber and vessel size and of left ventricular mass.[88] Chamber volumes and ejection fraction are also reliably detected by this technique.

Regional dysfunction is also detected by this technique. Myocardial scar leads to a reduction in signal intensity on the T2 image, due to a reduction in the water content. Acute infarction leads to increased signal intensity on T2 images due to edema formation within the infarcted tissue. Contrast agents such as gadolinium compounds have also been used to improve the detection of infarcted regions.[89] Contrast agents may help differentiate reversibly- from irreversibly-damaged myocardium in infarcted patients. Alterations in signal intensity and contrast enhancement aid in the detection of superimposed thrombus in areas of myocardial scar. MRI has also been used to screen for coronary disease by identifying changes in regional wall motion following pharmacological stress. Alterations in signal intensity have also been used to determine the presence of acute rejection following cardiac transplantation.

Magnetic resonance imaging has also been used to determine the presence and severity of valvular heart disease. Valvular regurgitation produces loss of signal within the receiving chamber which is readily detected[90–92] (Fig. 12). A semiquantitative assessment of severity is possible from the size of the area of signal loss. The severity of valvular stenosis is more difficult to assess with conventionally available MRI tech-

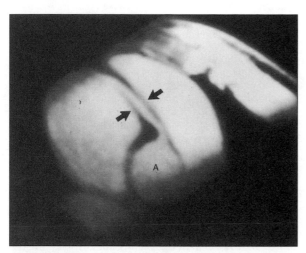

Figure 13. *Coronary magnetic resonance angiogram of a normal right coronary artery (arrows) as it originates from the aortic sinus of Valsalva (A) and courses between the right atrium and ventricle.*

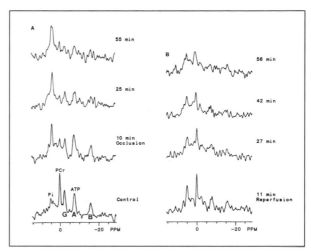

Figure 14. *Effects of occlusion and reperfusion on phosphorus-31 MR spectra of the myocardium in an experimental model. (A) Spectra acquired before and at the indicated stages after occlusion of the LAD. (B) Spectra acquired after release of occluder following a total of 63 min of LAD occlusion. A rapid loss of phosphocreatine (PCr) and a rise in inorganic phosphate (Pi) as well as more gradual depletion of adenosine triphosphate (ATP), during occlusion is apparent. During reperfusion, partial recovery of PCr and Pi is noted while the ATP levels continue to decline. The Gamma (G), Alpha (A), and Beta (B) peaks of ATP are labelled.*

niques due to the difficulty in obtaining instantaneous velocity maps across the valves. Advances in MR sequences and software may allow more precise determination of valvular stenotic lesions in the future.

Dynamic vascular imaging with magnetic resonance is increasingly applied to the aorta and more recently the coronary vasculature.[93] Two methods of generating contrast between blood flow and the vessel wall are possible. In spin-echo imaging, the blood appears dark compared to the vessel lumen, whereas in the gradient-echo technique, blood flow appears bright. The presence and volume of flow within a vessel can be reliably determined with these techniques. Three-dimensional display of dynamic vascular images is particularly valuable in the assessment of complex intravascular pathology such as aortic aneurysms or dissection. Dynamic imaging of the proximal coronary vessels is currently possible with MR angiographic techniques (Fig. 13).[94] Acquisition is performed during a breath hold in order to avoid motion artifact. Faster image acquisition times available in MR machines under development should extend the ability of MR to detect and localize coronary disease.

Magnetic resonance spectroscopy of the phosphorous nucleus has been used to detect metabolic abnormalities in specific diseases. Thus, in myocardial ischemia and infarction the relative proportion of high-energy phosphates is reduced compared to normal controls (Fig. 14).[95] Abnormalities in the distribution of phosphate metabolites as compared to controls have also been reported in dilated and hypertrophic cardiomyopathy, and in transplant rejection. Other nuclei such as carbon and hydrogen which are involved in glucose and lipid metabolism are currently under study.

ACKNOWLEDGMENTS

The authors wish to thank E. Murat Tuzcu, MD; Sebastian A. Cook, MD; Steven E. Nissen, MD; and Allen Klein, MD for providing illustrations.

REFERENCES

1. Seward JB, Khandheria BK, Edwards WD, et al. Biplanar transesophageal echocardiography: anatomic correlations, image orientation, and clinical applica-

tions. *Mayo Clin Proc.* 1990;65:1193-213.

2. Nissen SE, Gurley JC, Booth DC, et al. Intravascular ultrasound of the coronary arteries: Current applications and future directions. *Am J Cardiol.* 1992;69:18H-29H.

3. Tobis JM, Mallery J, Mahon D, et al. Intravascular ultrasound imaging of human coronary arteries in vivo. *Circulation.* 1991;83:913-926.

4. Tobis JM, Bessen M, Moriushi M, et al. Intravascular ultrasound cross-sectional arterial imaging before and after balloon angioplasty in vitro. *Circulation.* 1989;80:873-882.

5. St. Goar FG, Pinto FJ, Alderman EL, et al. Intravascular ultrasound imaging of angiographically normal coronary arteries: an in vivo comparison with quantitative angiography. *J Am Coll Cardiol.* 1991;18:952-958.

6. Nissen SE, Gurley JC, Grines CL, et al. Intravascular ultrasound assessment of lumen size and wall morphology in normal subjects and coronary artery disease patients. *Circulation.* 1991;84:1087-1099.

7. Keren G, Leon MB. Characterization of atherosclerotic lesions by intravascular ultrasound: Possible role in unstable coronary syndromes and in interventional therapeutic procedures. *Am J Cardiol.* 1991;68:85B-91B.

8. Pandian NG, Weintraub A, Kreis A, et al. Intracardiac, intravascular, two-dimensional, high-frequency ultrasound imaging of pulmonary artery and its branches in humans and animals. *Circulation.* 1990;81:2007-2012.

9. Weintraub AR, Schwartz SL, Pandian NG, et al. Evaluation of acute aortic dissection by intravascular ultrasonography. *N Engl J Med.* 1990;323:1566-1567.

10. Isner JM, Rosenfield K, Losordo DW, et al. Combination balloon-ultrasound imaging catheter for percutaneous transluminal angioplasty. *Circulation.* 1991;84:739-754.

11. Fitzgerald PJ, Koren J, McKenzie JR, et al. Combined catheter ultrasound imaging with online tissue characterization: feasibility study. *Circulation.* 1991;84:II-372.

12. Rosenfield K, Losordo DW, Ramaswamy K, et al. Three-dimensional reconstruction of human coronary and peripheral arteries from images recorded during two-dimensional intravascular ultrasound examination. *Circulation.* 1991;84:1938-1956.

13. Pandian NG, Weintraub A, Schwartz SL, et al. Intravascular and intracardiac ultrasound imaging: current research and future directions. *Echocardiography.* 1990;7:377-388.

14. Pandian NG, Hsu T. Intravascular ultrasound and intracardiac echocardiography: Concepts for the future. *Am J Cardiol.* 1992;69:6H-17H.

15. Moore CA, Smucker ML, Kaul S. Myocardial contrast echocardiography in humans: I. Safety—a comparison with routine coronary arteriography. *J Am Coll Cardiol.* 1986;8:1066-1072.

16. Reisner SA, Ong LS, Lichtenberg GS, et al. Myocardial - perfusion imaging by contrast echocardiography with use of intracoronary sonicated albumin in humans. *J Am Coll Cardiol.* 1989;14:660-665.

17. Feinstein SB, Cheirif J, Ten Cate F, et al. Safety and efficacy of a new transpulmonary ultrasound contrast agent: initial multicenter clinical results. *J Am Coll Cardiol.*1990;16:316-324.

18. Villaneuva FS, Glasheen WP, Sklenar J, et al. Successful and reproducible myocardial opacification during two-dimensional echocardiography from right atrial injection of contrast. *Circulation.* 1992;85:1577-1564.

19. Kaul S. Clinical applications of myocardial contrast echocardiography. *Am J Cardiol.* 1992;69:46H-55H.

20. Kaul S, Pandian NG, Okada RD, et al. Contrast echocardiography in acute myocardial ischemia: I. In-vitro determination of total left ventricular "area at risk." *J Am Coll Cardiol.* 1984;4:1272-1282.

21. Sabia P, Powers E, Jayaweera AR, et al. Functional significance of collateral blood flow in patients with recent myocardial infarction: a study using myocardial contrast echocardiography. *Circulation.* 1992;85:2080-2089.

22. Grill HP, Brinkner JA, Taube J, et al. Contrast echocardiographic mapping of collateralized myocardium in humans before and after coronary angioplasty. *J Am Coll Cardiol.* 1990;16:1594-1600.

23. Keller MW, Glasheen WP, Smucker ML, et al. Myocardial contrast echocardiography in humans: II. Assessment of coronary blood flow reserve. *J Am Coll Cardiol.* 1988;12:925-934.

24. Cheirif J, Zoghbi WA, Raizner AE, et al. Assessment of myocardial perfusion in humans by contrast echocardiography: I. Evaluation of regional coronary reserve by peak contrast intensity. *J Am Coll Cardiol.* 1988;11:735-743.

25. Goldman ME, Mindich BP. Intraoperative cardioplegic contrast echocardiography for assessing myocardial perfusion during open heart surgery. *J Am Coll Cardiol.* 1984;4:1029-1034.

26. Aronson S, Lee BK, Wiencek JF, et al. Assessment of myocardial perfusion during CABG surgery with two-dimensional transesophageal contrast echocardiography. *Anesthesiology.* 1991;75:433-440.

27. Skorton DJ, Miller JG, Wickline S, et al. Ultrasonic characterization of cardiovascular tissue. In: Marcus ML, Schelbert HL, Skorton DJ, et al (eds), Braunwald E (consulting ed). *Cardiac Imaging.* Philadelphia: WB Saunders, 1991; 538-556.

28. Hoyt RH, Collins SM, Skorton DJ, et al. Assessment of fibrosis in infarcted human heart by analysis of ultrasonic backscatter. *Circulation.* 1985;71:740-744.

29. Gluek RM, Mottley JG, Miller JG, et al. Effect of coronary artery occlusion and reperfusion on cardiac cycle dependent variation of myocardial ultrasonic backscatter. *Circ Res.* 1985;56:683-689.

30. Pérez JE, Miller JG, Wickline SA, et al. Quantitative ultrasonic imaging: Tissue characterization and instantaneous quantification of cardiac function. *Am J Cardiol.* 1992;69:104H-111H.

31. Pinamonti B, Picano E, Ferdeghini EM, et al. Quantitative texture analysis in 2-D echocardiography: Application to the diagnosis of myocardial amyloidosis. *J Am Coll Cardiol.* 1989;14:666-671.

32. Stuhlmuller JE, Fleagle SR, Burns TL, et al. Effects of instrument adjustments on quantitative echocardiographic gray level texture measurements. *J Am Soc Echo.* 1991;4:533-540.

33. Collins SM, Chandran KB, Skorton DJ. Three-dimensional cardiac imaging. *Echocardiography.* 1988;5:311-319.

34. Levine RA, Handschumacher MD, Sanfilippo AJ, et al. Three-dimensional echocardiographic reconstruction of

the mitral valve, with implications for the diagnosis of mitral valve prolapse. *Circulation.* 1989;80:589-598.

35. Flachskampf FA, Handschumacher M, Vandervoort PM, et al. Dynamic, three-dimensional reconstruction of the mitral annulus using a multiplane transesophageal echo-transducer. *Circulation.* 1991;84(suppl II):II-686. Abstract.
36. Recusani F, Bargiggia GS, Yoganathan AP, et al. A new method of quantification of regurgitant flow rate using color Doppler flow imaging of flow convergence region proximal to a discrete orifice: an in vitro study. *Circulation.* 1991;83:594-604.
37. Rodriguez L, Anconina J, Flachskampf FA, et al. Influence of flow rate, orifice size, and aliasing velocity on flow calculation using the flow convergence method. *Circ Res.* 1992;70:923-930.
38. Thomas JD, Thoreau DH, Vandervoort PM, et al. Automated analysis of flow convergence proximal to regurgitant orifices: flow rate calculation using digital Doppler velocity maps. *Computers in Cardiology.* Long Beach, CA: IEEE Computer Society;1991:13-16.
39. Bargiggia GS, Tronconi L, Sahn DJ, et al. A new method for quantitation of mitral regurgitation based on color flow Doppler imaging of flow convergence proximal to the regurgitant orifice. *Circulation.* 1991;84:1481-1489.
40. Rivera JM, Vandervoort P, Thoreau D, et al. Regurgitant orifice area, a fundamental measure of mitral incompetence; calculation by proximal acceleration. *J Am Coll Cardiol.* 1992;19:379A. Abstract.
41. Chen C, Rodriguez L, Guerrero JL, et al. Noninvasive estimation of instantaneous first derivative of left ventricular pressure using continuous wave Doppler echocardiography. *Circulation.* 1991;83:2101-2110
42. Chen C, Rodriguez L, Levine RA, et al. Noninvasive determination of the time constant of left ventricular relaxation using the continuous wave Doppler velocity profile of mitral regurgitation. *Circulation.* 1992;86:272-278.
43. Zaret BL, Wackers FJ. Nuclear Cardiology. I. *N Engl J Med.* 1993;329(11):775-783.
44. Dilsizian V, Bonow RO. Current diagnostic techniques of assessing myocardial viability in patients with hibernating and stunned myocardium. *Circulation.* 1993;87:1-20.
45. Gibson RS, Watson DD, Taylor GJ, et al. Prospective assessment of regional myocardial perfusion before and after coronary revascularization surgery by quantitative thallium-201 scintigraphy. *J Am Coll Cardiol.* 1983;1:804-815.
46. Cloninger KG, DePuey EG, Garcia EV, et al. Incomplete redistribution in delayed thallium-201 single photon emission computed tomographic images: An overestimation of myocardial scarring. *J Am Coll Cardiol.* 1988;12:955-963.
47. Kiat H, Berman DS, Maddahi J, et al. Late reversibility of tomographic myocardial thallium-201 defects: An accurate marker of myocardial viability. *J Am Coll Cardiol.* 1988;12:1456-1463.
48. Dilsizian V, Rocco TP, Freedman NMT, et al. Enhanced detection of ischemic but viable myocardium by reinjection of thallium after stress-redistribution imaging. *N Engl J Med.* 1990;323:141-146.
49. Maddahi J, Kiat H, Berman DS. Myocardial perfusion imaging with technetium-99m-labeled agents. *Am J Cardiol.* 1991;67:27D-34D.
50. Iskandrian As, Heo J, Kong B, et al. Use of technetium-99m isonitrile (RP-30A) in assessing left ventricular perfusion and function at rest and during exercise in coronary artery disease, and comparison with coronary arteriography and exercise thallium-201 SPECT imaging. *Am J Cardiol.* 1989;64:270-275.
51. Gibbons RJ, Verani MS, Behrenbeck T, et al. Feasibility of tomographic 99mTc-hexakis-2-methoxy-2-methyl-propyl-isonitrile imaging for the assessment of myocardial area at risk and the effect of treatment in acute myocardial infarction. *Circulation.* 1989;80:1277-1286.
52. Wackers FJT, Gibbons RJ, Verani MS, et al. Serial quantitative planar technetium-99m isonitrile imaging in acute myocardial infarction: efficacy for noninvasive assessment of thrombolytic therapy. *J Am Coll Cardiol.* 1989;14:861-873.
53. Christian TF, Gibbons RJ, Gersh BJ. Effect of infarct location on myocardial salvage assessed by technetium-99m isonitrile. *J Am Coll Cardiol.* 1991;17:1303-1308.
54. Baillet G, Mena IG, Kuperus JH, et al. Simultaneous Tc-99m-sestamibi angiography and myocardial perfusion imaging. *J Nucl Med.* 1989;30:38-44.
55. Lahiri A, Bhatta charya A, Carrio I. Antimyosin antibody imaging of myocardial necrosis. In: Zaret BL, Beller GA (eds). *Nuclear cardiology: state of the art and future directions.* Philadelphia: Mosby-Year Book; 1993:331-338.
56. Bhattacharya S, Liu XJ, Senior R, et al. 111In antimyosin antibody uptake is related to the age of myocardial infarction. *Am Heart J.* 1991;122:1583-1587.
57. Dec GW, Palacios I, Yasuda T, et al. Antimyosin antibody cardiac imaging: its role in the diagnosis of myocarditis. *J Am Coll Cardiol.* 1990;16:97-104.
58. Ballester M, Obrador D, Carrio I, et al. Indium-11-monoclonal antibody studies after the first year of heart transplantation: identification of risk groups for developing rejection during long-term follow-up and clinical implications. *Circulation.* 1990;82:2100-2107.
59. Stratton JR, Ritchie JL. 111In platelet imaging of left ventricular thrombi: predictive value for systemic emboli. *Circulation.* 1990;81:1182-1189.
60. Oster ZH, Srivastava SC, Som P, et al. Thrombus radioimmunoscintigraphy:an approach using monoclonal antiplatelet antibody. *Proc Natl Acad Sci USA.* 1985;82:3465-3468.
61. McGhie AI, Corbett JR, Akers MS, et al. Regional cardiac adrenergic function using i-123 meta-iodobenzylguanidine tomographic imaging after acute myocardial infarction. *Am J Cardiol.* 1991;67:236-242.
62. Henderson EB, Kahn JK, Corbett JR, et al. Abnormal I-123 metaiodobenzylguanidine myocardial washout and distribution may reflect myocardial adrenergic derangement in patients with congestive cardiomyopathy. *Circulation.* 1988;78:1192-1199.
63. Gould KL, Goldstein RA, Mullani NA, et al. Noninvasive assessment of coronary stenoses by myocardial perfusion imaging during pharmacologic coronary vasodilatation. *J Am Coll Cardiol.* 1986;7:775-789.
64. Isada L, Marwick TH, MacIntyre WJ. Physiologic evaluation of coronary flow: the role of positron emission

tomography. *Cleve Clin J Med.* 1993;60:19-24.

65. Go RT, Marwick T, MacIntyre WJ, et al. A prospective comparison of rubidium-82 PET and thallium-201 SPECT myocardial perfusion imaging utilizing a single dipyridamole stress in the diagnosis of coronary artery disease. *J Nucl Med.* 1990;31:1899-1905.

66. Schelbert HR. Myocardial ischemia and clinical applications of positron emission tomography. *Am J Cardiol.* 1989;64:46E-53E.

67. Brunken K, Schwaiger M, Grover-McKay M, et al. Positron emission tomography detects tissue metabolic activity in myocardial segments with persistent thallium perfusion defects. *J Am Coll Cardiol.* 1987;10:557-567.

68. Marshall RC, Tillisch JH, Phelps ME, et al. Identification and differentiation of resting myocardial ischemia and infarction in man with positron computed tomography, 18F-labeled fluorodeoxyglucose and N-13 ammonia. *Circulation.* 1983;67:766-778.

69. Braunwald E, Kloner RA. The stunned myocardium: Prolonged, postischemic ventricular dysfunction. *Circulation.* 1982;66:1146-1149.

70. Brundage BH. Myocardial imaging with ultrafast computed tomography. In: Zaret BL, Kaufman L, Berson AS, et al (eds). *Frontiers in Cardiovascular Imaging.* New York: Raven Press ; 1993;35-51.

71. Feiring AJ, Rumberger JA, Reiter SJ, et al. Determination of left ventricular mass in dogs in rapid acquisition cardiac computer tomography. *Circulation.* 1985;72:1355-1364.

72. Roig E, Georgiou D, Chomka EV, et al. Reproducibility of left ventricular myocardial volume and mass measurements by ultrafast computed tomography. *J Am Coll Cardiol.* 1991;18:990-996.

73. Hajduczok ZD, Weiss RM, Stanford W, et al. Determination of right ventricular mass in humans and dogs with ultrafast computed tomography. *Circulation.* 1990;82:202-212.

74. Roig E, Chomka EV, Castaner A, et al. Exercise ultrafast computed tomography for the detection of coronary artery disease. *J Am Coll Cardiol.* 1989;13:1073-1081.

75. Agatson AS, Janowitz WR. Coronary calcification: Detection by ultrafast computed tomography. In: Stanford W, Rumberger JA (eds). *Ultrafast computed tomography in cardiac imaging: Principles and practice.* Mount Kisco, NY: Futura Publishing; 1991:249-260.

76. Song SM, Leahy RM. Computation of 3-D velocity fields from 3-D cine CT images of a human heart. IEEE *Trans Med Imag.* 1991;10:295-306.

77. Rumberger JA, Weiss RM, Feiring AJ, et al. Patterns of regional diastolic function in the normal human left ventricle: An ultrafast computed tomographic study. *J Am Coll Cardiol.* 1989;14:119-126.

78. Song SM, Leahy RM. Computation of 3-D velocity fields from 3-D cine CT images of a human heart. IEEE *Trans Med Imag.* 1991;10:295-306.

79. Pettigrew RI. Magnetic resonance in cardiovascular imaging. In: Zaret BL, Kaufman L, Berson AS, et al (eds). *Frontiers in Cardiovascular Imaging.* New York: Raven Press; 1993;113-135.

80. Schaefer S. Cardiovascular applications of nuclear magnetic resonance spectroscopy. *Am J Cardiol.* 1989;64:38E-45E.

81. Edelman RR, Warach S. Magnetic resonance imaging. *N Engl J Med.* 1993;328(11):785-791.

82. MacMillan RM. Cardiac magnetic resonance imaging. *Cardiovasc Clin.* 1993:23;125-135.

83. Schaefer S. Clinical nuclear magnetic resonance spectroscopy: insight into metabolism. *Am J Cardiol.* 1990;66:45F-50F.

84. Schaefer S, Gober J, Valenza M, et al. Magnetic resonance imaging guided phosphorus-31 spectroscopy of the human heart. *J Am Coll Cardiol.* 1988;12:1449-1455.

85. Nienaber CA, von Kodolitsch Y, Nicolas V, et al. The diagnosis of thoracic aortic dissection by noninvasive imaging procedures. *N Engl J Med.* 1993;328:1-9.

86. Masui T, Finck S, Higgins CB. Constrictive pericarditis and restrictive cardiomyopathy: evaluation with MR imaging. *Radiology.* 1992;182:369-373.

87. Link KM, Lesko NM. Magnetic resonance imaging in the evaluation of congenital heart disease. *Magn Reson Q.* 1991;7:173-190.

88. Maddahi J, Crue J, Berman D, et al. Noninvasive quantification of left ventricular myocardial mass by gated proton nuclear magnetic resonance imaging. *J Am Coll Cardiol.* 1987;10:682-692.

89. Wolf GL. Role of magnetic resonance contrast agents in cardiac imaging. *Am J Cardiol.* 1990;66:59F-62F.

90. Sechtem U, Pflugfelder PW, Cassidy MM, et al. Mitral or aortic regurgitation: Quantification of regurgitant volumes with cine MR imaging. *Radiology.* 1988;167:425-430.

91. Aurigemma G, Reichek N, Schiebler M, et al. Evaluation of mitral regurgitation by cine MRI. *Am J Cardiol.* 1990;66:621-625.

92. Utz JA, Herfkens RJ, Heinsimer JA. Valvular regurgitation: Dynamic MR imaging. *Radiology.* 1988;168:91-94.

93. Pettigrew RI. Dynamic cardiac MR imaging: Techniques and applications. *Radiol Clin North Am.* 1989;1183-1203.

94. Manning WJ, Li W, Edelman RR. A preliminary report comparing magnetic resonance coronary angiography with conventional angiography. *N Engl J Med.* 1993;23;125-135.

95. Bottomley PA, Herfkins RJ, Smith LS, et al. Altered phosphate metabolism in myocardial infarction: P-31 NMR spectroscopy. *Radiology.* 1987;165:703-707.

12 Clinical Approach to Hyperlipidemia

Neil J. Stone, MD

LIPID/LIPOPROTEIN METABOLISM

ATHEROSCLEROSIS

Knowledge of lipid and lipoprotein metabolism is crucial for understanding atherosclerosis and clinical outcomes such as angina pectoris, myocardial infarction (MI), intermittent claudication, and thrombotic brain infarction. Atherosclerosis is the condition where the inner layers of the artery walls become thick and irregular due to fatty deposits whose striking component is cholesterol.[1] Whereas normal lining cells or intima of blood vessels contain less than 5% dry weight as lipid, the deposits or plaques of atherosclerosis contain 30%-65% dry weight as lipid (mainly in the form of cholesterol and phospholipid).

With the unaided eye, pathologists can divide the telltale signs of atherosclerosis into 2 major types. The earliest lesions are called *fatty streaks* which contain about 25% lipid. Fatty streaks can be seen in coronary arteries after puberty. During fatty streak development, cells are stimulated to take in more cholesterol than they can excrete. In diet-induced hypercholesterolemia, monocytes attach to endothelium and transform into cholesterol-filled macrophages/foam cells. The transformation to foam cells occurs through the unregulated uptake by scavenger receptors of low density lipoprotein (LDL) that has been oxidized. Plaque formation is aided by smooth muscle cells, platelets, and endothelial cells that release growth factors which hasten development of the fatty arterial plaques. Other factors, such as hypertension, cigarette smoke, and turbulence occurring at vessel branch points can injure the endothelium and also set this process

in motion.[2] The fatty streaks, however, do not invariably grow into cholesterol-laden plaques. They progress to intermediate lesions and, finally, to raised plaques in populations where either by individual genetic makeup or by diet-induced high blood-cholesterol levels, transformation through continuous buildup of cholesterol-laden cells to the fibrous plaque can occur. In other words, there is strong evidence based on experimental studies in animals that cholesterol plays a key role both in the initiation and the sustaining of atherosclerosis.

The second type and hallmark of coronary atherosclerosis is the atheromatous, lipid-rich *fibrous plaque*. These plaques are formed from progressive deposition of cholesterol in an orderly fashion, with the older cholesterol deposits at the base of the plaque and the newer ones at the surface. A simple atheroma may evolve into a complicated plaque with deposits of calcium and thrombus formation by ingrowth of the vessel into the plaque, setting the stage for hemorrhage into the plaque and resulting vessel blockage due to combined effects of plaque growth and thrombus. Fissuring of the plaque is considered the key event triggering abrupt arterial blockage and clinical ischemic syndromes.[3]

Physiologic changes also occur in arterial walls due to hypercholesterolemia (and other risk factors as well). Normally, acetylcholine dilates blood vessels by releasing a vasorelaxant substance from the endothelium (endothelium-derived relaxing factor). Paradoxical vasoconstriction induced by acetylcholine both early and late in the course of coronary atherosclerosis is seen, suggesting an association between endothelial dysfunction and atherosclerosis. Interestingly, treatment of hypercholesterolemia not only produces morphological improvement of the atherosclerotic lesion, but restores endothelium-dependent vascular relaxation to normal.[4]

Since lipids are established as playing a causal role in atherosclerosis, all physicians concerned with cardiovascular disease must understand the guidelines set forth by the Second Adult Treatment Panel Report of the National Cholesterol Education Program (NCEP).[5] These were designed to facilitate the detection, evaluation, and treatment of the high-risk patient in the population and should be viewed as complementary to population strategies designed to reduce the overall incidence of coronary artery disease (CAD).

DEFINITIONS

Cholesterol was discovered in bile by Chevreul in 1816 (*Chole* means "bile" and *steros* means "solid"). It has the multi-ring nuclear structure of the steroid family and is a key part of cell membranes, the D vitamins, and adrenal steroids. Most tissues synthesize cholesterol, but in humans this occurs chiefly in the liver and intestine. Plasma cholesterol concentrations are tightly regulated by removal processes keyed to specific liver and extrahepatic cell receptors. Cholesterol is cleared from the body by excretion into bile or conversion to bile acids. Cholesterol is only seen in animal fat; it is not found in plants. Blood cholesterol can be measured in a non-fasting state.

Triglycerides are storage forms of energy consisting of long-chain fatty acids attached to a glycerol backbone. These fatty acids can be saturated or unsaturated, a distinction important in determining whether a dietary fat can raise or lower the blood cholesterol level. Triglyceride levels rise postprandially and are affected by stress, which helps explain their great variability. Blood triglyceride levels must be measured with the patient fasting for 12-14 hrs, at stable weight for 3 weeks, and on a stable diet.

Lipids are insoluble in plasma water and must be transported on large macromolecules called *lipoproteins*. It is useful to characterize these as triglyceride-rich or cholesterol-rich lipoproteins. Examples of the former are chylomicrons, very low-density lipoproteins (VLDL), and intermediate-density lipoproteins (IDL). Examples of the latter are chylomicron remnants, low-density lipoproteins (LDL), and high-density lipoproteins (HDL). *Apoproteins* (apo) play key roles in the synthesis, processing, and disposal of lipoproteins. These are the protein subunits of the protein-phospholipid complex that packages lipids in the circulation. Knowledge of major apoproteins such as apo A1, A2 (major proteins of HDL); apo B100 or LDL B (major protein of LDL); apo CII and the isoforms of apo E (apoproteins needed for metabolism of VLDL and chylomicron remnants) is already important in the understanding genetic susceptibility to coronary atherosclerosis.

Long-chain dietary fat is broken down in the gut and repackaged in intestinal cells as *chylomicrons*. These large, triglyceride-laden particles are responsible for transient, postprandial lipemia. Chylomicrons are processed by aid of an enzyme called *lipoprotein lipase*. This is found in muscle and adipose tissue capillaries. Lipoprotein lipase levels are increased by exercise and decreased in insulinopenic diabetes and hypothyroidism.

Endogenously produced triglyceride from the liver and intestine circulates on VLDL. This family of particles is processed by lipoprotein lipase as well. When levels are sampled 12-14 hrs after a meal, the fasting triglyceride level reflects basal levels of VLDL. *Chylomicrons* have half-lives measured in minutes and VLDL have half-lives measured in hours; this explains the marked daily variations in triglyceride levels. Carbohydrate, fatty acids (raised due to increased catecholamines or uncontrolled diabetes), elevated basal insulin levels (obesity, estrogens), and augmented hepatic fatty acids (alcohol) stimulate VLDL overproduction from the liver. Nongenetic factors causing impaired clearance include uremia, myxedema, and poorly controlled diabetes.

VLDLs are metabolized to IDL or VLDL *remnants* whose apo E serves as a marker which can bind to the same LDL receptor that also recognizes apo B. Indeed, apo E is needed for the efficient conversion of VLDL remnants to LDL and the efficient disposal of chylomicron remnants by the liver. Moreover, genetic variation in apo E may play a role in susceptibility to coronary artery disease (CAD). The apo E[4] allele is associated with higher levels of LDL-cholesterol (LDL-c), as seen in Finns who have high levels of cholesterol and coronary artery disease (CAD), and is seen less frequently in octogenarians.[6] The opposite appears to be true for the apo E[2] allele.

Most of LDL is produced from the intravascular conversion of VLDL through IDL to LDL. Hepatic lipase assists in processing VLDL lipoprotein particles to LDL particles and helps determine LDL characteristics. The concentration of LDL is regulated by the LDL receptors, which recognize apo B. These LDL receptors are specified by commonly inherited genes. When a person inherits a mutant copy (or copies), deficient or absent LDL receptors are seen. This leads to hypercholesterolemia of a magnitude in proportion to the defect in LDL receptors. Another genetic defect leading to increased LDL occurs when there is a defect in apo B producing an LDL molecule that is not recognized by a normal LDL receptor. When plasma LDL levels rise, scavenger cells are needed to degrade LDL. These macrophages soon become swollen with cholesterol and convert to foam cells, which are prominently seen in arterial plaques.

Factors other than the absolute amount of native, circulating LDL may be important in the genesis of human atherosclerosis. Sniderman and colleagues[7] emphasize the coronary-prone situation of an elevated apo B in the face of a normal, or near-normal LDL-c. Indeed, when measured, apo B is shown to be superior to LDL-c in separating patients with angiographic CAD from those without CAD. Of particular interest to the cardiologist, LDL apo B along with HDL-cholesterol (HDL-c) were the most important predictors of subsequent atherosclerosis in saphenous vein bypass grafts.[8] In addition, those persons with a preponderance of small, dense LDL particles (usually in association with increased VLDL and IDL and reduced HDL) have a markedly increased risk of MI.[9] Finally, modified or oxidized LDL is highly cytotoxic and its uptake by macrophages to form fatty streaks could link the key elements of the lipid-infiltration and endothelial-injury hypotheses.[10]

Finally, HDLs are secreted from the liver and intestine and are also formed from surface materials generated by efficient triglyceride-rich lipoprotein metabolism. Apo Al is the major apoprotein and accounts for 30% of the mass of HDL. High-density lipoproteins play a key role in triglyceride metabolism by serving as a reservoir for apoproteins such as apo CII, which are needed to activate lipoprotein lipase. When triglyceride levels are high due to impaired catabolism, HDL levels are usually low. One mechanism is an increased transfer of cholesterol ester from HDL to VLDL/LDL due to increased cholesterol ester transfer protein. (CETP). Whereas increased CETP is associated with angiographic CHD, those with CETP deficiency have high HDL and longevity.[11] HDLs play a key role in cholesterol metabolism, as they function in reverse cholesterol transport and may also inhibit oxidative modification of LDL.[12] Moreover, since the initial observation that men with myocardial infarction (MI) had low levels of HDL-c, numerous epidemiologic and angiographic studies have confirmed that low HDL-c is a powerful, independent predictor of CAD. In the Framingham Study, a significant effect of HDL-c on MI can be seen, even among the group with the lowest values for cholesterol.[13] Because high HDL-c levels decrease risk of CAD, the new NCEP guidelines have you subtract one risk factor if the HDL-c level is ≥ 60 mg/dl.

RISK FACTORS FOR CHD: WHICH LIPIDS AND LIPOPROTEINS TO MEASURE

The recent NCEP guidelines rely for case finding on non-fasting blood cholesterol and HDL-c measurements. Elevated values must be confirmed at least once for greater precision. Risk-factor status for CAD is required to place the cholesterol results in perspective (Table 1). The intensity of evaluation and treatment depends then on both lipid values as well as risk of a coronary event. A blood cholesterol level <200 mg/dl is classified as "desirable." A level of 200-239 mg/dl is classified as "borderline-high" and a level of ≥ 240 is designated as "high blood cholesterol." The basis of these cutoffs is, in large part, derived from the large data set of more than 361,662 primary screenees from the Multiple Risk Factor Intervention Trial.[14] This landmark effort confirmed that with increasing cholesterol levels, the risk of CHD rises exponentially with highest rates above 240 mg/dl. Although coronary rates were lowest below 200 mg/dl, there did not appear to be a so-called "threshold" above which risk commenced. Values of HDL under 35 mg/dl or 2 or more risk factors also indicate increased risk and prompt lipoprotein analysis.

Risk factors are those personal traits or lifestyles that convey an increased risk of devel-

Table 1. Factors (other than LDL-c) Used to Determine High Risk Status

Age: Male ≥ 45 years
    Female ≥ 55 years or premature menopause
    without estrogen
Family history of premature CAD
Smoking
Hypertension
HDL-c <35 mg/dl
Diabetes

<u>Negative</u>
HDL-c ≥ 60 mg/dl

CAD=Coronary artery disease; HDL-c=High-density lipoprotein cholesterol; LDL-c=Low-density lipoprotein cholesterol.

oping CHD. Along with total cholesterol and HDL-c testing, all adults should be checked for the presence of hypertension, current cigarette smoking, diabetes mellitus, family history of CHD in a father or other male first-degree relative before age 55 or before 65 years in a mother or other female first-degree relative. To avoid excessive treatment of younger patients at lower risk, age 45 or more for males and 55 or more years for females are considered cutoffs for increased risk. Women who have had a premature menopause without estrogen replacement therapy are also considered to be at an increased risk. The new guidelines did not list obesity as a risk factor because it appears to operate through other risk factors (e.g., hypertension, lipids, low HDL-c, and diabetes mellitus). Also physical inactivity is not listed as a risk factor. Nonetheless, obesity and physical inactivity are clear targets for intervention to reduce one's risk of premature CAD. The pattern of

obesity appears to be particularly important in determining coronary risk. Abdominal or male-pattern obesity, which can be assessed clinically by a waist-to-hip ratio (>0.9 for men and >0.8 for middle-aged and elderly women), suggests insulin resistance and correlates strongly with increased hazard for coronary disease.[15]

Since the presence of CHD or risk factors for CHD increase the risk of CHD at any given cholesterol value, they can be expected to greatly influence decisions regarding further evaluation and treatment. For example, in the Multiple Risk Factor Intervention Trial (MRFIT), the risk of CHD for hypertensive smokers with the lowest cholesterol values is similar to the risk of CHD for normotensive, nonsmokers with the highest cholesterol values. Dietary studies showed that hypertensive smokers respond less well to cholesterol-lowering diets than their nonsmoking, normotensive counterparts.[16] If 2 values for cholesterol differ by more than 30 mg/dl, then a third determination should be performed. For those adults without evidence of CHD, subsequent classification and treatment is based on LDL-c values obtained from lipoprotein analysis (Tables 2–4).

Fortunately, total cholesterol, triglycerides and HDL-c can be measured on a single fasting blood sample. The following formula is used to calculate the LDL-c value: LDL-c = Total cholesterol – (HDL-c) – (triglyceride/5). [This assumes a specimen obtained after a 12-16 hr fast, a triglyceride less than 400 mg/dl and the absence of the rare familial Type III disorder.] Since risk assessment and therapy depend on LDL-c, its value should be repeated within 1-6 weeks. If values vary by more than 30 mg/dl, a third determination should be done. Tables 3 and 4 show how to proceed after LDL-c values are determined. Secondary causes of high blood cholesterol are grouped into categories of diet,

Table 2. Who Needs Lipoprotein Analysis

	TOTAL CHOLESTEROL	HDL-C	RISK FACTORS
Low-Risk Status	<200 mg/dl	≥ 35	<2 Risk Factors
High-Risk	≥ 240* mg/dl	<35*	≥ 2 Risk Factors*
Very High-Risk	CAD or Vascular Disease*		

*If present, proceed to lipoprotein analysis.

Table 3. Primary Prevention in Adults Without CHD

	LDL-C[†]	2 OR MORE RISK FACTORS	ACTION
Desirable LDL	<130	Absent	Repeat chol, HDL within 5 years. General education
	<130	Present	Re-evaluate yearly
Borderline High-Risk LDL	130-159	< 2 Risk Factors	Step I Diet; physical activity
	130-159	2 or more Risk Factors	Clinical evaluation* Initiate dietary therapy
High-Risk LDL	≥ 160	Absent or Present	Clinical evaluation* Initiate dietary therapy

* Do history, physical; evaluate for secondary causes; initiate family screening; and consider influence of age, sex, and other coronary heart disease (CHD) risk factors.
† Numerical values in mg/dl

Table 4. Secondary Prevention in Adults With Evidence of CHD

Optimal LDL	≤ 100 mg/dl	Individualize Rx on Diet & Physical Activity Level
	>100 mg/dl	Clinical evaluation* Initiate therapy

*Do history, physical; evaluate for secondary causes; initiate family screening; and consider influence of age, sex, and other CHD risk factors.

diseases, and drugs[17] to aid in their systematic appraisal as shown in Table 5. Family members should also be screened for blood cholesterol and risk factors. Conversely, screening relatives of those who present with CHD is particularly revealing as previously undetected risk factors were highly prevalent in siblings of such patients.[18]

SYNDROMES OF FAMILIAL DYSLIPIDEMIA

An enriched sample of cases of familial forms of hyperlipidemia is seen in survivors of MI. Goldstein and coworkers[19] in Seattle showed that 1 out of 5 survivors under 60 years of age had a simply inherited form of hyperlipidemia and one-third had either a cholesterol or triglyceride level above the upper 5% cut point for their age. Consideration of hyperlipidemia in patients with MI is important, but cholesterol values may under-represent the pre-event state if the patient is not sampled within the first 24 hours. After this time, triglyceride values begin to rise and cholesterol values fall over the next 4 weeks. Although family sampling is best accomplished at the time of MI, reliable lipid values are not obtained for at least 8-12 weeks when patients are recovered and again on stable diet and exercise regimens.

Several familial syndromes are worthy of review (Figures and Table 6). Familial hypercholesterolemia (FH), is a clinical disorder linked since the time of William Osler with premature CAD. It is a striking example of how valuable the sophisticated biochemical skills of the geneticist are to the cardiologist. Familial hypercholesterolemia is inherited as an autosomal dominant trait with a high degree of penetrance. Heterozygotes have a single dose of a mutant allele specifying a receptor protein with either absent or defective binding or faulty internalization. In the United States, the minimum gene frequency is estimated at 1 in 225. It accounts for 4.1% of survivors of MI under the age of 60 years.[19] Heterozygous FH is diagnosed when LDL-c values exceed the age-adjusted upper 5% cutoffs for the subject and first

Table 5. Secondary Causes of Altered Blood Lipids and Lipoproteins

		PRIMARY ALTERATION
Diet		
	Saturated fat	Raise LDL
	Dietary cholesterol	Raise LDL
	Excess calories	Raise LDL, HDL, TG
	Excess alcohol	Raise HDL, TG
Diseases		
	Hypothyroidism	Raise LDL
	Nephrosis	Raise LDL; lower HDL
	Obstructive liver disease	Raise LDL
	Chronic renal disease	Raise TG; lower HDL
	Diabetes mellitus	Raise TG; lower HDL
	Transplantation	Raise LDL, TG; lower HDL
Medications		
	Beta blockers*	Raise TG; lower HDL
	Estrogens	Raise TG, HDL; lower LDL
	Steroids	Raise TG, HDL
	Androgens	Lower TG, HDL; raise LDL
	Thiazides	Raise LDL
	Chlorthalidone	Raise LDL
	Cyclosporine	Raise LDL

*ß-blockers with intrinsic sympathomimetic activity have little effect on TG and may raise HDL-c.
TG=Triglycerides; LDL=Low density lipoprotein; HDL=High density lipoprotein.

Table 6. Familial Forms of Hyperlipidemia Associated With an Increased Risk of Coronary Artery Disease

GENETIC LIPID ABNORMALITY	% OF TOTAL
I. Survivors of myocardial infarction before age 60[24]	
Familial Combined Hyperlipidemia	11.3
Polygenic Hypercholesterolemia	5.5
Familial Hypertriglyceridemia	5.2
Familial Hypercholesterolemia	4.1
II. Patients with CAD at angiography before age 60[30]	
Lp (a) excess*	33.3%
Hypertriglyceidemia with low HDL-c**	14.5%
Combined Hyperlipidemia with low HDL-c	12.5%
Low HDL-c	7%
Combined Hyperlipidemia (Increased LDL + TG)	5%
Hypertriglyceridemia	3%
High LDL-c with low HDL-c	2%
Hypercholesterolemia only	1%

* 11.5% assoc with other dyslipidemias
**Low HDL-c=HDL below the 10th percentile; Hypertriglyceridemia=Triglycerides above the 90th percentile; Hypercholesterolemia=LDL above 90th percentile.

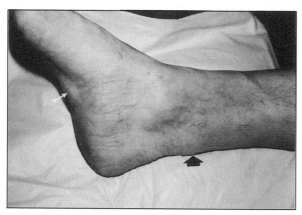

Figure 1. *Achilles and flexor hallicus longus tendon xanthomas (arrows) in a patient with heterozygous familial hypercholesterolemia.*

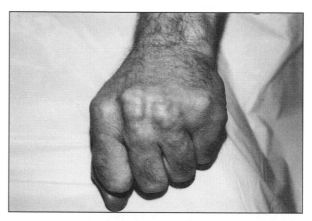

Figure 2. *Extensor tendon xanthomas occurring in tendons overlying the metacarpals in a patient with heterozygous familial hypercholesterolemia.*

degree relatives. Tendon xanthomas are found in about 80% of cases. They characteristically involve the Achilles tendons and tendons overlying the metacarpals (Figs. 1 and 2). Many patients recall episodes of acute tendonitis in their teens. Superior and inferior pole arcus in Caucasians under age 35 usually implies underlying FH, but corneal arcus in older and non-Caucasian populations has no predictive value. Xanthelasma (lipid deposits under the eyes) are inconsistent predictors of FH.

The patient with heterozygous FH typically has a cholesterol level of 325-450 mg/dl that does not respond to a cholesterol-lowering diet. Heterozygous FH must be recognized because of the predilection for premature CAD. In Framingham, 6 of 5,127 subjects had cholesterol values exceeding 400 mg/dl and detectable xanthomas. All of these subjects died from CAD before 50 years of age. The largest experience with FH was seen in 116 kindred comprising over 1,000 relatives studied at the National Institutes of Health.[20] For those with the FH trait, 29.5% were found to have CAD compared with only 10.5% of adult relatives without FH. The expectation of CAD by age 40 was 1 in 6; by age 60 it was more than 1 in 2. When compared with nonaffected men in the same kindred, it was as if CAD had developed 20 years earlier than expected (Fig. 3). Although CAD occurred less often and later in women than in men, affected female relatives also had a greater risk of CAD after age 45 (Fig. 4). A recent angiographic trial in men and women with FH has shown that intensive therapy with 2 or 3 drugs

to lower the markedly elevated LDL-c levels can result in decreased progression and even regression of existing coronary deposits.[21]

Homozygous cases, with a gene frequency of one in a million, have a double dose of 1 of the mutant alleles or, rarely, have 2 different mutant alleles. These severe defects result in LDL binding and internalization that is markedly impaired, preventing normal feedback of cholesterol synthesis by peripheral cells. The serum cholesterol exceeds 750 mg/dl and is often as high as 1,000 mg/dl. Affected homozygous children have characteristic interdigital web xanthomas and tuberous and tendon xanthomas. If untreated, these lesions are prominent by age 10. Homozygous children have distinctive cardiovascular findings. Basal systolic murmurs with time represent significant aortic stenosis. The aortic stenosis is unique due to intracellular lipid infiltration of aortic cusps. One informative patient had a peak systolic gradient of 108 mm Hg with plaquing extending from the highest part of the sinuses of Valsalva to the aortic ring! With respect to aortic plaquing, these cases invariably have the reverse of the usual situation with greater involvement of the ascending than the abdominal aorta. Two-dimensional echocardiography documents the stenosis of the supravalvular aortic ring. It is often associated with coronary ostial stenosis.[22] Since coronary disease is rapidly progressive and therapeutic options are limited due to insensitivity to lipid-lowering drugs, dramatic therapies are the rule rather than the exception. Therapeutic options include apheresis (effective, but expensive) and

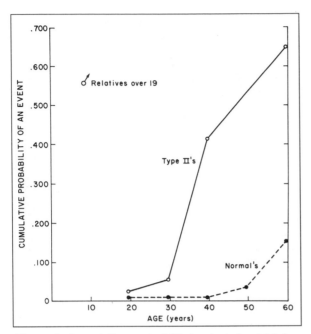

Figure 3. *Cumulative probability by decade of fatal or nonfatal coronary artery disease events in first-degree male relatives with heterozygous familial hypercholesterolemia. From Stone NJ, et al.[20] With permission of the American Heart Association.*

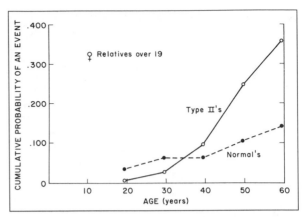

Figure 4. *Cumulative probability by decade of fatal or nonfatal coronary artery disease events in first-degree female relatives with heterozygous familial hypercholesterolemia. From Stone NJ, et al.[20] With permission of the American Heart Association.*

liver transplantation. The latter was used for a 6-year-old homozygous girl who underwent combined liver and heart transplantation. Her LDL-c declined by 81% from 988 to 184 mg/dl with a marked increase in her fractional catabolic rate. This remarkable case highlights the importance of hepatic LDL-receptors in controlling excess LDL-c levels.[23]

Familial combined hyperlipidemia (FCHL) is the most common monogenic lipid disorder among survivors of acute MI (Table 6).[24] The disorder appears to be inherited as an autosomal dominant trait. It is first expressed in adulthood, unlike FH, where affected children are easily detected. Elevated cholesterol and triglyceride values are common with relatives in successive generations having either or both lipids elevated. Xanthomas are not seen as the elevations are not as severe as in FH. Elevated apo B levels may also serve as a marker for this syndrome. In one study of those with hypertriglyceridemia, elevated plasma LDL apo B predicted those more likely to have CAD.[7] In the Familial Atherosclerosis Study (FATS) the authors evaluated 146 men with documented CAD who had elevated levels of apo B and a family history of vascular disease.[25] The study patients looked similar to those who have familial combined hyperlipidemia. Serial angiography showed that regression was associated with reduction in apo B or LDL levels. Intensive lipid-lowering therapy reduced the frequency of progression of coronary lesions and despite the small size of the study, reduced the incidence of coronary events.

Familial dyslipidemic hypertension occurs in families with early familial hypertension and multiple forms of lipid/lipoprotein abnormalities.[26] Elevated insulin levels appear to explain the interrelationships between the dyslipidemia (low HDL, high LDL-c and/or triglycerides) obesity, and hypertension found in these families.

Familial Type III or Familial Dysbetalipoproteinemia is a rare disorder. It results from an inherited apo E disorder resulting in accumulation of IDL in plasma. Affected relatives are homozygous for apo E2/E2 allele. This genotype is seen in 1% of the population. The diagnosis is confirmed by VLDL cholesterol/triglyceride ratio exceeding 0.3, and the clinical setting. The clinical disorder, however, characterized by tuboeruptive xanthomas along with digital and palmar crease xanthomas, striking elevations of both cholesterol and triglyceride levels, and premature CAD and vascular disease, is rarely seen. The clinical expression must depend on other environmental, genetic, or endocrine factors.

Familial hypertriglyceridemia (FHTG) was identified in 5.2% of survivors of MI under age 60 in the Seattle study. It has an autosomal dominant mode of inheritance and is expressed in adulthood. Genetic and clinical studies of FHTG are impaired, however, by absence of distinguishing clinical features and the common occurrence in the population of elevated triglyceride levels due to diet, obesity, alcohol intake and medications. The hypertriglyceridemia seen in these families occurs without low HDL, elevated apo B or LDL-c or associated vascular disease and are not associated with premature CAD.

Familial defective apo B 100 has an autosomal dominant mode of inheritance as well. The mutation causes a reduced affinity of LDL particles for the LDL receptor. Usually individuals do not have tendon xanthomas. This diagnosis requires sophisticated techniques available in specialized lipid clinics.

Familial low HDL or familial hypoalphalipoproteinemia occurs in those families where values of HDL-c below the 10% age-adjusted cutoffs are seen. Since low HDL-c is the most frequent lipid abnormality found in those with premature CAD, it is not surprising that familial low HDL increases risk of CAD. Genetic analysis using DNA probes has shown a strong association between the absence of a restriction site near apo Al and both premature CAD and familial hypoalphalipoproteinemia.[27]

Dramatic premature CAD is seen when apo AI is abnormal as in cases of apo Al and CIII deficiency and in some cases of Tangier's disease. Yet not all cases of genetic low HDL are associated with a predilection for early CAD. Although HDL-c can be as low as 11 mg/dl, premature CAD is not seen in apo Al Milano or in Fish-Eye Disease — HDL deficiency associated with severe corneal opacification.[28] Clinicians need to remember that vegetarian communities have low HDL, associated with low LDL-c and low systolic blood pressure and low rates of CAD.

In those with excess levels of the highly inherited Lp(a) the likelihood of early CAD increases several fold.[29,30] Apoprotein(a) is a plasminogen-like molecule that complexes to an LDL molecule which is called Lp(a). The levels of Lp(a) for an individual are remarkably stable and not sensitive to diet, exercise, age or most pharmaceutical interventions. An exception appears to be niacin. Lp(a) is still not completely understood; for example, case control compar-

Table 7. Hypertriglyceridemia (NIH Consensus Development Panel)	
TRIGLYERIDE LEVEL	DESIGNATION
>1000 mg/dl	Very high
400-1,000 mg/dl	High triglycerides
200-400 mg/dl	Borderline high
<200 mg/dl	Normal triglyerides

isons in the Helsinki trial and the Physician's Health Study showed that Lp(a) levels did not predict CHD events.[31,32] Thus, an elevated level suggests a heightened CHD risk of an individual rather than indicating specific therapy.[33]

SPECIAL ISSUES

HYPERTRIGLYCERIDEMIA

Normal triglycerides are considered to be <200 mg/dl. The gradation of hypertriglyceridemia is given in Table 7. Many studies have shown triglyceride levels per se not to be independent risk factors for CAD. Nonetheless, some have questioned this conclusion.[34] Although certain triglyceride-rich particles (small VLDL and remnants of chylomicrons or VLDL) are associated with increased atherogenicity, as has been noted previously, not all patients with high triglyceride levels are at risk for premature CAD. For example, fluffy or large VLDL created by alcohol, estrogen, or cholestyramine therapy is associated with a lower CAD risk. The association of triglycerides with atherogenic changes in LDL and HDL is another matter. In the Helsinki trial, those men with elevated LDL-c, low HDL-c, and high triglycerides were found to have the greatest likelihood of a coronary event.[35] Thus, a personal or family history of premature CAD indicates that the hypertriglyceridemia is probably deserving of specific therapy to lower risk of CAD. Physicians must be cautioned that when triglyceride levels exceed 1,000 mg/dl, the important risk is that of acute pancreatitis. Estrogen therapy in women as well as alcohol abuse, weight excess, or both can cause a patient with a mild genetic triglyceride abnormality to have the very high triglyceride values which can lead to acute pancreatitis. Control of triglyceride values is affected strongly by lifestyle. The first and often the most important therapeutic steps are an increase in physical activity and control of body weight along with a diet low in saturated fats and dietary cholesterol. Alcohol must be restricted in those patients with high triglycerides.

THE ELDERLY PATIENT

Few clinical trials have included persons above 65 years of age. The potential, however, for reducing CAD is quite high as the difference in rates of CAD between those with the highest cholesterol levels and the lowest (the "attributable risk") is quite high. For those at high-risk of CHD and without significant comorbidity such as malignancy, dementia, significant neuromuscular disability, or severe chronic lung disease, the treatment of high cholesterol seems a sensible concomitant to treating hypertension and advising cessation of cigarette smoking. When should clinicians stop treating older patients with high cholesterol? Framingham analyses show that relative risk (risk of the upper quartile divided by the risk of the lower quartile) of cardiovascular death associated with high cholesterol levels decreases continuously with age and inverts by the age of 80 years.[36] Until better data is available, clinical judgment is required in older individuals to be sure the potential benefits exceed the risks as well as the negative aspects (cost, convenience, side effects) of therapy. Although drug therapy may not be appropriate for some older patients, the prescription of a lower fat, well-balanced diet, and regular exercise such as walking is rarely inappropriate and often useful.

ISOLATED LOW HDL CHOLESTEROL

Low HDL-c is a major risk factor for CAD. For those with "isolated" low levels of HDL and other CHD risk factors, the goal of therapy is to lower the LDL-c below 130 mg/dl and treat other risk factors. Although changing from nonselective ß-blockers to lipid-neutral drugs in those with hypertension may be useful in raising HDL-c, the benefits of ß-blockers after an MI more than compensates for the decline in HDL-c seen. Thus, ß-blockers should not be withheld in the coronary patient for this reason.

For those with CHD and a low HDL-c, the use of niacin alone would seem to be the leading choice, although either a fibrate or a statin drug can be used. For patients with isolated low HDL-c levels and otherwise low-risk for CHD, the use of niacin or other HDL-raising drugs is not recommended.

DIABETES

Due to the high risk of premature CAD, aggressive treatment of all risk factors (particularly cigarette smoking, excess weight, and hypertension) as well as elevated LDL-c seems a sensible approach. The target for LDL-c is under 130 for both men and women since diabetic women share the same heightened risk as their male counterparts. Elevated levels of triglycerides are often seen in diabetics along with low levels of HDL-c and this influences drug therapy if non-pharmacologic approaches are maximized. Niacin is relatively contraindicated in Type II diabetic patients since it worsens glycemic control. Gemfibrozil is useful in those with higher triglyceride levels while statins are useful since they produce a marked decline in LDL-c as well as a moderate reduction in triglyceride values. Resins must be used cautiously and only when triglyceride excess is controlled first.

HYPERTENSION AND HYPERLIPIDEMIA

While treatment of hypertension is covered in another chapter, it is worth emphasizing three important points when high blood pressure is complicated by lipid abnormalities. First, weight control and increased physical activity can greatly help reduce abdominal obesity and its attendant hyperinsulinism which aggravates both conditions. Secondly, the adverse lipid effects of low-dose thiazides are probably overstated. Although in short-term studies, diuretics raise total cholesterol 5%-8%, triglycerides 15%-25%, and LDL-c 8%, significant elevations in total cholesterol are not seen at 1 year in most hypertension treatment trials.[37] Finally, lipid medications can affect antihypertensive drugs. Resins may decrease the absorption if taken concomitantly. Antihypertensives should be taken 1 hour before resins or 4 hours after. Niacin is a vasodilator and can cause hypotension if taken with vasodilators like nifedipine or angiotensin-converting enzyme inhibitors.

DIETARY TREATMENT

EFFECT OF DIET ON CAD

The link between diet and CAD was strongly suggested by observational data and recently confirmed by information from smaller studies using serial angiography to look at progression and regression of coronary plaques. The Seven Countries study suggested that dietary saturated fat intake was linked to both high blood cholesterol levels and high rates of CAD.[38] Two prospective studies, the Western Electric study[39] and the Zutphen trial[40] both with detailed dietary assessments, showed that 20-year rates of CAD were highly correlated with dietary cholesterol intake despite small effects on blood cholesterol values. These studies also showed that regular consumption of fish in the diet was associated with lower rates of CAD. While regular consumption of fish in place of highly saturated fatty meats seems sensible, there is still no compelling data to support taking fish oil capsules for primary prevention or for prevention of restenosis after angioplasty.

The observational data from olive oil-based diets in the Mediterranean countries has suggested that increased monounsaturated fats in the diet in place of saturated fats may be beneficial. On the other hand, a large prospective cohort study in women noted strong associations between the intake of fats which are converted from the natural "cis" form to the "trans" form.[41] Examples of foods high in trans-fatty acids are margarines, cookies, biscuits and white breads. Although polyunsaturated fats were used in early clinical trials to improve cholesterol lowering, there is no long-term population experience with a high polyunsaturated fat diet. Hence, intake of polyunsaturated fats is controlled, as excess use can promote obesity, gallstones, and low HDL-c.

Soluble fiber has been shown to be a useful adjunct to a cholesterol-lowering diet. In those with elevated cholesterol levels, there is small but significant cholesterol and LDL-c lowering independent of its replacement of saturated fat in the diet owing to the ß-glucan content.[42] Oat bran, rolled oats, broccoli, brussel sprouts, grapefruits, apples, and beans are good sources of such fiber.

Alcohol raises serum triglycerides and when ingested in excess is a common cause of secondary hyperlipidemia. A chronic, modest intake is associated with reduced death rates from CAD. This is explained in part by raised levels of HDL-c.[43] It also may have a salutary effect on coagulation with platelet aggregation inhibition and lower fibrinogen levels seen in some studies. Alcohol should not be recommended as part of an HDL-raising strategy due to its significant negative effects if its use cannot be controlled.[44] These include hypertension, stroke, accidents and violence, as well as alcoholism. Women should not drink if they are pregnant since fetal alcohol syndrome may occur and they may be more susceptible to alcoholic liver disease than their male counterparts.[45]

Recently, 2 large studies from Harvard showed that men and women in the top distribution for vitamin E had significant reductions in CAD.[46,47] These were observational cohort data. Clinical trial data is forthcoming. This area is of great interest because of the putative role of oxidized LDL in atherosclerosis.

Large clinical intervention trials on diet have not provided conclusive results. Their interpretation has been hampered by design problems. The best of the large trials was the Oslo Diet and Smoking Trial which looked at 1,232 men who were in the fifth decade of life and without overt CAD.[48] This was a randomized, double-blind trial where the treatment group received 8.2% of calories as saturated fat as compared with 18.3% in the control group. Blood cholesterol was lowered 13% in the treatment group and fatal and nonfatal myocardial infarctions were 47% lower in this group.

On the other hand, several angiographic trials have confirmed the anti-atherogenic effects of a cholesterol-lowering diet. The St. Thomas Atherosclerosis Trial looked at 90 men under 66 years of age with cholesterol levels exceeding 233 mg/dl.[49] The treatment groups included diet as well as diet plus cholestyramine resin. The diet group was given a 27% fat diet with 8% to 10% of calories from saturated fats. LDL-c fell 16% and only 15% showed progression on serial coronary angiography as compared with 46% progression in the control group. Even symptoms were improved. Likewise in the Heidelberg trial, men with angina who were assigned to a less than 20% fat diet and regular aerobic exercise had small improvements in LDL and HDL along with significantly less progression in treat-

Table 8. Treatment Goals for Primary and Secondary Prevention[5]			
STATUS	LDL-C START	MONITORING LDL-C	MONITORING TOTAL CHOLESTEROL
<2 risk factors and no CAD	≥ 160 mg/dl	<160 mg/dl	<240 mg/dl
2 or more risk factors and no CAD	>130 mg/dl	<130 mg/dl	<200 mg/dl
With CAD	>100 mg/dl	≤ 100 mg/dl	≤ 160 mg/dl
NCEP, 2nd Report of Adult Treatment Panel, 1993.			

ed versus controls as well as regression in 30% of treated versus only 4% of controls.[50] In the small, randomized Lifestyle Heart Trial, LDL-c was lowered impressively by a very low fat diet.[51] There were, however, fewer symptoms of CHD along with an average improvement in coronary diameter in those on the lifestyle modification regimen as compared with worsening of coronary diameters in those on the American Heart Association diet.

THE STEP 1 AND STEP 2 DIETS

The initiation and goal levels for dietary therapy are given in Table 8. While LDL-c values are needed to determine if diet is needed, in those with average values for HDL-c, a total cholesterol may serve as a surrogate. The Step 1 diet is recommended as the initial dietary intervention. The key components of this diet include a total fat intake of less than 30% calories, saturated fat intake of 8%-10% of calories, and dietary cholesterol of less than 300 mg/day. The Step 2 diet while still limiting fat to 30% of calories or less is stricter and serves as the therapeutic diet for the high-risk patient. In comparison to the Step 1 diet, saturated fat intake is restricted to less than 7% of calories and dietary cholesterol to less than 200 mg/day. Both diets limit polyunsaturated fats to up to 10% of calories, monounsaturated fats to up to 15% of calories, and carbohydrates to 55% or more of calories. In both diets, total calories are adjusted to achieve and maintain desirable weight.

The patient's cholesterol level should be measured at 6 weeks and at 3 months after starting the diet. If the goals of therapy are not met after 3 months on the Step 1 diet and reasonable adherence seems likely, the patient should begin the more intensive Step 2 diet. To promote long-term adherence to this regimen, involvement of a registered dietitian will most likely be needed to assure the individualization needed. Good diets are characterized by balance, variety, and taste, as well as simply meeting stated goals for dietary cholesterol and saturated fat.

Lower-risk patients who are unlikely to develop CAD in the ensuing 10-20 years should be given ample time to make the necessary behavioral changes. Motivation may come quickly, but knowledge, and skills (such as how to eat out, how to read labels, and low-fat meal preparation) take time and physicians should encourage the use of the excellent materials available in bookstores or from either the NCEP or the American Heart Association. Patients need to learn about dietary sources of saturated fats (Table 9). The decision to move to drug therapy can be delayed in such low-risk patients for some time. Yet some patients with hyperlipidemia should move more quickly to drug therapy. Individuals with very high LDL-c values over 220 mg/dl, those with multiple risk factors for CHD, or those with established CAD are among these patients. A recent study suggested that in patients seen in lipid clinics without CHD and with values for LDL-c from 160-200 mg/dl on their current diets, a Step 2 diet could be expected to lower LDL-c only 5% on average.[52] These patients also had lowered HDL-c on diet. This common occurrence after starting a low fat diet can be alleviated by adding regular aerobic exercise to the dietary prescription. This has the additional benefit of helping promote weight loss if the patient is overweight.

Table 9. Dietary Sources of Saturated Fats and Possible Substitutes

CATEGORY	ITEM	SATURATED FAT (G)	CHOLESTEROL (MG)
Meats	Ground beef patty Cooked, reg, 4 oz.	9.2	102
	Turkey, light, roasted skinless, 4 oz.	1.2	7.8
Eggs	One egg yolk	1.7	225
	Commercial egg substitute	0	0
Diary			
Cheese	American cheese 1 oz	6	30
	Substitute cheese	1	
Milk	Milk whole, 1 cup	5.1	33
	Milk skim, 1 cup	0.6	5
Cream	Ice cream, 1 cup	9.0	60
	Nonfat yogurt, 1 cup	0.3	Trace
Invisible Fats in Baked Goods, Snacks	Doughnut, 1 piece	5	20
	French fries, 1 order	7	15
	Fruits	0	0
Cooking/table fats			
	Butter, 1 T	7	30
	Soft diet margarine, 1 T	10	
	Hard margarine (stick)	2.1	0
	Coconut oil, 1 T	11.8	0
	Corn Oil, 1 T	1.7	0
Snacks	Peanuts, dry-roasted, 1/4 cup	3.1	0
	Popcorn, salted, buttered 3 cups	2.7	12
	Popcorn, 3 cups	Trace	0
	Chocolate chip cookies, 2	1.3	8

Values are approximate and taken from standard food tables.

If the LDL-c goals are unlikely to be met by dietary change alone, drug therapy should commence shortly after beginning dietary therapy. This does not imply that dietary therapy is not effective. It can be shown that to achieve LDL-c goals, dietary therapy can often reduce the amount of lipid-lowering medication needed.

Diet adherence and success vary greatly from patient to patient. Physician endorsement can be an important factor in inducing the patient to make this key behavioral change. The use of behavioral modification is particularly helpful when dealing with overweight patients.

Increased physical activity is also an essential component of the overall approach to lifestyle. Regular exercise not only lowers triglyceride levels and raises HDL levels, it can help promote weight reduction. Patients should be reminded of times when they were less active. Invariably they will remember that their weight did rise during those periods. Reasons for dietary failure include insufficient knowledge or skills or lack of motivation during high-stress periods of their lives. Periodic monitoring and feedback are invaluable here. Patients who prefer drug therapy without a reasonable dietary trial should be warned that cholesterol-lowering medication is never curative and the convenience of medication should be balanced by cost as well as potential side effects over an entire lifetime.

DRUG THERAPY (TABLES 10–12)

Initiation of drug therapy requires a consideration of benefits, risk of adverse effects and tolerability factors such as cost and convenience. Factors that argue for intense lowering of diet-resistant LDL include older age (≥ 45 years for men and ≥ 55 years for women), severity of LDL cholesterol elevation, severity of risk factor status (multiple risk factors and/or diabetes) or presence of atherosclerotic vascular disease.

Current NCEP guidelines recommend lipid-lowering drug therapy in men ≥ 45 years of age as well as women ≥ 55 years of age whose LDL-c exceeds 190 mg/dl despite an adequate trial of diet. If there are 2 or more risk factors, drug therapy should be considered if the LDL-c is 160 mg/dl or more. The goals of therapy are less than 160 mg/dl for those without 2 or more risk factors and less than 130 mg/dl for those with 2 or more risk factors (Table 11). For younger people, the severity of the LDL-c is a critical factor in the decision as to whether to begin drug therapy. For those with LDL-c above 220 mg/dl (usually heterozygotes for familial hypercholesterolemia), drug therapy is needed. On the other hand, if LDL-c is between 190-220 mg/dl and no other risk factors are present, use of lipid-lowering drugs may be delayed until the patient is older. Some lipid specialists believe that the relatively safe bile acid sequestrants should be considered for young men with high LDL levels and particularly so if they have a family history of premature CHD or hypercholesterolemia.

A lower target was set for those with established CHD because of the very high risk of recurrent CHD events. The Lipid Research Clinics follow-up study of men 40-69 years of age with cardiovascular disease at baseline, LDL cholesterol values above 160 mg/dl were almost 6 times as likely to cause death from CHD as those with values under 130 mg/dl. Several angiographic intervention trials employing varying methods for lowering LDL cholesterol showed overall regression with LDL values under 100 mg/dl on average. Thus, it is recommended that those with LDL-c of 130 mg/dl or

higher be considered for drug therapy. The optimal target level for this group with CHD is an LDL-c of 100 mg/dl or below.

If the LDL-c is between 100 and 129 mg/dl, clinical judgment must be used to decide whether lipid-lowering drugs should be started or whether a second drug should be initiated if the maximal level reached with diet and drug therapy has occurred. Moreover, the report suggests that consideration be given to starting lipid-lowering drug therapy at discharge after an acute coronary event if the LDL-c is 130 mg/dl or higher since LDL-c cholesterol values usually fall after a myocardial infarction. Certainly if LDL-c levels exceed 130 mg/dl three or more months after the acute coronary event despite dietary therapy, drug therapy should be strongly considered.

The major drugs are bile sequestrants or resins, niacin, and the HMG Coa Reductase Inhibitors or statins. Fibric acid drugs such as gemfibrozil were listed as other drugs because of their modest effects in lowering LDL-c. They are important, however, in patients with moderate to severe hypertriglyceridemia. Hormone replacement with estrogen, despite the lack of controlled clinical trials, is reasonable for postmenopausal women who qualify for lipid-lowering drug therapy (with the usual caveats regarding monitoring for uterine cancer and breast cancer). Estrogen therapy may not be appropriate for women with genetic hypertriglyceridemia. Estrogen replacement may cause LDL lowering along with an increase in HDL, and may render drug therapy unnecessary.

BILE SEQUESTRANTS OR RESINS

These are important drugs of first choice because they have an enviable record of safety. They are not absorbed, but bind bile acids in the intestine and prevent their reabsorption. This shrinks hepatic cholesterol pools and stimulates hepatic production of LDL receptors. These drugs are known as cholestyramine (Questran or Questran Lite©) or colestipol (Colestid©).The dosage form is a powder which as Questran contains 4 g of active medication and as Colestid contains 5 g. They lower cholesterol and LDL-c levels moderately and raise HDL-c levels slightly. Since triglyceride levels may rise, they should not be used in patients with baseline triglyceride

Table 10. Synopsis of Selected Diet and/or Drug Angiographic Trials Looking at Regression With Intensive Lipid Lowering

ANGIOGRAPHIC TRIALS	NO. OF SUBJECTS	CAD STATUS	TRIAL DESIGN	DIET OR DRUG THERAPY	LIPID CHANGE DURING TRIAL	CAD STATUS CHANGE IN TRIAL
CLAS Trial[56]	162 men selected to be compliant	Coronary bypass surgery survivors	Randomized; blinded; non-quantitative angiography	Controls given roughly Step I diet; treatment group on colestipol and niacin	LDL fell 43% TG fell 22% HDL rose 37% in group on drugs	Fewer lesions progressed in drug group; regression in 16.2% of those on drugs
Lifestyle Heart Trial[51]	28 to Rx 20 to control group; 36 males, 5 females	Angina; CAD at angiography	Quantitative angiography; randomization suboptimal	Controls: 30% total fat; <200 mg chol; Rx group averaged 6.8% total fat and no chol.	LDL fell to 95 in Rx group; control group LDL only 158	Rx had % diam. decline 2.2% vs an increase in controls to 3.4%
St. Thomas Atherosclerosis Trial (STARS)[49]	90 men under age 66; total cholesterol >233 mg/dl	Angina; CAD at angiography	Randomized; controlled; usual care vs diet vs meds and diet	Diet was 27% fat and 8%-10% saturated fat with increased fiber	LDL fell 16% with diet	Usual care showed 46% progression; only 15% with diet; symptoms better with diet
Familial Atherosclerosis Trial (FATS)[25]	146 men with familial vascular disease and increased apo B	CAD at angiography	Quantitative angiography; films blinded as to sequence and therapy	Controls on diet and/or resin; Rx was lovastatin 20 mg bid and colestipol 10 g tid or niacin 1 g qid + colestipol 10 g qid	LDL fell 46% HDL rose 15% with colestid and lovastatin; LDL fell 32% HDL rose 43% with colestid and niacin	Controls showed progression in 46%; only 21 and 25% in Rx; controls had regression only in 11%; Rx had 32% and 39%
Heidelberg Trial[50]	56 men Rx group; 57 to usual care; avg. age=53; avg. chol=239 avg. HDL=36	Angina; CAD at angiography	Randomized; Rx included low-fat diet and exercise	Treatment diet total fat under 20%; P/S >1.0; dietary cholesterol under 200 mg	LDL fell 8% HDL rose 3% TC/HDL fell 11% in Rx; weight also fell 5%	Controls showed 42% with progression; 20% with Rx regression in 4% controls vs 30% Rx
Monitored Atherosclerosis Regression Trial (MARS)[58]	270 patients; male and female; smoking and nonsmoking; total chol. from 190-295	CAD at angiography	Randomized; true double-blind trial; Rx diet and lovastatin	Diet: ≤ 27% fat; saturated fat ≤ 7%; diet chol ≤ 250; drug: lovastatin 40 mg bid	LDL fell 38% HDL rose in Rx group	If lesions >50% there was a significant decrease in % diam. stenosis vs diet alone

levels above 250 mg/dl.

In the Lipid Research Clinics Primary Prevention Trial, men assigned to the diet and cholestyramine arm had average reductions in total cholesterol and LDL-c of 8.5% and 12.6% as compared with those assigned to the placebo

Table 11. LDL-c Cutpoints for Drug Therapy*

STATUS	CONSIDER DRUG THERAPY	GOAL OF THERAPY
Without CHD and with fewer than 2 risk factors	≥ 190 mg/dl*	<160 mg/dl
Without CHD and with 2 or more risk factors	≥ 160 mg/dl	<130 mg/dl
With CHD	≥ 130 mg/dl**	<100 mg/dl

* In men <35 years old and premenopausal women with LDL-c 190-220 mg/dl, drug therapy probably should be delayed with the exception of high risk patients (e.g., diabetics)

** In CHD patients with LDL-c levels between100-130 mg/dl, clinical judgement is needed to decide whether drug therapy commences.

From the Second Report of the Expert Panel on Detection, Evaluation, and Treatment of High Blood Cholesterol in Adults (Adult Treatment Panel II). June 1993.

arm. The treatment group had a 19% reduction in fatal and nonfatal MI which was the primary endpoint. Importantly, incident rates for development of positive exercise tests, angina, and coronary bypass surgery were lowered 25%, 20%, and 21% as well. For every 1% lowering of cholesterol, there was a 2% reduction of CAD events.[53] The benefits were not seen initially, but were present after 2 years. There was a non-significant 7% reduction in all-cause mortality. This was not surprising as the study was not large enough to demonstrate such an effect. One of the earliest angiographic trials showed that in coronary patients with narrowings greater than 50%, resin and diet reduced progression on follow-up angiograms.[54]

Although remarkably safe, inconvenience and side effects limit adherence to these drugs. This is a gritty medication which is mixed with juice or a pulpy food like apple juice. It causes constipation, bloating, and aggravation of hemorrhoids in many patients. With careful patient education, patients can take these resins successfully for many years. For many patients with moderate hypercholesterolemia, 1 or 2 scoops per day may be all that is required. In this lower-dose form, the resin may be more easily tolerated.

Resins bind medications such as thyroxine, digoxin, antibiotics, diuretics, and statins. Patients should take other medications 1 hour before taking the resin or 4 or more hours after they have taken the resin. Despite these cautions, resins have been used safely for decades and should be considered in young patients with diet-resistant LDL-c levels between 190 and 220 mg/dl.

NIACIN

Niacin is also known as nicotinic acid or vitamin B3. Niacinamide (nicotinamide) is another form of the vitamin which does not lower lipids and should not be substituted for niacin. Niacin decreases liver synthesis of VLDL and LDL. Lower doses of niacin effectively lower triglycerides and raise HDL-c. Higher doses are needed for LDL-c lowering comparable to that of the statins.

In the Coronary Drug Project, niacin lowered cholesterol levels by 10% on average and significantly reduced risk of nonfatal MI by about 27%.[55] Fifteen years later, the niacin group had a highly significant 11% improvement in survival. Niacin was used with resin in both the Cholesterol Lowering Atherosclerosis Study (CLAS)[56] and Familial Atherosclerosis Treatment Study.[24] In both trials, the combination therapy lowered LDL-c levels to 100 mg/dl or less and raised HDL-c levels. This was associated with a decrease in coronary progression as well as an increased rate of regression of coronary plaques.

The usual initial dose of niacin is 100 or 250 mg. The dosage is increased gradually until the desired effects are seen. USP Niacin is inexpensive. Nonetheless, adherence can be difficult due to transient flushing after the dose is taken.

Table 12. Lipid-Lowering Therapy

NAME	MECHANISM	EFFECT	COMMENT
Resins Cholestyramine (Questran) or Colestipol (Colestid)	Binds bile acids in the gut; increases LDL catabolism	Major effect on total and LDL cholesterol; small rise in HDL; triglycerides rise as well. Caution: Do not use in patients with elevated triglycerides: >250 mg/dl	Constipation, bloating, and rectal irritation. Start at low doses; 1 scoop twice daily may be enough.
Niacin Nicotinc acid (both unmodified and sustained release); Nicotinamide is not a lipid lowering substitute for niacin.	Inhibits FFA release; decreased LDL and VLDL synthesis	Lowers cholesterol, triglycerides, and LDL; raises HDL	Flushing in all; an aspirin can prevent the flush; watch liver enzymes, FBS, and uric acid. Avoid in patients with ulcers. Sustained release with increase in liver enzymes when dose exceeds 1 g/day.
Statins or HMG Coa Reductase Inhibitors Lovastatin (mevacor) Pravastatin (pravachol) Simvastatin (zocor) Fluvastatin (leschol)	Inhibits cholesterol synthesis by competitive inhibition of HMG Coa Reductase; leads to increased LDL receptors	Marked lowering of total and LDL cholesterol; some rise in HDL-c; mild fall in TG; do not use to lower TG if TG is over 500 mg/dl	Monitor liver enzymes. If also on cyclosporine, niacin, gemfibrozil, or IV erythromycin there is risk of myositis. Advice of lipid specialist is crucial here. Only lovastatin is taken with food.
Fibrates Gemfibrozil (lopid)	Improves TG removal; increases cholesterol in bile	Major reductions in TG excess with rise in HDL-c. IF LDL-c only elevated, mild lowering of LDL-c. Drug of choice if TG over 800 mg/dl.	Low, but possible gall stone risk. Not recommended as monotherapy for patients with CAD as LDL lowering is not pronounced.
Probucol (lorelco)	Inhibits cholesterol synthesis; an anti-oxidant	Lowers cholesterol mildly; and also lowers HDL-c. Not listed as a major drug by the NCEP	Can decrease xanthomas; avoid in patients with abnormal ECG — especially prolonged QTc.

Although tachyphylaxis to this prostaglandin mediated effect occurs in about 80% over time, it can be uncomfortable enough to prompt patients to seek a different lipid-lowering drug. The flush can be lessened by taking a 5 grain aspirin about 1 hour before the niacin. In addition, niacin should be taken with food. Hot beverages or alcohol can make the flushing worse and should be minimized. Side effects commonly seen include aggravation of hyperuricemia and gout, hyperglycemia, and elevation of liver function tests. Many lipid specialists do not give niacin to diabetics as it aggravates blood-sugar control. Thus, lipids and a complete chemistry profile to include FBS, uric acid, and liver function tests should be performed frequently as the dose is titrated upward. Ulcer disease can be aggravated and when combined with statins, both liver-enzyme rise and myositis may be more common.

For young patients in whom cost is an issue, unmodified niacin is the drug of choice. It is particularly useful in combined hyperlipidemia or when high LDL-c is accompanied by a low HDL-cholesterol and high triglyceride levels. Sustained release forms make niacin easier to take, but there appears to be an increase in gastrointestinal side effects. If sustained release forms are given, many feel that the maximum dosage should be 2 g/day.

HMG Coa REDUCTASE INHIBITORS

These drugs or "statins" are the most effective drugs at lowering LDL-c. They are competitive inhibitors of cholesterol synthesis at the step where HMG Coa is converted to mevalonate. They lower total cholesterol and LDL-c cholesterol and raise HDL levels. Triglyceride values are also lowered. They are better tolerated and more convenient to take than resins, but long-term follow-up is limited to less than 10 years. Lovastatin (mevacor) was the first statin introduced. It has been followed by pravastatin (pravachol), simvastatin (zocor), and fluvastatin (leschol). Simvastatin is more potent and in patients with familial hypercholesterolemia, 10 mg of simvastatin has the same cholesterol-lowering effect as 20 mg of lovastatin. Lovastatin should be taken with food, whereas the other statins can be taken without food. Lower doses can be taken at night, but at higher dosages, a split dose of morning and evening is more effective. The dose response curve is not linear, but more logarithmic with the greatest effects seen at the lower dosages. Cardiologists can take advantage of this effect by adding resins as a second drug rather than giving the maximum dosage. For example, the benefits of going from 40 mg to 80 mg of lovastatin are much less than adding 8 g of cholestyramine to 40 mg of lovastatin.

The usual starting dosage is 10 or 20 mg of lovastatin, pravastatin, or fluvastatin. (The simvastatin dosage would be half of this). Statins have an excellent safety record. A large follow-up trial[57] showed that the frequency of elevated transaminases requiring discontinuation was 0.1% for both placebo and the 20-mg dose of lovastatin, 0.9% for the 40-mg dose, and 1.9% for the 80-mg dose. Myositis is defined as myalgia, soreness, or stiff-

ness associated with a CPK rise 10 times above the upper limit of normal. This is rarely seen in healthy persons on statins alone. It is most frequent in transplant patients who take cyclosporine with doses of lovastatin that exceed 20 mg/day and those with combined hyperlipidemia who take lovastatin with gemfibrozil or, less commonly, with niacin. The issue is not a trivial one. Severe rhabdomyolysis leading to renal failure has been reported. Eye exams are not needed as an increased incidence of cataracts has not been reported. Some of the statins can potentiate the effect of oral anticoagulants so the protime must be adjusted if these drugs are begun.

Statins are particularly useful in patients with severe LDL elevations (more than 220 mg/dl) as in familial hypercholesterolemia, in patients with CHD who need optimal LDL lowering below 100 mg/dl and in diabetics and hyperuricemics for whom niacin is a difficult drug to use. A recent angiographic trial using a large dose of lovastatin as single drug therapy confirmed the efficacy of lowering LDL-c in causing increased regression.[58] The Scandinavian Simvastatin Survival Study (4S) confirmed the value of secondary prevention. Simvastatin produced significant reductions in all-cause mortality as well as CHD morbidity in patients with CHD followed for a median of 5.4 years.[59]

FIBRATES

Fibric acid derivatives are the drugs of choice for patients with major problems in disposing of triglyceride-rich lipoproteins. They do this by increasing lipoprotein lipase. They also decrease VLDL production by the liver. They also partially inhibit the synthesis of cholesterol and bile acids and promote the secretion of cholesterol in the bile. Triglyceride reductions can be significant with declines of 20%-50%. In the Helsinki Heart Study of hypercholesterolemic middle-aged men, total cholesterol was reduced by 11% while HDL was increased by 10%.[33]

Clofibrate is a first generation fibrate which, owing to its significant lithogenicity and adverse safety profile is not recommended. Gemfibrozil is a second-generation fibrate that is recommended by the Food and Drug Administration for triglyceride lowering. In the Helsinki Heart Study it lowered fatal and nonfatal MI significantly as compared with placebo. As in the Lipid Research Clinics primary prevention trial, there was not a significant decrease in mortality (although these trials were not designed to show this effect). Gemfibrozil is Food and Drug Administration (FDA) approved for coronary prevention in those with elevated cholesterol, triglycerides, and low HDL-C. Since gemfibrozil alone reduces LDL-c only mildly, it is not recommended for patients with established CHD by the NCEP guidelines.

The usual dosage is 600 mg taken twice daily. The dose must be reduced or the drug avoided in patients with decreased renal function. Gemfibrozil is well-tolerated and mild gastrointestinal complaints are the most common side effects noted. It is not as lithogenic as clofibrate, but is still considered to slightly increase the risk of gallstones. Clinicians must be warned about an increased risk of myositis and rhabdomyolysis if gemfibrozil and a statin are combined.[60] This combination may be overused because there is no evidence that the gemfibrozil-plus-statin combination is more effective than a statin alone in familial or polygenic hypercholesterolemia.

PROBUCOL

This is not a first-line drug because clinical trial data showing efficacy is lacking. It has mild cholesterol-lowering action and does not affect triglyceride levels. HDL-c levels fall about 20% to 30% on average. Interestingly, studies in cases of severe FH have documented xanthoma regression. It is a powerful antioxidant and retards the oxidation of LDL particles. Despite this seemingly important effect, the lack of double-blind, randomized placebo-controlled trials prevent a clear clinical indication from emerging.

The recommended dosage is 500 mg twice daily. It is well-tolerated except for mild gastrointestinal side effects which include diarrhea. Prolongation of the QT interval has been seen and it should not be given to those with QT prolongation or who are given other drugs that can cause this to occur. Periodic electrocardiograms are necessary to monitor therapy.

ESTROGENS

When menopause occurs for any reason, there is an increase in the woman's risk of CHD. Postmenopausal estrogens can lower LDL-c lev-els and raise HDL-c levels. Their appropriate use may obviate the need for lipid-lowering therapy. Despite a number of prospective cohort observational studies showing benefit as great as 50% in rates of CHD for those who took estrogens as contrasted with those who did not, there have been no controlled clinical trials to date. Part of estrogen's beneficial actions appear to come from its salutary effects on LDL and HDL levels, while part may be due to its effect on the arterial wall.[61] In monkeys, estrogen decreases the accumulation of lipids in the arterial wall.

The putative benefits of estrogen must be counterbalanced with the evidence that estrogen increases risk for endometrial cancer and may be associated with a small increase in risk for breast cancer. The increase in endometrial cancer risk can probably be avoided by adding a progestin to the estrogen regimen for women who have a uterus. Accordingly, the use of estrogens in women who have a uterus and do not have greatly increased risk of CHD is unclear.[62] Clearly individualized judgment must be used and appropriate monitoring is required.

SPECIAL SITUATIONS

The patient with a normal LDL-C level but with an HDL level <35 presents a difficult dilemma. If asymptomatic, the best approach would be to encourage regular aerobic exercise, cessation of cigarette smoking, and caloric restriction with a low-fat diet to attain a normal weight. Patients must be counseled that the rise in HDL-c level will be slow. For patients with multiple risk factors, strong family histories of premature CHD or with existing CHD, a more aggressive approach seems reasonable. Niacin to raise HDL levels or a statin to lower LDL levels so that the ratio of LDL/HDL is improved are 2 theoretically attractive, but unproven approaches. Gemfibrozil therapy may cause a reciprocal rise in LDL levels in this situation.

Combination therapy should be considered with patients with very high levels of LDL-c, those with multiple lipid/lipoprotein abnormalities, or in those in whom higher dosages of 1 drug are not tolerable due to side effects or cost. For those with familial hypercholesterolemia, the drug combinations of choice are niacin and resin or statin and resin. Triple therapy can lower LDL-c levels into the normal range and has been shown in some cases to be associated with regression of xanthomas.[63] The most effective regimens take advantage of complementary mechanisms.[64]

REFERENCES

1. Small, DM. Progression and regression of atherosclerotic lesions. Insights from lipid physical biochemistry. *Arteriosclerosis*. 1988;8:103-129.
2. Ross R. The pathogenesis of atherosclerosis — An update. *N Engl J Med*. 1986;314:488-500.
3. Brown BG, Zhao X-Q, Sacco DE, et al. Lipid lowering and plaque regression. New insights into prevention of plaque disruption and clinical events in coronary disease. *Circulation*. 1993;87:1781-1791.
4. Harrison DG, Armstrong ML, Freiman PC, et al. Restoration of endothelium-dependent relation by dietary treatment of atherosclerosis. *J Clin Invest*. 1987;80,1808-1811.
5. Expert Panel on Detection, Evaluation, and Treatment of High Blood Cholesterol in Adults. Summary of the second report of the National Cholesterol Education Program (NCEP) expert panel on detection, evaluation, and treatment of high blood cholesterol in adults (Adult Treatment Panel II). *JAMA*. 1993,1269:3015-3023.
6. Davignon J, Gregg RE, Sing CF. Apolipoprotein E polymorphism and atherosclerosis. *Arteriosclerosis*. 1988;8:1-21.
7. Sniderman A, Shapiro S, Marpole D, et al. Association of coronary atherosclerosis with hyperapobetalipoproteinemia [increased protein but normal cholesterol levels in human plasma low density (B) lipoproteins]. *Proc Natl Acad Sci USA*. 1980;77:604-608.
8. Campeau L, Enjalbert M, Lesperance J, et al. The relation of risk factors to the development of atherosclerosis in saphenous-vein bypass grafts and the progression of disease in the native circulation. *N Engl J Med*. 1984;311:1329-1332.
9. Austin MA, Breslow JL, Hennekens CH, et al. Low density lipoprotein subclass patterns and risk of MI. *JAMA*. 1988;260:1917-1921.
10. Steinberg D, Parthasarathy S, Carew T, et al. Beyond - cholesterol: Modifications of low-density lipoprotein that increase its atherogenicity. *N Engl J Med*. 1989;320:915-924.
11. Bhatnagar D, Durrington PN, Channon KM, et al. Increased transfer of cholesteryl esters from high density lipoproteins to low density and very low density lipoproteins in patients with angiographic evidence of coronary artery disease. *Atherosclerosis*. 1993;98(1):25-32.
12. Parthasarathy S, Khoo JC, Miller E, et al. Low-density lipoprotein enriched in oleic acid is protected against oxidative modification: implications for dietary prevention of atherosclerosis. *Proc Natl Acad Sci USA*. 1990;87:3894-3898.
13. Abbott RD, Wilson PWF, Kannel WB, et al. High density lipoprotein cholesterol, total cholesterol screening, and myocardial infarction. *Arteriosclerosis*. 1988;8:207-211.
14. Martin MJ, Hulley SB, Browner WS, et al. Serum cholesterol, blood pressure, and mortality: Implications from a cohort of 361,662 men. *Lancet*. 1986;2:933-936.
15. Larsson B, Bengtsson C, Bjorntorp P, et al. Is abdominal body fat distribution a major explanation for the sex difference in the incidence of myocardial infarction? The study of men born in 1913 and the study of women. *Am J Epidemiol*. 1992;135(3):266-273.
16. Caggiula AW, Christakis G, Farrand M, et al, for the MRFIT. The Multiple Risk Factor Intervention Trial (MRFIT). *Preventive Medicine*. 1981;10:443-475.
17. Henkin Y, Como JA, Oberman A. Secondary dyslipidemia. Inadvertent effects of drugs in clinical practice. *JAMA*. 1992;267:961-968.
18. Becker DM, Becker LC, Pearson TA, et al. Risk factors in siblings of people with premature coronary heart disease. *J Am Coll Cardiol*. 1988;12:1-8.
19. Goldstein JL, Hazzard WR, Schrott HG, et al. Hyperlipidemia in coronary heart disease. I. Lipid Levels in 500 survivors of myocardial infarction. *J Clin Invest*. 1973;52:1533-1543.
20. Stone NJ, Levy RI, Fredrickson DS, et al. Coronary artery disease in 116 kindred with familial type II hyper lipoproteinemia. *Circulation*. 1974;49:476-488.
21. Kane JP, Malloy MJ, Ports TA, et al. Regression of coronary atherosclerosis during treatment of familial hypercholesterolemia with combined drug regimens. *JAMA*. 1990;264:3007-3012.
22. Beppu S, Minura Y, Sakakibara H, et al. Supravalvular aortic stenosis and coronary ostial stenosis in familial hypercholesterolemia: Two-dimensional echocardiographic assessment. *Circulation*. 1983;67:878-884.
23. Bilheimer, DW, Goldstein JL, Grundy SM, et al. Liver transplantation to provide low-density-lipoprotein receptors and lower plasma cholesterol in a child with homozygous familial hypercholesterolemia. *N Engl J Med*. 1984;311:1658-1664.
24. Goldstein JL. Genetic aspects of hyperlipidemia in coronary heart disease. *Hosp Pract*. 1973;2:53.
25. Brown G, Albers JJ, Fisher LD, et al. Regression of coronary artery disease as a result of interim lipid-lowering therapy in men with high levels of apoliprotein B. *N Engl J Med*. 1990;323:1289-1298.
26. Williams RB, Hunt SC, Hopkins PN, et al. Familial dyslipidemic hypertension: Evidence from 58 Utah families for a syndrome present in approximately 12% of patients with essential hypertension. *JAMA*. 1988; 259:3579-3586.
27. Ordovas JM, Schaefer EJ, Salem D, et al. Apolipoprotein A-1 gene polymorphism associated with premature coronary artery disease and familial hypoalphalipoproteinemia. *N Engl J Med*. 1986;314(11):671-677.
28. Schaefer EJ. Clinical, biochemical, and genetic features of familial disorders of high density lipoproteins. *Arteriosclerosis*. 1984;4:303-324.
29. Sandholzer C, Boerwinkle E, Saha N, et al. Apolipoprotein(a) phenotypes, Lp(a) concentration and plasma lipid levels in relation to coronary heart disease in a Chinese population: evidence for the role of the apo(a) gene in coronary heart disease. *J Clin Invest*. 1992;89(3):1040-1046.
30. Genest J, McNamara JR, Ordovas JM, et al. Lipoprotein cholesterol, apolipoprotein A-1 and B and lipoprotein

(a) abnormalities in men with premature coronary disease. *J Am Coll Cardiol*. 1992:19:792-802.

31. Jauhiainen M, Koskinen P, Ehnholm C, et al. Lipoprotein (a) and coronary heart disease risk: a nested case-control study of the Helsinki Heart Study participants. *Atherosclerosis*. 1991;89(1):59-67.

32. Ridker PM, Hennekens CH, Stampfer MJ. A prospective study of lipoprotein(a) and the risk of myocardial infarction. *JAMA*. 1993;270(18):2195-2199.

33. Scanu A, Lawn R, Berg K. Lipoprotein (a) and atherosclerosis. *Ann Intern Med*. 1991;115:209-218.

34. Brunzell JD, Austin MA. Plasma triglyceride levels and coronary disease. *N Engl J Med*. 1989;320:1273-1275.

35. Frick, MH, Eto O, Haapa K, et al. Helsinki Heart Study: Primary prevention trial with gemfibrozil in middle-aged men with dyslipidemia. *N Engl J Med*. 1987;317:1237-1245.

36. Kronmal RA, Cain KC, Ye Z, et al. Total serum cholesterol levels and mortality risk as a function of age: a report based on the Framingham data. *Arch Intern Med*. 1993;153:1065.

37. Moser M. Lipid abnormalities and diuretics. *Am Fam Physician*. 1989;40:213-220.

38. Keys A (ed). Seven Countries: A Multivariate Analysis of Death and Coronary Heart Disease. Cambridge, MA: *Harvard University Press*; 1980.

39. Shekelle RB, Shyrcck AM, Paul O, et al. Diet, serum cholesterol, and death from coronary heart disease: The Western Electric Study. *N Engl J Med*. 1981; 304:65-70.

40. Kromhout D, Bosschieter EB, de Lezzane Coulander C. The inverse relation between fish consumption and twenty year mortality from coronary heart disease. *N Engl J Med*. 1985;312:1205-1209.

41. Willett WC, Stampfer MJ, Manson JE. Intake of trans fatty acids and risk of coronary heart disease among women. *Lancet*. 1993;341:581-585.

42. Davidson MH, Dugan LD, Burns JH, et al. The hypocholesterolemic effects of B glucan in oatmeal and oat bran. A dose-controlled study. *JAMA*. 1991;265:1833-1839.

43. Rimm EB, Giovannucci EL, Willett WC, et al. Prospective study of alcohol consumption and risk of coronary disease in men. *Lancet*. 1991;338(8765):464-468.

44. Steinberg D, Pearson TA, Kuller LH. Alcohol and Atherosclerosis. *Ann Intern Med*. 1991;114:967-976.

45. Frezza M, di Padova C, Pozzato G, et al. High blood alcohol levels in women. *N Engl J Med*. 1990;322(2):95-99.

46. Stampfer MJ, Hennekens CH, Manson JE, et al. Vitamin E consumption and the risk of coronary disease in women. *N Engl J Med*. 1993;328:1444-1449.

47. Rimm EB, Stampfer MJ, Ascherio A, et al. Vitamin E consumption and the risk of coronary heart disease in men. *N Engl J Med*. 1993;328:1450-1456.

48. Hjermann I, Holme I, Velve Byre K, et al. Effect of diet and smoking intervention on the incidence of coronary heart disease. *Lancet*. 1981;2:1303-1310.

49. Watts GF, Lewis, B, Brunt JNH, et al. Effects of coronary artery disease of lipid lowering diet, or diet plus cholestyramine in the St. Thomas Atherosclerosis Regression Study (STARS). *Lancet*. 1992;339:563-569.

50. Schuler G, Hambrecht R, Schlierf G, et al. Regular physical exercise and low-fat diet. Effects of progression on coronary artery disease. *Circulation*. 1992;86:1-11.

51. Ornish D, Brown SE, Scherwitz LW, et al. Can lifestyle changes reverse coronary heart disease? The Lifestyle Heart Trial. *Lancet*. 1990;335:129-133.

52. Hunninghake DB, Stein EA, Dujovne CA, et al. The efficacy of intensive dietary therapy alone or combined with lovastatin in outpatients with hypercholesterolemia. *N Engl J Med*. 1993;328:1213-1219.

53. The Lipid Research Clinics Primary Prevention Trial Result I. Reduction in incidence of coronary heart disease. *JAMA*. 1984;251:351-364.

54. Brensike JF, Levy RI, Kelsey SF, et al. Effects of therapy with cholestyramine on progression of coronary arteriosclerosis: Results of the NHLBI Type II Coronary Intervention Study. *Circulation*. 1984;69:313-324.

55. Canner PL, Berge KG, Wenger NK, et al. Fifteen year mortality in coronary drug project patients: Long term benefit with niacin. *J Am Coll Cardiol*. 1986;8:1245-1255.

56. Blankenhorn DH, Nessim SA, Johnson RL, et al. Beneficial effects of combined colestipol-niacin therapy on coronary atherosclerosis and coronary venous bypass grafts. *JAMA*. 1987;257:3233-3240.

57. Bradford RH, Shear CL, Chremos AN, et al. I. Efficacy in modifying plasma lipoproteins and adverse event pro file in 8245 patients with moderate hypercholesterolemia. *Arch Intern Med*. 1991;151:43-49.

58. Blankenhorn DH, Azen SP, Kramsch DM, et al. Coronary angiographic changes with lovastatin therapy. The Monitored Atherosclerosis Regression Study (MARS). *Ann Intern Med*. 1993;119:969-976.

59. Scandinavian Simvastatin Survival Study Group. Randomised trial of cholesterol lowering in 4444 patients with coronary heart disease: the Scandinavian Simvastatin Survival Study (4S). *Lancet*. 1994;344:1383-1389.

60. Pierce R, Wysowski DK, Gross TP. Myopathy and rhab domyolysis associated with lovastatin-gemfibrozil combination therapy. *JAMA*. 1990;264:71-75.

61. Adams MR, Kaplan JR, Koritnik DR, et al. Pregnancy-associated inhibition of coronary atherosclerosis in monkeys. Evidence of a relationship with endogenous estrogen. *Arteriosclerosis*. 1987;7:378-384.

62. Grady D, Rubin SM, Petitti DB, et al. Hormone therapy to prevent disease and prolong life in postmenopausal women. *Ann Intern Med*. 1992;117:1016-1037.

63. Witzum JL, Simmons D, Steinberg D, et al. Intensive combination drug therapy of familial hypercholesterolemia with lovastatin, probucol, and colestipol hydrochloride. *Circulation*. 1989;79:16-28.

64. Malloy MJ, Kane JP, Kunitake ST, et al. Complementarity of colestipol, niacin, and lovastatin in treatment of severe familial hypercholesterolemia. *Ann Intern Med*. 1987;107:616-623.

13 Angina Pectoris

Edward J. Brown, Jr, MD
Robert A. Kloner, MD, PhD

DIAGNOSIS AND EVALUATION OF ANGINA PECTORIS: THE CLINICAL HISTORY

Chest pain is a frequent patient complaint, and its differential diagnosis is extensive (Table 1). A careful and thorough clinical history can provide important clues that may significantly narrow the diagnostic possibilities. The location, quality, and duration of the chest pain, as well as associated symptoms, can all help the clinician determine the cause of chest pain.

Angina pectoris is the subjective symptom patients experience with transient episodes of myocardial ischemia (Table 2). It is typically described as substernal chest discomfort, pressure, heaviness, squeezing, or burning, radiating to the shoulders, arms (left greater than right), neck, jaw, and epigastrium; it is exacerbated by exertion and relieved by rest or within a few minutes of use of sublingual nitroglycerin. The discomfort usually lasts at least 15 seconds and less than 15 minutes. Chest pain lasting only a few seconds is usually not angina pectoris. Angina pectoris is often a visceral sensation and, as such, may be difficult for the patient to describe and locate precisely. In fact, if a physician asks the patient to describe the "pain," the patient may correct the physician and use a description such as discomfort. A positive Levine's sign suggests angina; it is characterized by the patient's clenching his fist over his sternum when describing the sensation of discomfort. Occasionally, patients will describe angina as occurring initially in the arms, jaws, or shoulders and then radiating to the chest. Rarely, angina will occur only in those areas and not the chest. When trying to elicit a history of exercise-induced angina, it is often useful to ask the patient whether there are certain activities (such as walking up a hill, climbing stairs, or running) which reliably and predictably bring on the chest discomfort.

Angina pectoris can occur in the absence of exertion. This form of myocardial ischemia may be due to coronary artery spasm (Prinzmetal's angina) that results in an episodic decrease in coronary blood flow. Other factors can precipitate angina pectoris at rest, including severe anemia, which leads to decreased blood oxygen-carrying capacity; fever; arrhythmias, especially tachycardia; hyperthyroidism; and drugs, such as catecholamines, which increase myocardial oxygen consumption at rest. A history of cold- or emotion-induced angina should be sought, as these have been associated with vasospastic elements of coronary artery disease. Angina at rest may also be a presenting feature of unstable angina. In the history, it is important to establish the frequency and severity of angina. The patient should be asked to describe how many times angina occurs per day, per week, and per month; how many nitroglycerin tablets the patient uses during these times; and the severity of the angina on a 1+ to 10+ scale, with 1+ being very minimal sensation of chest discomfort and 10+ the most severe. In taking the history, it is important to ask the patient whether previous diagnostic procedures to evaluate coronary artery disease, such as exercise stress testing and cardiac catheterization, were performed.

Symptoms accompanying chest pain, as well as the way chest pain is relieved, can be helpful to know in establishing a diagnosis of angina pectoris. Angina pectoris precipitated by exertion is generally relieved after 1 to 5 minutes in a standing or sitting position. A supine position may aggravate angina pectoris because it promotes increased venous return, which results in increased myocardial wall stress, a major determinant of myocardial oxygen consumption.

Table 1. Conditions Causing Chest Pain and Differential Aspects

NONCARDIOVASCULAR DISORDERS	DIFFERENTIATING FEATURE
Neuromuscular	
Costochondritis and other chest wall syndromes	Pain exacerbated with inspiration Chest wall tenderness
Radicular syndromes	Radicular distribution to pain Rash of herpes zoster
Inflammatory syndromes of the shoulder joint	Pain on palpation and exacerbated by arm movement
Gastrointestinal	
Esophageal disease and hiatal hernia	Reflux of food Not exertionally related Eating may exacerbate pain Relief with antacids Note: Nitroglycerin may relieve esophageal spasm
Peptic ulcer or gastritis	Epigastric pain worse approximately 3 hours after eating Relieved by antacids, not exertionally related
Gallbladder disease	Right upper quadrant abdominal pain and tenderness. Not exertionally related
Psychologic	
Psychoneuroses	Panic disorders associated with hyperventilation Not exertionally related
Psychosomatic complaints	

CARDIOVASCULAR DISORDERS	
Coronary Artery Disease	
Fixed atherosclerotic disease	Exercise-induced angina
Prinzmetal's angina	Angina at rest. Transient ST elevation
Mixed angina	Elements of exertional angina plus vasospastic angina (cold-induced, emotion-induced, variable threshold angina)
Syndrome X	Typical angina without angiographic evidence of epicardial coronary artery disease or spasm. Presumably due to small vessel abnormality
Aortic Stenosis	Pain is typical of angina. Typical systolic ejection murmur. Delayed carotid upstrokes
Hypertrophic obstructive cardiomyopathy	Pain may be typical of angina. Characteristic murmurs, changes with maneuvers. Brisk carotid upstrokes
Primary myocardial disease	Pain may mimic angina
Pericarditis	Pain is sharper. Pleuritic component to pain. Pain worse with lying down, better with sitting up. Friction rub
Dissecting aortic aneurysm	Pain sharp, tearing, prolonged; often occurs in back or interscapular areas. Check for unequal pulses
Mitral valve prolapse syndrome	Transient pain, not necessarily related to exertion. Midsystolic click-murmur on physical exam

PULMONARY DISORDERS	
Pulmonary embolus, infarction	Tachypnea, dyspnea, cough, pleuritic pain Signs of RV failure if embolus is massive
Pulmonary hypertension	Pain may be exertional and mimic angina Signs of RV failure
Pneumothorax	Sudden onset of pain and dyspnea. Pain may have pleuritic component. Percussion reveals hyperinflation. Tracheal shift
Pleuritis	Pain is sharp and exacerbated by inspiration
Intrathoracic tumor	Not exertional

Table 2. Typical Features of Angina Pectoris

Clinical History
    Description
        Heavy, pressing, squeezing, or burning chest discomfort
    Location
        Substernal, anterior chest with or without radiation
    Duration
        >15 seconds, <15 minutes
    Radiation
        Jaw, arms (left>right), back, epigastrium, neck
    Precipitating factors
        Cold, exertion, anxiety, meals
    Associated symptoms
        Breathlessness, fatigue, nausea, palpitations, diaphoresis
    Pain relief
        Resting in a standing or sitting position; nitroglycerin, usually takes 1 to 5 minutes
    Associated risk factors
        Age, sex, cigarette smoking, hypertension, hypercholesterolemia, positive family history
        for atherosclerotic heart disease, diabetes mellitus

Physical Examination
    Physical findings present chronically
        Xanthelasma and xanthomas, carotid or femoral bruits, hypertension
    Physical findings present during active ischemia
        Cold and clammy skin, diaphoresis, transient S_4 gallops, transient mitral regurgitation murmur,
        pulsus alternans, transient precordial bulge, tachycardia, transient hypertension, paradoxical
        splitting of S_2
    Physical findings that suggest chest pain is not due to angina pectoris
        Tender precordium, systolic murmur consistent with mitral valve prolapse, a marfanoid body
        habitus, which increases the likelihood that chest pain is due to aortic dissection

Angina pectoris often abates within 1/2 to 2 minutes after the patient takes a nitroglycerin tablet. However, esophageal spasm, a condition that can cause chest pain, may also be relieved by the administration of nitroglycerin. Pain relieved when the patient leans forward or that limits respiratory excursion is generally not due to angina pectoris; it is more characteristic of pericarditis.

An assessment of cardiac risk factors can be helpful when evaluating patients with chest pain. Angina pectoris is a very unlikely cause of chest pain in patients in their 20s; it is a more likely explanation for chest pain in patients in their 60s. Similarly, a positive family history of heart disease or a diagnosis of diabetes mellitus, hyperlipidemia, hypertension, or cigarette smoking increases the chances that a patient with chest pain is suffering from angina pectoris. Young women who smoke cigarettes and use oral contraceptives have an increased risk of ischemic heart disease; in this group of patients with chest pain, the diagnosis of angina pectoris or myocardial ischemia should be seriously considered.

THE PHYSICAL EXAMINATION

In the absence of an active episode of chest pain there are physical findings that aid in differentiating ischemic chest pain from chest pain due to other causes. Xanthomas, if present, suggest hyperlipidemia and increase the likelihood that the patient has coronary artery disease (CAD). Carotid or renal bruits suggest the presence of peripheral vascular disease; if the peripheral arteries have atherosclerotic lesions, it is likely that the coronary arteries are also involved. As noted, hypertension is a risk factor for CAD and increases the likelihood that the patient has ischemia-related chest pain.

There may be transient physical findings during an attack of angina. The skin is typically cold and clammy, and the patient is often diaphoretic. S_3 (uncommon) and S_4 (common) diastolic gallops are sometimes heard during an attack of angina pectoris. A transient systolic murmur, which may result from ischemic papillary muscle dysfunction, is a helpful finding, if present.

Other physical findings that suggest chest pain secondary to ischemia are pulsus alternans, a precordial bulge (best appreciated if the patient is in the left lateral position), elevated blood pressure and heart rate, and a paradoxically split-second heart sound. Although these findings are not always present during angina pectoris, their transient presence during an episode of chest pain is diagnostically very helpful.[1]

Other physical signs suggest that chest pain is not angina pectoris. A tender area over the precordium that reproduces the chest pain when palpated suggests pain of musculoskeletal origin. A murmur of mitral valve insufficiency and/or a systolic click suggests mitral valve prolapse, a condition that can cause angina-like chest pain. A marfanoid body habitus should raise the suspicion that aortic dissection underlies chest pain. A typical systolic murmur and delayed carotid upstroke suggest significant aortic valve stenosis, which can cause angina.

SYNDROME X

"Syndrome X" refers to chest pain that suggests angina but occurs in the presence of angiographically patent coronary vessels and in the absence of spasm of the large epicardial coronaries. Some patients with this syndrome are thought to have an inadequate vasodilator reserve and do not exhibit a normal increase in coronary flow or a normal reduction in coronary vascular resistance during atrial pacing. The defect is thought to reside in small resistance vessels which cannot be seen on coronary angiography.

Beyond this broad description, there is no consensus on a basic definition of Syndrome X.[1a] The chest pain may or may not be due to myocardial ischemia. Several abnormalities have been associated with Syndrome X, including a positive exercise ECG, abnormal myocardial perfusion or energy metabolism measured with nuclear techniques, and abnormal wall motion during stress. While there is no precise definition, the prognosis of patients with Syndrome X is excellent. If psychiatric, musculoskeletal, and gastrointestinal causes of chest pain are excluded, atrial therapy with nitrates or calcium-channel blockers may provide symptomatic relief.[2]

INITIAL MANAGEMENT OF PATIENTS WITH CHEST PAIN

Most patients evaluated for chest pain are seen initially in a physician's office or an emergency room. Following the history and physical examination, a decision as to additional evaluation and therapy must be made (Fig. 1). The information gathered from the history and physical examination may allow the physician to exclude the diagnosis of angina pectoris with no further investigation. For example, the chest pain may clearly be due to a recently acquired chest-wall bruise. A second possible decision is that the chest pain may be due to angina pectoris; in this case, further diagnostic evaluation is necessary. A third possibility is that the chest pain is definitely angina pectoris. In this case, the next step is to classify the condition as either chronic stable (mild or severe) angina pectoris or unstable angina pectoris. Chronic stable angina pectoris is present in patients whose chest pain has remained unchanged in terms of severity, frequency, and duration over a period of several weeks to several months. Mild angina pectoris typically occurs only after unusual exertion and does not require the patient to alter lifestyle to prevent the pain. Severe chronic stable angina occurs frequently and causes the patient to modify daily routine in order to exclude strenuous activities.

When seen for the first time, patients with mild chronic stable angina usually do not require hospitalization, and evaluation and treatment can be performed on an outpatient basis. Patients with severe chronic stable angina, when seen for the first time, may or may not require hospitalization for evaluation and treatment. The decision to hospitalize depends on the severity of the disease and must be made on an individual basis. Certainly, patients having 5 to 10 daily episodes of angina pectoris precipitated by very minimal exertion would be most safely evaluated in the hospital.

Patients categorized by the history and physical exam as having unstable angina pectoris should be hospitalized. There is no precise definition of unstable angina that is universally accepted. However, all definitions have a common concern; the state of blood supply to the

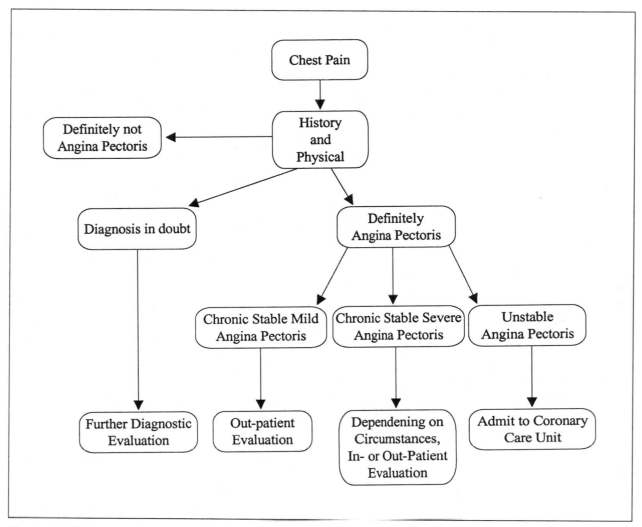

Figure 1. *Initial management strategy for patients with chest pain.*

myocardium is tenuous, and myocardial infarction is likely to follow if no treatment is instituted. Features common to all definitions of unstable angina include new onset of angina; more severe, prolonged or frequent episodes of angina superimposed on chronic stable angina; and angina occurring at rest.

Differentiating chest pain due to myocardial ischemia and myocardial infarction from chest pain due to other causes is one of the most difficult problems in clinical medicine (Table 1). Because the number of patients complaining of chest pain is large, it is impractical to admit all of them to coronary-care units for further cardiac evaluation. However, to send home a

patient actually suffering from a myocardial infarction or unstable angina with a diagnosis of chest pain of noncardiac origin can be a fatal mistake. Thus, one must have a low threshold for admitting patients when there is any reasonable doubt as to the correct diagnosis. An important point to remember is that patients with an acute myocardial infarction often have a vague feeling of uneasiness that is difficult for them to describe. For most people, an emergency visit is not a regular event, and the fact that they felt worried enough to come to an emergency room is itself an important sign that something is very wrong, whether or not the problem is well-stated.

LIMITATIONS OF THE HISTORY AND PHYSICAL EXAMINATION

Many important decisions about the evaluation and treatment of patients with angina pectoris are made on the basis of the initial history and physical exam. For this reason, it is important to be aware of how accurately these tools can reflect the presence and degree of coronary artery disease. Even the most skillfully and carefully conducted clinical history has limitations.[3,4] In a series of 188 patients classified clinically as having unstable angina pectoris, Alison et al[5] found that 10.6% had normal coronary arteries when coronary angiography was performed. Similar proportions of patients with normal coronary arteries have been found in other series of patients with the clinical diagnosis of unstable angina pectoris.[6,7]

At the other end of the spectrum are patients with silent myocardial ischemia. Some patients with severe CAD and frequent episodes of myocardial ischemia can be asymptomatic and beyond diagnosis by the clinical history.

Thus, classification of patients with angina pectoris from the history and physical examination may lead to inaccuracies in some cases. However, in spite of their shortcomings, the history and physical examination remain the most frequently used screening tests in cardiac diagnosis and, when properly done, are helpful in diagnosing and staging most patients with angina pectoris.

LABORATORY TESTS

Patients classified as having angina pectoris should undergo further studies to confirm the diagnosis and to stage the extent of their disease. Contemporary cardiology now offers the physician many noninvasive and invasive cardiac diagnostic procedures for this purpose. A proper understanding of the information that can be obtained from each of the available procedures, as well as their limitations, is necessary if the physician is to choose the proper test or combination of tests for each patient.

As shown in Figure 2, angina pectoris begins with a decrease in coronary blood supply usually caused by a stenotic lesion. Coronary arteriography allows visualization of the coronary artery and the extent of stenosis. Thallium-201 imaging is a measure of the amount of blood passing through a stenotic lesion, relative to blood passing through the remainder of the heart. Occasionally, regions of myocardium perfused by severely stenosed coronary arteries can have normal perfusion — perhaps because enough blood is passing through the stenosis to meet the regional myocardial oxygen demands, or perhaps because blood is reaching the area through collateral vessels. Thallium-201 imaging will detect the adequacy of perfusion to a region. Electrocardiography detects the electrical events associated with myocardial ischemia, which appear as ST-segment depression or elevation. Regional wall motion abnormalities that occur when myocardial tissue becomes ischemic can be detected and measured by M-mode and 2-dimensional echocardiography, radionuclide ventriculography, and gated magnetic resonance imaging techniques. Thus, the many tests available to the physician provide diagnostic and quantitative information in different forms. (See individual chapters addressing these tests.)

Because cardiologic diagnostic studies are expensive and in some cases are associated with risk to the patient, care and skill must be used when choosing the most appropriate means of evaluating each patient.

RESTING ELECTROCARDIOGRAM

The resting electrocardiogram should be a part of the evaluation of any patient with suspected or proven angina pectoris. The presence of Q waves indicates an old myocardial infarction, which is usually, although not always, secondary to CAD. (Emboli or trauma can also cause myocardial infarction.) Other abnormalities, such as intraventricular conduction delays, atrial or ventricular arrhythmias, or ST-T-wave changes are not specific and can be related to conditions other than coronary disease. However, in the presence of chest pain, they increase the suspicion that the pain is related to myocardial ischemia. Occasionally during an attack of angina pectoris, there will be transient ST-segment depression, which is a very specific finding for myocardial ischemia. A normal ECG, either during chest pain or between episodes of pain, does not exclude myocardial ischemia and is a frequent finding in patients with angina pectoris. Transient ST-segment elevation associated with rest pain is observed in Prinzmetal's variant angina due to vasospasm.

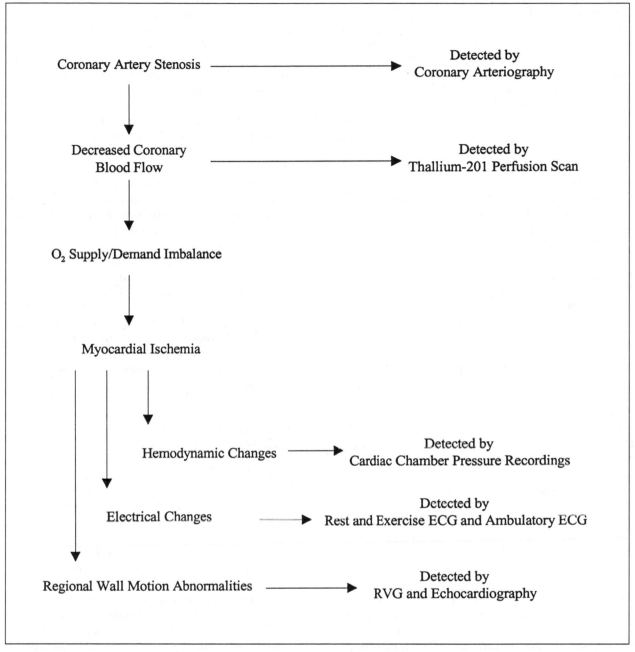

Figure 2. *Schematic showing the pathophysiology of myocardial ischemia and the type of information recorded by the various cardiac diagnostic techniques. RVG=Radionuclide ventriculography.*

EXERCISE STRESS TESTING

Patients categorized as having suspected or known stable CAD should undergo exercise stress testing as a part of their evaluation. In patients with chest pain of uncertain etiology, the exercise stress test is used as a diagnostic tool.

An exercise stress test which is positive for myocardial ischemia is good evidence that chest pain is angina pectoris. (See also Chapter 6.) A negative test does not entirely exclude angina pectoris but makes the diagnosis unlikely. Exercise tests are not simply negative or positive. A stress test that is negative after 10 minutes of vigorous exercise is more likely to exclude significant CAD than a "negative" exercise test that is terminated after only 2 or 3 minutes of exercise. "Positive" also encompasses a wide range of results. Stress tests that are positive with chest pain and 3 to 4 millimeters of ST depression after only 2 to 3 minutes of exercise are more likely to represent significant CAD than positive tests with 1 millimeter of upsloping ST depression after 10 minutes of exercise. The latter tests are more likely to represent false-positive results.

An exercise stress test must be interpreted in the context of the information obtained from the history and physical examination, because its predictive value varies with the population being studied (Bayes' theorem). In a population with a statistically low incidence of CAD, such as premenopausal nonsmoking women with chest pain, the predictive ability is very low.[8] However, in studies of patients with a high likelihood of CAD, such as men over the age of 60 with multiple risk factors, the predictive value is higher. Thus, in the latter group, a positive stress test is likely to be associated with the presence of CAD, while a negative test is likely to reflect the absence of CAD.

In patients with a diagnosis of angina pectoris, exercise stress testing can provide prognostic information and information about the extent of disease. The degree of positivity is related to the extent of CAD.[9,10] A patient with a very positive test (e.g., severe ST depression occurring early during exercise and exercise-induced hypotension) and, therefore, a high probability of left main or severe multivessel CAD should be considered for cardiac catheterization and possible revascularization. Alternatively, a patient who develops only 1 millimeter of ST depression after 10 minutes of exercise has a low likelihood of left-main or 3-vessel coronary disease and may not need to undergo cardiac catheterization.

Angina pectoris is a poor marker of the extent and severity of CAD. Many patients with known CAD and angina pectoris have frequent episodes of "silent ischemia." In this group of patients, exercise stress testing is particularly important for estimating disease severity. (See Chapter 14.)

AMBULATORY (HOLTER) ELECTROCARDIOGRAPHY

Ambulatory electrocardiography has been available for almost 30 years for the detection of cardiac arrhythmias. Recently, technological improvements have expanded the capabilities of Holter monitoring, and it is now possible to continuously record changes in ST segments. ST-segment depression is associated with myocardial ischemia and can be recorded during symptomatic angina pectoris or during episodes of asymptomatic or "silent ischemia." An ambulatory ECG can be useful for diagnostic purposes in patients with chest pain suggestive of Prinzmetal's angina and may establish the diagnosis in such cases. A second indication for this test is for diagnosis of chest pain in patients who are unable to perform a stress test. A third indication is the evaluation of postinfarction patients with angina, in order to look for a correlation between ventricular arrhythmias and ST depression — a combination believed to be associated with increased mortality. A fourth indication is to assess the efficacy of antianginal therapy.[11] Indications for ambulatory ECG may expand in the future. Evidence is accumulating that the technique may be useful for predicting future cardiac events, for the evaluation of asymptomatic patients with CAD, and for the diagnosis of patients with chest pain.[12]

THALLIUM-201 MYOCARDIAL PERFUSION SCINTIGRAPHY

Thallium-201 perfusion imaging is usually done in conjunction with exercise stress testing. (See also Chapters 5 and 6.) While exercise electrocardiography depends on ischemia-related electrical changes, thallium-201 depends on differences in myocardial perfusion. Areas of the myocardium supplied by stenotic vessels do not receive as much blood as surrounding, normally perfused areas and appear as thallium image defects or "cold spots." Infarcted myocardium receives very little blood and also appears as a "cold spot" on a thallium image. Thallium defects due to ischemia or infarct can be differentiated when repeat scans are obtained 3 hours or more after the initial exercise images. Infarcts will still appear as thallium defects, while defects due to reversible ischemia will "fill in" due to the redistribution phenomenon.

Thallium-201 stress imaging has a sensitivity of 85% to 90% and a specificity of 65% to 70% for the detection of significant coronary artery disease. Exercise testing without thallium-201 is generally reported to have a somewhat lower sensitivity and a lower specificity. The value of combining diagnostic techniques was demonstrated in a multicenter study that evaluated thallium-201 imaging and exercise ECG. Ritchie et al[12a] demonstrated that in a group of 190 patients, 148 of whom had significant CAD, the exercise ECG detected 73% of the patients with significant disease, and thallium-201 imaging detected 76%. Thus, sensitivities were similar; specificity was also found to be similar: 86% for exercise ECG and 88% for thallium-201 imaging. However, when the 2 studies were combined, sensitivity was significantly improved to 91%, better than either test alone. Specificity was not improved.

Due to the extra cost of adding thallium-201 imaging to an exercise stress test, it should not be routinely ordered. If a patient has a strongly positive exercise ECG, thallium-201 imaging adds little diagnostic information. One of the most common indications for thallium-201 perfusion imaging is the evaluation of patients with an abnormal resting ECG. In the presence of abnormal resting ST segments due to left bundle branch block, left ventricular hypertrophy, digoxin, or conduction abnormalities, the diagnostic value of exercise electrocardiography is greatly decreased, and thallium-201 imaging should be performed when exercise testing is done. Thallium-201 imaging is also indicated in patients undergoing evaluation for chest pain and for those who have equivocal ECG changes with exercise.

There are also indications for thallium-201 imaging in patients with known coronary artery disease. In patients with severe CAD, it is generally believed that resting coronary blood flow is normal in the absence of angina pectoris or an acute myocardial infarction, however, this may not always be true.[13,14] In patients with severe CAD, some defects that appear on initial images following injections at rest fill in on delayed images, suggesting decreased perfusion at rest. Although it is not clear what the best course is for patients with resting perfusion abnormalities, it is likely that they will benefit most from intensive medical therapy and should be strongly considered for revascularization surgery.

Patients with very severe left ventricular dysfunction and congestive heart failure due to diffuse CAD generally are not recommended for coronary artery bypass surgery because of the high mortality rate. This is particularly true in the absence of angina pectoris. Coronary angiography and left ventriculography usually reveal severe 3-vessel coronary artery disease with diffuse hypokinesis or akinesis. However, how much of the left ventricular dysfunction is due to scar tissue and how much to reversible ischemia is difficult to determine. Thallium-201 perfusion imaging that demonstrates perfusion defects that fill in over time or upon reinjection suggests reversibly ischemic tissue. If extensive areas of reversibly ischemic tissue can be demonstrated in this group of very ill patients, coronary artery bypass surgery may result in clinical improvement.[15]

Thallium-201 perfusion imaging can be useful in the evaluation of a stenosis of uncertain hemodynamic significance noted on coronary angiography. A lesion of 40% to 60% may or may not limit flow with exercise. A corresponding thallium-201 perfusion defect with exercise would support the hemodynamic significance of the lesion, while a negative scan would be good evidence that the lesion was not responsible for flow limitations or, by inference, ischemia.

Restenosis of coronary artery lesions following initially successful percutaneous transluminal angioplasty occurs in 1 of 4 patients. Early detection of restenosis frequently leads to second and even third or fourth attempts at successful angioplasty. Stress thallium-201 exams can be useful in detecting restenosis by revealing ischemia in the distribution of dilated coronary arteries.

For patients unable to exercise adequately, thallium examinations can be performed with dipyridamole. Dipyridamole blocks the uptake and degradation of adenosine, thus increasing the levels of adenosine, which is a coronary vasodilator. The vasodilation results in large increases in blood flow to myocardium supplied by normal coronary arteries. Blood flow to myocardium supplied by stenosed coronary arteries is either unchanged or decreases. The imbalance of flow to the heart can be detected by thallium imaging, and redistribution images can be used to differentiate ischemic from infarcted tissue. Image quality and the sensitivity and specificity of dipyridamole thallium imaging are comparable to results obtained during exercise thallium-stress testing.[16]

EXERCISE ECHOCARDIOGRAPHY

Exercise echocardiography is evolving rapidly and is employed as a regular diagnostic technique in many medical centers. Like radionuclide ventriculography, echocardiography detects changes in regional wall motion that occur during myocardial ischemia. The stress used to induce myocardial ischemia can be atrial pacing, pharmacologic (dopamine or dipyridamole), cold pressor, or, most commonly, exercise. Using upright bicycle stress, echocardiograms can be obtained during peak exercise; if treadmill stress is used, echocardiograms are obtained in the supine position immediately after exercise. Most exercise imaging is done with a 2-dimensional echocardiogram. The normal response to exercise is for all segments of the myocardium to become hyperdynamic. Myocardial segments that become hypokinetic or akinetic during exercise are consistent with ischemia. A major advantage to exercise echocardiography is that wall thickening, the most specific marker of myocardial ischemia, is evaluated. The major problem is the difficulty in obtaining adequate images. It is likely that exercise echocardiography will continue to evolve and eventually will be used routinely for the evaluation of cardiac patients.

AMBULATORY VENTRICULAR FUNCTION MONITORING

It is now possible to continuously monitor left ventricular function in patients using an ambulatory ventricular function monitor ("VEST"). The VEST can be worn by patients and is a nonimaging nuclear detector. Technetium-99m-labeled red blood cells are utilized and the detector, positioned over the heart, collects beat-to-beat variations in counts. Gated counts are summed over 15 to 30 seconds, and a continuous global left ventricular ejection fraction is reported. Patients can wear the VEST for a period of 4 to 6 hours. Experience with this new device is limited, but several clinical applications are possible. First, the VEST may be useful for the evaluation of patients with chest pain of unknown etiology. It appears that for the detection of myocardial ischemia, the VEST is more sensitive than stress or ambulatory electrocardiography. Second, the functional significance of coronary artery obstructions can be evaluated. Patients with CAD and multiple severe obstructions are more likely to experience large decreases in left ventricular ejection fraction with exercise. Third, data from a 4 to 6-hour VEST examination may provide important prognostic information that can help guide the therapy of patients with CAD. Fourth, VEST information

can help define the limits of exercise for patients with CAD. Fifth, VEST data can be used to assess the efficacy of antianginal therapy.

CARDIAC CATHETERIZATION

With the development of percutaneous transluminal coronary angioplasty (PTCA), cardiac catheterization evolved from a purely diagnostic tool to a therapeutic device. (See Chapters 9 and 17.) Cardiac catheterization is indicated for diagnostic reasons in patients with chest pain and to evaluate patients with known coronary artery disease. As noted earlier, most patients with chest pain can be diagnosed with a thorough history, physical examination, and noninvasive testing. However, in some patients, the results of noninvasive testing are equivocal. For example, some patients are unable to perform a stress test due to physical limitations. In this group, cardiac catheterization may be indicated to provide a diagnosis or at least to exclude CAD as a cause of chest pain.

Patients with severe angina pectoris that cannot be controlled with medications are candidates for revascularization with either surgery or angioplasty. This group needs catheterization to define coronary anatomy. Patients with strongly positive stress tests frequently undergo cardiac catheterization to exclude left-main CAD. Although it is difficult to predict cardiac events on the basis of coronary anatomy, knowledge about the coronary anatomy can be helpful in making therapeutic decisions. Patients with a left-main stenosis, a proximal left anterior descending coronary stenosis, or multiple lesions in all 3 major coronary arteries, are often considered for surgery. Lesser disease involving 1 or 2 vessels is more often treated medically or with coronary angioplasty.

Cardiac catheterization provides anatomic information and should only be interpreted in the context of other data derived from the history, physical exam, and noninvasive testing.

NATURAL HISTORY AND PATHOPHYSIOLOGY OF ANGINA PECTORIS

NATURAL HISTORY OF PATIENTS WITH ANGINA PECTORIS

The goals of therapy for angina pectoris are to relieve symptoms and to prolong life. To evaluate the effect of therapy on longevity, one must know the natural history of untreated angina pectoris. If coronary arteriography has been performed, natural-history studies of patients with angina pectoris that are based on coronary anatomy can be useful when dealing with individual patients. Follow-up studies in the 1960s, before the widespread use of current medical and surgical therapies, showed that patients with 1-vessel disease had an annual mortality rate of <4%. In patients with 2-vessel disease, this figure increased to 7% to 10%, and in those with three-vessel disease, to 10% to 12%. Patients with left-main coronary artery obstructions had a yearly mortality of 15% to 25%. Left ventricular dysfunction worsened the prognosis.[17]

Often, patients with angina pectoris are managed without knowledge of the coronary anatomy. In such patients, natural-history studies based on the clinical history or noninvasive criteria can be helpful. An example is the subset of patients with unstable angina pectoris. Using a definition of unstable angina that includes both accelerating symptoms and ST-segment changes during chest pain, Mulcahy et al[18] followed 101 patients treated with only bed rest and sublingual nitrates; they found a 9% rate of nonfatal myocardial infarction and a 4% incidence of death within the first 28 days. At the end of 1 year, the incidence of nonfatal myocardial infarction was 12%, and the incidence of cardiovascular death was 10%. Natural-history studies such as this are helpful as guidelines when making diagnostic and therapeutic decisions for patients presenting with unstable angina pectoris and unknown coronary anatomy.

PATHOPHYSIOLOGY OF ANGINA PECTORIS

Atherosclerotic coronary artery disease results from a buildup of lipid, foam cells, smooth muscle hyperplasia, fibrous tissue, and dystrophic calcification within the intima of the coronary vasculature, resulting in luminal narrowing. The luminal narrowing compromises blood flow to the heart, leading to myocardial ischemia and the clinical syndromes of angina pectoris, silent ischemia, myocardial infarction, or sudden death. Risk factors for the development of atherosclerotic heart disease include hypercholesterolemia, decreased high-density lipoprotein levels, tobacco smoking, hypertension, diabetes, male sex, older age, family history of CAD, obesity, and a sedentary lifestyle.

While fixed narrowing of the coronary arteries is due to atherosclerotic plaque, variable obstruction of the coronary arteries may occur with increased coronary artery tone and coronary vasospasm. Figure 3 shows the spectrum of coronary artery disease. On the left side of the figure is Patient A, who suffers from fixed atherosclerotic narrowing. This patient is likely to experience typical effort- or exercise-induced angina pectoris associated with ST-segment depression on the ECG. On the right-hand side of the figure is Patient C, who suffers from pure coronary artery vasospasm. This patient typically has focal vasospasm of a segment of a coronary artery and experiences angina at rest with transient ST elevation on the ECG (Prinzmetal's angina). Between these 2 ends of the spectrum are patients who experience mixed angina pectoris with elements of both exertion-related angina and rest angina (patient B). Clinical indications that a patient has a vasospastic component to angina pectoris include emotion-induced or cold-induced angina and variable-threshold exercise-induced angina. Such a patient has a mixture of fixed atherosclerotic narrowing plus vasospasm on top of the narrowing. Variable-threshold exercise-induced angina results when variable degrees of vasospasm alter the degree of narrowing of a coronary artery with a degree of fixed atherosclerosis. For example, a patient with a fixed atherosclerotic narrowing of 70% of a coronary lumen may be able to exercise on a treadmill for 7 minutes before developing angina on 1 day; on a second day, when the patient's vasomotor tone is high, and his 70% narrowing is now a 90% narrowing due to vasospasm on top of the atherosclerotic plaque, he may only be able to exercise for 3 minutes before experiencing angina.

What factors determine coronary tone? It has been appreciated that endothelial-derived relaxing factor (EDRF), believed to be nitric oxide,[18a] is released from the endothelium into the smooth muscle of the vessel to allow vascular relaxation. EDRF release is stimulated by exposure of normal coronary arteries to acetylcholine (Ach). In patients with atherosclerosis, local administration of Ach does not result in normal EDRF release, due to an abnormality or destruction of the endothelium, and vasoconstriction occurs instead of vasodilation. Thus, patients with atherosclerosis may have an abnormality in EDRF production or release which could predispose areas of the

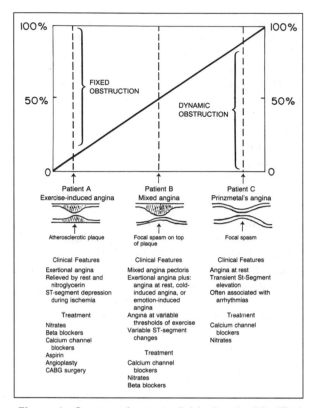

Figure 3. *Causes of myocardial ischemia. Modified from Muller J. Cardiology Reference Book, 2nd Edition. New York: CoMedica, Inc; 1984.*

coronary vasculature to spasm. In addition, an endothelial derived vasoconstricting agent (endothelin) has recently been discovered. Other possible explanations for changes in coronary tone include alterations in the sympathetic nervous system, spasm induced by thromboxane, and spasm induced by serotonin. Also, some patients with vasospasm in other arteries, such as those with Raynaud's phenomenon, have been observed to demonstrate coronary vasospasm. Finally, there may be interactions that occur between platelets and the endothelial wall and contribute to coronary vasospasm.

Coronary angioscopy has provided direct visualization of in vivo coronary arteries in patients and has helped to clarify the pathophysiology of coronary artery disease. Various coronary syndromes have been observed to correlate with specific lesions observed by coronary angioscopy. Forrester et al[19] demonstrated that the coronary arteries in patients diagnosed as

having stable angina had a smooth endothelial surface free of thrombus; those in patients with accelerating angina had ulcerations and a roughened endothelial lining; and those in patients with unstable rest angina often had thrombus. Intravascular ultrasound has also expanded our understanding of coronary lesions.

An understanding of the pathophysiology of myocardial ischemia must take into account that myocardial ischemia represents an imbalance of oxygen supply to the heart and the oxygen demand of the heart. Myocardial ischemia is exacerbated by decreases in oxygen supply and increases in oxygen demand. Conversely, antianginal therapy works primarily by improving oxygen supply or reducing oxygen demand.

FACTORS THAT INFLUENCE MYOCARDIAL OXYGEN SUPPLY

Delivery of oxygen to the myocardium depends on both the amount of blood flowing through the coronary arteries and the ability of the myocardial cells to extract oxygen from the blood. Unlike other organs of the body, the heart has the unique property of having nearly maximal oxygen extraction at rest; thus, there is little capability for increasing myocardial oxygen supply by increasing myocardial oxygen extraction. Myocardial oxygen supply can be adjusted to meet oxygen demands by changing coronary blood flow, which can and does fluctuate, depending on the needs of the myocardium.

The amount of blood flowing through the coronary arteries depends on both the perfusion pressure and the resistance across the coronary vascular bed:

$$CBF = \frac{Ao\ pressure - RA\ pressure}{Coronary\ vascular\ resistance}$$

where CBF = coronary blood flow; Ao = aortic; and RA = right atrial. Because of the high intramural pressures during systole, resistance to flow is high and relatively little blood is delivered to the left ventricular myocardium during systole. Most flow occurs during diastole; therefore, aortic diastolic pressure and the duration of diastole are important determinants of myocardial blood flow. Factors that increase the aortic diastolic pressure or prolong the time spent in diastole will increase the blood supply to the myocardium. Conversely, factors that reduce diastolic pressure or, as is true of tachycardia, shorten the time the ventricle spends in diastole, reduce the blood supply to the myocardium.

A second determinant of myocardial oxygen supply is coronary artery resistance. The coronary arteries are not rigid pipes; they are flexible tubes that exist in a state of tone. Relaxation of the vessels will decrease resistance to flow and increase coronary blood flow, while contraction (or spasm) of the vessels will increase resistance and decrease coronary blood flow. The factors that control coronary vascular resistance are incompletely understood. External compression of the vessels is important, particularly during systole, when the high intramyocardial pressure increases resistance almost to the point of stopping flow. During diastole, the end-diastolic ventricular pressure, if elevated, can increase intramyocardial pressure and, therefore, increase resistance and decrease flow through the coronary arteries.

Other influences that control coronary vascular resistance include neural, hormonal, local metabolic factors, EDRF and endothelin. Present and future investigations should increase our knowledge of the mechanism and relative contributions of these factors and lead to therapeutic interventions aimed at reducing coronary vascular resistance and increasing coronary blood flow.

FACTORS THAT INFLUENCE MYOCARDIAL OXYGEN DEMAND

Unlike the skeletal muscles, the heart depends almost exclusively on aerobic metabolism for its energy. Myocardial oxygen consumption is thus almost identical to the total metabolic requirements of the heart. There are 3 major determinants of myocardial oxygen consumption[20] (Fig. 4). The first is systolic wall tension development, which, when increased, increases myocardial oxygen demand. Systolic wall tension is directly related to systolic arterial pressure and intraventricular radius and inversely related to wall thickness. The second factor is heart rate, which, when faster, increases myocardial oxygen demand. The third major factor is contractility. Increased contractility leads to increased myocardial oxygen demand. A frequently used noninvasive index of myocardial oxygen demand is the "double product," which is obtained by multiplying the heart rate by the systolic blood

pressure. Inaccuracies arise when using this index because it does not consider contractility, intraventricular volume, or wall thickness.

TREATMENT OF ANGINA PECTORIS

When planning a treatment program, it is important to consider the factors that influence myocardial oxygen supply and those that influence myocardial oxygen demand. The ideal therapeutic regimen maximizes myocardial oxygen supply, minimizes myocardial oxygen demand, and is devoid of any adverse side effects.

Multiple treatment options exist for patients with angina pectoris. Over the past few years, treatment of angina pectoris has reduced patient symptomatology and improved survival. Choosing the best treatment or combination of treatment modalities for a given patient is an increasingly complicated task because of the many available options. Treatment goals should be to eradicate episodes of myocardial ischemia, decrease the progression of disease, and prevent future cardiac events.

GENERAL TREATMENT MEASURES

In all patients presenting with angina pectoris, there are some general measures that should be instituted (Table 3). Although the impact of altering risk factors is controversial, such measures should be recommended to all patients. A low-cholesterol, low-saturated fat diet should be started, particularly by patients with elevated serum lipids. There is accumulating evidence that reduction in serum cholesterol can prevent future cardiac events in patients with angina pectoris and perhaps cause atherosclerotic lesions to regress.

Hypertension, if present, should be controlled. There are 2 reasons to correct an abnormal blood pressure: first, to alter a risk factor and possibly slow the progress of coronary artery disease; and second, to decrease myocardial oxygen demand, which depends, in part, on the systolic blood pressure. Control becomes particularly important in severely hypertensive patients presenting with unstable angina pectoris.

Patients who smoke cigarettes should be encouraged to stop. It is clear that cigarette smoking leads to an increased incidence of atheroscle-

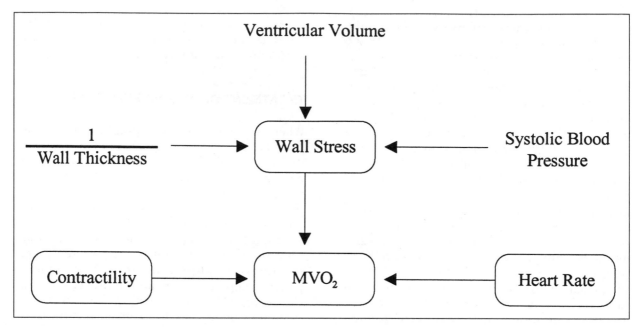

Figure 4. *Major determinants of myocardial oxygen demand (MVO_2).*

rotic heart disease. Thus, 1 reason to encourage patients to discontinue smoking is to reverse — or at least slow — the progress of atherosclerosis. A second reason is to halt the acute adverse effects of cigarette smoking on the heart. Nicotine released in cigarette smoke causes a release of endogenous catecholamines, which in turn step up myocardial oxygen demand by causing increases in heart rate, blood pressure, and myocardial contractility. Catecholamines can also decrease coronary blood supply by stimulation of coronary artery alpha receptors, which results in coronary artery vasoconstriction. An additional adverse effect of nicotine-related catecholamine release is increased platelet aggregation. Carbon monoxide, abundant in cigarette smoke, increases blood levels of carboxyhemoglobin and decreases the capacity of the blood to deliver oxygen to myocardial tissue. Thus, it is not surprising that cigarette smoking leads to decreased exercise tolerance, as measured by treadmill testing.[21]

The effect of exercise on patients with angina pectoris remains a controversial issue. Certainly, exercise that precipitates angina pectoris should be discouraged. Patients with unstable angina pectoris should not exercise at all; they should be restricted to bed rest. Exercise increases myocardial oxygen demand, which may exceed myocardial oxygen supply and, thus, precipitate

angina pectoris in patients with CAD. Although it is agreed that a long-term exercise program can improve a patient's sense of well-being, its ability to slow or reverse atherosclerosis or to improve collateral blood supply to the myocardium remains unknown.

A study by Kramsch et al[22] demonstrated a reduction in coronary atherosclerosis in exercised monkeys fed an atherogenic diet, as compared with sedentary monkeys also fed an atherogenic diet. Redwood et al[23] showed that patients with chronic stable angina participating in exercise programs can exercise for a longer period of time before developing angina pectoris. In part, this effect is due to the ability of the heart to maintain peripheral muscle oxygenation at a lower myocardial oxygen demand. This effect may be due to a decrease in systemic vascular resistance secondary to exercise and the ability of trained muscles to increase their oxygen extraction efficiency. The improved exercise tolerance following exercise training may also be due to an increase in collateral flow and, thus, an increase in oxygen supply.[24]

At present, exercise can be prescribed to angina patients at minimal risk with the promise that, at the very least, it can increase their sense of well-being. Before enrolling in an exercise program, the patient should have an exercise toler-

Table 3. General Treatment Measures for Patients With Angina Pectoris

Alter risk factors
   Lower cholesterol intake
   Control hypertension
   Discontinue smoking
   Lose weight
   Control diabetes mellitus
   Implement less stressful lifestyle
Avoid activity that precipitates angina pectoris
Exercise
Treat severe anemia
Treat hyperthyroidism

ance test to help determine the safety of such a program. Future studies should demonstrate whether or not exercise has an effect on collateral development and atherogenesis in humans.

Extensive experience with exercise stress testing has demonstrated the safety of exercise in patients with known or suspected coronary artery disease; the incidence of death or myocardial infarction during stress testing is less than 1 incident per 100,000 tests.

The risk that exercise will precipitate sudden death or a myocardial infarction is minimal. Therefore, particularly in cooperative patients, an exercise program can be an important component of a treatment program for angina pectoris.

Although it is difficult to alter patients' lifestyles, it is helpful to suggest that patients avoid stressful situations, particularly if these situations regularly precipitate angina pectoris.

Systemic conditions, such as severe anemia and hyperthyroidism, can worsen angina pectoris and should be treated if present.

NITRATES

Nitrates (Table 4) have been, and continue to be, the mainstay of pharmacologic treatment for angina pectoris. They are effective, relatively inexpensive, and are associated with very few side effects. Nitrates should be prescribed to patients with angina pectoris to relieve symptoms; there is no evidence that nitrates slow or reverse the progression of coronary artery disease or improve survival in patients with angina pectoris. Therefore, there is little reason to prescribe long-acting nitrates for asymptomatic patients unless they are experiencing episodes of silent myocardial ischemia.

Nitrates can be used to relieve an attack of angina pectoris or they can be used prophylactically before activities that predictably precipitate episodes of angina pectoris.

HEMODYNAMIC ACTIONS OF NITRATES

The major clinical benefit of nitrates for the treatment of angina pectoris is the result of relaxation of vascular smooth muscles. This effect is most pronounced in the venous circulation, where decreased venous tone decreases preload. This leads to decreased left ventricular volume and myocardial wall stress, a major determinant of myocardial oxygen demand, is reduced. To a lesser extent, nitrates reduce arterial tone and, therefore, afterload, which also reduces wall stress.

The clinical importance of nitrates' direct effect on the coronary vascular tone is controversial. Nitrates will dilate coronary stenoses, dilate coronary epicardial arteries, and prevent constriction of collateral vessels supplying ischemic myocardium.[25] Actions in the coronary vasculature can increase global and regional cardiac blood supply and may explain some of the benefits of nitrates in patients with angina pectoris.

In some patients, nitrates can have a detrimental effect. Decreased arterial tone, while beneficial for myocardial oxygen demand, can decrease coronary artery perfusion and, thus, myocardial oxygen supply. Therefore, caution should be observed when administering nitrates to patients with low blood pressure. Similarly, in patients with low falling pressures or preload, nitrates can further lower pressures and cause a dangerous decrease in cardiac output.

The effect of nitrates on the coronary vessels is less well understood than their effects on the peripheral vasculature. Cohn et al[26] showed that nitrates can increase flow to myocardium supplied by stenotic coronary arteries if the areas are also supplied by well-developed collateral vessels. The clinical importance of this increased flow, however, is not known. To the extent that coronary artery spasm contributes to atherosclerotic-related angina pectoris, nitrates may be helpful in relieving this spasm.

It is important to stress to patients that nitrates are not analgesics. Patients must be reassured that they will not develop a tolerance to the pain-relieving effects of intermittent therapy, and they should be encouraged to take nitrates whenever they experience angina pectoris.

Table 4. Dosage and Kinetics of Common Nitrate Preparations

MEDICATION	ROUTE OF ADMINISTRATION	RECOMMENDED DOSAGE (MG)	ONSET OF ACTION (MIN)	PEAK ACTION (MIN)	DURATION OF ACTION
Nitroglycerin					
	Sublingual	0.3-0.6		4-8	10-30 min
	lingual spray	0.4	2-5	4-8	10-30 min
	Buccal	1-3	2-5	4-10	30-300 † min
	Ointment (2%)	7.5-30	2-5	30-120	3-8 hr
	Transdermal Patches	7.5-10 mg/12 hr	30-60	60-180	8-12 hr
	Oral-extended release	2.6-6.5 mg	20-45	45-120	2-6 hr
Isosorbide Dinitrate					
	sublingual	2.5-10	5-20	15-60	45-120* min
	oral	10-40	15-45	15-60	2-6 hr ††
	slow release	40-80		45-120	8-12 hr
Isosorbide-5-Mononitrate	oral	20 mg			7-12 hr
Pentaerythritol tetranitrate	oral	40 mg	60	80-120	3-6 hr

† Effects persist as long as tablet is intact.
* Up to 3 to 4 hours in some studies.
†† Up to 8 hours in some studies.

BIOCHEMICAL/CELLULAR ACTIONS OF NITRATES

Recently, several discoveries have led to an understanding of nitrate actions at the cellular and molecular level. It is now realized that nitrates are metabolized to nitric oxide within vascular smooth muscle cells. Nitric oxide is EDRF, which may have efficacy in dilating coronary arteries with depressed endothelial function in conditions including coronary atherosclerosis and hypercholesterolemia. Thus, nitrates may act to restore EDRF depleted by disease and offset vasoconstrictor forces in the vessel walls. Debate continues over the importance of antiplatelet effects of nitrates, which may act to restore intrinsic antiplatelet and antithrombotic effects that are impaired in vascular endothelium damaged by the presence of coronary atherosclerosis.

One of the many functions of vascular endothelium is to regulate vascular tone. Endothelium-derived relaxing factor is a potent vasodilator released by the endothelium that is either nitric oxide or a compound that releases nitric oxide.[27] While treatment with nitroglycerin can replace EDRF in patients with nonfunctional endothelium due to atherosclerosis, hypertension, or diabetes mellitus, there are important differences between EDRF and nitroglycerin. EDRF will dilate all sizes of coronary vessels, while nitroglycerin has only minor effects on coronary microvessels <100 mm in diameter.[28] This property limits the effect of nitroglycerin on coronary flow but also prevents coronary steal. It appears that the smaller coronary vessels cannot convert nitroglycerin to nitric oxide.

Nitrates have substantial antiplatelet actions which may contribute to their effectiveness in the treatment of angina pectoris.[29] Nitrates are metabolized to nitric oxide, which activates platelet guanylate cyclase, and ultimately platelet aggregation is impaired.

NITRATE TOLERANCE

After many years of demonstrated antianginal efficacy with sublingual nitroglycerin, long-acting nitrate preparations were developed with the hope that even greater clinical benefits would result. However, it is now apparent that tolerance to the hemodynamic and antianginal effects develops rapidly with either isosorbide dinitrate 4 times per day or continuous applications of nitrate patches.[30] Tolerance is less likely to develop with twice-daily use of isosorbide-5-mononitrate.

While many questions remain, an understanding of the biochemical mechanism of nitrate action and nitrate tolerance is emerging. Nitrates are converted to nitric oxide (NO) in vascular smooth muscle cells. NO activates guanylate cyclase to produce cyclic guanosine 3', 5'-monophosphate (cGMP), which causes vasodilation. Although nitrate tolerance is incompletely understood, both intracellular mechanisms and systemic neurohumoral responses seem to be involved. The role of sulfhydryl groups in the development of nitrate tolerance has been the focus of many investigations. Sulfhydryl donors can partially reverse nitroglycerin-induced tolerance in patients. Among the sulfhydryl donors tested are N-acetyl cysteine, methionine, captopril, and cysteine. Very large doses of the above agents must be employed to be effective. If administration of sulfhydryl donors is to become clinically effective, more potent donors of sulfhydryl groups will have to be developed. However, this does not prove that intracellular sulfhydryl depletion is the reason for nitrate tolerance. Nonsulfhydryl compounds, such as hydralazine[31] and enalapril,[32] can also prevent the development of nitrate tolerance.

Systemic changes have been described during the development of nitrate tolerance and may partially contribute to the development of tolerance.[33] Nitrate rebound, which is difficult to explain with the sulfhydryl hypothesis, has been observed. Withdrawal of chronic nitrate therapy can result in a transient decrease in cardiac index, along with a transient increase in systemic and pulmonary pressures. During nitrate tolerance, several systemic biochemical changes have been noted. Increases in plasma volume, heart rate, plasma norepinephrine, renin activity, and body weight, along with decreases in renal blood flow, have all been observed with nitrate tolerance. Thus, systemic compensation to nitrate therapy may contribute to the development of nitrate tolerance.

While prevention of nitrate tolerance with sulfhydryl donors, such as acetylcystein, methionine, and captopril, is possible for the future,

the current approach to nitrate tolerance is to prescribe nitrates in a fashion that will not produce tolerance. The general principal is to provide daily nitrate-free intervals.

NITRATE PREPARATIONS

Nitrates are most effective when used to treat attacks of angina pectoris. The short-acting nitrates, either sublingual or oral spray nitroglycerin, are the most effective preparations because of the rapid onset of action. A second effective use of nitrates is prophylactic use prior to activities that predictably result in angina pectoris. For example, if a 1-block walk to a bus stop regularly precipitates angina pectoris, pretreatment with a nitrate preparation can prevent the attack. Depending on the predicted length of activity, a short- or longer-acting nitrate preparation can be prescribed. For patients with frequent or unpredictable episodes of angina pectoris, the longer-acting preparation can be helpful. However, because of tolerance to nitrate activity, long-term prophylaxis with nitrates is not always effective.

NITROGLYCERIN

The least expensive nitrate preparation and the drug of choice for an acute attack of angina pectoris is sublingual nitroglycerin. The usual dose is 0.3 to 0.6 mg. Patients with angina pectoris should be instructed to carry nitroglycerin with them at all times and to take the medication as soon as angina occurs. The onset of action is rapid and the effects persist for up to 30 minutes. If angina is not relieved, the dose may be repeated 1 or 2 times at 5-minute intervals. For more prolonged or unresponsive pain, patients should be instructed to seek medical attention. Because nitroglycerin decreases blood pressure, patients should be instructed to sit down when taking the medication, in order to avoid syncope. Nitroglycerin is light-sensitive and should be stored in dark containers. Nitroglycerin tablets should be discarded and replaced every 6 months. Buccal nitroglycerin can be given in a dose of up to 3 mg 3 times per day. In studies demonstrating efficacy for up to 5 hours, a nitrate-free interval of 15 hours was tested.

Nitroglycerin Patches

For patients with frequent episodes of angina pectoris, nitroglycerin patches can be considered. Like other long-acting preparations, patches should not be used to treat acute attacks of angina, but rather to prevent attacks in patients who experience frequent episodes of angina. Tolerance can be avoided by applying patches for only 12 hours followed by a nitrate-free interval of 12 hours. For patients awakening with angina pectoris or who experience early morning angina, the 12-hour interval should be overnight. However, most patients experience daytime exertion-related angina and can benefit most when the patches are applied for 12 hours during the day.

Intravenous Nitroglycerin

Intravenous nitroglycerin should be considered for patients with unstable angina pectoris. It has the advantage of rapid onset of action and certain absorption; the dose can be tailored to the needs of the particular patient to assure that blood pressure is not too severely lowered and that excessive reflex tachycardia does not occur. For acute ischemia, patients can be started on a continuous infusion of 5 to 15 μg/min. The rate of infusion can be increased every 3 to 5 minutes until the angina resolves, headache occurs, or the mean arterial blood pressure drops by more than 20 mm Hg. Major factors in the pathogenesis of unstable angina are fissuring and rupture of atheromatous plaques, which precipitate platelet aggregation and thrombus function. Platelets release vasoconstricting products and a deficiency of EDRF results in coronary artery spasm. Nitroglycerin's actions to limit platelet aggregation and enhance coronary vasodilation make it an important agent for the treatment of unstable angina. Because therapy must be continuous, nitrate tolerance rapidly diminishes the effectiveness of intravenous nitroglycerin. However, lower infusion rates may result in less tolerance, and therefore, infusion rates of intravenous nitroglycerin should be kept as low as possible. At high infusion rates, tolerance has been reported after as little as 24 hours of infusion.[34] Rates of <40 μg/min should be employed whenever possible. Because of the possibility that abrupt withdrawal may result in a rebound of anginal symptoms, patients should be tapered off intravenous nitroglycerin when they become asymptomatic.

Isosorbide Dinitrate

This relatively long-acting preparation comes in sublingual, oral-chewable, and slow-release forms. The onset of action is longer than that of nitroglycerin, and thus, this nitrate preparation should not be used for acute attacks of angina pectoris. Isosorbide dinitrate given more than 3 times per day has been associated with nitrate tolerance. Sustained release isosorbide dinitrate given at 8:00 AM and 8 PM did result in nitrate tolerance. When the same drug is given at 8:00 AM and 2 PM, tolerance to the 8:00 AM dose did not develop. However, whether or not tolerance follows the 2:00 PM dose is not known.[34a] In general, isosorbide dinitrate is most effective in preventing angina attacks during predictable activities. For example, it is a good medication to prescribe prior to a golf game that predictably precipitates attacks of angina pectoris.

Isosorbide-5-Mononitrate

Isosorbide-5-mononitrate is one of the principal active metabolites of isosorbide dinitrate. When used in an eccentric dosing schedule (8:00 AM and 2:00 PM), tolerance does not develop and both doses are effective. The slow-release formulation can be administered daily and remains effective for 12 hours without the development of tolerance.[35]

SIDE EFFECTS

Headache, flushing, and hypotension are the most common side effects and can often be relieved by lowering the dose of nitrate and, in the case of sublingual nitroglycerin, instructing the patient to sit when taking medication. Severe hypotension can be deleterious because of a lowered coronary perfusion pressure and decreased coronary blood supply. For these reasons, nitrates should be used with caution in hypotensive patients. Reflex tachycardia increases oxygen demand, and, therefore, excessive tachycardia should be avoided. Beta-blocking drugs can be helpful in abolishing the reflect tachycardia. With very high intravenous infusion rates, methemoglobinemia, ethanol intoxication, heparin resistance, and Wernicke's encephalopathy have been reported.

BETA-BLOCKADE

The ß-blocking drugs work by competing with endogenous catecholamines for ß-adrenergic receptor sites. The ß-receptors are subdivided into 2 types: $ß_1$ and $ß_2$. Beta$_2$ receptors, when stimulated, cause increased heart rate, increased contractility, and accelerated atrioventricular conduction. Other noncardiac effects include increased insulin release and increased muscle glycogenolysis. Beta$_2$ receptors, when stimulated, cause bronchodilation, dilation of peripheral blood vessels, and uterine smooth muscle relaxation.

Beta-blocking drugs affect the factors that influence both oxygen supply and oxygen demand, and not all of their effects are beneficial. Beta-blockade can actually decrease myocardial oxygen supply by blocking the vasodilating $ß_2$ receptors located in the walls of the coronary arteries, thereby increasing coronary vascular resistance and decreasing coronary blood flow. The hypotensive effect of ß-blockers can contribute to a reduction of coronary blood flow by reducing aortic pressure. Another potentially adverse effect is an increase in ventricular volume, which results in increased wall tension and, therefore, increased myocardial oxygen demand.

Beneficial effects of ß-blockade include decreases in heart rate and contractility, factors that lead to a decrease in myocardial oxygen demand. Schrumpf et al[36] demonstrated that ß-blocking drugs shift the oxygen-hemoglobin curve to the right, resulting in an increased delivery of oxygen to the myocardium. Back and associates[37] showed that ß-blockers may also have a beneficial effect on coronary blood flow in ischemic areas by redistributing blood flow from subepicardium to subendocardium. Overall, the effect of ß-blockade in most patients is favorable. Only in the failing or near-failing heart does ß-blockade sometimes have a detrimental effect. In such conditions, increases in left ventricular size and wall tension lead to an increase in myocardial oxygen demand and can also increase the severity of angina pectoris.

In addition to relieving angina pectoris, ß-blockers have been shown to reduce the morbidity and mortality in patients with coronary artery disease if administered following an acute myocardial infarction.[38] Timolol, used by the Norwegian Multicenter Study Group, was begun 7 to 28 days after the onset of myocardial infarction. Follow-up of 945 timolol-treated patients and 939 placebo-treated patients for a mean of 17 months demonstrated a reduction in both mortality and reinfarction in the drug-treated patients. In a similar study (BHAT) by the National Heart, Lung, and Blood Institute, propranolol or placebo was administered to 3,837 patients 5 to 21 days after acute myocardial infarction.[39] The propranolol-treated group had a reduced mortality compared to the placebo group. Metoprolol and atenolol have also been shown to reduce postinfarction mortality in large clinical trials. Early intravenous administration of metoprolol following the thrombolytic agent tissue plasminogen activator was shown to reduce the rate of reinfarction and ischemic events.[40]

Whether ß-blockade will reduce mortality and prevent myocardial infarctions in patients with coronary artery disease and a remote myocardial infarction or no history of a myocardial infarction is less clear . Because some patients receiving ß-blockers will suffer from side effects, it is probably not correct to administer ß-blockers to patients with CAD and mild or no angina pectoris who have not had a recent myocardial infarction. Rather, in this group of patients, ß-blockade should be reserved to treat symptoms when other methods of treatment are ineffective.

Beta-blocking drugs currently available in the United States are listed in Table 5. Four ß-blocking drugs have been approved for treatment of angina pectoris. Propranolol was the first ß-blocker available in the United States. It can be effectively administered twice daily in doses ranging from 40 to 320 mg/day; a long-acting preparation is available for once-daily dosing. Nadolol has a long half-life and can be administered once daily. Unlike propranolol, which is lipophilic, nadolol is hydrophilic. Hydrophilic substances do not easily penetrate the central nervous system and theoretically are associated with a decreased incidence of CNS side effects. Atenolol is another hydrophilic ß-blocking drug that can also be administered once daily in a dose of either 50 mg or 100 mg; it is selective for $ß_1$-receptors. Metoprolol, like propranolol, is lipophilic and is a twice-daily ß-blocker that is effective at doses ranging from 100 to 400 mg/day. At low doses, metoprolol is

Table 5. Dosages and Selected Pharmacologic Properties of Currently Available ß-Blocking Agents

DRUG GENERIC NAME (TRADE NAME)	USUAL DAILY ORAL DOSE (MG) RANGE	NO. OF DAILY DOSES	CARDIO-SELECTIVE	ISA*	LIPID SOLUBILITY	PLASMA HALF-LIFE (HR)	PRIMARY ROUTE OF ELIMINATION
Propranolol**° (Inderal)	160-480	2-4	No	No	High	3.2-6	Hepatic
Nadolol** (Corgard)	40-320	1	No	No	Low	12-24	Renal and biliary (90% unchanged)
Timolol° (Blocadren)	20-40	2	No	Minimal	Low to intermediate	3-5	Hepatic and renal (20% unchanged)
Metoprolol**° (Lopressor)	100-200	2-3	Yes	No	Intermediate	3-4	Hepatic
Atenolol**° (Tenormin)	50-200	1	Yes	No	Low	6-9	Renal (<40% unchanged) and hepatic
Pindolol (Visken)	7.5-22.5	3	No	Yes	Intermediate	3-4	Renal (~40% unchanged) and hepatic
Acebutolol (Sectral)	440-1,200	2-4	Yes	Yes	Low	4-6	Hepatic and renal
Labetalol† (Normodyne or Trandate)	300-1,200	3	No	(Yes)‡	Low to intermediate	3-4	Hepatic
Esmolol (IV)			Yes	No		9 min	Red blood cell

Note: The ß-blockers penbutolol (Levatol) and carteolol (Cartrol) were licensed recently by the FDA for the treatment of hypertension.
   ** Currently indicated for the treatment of angina pectoris.
   * ISA = intrinsic sympathomimetic activity
   † Labetalol possesses combined ß-blocking and relatively mild alpha-block activity (ß-blocking potency at least 4 times the alpha-blocking potency)
   †† Partial agonism of B$_2$ receptors
   ° Approved for long-term administration following myocardial infarction to reduce cardiac mortality and/or risk of reinfarction.
Modified from Shub C, Vlietstra RE, McGoon MD. Selection of optimal drug therapy for the patient with angina pectoris. *Mayo Clin Proc*. 1985;60:539.

cardioselective and blocks only ß$_1$-receptors. However, in doses above 100 mg/day, some degree of ß$_2$-receptor blockade is also present.

Seven additional ß-blocking drugs are available, but thus far none has been FDA-approved for treatment of angina pectoris. Timolol is a lipophilic ß-blocker that is administered twice daily at a dose range of 10 to 60 mg/day. Pindolol is a ß-blocker that has intrinsic sympathomimetic activity and has less of a tendency to lower heart rate than other ß-blocking drugs. Labetalol is a nonselective ß-blocking drug that also has selective α$_1$-receptor-blocking proper-

ties. Because of the latter property, a greater lowering of blood pressure would be expected with this drug than is seen with other ß-blocking drugs. Acebutolol is a third hydrophilic ß-blocker and also has mild sympathomimetic activity. Like metoprolol, at low doses acebutolol is a selective ß$_1$-receptor blocker. Esmolol is an intravenous ß-blocker with rapid onset of action and an elimination half-life of 9 minutes. Currently it is indicated only for treatment of supraventricular tachycardias. It has been used to safely treat stress tachycardia in patients with unstable angina as well as myocardial infarction.

Its advantage is that if side effects develop, they can be rapidly terminated by discontinuing the infusion of the drug. Carteolol and penbutolol, which became available in 1988, are indicated for hypertension. Both are nonselective ß-blockers with sympathomimetic activity.

In patients adequately ß-blocked, heart rate at rest should be in the 50s or 60s and should not go above 90 to 110 beats/min with moderate exercise. Increased doses of ß-blockers after these heart-rate goals are achieved can be beneficial because, while the negative chronotropic or heart-rate slowing effect may not increase, negative inotropy does increase.

The side effects of ß-blocking drugs are listed in Table 6. The negative inotropic effects that can lead to congestive heart failure in the failing or near-failing ventricle have been covered. In some patients, mild congestive heart failure precipitated by ß-blocking drugs can be reversed with digitalis; thus, the addition of digitalis may allow continuance of ß-blockade, and such patients can benefit, with improved exercise tolerance and reduced angina pectoris. Excessive heart-rate slowing can be a serious problem with ß-blocker administration. In some patients, probably those with intrinsic sinus node disease, rates at rest can fall to the 40s, 30s, and even lower. In these cases, either the ß-blocking drug must be discontinued or, in some instances, the heart rate can be supported with permanent cardiac pacing.

Abrupt withdrawal of ß-blockers can precipitate acute myocardial ischemia. The basis for this phenomenon is unclear, and different theories have been proposed. First, underlying coronary atherosclerosis may have progressed during therapy. Second, the patient may have increased his or her level of activity and not appropriately reduced it when the drug was stopped. Third, there may be a physiologic rebound effect involving increased sympathetic stimulation soon after the drug is stopped. If ß-blocker therapy is to be discontinued, it should be tapered gradually. In hospitalized patients with chronic stable angina pectoris, administering one half the usual dose for 24 hours and discontinuing it on day 2 is a safe approach. In patients with unstable angina pectoris, ß-blockade should not be discontinued without compelling reasons.

Other adverse effects can sometimes be avoided by changing from one ß-blocking drug to another.

CALCIUM-CHANNEL BLOCKERS

Calcium-channel blocking agents available in the United States are nifedipine, verapamil, diltiazem, nicardipine, bepridil, amlodipine, felodipine, and isradipine (Table 7). Calcium is important in the regulation of both myocardial and vascular smooth muscle contraction and relaxation and in the generation of the membrane action potential, particularly in the cells of the sinoatrial and atrioventricular nodes. The calcium-blocking drugs decrease the availability of intracellular calcium, which can result in decreased vasoconstriction in the coronary, peripheral, and pulmonary vasculature; decreased myocardial contractility; decreased rate of depolarization in the SA node; and slowed conduction in the AV node.

Several effects of calcium-channel blocking agents are potentially beneficial for patients with angina pectoris. First, by reducing the rate of SA node depolarization, heart rate is slowed and myocardial oxygen demand is decreased (seen with verapamil and diltiazem but not with nifedipine or nicardipine). Second, myocardial contractility and, subsequently, myocardial oxygen demand are decreased. Third, decreased smooth muscle tone in peripheral arteries results in vasodilation, decreased afterload, and decreased myocardial oxygen consumption. There also may be a small reduction in preload. Fourth, decreased coronary artery tone results

Table 6. Adverse Effects of ß-Blockade Therapy	
Cardiac	Congestive heart failure
	Excessive heart-rate slowing
	Propranolol withdrawal syndrome
Noncardiac	Fatigue
	Mental depression
	Insomnia
	Hallucinations
	Bad dreams
	Gastrointestinal upset
	Raynaud's phenomenon
	Bronchoconstriction
	Worsening of insulin-induced hypoglycemia
	Sexual dysfunction
	Further renal function deterioration in patients with renal disease

Table 7. Calcium-Channel Blockers Approved for Angina

	FREQUENCY OF ADMINISTRATION	COMMON TOTAL DAILY DOSAGE
Benzothiazepines		
Diltiazem	t.i.d. or q.i.d.	120-360 mg
Diltiazem CD	qd	120-480 mg
Phenylalkylamines		
Verapamil	t.i.d.	240-480 mg
Verapamil LA	qd	240 mg
Bepridil*	qd	300 mg
Dihydropyridines		
Nifedipine	t.i.d.	30-160 mg
Nifedipine XL	qd	30-90 mg
Nicardipine	t.i.d.	60-120 mg
Amlodipine	qd	2.5-10 mg

*Approved for chronic stable angina in patients who have failed to respond to other antianginal agents. May prolong QT interval and induce arrhythmias.

in increased coronary blood flow and increased myocardial oxygen supply. The control and movement of calcium in the myocardial cells, the smooth muscle cells in the coronary arteries, and smooth muscle cells in the peripheral arteries are different and are affected differently by various calcium-blocking agents.

These differences translate into varying clinical responses. Unlike the ß-blockers, which differ from each other primarily in side-effect profiles, the calcium blockers offer a range of therapeutic options, and selection of the appropriate calcium blocker should depend on the desired clinical response. Most of the calcium blockers are effective for the treatment of angina pectoris. They are particularly effective for angina pectoris caused by coronary spasm, but they are also effective for the treatment of angina caused purely by a fixed lesion or for angina due to fixed plus vasospastic narrowing (mixed angina pectoris).

Calcium-blocking agents can be used alone or combined with nitrates or ß-blocking drugs. For most patients, calcium blockers and ß-blockers are equally effective; frequently, the choice of which agent to use depends on other conditions the patient may have or on side effects (Table 8). For example, a patient with angina and asthma or peripheral vascular disease who is unable to tolerate ß-blockers can be successfully treated with calcium blockers. In a patient with a recent myocardial infarction and angina pectoris, a ß-

blocker would be a better choice, because ß-blockers, unlike the calcium blockers, have a prophylactic effect postinfarction, as discussed above.

Nifedipine is a potent coronary and peripheral artery vasodilator. Although, in vitro, nifedipine will block the SA and AV nodes, the lower in vivo doses usually do not have this effect. In vivo, the sympathetic reflex stimulation that results from vasodilation-induced hypotension may actually increase heart rate and conduction. The increase in heart rate after nifedipine administration tends to be a short-lived phenomenon and, with chronic administration of the drug, heart rate eventually returns to baseline. Similarly, although nifedipine's direct action is to decrease myocardial contractility, afterload reduction plus reflex sympathetic stimulation induced by peripheral vasodilation may increase myocardial contractility. The usual starting dose of nifedipine is 10 mg 3 times/day. The usual effective dose is 10 to 20 mg 3 times/day, which can be increased to 20 to 30 mg 3 to 4 times/day, if necessary. More than 180 mg daily is not recommended. A once-daily preparation of nifedipine (Procardia XL) has been shown to result in very steady plasma concentrations, which, by virtue of a unique gastrointestinal absorption system, may alleviate some of the previously observed vasodilator side effects such as headache, flushing, palpitations, and dizziness. Peripheral edema remains a side effect in the once-daily formulation. Tolerance to this form of therapy has not been observed.

Verapamil is a potent inhibitor of SA node depolarization and AV node conduction. Myocardial contractility is also decreased in vivo, with relatively less peripheral vasodilation than is seen with nifedipine. The usual starting dose of verapamil is 80 mg 3 times/day. The usual effective dose is 320 to 480 mg/day. More than 480 mg/day is not recommended. A once-daily formulation of verapamil is available. Verapamil may exacerbate AV conduction abnormalities, increase heart failure, and cause gastrointestinal side effects, including constipation and ileus.

Diltiazem has actions intermediate between those of nifedipine and verapamil. Compared to verapamil, diltiazem causes less reduction in myocardial contractility and less depression of the SA and AV nodes. Compared to nifedipine, diltiazem causes less peripheral vasodilation. Diltiazem appears to dilate both the coronary arteries and the peripheral arteries. The recommended starting dose of diltiazem is 30 mg 4 times/day. Many patients can tolerate a starting dose of 60 mg 3 or 4 times/day. The dose can be gradually increased to 360 mg daily in divided doses 3 or 4 times/day. Vasodilator side effects, as described above, may occur, and in some studies, diltiazem has exacerbated existing congestive heart failure. A twice-daily slow-release form is available.

Nicardipine is a dihydropyridine derivative which has similarities to nifedipine. The drug has a more selective vasodilatory effect in the coronary vasculature than in the systemic vasculature. It is more selective for vascular smooth muscle than cardiac muscle. Nicardipine is equally as effective in reducing angina pectoris as other calcium blockers and ß-blockers; it has been shown to reduce the frequency of rest angina. The drug also has been shown to be efficacious in the treatment of hypertension. Nicardipine has minimal negative inotropic and dromotropic effects. The usual starting dose is 20 mg 3 times/day, which can be increased to 40 mg 3 times/day. The most common side effects with this drug are pedal edema and dizziness (about 7% of patients), headache, asthenia, flushing, palpitations, nausea, and dyspepsia. Some patients (7%) developed increased angina in short-term trials when the drug was started or dosage increased.

Amlodipine is a dihydropyridine calcium antagonist with a prolonged duration of action

Table 8. Adverse Effects of Calcium-Channel Blockers

Cardiac	Congestive heart failure
	Palpitations
	Hypotension
	Bradycardia, conduction abnormalities (verapamil, diltiazem)
	Lightheadedness
	Prolong QT interval, arrhythmias (bepridil)
Noncardiac	Flushing
	Headache
	Weakness
	Nausea
	Constipation/diarrhea
	Nasal congestion
	Cough
	Wheezing
	Peripheral edema

that allows once-daily dosing. Its slow onset of action results in minimal vasodilator side effects. Amlodipine is indicated for patients with angina pectoris and has been demonstrated to be effective for vasospastic and stable angina pectoris.[39a] Two recent studies showed that amlodipine reduced both symptomatic and silent ischemia (assessed by Holter monitoring) in patients with chronic stable angina.[39b,c] The daily dose is from 2.5 to 10 mg. Amlodipine will improve the exercise capacity of some patients with mild to moderate congestive heart failure.[40a] The safety of amlodipine in a larger population of patients with congestive heart failure was recently confirmed by Packer et al.[40b]

ASPIRIN AND ANTICOAGULATION

There is now evidence to support the theory that atherosclerotic plaque rupture, platelet aggregation, and thrombus formation occur in the pathogenesis of unstable angina. Therefore, it is not surprising that antiplatelet and anticoagulant therapies are effective in the treatment of unstable angina. Large randomized trials have documented the benefit of aspirin for the treatment of unstable angina, and it is now evident that aspirin decreases the incidence of myocardial infarction, cardiac death, and refractory angina. The benefits of aspirin treatment continue for months after unstable angina is stabilized. Full-dose heparin in the first few days after the onset of unstable angina is also effective treatment—and probably more effective than aspirin during this time period. Heparin, like aspirin, decreases the incidence of myocardial infarction and refractory angina in unstable angina patients. A combination of aspirin plus heparin offers no advantage to heparin alone and increases the incidence of serious bleeding complications.[41] Thus, for unstable angina, heparin therapy for the first few days is appropriate. Before heparin is discontinued, aspirin should be started and continued indefinitely.[42] The optimal dose of aspirin appears to be ≤ 325 mg/day.[43] The evidence that aspirin is beneficial for patients with chronic stable angina is less impressive than the benefits for patients with unstable angina. However, there is ample evidence to support the routine use of daily aspirin for patients with chronic stable angina and patients with a prior myocardial infarction, even if they are asymptomatic,[44–46] unless they experience aspirin-related side effects.

INTRAAORTIC BALLOON COUNTERPULSATION

For patients with severe unstable angina pectoris not responding to the measures discussed above, intraaortic balloon counterpulsation can often be effective in relieving ischemia.[47] Intraaortic balloon counterpulsation relieves angina pectoris by decreasing systolic blood pressure and, therefore, myocardial oxygen demand; at the same time it increases diastolic blood pressure and, accordingly, increases coronary perfusion pressure and myocardial oxygen supply.

The problems with this technique are its frequent complications, most of which are due to vascular damage and thrombosis. More serious complications include perforation of the aortic wall and ischemia distal to the site of insertion in the aneurysms. Aortic insufficiency, and uncontrollable arrhythmias are all relative contraindications to use of intraaortic balloon counterpulsation. This technique should be reserved for patients who continue to have unstable angina pectoris in spite of other measures discussed. Because complications are more likely to occur,

the longer the balloon is in place, insertion of the balloon should be followed soon by coronary angiography and possibly by coronary artery bypass surgery.

PERCUTANEOUS TRANSLUMINAL CORONARY ANGIOPLASTY (PTCA)

The broad indications for PTCA are to treat patients with angina pectoris who have unacceptable symptoms, despite medical treatment, and to treat potentially life-threatening lesions. PTCA will relieve symptoms of angina, but there is little information comparing patients treated with medical therapy versus medical therapy plus PTCA.[47a] To establish a database in PTCA use, the NIH established a first registry in 1979[48] and a second one in 1985.[49] In the second registry, 2,500 patients in 16 centers were followed. When comparing the results from the early and late registries, success rates increased from 61% to 78%. In the later registry, complexity increased with 50% of the cases involving multivessel disease. Nonfatal myocardial infarction decreased from 4.9% to 4.3%, emergent coronary bypass surgery decreased from 5.8 to 3.4%, and the mortality rate was unchanged (1.2% vs 1.0%) when comparing results in the 2 registries.

Restenosis of dilated coronary arteries continues to be a problem. Symptomatic restenosis occurs in 20% to 25% of patients. Angiographic studies suggest that the restenosis rate may be 30% to 40%. Restenosis can be managed with repeat angioplasty. The rate of restenosis after a second angioplasty is similar to that after the first angioplasty. Many cardiologists consider repeat angioplasty for restenosis to be part of the long-term strategy for patients undergoing this form of therapy, and not necessarily a complication of the procedure.[50]

Medical therapy was compared to angioplasty in patients with single-vessel coronary artery disease. Angioplasty resulted in an improvement in symptoms and a modest improvement in exercise performance, but no difference in survival was noted.[51]

Many patients with coronary artery disease are candidates for either angioplasty or bypass surgery and the decision can be difficult. Several major trials comparing angioplasty to bypass surgery are underway.[52] Preliminary results support that the outcome is similar at 1 to 2 years.

However, those randomized to angioplasty are more likely to require repeat revascularization during follow-up. The CABRI trial randomized 1,054 patients with multivessel disease and ejection fractions over 35%. At 1 year, infarction rates (3.3% vs 2.9%), and death rates (2.1% vs 3.9%) were similar in the bypass surgery versus the angioplasty patients. However, while 8.6% of the bypass patients required revascularization, 40.3% of angioplasty patients underwent revascularization during the 1-year follow-up period. Revascularization in the angioplasty group was equally divided between bypass surgery and repeat angioplasty. Other randomized studies have reached similar conclusions. The GABI study randomized 359 patients to PTCA or bypass surgery. At 1 year, mortality and infarction rates were similar. While 6% of the bypass patients underwent revascularization during the year follow-up period, 40% of the angioplasty group required additional revascularization.[53] The RITA trial randomized 1,011 patients. Follow-up results have been reported at 2 to 2.5 years and are similar to results from the other trials. Death and infarction rates were similar, while the need for revascularization was higher in the angioplasty versus the bypass patients (37% vs 4%).[54] The longest follow-up reported is that of the EAST study, which followed 392 patients randomized to angioplasty or surgery for 3 years.[54a] Outcome, defined as death, infarction, or a thallium defect, was similar. Again, revascularization was more likely in the angioplasty patients than in the bypass patients (62% vs 13%). Overall, in-hospital costs were similar, as was quality of life. As the relatively small number of patients are followed for longer periods of time, additional guidelines to help patients and physicians choose between angioplasty and surgery will become available.

New devices, including lasers, stents, and atherectomy catheters, are under development. To date, early results have suggested little improvement over balloon angioplasty results. It is likely that a major improvement in the results of angioplasty will come not with new mechanical devices, but rather with an understanding and, hopefully, prevention of restenosis.

CORONARY ARTERY BYPASS SURGERY

As with any treatment strategy for patients with angina pectoris, coronary artery bypass surgery must be evaluated both for its ability to relieve symptoms and for its ability to alter the natural history of coronary artery disease and improve survival.

Compared to medical therapy, coronary bypass surgery can more effectively relieve symptoms, and it results in a greater improvement in quality of life. At the end of 5 years, 70% of patients undergoing coronary bypass surgery can expect a decrease in symptoms and 50% can expect to be asymptomatic. Patients should be considered for bypass surgery for relief of medically refractory angina pectoris. Individual patient lifestyles should also be considered. Patients who choose to lead inactive lives and who, on medical therapy, have only occasional episodes of angina pectoris should not be sent for bypass surgery for the purpose of symptom relief. However, patients with frequent angina pectoris, particularly those who are unable to perform their usual daily activities and who are not responding to maximal medical therapy and who are not candidates for angioplasty, are appropriate surgical candidates. The evolving role of coronary angioplasty for the relief of angina pectoris and the benefits and efficacy compared to coronary bypass surgery are currently being investigated.

To recommend coronary artery bypass surgery for the purpose of altering the natural history of coronary disease and improving survival is a more complex decision. Three large randomized trials that have provided useful guidelines for making this decision are the Veterans Administration Cooperative Trial,[55] the European Cooperative Surgery Study Group,[56] and the Coronary Artery Surgery Study (CASS).[57,58] Patients who can expect a survival benefit from coronary bypass surgery include those with left-main coronary stenosis, 3-vessel coronary disease (particularly if they have left ventricular dysfunction), severe symptoms, or a positive exercise test (Figs. 5, 6). There is less evidence that patients with 2-vessel coronary disease can expect a survival benefit. However, it appears that patients with mild to moderate angina, 2-vessel disease with a proximal left anterior descending coronary artery lesion, or a strongly positive exercise test can expect a survival benefit with surgery.[59]

When approaching the individual patient, a decision regarding coronary bypass surgery is often difficult. Medications and coronary angioplasty are also very effective therapies, and the large randomized trials comparing various treatments often do not include patients identical to the one you are caring for. Patients with left-main coronary disease or patients with 3-vessel disease, ischemia, and left ventricular dysfunction present the clearest indications and should undergo bypass surgery. Patients with 1- or 2-vessel coronary disease, particularly those with mild or no ischemic symptoms, present a treatment dilemma. If a given patient in this group has proximal left anterior descending coronary disease, substantial ischemia, and left ventricular dysfunction, a strong argument can be made for considering coronary bypass surgery, if angioplasty is not feasible.

For bypass surgery, the operative mortality rate is 1.3%, with a range of almost 0% in patients with 1-vessel disease and normal ventricular function to 3.5% in patients with 3-vessel disease and left ventricular dysfunction. Vein grafts have a patency rate of 70% to 86% 6 to 12 months after surgery. Graft failure during the first 6 months is most often due to thrombosis, while graft failure occurring beyond 1 year is usually due to fibrosis or atherosclerosis developing in the vein graft. At the end of 10 years, more than 50% of vein grafts are occluded. Compared with vein grafting, the use of internal mammary artery grafts has increased survival and decreased ischemic symptoms. The patency of internal mammary grafts is better than that of vein grafts; 90% are patent 10 years after surgery. A general approach to the management of angina is shown in Figure 7.

APPROACH TO UNSTABLE ANGINA PECTORIS

Unstable angina refers to a wide range of conditions triggered by severe transient myocardial ischemia. While a precise definition is lacking, Braunwald[60] has proposed a classification scheme that should provide uniformity to future studies (Table 9).

Goals of therapy are to decrease myocardial ischemia, prevent myocardial infarction, preserve left ventricular function, and prevent death. Patients with unstable angina should be admitted to the hospital and restricted to bed rest. Patients with transient ST-segment changes associated with angina are easily diagnosed. However, patients without ST changes frequent-

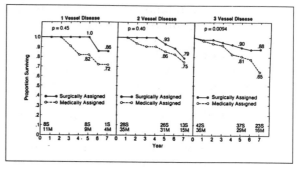

Figure 5. *Seven-year cumulative survival rates for medical (M) and surgical (S) patients with ejection fractions <0.50 (P = 0.012). From Passamani E, et al.[58]*

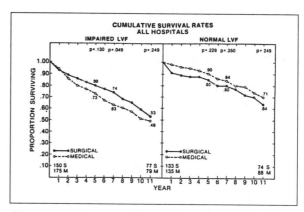

Figure 6. *Eleven-year cumulative survival for patients without left-main coronary artery disease, according to whether left ventricular function (LVF) was impaired or normal. Numbers of patients at risk at bottom of figure. Survival among patients with impaired LVF differed significantly at 7 years but not at 11 years. M=Medical; S=Surgical. From Detre K, et al. N Engl J Med. 1984;311:1333.*

ly require further diagnostic evaluation.

Medical management of unstable angina begins with bed rest and oxygen. Single therapy or combined therapy with ß blockers, nitrates, antiplatelet agents, antithrombotic agents, and calcium-channel blockers is frequently employed.[61] Nitrates decrease symptoms and the extent of myocardial ischemia, but there is no evidence that the incidence of major cardiac events—including myocardial infarction or death—is decreased. Intravenous nitroglycerin is commonly used for unstable angina but requires careful monitoring of blood pressure. Beta-blockers will also decrease ischemia and, although they will minimally decrease the risk of myocardial infarc-

Angina Diagnosis and Treatment

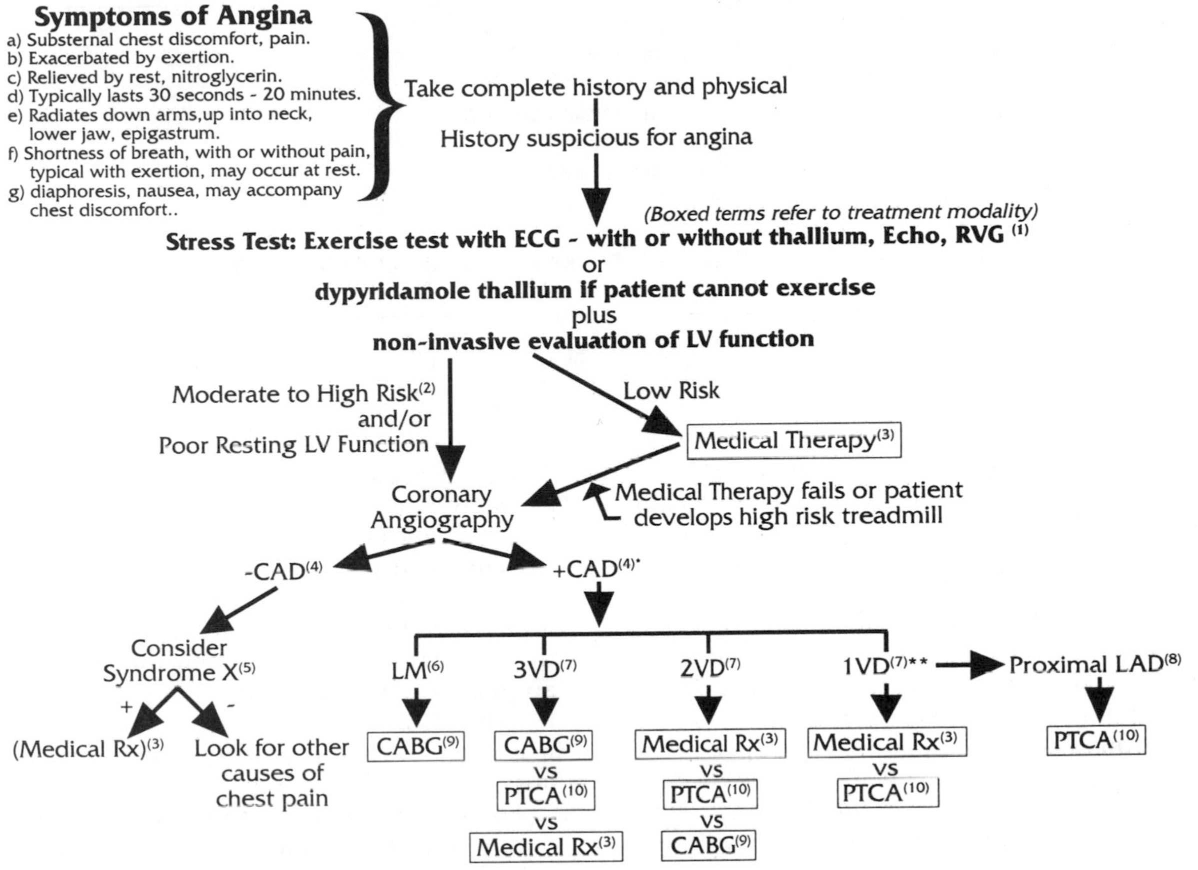

Symptoms of Angina
a) Substernal chest discomfort, pain.
b) Exacerbated by exertion.
c) Relieved by rest, nitroglycerin.
d) Typically lasts 30 seconds - 20 minutes.
e) Radiates down arms, up into neck,
   lower jaw, epigastrum.
f) Shortness of breath, with or without pain,
   typical with exertion, may occur at rest.
g) diaphoresis, nausea, may accompany
   chest discomfort..

Take complete history and physical

History suspicious for angina

(Boxed terms refer to treatment modality)

Stress Test: Exercise test with ECG - with or without thallium, Echo, RVG [1]
or
dypyridamole thallium if patient cannot exercise
plus
non-invasive evaluation of LV function

Moderate to High Risk[2]
and/or
Poor Resting LV Function

Low Risk

Medical Therapy[3]

Coronary
Angiography

Medical Therapy fails or patient
develops high risk treadmill

-CAD[4]   +CAD[4]*

Consider
Syndrome X[5]

LM[6]   3VD[7]   2VD[7]   1VD[7]** → Proximal LAD[8]

+   -

(Medical Rx)[3]   Look for other
causes of
chest pain

CABG[9]	CABG[9]	Medical Rx[3]	Medical Rx[3]	PTCA[10]
vs	vs	vs	vs	
	PTCA[10]	PTCA[10]	PTCA[10]	
	vs	vs		
	Medical Rx[3]	CABG[9]		

The treatment decision is based on LV function, symptom severity and response to Medical Rx.

**Other than Proximal LAD

(1) RVG: radionuclide ventriculography

(2) Moderate to high risk treadmill: exercise <6 minutes and stops due to symptoms of angina (see above), ST depression
multiple leads of ST depression >1-2 mm
exercise-induced hypotension
multiple and/or large areas of reversible thallium defects
decrease in LV function with echo and RVG

(3) Medical Therapy: reduce risk factors
nitrates
calcium channel blockers
beta blockers
aspirin

(4) CAD: coronary artery disease

(5) Syndrome X: chest pain with patent coronary vessels and absence of large epicardial coronary spasms

(6) LM: left main disease

(7) VD: vessel disease

(8) LAD: left anterior descending disease

(9) CABG: coronary artery bypass graft

(10) PTCA: percutaneous transluminal coronary angioplasty; may include atherectomy, stents, lasers

*In cases where coronary lesions are not ammenable to revascularization or patient is too high a risk for revascularization, Medical Rx is continued.

Figure 7. *Generalized guideline for management of angina. PTCA represents angioplasty; however, other interventional techniques including atherectomy and stents are also considered.*

Table 9. Braunwald Classification of Unstable Angina[60]

New onset of severe angina or accelerated angina. No rest pain.
Angina at rest within 1 month but not 48 hr (subacute).
Angina at rest within 48 hr (acute).
    Secondary – develops in the presence of extracardiac condition.
    Primary – absence of extracardiac conditions.
    Postinfarction – within 2 weeks of myocardial infarction.
        Absence or minimal antianginal therapy.
        Presence of appropriate therapy.
        Maximal tolerated doses, all 3 categories (ß-blocker, calcium antagonists, nitrates including intravenous).

---

tion, they do not decrease mortality. Calcium-channel blockers do not reduce the risk of death or myocardial infarction, and 1 study suggested that nifedipine used alone increases the incidence of myocardial infarction.[62]

Angioscopy has revealed plaque rupture, platelet activation, and thrombus formation at the site of unstable coronary artery lesions which produce unstable angina.[63,64] It is therefore not surprising that treatment of unstable angina with antiplatelet agents, including aspirin and ticlopidine, will reduce the incidence of death and myocardial infarction. Heparin will also provide benefits for patients with unstable angina.[65] Theroux et al[41] tested the usefulness of intravenous heparin therapy, aspirin 325 mg twice daily or a combination of both therapies administered over a 6-day period to patients with unstable angina pectoris. Heparin, but not aspirin, reduced the incidence of refractory angina. The incidence of myocardial infarction was reduced from 12% in the placebo group to 3% in the aspirin group, to <0.8% in the heparin group and to 1.6% in the aspirin plus heparin group. There were too few patients to evaluate the effect on mortality. Combining aspirin with heparin was no better than heparin alone, and the combination treatment was associated with a greater risk of bleeding. Heparin alone tended to be better than aspirin alone and has the benefit of a short half-life, which permits rapid discontinuation of therapy when more invasive procedures may necessitate a lower risk of bleeding.

Use of heparin provides the additional potential benefit of reduced complications and increased efficacy for patients who require acute coronary angioplasty.[66]

Thrombolytic therapy has been evaluated in patients, and no benefits have been observed. However, further studies on subsets of patients with unstable angina may establish a role for thrombolytics for some patients with unstable angina.[66a] New antithrombic agents, such as hirudin and hirulog, are being evaluated and may play a future role in the management of unstable angina.

For patients who continue to have angina despite medical treatment, intraaortic balloon pumping should be initiated, and patients should proceed to cardiac catheterization and, if appropriate, coronary artery revascularization with bypass surgery or coronary angioplasty.

Most patients with unstable angina will respond to initial treatment measures and, for this group, the need for interventional management is not clear. The difficulties defining unstable angina and the lack of trials comparing medical therapy to surgical therapy or angioplasty for the short or long term are lacking. For individual patients, attempts to stratify patient risk will often guide therapy decisions. Patients with transient ECG ST-segment changes are at a higher risk for infarction or death than patients with no ECG changes. Myocardial perfusion imaging can also provide important prognostic information. Patients with large, reversible thallium defects are at a greater risk for a significant cardiac event than patients with a normal thallium scan. Whether or not prognosis can be improved with revascularization is not clear, but patients who fall into a high-risk category

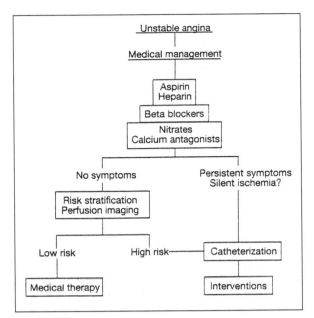

Figure 8. *Suggested approach to management of the patient with unstable angina. From McClellan JR.*[61]

should be considered for revascularization. Until more information is available for the management of patients with unstable angina, the treatment strategy outlined in Figure 8 is a good guide to follow.

CHOLESTEROL LOWERING, ATHEROSCLEROTIC REGRESSION, AND SLOWING OF PROGRESSION

Perhaps one of the most intriguing new concepts for treatment of coronary artery disease is that of slowing atherosclerotic progression or even causing atherosclerotic regression.

For patients with established coronary artery disease, several trials have evaluated cholesterol lowering as a means of preventing future coronary events (secondary prevention). A meta-analysis reported by Rossouw et al[67] evaluated the results of 8 secondary prevention trials. Cholesterol-lowering therapy reduced the incidence of myocardial infarction and cardiovascular deaths.

While hypercholesterolemia has long been recognized as a risk factor for coronary artery disease, it is only recently that convincing evidence has supported aggressive reduction of cholesterol as a means of reducing clinical events. Trials have utilized angiographic end points to evaluate cholesterol-lowering therapies. The Cholesterol-Lowering Atherosclerosis Study (CLAS) randomized men, aged 40 to 59 who had previous coronary bypass surgery, to placebo or colestipol-plus-niacin therapy, and statistically significant results were reported.[68] Coronary angiograms were reviewed over a 2-year period. The drug regimen lowered total plasma cholesterol by 26% and LDL cholesterol by 43%. Only 10% of patients receiving colestipol plus niacin developed new native coronary lesions while 22% of patients receiving placebo developed new lesions. Drug therapy also reduced the number of lesions that progressed in patients. Treated patients exhibited less progression of stenoses in bypass grafts as well. There was evidence of actual atherosclerotic regression in coronary arteries in 16% of treated patients versus only 2% of placebo patients.

The Familial Atherosclerosis Treatment Study (FATS) enrolled patients with angiographic evidence of coronary artery disease but no coronary bypass surgery.[69] Patients were assigned to placebo, colestipol plus nicotinic acid, or colestipol plus lovastatin. Treatment lowered cholesterol compared to placebo. Pre- and posttreatment angiograms in treated patients showed regression and less progression of atherosclerotic lesions, compared to placebo-treated patients.

The above studies and others have demonstrated that cholesterol lowering treatment can lessen progression of atherosclerotic lesions, but the overall effect on luminal diameters of coronary arteries is minimal. However, the Scandinavian Simvastatin Survival Study (4S)[69a] demonstrated that cholesterol reduction therapy has an important impact on clinical events. Patients with a history of coronary artery disease, with moderately high total cholesterol levels (212–309 mg/dl), were randomized to placebo or the HMG CoA reductase inhibitor, simvastatin. Treatment resulted in a 25% reduction in total cholesterol. Over a median follow-up period of 5.4 years treatment was associated with a reduction in coronary deaths, acute myocardial infarctions, cardiac arrests and the frequency of revascularization procedures (also see Chapter 12).

The apparent paradox between minimal

changes in the luminal diameter with cholesterol lowering therapy and the more dramatic reduction in clinical events may be explained by effects of cholesterol lowering therapy on the vessel wall. It may be that cholesterol plaques become stabilized and are less likely to rupture and produce clinical events when serum cholesterol levels are lowered. With the publication of the 4S trial, the cholesterol hypothesis has become the cholesterol theory. It is now clear that patients with coronary artery disease and elevated cholesterol can benefit when cholesterol levels are lowered. Further research is focusing on the benfits of lowering cholesterol in patients who do not have elevated cholesterol levels and in subjects with no symptomatic coronary desease (primary prevention).

Several animal studies have demonstrated that calcium-channel blockers retard atherogenesis associated with a high-cholesterol diet. In clinical trials involving small numbers of patients, there is also evidence that certain calcium blockers may slow the progression of atherosclerosis.[70–73] Loaldi et al[74] studied the effects of propranolol, nifedipine, and isosorbide dinitrate on atherosclerosis in patients with effort angina and known coronary artery disease. Over a 2-year period, they observed that progression of old narrowings and the appearance of new narrowings were fewer in the nifedipine-treated patients (31% and 10%, respectively) than in propranolol (53% and 34%, respectively) or isosorbide dinitrate (47% and 29%, respectively) patients. Nifedipine also was associated with regression of percent stenosis in a larger number of lesions than the other drugs.

The concept of atherosclerotic regression and slowing of progression with cholesterol-lowering agents and calcium blockers will likely continue to be tested in large multicenter trials.

REFERENCES

1. Martin CE, Shaver JA, Leonard JJ. Physical signs, apexcardiography, phonocardiography, and systolic time intervals in angina pectoris. *Circulation.* 1972;46:1098-1114.
1a. Conti CR. What is Syndrome X? *Clin Cardiol.* 1993;16:1-3. Editorial.
2. Assey ME. The puzzle of normal coronary arteries in the patient with chest pain: What to do? *Clin Cardiol.* 1993;16:170-180.
3. Proudfit WL, Hodgman JR. Physical signs during angina pectoris. *Prog Cardiovasc Dis.* 1968;10:283.
4. Banks DC, Raftery ED, Oran S. Clinical significance of the coronary arteriogram. *Br Heart J.* 1971;33:863-870.
5. Alison HW, Russel RO Jr, Mantle FA, et al. Coronary anatomy and arteriography in patients with unstable angina pectoris. *Am J Cardiol.* 1978;41:204-209.
6. Fischl SJ, Herman MV, Gorlin R. The intermediate coronary syndrome: Clinical, angiographic and therapeutic aspects. *N Engl J Med.* 1973;228:1193-1198.
7. Conti CR, Brawley RK, Griffith LS, et al. Unstable angina pectoris: Morbidity and mortality in 57 consecutive patients evaluated angiographically. *Am J Cardiol.* 1973;32:745-750.
8. Rifkin RD, Hood WB Jr. Bayesian analysis of electrocardiographic exercise stress testing. *N Engl J Med.* 1977;297:681-686.
9. Goldman S, Tselos S, Cohn K. Marked depth of ST-segment depression during treadmill exercise test: Indicator of severe coronary artery disease. *Chest.* 1976;69:729-733.
10. Cheitlin MD, Davia JE, deCastro CM, et al. Correlations of "critical" left coronary artery lesions with positive exercise tests in patients with chest pain. *Am Heart J.* 1975;89:305-310.
11. Fisch C, DeSanctis RW, Dodge HT, et al. ACC/AHA Task Force Report. Guidelines for ambulatory electrocardiography. *J Am Coll Cardiol.* 1989;13:249-258.
12. Kennedy HL, Wiens RD. Ambulatory (Holter) electrocardiography and myocardial ischemia. *Am Heart J.* 1989;117:164-176.
12a. Ritchie JL, Zaret BL, Strauss HW, et al. Myocardial imaging with thallium-201: A multicenter study in patients with angina pectoris or acute myocardial infarction. *Am J Cardiol.* 1978;42:345-350.
13. Gerstenblith G, Ouyang P, Achuff SC, et al. Nifedipine in unstable angina: A double blind, randomized trial. *N Engl J Med.* 1982;306:885-889.
14. Wackers FJ, Lie KL, Liem KL, et al. Thallium-201 scintigraphy in unstable angina pectoris. *Circulation.* 1978;57:738-742.
15. Atkins GW, Pohost GM, DeSanctis RW, et al. Selection of angina-free patients with severe left ventricular dysfunction for myocardial revascularization. *Am J Cardiol.* 1988;46:697.
16. Iskandrian AS, Heo J, Askenase A, et al. Dipyridamole cardiac imaging. *Am Heart J.* 1988;115:432-443.
17. Humphries JO. Expected course of patients with coronary artery disease. In: Rahimtoola SH (ed). *Coronary Bypass Surgery.* Philadelphia: FA Davis; 1977:48.
18. Mulcahy R, Daly L, Graham I, et al. Unstable angina: Natural history and determinants of prognosis. *Am Cardiol.* 1981;48:525-528.
18a. Meredith IT, Anderson TJ, Uehata A, et al. Role of endothelium in ischemic coronary syndromes. *Am J Cardiol.* 1993;72:27C-32C.
19. Forrester JS, Litvack F, Grundfest W, et al. A perspective of coronary disease seen through the arteries of a living man. *Circulation.* 1987;75:505-513.
20. Braunwald E, Ross J Jr, Sonnenblick EH. Myocardial energetics. In: Braunwald E, Ross J Jr, Sonnenblick EH (eds). *Mechanisms of Contraction of the Normal and Failing Heart.* Boston: Little Brown; 1976:171.

21. Aronow WS. Editorial. Smoking, carbon monoxide, and coronary heart disease. *Circulation.* 1973; 48:1169-1172.

22. Kramsch DM, Aspen AJ, Abramowitz BM, et al. Reduction of coronary atherosclerosis by moderate conditioning exercise in monkeys on an atherogenic diet. *N Engl J Med.* 1981;305:1483-1489.

23. Redwood DR, Rosing DR, Epstein SE. Circulatory and symptomatic effects of physical training in patients with coronary artery disease and angina pectoris. *N Engl J Med.* 1972;286:959-965.

24. Sim DN, Neill WA. Investigation of the physiological basis for increased exercise threshold after physical conditioning. *J Clin Invest.* 1974;54:763-770.

25. Abrams J. Transdermal nitroglycerin and nitrate tolerance. *Ann Intern Med.* 1986;104:424-426.

26. Cohn PF, Maddox DE, Holman BL, et al. Effect of sublingually administered nitroglycerin on regional myocardial blood flow in patients with coronary artery disease. *Am J Cardiol.* 1977;39:672-678.

27. Harrison DG, Kurz MA, Quillen JE, et al. Normal and pathophysiologic considerations of endothelial regulation of vascular tone and their relevance to nitrate therapy. *Am J Cardiol.* 1992;70:11B-17B.

28. Sellke FW, Myers PR, Bates JN, et al. Influence of vessel size on the sensitivity of porcine coronary microvessels to nitroglycerine. *Am J Physiol.* 1990;258 (Heart and Circ Physiol 27):H515-H520.

29. Loscalzo J. Role of nitrates in angina pectoris. *Am J Cardiol.* 1992;70:18B-22B.

30. Thadani U. Role of nitrates in angina pectoris. *Am J Cardiol.* 1992;70:43B-53B.

31. Bauer JA, Fung H-L. Concurrent hydralazine administration prevents nitroglycerine-induced hemodynamic tolerance in experimental heart failure. *Circulation.* 1991;84:35-39.

32. Katz RJ, Levy WS, Buff L, et al. Prevention of nitrate tolerance with angiotensin converting enzyme inhibitors. *Circulation.* 1991;83:1271-1277.

33. Parker JO, Parker JD. Neurohormonal activation during nitrate therapy: a possible mechanism for tolerance. *Am J Cardiol.* 1992;70:93B-97B.

34. Horowitz JD. Role of nitrates in unstable angina pectoris. *Am J Cardiol.* 1992;70:64B-71B.

34a. Silber S, Vogler AC, Krause KH, et al. Induction and circumvention of nitrate tolerance applying different dosage intervals. *Am J Med.* 1987;83:860-870.

35. Chrysant SG, Glasser SP, Bittar N, et al. Efficacy and safety of extended-release isosorbide mononitrate for stable effort angina pectoris. *Am J Cardiol.* 1993;72:1249-1256.

36. Schrumpf JD, Sleps DS, Wolfson S, et al. Altered hemoglobin-oxygen affinity with long-term propranolol therapy in patients with coronary artery disease. *Am J Cardiol.* 1977;40:76-82.

37. Buck JD, Gross GJ, Warltier DC, et al. Comparative effects of cardioselective versus noncardioselective beta blockade on subendocardial blood flow and contractile function in ischemic myocardium. *Am J Cardiol.* 1979;44:657-663.

38. The Norwegian Multicenter Study Group. Timolol-induced reduction in mortality and reinfarction in patients surviving infarction. *N Engl J Med.* 1981;304:801-807.

39. National Heart, Lung, and Blood Institute Cooperative Trial. Preliminary report. The beta-blocker heart attack trial. *JAMA.* 1981;246:2073-2074.

39a. Frishman WH (ed). A Supplement: Second-generation calcium antagonism in cardiovascular disease. *Am J Cardiol.* 1994;73:1A-58A.

39b. Deanfield JE, Detry J-M, Lichtlen PR, et al. Amlodipine reduces transient myocardial ischemia in patients with coronary artery disease: Double-blind circadian anti-ischemia program in Europe (CAPE Trial). *J Am Coll Cardiol.* 1994;24:1460-1467.

39c. Ezekowitz MD, Hossack K, Mehta JL, et al. Amlodipine in chronic stable angina: Results of a multi-center double-blind crossover trial. *Am Heart J.* 1995:129:527-535.

40. TIMI Study Group. Comparison of invasive and conservative strategies after treatment with intravenous tissue plasminogen activator in acute myocardial infarction: results Thrombolysis in Myocardial Infarction (TIMI) phase II Trial. *N Engl J Med.* 1989;320:618-627.

40a. Packer M, Nicod P, Khandheria BR, et al. Randomized, multicenter, double-blind, placebo-controlled evaluation of amlodipine in patients with mild-moderate heart failure. *J Am Coll Cardiol.* 1991;17:274A.

40b. Packer M. The PRAISE Trial (Prospective Randomized Amlodipine Survival Evaluation): Background and Main Results. Presented at the 44th Annual Scientific Session, American College of Cardiology, New Orleans, March 1995.

41. Theroux P, Oulmet H, McCums J, et. al. Aspirin, heparin, or both to treat acute unstable angina. *N Engl J Med.* 1989;319:1105-1111.

42. Theroux P, Waters D, Lam J, et al. Reactivation of unstable angina after the discontinuation of heparin. *N Engl J Med.* 1992;327:141-145.

43. Kearon C, Hirsh J. Optimal dose for starting and maintaining low-dose aspirin. *Arch Intern Med.* 1993;153:700-701.

44. Ridker PM, Manson JE, Gaziano M, et al. Low-dose aspirin therapy for chronic stable angina. *Ann Int Med.* 1991;114:385-389.

45. Juul-Moller S, Edvardsson N, Jahnmatz B, et al. Double blind trial of aspirin in primary prevention of myocardial infarction in patients with stable chronic angina pectoris. *Lancet.* 1992;340:1421-1425.

46. Antiplatelet Trialists' Collaboration. Secondary prevention of vascular disease by prolonged antiplatelet treatment. *Br Med J.* 1988;296:320-331.

47. Weintraub RM, Voukydia PC, Aroesty JM, et al. Treatment of preinfarction angina with intraaortic balloon counterpulsation and surgery. *Am J Cardiol.* 1974;34:809-814.

47a. Landar C, Lange RA, Hillis LD. Percutaneous transluminal coronary angioplasty. *N Engl J Med.* 1994; 330:981-993.

48. Kent KM, Bentivoglio LG, Block PC, et al. Percutaneous transluminal coronary angioplasty:

report from the Registry of the National Heart, Lung, and Blood Institute Registry. *Am J Cardiol.* 1982; 49:2011-2020.

49. Detre K, Holubkov R, Kelsey S, et al. Percutaneous transluminal coronary angioplasty in 1985-1986 and 1977-1981: the National Heart, Lung, and Blood Institute Registry. *N Engl J Med.* 1988;318:265-270.

50. ACC/AHA Task Force Report. Guidelines for percutaneous transluminal coronary angioplasty. *J Am Coll Cardiol.* 1993;22:2033-2054.

51. Parisi AF, Folland ED, Hartigan P. A comparison of angioplasty with medical therapy in the treatment of single-vessel coronary artery disease: Veterans Affairs ACME Investigator. *N Engl J Med.* 1992;326:10-16.

52. Lembo NJ, King SB III. Randomized trials of percutaneous transluminal coronary angioplasty, coronary artery bypass grafting surgery, or medical therapy in patients with coronary artery disease. *Cor Art Dis.* 1990;1:449-454.

53. Hamm CW, Reimers J, Ischinger T, et al. A randomized study of coronary angioplasty compared with bypass surgery in patients with symptomatic multivessel coronary disease. *N Engl J Med.* 1994;331:1037-1043.

54. RITA Trial participants. Coronary angioplasty versus coronary artery bypass surgery: the Randomized Intervention Treatment of Angina (RITA) trial. *Lancet.* 1993;341:573-580.

54a. King SB, Lembo NJ, Weintraub WS, et al. A randomized trial comparing coronary angioplasty with coronary bypass surgery. *N Engl J Med.* 1994;331:1044-1050.

55. The Veterans Administration Coronary Artery Bypass Surgery Cooperative Study Group. Eleven-year survival in the Veterans Administration randomized trial of coronary bypass surgery for stable angina. *N Engl J Med.* 1984;311:1333-1339.

56. European Coronary Surgery Study Group. Long-term results of prospective randomized study of coronary artery bypass surgery in stable angina pectoris. *Lancet.* 1982;2:1173-1180.

57. CASS Principal Investigators and their Associates. Coronary artery surgery study (CASS): A randomized trial of coronary artery bypass surgery. Survival data. *Circulation.* 1983;68:939.

58. Passamani E, Davis KB, Gillespie MJ, et al, and the CASS Principal Investigators and their Associates. A randomized trial of coronary artery bypass surgery: Survival of patients with a low ejection fraction. *N Engl J Med.* 1985;312:1665-1671.

59. Rahimtoola SH. A perspective on the three large multicenter randomized clinical trials of coronary bypass surgery for chronic stable angina. *Circulation.* 1985;72(suppl V):V-123-135.

60. Braunwald E. Unstable angina: A classification. *Circulation.* 1989;80:410-414.

61. McClellan JR. Unstable angina: Prognosis, noninvasive risk assessment, and strategies for management. *Clin Cardiol.* 1994;17:229-238.

62. Holland Interuniversity Nifedipine/Metoprolol Trial (HINT) Research Group. Early treatment of unstable angina in the coronary care unit: A randomized, double-blind, placebo controlled comparison of recurrent ischemia in patients treated with nifedipine or metoprolol, or both. *Br Heart J.* 1986;56:400-413.

63. Fuster V, Badimon JJ, Chesebro JH. Mechanisms of disease: The pathogenesis of coronary artery disease and the acute coronary syndromes (first of two parts). *N Engl J Med.* 1992;326:242-250.

64. Fuster V, Badimon L, Badimon JJ, et al. Mechanisms of disease: The pathogenesis of coronary artery disease and acute coronary syndromes (second of two parts). *N Engl Med.* 1992;326:310-318.

65. The RISC Group. Risk of myocardial infarction and death during treatment with low-dose aspirin and intravenous heparin in men with unstable coronary artery disease. *Lancet.* 1990;336:827-830.

66. Laskey MAL, Deutsch E, Barnathan E, et al. Influence of heparin therapy on percutaneous transluminal angioplasty outcome in unstable angina pectoris. *Am J Cardiol.* 1990;65:1425-1429.

66a. Borzak S, Verter J, Bajwa H et al. Thrombolytic therapy for unstable angina. *Clin Cardiol.* 1993;16:637-642.

67. Rossouw J, Lewis B, Rifkind B. The value of lowering cholesterol after myocardial infarction. *N Engl J Med.* 1990;323:1112-1119.

68. Blankenhorn DH, Nessin SA, Johnson RL, et al. Beneficial effects of combined colestipol-niacin therapy on coronary atherosclerosis and coronary venous bypass grafts. *JAMA.* 1987;257:3233-3240.

69. Brown G, Albers JJ, Fisher LD, et al. Regression of coronary artery disease as a result of intensive lipid lowering therapy in men with high levels of apolipoprotein B. *N Engl J Med.* 1990;323:1289-1298.

69a. Scandinavian Simvastatin Survival Study Group. Randomized trial of cholesterol lowering in 4444 patients with coronary heart disease: The Scandinavian Simvastatin Survival Study (4S). *Lancet.* 1994;344:1383-1389.

70. Kober G, Schneider W, Kaltenback M. Can the progression of coronary sclerosis be influenced by calcium antagonists? *J Cardiovasc Pharmacol.* 1989; 13(suppl 4):S2-S6.

71. Lichtlen PR, Hugenholtz PG, Rafflenbeul W, et al. Retardation of angiographic progression of coronary artery disease by nifedipine. Results of the International Nifedipine Trial on Antiatherosclerotic Therapy (INTACT). *Lancet.* 1990;335:1109-1113.

72. Walters D, Lesperance J, Francetich M, et al. A controlled clinical trial to assess the effect of a calcium channel blocker on the progression of coronary atherosclerosis. *Circulation.* 1990;82:1940-1953.

73. Walters D, Lesperance J, Francetich M, et al. A controlled clinical trial to assess the effect of a calcium channel blocker on the progression of coronary atherosclerosis. *Circulation.* 1990;82:1940-1953.

74. Loaldi A, Polese A, Montursi P, et al. Comparison of nifedipine, propranolol and isosorbide dinitrate on angiographic progression and regression of coronary arterial narrowings in angina pectoris. *Am J Cardiol.* 1989;64:433-439.

CHAPTER 14

Silent Myocardial Ischemia

Thomas L. Shook, MD

Myocardial ischemia occurs when myocardial oxygen demand exceeds myocardial oxygen supply. Angina pectoris is the symptom complex classically associated with transient myocardial ischemia. However, ischemia can occur with or without angina. *Silent* myocardial ischemia is simply myocardial ischemia occurring in the absence of chest pain or anginal equivalents (dyspnea, nausea, or pain in locations other than the chest).[1-5] Symptoms occur late (or not at all) in a series of events beginning with the initiation of anaerobic metabolism and followed by: 1) impairment of myocardial cellular function and local electrophysiologic disturbances, 2) abnormal left ventricular diastolic performance, 3) abnormal left ventricular systolic performance, and 4) surface electrocardiographic abnormalities.

Clinical understanding of the inconstant relationship between myocardial ischemia and symptoms has been markedly enhanced by recent epidemiologic and methodologic discoveries. First, ischemia severe enough to cause completed myocardial infarction (MI) can be entirely silent. Follow-up data from the Framingham Study suggest that 35% of MIs in women and 28% in men are clinically unrecognized.[6] About one-half of these are entirely asymptomatic, and one-half are accompanied by few or atypical symptoms. These data doubtless underestimate the true incidence of silent MI, since non–Q-wave MIs, those manifested by development of new conduction disturbance, and silent MIs followed by sudden cardiac death are not included. Very likely, one-third of all MIs are truly asymptomatic.

A second major advance in the understanding of myocardial ischemia has been the development of methods to accurately monitor ST-segment changes during ambulatory ECG (or Holter monitoring). Use of these techniques has revealed that patients with coronary artery disease have frequent episodes of characteristic ischemic ST-segment change during daily activity. Approximately 75% of all episodes of myocardial ischemia detected by ambulatory ECG are silent.[7-9] Moreover, these episodes tend to occur at relatively low heart rates and during sedentary activities. Prompted by these findings, additional important observations have followed from the use of conventional exercise ECG testing, radionuclide scintigraphy, exercise echocardiography, and other techniques. These studies are beginning to have important prognostic and therapeutic implications.

PATHOPHYSIOLOGY

General features of the pathophysiology of myocardial ischemia have been discussed. Myocardial ischemia occurs when myocardial oxygen demand exceeds myocardial oxygen supply. When 1 or all of the determinants of myocardial oxygen demand (systolic wall stress, heart rate, and myocardial contractility) increase(s), myocardial blood supply normally increases to meet demand. The presence of flow-limiting atheromatous plaque in epicardial coronary arteries limits increases in flow, resulting in inadequate perfusion and conversion from aerobic to anaerobic metabolism. Subsequently, abnormalities of cellular function are manifested by impaired ion flux and local electrophysiologic disturbances. Next, elevation of left ventricular end-diastolic pressure and a fall in the rate of ventricular relaxation occur, indicative of ventricular diastolic impairment. This is followed by impaired systolic performance as manifested by regional or global contractile failure. Surface ECG abnormalities—ST-segment depression or elevation—occur late in this sequence of events. Generally, angina is an even later manifestation of ischemia. However, all of the above ischemic events may be present without any symptoms whatsoever.

Why are some episodes of myocardial ischemia symptomatic and others not? Silent ischemia may simply represent brief or less severe ischemia. Also, the difference in pain perception or central transmission of pain may vary from individual to individual or within the same individual during different circumstances. For example, patients with diabetes may have a neuropathic basis for painless ischemia. Also, MI may destroy or alter cardiac nerve endings. Finally, different relationships between disturbed myocardial blood supply and superimposed, changing myocardial demand may determine whether an episode is symptomatic.

The observation that silent myocardial ischemia occurs during daily activities and at heart rates considerably lower than those provoking ischemia during treadmill exercise has fostered speculation that changing myocardial blood supply may also be important in the pathophysiology of silent myocardial ischemia. Normal coronary arteries are capable of both dilation and constriction in response to multiple neurohumoral stimuli. It is now apparent that diseased epicardial coronary arteries retain the capacity for changing coronary vasomotor tone in spite of their involvement with atherosclerosis. Unfortunately, while atherosclerotic coronary arteries may still respond normally to direct vasodilators, such as nitroglycerin and calcium-channel blockers, certain neurohumoral substances depend on normal endothelium to mediate their vasodilating properties. When endothelium is damaged, these substances may have paradoxical vasoconstrictor properties.[10]

In addition to demonstrating that most episodes of myocardial ischemia during daily activities are asymptomatic and that they tend to occur at relatively low heart rates, ambulatory ECG recordings show a marked circadian variation in frequency and duration of silent ischemia.[11] Ambulatory ECG recordings demonstrate a significant peak of events in the morning hours. This circadian peak closely

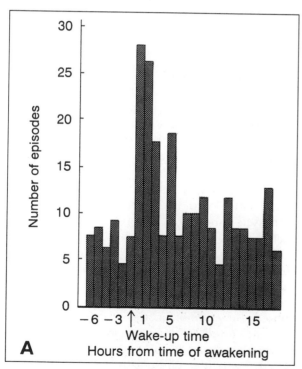

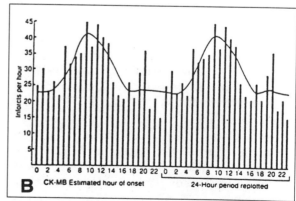

Figure 1. (A) Hourly distribution of number of episodes of myocardial ischemia, corrected for time of awakening. The peak incidence of ischemia occurs within the first 2 hours of awakening. Reprinted from Rocco MB et al.[11] (B) Hourly frequency of onset of myocardial infarction in 703 patients. A prominent circadian rhythm is present, with primary peak incidence at 9 AM and secondary peak at 8 PM. Reprinted from Muller JE et al.[12] With permission.

parallels the peak time of onset of MI (Fig. 1),[12] and circadian peaks of endogenous catecholamines, platelet aggregability,[13] and platelet α2-adrenoreceptor affinity.[14] Coronary arteries already narrowed by atherosclerotic plaque may have heightened vasoconstrictor sensitivity resulting from the loss of endothelial-mediated vasodilation at certain times of the day. These findings have also supported speculation that many episodes of silent myocardial ischemia are prompted by reductions in myocardial blood supply as much as by increases in myocardial oxygen demand.

METHODS OF DETECTION OF SILENT MYOCARDIAL ISCHEMIA

Detection of silent myocardial ischemia has relied heavily on ECG (exercise and ambulatory) and radionuclide studies.

AMBULATORY ECG

ST-segment changes suggestive of myocardial ischemia were demonstrated in Norman Holter's original description of ambulatory ECG monitoring in 1961.[15] However, the early use of ambulatory monitoring was primarily limited to detection of arrhythmias until the studies of Stern and Tzivoni.[16,17] These studies demonstrated frequent asymptomatic ischemic ST-segment changes on ambulatory ECG monitor recordings in patients with known or suspected coronary artery disease (CAD). However, these early studies were criticized because of concerns about technical aspects of the recording and playback systems utilized. Specifically, poor frequency-response characteristics or marked phase-shift of some Holter recording and playback systems may cause artifactual ST-segment deviations.[18] With the advent of frequency-modulated (FM) systems and improved direct recording (AM) systems, these limitations can be overcome.[19]

When patients with known CAD are monitored, they are frequently observed to have multiple episodes of characteristic ischemic ST-segment depression, 70% to 90% of which are asymptomatic (Fig. 2). Studies suggest that most patients with CAD and angina also have

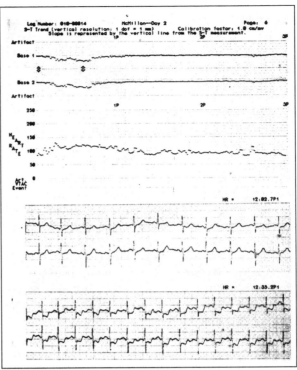

Figure 2. *Episodes of ST-segment depression by ambulatory ECG in a patient with known coronary artery disease. These episodes were asymptomatic.*

episodes of silent myocardial ischemia. There is, however, a very wide range of episode duration, number, and total time of ischemia. It is difficult to predict from clinical features which patients will have silent myocardial ischemia. Similarly, it is very difficult to predict from exercise testing the frequency or severity of myocardial ischemia as assessed by ambulatory recording.[20] Radionuclide studies also appear to predict poorly the presence of silent ischemia on ambulatory ECG recording.[21]

EXERCISE ECG TESTING

Graded exercise accompanied by transient ST-segment depression on the ECG is widely accepted as a sign of myocardial ischemia. The presence of angina is useful as confirmation, but ECG evidence alone is sufficient to diagnose ischemia. Such changes and their "severity" are commonly believed to be important indicators of the severity of obstructive CAD and its prognosis. Approximately one-third to one-half of exercise tests in patients with known CAD are not accompanied by angina. Clinical characteristics (age, sex, previous MI, extent of CAD, presence or absence or type of drug therapy) are similar in patients with silent and symptomatic positive exercise tests.[17] There appears to be no difference in the number or sequence of ECG leads involved or the degree of maximal ST-segment depression in silent and symptomatic patients with strongly abnormal treadmill tests (ST-segment depression >2.0 mm). There are few differences in treadmill characteristics (heart rate, blood pressure, double product, duration of exercise, etc.) when silent and symptomatic patients are compared, although patients with silent ischemia appear to have slightly longer exercise duration, slightly higher heart rate at onset of ST-segment depression, higher peak heart rate, and slightly longer duration of ST depression.

In patients without known CAD, the presence of asymptomatic exercise-induced ST-segment depression is less reliable as an indicator of ischemia. As the pretest probability of CAD decreases, the frequency of false-positive test responses increases (Bayes' theorem). Thus, an abnormal exercise ECG response in patients who have a low pretest probability of CAD may represent a false-positive, nonischemic response. In this circumstance, such ST-segment depression should not be termed silent ischemia unless additional confirmatory evidence is available. However, such patients are at increased risk (3–5-fold) for subsequent cardiac events and should have additional follow-up testing.[22]

RADIONUCLIDE AND STRESS ECHO STUDIES

Thallium stress-redistribution scintigraphy, exercise radionuclide ventriculography, and stress echocardiography improve the sensitivity and specificity of exercise ECG for detection of exercise-induced myocardial ischemia. This is the case regardless of whether symptoms are present. As discussed in earlier chapters, the utility of these studies for the diagnosis of CAD is also dependent on the pretest likelihood. In patients with known coronary artery disease, however, additional confirmatory and quan-

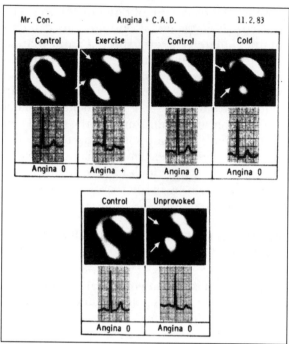

Figure 3. *Tomographic slices through the mid-left ventricle showing the regional myocardial uptake of rubidium-82 (^{82}Rb) in the posterior wall, free wall, anterior wall, and interventricular septum. This demonstrates the distribution of regional perfusion during control, cold pressor test, unprovoked ST depression, and exercise. Evidence of regional ischemia occurred during all 3 tests and supported the ST-segment changes as evidence of ischemia whether or not chest pain occurred. CAD=Coronary artery disease. Reprinted from Deanfield JE et al.[8]*

titative evidence of physiologically significant ischemia can be obtained by imaging studies. In the absence of angina, additional confirmation of ischemia can be very helpful clinically. The results of exercise testing, even when confirmed by radionuclide studies, do not clearly predict the frequency and extent of silent ischemia detected by ambulatory monitoring.[21]

Important studies using positron emission tomography (PET) confirmed the presence of transient hypoperfusion during spontaneous episodes of asymptomatic ST-segment depression in patients with typical angina and a positive exercise test (Fig. 3).[8] These findings validated the concept of significant ischemia accompanied by painless ST depression. In particular, PET defects indicative of spontaneous asymptomatic reductions in myocardial blood flow were found to be readily provoked by mental stress. These studies support the hypothesis that ambulatory ischemia is often triggered by decrements in blood supply, as well as increases in myocardial oxygen demand. Clinical application of PET scanning is promising but largely undeveloped.

PREVALENCE OF SILENT MYOCARDIAL ISCHEMIA

As previously noted, approximately one-third of all MIs are truly asymptomatic. Findings from ambulatory ECG studies were reviewed by Rozanski and Berman.[1] In 10 studies, 75% (range, 61%–81%) of all episodes of ambulatory ischemia detected by monitoring were silent. The methods used for analysis and definition of ischemic changes have changed somewhat over the course of these studies. Nonetheless, patients with known CAD appear to have approximately a 3:1 ratio of silent:symptomatic episodes of ischemia during daily activity. Episodes characteristically last for approximately 24 minutes and demonstrate a mean of 1.5 mm of ST-segment depression. Depending on the patient population studied, there is a wide range in the number of episodes and total duration of ischemia per 24 hours of monitoring. Most patients with chronic, stable angina have some evidence of silent ischemia. About one-third have frequent episodes (>6 episodes/48 hr).

Hospitalized patients with unstable angina have a high frequency of asymptomatic ST-segment depression during continuous ambulatory ECG monitoring. Almost 90% of episodes occur silently. In one study, 37 of 70 patients hospitalized for unstable angina had ST-segment depression detected on continuous monitoring.[4] They had a mean daily duration of 157 minutes of ST-segment change.

Cohn[3] has proposed a classification scheme describing three types of patients with transient myocardial ischemia: 1) type I—totally asymptomatic persons, 2) type II—patients asymptomatic after MI, 3) and type III— patients with coexisting angina and silent myocardial ischemia. His estimates suggest that 2% to 4% of totally asymptomatic middle-aged men have provocable silent myocardial ischemia. Thus, there are probably 1 million to 2 million men (and probably a similar number of women) in the United States who have totally asymptomatic, significant myocardial ischemia. Approximately 20% to 30% of patients post-MI have evidence of provocable asymptomatic myocardial ischemia (type II). Thus, 50,000–100,000 persons/yr are found to have silent ischemia after MI. Probably 80% to 90% of patients with angina (type III) have coexistent silent myocardial ischemia (approximately 3 million persons in the United States).

PROGNOSIS

Assessment of prognosis governs many important management decisions in patients with known or suspected CAD. Much is known about the determinants of prognosis in such patients. Until recently, little has been known about the prognostic implications of the presence of silent myocardial ischemia. There is growing concern that the presence of ischemia, regardless of accompanying symptoms, may significantly affect prognosis.

The degree of resting left ventricular dysfunction (ejection fraction) is the most powerful determinant of prognosis in patients who have had an MI; however, in these patients and, more specifically, in patients without prior MI, a number of other features are also important. The extent of CAD as assessed by coronary angiography can be an important predictor of prognosis. For example, high-grade stenosis of the left main coronary artery was shown early on in the Coronary Artery Surgery Study to be a significant determinant of prognosis. Angiography alone, however, is limited because visual interpretation of the coronary angiogram often reflects poorly the pressure gradient across the coronary stenosis and, accordingly, coronary blood flow reserve. Thus, it provides limited physiologic information. Exercise testing has proved to be an important predictor of subsequent cardiac events, largely because of its ability to quantify the extent of inducible myocardial ischemia. A number of exercise test variables have been shown to predict adverse events. The depth, duration, and time of onset of ST-segment depression and total exercise time have been found to predict an adverse prognosis. Recently, it was observed that the presence of inducible ischemia on exercise testing, regardless of the presence of symptoms, affects prognosis.[22] Follow-up data from the Coronary Artery Surgery Study suggest that the prognosis of patients with the same angiographic extent of CAD and the same extent of abnormality on exercise testing is independent of the presence of angina.[23]

Abnormal exercise findings in patients after MI have been shown in multiple studies to define a group at high risk for cardiac death, recurrent MI, and unstable angina. This unfavorable prognosis applies equally to patients with silent or symptomatic ischemia on exercise testing.

Studies using thallium scintigraphy also support the concept that patients with exercise-induced ischemia have an adverse prognosis regardless of the presence of chest pain. Asymptomatic patients after MI have widely different rates of subsequent cardiac events depending on whether inducible myocardial hypoperfusion is present during exercise (59% event rate in the next 15 months) or absent (6% event rate).[24] In another group of patients with typical angina and ischemia as observed with thallium scintigraphy at low work load, the cardiac event rate was equivalent in patients without symptoms or with typical angina. Thus, both conventional exercise testing and thallium scintigraphy indicate adverse prognosis if exercise-inducible ischemia is present, whether silent or symptomatic.

Does the presence of spontaneous silent ischemia on ambulatory monitoring affect prognosis? Stern and Tzivoni's[16] early studies found an increased rate of subsequent cardiac events in follow-up of patients who were observed to have out-of-hospital ischemic changes on ambulatory ECG recording, as compared with patients who had no such changes. A markedly worse prognosis has also been observed in patients with silent ischemia hospitalized for unstable angina.[4,5] Forty-three percent of patients with evidence of silent

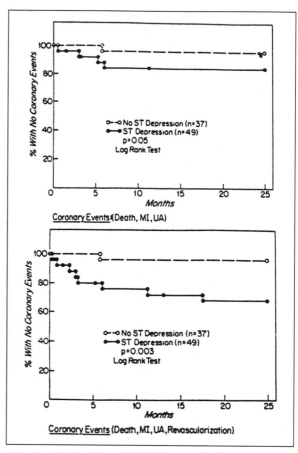

Figure 4. *Kaplan–Meier curves comparing the probability of not experiencing (top) an acute ischemic event (death, myocardial infarction [MI], unstable angina), or (bottom) a progressive ischemic event (death, MI, unstable angina, or revascularization). Follow-up of 37 patients without ST-segment depression (open circles) and 49 patients with ST-segment depression (closed circles) on ambulatory monitoring. Reprinted from Rocco MB et al.[23]*

ischemia developed subsequent MI or required surgery or balloon angioplasty, compared with 12% of patients without silent ischemia. Multiple logistic regression analysis revealed that ST-segment depression was the most potent prognostic variable for the prediction of long-term mortality in this group of patients. Rocco et al[25] followed 86 patients with chronic stable angina for an average of 12.5 months after ambulatory ECG recording. Patients with ST depression during monitoring had a significantly increased incidence of cardiac death, infarction, or unstable angina compared with patients who did not exhibit any ST depression (Fig. 4). Similarly, DeWood and Rozanski[26] reported 3-year follow-up with 59 patients who had ambulatory ECG monitoring. Those patients who demonstrated silent ischemic ST-segment changes had a 5-fold increase in the incidence of subsequent events. Silent ischemia on ambulatory monitoring appears to adversely affect prognosis. Multiple other studies have confirmed these findings.[27–41]

THERAPY FOR SILENT MYOCARDIAL ISCHEMIA

Several studies have demonstrated that drug therapy using conventional antianginal agents can markedly reduce or eliminate silent ischemia detected by ambulatory ECG recording. Nitrates (hourly sublinguinal nitroglycerin, transdermal nitroglycerin), ß-blockers (propranolol, atenolol, labetalol, and metoprolol), and calcium-channel blockers (nifedipine, verapamil, amlodipine, and diltiazem) have all been shown to be effective in reducing episodes of silent ischemia. In 1 study, a combination of propranolol and nifedipine was superior to either drug alone in reducing the total number of ischemic episodes. Not unexpectedly, successful balloon coronary angioplasty has also been documented to abolish silent myocardial ischemia as detected by ambulatory ECG monitoring.

The observation that asymptomatic ST depression detected during ambulatory monitoring occurs at relatively low heart rates has prompted the hypothesis that silent myocardial ischemia is a consequence of reduced myocardial oxygen supply caused by enhanced coronary vasomotor tone. Theoretically, treatment strategies with nitrates or calcium-channel blockers should prove superior; to date, however, clinical studies appear to favor use of ß-blockers, at least as single-agent therapy. In the Angina and Silent Ischemia Study, long-acting propranolol was significantly more effective than either diltiazem or nifedipine in suppressing both total ischemic time and number of ischemic events on 24-hour ambulatory ECG monitoring.[42] Other studies have had similar findings.[43,44]

The marked circadian variation in ischemic activity is another important consideration in the design of potential therapies for silent ischemia. Long-acting ß-blockers, and long-acting calcium-channel blockers (including amlodipine[45] and the slow-release form of nifedipine,[46] for example), have been demonstrated to suppress both morning and evening peaks in myocardial ischemic activity. Ultimately, drugs or drug preparations found to be successful in suppressing the morning surge of ischemia may be preferred.

The precise role for drug, percutaneous interventional, or surgical therapy of silent myocardial ischemia awaits demonstration that the adverse prognosis associated with the presence of silent ischemia can be altered. As is true for any asymptomatic disorder, general recommendations for therapy (and attendant costs, risks, and morbidity) await a consensus that there are significant prognostic benefits. Substantial evidence that silent ischemia adversely affects prognosis has been reviewed; however, no trials have yet demonstrated that medical treatment of active ischemia improves prognosis. One short-term (4 wk) study demonstrated reduced risk for adverse cardiac events in asymptomatic or mildly symptomatic patients with ambulatory ischemia treated with atenolol versus placebo (Fig. 5).[47] Surgical treatment has been demonstrated to improve survival in certain groups of patients with CAD. Importantly, patients with 3-vessel CAD and evidence of inducible ischemia do derive benefit from surgery; patients with equivalent CAD but no ischemia do not.[23] Since the presence of ischemia on exercise testing or ambulatory monitoring alters prognosis, independently of symptoms, a logical conclusion is that medical therapy designed to eliminate or decrease ischemia should favorably affect prognosis. At present, however, no studies have clearly demonstrated that treatment tailored to suppress active, asymptomatic ischemia improves prognosis. In the Asymptomatic Cardiac Ischemia Pilot Study, no differences were observed in the incidence of death or MI between groups treated specifically for abolition of asymptomatic ischemia and those treated only for angina.[48] The study, however, was of

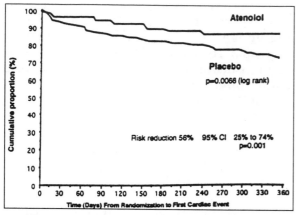

Figure 5. *Event-free survival: Kaplan–Meier curves comparing the cumulative probabilities of not experiencing an adverse event during follow-up for patients with ambulatory ECG-monitored silent ischemia randomized to atenolol (upper curve) and placebo (lower curve). Adverse events included death, resuscitated ventricular tachycardia/fibrillation, myocardial infarction, hospitalization for unstable angina, aggravation of angina, or revascularization. Reprinted from Pepine CJ et al.[47] With permission from the American Heart Association.*

insufficient sample size to definitively answer this question, and a larger randomized trial has been planned.

Indications for the use of ambulatory ECG as a guide to therapy remain unclear. Ultimately, ambulatory ECG may be used as a routine tool to "tailor" therapy to assure adequate control of daily ischemia for an individual's level of activity and lifestyle.

CONCLUSION

Silent myocardial ischemia has become recognized as an important manifestation of CAD. The presence of provoked or spontaneous silent ischemia appears to adversely effect the prognosis of patients with CAD. Improved methods of detection of silent ischemia have shed new light on the place of this phenomenon in the pathophysiology and clinical course of the disease. The precise role of these techniques in clinical decision-making remains somewhat uncertain.

REFERENCES

1. Rozanski A, Berman DS. Silent myocardial ischemia:. I. Pathophysiology, frequency of occurrence, and approaches toward detection. *Am Heart J.* 1987; 114:615-626.
2. Tzivoni D Gavish A, Zin D, et al. Prognostic significance of ischemic episodes in patients with previous myocardial infarction. *Am J Cardiol.* 1988;62:661-664.
3. Cohn PF. The concept and pathogenesis of active but asymptomatic coronary artery disease. *Circulation.* 1987;75(suppl II):2-3.
4. Gottlieb SO, Weisfeldt ML, Ouyang P, et al. Silent ischemia as a marker for early unfavorable outcomes in patients with unstable angina. *N Engl J Med.* 1986;314:1214-1219.
5. Gottlieb SO, Weisfeldt ML, Ouyang P, et al. Silent ischemia predicts infarction and death during 2 year follow-up of unstable angina. *J Am Coll Cardiol.* 1987;10:756-760.
6. Kannel WB, Abbott RD. Incidence and prognosis of unrecognized myocardial infarction: An update on the Framingham study. *N Engl J Med.* 1984; 311:1144-1147.
7. Maseri A, Mimmo R, Chierchia S, et al. Coronary artery spasm as a cause of acute myocardial ischemia in man. *Chest.* 1975;68:625-633.
8. Deanfield JE, Shea M, Ribiero P, et al. Transient ST-segment depression as a marker of myocardial ischemia during daily life. *Am J Cardiol.* 1984;54:1195-1200.
9. Selwyn AP, Fox K, Eves M, et al. Myocardial ischaemia in patients with frequent angina pectoris. *Br Med J.* 1978;2:1594-1596.
10. Ludmer PL, Selwyn AP, Shook TL, et al. Paradoxical vasoconstriction induced by acetylcholine in athero-sclerotic coronary arteries. *N Engl J Med.* 1986; 315:1046-1051.
11. Rocco MB, Barry J, Campbell S, et al. Circadian variation of transient myocardial ischemia in patients with coronary artery disease. *Circulation.* 1987;75:395-400.
12. Muller JE, Stone PH, Turi ZG, et al, and the MILIS Study Group. Circadian variation in the frequency of onset of acute myocardial infarction. *N Engl J Med.* 1985; 313:1315-1322.
13. Tofler GH, Brezinski D, Schafer AL, et al. Concurrent morning increase in platelet aggregability and the risk of myocardial infarction and sudden cardiac death. *N Engl J Med.* 1987;316:1514-1518.
14. Mehta J, Malloy M, Lawson D, et al. Circadian variation in platelet alpha 2-adrenoceptor affinity in normal subjects. *Am J Cardiol.* 1989;63:1002-1005.
15. Holter NJ. New method for heart studies: Continuous electrocardiography of active subjects over long periods is now practical. *Science.* 1961;134:1214-1220.
16. Stern S, Tzivoni D. Early detection of silent ischemic heart disease by 24-hour electrocardiogram monitoring of active subjects. *Br Heart J.* 1974;36:481-486.

17. Stern S, Weisz G, Gavish A, et al. Comparison between silent and symptomatic ischemia during exercise testing in patients with coronary artery disease. *J Cardiopulmonary Rehab.* 1988;12:507.

18. Bragg-Remschel DA, Anderson CM, Winkle RA. Frequency response characteristics of ambulatory ECG monitoring systems and their implications for ST segment analysis. *Am Heart J.* 1982;103:20-31.

19. Shook TL, Balke CW, Kotilainen PW, et al. Comparison of amplitude-modulated (direct) and frequency-modulated ambulatory techniques for recording ischemic electrocardiographic changes. *Am J Cardiol.* 1987;60:895-900.

20. Shook TL, Glasser SP, Crawford MH, et al. Discordance between ambulatory electrocardiography and exercise testing for assessment of the severity of ischemia. *Circulation.* 1987;76(suppl IV):362.

21. Reed DC, Stone PH, Shook TL, et al. Discordance between radionuclide, Doppler echo, angiographic and ambulatory ECG markers of ischemia. *J Am Coll Cardiol.* 1989;13:2A. Abstract.

22. Giagnoni E, Secchi MB, Wu SC, et al. Prognostic value of exercise EKG testing in asymptomatic normotensive subjects: A prospective matched study. *N Engl J Med.* 1983;309:1085-1089.

23. Weiner DA, Ryan T J, McCabe CH, et al. Significance of silent myocardial ischemia during exercise testing in patients with coronary artery disease. *Am J Cardiol.* 1987;59:725-729.

24. Gibson RS, Watson DD, Craddock GB, et al. Prediction of cardiac events after uncomplicated myocardial infarction: A prospective study comparing predischarge exercise thallium-201 scintigraphy and coronary angiography. *Circulation.* 1983;68:321-336.

25. Rocco MB, Nabel EG, Campbell S, et al. Prognostic Importance of myocardial ischemia detected by ambulatory monitoring in patients with stable coronary artery disease. *Circulation.* 1988;78:877-884.

26. DeWood MA, Rozanski A. Long-term prognosis of patients with and without silent ischemia. *Circulation.* 1986;74:II-59. Abstract.

27. Egstrup K. Asymptomatic myocardial ischemia as a predictor of cardiac events after coronary artery bypass grafting for stable angina pectoris. *Am J Cardiol.* 1988;61:248-252.

28. V Arnim T, Gerbig HW, Krawietz W, et al. Prognostic implications of transient predominantly silent ischaemia in patients with unstable angina pectoris. *Eur Heart J.* 1988;9:435-440.

29. Aronow WS, Epstein S. Usefulness of silent myocardial ischemia detecting by ambulatory electrocardiographic monitoring in predicting new coronary events in elderly patients. *Am J Cardiol.* 1988;62:1295-1296.

30. Hedblad B, Juul-Moller S, Hanson BS, et al. Increased mortality in men with ST segment depression during 24h ambulatory long-term recording. *Eur Heart J.* 1989;10:149-158.

31. Nademanee K, Intarachot V, Josephson MA, et al. Prognostic significance of silent myocardial ischemia in patients with unstable angina. *J Am Coll Cardiol.* 1987;10:1-9.

32. Langer A, Freeman MR, Armstrong PW. ST segment shift in unstable angina:pathophysiology and association with coronary anatomy and hospital outcome. *J Am Coll Cardiol.* 1989;13:1495-1502.

33. Johnson SM, Mauritson Dr, Winniford MD, et al. Continuous electrocardiographic monitoring in patients with unstable angina pectoris:identification of high-risk subgroup with severe coronary disease, variant angina, and/or impaired early prognosis. *Am Heart J.* 1982;103:4-12.

34. Deedwania P, Carbajal EV. Silent ischemia during daily life is an independent predictor of mortality in stable angina. *Circulation.* 1990;81:748-756.

35. Yeung AC, Barry J, Orav J, Bonassin E, et al. Effects of symptomatic ischemia on long-term prognosis in chronic stable coronary disease. *Circulation.* 1991;83:1598-1604.

36. Bugiardina R, Pozzati A, Borghi A, et al. Angiographic morphology in unstable angina and its relation to transient ischemia and hospital outcome. *Am J Cardiol.* 1991;67:460-464.

37. Pozzati A, Bugiardini R, Borghi A, et al. Transient ischaemia refractory to conventional medical treatment in unstable angina: Angiographic correlates and prognostic implications. *Eur Heart J.* 1992;13:360-365.

38. Langer A, Minkowitz J, Dorian P, et al. Pathophysiology and prognostic significance of Holter-detected ST segment depression after myocardial infarction. *J Am Coll Cardiol.* 1992;20:1313-1317.

39. Currie P, Ashby D, Saltissi S. Prognostic significance of transient myocardial ischemia on ambulatory monitoring after acute myocardial infarction. *Am J Cardiol.* 1993;71:773-777.

40. Bonaduce D, Petretta M, Lanzillo T, et al. Prevalence and prognostic significance of silent myocardial ischaemia detected by exercise test and continuous ECG monitoring after acute myocardial infarction. *Eur Heart J.* 1991;12:186-193.

41. Raby KE, Barry J, Vita G, et al. Prognostic significance of asymptomatic ischemia's response to medical therapy. *Circulation.* 1993;88(suppl I):298. Abstract.

42. Stone PH, Gibson RS, Glasser SP, et al. Comparison of propranolol, diltiazem and nifedipine in the treatment of ambulatory ischemia in patients with stable angina: Differential effect on ambulatory ischemia, exercise performance and anginal symptoms. *Circulation.* 1990;82:1962-1972.

43. Deedwania PC, Carbajal EV. Anti-ischemic effects of atenolol versus nifedipine in patients with coronary artery disease and ambulatory silent ischemia. *J Am Coll Cardiol.* 1991;17:963-969.

44. Pepine CJ. Beta-blockers or calcium antagonists in silent ischaemia? *Eur Heart J.* 1993;14 (suppl F):7-14.

45. Deanfield JE, Detry J-MRG, Lichtlen PR, et al. Amlodipine reduces transient myocardial ischemia in patients with coronary artery disease: Double-blind circadian anti-ischemic program in Europe (CAPE Trial). *J Am Coll Cardiol.* 1994;24:1460-1467.

46. Parmley WW, Nesto RW, Singh BN, et al. Attenuation of the circadian patterns of myocardial ischemia with nifedipine GITS in patients with chronic stable angina. *J Am Coll Cardiol.* 1992;19:1380-1389.

47. Pepine CJ, Cohn PF, Deedwania PC, et al. Effects of treatment on outcome in mildly symptomatic patients with ischemia during daily life. *Circulation.* 1994; 90:762-768.

48. Knatterud GL, Bourassa MG, Pepine CJ, et al. Effects of treatment strategies to suppress ischemia in patients with coronary artery disease: 12-week results of the Asymptomatic Cardiac Ischemia Pilot (ACIP) Study. *J Am Coll Cardiol.* 1994;24:11-20.

15 Acute Myocardial Infarction

James M. Hagar, MD
Harold G. Olson, MD
Robert A. Kloner, MD, PhD

Acute myocardial infarction (MI) is one of the most common serious health problems in Western society. In the United States alone, approximately 1,500,000 persons develop myocardial infarction annually. Approximately 500,000 deaths annually are attributable to acute myocardial infarction, amounting to one-fourth of all deaths in the United States.[1]

Sixty percent of MI-related deaths occur suddenly in the first hour of infarction, before medical attention is sought. Sudden death often occurs before histologic evidence of necrosis has developed, and is usually due to ventricular arrhythmias, chiefly ventricular fibrillation. The advent of pre-hospital resuscitation, coronary care units, and defibrillators in the early 1960s has markedly reduced the in-hospital mortality and lowered the overall case fatality rate for acute myocardial infarction, mostly by treating arrhythmias. Trials of ß-blocking drugs since the 1970s have demonstrated improved survival following infarction in patients treated with these agents. The incidence of acute myocardial infarction has also begun to decline.[2] However, until the advent of thrombolytic therapy no therapeutic intervention had the ability to limit infarct size in humans.

It is now generally accepted that acute thrombotic coronary artery occlusion is present in most cases of myocardial infarction, ushering in another revolution in treatment. Thrombolytic therapy and other methods to reperfuse infarcting myocardium have been demonstrated to decrease infarct size, wall motion abnormalities, complications, and mortality. Reperfusion therapy has become the standard of care for acute myocardial infarction in appropriate patients, as the ability to salvage infarcting myocardium has become a clinical reality.

DIAGNOSIS OF MYOCARDIAL INFARCTION

HISTORY

The typical history of a patient with acute myocardial infarction is one of severe substernal chest pressure, described as an intolerable crushing or constricting pain. The sensation of myocardial ischemia, transmitted via visceral afferent sympathetic nerves, is often difficult for the patient to describe precisely, in spite of the severe nature of the discomfort. Typically the pain is localized beneath the sternum with radiation to the inner aspect of the left arm, but pain in the jaw, neck, epigastrium, arm only, or back is also common. Retrospectively, a history of new or worsening angina preceding the infarction by hours to weeks can be elicited in approximately half of patients. Such symptoms may be mild, however, and medical attention is often not sought. The pain is distinguished from angina pectoris by a duration of longer than 30 minutes and lack of complete relief with rest or nitroglycerin. There are often associated symptoms of diaphoresis, weakness, or a feeling of impending doom. Vagal symptoms of nausea, vomiting, and abdominal cramps often occur, particularly in the setting of inferior wall infarction. When heart failure supervenes, dyspnea and cough, rarely with pink frothy sputum, are prominent. When diminished forward cardiac output occurs due either to extensive right or left ventricular infarction weakness and altered mentation may be noted. Syncope may be the presenting symptom in 5% of infarction patients. Some patients, especially the elderly, experience only nonspecific symptoms and perceive only that they have "indigestion." In 20% of patients, particularly diabetics, myocardial infarction is completely silent and is diagnosed only by routine electrocardiography or when complications (heart failure, arrhythmias) later develop.[3]

ACUTE RISK FACTORS FOR MYOCARDIAL INFARCTION

Multiple large studies have found that Q-wave myocardial infarction occurs in a circadian rhythm, with the peak incidence occurring between 6:00 AM and 12:00 PM. Some studies have also found a late afternoon peak. This early morning peak appears to be related to the catecholamine surge, enhanced platelet aggregability, and reduced fibrinolytic activity which are observed when first rising in the morning. Patients treated with aspirin or ß-blockers do not show this early morning peak of MI onset.[4,5] Such triggers of acute MI, termed acute risk factors, may cause sudden fracture of atherosclerotic plaque, leading to thrombosis and acute MI. In addition to "the early morning peak," heavy physical exertion and emotional stress such as anger have been correlated with the onset of infarction. In one study 4.4% of acute MI patients reported heavy exertion within 1 hour of the onset of their infarctions, with a relative risk of infarction within 1 hour after heavy exertion of 5.9 compared to less heavy exertion or no exertion.[6]

PHYSICAL EXAMINATION

The patient typically appears anxious, restless, and diaphoretic. The skin often is cool and clammy. Bradycardia may be present in patients with vagal reactions and in those with heart block, and the pulse is irregular if atrial or ventricular arrhythmias are present. In patients with severe pump failure, hypotension, tachycardia, oliguria, cool extremities, and peripheral cyanosis are noted. Low-grade fever is common in the first few days following infarction but rarely exceeds 102° F. Lung examination may reveal basilar rales or wheezes indicating congestive heart failure, though absence of rales does not exclude significant pulmonary venous congestion. Jugular venous distention and hepato-jugular reflux can be seen

in patients with biventricular failure, but if found without evidence of left-sided heart failure, suggest the diagnosis of right ventricular infarction. The cardiac impulse is often faint and diffuse, or systolic bulging along the sternal border can be felt when a large segment of anterior wall is dyskinetic. A loud fourth heart sound is invariably present and is often palpable; a third heart sound may be audible if congestive failure is present. A blowing, usually holosystolic, murmur of mitral insufficiency is sometimes heard, indicative of papillary muscle ischemia or infarction. Pericardial friction rubs occur frequently in the first days of myocardial infarction, are transient and intermittent, and usually indicate transmural infarction.

DIFFERENTIAL DIAGNOSIS

There are a number of disorders that may be confused with acute myocardial infarction (Table 1). These usually can be suspected from a careful history and physical examination. The clinician must maintain a high level of suspicion for potentially life-threatening disorders for which specific therapy must be given. In particular these include aortic dissection, which is frequently fatal within hours if not recognized, and pulmonary embolism. In cases of pericarditis, peptic ulcer disease, or aortic dissection, a mistaken diagnosis of myocardial infarction could lead to administration of thrombolytic therapy, with disastrous results. Distinguishing features of these disorders are listed in Table 1.

ELECTROCARDIOGRAPHIC FINDINGS

The electrocardiogram is of central importance in the diagnosis of acute myocardial infarction (Table 2, Fig. 1). Evolutionary changes diagnostic of myocardial infarction will be seen on serial tracings in approximately two-thirds of patients with acute myocardial infarction, with the remainder having only ST and T wave depression. The initial electrocardiogram (ECG), however, will show only mild or nonspecific abnormalities as much as half the time, and is normal in about 20% of cases.[7]

Table 1. Disease Entities That May Be Confused With Myocardial Infarction	
Angina pectoris	Pain less severe and of shorter duration than myocardial infarction; usually less than 20 minutes; relieved with rest and nitroglycerin
Aortic dissection	Pain is sharp, tearing and extremely severe; typically radiates to back. Neurologic signs, loss of pulses or aortic insufficiency often develop; mediastinum widened on chest x-ray; myocardial infarction may occur if dissection extends into coronary artery; diagnosis confirmed by CT scan, transesophageal echocardiogram, or aortography.
Pulmonary embolism	Dyspnea, tachycardia and hypoxemia are prominent; pain is usually pleuritic, especially when pulmonary infarction develops but may resemble angina in bland infarction; ECG is nonspecific, LDH may be elevated but not CK; diagnosis confirmed by lung scan or pulmonary angiogram
Pericarditis	May be preceded by viral illness; pain is sharp, positional, pleuritic and relieved by leaning forward; pericardial rub often present; diffuse ST elevation occurs without evolution of Q waves; CK ususally normal but rises in some cases; responds to antinflammatory agents
Myocarditis	May be preceded by viral illness; pain is generally vague and mild if present; CK total and MB often elevated; conduction abnormalities and sometimes Q waves can occur
Musculoskeletal disorders	Includes costochondritis, cervical osteoarthritis; pain is atypical, stabbing, localized, may be pleuritic; reproduced by motion or palpation; ECG changes absent
Gastrointestinal disorders	Esophageal reflux is often made worse with recumbency or after meals, may be associated with regurgitation and relieved by antacids. Episodes of spasm may be brought on by cold liquids, relieved by nitroglycerin, and may closely resemble angina or infarction. Diagnosis may be confirmed by upper GI series, endoscopy or esophageal manometry. Peptic ulcer disease, pancreatitis and cholecystitis may occasionally mimic infarction; abdominal tenderness is present, with radiation to back and elevated amylase in pancreatitis; sonography can confirm cholecystitis
Pneumothorax	Onset abrupt with sharp pleuritic chest pain and dyspnea; breath sounds absent, chest x-ray confirms
Pleuritis	Pain is sharp and increases on inspiration; friction rub or dullness may be present; other respiratory symptoms and underlying pulmonary infection usually present

In the classic pattern, initial hyperacute T wave peaking followed by ST-segment elevation develops promptly following onset of ischemia in the leads facing the area of injury. As cell death occurs, R-wave height is lost and pathologic Q waves, defined as greater than 0.04 seconds in duration and 25% of total QRS height, develop over hours to days. ST-segment elevation decreases toward baseline and finally returns to normal simultaneous with the development of symmetrical T-wave inversion over subsequent days. Posterior infarction

Table 2. Localization of Myocardial Infarction

LOCATION	ECG LEADS INVOLVED	PROBABLE ARTERY INVOLVED
Anteroseptal	V_1-V_2	Proximal left anterior descending (LAD) septal perforators
Anteroapical	V_2-V_4	LAD or its branches
Anterolateral	V_4-V_6, I, aVL	Mid LAD or circumflex
Extensive anterior	V_1-V_6	Proximal LAD
High lateral	I, aVL	Circumflex or first diagonal branch of LAD
Inferior	II, III, aVF	Right coronary; less often circumflex or distal LAD
Posterior	Mirror image in V_1 and V_2	Posterior descending
Right ventricular	V_1 and reversed chest leads rV_3-rV_4	Right coronary

produces an "inverted" pattern, with ST depression instead of elevation, T-wave peaking and development of R waves in V_1 and V_2. Right ventricular infarction is manifested electrocardiographically as ST elevation in right-sided precordial leads, especially V_{3R}-V_{4R}, and sometimes in V_1. These changes should be sought in all cases of inferior infarction, with which they are frequently associated. Some patients may present with new left bundle branch block. This finding usually indicates extensive anterior wall infarction.

ST depression may be seen in leads remote from the area of infarction, usually anterior ST depression with inferior infarctions or inferior ST depression with anterior infarction. Such ST-segment changes have traditionally been thought not to indicate remote ischemia, and are commonly referred to as "reciprocal" ST changes. Reciprocal anterior ST depression in inferior infarction appears to indicate posterolateral extension of infarction[8] but is difficult to distinguish from "ischemia at a distance" due to obstruction of the left anterior descending coronary artery.[9] Regardless of its cause, such ST-segment depression is associated with a higher mortality rate.[10] Following early and complete reperfusion, such as that associated with thrombolytic therapy, ST elevation resolves rapidly, development of Q waves is accelerated, and arrhythmias such as accelerated idioventricular rhythm may occur.

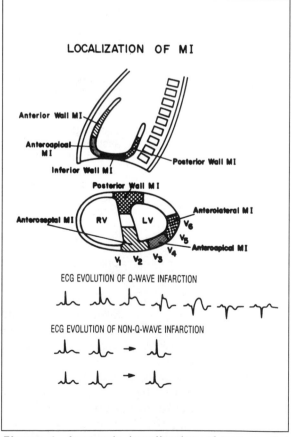

Figure 1. *Anatomic localization of myocardial infarction by ECG.*

Acute bundle branch blocks or hemiblocks may also resolve following successful reperfusion. When ST-segment elevation persists, a large area of dyskinesis is suggested[11] and when still present 3-6 months after recovery from infarction, it is likely that a ventricular aneurysm has developed. T-wave inversion may persist for weeks or months. Months to years after infarction, Q waves sometimes diminish in size or may disappear, particularly with inferior wall infarction.

In many cases, ST-segment depression or elevation is initially noted on ECG, which persists for 48 hours or more with enzyme release and T-wave changes but without development of pathologic Q waves. This usually indicates non-transmural necrosis. The finding of non–Q-wave infarction, previously called non-transmural or subendocardial infarction, has important diagnostic and therapeutic implications, as discussed later in this chapter.

The suggested nomenclature for localizing infarct site by ECG is shown in Figure 1 and Table 2. Useful inferences concerning the involved coronary artery can often be made (Fig. 1)[12,13] but anatomic variation and collateral flow in the presence of multivessel disease frequently make such estimations inexact.

The electrocardiographic diagnosis of acute myocardial infarction may be mimicked by a variety of conditions. ST-segment elevation occurs without infarction in coronary spasm, where it is rapidly reversible, and in pericarditis, which produces diffuse ST elevation. In distinction from myocardial infarction, the ST elevation in pericarditis returns to baseline before T inversion occurs, and PR-segment depression is often seen. J-point elevation seen in early repolarization, a normal variant, is sometimes confused with acute infarction, but evolutionary changes and cardiac enzyme elevations do not occur. ST-segment depression and T-wave changes from left ventricular hypertrophy, digitalis, hypokalemia, hyperventilation and many other conditions may suggest ischemia.[14] Q waves are found without infarction in patients with bypass tracts, hypertrophic cardiomyopathy, and dilated cardiomyopathy, as well as chronic lung disease and neuromuscular disorders.[15] Likewise, the typical changes of infarction may be masked by other ECG abnormalities, particularly left (but not right) bundle branch block.

It has been traditional to equate ST elevation with transmural myocardial injury, ST depression with subendocardial ischemia, T-wave inversion with transmural ischemia and development of Q waves with transmural necrosis of myocardium. While these concepts are clinically useful, the actual situation is more complex. For example, development of transient Q waves has been documented after reversible ischemia and following thrombolytic therapy.[16] In particular, it has been appreciated that anatomically transmural infarction may not develop Q waves on ECG, and that many nontransmural infarctions do manifest Q waves on surface ECG, usually when they encompass greater than 50% of the thickness of the ventricular wall.[17] Thus, the terms Q wave and non–Q-wave infarction should be used clinically, and transmural or non-transmural applied pathologically.

LABORATORY DIAGNOSIS

Determination of serum levels of enzymes released from damaged myocytes is crucial to the diagnosis of myocardial infarction. Each enzyme has its own time course, use and limitations. These tests[18,19] and the strategies for their use[20] have been the subject of excellent reviews.

1. Creatine kinase (CK) is present in high concentration in muscle cells. Serum levels rise within 6-8 hours after onset of infarction, peak within 24 hours, and return to normal within 48-96 hours. Peak level is higher and occurs earlier (8-12 hrs) when coronary reperfusion is achieved. Peak and duration of elevation are increased in larger infarcts, but peak level does not correlate with infarct size following reperfusion due to enzyme "washout." Total CK rises following any form of muscle trauma, such as intramuscular injections or rhabdomyolysis, as well as in hypothyroidism, renal failure or stroke. CK is optimally sampled on admission, 12 and 24 hours later.

2. The MB isoenzyme of CK is currently the mainstay in the diagnosis of myocardial infarction. It is found only in minute amounts in non-cardiac tissues, and usually does not increase following muscle trauma. Its levels rise and peak slightly earlier than the total CK, and normalize in 36-72 hours. The usual electrophoretic assay reliably detects levels greater than 5 IU/ml, but optimum specificity is achieved when a cutoff of 5% of total CK or 13 IU/ml is used. The subset of patients (15%-20%) with elevated CK-MB but normal total CK should be considered to have myocardial infarction if a typical rise and fall in total CK levels is seen and clinical presentation is compatible, as their mortality is increased.[21] Cardiac release of CK-MB may occur with perimyocarditis, defibrillation, cardiac surgery, cardiac contusion, or prolonged severe ischemia without infarction. Elevations of CK-MB have also been noted in myopathies, hypothyroidism, and following strenuous exercise. False positive tests sometimes occur in the setting of chronic renal failure, rhabdomyolysis, isoenzyme variants, or with some immunoassay methods which detect BB isoenzyme from brain and kidney.

3. Lactate dehydrogenase (LD) and its five isoenzymes rise within 24-48 hours of infarction, peak in 3-5 days and persist for 7-10 days. LD is present ubiquitously and is elevated in disorders of muscle, kidney, liver, brain, pancreas, and in hematologic disorders. The ratio of LD1/LD2, of greater than 1.0 (or .76 if lower specificity is acceptable) is relatively specific for myocardial necrosis, though hemolysis also raises LD1. LD isoenzymes are useful when CK-MB is negative and it is believed that infarction may have occurred 2-4 days previously or more.

4. Serum glutamic oxaloacetic transferase (SGOT) is another non-specific marker for myocyte necrosis, peaking 48-72 hours after infarction. It is of little or no clinical utility.

5. The MB and MM isoenzymes each exist in 3 isoforms, and assays for these isoforms are becoming available. The pattern of isoforms becomes abnormal before the total CK-MB rises, making early enzymatic confirmation of acute infarction possible. The presence of elevated CK-MB subforms has a 97% sensitivity for diagnosis of acute myocardial infarction at 6 hours of chest pain compared with a sensitivity of 48% for conventional CK-MB assay.[22] Isoforms of CK-MM have also been employed. These tests may be of value in assessing early infarction, reperfusion, infarct extension, and postoperative infarction.

6. Cardiac troponin-T and troponin-I, regulatory proteins which modulate the calcium-mediated interaction of actin and myosin in striated muscle, are released into the plasma following myocardial injury. Elevated levels appear 3 hours after onset of infarction and peak at 24 hours.[23] Levels remain elevated for 5 to 7 days, which allows the diagnosis of infarction to be made after CK-MB levels have returned to normal. Recent studies suggest that troponin levels are sensitive and specific in the diagnosis of acute MI. Cardiac troponin determination may also be useful in situations where CK-MB levels may be falsely elevated, such as in skeletal muscle injury or renal failure.[24]

7. Myosin light chains are detected in the plasma beginning 6 hours after the onset of myocardial infarction and remain elevated for at least 7 days. This structural protein marker seems to be less dependent on myocardial blood flow than CK, and is therefore useful for measurement of myocardial infarct size following reperfusion therapies.

8. Myoglobin appears and disappears in serum and urine very early in infarction, and peaks in 3-20 hours. Its place in clinical practice is unclear, but as with CK isoforms it is potentially useful in the early diagnosis of infarction.

9. Other laboratory abnormalities are associated with acute myocardial infarction. Marked hyperglycemia or ketoacidosis are frequent in diabetics, are sometimes the only symptom of myocardial infarction, and can occur even in non-insulin-requiring or borderline diabetics. Leukocytosis, sometimes with increased band forms, may persist for up to a week. Serum lipids are altered variably and do not accurately reflect the true profile for weeks after myocardial infarction.

CHEST X-RAY

The chest roentgenogram is of value in the initial assessment of the myocardial infarction patient, but has limitations. Cardiomegaly, when present, could indicate pre-existing heart disease which has led to ventricular dilatation or hypertrophy. When pulmonary artery wedge pressure acutely exceeds 18 mm Hg or more, pulmonary vascular redistribution is noted, and interstitial and alveolar edema become manifest above wedge pressures of 22-25 mm Hg. Though important findings, the presence of pulmonary congestion or pulmonary edema does not always correlate with the patient's current hemodynamic status. Radiographic findings lag behind the clinical picture by up to 12 hours when the onset of heart failure has been abrupt, and persist for up to several days after heart failure has been treated.

RADIONUCLIDE STUDIES

Radionuclide imaging studies are of value in cases where the triad of history, ECG and enzymes are insufficient to confirm the diagnosis of acute myocardial infarction, or when infarct location is uncertain as in association with left bundle branch block. These are described in detail in chapter 5. 99mTechnetium-pyrophosphate scanning may be useful in this setting, particularly in patients presenting 48 hours or more after suspected infarction after CK levels have returned to normal. The tracer binds to accumulated calcium within irreversibly damaged myocardium. Sensitivity is highest when performed between 24-72 hours after infarction, and in transmural infarcts, and is significantly lower in nontransmural infarction. In Q-wave infarcts scintigraphic abnormalities may be present for 5 to 7 days after infarction. Newer infarct-avid agents, particularly imaging with 111Indium labeled antimyosin Fab fragments, have improved sensitivity for detecting Q wave infarcts.[25] However, infarct size after thrombolytic therapy may be overestimated, and false positive tests have been noted in cases of dilated cardiomyopathy. Radionuclide angiography with 99mTc-RBC is useful to localize and quantify left or right ventricular wall motion abnormalities and ventricular function, which are related to prognosis.

Myocardial perfusion imaging agents, 201Thallium and the newer 99mTechnetium sestamibi and related compounds, accumulate within myocardium in proportion to regional blood flow and localize defects in ischemic or infarcted areas. The very slow washout and minimal redistribution characteristics of 99mTechnetium sestamibi make it ideal for quantitative assessment of infarct size in clinical trials of reperfusion therapy. The tracer is administered prior to therapeutic interventions and imaging performed several hours later, thereby not delaying treatment. This allows quantitative assessment of the amount of non-perfused myocardium present prior to thrombolysis (i.e., the area at risk). A second study is performed a week later, which allows assessment of the ultimate size of the infarction. Comparison of the studies provides a measure of infarct salvage by the therapeutic intervention.[26] In routine clinical practice, the most important use of the perfusion agents is in conjunction with exercise in the post-infarct assessment of inducible ischemia.

Positron-emission tomography (PET), which provides information on regional myocardial metabolism and uptake of glucose, fatty acids, as well as regional blood flow, has provided exciting insights into the pathophysiology of myocardial infarction and reperfusion not available by other modalities. Positron-emission tomography imaging is capable of differentiating viable from infarcted myocardium, quantifying infarct size, and assessing residual ischemia following infarction. Mismatch between regional myocardial blood flow (N-13 ammonia uptake) and oxidative metabolism (fluorine-18 fluorodeoxyglucose uptake) on serial PET imaging predicts myocardial viability ("stunned" and "hibernating" myocardium) after infarction.[27] Matched reductions of flow and metabolism generally indicate that revascularization will not restore regional function. It has been confirmed that the presence of viable myocardium detected by PET is associated with better 3-year survival, and that among patients with reduced ventricular function only those with viable myocardium had improved survival after revascularization.[28] Development of longer-lived radionuclides and availability of nuclides such as rubidium-82 that do not require a cyclotron for production may allow dissemination of this technique beyond a few research centers.

ECHOCARDIOGRAPHY

Two-dimensional and doppler echocardiography are of considerable value in the diagnosis of essentially all the complications of acute myocardial infarction,[29] and can provide prognostic information as well. A regional wall motion abnormality can be demonstrated in nearly all patients with acute myocardial infarction. Accordingly, echocardiography has a high sensitivity for the early diagnosis of acute myocardial infarction when the ECG is nondiagnostic and results of cardiac enzyme tests are pending. It is therefore particularly useful in the emergency department to evaluate patients with acute chest pain.[30] Using echocardiography, the location and extent of infarction and the degree of left and right ventricular dysfunction can be reliably assessed.[31] In addition, echocardiography is an essential aid in the diagnosis of the mechanical complications of myocardial infarction, including papillary muscle rupture, ventricular septal rupture, ventricular aneurysm and pseudoaneurysm, ventricular mural thrombus, pericardial effusion, and infarct extension and expansion. Preliminary studies suggest that echocardiographic criteria can be used to identify low risk myocardial infarction patients who can be safely discharged after 5 days.[32] Newer uses of echocardiography include tissue characterization using myocardial contrast agents, visualization of coronary artery lumina, and the detection of coronary reperfusion and myocardial viability after thrombolytic therapy.

Stress echocardiography using exercise or intravenous dobutamine can detect residual or remote ischemia after myocardial infarction and/or thrombolytic therapy. Viability of akinetic segments after thrombolysis (myocardial stunning) can be detected by the improvement of their wall motion with low dose dobutamine infusion, and inducible ischemia by new or increased severity of wall motion abnormalities at high doses.[33] The sensitivity and specificity of dobutamine stress echocardiography is probably comparable to stress myocardial perfusion scintigraphy.

OTHER STUDIES

Magnetic resonance imaging (MRI) of the cardiovascular system is increasingly recognized as valuable in a variety of disease states and is available at many centers. Using gated cine images, assessment of ventricular volumes, global and regional wall motion, and ventricular mass can be measured accurately. Infarcted and viable myocardium can be distinguished and infarct size estimated.[34] Flow imaging allowing visualization of flow velocities, and perfusion imaging using tracers hold promise as well. As these advanced MRI techniques continue to develop and become widely available, their role in managing myocardial infarction will further expand.

There are presently many different methods available for imaging myocardial infarct size, wall motion, ventricular function, and myocardial perfusion after infarction. There is no agreement on the use of these imaging methods, and their indications and cost-effectiveness need to be critically assessed. As a general rule, most or all patients with myocardial infarction will require an assessment of left ventricular function and some assessment of residual ischemia after infarction, which are major determinants of prognosis.

PATHOLOGY AND PATHOGENESIS OF MYOCARDIAL INFARCTION

Most myocardial infarctions occur in the territory of an atherosclerotic coronary artery, when plaque disruption leads to platelet aggregation, thrombus formation and spasm, causing acute reduction of blood flow and myocardial ischemia. When ischemia is sufficiently severe and prolonged, infarction results. Because therapeutic interventions in modern cardiology are increasingly directed toward modifying the cellular and molecular events of ischemia and infarction, a sound understanding of these events is important.

Within seconds of coronary artery occlusion, cellular metabolism shifts to anaerobic glycolysis. Contraction ceases and high energy stores of creatine phosphate, then adenosine triphosphate (ATP), become depleted.[35] Eventually injury becomes irreversible, proceeding as a wavefront of cell death from subendocardium toward subepicardium,[36] and culminating in a transmural infarct. The duration of ischemia necessary for completion of cell death averages from 2 to 6 hours in experimental studies; it may be longer in vivo if infarction progresses in a "stuttering" fashion. The rate of necrosis and infarct size is determined by 1) the size of the coronary bed at risk, 2) the amount of collateral flow and residual antegrade flow to the ischemic region, and 3) the duration of infarct-artery occlusion before reperfusion occurs, if reperfusion occurs at all.[37] An intervention that lessens cardiac work and heart rate during ischemia (for example a ß-blocking or negative inotropic drug) might delay the rate of progression of necrosis but does not limit ultimate infarct size if there is no reperfusion.

In the absence of reperfusion, light microscopic evidence of cellular injury is first seen within 6-8 hours. Mild white cell infiltration begins at the edge of the infarct within 12 hours, and by 24 hours, clear myocyte disruption and coagulative necrosis are evident. Mononuclear cell infiltration and myocyte removal begin by the fourth day, making the infarct susceptible to expansion or rupture. Collagen deposition begins at the periphery after 10-12 days, and healing with dense scar formation is essentially complete in 4-6 weeks in all but very large infarcts.

Functionally, the onset of severe ischemia first results in increased diastolic stiffness and elevation of end-diastolic pressure. The involved wall becomes akinetic or dyskinetic, compromising systolic function, though compensatory hyperkinesis of the remaining myocardium acutely preserves global function in smaller infarcts. Greater losses of functioning myocardium lead to progressively more severe

ventricular dysfunction, with subsequent dilatation and remodeling due to abnormal wall stress within the infarcted segment. Based on pathologic studies, infarction without reperfusion of greater than 10% of ventricular mass leads to a reduced ejection fraction, to dilatation and congestive failure when 25% or more is lost, and to cardiogenic shock or death with loss of 40% or more, whether this loss results from single or multiple insults.

CONSEQUENCES OF CORONARY REPERFUSION

When reperfusion occurs early in the course of infarction, either spontaneously or due to therapeutic revascularization, a different sequence of events ensues. Restoration of the flow of oxygenated blood leads to large increases in tissue water, sodium, and calcium and explosive disruption of irreversibly injured myocytes, which are unable to regulate their cell volume. Ventricular arrhythmias often increase, white cell infiltration is accelerated, and microvascular damage leads to intramural hemorrhage within the infarct zone.[38] Central portions of the infarct may not reperfuse as a result of microvascular injury, the so-called "no-reflow phenomenon."[39] "No-reflow" has been documented in humans, and is associated with poor recovery of left ventricular function.[40] Ultimately, salvage of ischemic but viable myocardial cells occurs in the midmyocardial and supepicardial layers of the ventricular wall resulting in a smaller and largely subendocardial infarction. The rate of infarct healing is also accelerated by reperfusion. However, the process of accelerated tissue injury that occurs initially upon reperfusion might be modifiable with adjunctive pharmacologic agents. Therapy directed at the mediators of this "reperfusion injury" could potentially enhance the myocardial salvage that occurs with reperfusion and has been the subject of much investigation.[41]

Beside risk zone size, collateral blood flow, and timely reperfusion, the presence of antecedent ischemia may also influence infarct size. Transient episodes of reversible ischemia paradoxically protect against subsequent prolonged ischemia and markedly reduce infarct size in experimental models. This phenomenon is known as ischemic preconditioning, and is mediated at least in part by endogenous adenosine.[42] Such episodes of transient ischemia frequently precede myocardial infarction in humans and could cause preconditioning. Patients in the TIMI-4 trial having angina within the 48 hours preceding infarction had lower hospital mortality and smaller infarcts than those without it.[43] During percutaneous transluminal coronary angioplasty (PTCA) it has been observed that the second balloon inflation is associated with less ischemia than the initial inflation.[44] These data suggest that preconditioning occurs in human myocardial infarction and is an important determinant of infarct size and prognosis. Whether the molecular mechanisms underlying preconditioning can be harnessed for clinical use remains to be determined.

Global and regional left ventricular function are also profoundly affected by coronary reperfusion. Persistent total occlusion of an infarct artery will result in progressive functional deterioration of segmental wall motion in that region, unless mitigated by spontaneous reperfusion or collateral blood flow. When reperfusion halts the progression of myocardial infarction, wall motion in the viable but injured portions of the previously ischemic area does not recover immediately. This prolonged postischemic dysfunction, termed myocardial "stunning," persists for days to weeks after restoration of flow.[45] Stunned myocardium can be recruited with inotropic agents. Segmental wall motion ultimately recovers unless flow is inadequate, for example if a severe stenosis remains in the infarct artery. Myocardium that is viable but noncontracting because of a chronic reduction in resting blood flow is termed hibernating myocardium. The distinction between viable, either stunned or hibernating, from nonviable myocardium is an important task of the clinician caring for the post-infarction patient, as it is a major determinant of prognosis and may dictate the need for revascularization.

PATHOPHYSIOLOGY OF CORONARY THROMBOSIS

Early angiography in acute myocardial infarction[46] and angioscopy[47] have provided a great deal of insight into the complex events that occur within an infarct-related coronary artery. Acute thrombotic occlusion is found in 80%-90% of cases of Q-wave infarction studied within 4-6 hours of onset, and in fewer non–Q-wave infarcts.[48,49] Coronary occlusion is usually the result of instability of an underlying atherosclerotic plaque and its dynamic interaction with mediators of vascular tone, platelets, and the clotting cascade, as shown in simplified form in Figures 2 and 3. Fissuring, rupture, or hemorrhage into an atheromatous plaque[50] is the event which usually initiates myocardial infarction. Atheroma, collagen, and tissue thromboplastins within the plaque are thereby exposed to circulating platelets and clotting factors (Fig. 3). Platelet aggregation further promotes thrombosis and leads to vasoconstriction via release of thromboxane A2, overwhelming endogenous vasodilators such as prostacyclin and endothelial-derived nitric oxide. Activation of the intrinsic and extrinsic coagulation cascades lead ultimately to thrombin activation, fibrin deposition, and entrapment of erythrocytes into an expanding thrombus. Luminal obstruction results from the combination of atheromatous plaque, intraluminal thrombus, aggregated platelets, and variable degrees of spasm (Fig. 2).

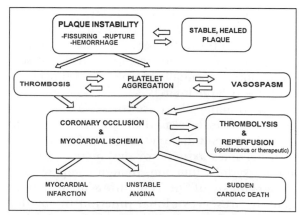

Figure 2. Pathogenic mechanisms in unstable coronary syndromes.

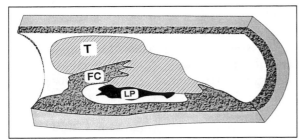

Figure 3. *Pathophysiology of acute myocardial infarction. Rupture of the fibrous cap (FC) of atherosclerotic plaque exposes lipid pool (LP) within plaque to circulating platelets and coagulation factors, resulting in formation of intraluminal thrombus (T).*

Plaque rupture typically occurs at the edge of the plaque's fibrous cap overlying a lipid pool, where shear forces are greatest. Plaques with relatively large lipid cores and thin fibrous caps appear to be more vulnerable to rupture. The cholesterol content of a given plaque, and thus its fluidity, may also determine its susceptibility to rupture. In addition, activated macrophages are frequently found at sites of plaque rupture. It is believed that collagenases and other proteases elaborated by these macrophages may degrade the fibrous cap and initiate plaque rupture.[51]

A totally occluding thrombus is the usual proximate cause of myocardial infarction. When subtotal, unstable angina is more often the result. Spontaneous thrombolysis occurs in a third to a half of infarct arteries over hours to days following infarction.[52] Non–Q-wave infarction is often the result of such spontaneous lysis, though such an infarct may also result from an initially subtotal occlusion or a transmural infarct that fails to produce a Q wave. Clot lysis leaves behind a fixed stenosis of varying severity and unstable morphology which is prone to reocclusion or may heal with incorporation of thrombus and progression of stenosis.

NON-ATHEROSCLEROTIC ETIOLOGIES

A wide variety of disorders other than atherosclerosis can occasionally lead to myocardial infarction, accounting for a few percent of cases, and are shown in Table 3.[53]

Table 3. Causes of Myocardial Infarction Without Coronary Atherosclerosis

Vasculitis
    Systemic lupus eyrthematosus
    Polyarteritis nodosa
    Takayasu's arteritis
    Mucocutaneous lymph node syndrome
    Luetic aortitis
Anomalous Origin of Coronary Artery
Acquired Coronary Artery Abnormalities
    Trauma
    Aortic dissection
    Spontaneous coronary artery dissection
    Iatrogenic
Coronary Spasm
    Variant angina
    Cocaine abuse
    Nitroglycerin withdrawal
Coronary Artery Embolus
    Infective endocarditis
    Mitral valve prolapse
    Atrial myxoma
    Left atrial or ventricular thrombus
Hypercoagulable States
    Polycythemia vera
    Thrombocytosis

Vasculitides have been reported to produce coronary occlusion, including lupus erythematosus, polyarteritis nodosa and Kawasaki disease (which leads to the late sequela of coronary artery aneurysm). Coronary anomalies, emboli, hypercoagulable states and aortic diseases involving the coronary arteries also cause myocardial infarction on occasion. Myocardial infarction sometimes occurs in persons with normal coronaries without evidence of any of these disorders, usually in heavy smokers or cocaine users.

Cases of myocardial infarction and sudden death associated with cocaine abuse are not infrequent. Coronary spasm, often with resultant thrombus formation, may be the cause,[54] although arterial intimal hyperplasia has also been reported in a few cases. Intranasal cocaine causes vasoconstriction of coronary arteries and reduces coronary blood flow, probably via an α-adrenergic effect.[55] Cocaine also has direct myocardial depressant effects and can directly cause myocyte necrosis. Coronary arteriography and ergonovine testing in these patients are usually normal, and recurrent infarction can occur with continued drug use.

REPERFUSION THERAPY FOR MYOCARDIAL INFARCTION

Since the 1960s, management of the patient with known or suspected myocardial infarction has focused on early prehospital supportive care and coronary care unit monitoring. This has reduced the mortality associated with acute MI by one-half or more, almost entirely due to treatment of primary ventricular arrhythmias.[56] However, most sudden death still occurs before medical attention is sought. Mortality due to pump failure and cardiogenic shock, related to infarct size, have not been appreciably altered by such conventional therapy, and pharmacologic limitation of infarct size has proved disappointing.[57] However, with the recognition of the importance of thrombosis in the pathogenesis of myocardial infarction and the wide availability of thrombolytic therapy, there has been a paradigm shift in the treatment of myocardial infarction, toward a primary goal of minimizing infarct size.

THE FIBRINOLYTIC SYSTEM

Under normal circumstances, the endogenous fibrinolytic system is responsible for the dynamic equilibrium between thrombosis and thrombolysis. When fibrin is formed and polymerized into thrombus, circulating plasminogen is bound to it. Locally produced tissue plasminogen activator (t-PA) eventually induces clot-specific lysis by cleaving this bound plasminogen to its active form, plasmin, which specifically degrades fibrin to degradation products. Tissue plasminogen activator acts selectively on plasminogen bound to fibrin rather than free circulating plasminogen (fibrin

specificity). The fibrinolytic process remains localized because of t-PA's fibrin specificity, the relative specificity of plasmin for fibrin rather than fibrinogen, and a plasminogen activator inhibitor derived from endothelium. When plasmin becomes activated systemically, circulating fibrinogen is also degraded, leading to a hemorrhagic state brought on by fibrinogen depletion and fibrin/fibrinogen degradation products having anticoagulant and platelet inhibiting properties. Such a systemic lytic state may lead to bleeding at any site. Even when a fibrin-specific agent is administered, dissolution of hemostatic plugs occurs in wounds and puncture sites and within arterial thrombi in coronary and cerebral vessels. Thus the incidence of intracranial hemorrhage and major bleeding at catheterization sites, which accounts for most bleeding episodes in thrombolytic patients, does not differ significantly between intravenous fibrinolytic agents.

Available fibrinolytic drugs act at different points in the clotting cascade. Recombinant single-chain tissue plasminogen activator (rt-PA) and its double-chain counterpart (dt-PA) maintain the same relative fibrin specificity of the native protein, though at the massive intravenous doses used clinically, a mild lytic state can be observed. Streptokinase, a bacterial protease, combines with both fibrin-bound and circulating plasminogen to form an active complex which activates other plasminogen molecules and leads to degradation of both fibrin and fibrinogen. Anisoylated plasminogen-streptokinase activator complex (anistreplase, also known as APSAC), is initially inactive, binds to fibrin, and is then deacylated to the active complex. This confers some fibrin specificity at low doses, but fibrinogenolysis equal to streptokinase occurs at the doses used for coronary thrombolysis. Urokinase activates plasminogen directly. It is not antigenic and produces a slightly less severe lytic state than streptokinase. Its inactive precursor, called pro-urokinase is converted to urokinase by plasmin. Both agents have some degree of fibrin specificity.

The ideal fibrinolytic agent would combine very high fibrinolytic activity, fibrin specificity, low antigenicity, and a long duration of action, in order to allow rapid and sustained action after single bolus administration and the potential for readministration. Newer thrombolytic drugs and a mutant human plasminogen activator with improved pharmacologic profiles and lower cost are undergoing early clinical trials. Their thrombolytic efficacy is probably only modestly greater than previous agents. The major limitation of all available plasminogen activators is that they generate active thrombin and stimulate platelet aggregation, which necessitates adjunctive therapy with antithrombin and antiplatelet drugs to sustain arterial patency.

THROMBOLYTIC THERAPY

The clinical and pharmacologic features of intravenous thrombolytic regimens that have undergone clinical trials are compared in Table 4. Streptokinase and APSAC, being antigenic, induce hypotension with rapid infusion and occasional allergic phenomena; hypotension is less frequent and severe with APSAC, permitting it to be given by bolus injection. Neutralizing antibodies also develop after administration of these agents, making them ineffective if readministered within 3-6 months, and causing relative resistance to their action for up to 4 years. Systemic fibrinogenolysis, as expected, is severe with streptokinase, anistreplase, and urokinase lasting from 12-36 hours; it is mild, usually clinically insignificant, with rt-PA. Agents differ in circulating half life, being very brief with rt-PA (though activity at the site of thrombus may be longer), and more prolonged with other agents. Based on the results of the Global Utilization of Streptokinase or Tissue Plasminogen Activator for Occluded Coronary Arteries (GUSTO) trial,[58] it is currently recommended that a 100 mg dose of rt-PA be given as an initial bolus of 15 mg, followed by an infusion of 0.75mg/kg over the next 30 minutes (up to 50 mg), and an additional 0.5 mg/kg (up to 35 mg) during the next hour. Heparin (5,000 units) precedes the initiation of rt-PA, followed by an intravenous infusion for at least 48 hours. The activated partial thromboplastin time should be monitored initially 60-90 minutes after initiation of therapy to reduce the chance of early reocclusion. Urokinase and APSAC can

be given as an intravenous bolus, and streptokinase is given over 1 hour to avoid hypotension; anticoagulation is delayed 4-8 hours with these agents to prevent excess bleeding. APSAC, because of its ease of administration, offers the potential additional advantage of earlier or even prehospital administration. Administration of rt-PA using 2 bolus injections of 50 mg each 30 minutes apart is another method suitable for prehospital administration.[59]

Intravenous rt-PA achieves vessel patency in 80%-85% of patients within 90 minutes of treatment when given over 90 minutes. Patency rate at 90 minutes is 70%-75% with the older 3-hour infusion regimen. There is relatively little systemic fibrinogen depletion and a minimal systemic lytic state with rt-PA relative to other agents. Other available intravenous fibrinolytic agents have somewhat lower efficacy, at least in terms of initial patency. With streptokinase, arterial patency rate (assessed at end of infusion) is 50%-60%, for urokinase and APSAC, it is in the 60%-70% range. Efficacy of streptokinase and APSAC is dependant upon how long after onset it is given; in the first Thrombolysis In Acute Myocardial Infarction (TIMI-1) trial patency with streptokinase was achieved in 50% of arteries when given within 3 hours after symptom onset, but was substantially less when given later. With all intravenous agents, successful reperfusion occurs typically about 45 minutes after treatment. The effectiveness of thrombolytic therapy also depends on the completeness of initial reperfusion. Prompt and complete restoration of normal (TIMI grade 3) flow is necessary for the maximal clinical benefit of thrombolysis to be derived.[60]

Restoration of coronary flow is often associated with a decrease in ST-segment elevation (often to normal), marked improvement or resolution of chest pain, early rise in the total CK or CK-MB, and increased incidence of arrhythmias. Arrhythmias include increased numbers of ventricular premature beats, ventricular tachycardia or fibrillation, paroxysmal sinus bradycardia, or accelerated idioventricular rhythm.[61] Accelerated idioventricular rhythm in particular has been thought

Table 4. Comparison of Thrombolytic Agents

	IV SK	APSAC	UK	PRO-UK	rt-PA
Half Life (min)	23	90	16	7	5
Systemic Lytic State	4+	4+	3+	2+	1+
Dose: Bolus	none	30 mg	2,000,000 U	?	15 mg
Infusion	1 hr	—	—		90 min*
Total Dose	1,500,000 U	30 mg	2,000,000 U		100 mg
Reperfusion Rate (%)	50-60	60-70	60	60-70	75-85*
Reocclusion Rate (%)	15	10	10	NA	20
Antigenicity	yes	yes	no	no	no
Simultaneous Heparin	no	no	no	no	yes
Cost Per Dose	$340	$2,060	$2,750	NA	$2,750

IV SK=Intravenous steptokinase; APSAC=Anisoylated plasminogen streptokinase activator complex; UK=Urokinase; pro-UK=Single chain urokinase plasminogen activator; rt-PA=recombinant tissue-type plasminogen activator; NA=Data not available.

Reperfusion rate assessed at 90 minutes following infusion if agent given within 4 hours. Lytic state is arbitrary scale, 1+ to 4+. Cost is June 1994 drug Facts and Comparisons and 1993 Red Book average wholesale price.

*See text.

Adapted in part from Marder VJ, Sherry S. Thrombolytic therapy: Current status. *N Engl J Med.* 1988;318:1512-1520. With permission.

to be characteristic of reperfusion. However, ST segments, chest pain, or arrhythmias are not able to discriminate between those who have and have not achieved reperfusion with enough accuracy to be clinically useful[62] except in patients having complete resolution of ST-segment elevation within 90 minutes of treatment. An early rise in total CK, to at least 20% of its ultimate peak within 3 hours, has been correlated with early arterial patency and improved survival after thrombolytic therapy.[63] More recently, a rapid and progressive decrease in pain and ST elevation has been shown to be a reliable marker of reperfusion with TIMI grade 3 flow, but only if ST segments are monitored frequently or continuously.[64]

Selection of patients for thrombolytic therapy involves weighing the anticipated benefit against the risk of serious adverse effects of treatment for any given patient. Patient selection is therefore somewhat individualized and indications continue to evolve. In general,

patients to be considered for thrombolytic therapy should present with chest pain lasting longer than 30 minutes and not relieved by nitroglycerin in association with ST-segment elevation, in order to distinguish patients with unstable angina and variant angina. Patients with chest pain and a new left bundle branch block have also been shown to benefit from thrombolytic therapy. More than 80% of patients meeting these criteria will have completely occluded infarct arteries at initial presentation. Multiple trials of thrombolytic therapy in patients with ST depression infarcts and in unstable angina have failed to demonstrate clinically significant benefit.[65] It has been suggested from angioscopic studies that the usually nonocclusive thrombi present in unstable angina may contain more fibrin and fewer platelet aggregates than in myocardial infarction[66] and are relatively resistant to thrombolytic therapy.[67] Among those with ST elevation, patients with anterior infarctions have shown the greatest survival benefit from thrombolysis. Those with inferior infarctions have a less impressive survival benefit when given thrombolysis, since smaller infarct size and low mortality makes it difficult to demonstrate improved survival in this group. Nevertheless, preservation of ventricular function and mortality reduction do accrue to patients with inferior infarcts given thrombolytic therapy, particularly when posterior or lateral extension, reciprocal precordial ST depression, or ST elevation in greater than 3 leads are present. Thus, all patients having acute ST elevation on ECG or new (or presumably new) left bundle branch block in the clinical setting of acute myocardial infarction should be considered potential candidates.

The time from onset of infarction to initiation of treatment is critical in determining whether any benefit will be derived from treatment. Consistent with experimental models, clinical trials demonstrate the greatest benefit in patients treated within the first 2 hours after infarction. Those treated within 4 hours uniformly demonstrate benefit in most studies, and when treatment is given from 4-6 hours after onset, treatment benefit is reduced, though present. Late treatment, from 6-12 hours after symptom onset has been shown to have a modest clinical benefit.[68] Treatment 12-24 hours after onset of symptoms has generally not shown a statistically significant survival benefit, except in the ISIS-2 trial. Such late treatment may be considered on a case-by-case basis for patients with intermittent or "stuttering" symptoms, on the supposition that the presence of ongoing pain indicates the presence of ischemic but viable myocardium.

Since early administration of thrombolytic therapy is critical to its success, treatment in the prehospital phase of infarction might yield additional benefits. Two randomized clinical trials have shown that it is feasible to administer thrombolytics to suspected infarction patients in the prehospital setting. Both the European Myocardial Infarct Project Group (EMIPG)[69] and the Myocardial Infarction and Triage and Intervention Trial (MITI)[70] found that prehospital administration of thrombolytics reduced the time to treatment from symptom onset by 30-60 minutes, compared to patients treated in hospital. Both studies showed a nonsignificant trend toward improved survival in patients receiving prehospital compared with in-hospital thrombolysis. More impressive, a subgroup analysis of the MITI trial showed that if treatment could be initiated within 70 minutes of symptom onset, mortality could be reduced to a rate of 1.2% compared to 8.7%, and infarct size reduced by 50% compared to patients treated later. Using data from the GUSTO trial, it has been calculated that for each hour of delay in treatment with thrombolytic therapy there are 10 lives lost per thousand treated.

Contraindications to thrombolytic therapy include any condition predisposing to major bleeding complications, and are listed in Table 5. Hypertension can usually be rapidly controlled, but if not, would contraindicate thrombolytic therapy. A recent history of cerebral ischemia markedly predisposes to bleeding and is a strong contraindication. Cardiopulmonary resuscitation may not lead to increased bleeding risk if it is brief (<10 minutes) and without significant trauma.

Table 5. Contraindications for Thrombolytic Therapy

Absolute

- Major trauma or surgery within 2 months
- History of cerebrovascular accident within 6 months
- History of intracranial tumor or neurosurgery
- Active internal bleeding
- Severe uncontrolled hypertension
- Active peptic ulcer disease
- Puncture of a non-compressible vessel

Relative

- History of remote stroke or any cerebral pathology
- History of recent transient ischemia attacks
- Prolonged (greater than 10 min) or traumatic cardiopulmonary resuscitation
- Impaired hemostasis
- History of peptic ulcer disease
- Hemorrhagic diabetic retinopathy

Major bleeding, especially cerebral bleeding, is the most serious complication of thrombolytic therapy. While fibrin-specific agents produce little systemic lytic effect, major bleeding complications, due to disruption of hemostatic plugs at the sites of invasive procedures, in the CNS and other sites, are no less likely. In studies where invasive procedures are employed within the study protocol, bleeding episodes occur in most patients, and bleeding requiring transfusions in 11%-30%. Administration of heparin simultaneous with infusion of the thrombolytic agent also predisposes to excessive bleeding without improving efficacy. When invasive procedures are minimized, bleeding episodes are uncommon; the incidence of any bleeding episodes can be expected to be 3.5%-5% with bleeding requiring transfusion in 0.3%-0.5%. Intracerebral bleeding has varied in incidence from 0.1% to 0.2% in the largest trials of streptokinase to 0.5% in the TIMI-2 trial among patients receiving 100 mg rt-PA and 1.9% in the subset of patients treated with 150 mg rt-PA. Hypertension, age over 65 years, female gender, weight less than 70 kg, and previous cerebrovascular disease are potent risk factors for intracerebral hemorrhage, which is often fatal when it occurs. However, the increased incidence of hemorrhagic stroke in patients given thrombolytic therapy is largely offset by a reduction in thrombotic and embolic stroke. Overall, thrombolytic therapy is associated with an excess of 4 total strokes for 1000 patients treated. There is also a slightly higher risk of intracranial hemorrhage with rt-PA than with streptokinase treatment.[71]

An overview of the large randomized trials comparing thrombolytics to placebo has revealed a phenomenon that has been termed "early hazard." During the first 24 hours following treatment, patients assigned to thrombolytics have an increased mortality compared to patients assigned to placebo. After 24 hours, the thrombolytic patients demonstrate a substantial survival benefit.[72] Most early deaths are due to shock, congestive heart failure, or cardiac rupture.[73] While the mechanism behind this early hazard is unclear, it may represent a form of myocardial reperfusion injury. Hemorrhagic stroke is another important cause of early death. Reduction of the early hazard would further augment the survival advantage of patients receiving thrombolytic therapy. For example, early ß-blockade may reduce the incidence of cardiac rupture, though such a benefit has not been clearly demonstrated. It should be emphasized that the survival benefit of thrombolytic therapy unequivocally surpasses these risks in nearly all patients meeting current eligibility criteria.

Reocclusion, reinfarction, and recurrent ischemia after thrombolytic therapy are significant complications of treatment. Studies utilizing repeat angiography have demonstrated reocclusion of initially reperfused arteries in about 15%-20% of patients after intravenous streptokinase, though this varies markedly between studies. The reocclusion rate may be slightly higher, about 20%-25% using rt-PA or other fibrin-selective agents. It should be emphasized that 3 randomized studies have shown a higher rate of sustained vessel patency when rt-PA is given with adequate doses of intravenous heparin[74,75] compared to subcutaneous or no heparin.[76] Adequate anticoagulation with intravenous heparin is therefore essential to preventing reocclusion after rt-PA treatment. Prolonged maintenance infusion of the thrombolytic agent[77] or combination therapy with streptokinase plus rt-PA have also been employed to reduce residual intraluminal thrombus, reocclusion, and recurrent ischemia. It is hoped that newer antithrombin drugs and antiplatelet agents will further reduce the incidence of reocclusion.

While reocclusion occurs in about 20% of thrombolytic patients, reinfarction develops in only 4%-6% of patients, indicating that many reocclusions are silent or associated with angina rather than reinfarction. Symptomatic or not, it is important to identify patients with early reocclusion, because the short- and long-term benefits of thrombolytic therapy are greatest in those with prompt and sustained infarct-artery patency. However, reocclusion is often difficult to identify noninvasively based on symptoms and routine electrocardiography. More sensitive methods including continuous ST-segment analysis, CK-MB and CK isoform determinations, and echocardiography have been employed to detect reocclusion noninvasively with better results.[78]

There is no doubt that thrombolytic therapy reduces mortality from myocardial infarction. Hospital mortality is reduced by 30%, and further still in patients treated within the first 90 minutes, those with anterior infarctions, and when antiplatelet therapy is also given. The incidence of congestive heart failure and other complications is also reduced. It has been demonstrated repeatedly that successful thrombolysis results in improved recovery of both global and regional left ventricular function, especially when infarct-artery flow is normal and when a severe residual stenosis is not present or is corrected by angioplasty. This is true both in inferior as well as anterior infarctions.

While preservation of ventricular function after infarction is a powerful determinant of long-term survival and is the presumed mechanism of mortality benefit from thrombolysis, the presence of a patent infarct-related artery itself may enhance survival. The initial survival benefit of thrombolytic therapy is maintained only when there is sustained patency of the infarct artery, while unsuccessful thrombolysis or failure to maintain arterial patency is associated with increased mortality. In fact, both patency of the infarct-related artery and preservation of ventricular function independently predict long-term survival after thrombolytic therapy.[79] This "open artery" hypothesis suggests that reperfusion per se, even late reperfusion, might have benefits on ventricular remodeling, late development of arrhythmias, or collateral blood flow that improve long-term survival.[80]

Recurrent ischemia, usually postinfarction angina, develops in 20%-30% of patients following thrombolytic therapy, which is not more frequent than in those not given thrombolytic therapy. However, recurrent angina is more frequent in those who successfully reperfuse. Plaque instability and residual thrombus will lead to reocclusion in some patients, but plaque healing occurs in many others leaving behind a stable lesion and a fixed stenosis varying from insignificant to severe in

extent. The likelihood of reocclusion and recurrent angina depends to a large extent on how severe and unstable this underlying stenosis is, and the total extent of coronary artery disease. Such considerations have led to the investigation of expectant or "noninvasive" strategies for uncomplicated patients after thrombolysis.

CLINICAL TRIALS OF THROMBOLYTIC THERAPY

There have been dozens of randomized and nonrandomized clinical trials of thrombolytic therapy published, and many more are in progress. Understanding the lessons of each major trial is important to grasping the basis for current recommendations and their limitations. There are many excellent in-depth reviews of such trials to which the reader is encouraged to refer.[81,82] The design and conclusions of the major trials are summarized in Table 6. Thrombolytic trials in acute myocardial infarction can be categorized historically and conceptually into 4 groups: 1) trials to investigate the efficacy of thrombolytic therapy; 2) trials to determine the most effective clinical strategy for administration of a thrombolytic agent and management of patients receiving thrombolytic therapy; 3) trials directly comparing different thrombolytic regimens or agents; and 4) trials to determine the incremental value of adjunctive pharmacologic therapy in patients receiving thrombolytic therapy.

Early trials of intracoronary streptokinase with small numbers of patients established that patency rates of 70%-75% could be achieved, and that efficacy was strongly time-dependent. No survival benefit could be demonstrated, however, unless results of multiple trials were pooled.[83] The exception was the Western Washington trial[84] which showed improved survival in treated patients at 1 month, which persisted at 1 year in the subgroup with patent infarct arteries.[85] Intravenous thrombolysis, first with streptokinase, then with other agents was then studied. With larger numbers of patients enrolled and treatment given earlier, significantly improved survival has been repeatedly demonstrated, averaging 35%-50% mortality reduction.

Table 6. The Major Thrombolytic Clinical Trials

ACRONYM	TRANSLATION	ENTRY CRITERIA	DESCRIPTION OF STUDY	NO. OF PATIENTS	MAJOR FINDINGS
AIMS	APSAC Intervention Mortality Study	ST↑MI<6hr	APSAC vs placebo	1,258	↓mortality with APSAC
ASSET	Anglo Scandinavian Study of Early Thrombolysis	MI<5hr	rt-PA vs placebo	5,011	↓mortality with rt-PA
ECSG	European Cooperative Study Group				
	1	ST↑MI<6hr	rt-PA vs SK	129	↑patency with rt-PA
	2	ST↑MI<6hr	rt-PA vs palcebo	129	↑patency with rt-PA
	3	ST↑MI<4hr	6hr rt-PA infusion vs placebo if patent artery	123	no difference in late reocclusion
	4	ST↑MI<5hr	rt-PA ± emergency PTCA at 2hr	367	emergency PTCA detrimental
	5	ST↑MI<5hr	rt-PA vs placebo	721	NS ↓mortality, ↓infarct size with rt-PA
	6		rt-PA ± heparin	652	heparin sl better patency
GISSI	Gruppo Italiano per lo Studio della Sopravvivenza nell'Infarto Miocardio				
	1	MI<12hr	SK vs placebo	11,806	↓mortality with SK
	2	ST↑MI<6hr	rt-PA vs SK; heparin vs none	12,490	no difference in mortality
	3		± IV + TD nitrate; ± lisinopril + any thrombolytic	19,394	nitrate no effect; lisinopril minimal positive effect
GUSTO	Global Utilization of Streptokinase or Tissue Plasminogen Activator for Occluded Coronary Arteries				
	1	↑ST MI<6hr	front-loaded t-PA vs SK vs both; early IV heparin (also SC heparin for SK)	41,021	t-PA slightly lower mortality. no diff heparin SC or IV with SK
	2	nonQ MI + unstable angina	heparin vs hirudin	12,000	just begun
	2 substudy	nonQ MI + unstable angina	t-PA vs direct PTCA vs heparin	1,200	just begun
HART	Heparin Aspirin Reperfusion Trial	ST↑MI<6hr	rt-PA + heparin vs aspirin	205	↑patency with heparin

continued

Table 6. The Major Thrombolytic Clinical Trials (continued)

ACRONYM	TRANSLATION	ENTRY CRITERIA	DESCRIPTION OF STUDY	NO. OF PATIENTS	MAJOR FINDINGS
ISIS	International Study of Infarct Survival				
	1	suspected MI <12hr	atenolol vs placebo	16,027	↓mortality with atenolol
	2	suspected MI <24hr	SK vs placebo ± ASA	17,187	↓mortality with SK, ASA, lowest with both
	3	suspected MI <24hr	d-TPA va SK vs APSAC	39,713	no diff in mortality
	4	suspected MI <24hr	rt-PA ± magnesium ± nitrates ± captopril	58,000	magnesium no effect; nitrates minimal or no effect; captopril small but significant ↓mortality
ISAM	Intravenous Streptokinase in Acute Myocardial Infarction	ST↑MI<6hr	SK vs placebo	1,741	↓infarct size, NS ↓ mortality
	International Study (GISSI-2 + non-Italian addition)	ST↑MI<6hr	rt-PA vs SK, heparin vs none	20,891	no difference mortality any group
LATE	Late Assessment of Thrombolytic Efficacy	MI 6-24hr	rt-PA vs placebo	5,711	↓mortality with rt-PA treated 6-12hr post symptom onset, no diff 12-24hr
MITI	Myocardial Infarction Triage and Intervention	Chest pain suspected cardiac <6hr	feasibility of pre-hospital thrombolysis	2,472	prehospital Rx possible ~1hr earlier than in-hospital
PAMI	Primary Angioplasty in Myocardial Infarction	ST↑MI<12hr	Primary PTCA vs t-PA	395	susbstantial but just NS (*P* = .06) ↓mortality PTCA vs rt-PA; sig↓ death + reinfarct PTCA vs rt-PA
TAMI	Thrombolysis and Angioplasty in Myocardial Infarction Study				
	1	ST↑MI<4-6hr	rt-PA + immediate vs late PTCA	386	no advantage of immed PTCA

continued

Table 6. The Major Thrombolytic Clinical Trials (continued)

ACRONYM	TRANSLATION	ENTRY CRITERIA	DESCRIPTION OF STUDY	NO. OF PATIENTS	MAJOR FINDINGS
TAMI (cont.)	2	ST↑MI<4-6hr	rt-PA + UK, various doses	140	↓reocclusion with combined activators
	3	ST↑MI<4-6hr	rt-PA + IV heparin immed vs delayed 90 min	170	no difference
	4	ST↑MI<6hr	rt-PA ± PGI2	50	negative pharmacokinetic interaction
	5	ST↑<6hr	rt-PA vs UK vs both; early vs late cardiac catheterization	575	acute angiography and PTCA potentiate infarct wall motion improvement and late patency
	6	ST↑<6hr -24hr	late reperfusion	200	improved patency and infarct vessel remodeling in late entry patients
	7		accelerated t-PA regimens	180	no regimen better than Neuhaus front-loading
TAPS	TPA APSAC Patency Study	ST↑MI	front-loaded rt-PA vs APSAC	421	↓mortality and bleeding with rt-PA
TIMI	Thrombolysis in Myocardial Infarction				
	I(1)	ST↓MI<6hr	rt-PA vs SK	290	↑reperfusion with rt-PA
	II(2)	ST↑MI<4hr	rt-PA + early PTCA vs conservative Rx; also early vs late ß-blocker	3,262	no benefit from early PTCA; ↓reinfarction, ischemia with early ß-blocker
	IIIa	unstable angina + nonQ MI	rt-PA vs placebo, routine early catheterization	306	small benefit rt-PA in stenosis severity
	IIIb	unstable angina + nonQ MI	rt-PA vs placebo; early PTCA vs conservative Rx		no benefit rt-PA; minimal benefit early PTCA but no diff death or recurr MI
	4	ST↑MI<6hr	rt-PA vs APSAC vs both (angiographic trial)	367	better patency at 60 min with rt-PA; ↓6 week mortality

continued

Table 6. The Major Thrombolytic Clinical Trials (continued)

ACRONYM	TRANSLATION	ENTRY CRITERIA	DESCRIPTION OF STUDY	NO. OF PATIENTS	MAJOR FINDINGS
TIMI (cont.)	5	ST↑MI<6hr	rt-PA vs heparin vs hirudin (pilot for TIMI 9)	214	↑patency with hirudin at 18-36hr; ↓death and recurrent MI
	6	ST↑MI<6hr	SK + heparin vs hirudin (pilot for TIMI 9)		trend for ↓recurrent MI, CHF; ↑EF with hirudin
	7	unstable angina + nonQ MI	dose finding for hirulog (pilot for TIMI 8)		?
	8	unstable angina + nonQ MI	hirulog vs heparin	~5,000	about to begin
	9	ST↑MI<12hr	any thrombolytic + hirudin vs heparin	~4,000	in progress, no results yet

APSAC=Anisoylated plasminogen streptokinase activator complex; SK=Streptokinase; rt-PA=Recombinant tissue-type plasminogen activator; d-tPA=Duteplase; UK=Urokinase; CHF=Congestive heart failure; TD=Transdermal; EF=Ejection fraction; PTCA=Percutaneous transluminal coronary angioplasty; SC=Subcutaneous; IV=Intravenous; NS=Non-significant; ST↑MI=Acute myocardial infarction with ST segment elevation, in remaining trials less specific ECG criteria employed; PGI2=Prostaglandin I_2; sl=Slightly; diff=Difference; "<6hr" or similar refers to time from onset of symptoms to randomization. Adapted with permission from Scheidt S, Adgey AA, Braunwald E, et al. Thrombolytic therapy after GUSTO: Medical roundtable discussion. *Cardiovasc Rev Rep.* January 1994;15:45-46.

The first trial of the Italian Group for the Study of Streptokinase in Myocardial Infarction (GISSI-1)[86] enrolled nearly 12,000 patients within 12 hours of onset of symptoms. Mortality was reduced from 12% to 9% in patients treated within 3 hours. A striking 47% decrease in mortality occurred in patients receiving treatment within 1 hour. Benefit was also seen with treatment up to 6 hours, and a trend from 6 to 9 hours; benefit persisted at 1-year follow-up. Subgroup analysis in this study could not show statistically significant survival benefit in patients over age 65 or those with inferior infarction, however.

The TIMI trials have compared various strategies for administration of thrombolytic therapy. The Phase I trial[87] compared intravenous streptokinase with rt-PA, following angiography to document an occluded infarct artery, in patients with symptoms of less than 7 hours duration. Reperfusion occurred in 56% of those treated with rt-PA, and in 31% of streptokinase treated patients. The much reduced efficacy of streptokinase after 3 hours of symptoms was demonstrated; even when given in less than 3 hours, the reperfusion rate was only 47%. Bleeding complications were comparable between groups and frequent at catheterization sites. At 12-month follow-up, mortality was comparable between groups; mortality was less in patients with successful reperfusion and sustained arterial patency.[88]

The role of immediate angioplasty was then studied in the TIMI phase 2A trial. Patients within 4 hours of infarction received thrombolysis with rt-PA followed either by immediate (2 hrs) or delayed (18-48 hrs) catheterization and angioplasty.[89] Patients having delayed angioplasty had lower bleeding rates, transfusion requirements, need for emergent bypass surgery and overall adverse clinical event rate. Mortality, arterial patency at discharge and ventricular function were equal in both groups. It was concluded that immediate angioplasty after thrombolysis as a routine strategy is not necessary and increases complication rates. The European Cooperative Study,[90] utilizing a similar study design, reached the same conclusion and noted increased mortality as well in the immediate angioplasty group. The first Thrombolysis and Angioplasty in Myocardial Infarction (TAMI-1) trial,[91] randomizing patients after successful thrombolysis, was also unable to show a benefit with immediate compared to delayed (7-10 days) angioplasty. In addition, 14% of patients in the delayed group no longer had a significant stenosis by 7 days, obviating the need for angioplasty.

This delayed strategy was then compared to a "noninvasive" strategy in the TIMI 2B study,[92] involving 3,262 patients. Following thrombolysis, patients received either catheterization at 18-48 hours with PTCA of suitable lesions as before (invasive group), or catheterization and angioplasty only if spontaneous or exercise induced ischemia recurred (noninvasive group). Thirty-three percent of the noninvasively treated patients required cardiac catheterization, and 13% had PTCA. The noninvasive patients had fewer transfusions, less emergency bypass surgery following PTCA, and fewer adverse endpoints than the invasively treated patients, but also had more positive discharge treadmill exercise tests. Reinfarction, death and ventricular function were comparable between groups. It was concluded that the strategy of deferring angiography and revascularization for spontaneous or inducible ischemia does not subject the patient to increased risk of death or reinfarction, with fewer complications and reduced cost.

The Second International Study of Infarct Survival (ISIS-2)[93] was a massive study involving 17,187 patients randomized to treatment with streptokinase, aspirin, both, or neither commencing up to 24 hours after symptom onset; some of the patients undoubtedly had non–Q-wave infarctions or unstable angina. Mortality was reduced 25% by aspirin or streptokinase alone, and 42% by the combination. Remarkably, survival benefit was evident even when treatment began 13-24 hours after admission. Aspirin given alone prevented reinfarction and eliminated the increased reinfarction rate noted in streptokinase treated patients, without increasing the incidence of serious bleeding. The implications of the ISIS-2 study were profound. The important adjuvant role of aspirin was convincingly demonstrated, and lent the first firm support to the concept that even delayed reperfusion may be beneficial.

Late initiation of thrombolytic therapy, given 6-24 hours after symptom onset, has not consistently resulted in infarct size limitation, mortality reduction or preservation of ventricular function in individual randomized trials. This is consistent with animal models in which little salvage of myocardium occurs when reperfusion is delayed more than 3 hours. However, the LATE[68] trial, ISIS-2, and pooled data from the Fibrinolytic Trialists study[72] support the notion that treatment 6-12 hours after symptom onset offers a significant survival advantage compared to placebo.[94] The ISIS-2 trial was the first to show mortality reduction in the subgroup of patients treated after 12 hours. Along with the Western Washington trial, showing marked mortality benefit in spite of no improvement of ventricular function, the possibility is raised that there are other mechanisms by which delayed reperfusion may be beneficial. Subepicardial myocardium supplied by collateral vessels and at infarct borders may be salvaged by late reperfusion and can lead to some preservation of ventricular function.[95] There is increasing evidence that the presence of a persistently patent infarct artery, while not reducing infarct size or preserving ejection fraction, prevents infarct expansion,[96] progressive left ventricular dilatation and remodeling,[97] and aneurysm formation, analogous to the beneficial effects of spontaneous thrombolysis and collateral blood flow. It can also be argued that a patent infarct artery increases potential collateral blood flow to other diseased vessels, and might reduce the incidence of late ventricular arrhythmias.

The most important, and as yet unanswered question, is whether sustained patency of infarct-related arteries actually reduces long-term mortality after infarction. In this regard the "open artery hypothesis" receives strong support from the SAVE trial which found that sustained arterial patency is a predictor of long-term survival independent of left ventricular function. The importance of arterial patency on survival has also been demonstrated in a subset of patients in the GUSTO trial. This strongly suggests that while successful initial reperfusion reduces mortality from myocardial infarction, sustained arterial patency, whether spontaneous or due to thrombolysis or angioplasty, independently improves long-term survival. The mechanism of this benefit awaits further investigation and has important consequences for management of post-infarction patients.

CHOICE OF THROMBOLYTIC AGENTS

The choice of thrombolytic agent in a given circumstance has been a difficult issue to resolve. Angiographic trials have shown that higher initial patency rates can be achieved with rt-PA than with other intravenous agents, though patency rate at discharge is equal. Whether this translates into a greater mortality reduction and preservation of ventricular function required very large "megatrials" because the anticipated differences between treatments are small. To date there are 3 randomized clinical trials that have directly compared streptokinase to rt-PA, and 1 comparing APSAC to rt-PA.

The GISSI-2 trial, part of the larger International rt-PA/SK Mortality Trial[98,99] together randomized 20,891 patients within 6 hours of onset to rt-PA or streptokinase, and to subcutaneous heparin started 12 hours after thrombolysis or no heparin.[100] This study found no significant mortality difference between rt-PA and streptokinase (8.9% compared to 8.5% respectively), with more strokes in the rt-PA-treated patients (1.3% and 1.0% respectively). There was no significant reduction in mortality, reinfarction, or stroke in patients given subcutaneous heparin compared to no heparin, while major bleeding complications were increased. The ISIS-3 trial randomized 41,299 patients within 24 hours after onset of suspected myocardial infarction to either rt-PA, APSAC or streptokinase, and to either subcutaneous or no heparin.[100] This study also found no difference in 35 day survival between thrombolytic agents. There was a comparable increase in stroke in the rt-PA group, most likely due to cerebral

hemorrhage. Patients receiving heparin were slightly more likely to suffer cerebral hemorrhage or noncerebral bleeding.

Both of these trials seemed to indicate unequivocally that there was no difference between thrombolytic agents in survival and that rt-PA was associated with a higher incidence of hemorrhagic stroke. Nevertheless, ardent proponents of rt-PA argued that these studies were flawed because intravenous heparin was not routinely used. Administration of intravenous, rather than subcutaneous, heparin had resulted in a higher rate of sustained arterial patency in smaller angiographic trials. Without concomitant intravenous heparin, the earlier and higher rate of reperfusion with rt-PA, and therefore any survival advantage, would be mitigated by a higher early reocclusion rate. Furthermore, it was found that infarct-related arteries could be opened more rapidly with accelerated, or front loaded, rt-PA administration given over 90 minutes instead of 3 hours.[101] This regimen resulted in an infarct-artery patency rate of 85% at 90 minutes, compared to 70% with the conventional method.

To address these issues, the GUSTO study was carried out, to determine whether earlier and sustained infarct artery patency would result in improved survival. In 15 countries, 41,021 patients with acute infarction presenting within 6 hours of symptom onset were treated in one of 4 ways: streptokinase with subcutaneous heparin, streptokinase with intravenous heparin, accelerated rt-PA with intravenous heparin, or streptokinase plus rt-PA with intravenous heparin. Thirty day mortality in the rt-PA group was 6.3% compared to 7.2% and 7.4% in the 2 streptokinase groups, respectively, and 7.0% in the combination group. This represents a 14% relative reduction in mortality (confidence intervals 5.9%-21.3%) with rt-PA treatment compared to either streptokinase regimen. While all subsets of patients showed a benefit from rt-PA compared to streptokinase, those less than 75 years old, those with anterior wall infarction, and those treated less than 4 hours after onset of infarction received the greatest benefit. An angiographic substudy of the GUSTO trial demonstrated that earlier and more complete reperfusion consistently occurred in rt-PA treated patients, confirming that this was the most likely mechanism for their improved survival.[102] Hemorrhagic stroke developed significantly more often in patients treated with accelerated rt-PA (0.72%) and combination therapy (0.94%) than with either streptokinase regimen (approximately 0.5%). However, the higher risk of stroke did not outweigh the survival advantage of rt-PA. The combined endpoint of death or disabling stroke was slightly but significantly lower with rt-PA treatment.

From the perspective of the GUSTO trials, it therefore appears that rt-PA is a somewhat more effective thrombolytic agent for most patients. However, because of the extreme cost difference between rt-PA and streptokinase, cost-effectiveness considerations may also enter into treatment strategies. Using GUSTO data it has been estimated that it would cost slightly less than a quarter-million dollars to save 1 additional life if one chooses to use rt-PA routinely instead of streptokinase.[103]

ANGIOPLASTY IN MYOCARDIAL INFARCTION

The use of coronary angioplasty (PTCA) in myocardial infarction actually comprises 5 different treatment strategies, each one with differing indications and safety profiles, and each the subject of randomized trials. These strategies are: 1) primary revascularization by angioplasty, 2) emergent catheterization and angioplasty following thrombolytic therapy, 3) "salvage" angioplasty after failed thrombolysis, 4) delayed, "routine" angioplasty of residual stenoses after thrombolytic therapy, and 5) deferred angioplasty, for indications of spontaneous or inducible ischemia after thrombolysis.

Primary revascularization by means of PTCA in acute myocardial infarction is a very attractive alternative to thrombolytic therapy when facilities can be made available in a timely manner. Several randomized trials comparing primary angioplasty with thrombolytic therapy have shown that primary angioplasty results in an initial patency rate of well over 90%, a higher sustained patency rate, a lower incidence of reinfarction and recurrent ischemia, and

minimal risk of intracranial hemorrhage. In these trials the combined occurrence of cardiac death and nonfatal reinfarction was also lower with primary angioplasty, especially in high risk patients.[104] Reocclusion occurs in approximately 12% of cases, which is higher than elective PTCA but is lower than that expected after thrombolytic therapy. The rate of restenosis may be lower than after elective PTCA.[105] However, primary angioplasty does not reduce infarct size or preserve left ventricular function to any greater extent than thrombolytic therapy alone followed by conservative treatment.[106] In these studies primary PTCA delayed the time to treatment an average of 45-60 additional minutes, which may have tended to offset some of its anticipated benefit on ventricular function. The total cost of treatment by primary PTCA is comparable to that of thrombolytic therapy.[107]

Primary angioplasty is therefore an excellent therapy for acute myocardial infarction, provided that it does not introduce excessive delay in treatment. However, its use is limited to facilities where catheterization and bypass surgery are immediately available, estimated to be approximately 8% of hospitals. It should be strongly considered in patients who have contraindications to or are less likely to benefit from intravenous thrombolytic therapy, such as patients with previous stroke, bleeding disorders, extensive anterior infarction, cardiogenic shock, and those over 75 years of age. In cardiogenic shock, the prognosis is poor even with thrombolytic therapy, and retrospective data indicate that outcome may be improved by primary angioplasty.[108]

Immediate angioplasty as a routine strategy after thrombolysis, studied in the TIMI-2A, TAMI-1 and ECSG trials, has uniformly been found to be of no benefit to stable patients compared to delayed PTCA. The risks of reocclusion and bleeding are increased with such a strategy, and mortality is increased.[109] However, immediate angiography and revascularization did improve the recovery of wall motion in some patients, and immediate PTCA is a reasonable and effective treatment when clinical instability warrants its use. Salvage angioplasty after failed thrombolysis has been well studied in the TAMI trials. This subset of high-risk patients had a 14% mortality, 29% reocclusion rate, and no improvement in ventricular function in the TAMI-1 trial.[110] The higher rate of reocclusion when angioplasty follows thrombolysis, compared to primary angioplasty, may be due to bleeding within the plaque.[111] This problem would tend to limit the use of salvage angioplasty to patients in the highest risk subsets.

Whether angioplasty is desirable for all patients having a residual stenosis after thrombolysis is less clear. The findings of the TIMI-2B trial suggest that expectant management and conventional risk stratification are able to detect most patients at high risk after thrombolysis. The corollary of this is that all residual lesions after thrombolysis do not seem to require angioplasty. When stable patients are managed conservatively after thrombolytic therapy, their outcome and ventricular function after 1 year are identical to those receiving routine delayed PTCA of residual stenoses, with significantly fewer procedure-related complications.[112] Long-term arterial patency rate is the same whether PTCA is performed or not, because of reocclusion in PTCA-treated patients and spontaneous recanalization in non–PTCA-treated patients.[113] This does not mean, however, that diagnostic angiography in stable patients after thrombolysis does not have value. The anatomic and prognostic information obtained is very useful, even if PTCA is not performed, and it remains a useful method of risk stratification for many patients.

BYPASS SURGERY IN MYOCARDIAL INFARCTION

Coronary artery bypass grafting (CABG) is sometimes required in the setting of acute or recent myocardial infarction. Patients with early recurrence of rest ischemia in spite of medical therapy are candidates for early surgical intervention if they have 3 vessel or left main disease, or other anatomy not suitable for PTCA. Patients failing primary angioplasty having large areas of jeopardized myocardium or hemodynamic instability are also candidates. Coronary artery bypass grafting is more often required when PTCA is performed early after

infarction. Patients stabilized medically or having inducible but not rest ischemia can usually undergo bypass surgery electively. Twenty-two percent of patients in the TAMI trials underwent CABG after thrombolysis. Patients requiring CABG had the same total mortality and better left ventricular function at subsequent follow-up than non-operated patients in spite of worse baseline characteristics.[114] While the operative mortality in such patients is higher than in those without recent infarction, the increased mortality is limited to those with poor ventricular function, shock, and advanced age.[115] Recent myocardial infarction per se does not appear to increase surgical mortality when these other factors are accounted for.[116]

Primary revascularization by coronary bypass grafting in the first hours of infarction has also been performed, with acceptable mortality rates and long-term results better than no reperfusion.[117] While intriguing to consider that such therapy both limits infarct size and offers definitive revascularization, it is clearly impractical for widespread use, and its safety and effectiveness are unlikely to be equal to that of thrombolysis with PTCA in unselected patients.

RECOMMENDATIONS

It must be kept in mind that because of delay in seeking medical attention, contraindications to thrombolytic therapy, or a nondiagnostic initial electrocardiogram, less than half of patients with acute myocardial infarction are candidates for thrombolytic therapy. Furthermore, many patients who are candidates for such therapy do not receive it. A great deal of additional benefit can be derived from administration of thrombolytic therapy to a larger proportion of eligible patients and shortening the time to treatment.

At the present time it is recommended that intravenous thrombolysis be administered immediately to all patients 75 years and younger with acute myocardial infarction having ST elevation or left bundle branch block on their ECG who present within 12 hours of onset of symptoms if no contraindications exist. Patients over 75 years old also benefit from thrombolytic therapy, particularly those with high-risk features. Treatment of patients more than 12 hours after symptom onset should be considered on a case-by-case basis. Thrombolytic treatment for ST depression or non–Q-wave infarcts has not been found effective. If facilities are available, emergent catheterization with coronary angioplasty is a highly effective alternative, especially in large infarctions or when contraindications to intravenous thrombolysis exist. When thrombolytic therapy is unsuccessful (judged clinically and by ECG) emergent "salvage" PTCA might benefit selected high-risk patients, but high bleeding and reocclusion rates preclude this as a routine strategy. Delaying angioplasty of significant residual lesions for several days in stable patients reduces complications and does not increase morbidity due to recurrent ischemia. In the 20%-30% of patients having spontaneous recurrent ischemia after thrombolysis, and in those having inducible ischemia prior to discharge, coronary angiography and revascularization are indicated. In those who remain stable and without inducible ischemia conservative treatment does not subject the patient to increased short term risk. Although diagnostic angiography is a reasonable method of risk stratifying patients after thrombolytic therapy, routine angioplasty of residual stenoses in asymptomatic patients does not improve their outcome or ventricular function.

ADJUNCTIVE PHARMACOLOGIC THERAPY

Every patient with acute myocardial infarction (AMI), whether receiving reperfusion therapy or not, is a candidate for "conventional" therapies. These include bed rest in the first days of infarction, supplemental oxygen if hypoxemia is known or suspected, narcotics or anxiolytics if needed for uncontrolled pain or anxiety, low dose aspirin, and low dose subcutaneous heparin for prevention of thromboembolism.

There are many additional pharmacologic agents that are potentially beneficial during myocardial infarction. The rationale for such therapies might be to:

1) Delay the progression of myocardial necrosis in order to prolong the time window for effective thrombolysis and enhance salvage of myocardium. Maneuvers to decrease afterload and heart rate, and to increase collateral blood flow, such as ß-blockers and nitrates, may be useful when given both before as well as after reperfusion.

2) Limit myocyte injury at the time of reperfusion (discussed in pathobiology section). Many agents have been investigated, including calcium blockers, oxygen radical scavengers, adenosine agonists, metabolic substrates, white cell inhibitors, and thromboxane antagonists, but none has shown sufficient promise to warrant clinical use.

3) Enhance the return of function of viable but "stunned" myocardium.

4) Prevent coronary reocclusion following thrombolysis or angioplasty. Antiplatelet therapy with aspirin and anticoagulation with heparin are in routine clinical use for this purpose and are discussed subsequently.

5) Prevent long-term complications of myocardial infarction, such as recurrent infarction, ventricular remodeling, and late arrhythmic death.

As will be discussed, none of these treatments can be thought of as standard treatment for all patients. Treatment must be individualized based on known pathogenic mechanisms, the risks and benefits of treatment, and the results of large clinical trials.

BETA-BLOCKERS

There are many published trials of ß-blockade both early and late after MI. Short-term trials utilizing intravenous then oral dosing beginning in the first hours of infarction have shown reductions in 7-day mortality and reinfarction rates averaging 15%[118] in relatively uncomplicated patients who mostly did not receive thrombolytic therapy. The benefit versus risk of applying this therapy to all patients remains controversial. Immediate and delayed initiation of beta blockade were directly compared, among patients receiving thrombolytic therapy, in the TIMI-2B trial where immediate ß-blockade reduced the incidence of reinfarction and recurrent ischemia within the first 6 days, especially in patients receiving thrombolysis within 4 hours and those in the low risk subset.[92] However, ß-blockers did not reduce ultimate infarct size, and early and late mortality were not reduced compared to starting the drug on the sixth day.

Longer-term trials with ß-blockers, the ISIS-1[119] and the Beta Blocker Heart Attack Trial (BHAT)[120] trials have shown unequivocally that these agents reduce mortality by an average of 20%. This survival benefit persists during at least 3 years of treatment. Both sudden and non-sudden cardiac mortality is decreased, which suggests that ß-blockers exert their beneficial effect both by relief of ischemia and by preventing arrhythmias. Only agents without intrinsic sympathomimetic activity are effective for this purpose. Currently recommended regimens include timolol 20 mg, propranolol 180-240 mg, metoprolol 200 mg, and atenolol 100 mg, daily in divided doses. Contraindications include heart failure, heart block, bradycardia or obstructive lung disease.

High-risk patients, those with large infarcts or transient heart failure, are the ones most likely to benefit from ß-blockade but are also the ones most likely to suffer side-effects of treatment. Congestive heart failure develops with treatment in 5%-15% of patients if there is a history of previous heart failure.[121] Experience has shown, however, that most patients with compensated ventricular dysfunction tolerate ß-blockade well if monitored carefully. On the other hand, the cost effectiveness of administering ß-blockers to all low-risk patients has been questioned, as the incremental benefit is small. Nevertheless, ß-blockade remains an effective prophylactic treatment after myocardial infarction, and is a reasonable option for most patients. If desired it can be given safely early after infarction in selected patients, and when given should be continued for at least 2-3 years, and probably indefinitely.

ANTIPLATELET DRUGS

The value of aspirin alone and in conjunction with thrombolytic therapy has been most convincingly demonstrated in the ISIS-2 trial. An independent decrease in mortality and reinfarction was found which was synergistic with the benefit of thrombolysis, even when treatment was initiated 12-24 hours after symptom onset. Remarkably the magnitude of the survival benefit from aspirin therapy was equal to that of thrombolytic therapy. The risk of major bleeding complications is not increased significantly by aspirin therapy. Aspirin probably does not improve early arterial patency after thrombolytic therapy.[122] Instead, it is believed that active thrombin exposed at the clot surface by therapeutic thrombolysis triggers further platelet aggregation and subsequent reocclusion, which can be prevented by antiplatelet agents. This explains the marked clinical benefits of aspirin in myocardial infarction as well its synergism with thrombolytic therapy. Aspirin treatment is also of unequivocal benefit for prevention of myocardial infarction in patients with both stable and unstable angina,[123,124] and in secondary prevention of death and recurrent infarction after a first myocardial infarction.[125] Aspirin may even prevent infarction in healthy individuals over age 50.[126] Though it may help prevent early complications after PTCA, aspirin does not appear to influence restenosis. Thus, low dose aspirin treatment should be initiated immediately upon admission to all patients with myocardial infarction or unstable angina and continued indefinitely thereafter, unless surgery is planned or a contraindication for its use exists. A dose of 160–325 mg per day is as effective as higher doses and is better tolerated; doses as low as 80 mg per day are also effective.

Though aspirin is a clinically effective antiplatelet agent, its ability to inhibit platelet aggregation is relatively modest. This has prompted the development of more powerful antiplatelet drugs which block the platelet IIb/IIIa receptor involved in platelet aggregation. A monoclonal antibody (7E3) directed against this receptor and integrelin, a peptide blocker of the receptor, have been utilized in pilot studies. The monoclonal antibody 7E3 effectively reduces the incidence of reocclusion in association with thrombolytic therapy[127] and in high-risk coronary angioplasties.[128] The clinical value and safety of these and other promising agents is the subject of ongoing trials. The combination of a platelet inhibitor and antithrombin agent may be particularly effective[129] if its safety profile can be established.

ANTITHROMBINS AND ANTICOAGULANTS

Possible uses for anticoagulants in myocardial infarction include: 1) low dose heparin for prophylaxis of deep venous thrombosis, 2) full anticoagulation with heparin and warfarin as routine treatment of infarction, 3) use of heparin after thrombolysis or angioplasty, 4) use of heparin in patients with unstable coronary syndromes and recurrent ischemia after infarction, and 5) treatment of patients with known mural thrombosis or embolic stroke after infarction. The use of anticoagulants in cardiovascular disease has been recently reviewed.[130]

It is generally accepted that low dose subcutaneous heparin is effective in preventing deep venous thrombosis in bed-bound infarction patients; along with early mobilization, this treatment has dramatically reduced the incidence of thromboembolic events in the modern era. Routine anticoagulation for myocardial infarction was a common therapy in the past and has been debated for decades. Trials of anticoagulation with heparin and coumadin in the 1960s and 1970s did not show clear-cut survival benefits, but have been criticized for methodologic flaws. Two more recent trials found a 10%-24% reduction in death, 34%-53% less reinfarction and a 40%-55% reduction in stroke among warfarin-treated patients after infarction.[131,132] The obvious question is whether warfarin is as good as aspirin at reducing these same endpoints. A trial of warfarin treatment following thrombolytic therapy found that it is less effective than aspirin in preventing reinfarction or recurrent ischemia.[133] Disappointingly, neither treatment was able to reduce the 30% rate of reocclusion, highlighting the need for more effective antithrombotic drugs. Ease of use and lower rate of bleeding complications make aspirin preferable in most patients, but warfarin is a reasonable alternative for secondary prevention in those unable to tolerate aspirin after

thrombolytic therapy, those with extensive anterior infarction with or without an apical mural thrombus, those with atrial fibrillation, and those with severe left ventricular dysfunction. Combined treatment with aspirin and low-dose warfarin might produce additional clinical benefits; this is the subject of ongoing trials.

Anticoagulation with heparin is important adjunctive treatment in patients with spontaneous ischemia following infarction, unstable coronary syndromes, and immediately following angioplasty, situations where intraluminal thrombus and unstable plaque are likely to be present. Following successful thrombolytic therapy, intravenous heparin is administered routinely in order to reduce the rate of reocclusion. With shorter acting agents such as rt-PA, anticoagulation is initiated prior to the conclusion of the thrombolytic infusion. Prompt administration of heparin in adequate doses results in higher rates of arterial patency: inadequate heparin therapy may have obscured differences between rt-PA and streptokinase in several large trials.[134] With streptokinase and APSAC, heparin is initiated several hours following the end of infusion; earlier treatment increases bleeding complications without further benefit.[135] Whether heparin is necessary after streptokinase treatment, and the nature of the interaction between heparin and aspirin, has not yet been the subject of a randomized trial; in the GISSI-1 trial which did not require heparin therapy, the incidence of reinfarction was similar to that reported in other trials. Heparin is continued for 24-48 hours in patients undergoing deferred or no catheterization. There is currently no data to suggest that longer duration of anticoagulation benefits stable patients. After angioplasty, aspirin therapy plus heparin for 6-24 hours after the procedure remains fairly routine treatment.

Hirudin derived from the leech Hirudo Medicinalis, and its synthetic relative hirulog, are direct thrombin antagonists with significant advantages over heparin. Unlike heparin, which is bound by platelet factor 4 and heparinases and which requires antithrombin-3 for activity, hirudin directly combines with thrombin and has no known circulating inhibitor. Another advantage of hirudin is that it can inactivate clot-bound thrombin as well as circulating thrombin, which heparin cannot do because of its indirect action. Early clinical studies comparing hirudin with heparin have shown that hirudin is superior in sustaining infarct-related arterial patency and reduces post-infarction angina and reinfarction.[136] Ongoing large clinical trials of hirudin and hirulog will determine their place in the therapy of ischemic heart disease. These promising agents may one day replace heparin in the treatment of myocardial infarction and unstable coronary syndromes if excessive bleeding does not limit their use.

NITRATES

Oral and intravenous nitrates are essential initial therapy in patients with acute myocardial ischemia including suspected myocardial infarction, and in those with recurrent ischemia or congestive heart failure complicating infarction. There is no definite evidence in humans that nitrates alone can limit infarct size in the face of a persistently occluded infarct artery, but they exert potentially beneficial effects by relieving coronary spasm, increasing collateral flow, and reducing subendocardial ischemia by lowering end-diastolic pressure. Small trials of intravenous nitrates in myocardial infarction both with and and without thrombolytic therapy have shown a trend toward reduced mortality in treated patients which has led to their widespread use. However, in the ISIS-4 and GISSI-3 trials the routine use of intravenous oral and/or transdermal nitrates, with or without angiotensin converting enzyme inhibition, in patients receiving thrombolytic therapy had no effect on any endpoint or subgroup.[137,138] Nevertheless, they remain valuable in myocardial infarction patients for the treatment of symptomatic ischemia or congestive heart failure and do not adversely affect survival. Intravenous nitroglycerin should be given with intensive care unit monitoring as hypotension may occur, especially when hypovolemia or right ventricular infarction is present. Nitrate therapy is then continued with oral nitrates within 24-36 hours to avoid development of tolerance.

CALCIUM-CHANNEL BLOCKADE

Experimental evidence has indicated potential benefits of calcium-channel blockers administered early during infarction or at reperfusion. However, numerous clinical trials have shown that routine treatment with calcium-channel blockers does not decrease mortality after myocardial infarction,[139] even when begun very early and in conjunction with thrombolytic therapy.[140] This stands in marked contrast to the ß-blocking drugs with their clear-cut benefits. Trials employing short-acting forms of nifedipine, but not diltiazem or verapamil, have actually shown higher mortality in treated patients, probably related to increased heart rate. Trials using slow-release nifedipine or newer long-acting dihydropyridines (which are associated with fewer vasodilator side-effects and less reflex tachycardia) have not been performed in acute MI. One short-term trial of diltiazem after non–Q-wave infarction suggested a lower reinfarction rate, though mortality was not decreased.[141] It was found that treatment was harmful in the subset of patients having pulmonary congestion or ventricular dysfunction, and beneficial in the remainder of patients, which could account for no overall benefit. At the present time, it is not recommended that calcium blockers be administered routinely to any subset of patients, but only if a valid indication for their use exists, such as recurrent angina, hypertension, or rate control of atrial fibrillation.

INOTROPIC DRUGS

The use of digitalis in acute myocardial infarction has been debated for many years. In experimental models of infarction, digitalis worsens ischemia when heart failure is not present by increasing oxygen demand, though when heart failure is present this is offset by a beneficial reduction in wall stress. Detrimental effects are harder to prove in humans. Retrospective studies show increased mortality in infarction patients treated with the drug,[142] but when adjusting for the increased numbers of poor prognostic variables present in treated patients, higher mortality is not clearly demonstrated.[143] Digitalis is a mainstay of therapy for patients developing atrial fibrillation or flutter. In patients with heart failure due to systolic dysfunction, digitalis is a reasonable option. For critically ill patients requiring immediate treatment of pulmonary edema or cardiogenic shock, the delayed onset of action and relatively mild inotropic effect of digitalis make it an agent of second choice. Adverse effects included exacerbation of arrhythmias if hypokalemia or hypomagnesemia are present and vasoconstriction with excessively rapid intravenous administration.

Intravenous catecholamines are indicated for treatment of low cardiac output states complicating myocardial infarction when the patient is symptomatic (oliguria, altered mentation, heart failure with hypotension, shock) and intravascular volume is adequate. Contractility of both nonischemic and reversibly injured "stunned" myocardium can be enhanced with these agents. Combination therapy with a vasodilator is often useful if systemic vascular resistance is increased and blood pressure is adequate. The possibility of worsening ischemia and arrhythmias must be weighed against the anticipated benefit, but are infrequent if high doses and excessive tachycardia are avoided. Dopamine, with potent ß-agonist effects, increases cardiac output and blood pressure as well as renal blood flow; α-adrenergic vasoconstriction at high doses can be harmful, however. Dobutamine lacks both the renal and α-adrenergic effects of dopamine; it increases heart rate and blood pressure less and lowers pulmonary artery wedge pressure more than dopamine. Dopexamine is a relatively pure ß-agonist like dobutamine, but retains the beneficial renal effects of dopamine. All these agents should be administered with invasive hemodynamic monitoring.

The phosphodiesterase inhibitors are a newer class of non-catecholamine inotropic drugs, which have both inotropic and arterial vasodilating properties and produce little or no increase in myocardial oxygen demand or arrhythmias. Amrinone, given by intravenous infusion, may be useful in patients requiring both an inotrope and a vasodilator. Tolerance to its effects occurs with prolonged infusion, and thrombocytopenia is a frequent side effect.

MAGNESIUM

Although small placebo controlled trials suggested that intravenous magnesium given early after acute myocardial infarction markedly improved survival, the findings of the ISIS-4 and GISSI-3 studies show unequivocally that routine treatment with magnesium has no effect on survival. Magnesium therapy should not be given routinely in myocardial infarction patients, but only for treatment of hypomagnesemia or magnesium-responsive arrhythmias.

ARTERIAL VASODILATORS

Arterial vasodilators are valuable adjunctive therapy for congestive heart failure complicating myocardial infarction, and also for treatment of severe hypertension in this setting. Intravenous agents, nitroglycerin or nitroprusside, are preferred for initial treatment because of their rapidity of action and ease of titration. Intravenous nitroprusside, with its balanced arterial and venodilating properties, is particularly useful. Excessive reductions in blood pressure, however, may lead to "coronary steal" and worsening of ischemia by diverting blood flow away from ischemic areas. Thiocyanate toxicity is a problem with prolonged use. Intravenous nitroglycerin is very effective for relieving pulmonary congestion and has milder arteriolar effects. Serious hypotension can occur with either agent, but is more likely with nitroprusside. Neither agent has been found beneficial for routine use in uncomplicated patients.

Treatment with an angiotensin-converting enzyme (ACE) inhibitor beginning within 24 hours of infarction was found to modestly improve survival (by 4.5/1,000) in the ISIS-4 trial, as well as in the GISSI-3 trial. The benefit is greatest in anterior infarction and in those with transient or persistent congestive heart failure, reducing mortality by 27% when begun 2-9 days after infarction in these patients.[144] Long-term treatment with an oral ACE inhibitor is indicated after anterior myocardial infarction and when heart failure or significant systolic dysfunction is present after infarction. Their use in such patients reduces left ventricular remodeling, development of congestive heart failure, and long-term mortality, as discussed in the following chapter.

COMPLICATIONS OF MYOCARDIAL INFARCTION

CONGESTIVE HEART FAILURE

The onset of myocardial infarction brings with it a prompt decrease both in systolic contractile force in the ischemic zone and diminished ventricular compliance, which may lead to clinically evident congestive heart failure. More than half of infarction patients have an elevated pulmonary capillary wedge pressure on admission, often not recognized clinically. This is frequently due only to diastolic dysfunction, requiring elevated pulmonary wedge pressure (15-18 mm Hg or more) to maintain cardiac output. When more severe, pulmonary rales, dyspnea and radiographic vascular congestion occur, but these findings lag behind the hemodynamic changes. A smaller number of patients, about 15%, present with frank pulmonary edema. Hypotension, when it occurs, may be a manifestation of hypovolemia, increased vagal tone, right ventricular infarction, or cardiogenic shock.

It was observed very early that patients with heart failure and shock had a worse outcome, and the classification system of Killip made use of this fact. Those with rales encompassing 50% of the lung fields or a third heart sound (class II) had 17% mortality, pulmonary edema (class III) a 38% mortality, and cardiogenic shock a mortality more than 80% compared to those with none of these findings (class I) who had a 6% mortality. Recognizing that there is considerable heterogeneity among patients within each Killip class and that clinical indicators sometimes fail to detect significant hypoperfusion or heart failure, classification based on hemodynamics (Table 7) has proven more useful in clinical practice.[145] Patients with pulmonary congestion are treated with diuretics and oral or intravenous nitrates to reduce preload, if they are not hypotensive. Arterial vasodilators and possibly digitalis are added if congestion fails to respond. Those with hypoperfusion and low or "normal" filling pressures may improve with careful volume expansion, while those with severely depressed cardiac output and pulmonary congestion, who have the highest mortality, may require inotropic support or intraaortic balloon

Table 7. Clinical and Hemodynamic Subsets in Acute Myocardial Infarction

	CLINICAL FINDING	HEMODYNAMIC FINDING		HOSPITAL MORTALITY	
		CI	PCW	CLINICAL	HEMODYNAMIC
I	No pulmonary congestion or hypoperfusion	>2.2	<18	1	3
II	Pulmonary congestion only	>2.2	>18	11	9
III	Peripheral hypoperfusion only	<2.0	<18	18	23
IV	Pulmonary congestion and peripheral hypoperfusion	<2.2	>18	60	51

CI=Cardiac index (L/min/m^2); PCW = Pulmonary capillary wedge pressure (mm Hg). Adapted from Forrester JS, et al.[145] With permission.

counterpulsation. Invasive hemodynamic monitoring with a pulmonary artery catheter is valuable in the diagnosis and management of some subsets of infarction patients, and suggested indications for its use are shown in Table 8. It is, however, neither indicated nor desirable in the treatment of uncomplicated patients or those with mild pulmonary congestion resolving rapidly with diuretics.

POST INFARCTION ANGINA AND INFARCT EXTENSION

Recurrence of angina during recovery from myocardial infarction is associated with higher rates of death and reinfarction, both in the short and long term[9] and should be considered a strong indication for urgent catheterization and potential revascularization. Early recurrence of angina may indicate instability within a reperfused infarct-related artery, instability in a vessel remote from the infarct, or jeopardized collateral flow, and often portends infarct extension.

Infarct extension occurs in approximately 10% of patients managed conventionally. It is

---

Table 8. Indications for Hemodynamic Monitoring in Acute Myocardial Infarction

Diagnosis
   Diagnosis of suspected left ventricular failure
   Hypotension
   Right ventricular infarction
   Persistent oliguria or azotemia
   Acute mitral regurgitation
   Suspected ventricular septal rupture
   Uncertain volume status

Treatment
   Persistent congestive heart failure or pulmonary edema
   Cardiogenic shock
   Intravenous inotropic support

---

diagnosed by the finding of reappearance of CK-MB after infarction. Prolonged chest pain and new ECG changes are characteristic, but found in only half of patients.[146] Infarct extension may lead to cardiogenic shock, and is associated with a four-fold increased hospital mortality. It is more likely to occur in patients with non–Q-wave infarction, diabetes, early recurrence of chest pain, prior infarction and in women.[147] Analogous to reocclusion and reinfarction following thrombolysis, infarct extension usually results from reocclusion of a spontaneously reperfused or subtotally occluded infarct artery.

CARDIOGENIC SHOCK

Cardiogenic shock results from loss of a critical amount of contractile function, leading to hypotension and inadequate tissue perfusion. The resultant decrease in coronary blood flow and increase in vascular resistance further increase ischemia, leading to ongoing necrosis and further worsening of ventricular function, in a vicious cycle that is usually fatal. Patients dying from cardiogenic shock uniformly have infarction of 40% or more of the left ventricle,[148] and most have severe 3-vessel coronary disease. Cardiogenic shock usually results from extension of the initial infarction at its borders, and expansion of the infarct, with resultant deterioration of ventricular function. It complicates 7%-15% of infarctions in the first days after admission, often heralded by persistent CK-MB release and recurrent chest pain suggesting infarct extension. It is diagnosed when arterial hypotension (<90 mm Hg systolic) and depressed cardiac index (below 1.8 l/min/M^2) occur with elevated pulmonary artery wedge pressure and signs of hypoperfusion. Other causes of shock such as papillary muscle rupture, free wall rupture and ventricular septal defect must be excluded clinically and by echocardiography. Cardiogenic shock occurs more frequently among those with large infarcts, previous infarction, admission ejection fraction below 35%, diabetes, and advanced age.[149]

Treatment of cardiogenic shock is aimed at maintaining cardiac output and perfusion pressure and minimizing ischemia. The inotropic drugs dopamine and dobutamine, as well as amrinone, alone or in combination, will improve contractility. Vasodilators often further improve cardiac output but may worsen coronary perfusion pressure. Intraaortic balloon counterpulsation improves the hemodynamic profile by reducing afterload and increasing cardiac output while simultaneously increasing diastolic blood pressure. None of these treatments by themselves diminish the abysmal mortality from cardiogenic shock, which is 85%-90% without aggressive revascularization.

It might be expected that timely reperfusion with thrombolytic therapy would decrease the incidence of cardiogenic shock complicating myocardial infarction. In meta-analyses a survival benefit is found in patients with systolic blood pressure less than 100 mm Hg at presentation. The incidence of cardiogenic shock was reduced in the European Cooperative trial,[150] one of the few trials to show this. However, numerous other trials have demonstrated neither a decreased incidence of cardiogenic shock nor decreased mortality when it occurs. It appears that the benefits of thrombolytic therapy are limited in this high-risk group.

On the other hand, the current aggressive interventional approach to revascularization using thrombolytic therapy, circulatory support, primary angioplasty, and/or bypass surgery appears to have improved the prognosis of patients who develop cardiogenic shock. Overall mortality in such patients is about 50%, and is 33% when patency of the infarct artery is achieved.[151] Early and late survival are related to arterial patency, age, and infarct size. This is lower than the mortality rate of more than 85% found in historical controls, suggesting that acute revascularization by these means has decreased mortality. Cardiogenic shock patients having evidence of reversible or ongoing ischemia or reversible myocardial injury will probably benefit most from revascularization, while those with shock due to necrosis of a critical mass of myocardium without ongoing ischemia will probably not. Unfortunately this distinction is often difficult or impossible to make in individual cases.

INTRAAORTIC BALLOON COUNTERPULSATION

Intraaortic balloon counterpulsation (IABP) is indicated for the following conditions: 1) stabilization of the hemodynamically unstable patient prior to angiography and bypass surgery, 2) cardiogenic shock unresponsive to medical therapy, 3) acute severe mitral regurgitation or ventricular septal rupture, and 4) persistent angina refractory to maximal medical therapy, pending definitive therapy. Inserted either percutaneously or surgically through the femoral artery, preferably under fluoroscopic guidance, the balloon is positioned in the descending aorta, beyond the left subclavian artery and above the renal arteries. The balloon is adjusted to inflate at aortic closure (dicrotic notch) and deflate prior to aortic valve opening. Systolic pressure (afterload) and pulmonary wedge pressure (preload) are reduced, while diastolic pressure (coronary perfusion) is raised. Stroke volume rises, myocardial oxygen demand falls and ischemia is reduced. Pulmonary shunting from septal rupture and mitral regurgitation, if present, are reduced. Intraaortic balloon counterpulsation appears to facilitate thrombolysis when hypotension is present,[152] and its use may reduce mortality from cardiogenic shock in patients receiving thrombolytic therapy.[153] Complications include aortic dissection, embolization, and femoral artery occlusion.

MECHANICAL COMPLICATIONS OF INFARCTION

The so-called mechanical complications of infarction have a common pathogenesis, involving disruption of necrotic cardiac tissues, usually with dramatic consequences. The most common form is infarct expansion, which occurs in approximately 30% of infarctions, particularly anterior infarcts, and is characterized by regional dilatation and thinning of the infarcted wall segment. It develops most commonly 3-7 days following infarction when the infarct tissues are weakest and scar formation has not begun, and is found near the edge of the infarct where shearing forces are greater. Infarct expansion results in ventricular dilatation, further impairment of left ventricular systolic function, and may lead to the development of overt congestive heart failure. Progression of the expansion process may lead ultimately to ventricular free wall rupture in some patients.[154]

Cardiac rupture is most common following first, large, and transmural infarctions, usually anterior, without collateral flow; it is somewhat more common in women and in those with a history of hypertension, and is usually located in the free wall of the ventricle. Early ß-blockade may decrease the incidence of cardiac rupture, and it is possible that early vasodilator therapy may do so as well. When thrombolytic therapy is administered within 12 hours of symptom onset the incidence of cardiac rupture is reduced. When thrombolytic therapy is administered after more than 12 hours the incidence of cardiac rupture is increased, even though overall mortality is reduced.[155] Thrombolysis in these cases might serve to exacerbate intramural hemorrhage in areas where there has been irreversible injury to myocardium and microvessels.

The patient with cardiac rupture suddenly develops shock and circulatory collapse with electromechanical dissociation and signs of tamponade. Death is often immediate, but if the diagnosis can be made and the patient stabilized with pericardiocentesis, inotropes and intraaortic balloon pump, operative repair, usually with coronary artery bypass, is lifesaving. Occasionally incomplete rupture occurs, in which pericardium and thrombus seal a site of rupture, forming a pseudoaneurysm which communicates with the ventricular cavity through a narrow neck. Pseudoaneurysms can be visualized by echocardiography or left ventriculography. Death is not immediate in such cases, thus survival is more likely; treatment is the same.

The pathogenesis of ventricular septal rupture is similar to that of rupture of the free wall. The septal defect is located near the apex in patients with anterior infarction, and in the basal septum following inferior infarction. Clinically, there is abrupt onset of heart failure ranging from mild to profound in a previously stable patient, associated with a new holosystolic murmur at the left sternal border, sometimes with a thrill. The diagnosis is confirmed by doppler echocardiography. Right-heart catheterization rapidly diagnoses septal rupture by demonstrating a step-up in oxygen saturation from right atrium to pulmonary artery, distinguishing it from papillary muscle rupture and allowing shunt calculations. Treatment with inotropes and vasodilators is useful, and intraaortic balloon counterpulsation can decrease the degree of shunting. Immediate surgical repair is recommended if the shunt flow is large (>2:1 flow) or if circulatory support is required. In patients who are clinically stable with small shunts, delaying surgery 4-6 weeks to allow infarct healing is appropriate.

Papillary muscle rupture results in acute mitral regurgitation and variable hemodynamic compromise depending on whether rupture is partial or complete, and may occur with relatively small infarctions. Rupture of the posteromedial papillary muscle, in the setting of inferoposterior infarction, is more common than anterolateral rupture, which results from anterolateral infarction. Complete rupture of a papillary muscle is rapidly fatal; when partial, stabilization is possible. The patient develops abrupt onset of pulmonary edema, hypotension and tachycardia. If hypotension is severe, the murmur of mitral insufficiency may be soft and short; in less severe cases a typical loud holosystolic apical murmur is heard. Pulmonary artery catheterization demonstrates markedly increased pulmonary wedge pressure with very large V waves. Echocardiography can distinguish rupture from dysfunction of a papillary muscle. Treatment with vasodilators and intraaortic balloon counterpulsation are particularly useful in treating this condition. Urgent mitral valve repair or replacement, often with bypass grafting, is then indicated.

When mitral regurgitation is due to ischemia or infarction of a papillary muscle without rupture, the clinical presentation is variable. The patient may present days to weeks after infarction with symptoms of congestive heart failure and a murmur of mitral regurgitation. If dysfunction is related to intermittent ischemia, repeated bouts of pulmonary edema may occur, with relatively few symptoms between episodes.

Many of these patients can be managed medically or undergo revascularization without valve replacement. In other cases, severe chronic mitral regurgitation leads to ventricular dilatation and chronic heart failure. In such patients, coronary bypass alone will not improve the regurgitation, and valve repair or replacement is necessary.

VENTRICULAR ANEURYSM AND MURAL THROMBOSIS

Ventricular aneurysm formation is a late sequela of myocardial infarction. They develop most often in the first 3 months following anterior infarction[156] in patients with poor collateral flow, probably as a result of infarct expansion. An aneurysm consists of a thin fibrotic wall which bulges in both diastole and systole; this can sometimes be detected as a precordial bulge or abnormal cardiac silhouette on chest radiograph. Persistent ST-segment elevation on the electrocardiogram indicates dyskinetic wall motion, but a true aneurysm may not be present in all such cases. The diagnosis is best made by echocardiography or ventriculography. The presence of an aneurysm, especially when developing early after infarction, is associated with a markedly increased risk of death, heart failure, angina, ventricular arrhythmias, and embolization. Surgical resection is indicated for patients having intractable heart failure, angina or arrhythmias, but only if function of the remaining myocardium is good.

Mural thrombus adherent to the infarcted wall is found in a large proportion of necropsy cases of infarction; in clinical series, a third of anterior infarctions have demonstrable mural thrombi, but they are rare in inferior infarction. The thrombi are usually found in areas of severe wall motion abnormality or in ventricular aneurysms, and can be reliably diagnosed by echocardiography, though false positive studies sometimes occur. The embolic potential of such thrombi is controversial, with a reported incidence of embolic events ranging from 4%-52%. Embolization is more likely to occur with protruding and mobile thrombi[157] and during the first 6 weeks following infarction. Overall, the risk of systemic embolization is more than 5-fold increased in patients with mural thrombi after anterior infarction and the risk of stroke averages 2%-6%. Anticoagulation with warfarin markedly reduces the risk of stroke. Both thrombolytic therapy and early treatment with high-dose heparin reduce the incidence of mural thrombus by one-half and two-thirds, respectively, while aspirin and warfarin are ineffective to prevent thrombus formation.[158] Some authorities recommend that all patients with Q-wave anterior myocardial infarction be treated with a course of full-dose heparin. If echocardiography prior to discharge shows a mural thrombus, warfarin is begun and continued for at least 3 months, after which the echocardiogram is repeated. Although persistence of thrombus by echocardiography is common after treatment, this does not necessarily indicate continued embolic potential. Some authorities recommend a course of warfarin treatment for all anterior infarction patients who have extensive wall motion abnormalities or left ventricular dysfunction.

VENTRICULAR REMODELING

Beginning 1-2 weeks after large Q-wave infarction, left ventricular dilation and dysfunction often begin to occur and worsen progressively over subsequent months to years. Distinct from infarct expansion alone, this ventricular "remodeling" involves lengthening of both infarct and noninfarct segments and a change in shape of the ventricle to a more globular configuration. This process initially serves to restore stroke volume to normal, but the resulting elevation of systolic and diastolic wall stress ultimately leads to severe ventricular dysfunction and congestive heart failure. Remodeling does not occur in small infarcts and is thus most common after anterior infarction. Remodeling occurs when there is persistent occlusion or a high-grade stenosis of the infarct artery, and can be largely prevented by timely reperfusion and sustained infarct artery patency. It is likely that late reperfusion with thrombolytics or angioplasty also reduces ventricular remodeling.[159]

Treatment with an ACE inhibitor reduces early infarct thinning and expansion and prevents later ventricular remodeling in experimental animals and in humans. In patients with asymptomatic ventricular dysfunction after either anterior or inferior infarction, progressive ventricular enlargement is prevented by ACEI treatment,[160] and is greatest in patients with persistently occluded arteries.[161] To determine their effect on survival, the Survival and Ventriular Enlargement (SAVE) trial randomized more than 2,200 patients with left ventricular dysfunction after infarction to early ACE inhibitor or placebo. Death, congestive heart failure, and all cardiovascular events were strikingly reduced by an ACE inhibitor, even in patients receiving thrombolytic therapy, aspirin, and/or ß-blockers.[162] In patients receiving thrombolytic therapy in the GISSI-3 study, early treatment with an ACE inhibitor also reduced mortality and the development of severe ventricular dysfunction.[138] Unexpectedly, the incidence of reinfarction was also reduced in the SAVE trial, and evidence is emerging that ACE inhibitors might have antiischemic effects as well.[163] Long-term treatment with an ACE inhibitor is indicated after Q-wave MI when associated with left ventricular dysfunction or anterior location. (See the following chapter.)

It has also been suggested that long-term use of oral nitrates after infarction may have beneficial effects on left ventricular function and ventricular remodeling[164] but this has not been subjected to a large randomized trial.

RIGHT VENTRICULAR INFARCTION

Involvement of the right ventricle occurs in roughly a third of inferior wall infarctions when studied pathologically[165] or noninvasively, but is infrequent in anterior infarction. Hemodynamically significant right ventricular infarction is seen only in about 10% of inferior infarcts, and is characterized by elevated right atrial pressure and depressed cardiac index with normal or low pulmonary wedge pressure. Kussmaul's sign, "square root" right ventricular pressure tracing and diastolic equalization of pressures are frequent findings, resembling pericardial disease. In fact, it is the restraining action of the pericardium and shifting of the septum that

probably contribute most to impairment of left ventricular filling when the right ventricle dilates acutely. The finding of ST elevation in the right precordial leads is highly specific for right ventricular infarction, but is transient and is easily missed.[166] Hemodynamic monitoring is useful both in diagnosis and treatment.

The manifestations of right ventricular infarction range from mild jugular venous distention to frank shock. Profound hypotension after administration of nitrates is not uncommon. Initial treatment of the hypotensive patient with right ventricular infarction consists of volume expansion, which may be sufficient in mild cases. When equalization of left and right sided pressures occurs, no further effect of volume expansion is likely and treatment with dobutamine, which is more effective, becomes necessary if hypoperfusion persists.[167] Brady-arrhythmias are best treated by dual-chamber pacing; ventricular pacing alone is ineffective. Though shock may be severe, and inotropic support required for several days, both short- and long-term prognoses are good with appropriate therapy, in marked contrast to shock due to left ventricular failure.

NON–Q-WAVE INFARCTION

The subset of patients presenting with MI without development of Q waves represents a distinct group of particular concern to the clinician.[168] Non–Q-wave infarction, which pathologically is often subendocardial, tends to be smaller in size than Q-wave infarction. In the pre-thrombolytic era, non–Q-wave infarction was associated with a lower hospital mortality than Q-wave infarction. In the thrombolytic era the mortality from Q-wave infarction has markedly decreased. While death rate from non–Q-wave infarction is low, it now comprises a higher percentage of total hospital deaths due to myocardial infarction. Non–Q-wave infarction is associated with a higher in-hospital morbidity and mortality than unstable angina, regardless of medical or antithrombotic therapy.[169] Reinfarction and recurrent angina are nearly twice as frequent after non–Q- versus Q-wave infarction.[170] As a result, ultimate mortality is equal to that of transmural infarction. In these patients there is a high incidence of multi-vessel disease, the infarct related artery is typically patent, usually with a high grade stenosis, and treadmill testing is often positive. These factors argue for early angiography in most or all patients with non–Q-wave infarcts. In particular those with anterior ECG changes, spontaneous or inducible ischemia after infarction, and those with a history of prior infarction warrant angiography. Most studies of non–Q-wave infarction were performed in the pre-thrombolytic era; the nature and prognosis of non–Q-wave infarction at the present time may be different and requires further study.

PERICARDITIS

Pericarditis, developing in 10% or less of infarctions, occurs most commonly in the first 2-4 days and is due to inflammation associated with transmural necrosis. It occurs more frequently in those with Q wave infarctions, as well as those with larger and more complicated infarctions,[171] and is uncommon after successful thrombolytic therapy. The patient has pain of a positional and pleuritic nature, often with a transient pericardial rub and sometimes with fever or leukocytosis. Electrocardiographic changes are difficult to distinguish from those of the underlying infarction. The syndrome is brief and self-limited, responds to anti-inflammatory agents, and is important to distinguish from recurrent ischemia. The authors prefer aspirin therapy, which has not been shown to inhibit infarct healing, while corticosteroids and other nonsteroidal anti-inflammatory agents have been shown to cause scar thinning in experimental animals. The presence of a small pericardial effusion by echocardiography is seen in 25% of infarction patients and does not indicate pericarditis. The finding of a large effusion or tamponade is more likely to indicate subacute ventricular rupture than pericarditis.

Pericarditis occurring later, from 2 weeks to 3 months after infarction is known as Dressler's syndrome.[172] Pericardial rub, fever, pleural effusions and sometimes pneumonitis can be found. Small pericardial effusions are often noted by echocardiography; large effusions or tamponade are infrequent. The syndrome is probably an autoimmune disorder. Treatment with anti-inflammatory agents is usually necessary; recurrence is not uncommon and corticosteroids are sometimes required, though the ability of these agents to impair infarct healing should be kept in mind. For reasons that are unclear, Dressler's syndrome is now extremely rare.

ARRHYTHMIAS IN MYOCARDIAL INFARCTION

SUPRAVENTRICULAR ARRHYTHMIAS

Sinus bradycardia occurs in about 20% of cases of acute MI. It is most common in inferior infarction, related to sinoatrial node ischemia, and is not associated with a poorer prognosis. It is often asymptomatic but when severe, accompanied by hypoperfusion or increased ventricular ectopy, chronotropic agents or temporary pacing can be used. Sinus bradycardia is sometimes seen in patients following successful thrombolytic therapy or abrupt reperfusion of the right coronary artery, known as the Bezold-Jarish reflex.

Sinus tachycardia is also common, and can be caused by pain, anxiety, left ventricular dysfunction (which may be otherwise unsuspected), congestive heart failure, hypovolemia, pericarditis, exogenous catecholamines, or atrial infarction. Its recognition is important, in order that the underlying process be addressed, since tachycardia can increase myocardial oxygen demand, increase infarct size and raise mortality. Treatment with ß-blockers is advised if tachycardia is attributable to hyperdynamic circulation and not to ventricular dysfunction; invasive hemodynamic monitoring is often necessary to make this distinction.

Atrial premature beats are relatively common, and may indicate atrial dilatation or congestive failure. Atrial fibrillation occurs in about 15% of infarction patients and may be related to atrial ischemia. It is more common in anterior infarction and in association with ventricular dysfunction; patients manifesting this arrhythmia have a worse prognosis. Atrial fibrillation tends to occur most frequently in the first day of infarction, is transient but often recurrent, and can lead to profound hemodynamic compromise. Supraventricular tachycardia and atrial flutter are also occasionally seen during infarction. Treatment of these arrhythmias is the same as when they occur in other settings, but must be prompt to avoid the detrimental effects of the tachycardia.

VENTRICULAR ARRHYTHMIAS

Ventricular arrhythmias are major causes of mortality during and after MI. Sudden arrhythmic death occurs in approximately 15% of patients with acute MI in the first hour, accounting for about 60% of all infarction-related mortality. The cause is usually ventricular fibrillation (VF) or ventricular tachycardia (VT). Most of these events occur prior to hospital admission, but will develop in 3%-9% of patients following admission, usually within 12 hours of infarction. Ventricular fibrillation occurring within the first 24-48 hours of infarction is usually not associated with severe pump failure or shock and is termed primary. Ventricular fibrillation occurring later during the hospital phase of infarction usually occurs in the setting of infarct extension, severe pump failure or shock, and is termed secondary.

Premature ventricular beats occur in more than 90% of patients with acute MI, and do not predict subsequent VF, even when frequent, early or paired. In fact, 50%-60% of cases of VF occur without preceding high grade arrhythmias. Primary VF occurs more frequently in younger patients, patients with first infarction, and almost always within the first 12-24 hours of infarction. Survival after VF in the prehospital phase of infarction depends upon the rapid initiation of cardiopulmonary resuscitation. Ventricular fibrillation occurring after hospital admission is associated with a somewhat higher in-hospital mortality in some studies, and in thrombolytic-treated patients is more frequent in patients who fail to reperfuse.[173] It does not, however, signify a poor long-term prognosis among those who survive it. Secondary, VF on the other hand, is associated with an extremely high in-hospital and late mortality.

The issue of prophylactic antiarrhythmic therapy in MI has changed greatly in recent years. In the past it has been common practice to routinely administer lidocaine to all patients with diagnosed or suspected MI. Lidocaine had been thought to reduce the incidence of primary VF in the prethrombolytic era.[174] However, its use has not been consistently shown to decrease mortality. Furthermore, the incidence of prehospital VF has declined markedly in the modern era[175] and immediate defibrillation is routinely available when VF or sustained VT do occur in the hospital setting. Disturbingly, recent randomized trials and meta-analyses of other trials have shown a trend toward increased mortality in patients receiving prophylactic lidocaine, usually due to asystole.[176] Therefore, routine prophylactic therapy with lidocaine cannot be recommended at the present time. It might be considered on a case-by-case basis in settings where close monitoring and immediate defibrillation are not available, restricted to patients younger than age 70 and when begun within 6 hours of infarction.

In the late hospital phase and following hospital discharge, life-threatening ventricular arrhythmias or sudden cardiac death occur in 3%-8% of patients in the first year. The risk is greatest in the first months after infarction, and declines after the first year. Patients having such spontaneous arrhythmic events are at grave risk of recurrence and death, and aggressive intervention is warranted in all such cases. The ability to predict in whom arrhythmic events will occur would further improve mortality. It is well established that the presence of frequent ventricular premature beats after infarction, especially in couplets and nonsustained runs, is associated with a higher incidence of late sudden death[177] and the risk is greater with increasing degrees of ventricular dysfunction. However, ambulatory ECG monitoring is a poor predictor of future arrhythmic death after infarction. Only about one-fourth of the 5%-15% of patients ultimately developing sudden death after discharge have serious arrhythmias detected on ambulatory monitoring, limiting its utility.

The signal averaged ECG has better sensitivity for identifying patients at increased risk of late arrhythmias. Approximately 30% of survivors of MI have ventricular late potentials, indicating continuous slow electrical activity that predisposes to reentrant arrhythmias. These patients have a moderate risk of arrhythmic events, approximately 15% in the first year. Those without late potentials have a less than 5% incidence of serious arrhythmias in the first year and require no further investigation.[178] This prognostic information is independent of left ventricular dysfunction. The combination of late potentials and low ejection fraction identified a group at high risk for arrhythmic events.[179] A strategy of referring this subgroup of patients for programmed ventricular stimulation is a reasonable and cost-effective clinical strategy. Other combinations of clinical factors and detection methods can also be used to select high-risk patients for programmed stimulation.[180]

Survivors of MI in whom programmed ventricular stimulation induces sustained VT or VF are at high risk of spontaneous ventricular tachyarrhythmias during follow-up, especially when left ventricular dysfunction is present. In a large study of ventricular arrhythmias after infarction, sustained monomorphic VT was inducible by programmed electrical stimulation in 6%. During 28 month follow-up, 25% of those with inducible VT had an arrhythmic event, compared to 4% in noninducible patients. It was suggested that electrophysiologic testing should be limited to patients with ejection fraction less than 40%, and consideration of antiarrhythmic treatment only to those with inducible VT.[181]

Even when post-infarction patients at high risk for life-threatening arrhythmias are identified, there is no evidence that anti-arrhythmic drug treatment prevents late arrhythmic death. The now famous Cardiac Arrhythmia Suppression Trial (CAST) study found that treatment of post-infarction patients having frequent ventricular ectopy with encainide or flecainide significantly increased mortality from arrhythmias.[182] Antiarrhythmic therapy was not beneficial in any subset, and there was a substantial harm overall. Most other antiarrhythmic drugs have likewise proven disappointing,[183] with the exception of amiodarone. In high-risk patients after infarction low-dose amiodarone (200 mg/day after initial oral loading) has been found to reduce the incidence of arrhythmic events and death in early studies,[184] and larger trials are now ongoing. However, amiodarone may improve survival only in patients without left ventricular dysfunction.[185] Amiodarone is typically given for 1 year after infarction, after which the risk of sudden death is very low.

The disappointing results of treatment with Type I antiarrhythmics contrast sharply with the proven effectiveness of ß-blockers after infarction, which reduce long-term mortality largely by preventing arrhythmic death. Essentially they are the only class of anti-arrhythmic agent proven to reduce arrhythmic death after infarction, and should be used whenever possible in high-risk patients.

The management of patients at high risk of late arrhythmias is clearly problematic at the present time. It is believed by many authorities that "guided" antiarrhythmic therapy that results in suppression of VT inducible by programmed ventricular stimulation is superior to empiric or noninvasively guided anti-arrhythmic therapy and reduces the incidence of subsequent arrhythmic events.[186] However, the evidence for this is still inconclusive. Accordingly, patients who have manifested life-threatening arrhythmias after myocardial infarction may be best managed by automatic implantable defibrillator placement or by arrhythmia mapping and ablation, in conjunction with definitive revascularization.

EFFECT OF THROMBOLYTIC THERAPY ON VENTRICULAR ARRHYTHMIAS

Abrupt coronary reperfusion can lead to increased ventricular arrhythmias, including VT, VF, or accelerated idioventricular rhythm. Once believed useful to noninvasively predict reperfusion after thrombolysis, it has been shown that such arrhythmias are nearly as frequent in the absence of reperfusion and thus are not useful for this purpose.[187] Likewise, the routine administration of lidocaine to patients receiving thrombolytic therapy, though common practice, is of no known value because the incidence of life-threatening arrhythmias directly attributable to reperfusion is clinically insignificant and the effectiveness of lidocaine against such arrhythmias is uncertain.

In patients who have received thrombolytic therapy, the incidence of late potentials (measured days to weeks after infarction) is reduced.[188] Those who do have late potentials after thrombolytic therapy have a 7-fold higher risk of serious arrhythmias than those who do not. Paradoxically, having received thrombolytic therapy probably does not result in fewer arrhythmic events during long-term follow up.[189] This is explained by the finding that late potentials are most strongly associated with a persistently occluded infarct artery.[190] Since late patency rates in thrombolytic versus non-thrombolytic patients are similar, the lack of reduction in late arrhythmias is understandable, and further supports the "open artery hypothesis." It has also been found that late PTCA of occluded vessels after thrombolytic therapy does not reduce the incidence of late potentials.[191] Apparently late reperfusion does not improve the electrical stability of the infarct and peri-infarct regions.

Overall, the incidence of late arrhythmic events among patients with remote MI has declined markedly over the past decade. This is most likely to be the result of an overall trend toward aggressive revascularization, rather than to thrombolytic therapy per se. Sadly, little progress has been made toward the prevention of prehospital death in acute MI, which has not decreased in the modern era and constitutes an increasingly large proportion of myocardial infarction-related death as other causes of mortality have decreased.

CONDUCTION ABNORMALITIES

New abnormalities of atrioventricular conduction develop in 16%-25% of patients with MI. Patients having a new conduction abnormality during MI often progress to complete atrioventricular block and have twice the hospital mortality rates than those who do not.[192] The increased mortality is related to more extensive infarction as well as brady-arrhythmias. Complete heart block in anterior infarction is usually due to extensive necrosis of the conducting system below the bundle of His and is therefore associated with bundle branch blocks. Heart block complicating inferior infarction is usually due to ischemia of the atrioventricular node, in which case the QRS width is normal.

Temporary ventricular pacing is required when a bradyarrhythmia or conduction abnormality results in hypoperfusion (Table 9). Sinus bradycardia and symptomatic type I second degree AV block usually respond to atropine but occasionally require pacing. Third degree block, and type II second degree block in anterior infarction (and in inferior infarction with wide QRS) require pacing in all cases. Complete heart block often develops suddenly and is somewhat more frequent after anterior infarctions. Transient complete heart block developing during acute inferior infarction does not usually recur. About 30% of patients with high-risk patterns of bundle branch block (Table 9) will progress to high-grade heart block, and prophylactic temporary pacing should be considered. Risk of complete heart block is less than 10% in other groups, such as in bifascicular block not known to be new, or new unifascicular block. The availability of reliable external pacing may obviate the need for temporary transvenous pacing in moderate risk patients.

Resolution of high-grade AV block occurs in more than 90% of the patients who develop it. Nevertheless, permanent ventricular pacing is required if symptomatic bradyarrhythmias, third-degree block, or type II second-degree blocks persist during recovery from infarction. In patients with transient complete heart block in whom a bundle branch block persists, permanent ventricular pacing should at least be considered or electrophysiologic studies performed.

POST-MYOCARDIAL INFARCTION CARE

PROGNOSIS AFTER INFARCTION

Discharge of the patient surviving uncomplicated MI typically takes place after 7 hospital days and the safety of this approach has been

Table 9. Indications for Temporary Transvenous Pacing in Acute Myocardial Infarction

Definite

    Complete heart block

    Second degree AV block Type II

    Second degree AV block Type I with hypoperfusion

    Sinus bradycardia despite atropine with hypoperfusion

    Junctional or idioventricular rhythm with slow ventricular rate and hypoperfusion

    "High risk" bundle branch block:

        Bifascicular block with first degree AV block

        New bifascicular block

Possible

    Second degree AV block Type I with wide QRS

    Overdrive pacing of ventricular tachycardia

    AV synchronous pacing for right ventricular infarction with hypoperfusion

Table 10. Adverse Risk Factors After Acute Myocardial Infarction

Clinical

    Anterior infarction

    Reinfarction or infarct extension

    Postinfarction angina

    Age >70 years

    Female gender

    Diabetes mellitus

    Angina pectoris, ST segment elevation or depression, abnormal blood pressure response, or ventricular ectopy induced by exercise testing

    Inability to perform exercise testing

    ST depression on ECG

    New bundle branch block (any type, including fascicular blocks)

    Hypertension or loss of preexisting hypertension

Hemodynamic/Angiographic

    Congestive heart failure (clinical, hemodynamic, or radiographic)

    Left ventricular ejection fraction less than 0.40

    Occluded infarct-related artery

    Increased left ventricular end-diastolic volume

    Large infarct size (estimated by enzymes, ^{99m}Technetium radionuclide scan, electrocardiographic QRS mapping, or echocardiography)

Arrhythmic

    Mobitz II second-degree or third-degree heart block

    Ventricular fibrillation or ventricular tachycardia more than 24 hours after infarction

    Frequent ventricular premature beats (especially nonsustained ventricular tachycardia)

    Atrial fibrillation

    Abnormal signal-averaged electrocardiogram

    Spontaneous ST segment depression on ambulatory ECG

    Decreased heart rate variability

    Inducible sustained monomorphic ventricular tachycardia during electrophysiologic study

Modified from Hessen SE, Brest AN. Risk profiling the patient after acute myocardial infarction. *Cardiovasc Clin.* 1989:20:284. With permission.

demonstrated repeatedly. Earlier discharge 3 or 4 days after thrombolytic therapy and/or PTCA may be possible in highly selected patients.[193] Approximately 50% of patients surviving myocardial infarction have 3 vessel or left main coronary artery disease, and are at increased risk of further cardiac events. Without further intervention, death occurs in 5%-15% of patients in the first year after infarction, and reinfarction in about the same number. In patients receiving thrombolytic therapy, most of this mortality, as well the survival benefit, occurs in the first 30 days. Mortality in the GUSTO trial during the following 11 months was less than 3%. This reflects appropriate "risk stratification": identification of those patients who are at the greatest risk after infarction and targeting them for early intervention.

Many factors have been associated with a poor prognosis, and these are listed in Table 10. Left ventricular dysfunction, severity of coronary disease, a large amount of jeopardized myocardium, and early recurrence of ischemia are the most powerful predictors of subsequent cardiac events. The prognostic importance and evaluation of arrhythmias has been previously discussed. Combinations of clinical factors can stratify patients into subgroups with 2-year mortality ranging from 3%-60%.[194]

Other groups of infarction patients have clinical characteristics that might influence their management. Patients with previous bypass surgery constitute an increasing fraction of patients with suspected MI. These patients are more likely to develop a non–Q-wave infarction, are less likely to have ST-segment elevation and receive thrombolytic therapy, and are more likely to suffer recurrent angina and reinfarction.[195] Patients with diabetes, especially diabetic women, have more extensive coronary artery disease and a high mortality both during hospitalization and in the first year.[196] Women in general have a much higher early mortality rate and much poorer long-term survival than men after MI.[197] In spite of this, women less often undergo coronary arteriography than men after infarction, though this difference might be attributible to other clinical features.[198] In the elderly, mortality after infarction increases markedly with age.[199] Available studies have not documented that an aggressive interventional approach prolongs survival in the elderly. On the other hand, carefully selected patients in their 80s can undergo PTCA and CABG with reasonable complication rates. The authors recommend a more selective approach to intervention in these patients.

RISK STRATIFICATION AFTER MYOCARDIAL INFARCTION

The most common strategy for stratifying patients following infarction is to use clinical criteria coupled with low-level treadmill exercise prior to discharge. Left ventricular function is assessed by echocardiography or radionuclide ventriculography. A symptom-limited exercise test is performed after 4-6 weeks and identifies additional patients at increased risk.[200] Return to work is then recommended at this point for patients without marked ischemia or functional impairment. Inability to complete a low-level exercise test or abnormal hemodynamic response (rise of systolic blood pressure of <30

mm Hg) are predictors of death and reinfarction, even more so than ST-segment response.[195] Exercise-induced ST elevation in infarct leads associated with reciprocal ST depression after thrombolytic therapy indicate persistent infarct artery occlusion and not ischemia.[201] With no abnormalities and normal functional capacity, 1 year mortality is 1%, compared to 13% with an abnormal test; this prognostic information has additive value beyond clinical assessment alone.[202] Such an approach leads to coronary angiography in about one-half of infarction patients and identifies a group of patients with moderate high risk and a group at extremely low risk.

Survival after MI has greatly improved in the past 30 years.[203] Mortality during the first year has been reduced from 30% or more to 2%-5%. As a result, studies of prognosis and risk stratification in the prethrombolytic era may not have the same clinical utility in the patients seen today, where mortality is low and revascularization therapies are widely applied. In fact it is now being recognized that exercise testing is of limited value for the assessment of prognosis in patients who have received thrombolytic therapy. Exercise testing predicts only 50%-70% of patients who will suffer subsequent ischemic events, while only about 25% of those with positive tests have subsequent events.[204] The sensitivity of low-level exercise testing is greatly enhanced by thallium perfusion imaging, as well its predictive value for multivessel disease.[205] It remains to be seen whether routine use of this approach, which results in a greater use of angiography and angioplasty, is cost-effective. Performing symptom-limited rather than low-level exercise testing after infarction appears to be safe and has twice the sensitivity of a low-level study for detecting ischemia.[206] Its safety and utility are being evaluated in large scale trials. Considering the poor performance of exercise testing in thrombolytic patients, symptom-limited exercise may become the standard of care.

A sensible strategy of risk stratification, such as that outlined above using clinical findings and exercise testing, identifies patients in whom coronary angiography is warranted. Patients with a complicated course, early recurrence of spontaneous ischemia, reduced ejection fraction, heart failure, previous infarction, abnormal low-level exercise test, and other factors should be considered high risk and referred for angiography as well (Table 11). Patients having angina prior to infarction are also more likely to have recurrent symptoms and cardiac events after thrombolytic therapy.[207] Coronary angiography in asymptomatic patients without any of these factors, constituting slightly less than half of post-infarction patients, does not add additional prognostic information and is not beneficial.[208]

Other strategies and combinations of tests may be used to stratify patients after MI. A given strategy is reasonable if it provides effective risk stratification and prognostic information beyond clinical assessment alone at a reasonable cost and risk. The management of patients after MI and thrombolytic therapy has been recently reviewed.[209]

RISK FACTOR MODIFICATION AND REHABILITATION

In addition to secondary prevention with antiplatelet drugs and ß-blockers, intensive effort should be made to modify coronary risk factors in the postinfarction patient. Progression of disease and death after infarction is more common among those with elevated cholesterol, smokers, and women, and is reduced by smoking cessation. Lipid-lowering drugs have been shown to reduce mortality in patients after infarction.[210,211] Decreased rate of progression, and in some cases regression, of coronary atherosclerosis has also been observed in patients with prior bypass surgery.[212] Diabetes and hypertension contribute to increased late mortality as well, and should be controlled optimally. Continued smoking is a powerful predictor of late mortality in angina, MI, and particularly after bypass surgery. Long-term survival and quality of life are reduced in smokers, who have more angina, more unemployment, a greater limitation of physical activity, and more hospital admissions.[213] Overall there is a sound conceptual basis for believing that intensive multiple risk factor intervention will improve long-term prognosis

Table 11. Indications for Coronary Angiography After Acute Myocardial Infarction

Definitely Indicated
  Large infarction
  Non–Q-wave infarction
  Reduced ejection fraction after infarction
  Congestive heart failure
  Postinfarction angina or reinfarction
  Previous infarction
  Inability to complete a low-level exercise test
  Angina or ST-segment depression on exercise test
  Abnormal blood pressure response to exercise

Possibly Indicated
  Uncomplicated anterior wall infarction
  Infarction with reciprocal ST-segment depression

Not Recommended
  Uncomplicated course with normal left ventricular function and negative exercise test
  Thrombolytic therapy, without other indications

after MI, and in virtually all patients with coronary artery disease as well.

Exercise training of the stable post-infarction patient is intended mainly to avoid the complications of prolonged bed rest and return the patient to a maximum level of functional capacity following discharge. It hastens and augments the spontaneous improvement in functional capacity that occurs during convalescence. Structured exercise programs are especially beneficial in patients with marked impairment of exercise capacity on pre-discharge exercise testing.[214] Comprehensive programs of cardiac rehabilitation involving exercise, dietary modification, and lifestyle modification have not been shown to improve long-term mortality but do result in fewer nonfatal cardiac events, less disability, and improved quality of life.[215] For the uncomplicated infarction patient with a negative low-level stress test, a program of graded walking, swimming, or other exercise can be safely prescribed. Exercise training in cardiac patients is discussed further in chapter 37. Though such training is clearly safe for most patients, early exercise may have deleterious effects on infarct healing and ventricular remodeling in patients with large anterior infarctions.[216] When training is begun 4-8 weeks after infarction in these patients, no such deterioration occurs.[217]

Education of the post-infarction patient in the outpatient setting is of great importance. Lifestyle and dietary changes must be reinforced, and guidelines concerning return to work given. The post-discharge exercise test is useful for disability assessment in this setting. Patients may exhibit either excessive anxiety or excessive denial that can hinder their recovery. The physician should be alert for symptoms of depression and of social and sexual dysfunction which are common even after uncomplicated infarction.

THE PATIENT IN WHOM MYOCARDIAL INFARCTION IS RULED OUT

Many patients presenting to emergency departments have chest pain of a nonspecific nature and ECGs that are nondiagnostic. Such patients are typically admitted to a coronary care unit for 24 hours to obtain serial ECGs and CK isoenzymes, since many cases of MI would otherwise be missed. Increasingly however, such patients are being evaluated in "chest pain areas" within emergency departments to determine whether hospital admission is warranted. Patients are held in a designated monitored area. Electrocardiograms are obtained every 30 minutes and CK-MB is obtained initially and at 3, 6, and 9 hours after emergency room admission and an echocardiogram is obtained. After 9-12 hours, if all tests are negative, the patient undergoes an exercise stress test.[218] If this study is negative the patient is discharged home and referred to a private physician. This efficient approach has resulted in fewer coronary care unit admissions of patients with noncardiac chest pain, and reduced costs for hospitalization.[219]

On the other hand, many patients are admitted to coronary care units who clearly have acute myocardial ischemia but do not develop myocardial infarction. It must be kept in mind that many of these "ruled-out" patients have extensive heart disease and a prognosis as bad as or worse than those with infarction.[220] Risk is particularly high among patients presenting with ischemia-related pulmonary edema, who have a 60% mortality within 2 years.[221]

SUMMARY

Newer therapies for MI have led to a revolution in the treatment of this condition. The reduction in both early and late mortality with thrombolytic therapy, ß-blockade, aspirin and revascularization has radically altered the natural history of myocardial infarction. Further progress needs to be made in the earlier or prehospital administration of thrombolytic therapy and its administration to a larger fraction of infarction patients, prevention of reocclusion with antithrombin agents, risk stratification, prevention of prehospital cardiac arrest, and prevention of late arrhythmic death. Primary prevention of atherosclerotic heart disease[222] is the final and ultimately attainable goal.

REFERENCES

1. American Heart Association. *Heart and Stroke Facts.* Dallas: American Heart Association, National Center, 1994.
2. Gillum RF. Acute myocardial infarction in the United States, 1970-1983. *Am Heart J.* 1987:113:804-811.
3. Kannel WB, Abbott RD. Incidence and prognosis of unrecognized myocardial infarction. *N Engl J Med.* 1984;311:1144-1147.
4. Ridker PM, Manson JE, Buring JE, et al. Circadian variation of acute myocardial infarction and the effect of low-dose aspirin in a randomized trial of physicians. *Circulation.* 1990;82:897-902.
5. Willich SN, Pohjola-Sintonen S, Bhatia SJ, et al. Suppression of silent ischemia by metoprolol without alteration of morning increase of platelet aggregability in patients with stable coronary artery disease. *Circulation.* 1989;79:557-565.
6. Mittleman MA, Maclure M, Tofler GH, et al, and the determinants of Myocardial Infarction Onset Study Investigators. Triggering of acute myocardial infarction by heavy physical exertion. Protection against triggering by regular exertion. *N Engl J Med.* 1993:329:1677-1683.

7. Adams J, Trent R, Rawles J. Earliest electrocardiographic evidence of myocardial infarction: implications for thrombolytic treatment. The GREAT Group. *Br Med J.* 1993;307:409-413.

8. Goldberg HL, Borer JS, Jacobstein JG, et al. Anterior ST segment depression in acute myocardial infarction: Indicator of posterolateral infarction. *Am J Cardiol.* 1981;48:1009-1015.

9. Schuster EH, Bulkley BH. Early post-infarction angina: Ischemia at a distance and ischemia in the infarct zone. *N Engl J Med.* 1981;305:1101-1105.

10. Krone RJ, Greenberg H, Dwyer EM Jr, et al. Long-term prognostic significance of ST segment depression during acute myocardial infarction. The Multicenter Diltiazem Postinfarction Trial Research Group. *J Am Coll Cardiol.* 1993;22:361-367.

11. Arvan S, Varat MA. Persistent ST-segment elevation and left ventricular wall abnormalities: a two-dimensional echocardiographic study. *Am J Cardiol.* 1984;53:1542-1546.

12. Blanke H, Cohen M, Schlueter GV. Electrocardiographic and coronary arteriographic correlations during acute myocardial infarction. *Am J Cardiol.* 1984;54:249-255.

13. Fuchs RM, Achuff SC, Grunwals L, et al. Electrocardiographic localization of coronary artery narrowings: studies during myocardial ischemia and infarction in patients with one-vessel disease. *Circulation.* 1982;66:1168-1176.

14. Marriott HJ. Coronary mimicry: normal variants, and physiologic, pharmacologic and pathologic influences that simulate coronary patterns in the electrocardiogram. *Ann Intern Med.* 1960;52:411-427.

15. Goldberger AL. ECG simulators of myocardial infarction. Pathophysiology and differential diagnosis of psuedo-infarct Q wave patterns (Part I) and pseudo-infarction ST-T patterns (Part II). *PACE.* 1982;5:106-119, 414-430.

16. Bateman TM, Czer LSC, Gray RJ, et al. Transient pathologic Q waves during acute ischemic events: An electrocardiographic correlate of stunned but viable myocardium. *Am Heart J.* 1983;106:1421-1426.

17. Raunio H, Rissanen V, Roppanen T, et al. Changes in the QRS complex and ST segment in transmural and subendocardial myocardial infarctions. A clinico-pathologic study. *Am Heart J.* 1979;98:176-184.

18. Lee TH, Goldman L. Serum enzyme assays in the diagnosis of acute myocardial infarction. Recommendations based on a quantitative analysis. *Ann Intern Med.* 1986:102:221-233.

19. De Zwaan C, Willems GM, Vermeer F, et al. Enzyme tests in the evaluation of thrombolysis in acute myocardial infarction. *Br Heart J.* 1988;59:175-183.

20. Roberts R, Kleiman NS. Earlier diagnosis and treatment of acute myocardial infarction necessitates the need for a "new diagnostic mind-set". *Circulation.* 1994;89:872-881.

21. Hong RA, Licht JD, Wei JY, et al. Elevated CK-MB with normal creatine kinase in suspected myocardial infarction: associated clinical findings and early prognosis. *Am Heart J.* 1986;111:1041-1047.

Puleo RR, Meyer D, Wathen C, et al. Use of a rapid assay of subforms of creatine kinase MB to diagnose or rule out acute myocardial infarction. *N Engl J Med.* 1994;331:561-566.

23. Katus HA, Remppis A, Neumann FJ, et al. Diagnostic efficiency of troponin T measurements in acute myocardial infarction. *Circulation.* 1991;83:902-912.

24. Adams JE III, Bodor GS, Davilla-Roman VG, et al. Cardiac troponin-I. A marker with high specificity for cardiac injury. *Circulation.* 1993;88:101-106.

25. Volpini, M, Giubbini R, Gei P, et al. Diagnosis of acute myocardial infarction by indium-111 antimyosin antibodies and correlation with the traditional techniques for the evaluation of extent and localization. *Am J Cardiol.* 1989;63:7-13.

26. Gibbons RJ. Perfusion imaging with 99mTc-sestamibi for the assessment of myocardial area at risk and the efficacy of acute treatment in myocardial infarction. *Circulation.* 1991;84:137-142.

27. Czernin J, Porenta G, Brunken R, et al. Regional blood flow, oxidative metabolism, and glucose utilization in patients with recent myocardial infarction. *Circulation.* 1993;88:884-895.

28. Yoshida K, Gould KL. Quantitative relation of myocardial infarct size and myocardial viability by positron emission tomography to left ventricular ejection fraction and 3-year mortality with and without revascularization. *J Am Coll Cardiol.* 1993;22:984-997.

29. Feigenbaum H. Coronary Artery Disease. In: Feigenbaum H. *Echocardiography*, 5th ed. Philadelphia: Lea and Febinger, 1994:447-510.

30. Sabia P, Afrookteh A, Touchstone DA, et al. Value of regional wall motion abnormality in the emergency room diagnosis of acute myocardial infarction. A prospective study using two-dimensional echocardiography. *Circulation.* 1991;84:185-192.

31. Shen WK, Khandheria BK, Edwards WD, et al. Value and limitations of two-dimensional echocardiography in predicting myocardial infarct size. *Am J Cardiol.* 1991;68:1143-1149.

32. Launberg J, Berning J, Fruergaard P, et al. Sensitivity and specificity of echocardiographic identification of patients eligible for safe early discharge after acute myocardial infarction. *Am Heart J.* 1992;124:846-853.

33. Previtali M, Poli A, Lanzarini L, et al. Dobutamine stress echocardiography for assessment of myocardial viability and ischemia in acute myocardial infarction treated with thrombolysis. *Am J Cardiol.* 1993;72:124G-130G.

34. Sechtem U, Voth E, Baer F, et al. Assessment of residual viability in patients with myocardial infarction using magnetic resonance techniques. *Int J Card Imaging.* 1993;9(suppl 1):31-40.

35. Jennings RB, Reimer KA. Pathobiology of acute myocardial ischemia. *Hosp Pract.* 1989;24:89-107.

36. Reimer KA, Jennings RB. The wavefront phenomenon of myocardial ischemic cell death: II. Transmural progression of necrosis within the framework of ischemic bed size (myocardium at risk) and collateral flow. *Lab Invest.* 1979;40:663-644.

37. Christian TF, Schwartz RS, Gibbons RJ. Determinants of infarct size in reperfusion therapy for acute myocardial infarction. *Circulation*. 1992;86:81-90.

38. Reimer KA, Vander Heide RS, Richard VJ. Reperfusion in acute myocardial infarction; effect of timing and modulating factors in experimental models. *Am J Cardiol*. 1993;72:13-21.

39. Piana RN, Paik GY, Moscucci M, et al. Incidence and treatment of "no-reflow" after percutaneous coronary intervention. *Circulation*. 1994;89:2514-2518.

40. Ito H, Tomooka T, Sakai N. Lack of myocardial perfusion immediately after successful thrombolysis. A predictor of poor recovery of left ventricular function in anterior myocardial infarction. *Circulation*. 1992; 85:1699-1705.

41. Kloner RA. Does reperfusion injury exist in humans? *J Am Coll Cardiol*. 1993;21:537-545.

42. Lawson CS, Downey JM. Preconditiong: state of the art myocardial protection. *Cardiovasc Res*. 1993: 27:542-550.

43. Kloner RA, Shook T, Przyklenk K, et al, and the TIMI 4 Study Group. Previous angina alters in-hospital outcome in TIMI 4. A clinical correlate to preconditioning? *Circulation*. 1995;91:37-45.

44. Deutsch E, Berger M, Kussmaul WG, et al. Adaptation to ischemia during percutaneous transluminal coronary angioplasty. Clinical, hemodynamic, and metabolic features. *Circulation*. 1990;82:2044-2051.

45. Kloner RA, Przyklenk K. Stunned and hibernating myocardium. Ann Rev Med. 1991;42:1-8.

46. deFeyter PJ, Serruys PW, Wijns W. Early angiography after myocardial infarction: what have we learned. *Am Heart J*. 1985;109:194-199.

47. Forrester JS, Litvack F, Grundfest W, et al. A perspective of coronary disease seen through the arteries of a living man. *Circulation*. 1987;75:505-513.

48. De Wood MA, Stifter WF, Simpson CS, et al. Coronary arteriographic findings soon after non-Q wave myocardial infarction. *N Engl J Med*. 1986; 315:417-423.

49. De Wood MA, Spores J, Notske R, et al. Prevalence of total coronary occlusion during the early hours of transmural myocardial infarction. *N Engl J Med*. 1980;303:897-902.

50. Davies MJ, Thomas AC. Plaque fissuring—the cause of acute myocardial infarction, sudden ischemic death, and crescendo angina. *Br Heart J*. 1985; 53:363-373.

51. van der Wal AC, Becker AE, van der Loos CM, et al. Site of intimal rupture or erosion of thrombosed coronary atherosclerotic plaques is characterized by an inflammatory process irrespective of the dominant plaque morphology. *Circulation*. 1994;89:36-44.

52. Ong L, Reiser P, Coromilas J, et al. Left ventricular function and rapid release of creatine kinase MB in acute myocardial infarction. Evidence for spontaneous reperfusion. *N Engl J Med*. 1983;309:1-6.

53. Cheitlin MD, McAllister GA, de Castro CM. Myocardial infarction without atherosclerosis. *JAMA*. 1975; 231:951-955.

54. Isner JM, Estes NA, Thompson PD, et al. Acute cardiac events temporally related to cocaine abuse. *N Engl J Med*. 1986;315:1438-1443.

55. Lange RA, Cigarroa RG, Yancy CW, et al. Cocaine-induced coronary-artery vasoconstriction. *N Engl J Med*. 1989;321:1557-1562.

56. Goldman L. Coronary care units: A perspective on their epidemiologic impact. *Int J Cardiol*. 1982; 2:284-287.

57. Rude RE, Muller JE, Braunwald E. Efforts to limit the size of myocardial infarcts. *Ann Intern Med*. 1981;95:736-761.

58. The GUSTO Investigators. An international randomized trial comparing four thrombolytic stategies for acute myocardial infarction. *N Engl J Med*. 1993;329:673-682.

59. Purvis JA, McNeill AJ, Siddiqui RA, et al. Efficacy of 100 mg of double-bolus alteplase in achieving complete perfusion in the treatment of acute myocardial infarction. *J Am Coll Cardiol*. 1994;23:6-10.

60. Anderson JL, Karagounis LA, Becker LC, et al. TIMI perfusion grade 3 but not grade 2 results in improved outcome after thrombolysis for myocardial infarction. Ventriculographic, enzymatic, and electrocardiographic evidence from the TEAM 3 study. *Circulation*. 1993;87:1829-1839.

61. Goldberg S, Greenspoon AJ, Urban PL, et al. Reperfusion arrhythmia: a marker of restoration of antegrade flow during intracoronary thrombolysis for acute myocardial infarction. *Am Heart J*. 1983; 105:26-32.

62. Califf RM, O'Neill W, Stack RS, et al, and the TAMI Study Group. Failure of simple clinical measurements to predict perfusion status after intravenous thrombolysis. *Ann Intern Med*. 1988;108:658-662.

63. Norris RM, White HD, Cross DB, et al. Non-invasive diagnosis of arterial patency after thrombolytic treatment and its relation to prognosis. *Br Heart J*. 1993;69:485-491.

64. Shah PK, Cercek B, Lew AS, et al. Angiographic validation of bedside markers of reperfusion. *J Am Coll Cardiol*. 1993;21:55-61.

65. Effects of tissue plasminogen activator and a comparison of early invasive and conservative strategies in unstable angina and non-Q-wave myocardial infarction. Results of the TIMI IIIB Trial. Thrombolysis in Myocardial Ischemia. *Circulation*. 1994;89:1545-1556.

66. Mizuno K, Satomura K, Miyamoto A, et al. Angioscopic evaluation of coronary-artery thrombi in acute coronary syndromes. *N Engl J Med*. 1992;30;326:287-291.

67. Ambrose JA. Plaque disruption and the acute coronary syndromes of unstable angina and myocardial infarction: if the substrate is similiar, why is the clinical presentation different? *J Am Coll Cardiol*. 1992;19:1653-1658.

68. Late Assessment of Thrombolytic Efficacy (LATE) study with alteplase 6-24 hours after onset of acute myocardial infarction. *Lancet*. 1993;342:759-766.

69. The European Myocardial Infarct Project Group. Prehospital thrombolytic therapy in patients with suspected acute myocardial infarction. *N Engl J Med*. 1993;326:383-389.

70. Weaver WD, Cerqueira M, Hallstrom AP, et al. Prehospital-initiated vs hospital-initiated thrombolytic therapy. The Myocardial Infarction Triage and Intervention Trial. *JAMA*. 1993;270:1211-1216.

71. Maggioni AP, Franzosi MG, Santoro E, et al. The risk of stroke in patients with acute myocardial infarction after thrombolytic and antithrombotic treatment. Gruppo Italiano per lo Studio della Sopravvivenza nell'Infarto Miocardico II (GISSI-2), and The International Study Group. *N Engl J Med*. 1992;327:1-6.

72. Fibrinolyic Therapy Trialists' Collaborative Group. Indications for fibrinolytic therapy in suspected acute myocardial infarction: a collaborators overview of mortality and major morbidity results from all randomized trials of more than 1000 patients. *Lancet*. 1994;343:311-322.

73. Ohman EM, Topol EJ, Califf RM, et al. An analysis of the cause of early mortality after administration of thrombolytic therapy. The Thrombolysis Angioplasty in Myocardial Infarction Study Group. *Coron Artery Dis*. 1993;4:957-964.

74. Bleich SD, Nichols TC, Schumacher RR, et al. Effect of heparin on coronary artery patency after thrombolysis with tissue plasminogen activator in acute myocardial infarction. *Am J Cardiol*. 1990;66:1412-1417.

75. de Bono DP, Simoons ML, Tijssen J, et al. Effect of early intravenous heparin on coronary patency, infarct size, and bleeding complications after alteplase thrombolysis; results of a randomized double blind European Cooperative Study Group (ECSG-6). *Br Heart J*. 1992;67:122-128.

76. Hsia J, Hamilton DP, Kleiman N, et al. A comparison between heparin and low-dose aspirin as adjunctive therapy with tissue plasminogen activator for acute myocardial infarction. *N Engl J Med*. 1990;323:1423-1437.

77. Johns JA, Gold HK, Leinbach RC, et al. Prevention of coronary artery reocclusion and reduction in late coronary artery stenosis after thrombolytic therapy in patients with acute myocardial infarction. *Circulation*. 1988;78:546-556.

78. Klootwijk P, Cobbaert C, Fioretti P, et al. Noninvasive assessment of reperfusion and reocclusion after thrombolysis in acute myocardial infarction. *Am J Cardiol*. 1993;72:75G-84G.

79. White HD, Cross DB, Elliott JA, et al. Long-term prognostic importance of patency of the infarct-related coronary artery after thrombolytic therapy for acute myocardial infarction. *Circulation*. 1994;89:61-67.

80. Kim CB, Braunwald E. Potential benefits of late reperfusion of infarcted myocardium. The open artery hypothesis. *Circulation*. 1993;88:2426-2436.

81. Cairns JA, Fuster V, Kennedy JW. Coronary thrombolysis. *Chest*. 1992;102:482-507.

82. Anderson HV, Willerson JT. Thrombolysis in acute myocardial infarction. *N Engl J Med*. 1993;329:703-709.

83. Yusuf S, Collins R, Peto R, et al. Intravenous and intracoronary fibrinolytic therapy in acute myocardial infarction: Overview of results on mortality, reinfarction, and side effects from 33 randomized controlled trials. *Eur Heart J*. 1985;6:556-585.

84. Kennedy JW, Ritchie JL, Davis KB, et al. Western Washington randomized trial of intracoronary streptokinase in acute myocardial infarction. *N Engl J Med*. 1983;309:1477-1482.

85. Kennedy JW, Ritchie JL, Davis KB, et al. The Western Washington randomized trial of intracoronary streptokinase in acute myocardial infarction. *N Engl J Med*. 1985;312:1073-1078.

86. Gruppo Italiano per lo Studio della Streptochinasi nell'Infarto Miocardico II (GISSI). Effectiveness of intravenous thrombolytic treatment in acute myocardial infarction. *Lancet*. 1986;1:397-402.

87. Chesebro JH, Knattrud G, Roberts R, et al. Thrombolysis in Acute Myocardial Infarction (TIMI) Trial, Phase I: A comparison between intravenous tissue plasminogen activator and intravenous streptokinase: clinical findings through hospital discharge. *Circulation*. 1987;76:142-154.

88. Dalen JE, Gore JM, Braunwald E, et al. Six and twelve month follow-up of the Phase I Thrombolysis in Myocardial Infarction (TIMI) Trial. *Am J Cardiol*. 1988;62:179-185.

89. TIMI Research Group. Immediate versus delayed catherization and angioplasty following thrombolytic therapy for acute myocardial infarction. TIMI II A Results. *JAMA*. 1988;260:2849-2858

90. Simoons ML, Betriu A, Col J, et al, for the European Cooperative Study Group for Recombinant Tissue-Type Plasminogen Activator. Thrombolysis with tissue plasminogen activator in acute myocardial infarction: no additional benefit from immediate percutaneous coronary angioplasty. *Lancet*. 1988;1:197-202.

91. Topol EJ, Califf RM, George BS, et al. A randomized trial of immediate versus delayed elective angioplasty after intravenous tissue plasminogen activator in acute myocardial infarction. *N Engl J Med*. 1987;317:581-588.

92. TIMI Study Group. Comparison of invasive and conservative strategies after treatment with intravenous tissue plasminogen activator in acute myocardial infarction. *N Engl J Med*. 1989;320:618-627.

93. ISIS-2 (Second International Study of Infarct Survival) Collaborative Group. Randomised trial of intravenous streptokinase, oral aspirin, both, or neither among 17,187 cases of suspected acute myocardial infarction: ISIS-2. *Lancet*. 1988;2:349-360.

94. Late Assessment of Thrombolytic Efficacy (LATE) study with alteplase 6-24 hours after onset of acute myocardial infarction. *Lancet*. 1993;342:759-766.

95. Rentrop KP, Feit F, Sherman W, et al. Late thrombolytic therapy preserves left ventricular function in patients with collateralized total coronary occlusions: Primary end point findings of the second Mount Sinai-New York University Reperfusion Trial. *J Am Coll Cardiol*. 1989;14:58-64.

96. Hochman JS, Choo H. Limitation of myocardial infarct expansion by reperfusion independent of myocardial salvage. *Circulation*. 1987;75:299-306.

97. Hirayama A, Adachi T, Asada S, et al. Late reperfusion for acute myocardial infarction limits the dilatation of left ventricle without the reduction of infarct size. *Circulation*. 1993;88:2565-2574.

98. Gruppo Italiano per lo Studio della Sopravvivenza nell'Infarcto Miocardico (GISSI). GISSI-2: A factorial randomized trial of alteplase versus streptokinase and heparin versus no heparin among 12,490 patients with acute myocardial infarction. *Lancet*. 1990;336:65-71.

99. International Study Group. In-hospital mortality and clinical course of 20,891 patients with suspected acute myocardial infarction randomised between alteplase and streptokinase with or without heparin. *Lancet*. 1990:336:71-75.

100. Third International Study of Infarct Survival Collaborative Group. ISIS-3. A randomised comparison of streptokinase vs. tissue plasminogen activator vs. anistreplase and of aspirin plus heparin vs. aspirin alone among 41,299 cases of suspected acute myocardial infarction. *Lancet*. 1992;339:753-770.

101. Neuhaus K-L, von Essen R, Tebbe U, et al. Improved thrombolysis in acute myocardial infarction with front-loaded administration of alteplase: results of the rt-PA-APSAC patency study (TAPS). *J Am Coll Cardiol*. 1992;19:885-891.

102. The GUSTO Angiographic Investigators. The effects of tissue plasminogen activator, streptokinase, or both on coronary-artery patency, ventricular function, and survival after acute myocardial infarction. *N Engl J Med*. 1993;329:1615-1622.

103. Farkouh ME, Lang JD, Sackett DL. Thrombolytic agents: The science of the art of choosing the better treatment. *Ann Intern Med*. 1994;120:886-888.

104. Grines CL, Browne KF, Marco J, et al. A comparison of immediate angioplasty with thrombolytic therapy for acute myocardial infarction. *N Engl J Med*. 1993; 328:673-679.

105. Simonton CA, Mark DB, Hinohara T, et al. Late restenosis after emergent coronary angioplasty for acute myocardial infaction: comparison with elective coronary angioplasty. *J Am Coll Cardiol*. 1988; 11:698-705.

106. Gibbons RJ, Holmes DR, Reeder GS, et al. Immediate angioplasty compared with the administration of a thrombolytic agent followed by conservative treatment for myocardial infarction. The Mayo Coronary Care Unit and Catheterization Laboratory Groups. *N Engl J Med*. 1993;328:685-691.

107. Reeder GS, Bailey KR, Gersh BJ, et al. Cost comparison of immediate angioplasty versus thrombolysis followed by conservative therapy for acute myocardial infarction: a randomized prospective trial. The Mayo Coronary Care Unit and Catheterization Laboratory Groups. *Mayo Clin Proc*. 1994;69:5-12.

108. Califf RM, Bengston JR. Cardiogenic shock. *N Engl J Med*. 1994;330:1724-1730.

109. Arnold AE, Simoons ML, Van de Werf F, et al. Recombinant tissue-type plasminogen activator and immediate angioplasty in acute myocardial infarction. One-year follow-up. The European Cooperative Study Group. *Circulation*. 1992:86:111-120.

110. Califf RM, Topol EJ, George BS, et al, and the TAMI Study Group. Characteristics and outcome of patients in whom reperfusion with intravenous tissue-type plasminogen activator fails: results of the Thrombolysis and Angioplasty in Myocardial Infarction (TAMI) I trial. *Circulation*. 1988;77:1090-1099.

111. Waller BF, Rothbaum DA, Pinkerton CA, et al. Status of the myocardium and infarct-related coronary artery in 19 necropsy patients with acute recanalization using pharmacologic (streptokinase, r-tissue plasminogen activator), mechanical (percutaneous transluminal coronary angioplasty) or combined types of reperfusion therapy. *J Am Coll Cardiol*. 1987;9:785-801.

112. Ellis SG, Mooney MR, George BS, et al. Randomized trial of late elective angioplasty versus conservative management for patients with residual stenoses after thrombolytic treatment of myocardial infarction. Treatment of Post-Thrombolytic Stenoses (TOPS) Study Group. *Circulation*. 1992;86:1400-1406.

113. Topol EJ, Califf RM, Vandormael M, et al, and the Thrombolysis and Angioplasty in Myocardial Infarction-6 Study Group. A randomized trial of late reperfusion therapy for acute myocardial infarction. *Circulation*. 1992;85:2090-2099.

114. Kereiakes DJ, Califf RM, George BS, et al. Coronary bypass surgery improves global and regional left ventricular function following thrombolytic therapy for acute myocardial infarction. *Am Heart J*. 1991; 122:390-399.

115. Applebaum R, House R, Rademaker A, et al. Coronary artery bypass grafting within thirty days of acute myocardial infarction. Early and late results in 406 patients. *J Thorac Cardiovasc Surg*. 1991;102:745-752.

116. Sintek CF, Pfeffer TA, Khonsari S. Surgical revascularization after acute myocardial infarction. Does timing make a difference? *J Thorac Cardiovasc Surg*. 1994;107:1317-1321.

117. De Wood MA, Notske RN, Berg R Jr, et al. Medical and surgical management of early Q wave myocardial infarction. I. Effects of surgical revascularization on survival, recurrent myocardial infarction, sudden death and functional class at 10 or more years of follow-up. II. Effects on mortality and global and regional left ventricular function at 10 or more years of follow-up. *J Am Coll Cardiol*. 1989;14:65-90.

118. Furberg CD, Byington RP. Beta-adrenergic blockers in patients with acute myocardial infarction. *Cardiovasc Clin*. 1989;20:235-247.

119. ISIS-1 Collaborative Group. A randomized trial of intravenous atenolol among 16,027 cases of suspected acute myocardial infarction. *Lancet*. 1986;2:57-66.

120. Beta-blocker Heart Attack Trial (BHAT) Research Group. Randomized trial of propranolol in patients with acute myocardial infarction. *JAMA*. 1982; 247:1707-1714.

121. Chadda K, Goldstein S, Byington R, et al. Effect of propranolol after acute myocardial infarction in patients with congestive heart failure. *Circulation*. 1986;73:503-510.

122. Norris RM, White ED, Cross DB, et al. Aspirin does not improve early arterial patency after streptokinase treatment for acute myocardial infarction. *Br Heart J*. 1993;69:492-495.

123. Juul-Moller S, Edvardsson N, Jahnmatz B, et al. Double-blind trial of aspirin in primary prevention of myocardial infarction in patients with stable chronic angina pectoris. The Swedish Angina Pectoris Aspirin Trial (SAPAT) Group. *Lancet*. 1992;340:1421-1425.

124. Theroux P, Waters D, Qui S, et al. Aspirin versus heparin to prevent myocardial infarction during the acute phase of unstable angina. *Circulation*. 1993;88:2045-2048.

125. Antiplatelet Trialists' Collaboration. Collaborative overview of randomised trials of antiplatelet therapy—I: Prevention of death, myocardial infarction, and stroke by prolonged antiplatelet therapy in various categories of patients. *Br Med J*. 1994;308:81-106.

126. Physicians' Health Study Research Group Steering Committee. Final report on the aspirin component of the ongoing physicians' health study. *N Engl J Med*. 1989;321:129-135.

127. Klieman NS, Ohman EM, Califf RM, et al. Profound inhibition of platelet aggregation with monoclonal antibody 7E3 Fab after thrombolyic therapy. Results of the Thrombolysis and Angioplasty in Myocardial Infarction (TAMI) 8 Pilot Study. *J Am Coll Cardiol*. 1993;22:381-389.

128. EPIC Investigators. Use of a monoclonal antibody directed against the platelet glycoprotein IIb/IIIa receptor in high-risk coronary angioplasty. The EPIC Investigation. *N Engl J Med*. 1994;330:956-961.

129. Nicolini FA, Lee P, Rios G, et al. Combination of platelet fibrinogen receptor antagonist and direct thrombin inhibitor at low doses markedly improves thrombolysis. *Circulation*. 1994;89:1802-1809.

130. Hirsh J, Fuster V. Guide to anticoagulant therapy. Part 1: Heparin. Part 2: Oral anticoagulants. American Heart Association. *Circulation*. 1994;89:1449-1480.

131. Smith P, Arnesen H, Holme I. The effect of warfarin on mortality and reinfarction after myocardial infarction. *N Engl J Med*. 1990;323:147-152.

132. Anticoagulants in the Secondary Prevention of Events in Coronary Thrombosis (ASPECT) Research Group. Effect of long-term oral anticoagulation treatment on mortality and cardiovascular morbidity after myocardial infarction. *Lancet*. 1994;343:499-503.

133. Meijer A, Verheugt FW, Werter CJ, et al. Aspirin versus coumadin in the prevention of reocclusion and recurrent ischemia after successful thrombolysis: a prospective placebo-controlled angiographic study. Results of the APRICOT Study. *Circulation*. 1993; 87:1524-1530.

134. Arnout J, Simoons M, de Bono D, et al. Correlation between level of heparinization and patency of the infarct-related coronary artery after treatment of acute myocardial infarction with alteplase (rt-PA). *J Am Coll Cardiol*. 1992;20:513-519.

135. Topol EJ, George BS, Kereiakes DJ, et al, and the TAMI Study Group. A randomized controlled trial of intravenous tissue plasminogen activator and early intravenous heparin in acute myocardial infarction. *Circulation*. 1989;79:281-286.

136. Cannon CP, McCabe CH, Henry TD, et al. A pilot trial of recombinant desulfatohirudin compared with heparin in conjunction with tissue-type plasminogen activator and aspirin for acute myocardial infarction: results of the Thrombolysis in Myocardial Infarction (TIMI) 5 trial. *J Am Coll Cardiol*. 1994;23:993-1003.

137. ISIS Collaborative Group. ISIS-3: Randomised study of oral isosorbide mononitrate in over 50,000 patients with suspected acute myocardial infarction. *Circulation*. 1993;88:I-394. Abstract.

138. Gruppo Italiano per lo Studio della Sopravvivenza nell'Infarto Miocardico (GISSI). GISSI-3: effects of lisinopril and transdermal glyceryl trinitrate singly and together on 6-week mortality and ventricular function after acute myocardial infarction. *Lancet*. 1994; 343:1115-1122.

139. Held PH, Yusuf S. Calcium antagonists in the treatment of ischemic heart disease: myocardial infarction. *Coron Artery Dis*. 1994;5:21-26.

140. Erbel R, Pop T, Meinertz T, et al. Combination of calcium channel blocker and thrombolytic therapy in acute myocardial infarction. *Am Heart J*. 1988;115:529-538.

141. Multicenter Diltiazem Postinfarction Trial Research Group. The effect of diltiazem on mortality and reinfarction after myocardial infarction. *N Engl J Med*. 1988;319:385-392.

142. Moss AJ, Davis HT, Conrad DL, et al. Digitalis-associated cardiac mortality after myocardial infarction. *Circulation*. 1981;64:1150-1156.

143. Muller JE, Turi ZG, Stone PH, et al, and the MILIS Study Group. Digoxin therapy and mortality after myocardial infarction. Experience in the MILIS study. *N Engl J Med*. 1986;314:265-271.

144. The Acute Infarction Ramipril Efficacy (AIRE) Study Investigators. Effect of ramipril on mortality and morbidity of survivors of acute myocardial infarction with clinical evidence of heart failure. *Lancet*. 1993;342:821-882.

145. Forrester JS, Diamond G, Chartterjee K, et al. Medical therapy of acute myocardial infarction by application of hemodynamic subsets (two parts). *N Engl J Med*. 1876;295:1356-1362, 1404-1413.

146. Weisman HF, Healy B. Myocardial infarct expansion, infarct extension, and reinfarction: pathophysiologic concepts. *Prog Cardiovasc Dis*. 1987;30:73-110.

147. Muller JE, Rude RE, Braunwald E, et al, and the MILIS Study Group. Myocardial infarct extension: occurrence, outcome, and risk factors in the Multicenter Investigation of Limitation of Infarct Size. *Ann Intern Med*. 1988;108:1-6.

148. Page DL, Caulfield JB, Kastor JA, et al. Myocardial changes associated with cardiogenic shock. *N Engl J Med*. 1971;285:133-137.

149. Hands ME, Rutherford JA, Muller JE, et al, and the MILIS Study Group. The in-hospital development of cardiogenic shock after myocardial infarction: incidence, predictors of occurence, outcome and prognostic factors. *J Am Coll Cardiol*. 1989;14:40-46.

150. Van de Werf F, Arnold AE. Intravenous tissue plasminogen activator and size of infarct, left ventricular function, and survival in acute myocardial infarction. *Br Med J*. 1988;297:1374-1379.

151. Bengtson JR, Kaplan AJ, Pieper KS, et al. Prognosis in cardiogenic shock after acute myocardial infarction in the interventional era. *J Am Coll Cardiol*. 1992; 20:1482-1489.

152. Gurbel PA, Anderson RD, MacCord CS, et al. Arterial diastolic pressure augmentation by intra-aortic balloon counterpulsation enhances the onset of coronary artery reperfusion by thrombolytic therapy. *Circulation*. 1994;89:361-365.

153. Waksman R, Weiss AT, Gotsman MS, et al. Intra-aortic balloon counterpulsation improves survival in cardiogenic shock complicating acute myocardial infarction. *Eur Heart J*. 1993;14:71-74.

154. Schuster EH, Bulkley BH. Expansion of transmural myocardial infarction: A pathophysiologic factor in cardiac rupture. *Circulation*. 1979;60:1532-1538.

155. Honan MB, Harrell FE, Reimer KA, et al. Cardiac rupture, mortality and the timing of thrombolytic therapy: a meta-analysis. *J Am Coll Cardiol*. 1990; 16:359-367.

156. Visser CA, Kan G, Meltzer RS, et al. Incidence, timing and prognostic value of left ventricular aneurysm formation after myocardial infarction: a prospective, serial echocardiographic study of 158 patients. *Am J Cardiol*. 1986;57:729-732.

157. Visser CA, Kan G, Meltzer RS, et al. Embolic potential of left ventricular thrombus after myocardial infarction: a two-dimensional echocardiographic study of 119 patients. *J Am Coll Cardiol*. 1985;5:1276-1280.

158. Vaitks PT, Barnathan ES. Embolic potential, prevention and management of mural thrombus complicating anterior myocardial infarction: a meta-analysis. *J Am Coll Cardiol*. 1993;22:1004-1009.

159. Leung WH, Lau CP. Effects of severity of the residual stenosis of the infarct-related coronary artery on left ventricular dilation and function after acute myocardial infarction. *J Am Coll Cardiol*. 1992;20:307-313.

160. Sharpe N, Smith H, Murphy J, et al. Treatment of patients with symptomless left ventricular dysfunction after myocardial infarction. *Lancet*. 1988;1:255-259.

161. Pfeffer MA, Lamas GA, Vaaughan DE, et al. Effect of captopril on progressive ventricular dilatation after anterior myocardial infarction. *N Engl J Med*. 1988;319:80-86.

162. Pfeffer MA, Braunwald E, Moye LA, et al. Effect of captopril on mortality and morbidity in patients with left ventricular dysfunction after myocardial infarction. Results of the Survival and Ventricular Enlargement Trial. *N Engl J Med*. 1992;327:669-677.

163. Sogaard P, Nogaard A, Gotzsche CO, et al. Therapeutic effects of captopril on ischemia and dysfunction of the left ventricle after Q-wave and non-Q-wave infarction. *Am Heart J*. 1994;127:1-7.

164. Jugdutt BI. Effects of nitrate therapy on ventricular remodeling and function. *Am J Cardiol*. 1993;72:161-168.

165. Isner JM, Roberts WC. Right ventricular infarction complicating left ventricular infarction secondary to coronary heart disease: Frequency, location, associated findings and significance from analysis of 236 necropsy patients with acute or healed myocardial infarction. *Am J Cardiol*. 1978;42:885-894.

166. Bellamy GR, Rasmussen HH, Nassar FN, et al. Value of two-dimensional echocardiography, electrocardiography, and clinical signs in detecting right ventricular infarction. *Am Heart J*. 1986;112:304-309.

167. Dell'Italia LJ, Starling MR, Blumhardt R, et al. Comparative effects of volume loading, dobutamine and nitroprusside in patients with predominant right ventricular infarction. *Circulation*. 1985;72:1327-1335.

168. Klien LW, Helfant RH. The Q-wave and non-Q wave myocardial infarction: differences and similarities. *Prog Cardiovasc Dis*. 1986;29:205-220.

169. Cohen M, Xiong J, Parry G, et al. Prospective comparison of unstable angina versus non-Q wave myocardial infarction during antithrombotic therapy. Antithrombotic Therapy in Acute Coronary Syndromes Research Group. *J Am Coll Cardiol*. 1993;22:1138-1343.

170. Berger CJ, Murabito JM, Evans JC, et al. Prognosis after first myocardial infarction. Comparison of Q-wave and non Q-wave myocardial infarction in the Framingham Heart Study. *JAMA*. 1992;268:1545-1551.

171. Tofler GH, Muller JE, Stone PH, et al. Pericarditis in acute myocardial infarction: characterization and clinical significance. *Am Heart J*. 1989;117:86-90.

172. Dressler W. The post-myocardial infarction syndrome: a report of fourty-four cases. *Arch Intern Med*. 1959;103:28-42.

173. Berger PB, Ruocco NA, Ryan TJ, et al. Incidence and significance of ventricular tachycardia and fibrillation in the absence of hypotension or heart failure in acute myocardial infarction treated with recombinant tissue-type plasminogen activator: results from the Thrombolysis in Myocardial Infarction (TIMI) Phase II trail. *J Am Coll Cardiol*. 1993;22:1773-1779.

174. Lie KI, Wellens HJ, Van Capelle FJ, et al. Lidocaine in the prevention of primary ventricular fibrillation: A double-blind randomized study of 212 consecutive patients. *N Engl J Med*. 1974;291:1324-1326.

175. Antman EM, Berlin JA. Declining incidence of ventricular fibrillation in myocardial infarction. Implications for the prophylactic use of lidocaine. *Circulation*. 1992;86:764-773.

176. Berntsen RF, Rasmussen K. Lidocaine to prevent ventricular fibrillation in the prehospital phase of suspected acute myocardial infarction: the North-Norwegian Lidocaine Intervention Trial. *Am Heart J*. 1992;124:1478-1483.

177. Bigger JT Jr, Fleiss JL, Kleiger R, et al. The relationships among ventricular arrhythmias, left ventricular dysfunction, and mortality in the two years after myocardial infarction. *Circulation*. 1984;69:250-258.

178. Steinberg JS, Regan A, Sciacca RR, et al. Predicting arrhythmic events after acute myocardial infarction using the signal-averaged electrocardiogram. *Am J Cardiol.* 1992;69:13-21.

179. Mcclements BM, Adgey AAJ. Value of signal-averaged electrocardiography, radionuclide angiography, Holter monitoring and clinical variables for the prediction of arrhythmic events in survivors of acute myocardial infarction in the thrombolytic era. *J Am Coll Cardiol.* 1993;21:1419-1423.

180. Pedretti R, Etro MD, Laporta A, et al. Prediction of late arrhythmic events after acute myocardial infarction from combined use of noninvasive prognostic variables and inducibility of sustained monomorphic ventricular tachycardia. *Am J Cardiol.* 1993;71:1131-1141.

181. Bourke JP, Richards DA, Ross DL, et al. Routine programmed electrical stimulation in survivors of acute myocardial infarction for prediction of spontaneous ventricular tachyarrhythmias during follow-up: results, optimal stimulation protocol and cost-effective screening. *J Am Coll Cardiol.* 1991;18:780-788.

182. Echt DS, Liebson PR, Mitchell LB, et al. Mortality and morbidity in patients receiving encainide, flecainide, or placebo. The Cardiac Arrhythmia Suppression Trial. *N Engl J Med.* 1991;324:781-788.

183. Teo KK, Yusuf S, Furberg CD. Effects of prophylactic antiarrhythmic drug therapy in acute myocardial infarction. An overview of results from randomized controlled trials. *JAMA.* 1993;270:1589-1595.

184. Ceremuzynski L, Kleczar E, Krzeminska-Pakula M, et al. Effect of amiodarone on mortality after myocardial infarction: a double-blind, placebo-controlled, pilot study. *J Am Coll Cardiol.* 1992;20:1056-1062.

185. Pfisterer M, Kiowski W, Burckhardt D, et al. Beneficial effects of amiodarone on cardiac mortality in patients with asymptomatic complex ventricular arrhythmias after acute myocardial infarction and preserved but not impaired left ventricular function. *Am J Cardiol.* 1992;69:1399-1402.

186. Mitchell LB, Duff JH, Manyari DE, et al. A randomized trial of the noninvasive and invasive approaches to drug therapy of ventricular tachycardia. *N Engl J Med.* 1987;317:1681-1687.

187. Miller FC, Krucoff MW, Satler LF, et al. Ventricular arrhythmias during reperfusion. *Am Heart J.* 1986;112:928-932.

188. Gang ES, Lew AS, Hong M, et al. Decreased incidence of ventricular late potentials after successful thrombolytic therapy for acute myocardial infarction. *N Engl J Med.* 1989;321:712-716.

189. Tobe TJ, de Langen CD, Crijns HJ, et al. Effects of streptokinase during acute myocardial infarction on the signal-averaged electrocardiogram and on the frequency of late arrhythmias. *Am J Cardiol.* 1993;72:647-651.

190. Pedretti R, Laporta A, Etro MD, et al. Influence of thrombolysis on signal-averaged electrocardiogram and late arrhythmic events after acute myocardial infarction. *Am J Cardiol.* 1992;69:866-872.

191. Ragosta M, Sabia PJ, Kaul S, et al. Effects of late (1 to 30 days) reperfusion after acute myocardial infarction on the signal-averaged electrocardiogram. *Am J Cardiol.* 1993;71:19-23.

192. Hindman MC, Wagner GS, JaRo M, et al. The clinical significance of bundle branch block complicating acute myocardial infarction. 1. Clinical characteristics, hospital mortality, and one year follow-up; 2. Indications for temporary and permanent pacemaker insertion. *Circulation.* 1978;58:679-699.

193. Topol EJ, Burek K, O'Neill WW, et al. A randomized controlled trial of hospital discharge three days after myocardial infarction in the era of reperfusion. *N Engl J Med.* 1988;318:1083-1088.

194. Krone RJ, Gillespie JA, Weld FM, et al, and the Multicenter Postinfarction Study Group. Low-level exercise testing after myocardial infarction: usefulness in enhancing clinical risk stratification. *Circulation.* 1985;71:80-89.

195. Dittrich HC, Gilpin E, Nicod P, et al. Outcome after acute myocardial infarction in patients with prior coronary artery bypass surgery. *Am J Cardiol.* 1993;72:507-513.

196. Zuanetti G, Latini R, Maggioni AP, et al. Influence of diabetes on mortality in acute myocardial infarction data from the GISSI-2 study. *J Am Coll Cardiol.* 1993;22:1788-1794.

197. Greenland P, Reicher-Reiss H, Goldbourt U, et al. In-hospital and 1-year mortality in 1,524 women after myocardial infarction. Comparison with 4,315 men. *Circulation.* 1991;83:484-491.

198. Mark DB, Shaw LK, DeLong ER, et al. Absence of sex bias in the referral of patients for cardiac catheterization. *N Engl J Med.* 1994;330:1101-1106.

199. Maggioni AP, Maseri A, Fresco C, et al. Age-related increase in mortality among patients with first myocardial infarctions treated with thrombolysis. The Investigators of the Gruppo Italiano per lo Studio della Sopravvivenza nell'Infarto Miocardico (GISSI-2). *N Engl J Med.* 1993;329:1442-1448.

200. DeBusk RF, Blomqvist CG, Kouchoukos NT, et al. Identification and treatment of low-risk patients after acute myocardial infarction and coronary-artery bypass graft surgery. *N Engl J Med.* 1986;314:161-166.

201. Stevenson RN, Umachandran V, Ranjadayalan K, et al. Early exercise testing after treatment with thrombolytic drugs for acute myocardial infarction: importance of reciprocal ST segment depression. *Br Med J.* 1994;308:1189-1192.

202. Stone PH, Turi ZG, Muller JE, et al. Prognostic significance of the treadmill exercise test performed 6 months after myocardial infarction. *J Am Coll Cardiol.* 1986;8:1007-1019.

203. de Vreede JJ, Gorgels AP, Verstraaten GM, et al. Did prognosis after acute myocardial infarction change during the past 30 years? A meta-analysis. *J Am Coll Cardiol.* 1991;18:698-706.

204. Stevenson R, Umachandran V, Ranjadayalan K, et al. Reassessment of treadmill stress testing for risk stratification in patients with acute myocardial infarction treated by thrombolysis. *Br Heart J.* 1993;70:415-420.

205. Haber HL, Beller GA, Watson DD, et al. Exercise thallium-201 scintigraphy after thrombolytic therapy with or without angioplasty for acute myocardial infarction. *Am J Cardiol*. 1993;71:1257-1261.

206. Jain A, Myers GH, Sapin PM, et al. Comparison of symptom-limited and low level exercise tolerance tests early after myocardial infarction. *J Am Coll Cardiol*. 1993;22:1816-1820.

207. Barbash GI, White HD, Modan M, et al. Antecedent angina pectoris predicts worse outcome after myocardial infarction in patients receiving thrombolytic therapy. Experience gleaned from the International Tissue Plasminogen Activator/Streptokinase Mortality Trial. *J Am Coll Cardiol*. 1992;20:36-41.

208. Leroy F, Lablanche JM, McFadden EP, et al. Relative prognostic value of clinical, exercise, and angiographic data after a first myocardial infarction. *Coron Artery Dis*. 1993;4:727-736.

209. O'Rourke RA. Management of patients after myocardial infarction and thrombolytic therapy. *Curr Probl Cardiol*. 1994;19:179-226.

210. Carlson LA, Rosenhamer G. Reduction of mortality in the Stockholm Ischaemic Heart Disease Secondary Prevention Study by combined treatment with clofibrate and nicotinic acid. *Acta Med Scand*. 1988; 223:405-418.

211. Coronary Drug Project Research Group. Natural history of myocardial infarction in the coronary drug project: long-term prognostic importance of serum lipid levels. *Am J Cardiol*. 1978;42:489-498.

212. Blankenhorn DH, Nessim SA, Johnson RL, et al. Beneficial effects of combined colestipol-niacin therapy on coronary atherosclerosis and coronary venous bypass grafts. *JAMA*. 1987;257:3233-3240.

213. Cavender JB, Rogers WJ, Fisher LD, et al, and the CASS Investigators. Effects of smoking on survival and morbidity in patients randomized to medical or surgical therapy in the Coronary Artery Surgery Study (CASS): 10-year follow-up. *J Am Coll Cardiol*. 1992;20:287-294.

214. Greenland P, Chu JS. Efficacy of cardiac rehabilitation services, with emphasis on patients after myocardial infarction. *Ann Intern Med*. 1988;109:650-663.

215. Hedback B, Perk J, Wodlin P. Long-term reduction of cardiac mortality after myocardial infarction: 10-year results of a comprehensive rehabilitation programme. *Eur Heart J*. 1993;14:831-835.

216. Jugdutt BI, Michorowski BL, Kappagoda CT. Exercise training after anterior Q wave myocardial infarction: importance of regional left ventricular function and topography. *J Am Coll Cardiol*. 1988;12:362-372.

217. Giannuzzi P, Tavazzi L, Temporelli PL, et al. Long-term physical training and left ventricular remodeling after anterior myocardial infarction. *J Am Coll Cardiol*. 1993;22:1821-1829.

218. Gibler WB, Runyon JP, Levy RC, et al. A rapid diagnostic and treatment center for patients with chest pain in the emergency department. *Ann Emerg Med*. 1995;25:1-8.

219. Lee TH, Juarez G, Cook EF, et al. Ruling out acute myocardial infarction. A prospective multicenter validation of a 12-hour strategy for patients at low risk. *N Engl J Med*. 1991;324:1239-1246.

220. Schroeder JS, Lamb IH, Hu M. Do patients in whom myocardial infarction has been ruled out have a better prognosis after hospitalization than those surviving infarction? *N Engl J Med*. 1980;303:1-5.

221. Clark LT, Garfein OB, Dwyer EM. Acute pulmonary edema due to ischemic heart disease without accompanying myocardial infarction: natural history and clinical profile. *Am J Med*. 1983;75:332-336.

222. Manson JE, Tosteson H, Ridker PM, et al. The primary prevention of myocardial infarction. *N Engl J Med*. 1992;326:1406-1416.

16 Left Ventricular Remodeling After Myocardial Infarction

Gary F. Mitchell, MD
Marc A. Pfeffer, MD, PhD

Left ventricular (LV) enlargement and distortion of regional and global ventricular geometry occur to a variable degree in a significant proportion of patients following acute, transmural MI (MI). In general, this "ventricular remodeling" represents an important adaptive mechanism that helps to compensate for loss of contractile function. However, in a subset of patients, volume enlargement, with changes in wall thickness and chamber geometry, continues for months or years after infarction, and may contribute to an adverse clinical outcome even in the absence of further myocardial necrosis.

Though truly a continuum over time and severity, a distinction can be drawn between the patterns of ventricular remodeling observed early and late post-MI. Early remodeling, within hours to days after the onset of ischemia, involves predominantly the zone of myocardial necrosis. In the absence of further ischemic damage, the infarct zone can undergo extensive dilatation and thinning—a process known as infarct expansion. The resultant marked lengthening of the infarct zone distorts the LV apex and creates a region of abnormal curvature at the interface between infarcted and residual functioning tissue. There are several lines of evidence to suggest that this geometry may place an abnormally high load on the myocardium at this interface, thereby adversely influencing late ventricular remodeling. In the late phase of ventricular remodeling, continuing for months after MI, scar formation is finalized, and depending on the outcome of early compensatory mechanisms, ventricular remodeling either stabilizes or, in a significant proportion of patients, enters a phase of progressive chamber enlargement and shape distortion primarily involving the residual myocardium. These early and progressive alterations in ventricular volume bear a direct association with long-term survival post-infarction.

INFARCT EXPANSION

The process of infarct expansion was first described by Hutchins and Bulkley,[1] who carefully distinguished infarct extension from expansion. They defined infarct expansion as acute dilatation and thinning of the area of infarction not explained by additional myocardial necrosis, resulting in an infarcted region that occupies a greater proportion of the surface area of the ventricle. Infarct extension, in contrast, involves additional myocyte necrosis usually within the same vascular bed. In their autopsy study of 76 patients who died within 30 days of acute MI, they found that infarct extension, a more frequent clinical diagnosis, was less common pathologically, occurring in only 13 (17%) patients. Conversely, infarct expansion was infrequently diagnosed but pathologically quite common, with the majority (59%) of these nonsurvivors of acute MI having infarct expansion. Marked expansion was found to occur only in transmural infarctions, where the incidence was 72%, and was more common with first infarctions.

Much of our knowledge of the clinical course of infarct expansion is derived from serial echocardiographic studies. Eaton et al,[2] using the papillary muscles as a fixed internal landmark on short-axis views of the heart, measured the circumferential lengths of the infarct-containing and noninfarcted segments of the left ventricle (Fig. 1). In this early noninvasive study of 28 consecutive patients with acute anterior or inferior MI, evidence of

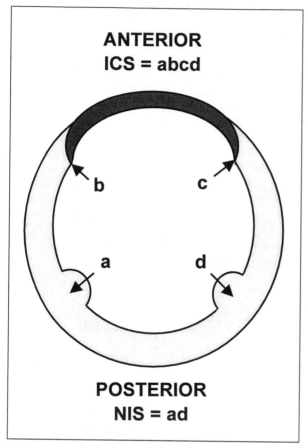

**ANTERIOR
ICS = abcd**

b   c

a   d

**POSTERIOR
NIS = ad**

Figure 1. *Echocardiographic definitions of infarct-containing segment (ICS) and the noninfarcted segment (NIS) for an anterior infarction. The endocardial length anterior to the papillary muscles (at points a and d) corresponds to the infarct-containing segment (length of the endocardial line clockwise from a through b and c to d). The length of the noninfarcted segment would be measured along the line from d clockwise to a to finish the endocardial circumference. Note that the infarct-containing segment also contains a significant proportion of normal myocardium (segments ab and cd) so that changes in this segment represent a mixture of changes in infarcted and noninfarcted tissue.*

infarct expansion was found in 8 patients, all with anterior infarctions. In patients with infarct expansion, a 25% increase in LV circumference was attributed to changes in the infarct-containing segment, which, at 2 weeks, had lengthened an average of almost 50% above baseline, without change in the noninfarcted segment. This acute remodeling of the infarct zone dramatically increases LV chamber volume. For example, a 25% increase in total circumference, as noted by Eaton and colleagues, would nearly double ventricular volume even in the absence of changes in chamber geometry. This marked ventricular enlargement was accompanied by a significantly increased mortality at 8 weeks of follow-up.

In a subsequent study of 27 patients with anterior MI, the same investigators demonstrated that infarct expansion occurs in the early hours of transmural MI, without any difference found in infarct-containing segment lengths obtained at 24, 48, or 72 hours after the onset of symptoms.[3] There was no further lengthening of the infarct segment over the ensuing 9 to 21 day follow-up period. Together, these studies established that the process responsible for early ventricular enlargement is the lengthening and thinning of the infarct zone that characterizes infarct expansion, suggesting that attempts to intervene in the process of infarct expansion will need to be initiated early in the course of MI.

Grossly, infarct expansion results in a markedly thinned zone of infarction that occupies a larger percentage of the ventricular surface area. The predominant structural correlate of infarct expansion is disruption of the interstitial collagen network, with slippage of necrotic myocyte bundles alongside one another, leading to a decreased number of myocytes across the wall of the necrotic zone.[4] Additional thinning and geometric distortion occur as a result of lesser contributions from overstretching of myocytes and from loss of intramyocardial vascular volume if the infarct-related vessel is persistently occluded. This distortion in local geometry forms the substrate for aneurysm development[5,6] or, in the most extreme cases, myocardial rupture.[7]

In an autopsy study of 204 patients with a single MI, a number of important risk factors for infarct expansion were identified.[8] Patient selection for this study was based on the earlier work of Hutchins and Bulkley, who showed that infarct expansion is more likely to occur in patients without a previous MI. Again, infarct expansion was relatively common in this autopsy series, with moderate-to-marked infarct expansion occurring in 45% of the patients.

Expansion was found in large, transmural infarcts and was twice as likely to occur in patients with left anterior descending (LAD) coronary artery lesions and infarction involving the LV apex as opposed to those with right coronary or left circumflex coronary artery lesions. One reason for this association was that LAD lesions produced larger infarcts. However, multivariate analysis demonstrated an association with LAD lesions independent of infarct size. They noted that regions of myocardium supplied by the LAD, such as the apex, are more curved and are normally thinner than the septum or free wall. They suggested that the baseline wall thickness may account for the increased tendency for apical infarctions to expand. They also noted a negative correlation between the presence of LV hypertrophy and the occurrence of infarct expansion, reinforcing the concept of an inverse relationship between baseline wall thickness and expansion. Other investigators have added persistent occlusion of the infarct-related artery (see below), peri-infarct hypertension, administration of glucocorticoids, and nonsteroidal anti-inflammatory usage to the growing list of risk factors for infarct expansion.[9,10]

As noted above, an important risk factor for infarct expansion is involvement of the LV apex in the infarction. From the law of LaPlace, wall tension is proportional to the product of chamber pressure and radius of curvature (Fig. 2). The normal LV apex has the smallest radius of curvature of the left ventricle, especially during systole, and thus has a relatively low wall tension. Wall stress (wall tension divided by wall thickness) is more or less uniformly distributed throughout the myocardium. Under normal circumstances, the myocardium at the apex is therefore thinner than in the remainder of the ventricle.[11,12] Additionally, the decrease in radius of curvature in the LV apex during systole normally exceeds the increase in chamber pressure, so that wall stress actually decreases in mid and late systole despite an increasing intracavitary pressure.[13]

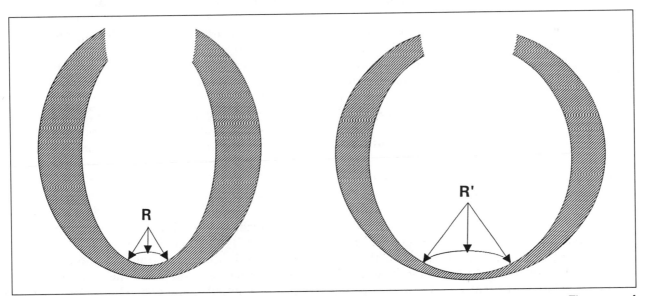

Figure 2. Schematic representation of the relationship between apical curvature and wall thickness. The apex of the left ventricle is the region with the shortest radius of curvature (R). The law of LaPlace states that tension is directly related to radius of curvature. Therefore, at a given pressure the apex will have a relatively low wall tension. Wall stress is the ratio of wall tension to wall thickness. Since wall stress is relatively uniform throughout the ventricle, low wall tension in the normal apex is associated with decreased myocardial wall thickness, as seen on the left. After apical infarction, global sphericity increases, wall thinning occurs both within and remote from the infarct zone, and the radius of curvature increases substantially at the apex (right panel). This unfavorable change in apical geometry (R' > R) superimposed on the already thin apical myocardium amplifies wall stress at the apex, possibly facilitating infarct expansion.

With the onset of ischemia, contractile function is lost within seconds and diastolic and paradoxical systolic lengthening follow within minutes. In the acutely ischemic apex, the unfavorable increase in radius of curvature accompanying loss of contraction will amplify systolic forces on the normally thin myocardium and may set up the milieu for infarct expansion. Once infarct expansion is initiated, further geometric distortion and thinning will greatly increase local systolic and diastolic wall stress and may promote additional expansion and aneurysm development or myocardial rupture. Picard et al,[14] have demonstrated that endocardial surface area may increase dramatically within 10 minutes after occlusion of a coronary artery in the dog. Despite comparable areas of abnormal wall motion initially after circumflex or left anterior descending coronary artery occlusion, subsequent surface area expansion was greater for left anterior descending occlusions involving the apical region. These experimental findings underscore the susceptibility of the apical region to distortion after ischemic insults.

This marked geometric distortion of the normally tightly curved apex allows for substantial increases in chamber volume, even with a minimal change in chamber circumference, as the apex assumes a more spherical configuration. We have evaluated this process by defining a "sphericity index," which is the ratio of the observed biplane ventricular volume divided by the volume of a theoretical ventricle with the same biplane circumference but perfectly spherical geometry.[15] Normal hearts, being somewhat ellipsoidal, have a diastolic sphericity index of 0.66, implying that the normal ventricular chamber would occupy only two-thirds of the volume of a sphere with the same circumference. As a result, diastolic volume could theoretically increase by up to 50% based on a change from an elliptical to a spherical geometry alone, without an increase in perimeter. The systolic chamber is even less spherical with a sphericity index of about 0.50. In a population of 52 patients 3 weeks after a large, first anterior Q-wave MI, sphericity index was increased at a baseline compared with healthy subjects both in diastole and in systole.

This suggested that volume enlargement within the first 3 weeks after infarction was not only a result of increased circumference, but also increased sphericity. We estimated that of the 88 mL increase in end-diastolic volume, 66 mL was the result of increased circumference and 22 mL could be attributed to increased chamber sphericity.

Lamas and colleagues,[16] have shown that those patients with the most abnormal global shape (sphericity index) as they enter the chronic phase of remodeling have a significantly longer akinetic/dyskinetic segment (reflecting infarct size plus the effects of early infarct expansion), higher filling pressures, larger volumes, and lower ejection fractions. They are also more likely to experience a reduction in exercise capacity and a higher heart failure score in the ensuing year. Of the various ventriculographic parameters tested, only sphericity index independently predicted reduced exercise capacity and accumulation of heart failure score points. Thus, early distortion of ventricular geometry appears to have an important effect on subsequent events both in terms of ventricular remodeling and progression to clinical heart failure.

Although critical changes occur in the infarct zone during the early phase of remodeling, important structural changes also occur in the adjacent and remote myocardium.[17] The infarct zone, which is significantly more compliant than contracting adjacent tissue, expands paradoxically during systole, creating a transitional rim of concavity or negative (anticlastic) curvature encircling the infarct[15] (Fig. 3). Wall stress in this region will be markedly elevated by this mechanically disadvantageous configuration.[15,18–21] This may lead to reduced systolic excursion in the border zone despite normal or near normal perfusion,[22] further compromising global ventricular function. Thus, apparent loss of function in the noninfarcted border zone may represent stunning, or it may simply represent regional loading that exceeds the otherwise normal contractile reserve of the border zone myocardium.

Important changes also occur in the remote myocardium in the acute phase. In the peri-infarct period, increased catecholamine levels

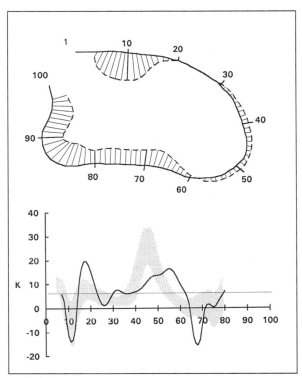

Figure 3. *Regional function and geometry. Illustrated are the diastolic (solid line) and systolic (broken line) left ventricular silhouettes in a patient 3 weeks after anterior myocardial infarction. Centerline wall-motion chords are shown. Below is a plot of the systolic curvature values measured at the intersection of each of the centerline chords with the systolic silhouette. Curvature is defined as the inverse of the radius of a "best fit" circle along a small arc at each point on the silhouette. Areas of concavity where the best fit circle would be outside of the chamber, such as at chord 10 on the systolic silhouette, are assigned a negative value by convention. Juxtaposition of contractile and noncontractile tissue forms a rim of negative curvature encircling the ventricular chamber at the interface. This is seen as 2 regions of negative curvature (centered at chords 12 and 68) in this 2-dimensional image.*

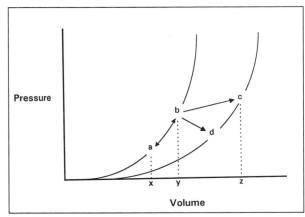

Figure 4. *Changes in the pressure–volume relationship after infarction. This figure presents 2 theoretical diastolic pressure–volume curves that might be observed after myocardial infarction. Acutely, much of the volume increase is passive, as a result of an increase in end-diastolic pressure. This corresponds to movement from point a to point b on an otherwise normal pressure–volume curve, leading to an increase in volume from x to y. The increase in filling pressure and resultant increase in contractility through a Frank–Starling mechanism, together with an increase in heart rate, may fully compensate for loss of contractile function in small infarcts. Such patients may experience no remodeling and return to the normal operating point, a. In larger infarctions, infarct expansion plus late remodeling of the ventricular chamber leads to a shift in the pressure–volume relationship to larger volumes at a given pressure. As a result, volume can increase even though filling pressure is unchanged (point c) or actually decreases (point d).*

augment contractility in noninfarcted myocardium and thereby partially restore global contractile performance.[23] The loss of global systolic function leads to an elevation in filling pressure that serves to enhance contractility in the residual myocardium by a Frank–Starling mechanism (Fig. 4). Thus, some lengthening and thinning of remote myocardium is to be expected based on distention alone. In addition, Weissman and associates[17] have demonstrated

thinning and increased radius of curvature in the remote zone of the infarcted rat ventricle even at 0 mm Hg distending pressure. Such thinning and regional enlargement, also the result of myocyte slippage, results in a reduced number of cells distributed across the wall, and represents true chamber remodeling with a shift in the pressure–volume relationship to the right (higher volume for a given pressure).[17,24] One important consequence of the foregoing events is marked elevation of diastolic wall stress, as each of the major determinants of wall stress (pressure, radius of curvature, and wall thickness) has changed in an unfavorable direction. Anversa et al[24] have estimated increases in diastolic wall stress of 2 to 9 fold after small or large infarctions, respectively, in the rat. These early changes in ventricular volume may, however, provide partial compensation for the loss of contractile function. Since chamber volume increases roughly with the cube of radius, while stress is related directly to radius, a comparable degree of shortening will eject a larger stroke volume from a larger chamber at only a moderate increase in wall stress.[13]

As remodeling enters an intermediate phase, days-to-weeks postinfarction, additional lengthening may occur in the infarct zone, although a shift towards quantitatively more significant changes in the residual myocardium is seen.[25] With the onset of eccentric hypertrophy, or series replication of contractile elements, chamber volume and compliance will increase,[26] producing a rightward shift in the diastolic pressure–volume relationship (Fig. 4). Filling pressures are, therefore, stable or reduced despite a further increase in diastolic volume. Additionally, concentric hypertrophy, or parallel replication of sarcomeres, begins in regions of increased systolic wall stress. Thus, a mixture of eccentric and concentric hypertrophy will be initiated during this phase. The distribution of each will be variable as a result of the marked heterogeneity of geometric distortion and wall thinning and, therefore, of wall stress within the ventricle.[27,28] For example, at the border zone where the rim of anticlastic curvature is found, high systolic wall stress is predicted by theoretical considerations, and maximal concentric hypertrophy develops in this region in the rat.[29] Volume enlargement is not found in all patients during this intermediate phase of remodeling. Over half of the post-infarction patients will have no change or a reduction in ventricular volume. Jeremy and co-workers[30] have suggested that those patients who experience a return to normal stroke volume through compensatory enlargement during the early phase of postinfarction remodeling enter a period of stable or decreasing LV volume in the late phase.

The clinical implications of these early changes in ventricular volume and geometry deserve comment. In a study of predictors of prognosis after MI, Hammermeister and associates[31] demonstrated a strong relationship between systolic and diastolic volume and subsequent mortality. Relatively small increases in end-diastolic or end-systolic volume index were associated with a 4- to 5-fold increased risk of cardiovascular death. White et al[32] have also shown that end-systolic and end-diastolic volumes determined 1 month after infarction are powerful predictors of mortality, surpassing even ejection fraction and extent of coronary artery disease in this regard using multivariate analysis. This was especially true in patients with a reduced ejection fraction. Early enlargement and distortion are, thus, of more than cosmetic interest, and it stands to reason that preventing enlargement may improve outcome.

LATE REMODELING

Not only does infarct expansion produce substantial early changes in ventricular volume and geometry, it also tends to predispose to additional late ventricular remodeling during the chronic phase of healing.[33] In an echocardiographic study of patients with acute anterior MI, patients without infarct expansion on the initial study at 3 weeks post-MI did not exhibit further enlargement at 13 months. In contrast, patients with infarct expansion at the time of the initial study had late increases in both the infarct-containing and especially the noninfarcted segments. Note that the late increase in the length of the infarct-containing segment does not necessarily imply progressive infarct expansion in the late phase. Even with large infarctions, the infarct-containing segment, as defined echocardiographically, contains roughly equal amounts of infarcted and noninfarcted tissue (Fig. 1). As a result, changes in this segment represent a mixture of changes in the true infarct zone and in adjacent viable myocardium. In this study, for example, late lengthening of the infarct-containing segment was about half that of the noninfarcted segment. This suggests that all of the lengthening in this segment could have been the result of lengthening of viable tissue. The effect on overall lengthening, when expressed as a percentage of initial length, may have been diluted by the infarct zone, which did not change. In an angiographic study of patients with anterior MIs, using the length of the akinetic or dyskinetic segment as an index of the size of the actual zone of infarction, we did not find any evidence for progressive infarct expansion during the late phase of healing after infarction.[34]

Gaudron and colleagues[35] have shown a similar tendency to progressive ventricular enlargement in a substantial proportion of patients followed for 3 years after large, first transmural infarctions. They found a progressive deterioration in ventricular function and hemodynamics at rest and with exercise in the subset of patients with "noncompensatory" enlargement. In contrast, patients with limited enlargement had an early phase of "compensatory" enlargement that restored stroke volume and hemodynamics to normal within 4 weeks, after which LV function and resting hemodynamics were stable. Predictors of late enlargement included extent of akinesis/dyskinesis, baseline ejection fraction and stroke index, anterior infarct location, and patency of the infarct-related vessel. Thus, it appears that late remodeling may be dependent on changes in the critical early phase. If these early changes are sufficiently severe, compensatory enlargement may be inadequate. Filling pressures and wall stress remain high and a vicious cycle of increasing stress leading to increasing volume enlargement ensues. The final result is the insidious onset of congestive heart failure weeks to months later in those patients who develop progressive enlargement, even in the absence of further ischemic insults and despite a lack of symptoms at the time of discharge from the hospital after infarction.

Anatomically, the late period of LV remodeling corresponds to formation of a firm, fibrous scar in the infarct zone. Studies in experimental models[36–38] and in humans[34] suggest that the infarct zone may actually shrink during this late phase, as formation of the relatively noncompliant scar is completed. Shrinkage of the scar may be accompanied by a favorable redistribution of wall stress away from the critical interface between infarcted and viable myocardium. As noted above, this region may be under increased wall stress shortly after infarction because of an abnormal local geometry (Fig. 3). Formation of a smaller, less-compliant scar would produce less geometric distortion at this interface, since the size of the aneurysmal infarct zone and the contracting base would be more closely matched.[39] Therefore, recovery of contractile function may simply represent remodeling to a more favorable geometry (regional unloading).

As the infarct shrinks and/or function is recovered, there is a proportionate increase in length of the contractile segment, whereas total biplane circumference remains relatively unchanged. It is difficult to determine the extent to which lengthening of the contractile segment represents true eccentric hypertrophy versus reclaimed function at the border zone. However, the echocardiographic data presented above, using the papillary muscles as fixed internal landmarks in the midst of a zone of normal myocardium, suggest that at least a component of the late increase in noncontractile segment length represents true eccentric hypertrophy.[33] Despite the stable biplane circumference, volume continues to increase in an anterior Q-wave MI population as the ventricle becomes progressively more spherical in the chronic phase.[15] Once symptoms develop in these patients with progressive enlargement, ventricular volumes are markedly increased and function severely depressed. Therapy initiated at that time is generally palliative in nature and 5-year mortality is quite high.

PATENCY OF THE INFARCT-RELATED VESSEL

Observations both in experimental animals and in humans support the hypothesis that patency of the infarct-related vessel has a protective effect against infarct expansion and early chamber remodeling, independent of myocardial salvage.[40] Possible mechanisms include the erectile effect of tissue perfusion and vessel distention and the promotion of hemorrhage and edema, each of which stiffens the acutely infarcted region. Perfusion of the infarct-related vessel may also provide collaterals to the border zone or may salvage islets of viable myocardium within the infarct or in the epicardial region. Limitation of early infarct expansion may then lead to diminished late ventricular remodeling.

In addition, infarct healing in the subacute and chronic phases may be promoted by patency of the infarct-related vessel. It is possible that the intercellular collagen and vascular framework in the infarct zone is preserved if patency of the infarct-related vessel is reestablished. Healing can then proceed more expeditiously, as inflammatory cells are distributed directly to infarcted myocytes via the native blood vessels rather than through the much slower formation of granulation tissue. The latter process, which starts at the margins of the infarct and progresses to the center of the zone of necrosis via neovascularization, may require weeks in large infarcts,[41] thereby lengthening the period of susceptibility to further distortion. The result is that infarcts perfused by a patent infarct-related vessel or by well-developed collaterals have less infarct expansion,[42] and the patients are less likely to develop aneurysms,[43] late volume enlargement,[44-48] and an adverse clinical outcome.[49]

Jeremy et al[44] examined the effects of spontaneous reperfusion of the infarct-related vessel in patients with anterior or inferior MIs not treated with lytic agents. All patients had quantitative radionuclide ventriculograms 48 hours and 1 month after infarction. Patency of the infarct-related vessel was assessed by coronary angiography performed 7 to 10 days after infarction. Left ventricular enlargement occurred in 14 of 14 patients with a persistently occluded vessel as opposed to 2 of 26 patients with a patent vessel or well-developed collateral circulation.

We have previously reported that persistent occlusion of the infarct-related vessel is a risk factor for late ventricular enlargement.[45] In that placebo-controlled, double-blind trial of captopril after anterior MI, persistent occlusion of the infarct-related LAD coronary artery was present in 36 of 52 patients at 3 weeks post-infarction. Patients with a persistently occluded left anterior descending coronary artery had end-diastolic volumes at baseline that were not significantly different from those of patients with a patent vessel. However, the occlusion group had lower ejection fractions, a greater extent of dyskinesis, and more pronounced abnormalities of regional geometry, especially at the apex. Over the ensuing year in the placebo group, patients with a patent infarct-related vessel did not have further ventricular remodeling. In contrast, patients with an occluded vessel had progressive diastolic chamber enlargement that was attributable to development of a more spherical geometry. This late remodeling was not observed in patients with an occluded vessel randomized to captopril.[15]

It appears, then, that reperfusion of the infarct-related vessel favorably affects the remodeling process, possibly independent of any effect on myocardial salvage. It is important to note that the foregoing observations, although suggestive, do not prove that late revascularization by mechanical means will affect clinical outcome. It is possible, for example, that spontaneous reperfusion of the infarct-related vessel is merely a marker for some other biologic characteristic, such as the balance between endogenous lytic and thrombotic pathways, which is ultimately responsible for the difference in clinical outcome. Similarly, early remodeling while the artery is occluded may provide the stimulus to late remodeling even if the artery is subsequently opened beyond the period of risk for infarct expansion. Clearly, a large, prospective randomized clinical trial of late reperfusion is needed in which patients without conventional indication for delayed revascularization (such as persistent ischemia) are randomized to mechanical revascularization or conventional therapy.

MODIFICATION OF THE REMODELING PROCESS

Considerable attention has been focused on interrupting the deleterious, progressive component of LV remodeling after MI. Certain risk factors for infarct expansion and progressive enlargement, such as infarct location, cannot be modified. However, limitation of infarct size, restoration of patency of the infarct-related vessel, and control of ventricular preload and afterload present possible opportunities to intervene in the remodeling process. It is unequivocally clear that the most effective intervention is to control the extent of initial damage in order to prevent initiation of the remodeling cascade. Small, nontransmural infarcts do not undergo infarct expansion and are therefore unlikely to exhibit progressive shape distortion and volume enlargement. If coronary blood flow can be reestablished within the conventionally accepted time-frame for myocardial salvage (within 6 hours), it is less likely that significant deleterious remodeling and progression to heart failure will ensue.

Substantial work has been done in the area of modification of ventricular loading conditions in the acute and chronic phase after infarction. In the rat infarct model, a favorable effect of captopril on ventricular remodeling and long-term survival has been demonstrated in the group of animals with moderate-to-large MIs.[50,51] Whether this beneficial effect was primarily related to a decrease in preload or afterload is not clear, since both blood pressure and filling pressure were reduced. In a study comparing captopril and the selective arterial vasodilator, hydralazine, venous pressures remained elevated and attenuation of ventricular enlargement was not observed in the hydralazine group, suggesting that reduction of preload is important in the remodeling process.[52] Through analysis of diastolic pressure–volume relationships, the decreased operating volume in rats treated with captopril was shown to be the result of a combination of true remodeling (shift in the pressure–volume curve to the left) and decreased distention.

These experimental observations were extended to humans in a double-blind, placebo-controlled clinical trial designed to test the effects of captopril on late volume enlargement after infarction.[15] Fifty-two patients with large, first anterior myocardial infarctions (ejection fraction <45%) were randomized to treatment with standard therapy plus either captopril or placebo from 3 weeks to 1 year post-MI. Late volume enlargement was seen in the placebo group but not in those treated with captopril. Similar attenuation of late volume enlargement by converting enzyme inhibition has been reported by other investigators.[53,54]

The important issue of whether limitation of late volume enlargement after MI would translate to a long-term improvement in clinical outcome was subsequently addressed by the Survival and Ventricular Enlargement (SAVE) study.[55] This study randomized 2,231 patients to captopril or placebo therapy during the subacute phase of recovery, 3 to 16 days post-infarction. Patients randomized to active therapy had a 19% reduction in total mortality as a result of a significant reduction in cardiovascular mortality. They were less likely to experience the development of congestive heart failure or recurrent MI—events associated with a markedly increased risk of death during the 2- to 5-year follow-up period. Furthermore, the pathophysiologic premise of this study was confirmed in an echocardiographic substudy that established a link between ventricular enlargement and adverse events.[56] Patients with adverse cardiac events, regardless of therapy assignment, were found to have progressive ventricular enlargement. However, the proportion of patients experiencing ventricular enlargement was significantly reduced by active therapy.

As data continue to accumulate on the utility of converting enzyme inhibitors in the late phase of recovery from MI, considerable interest in much earlier use of these and other agents has developed. The rationale behind such an approach is that if the inciting events in the acute phase (infarct expansion) can be controlled, late progressive remodeling and enlargement culminating in an adverse outcome will be less likely. It is important to note, however, that pharmacologic modification of loading conditions in the acute phase of MI raises a number of additional safety issues such as exacerbation of ischemia or promotion of infarct extension. It is conceivable that worsening of ischemia in the presence of multivessel disease or production of clinically significant hypotension in the face of limited contractile reserve may offset a potential long-term beneficial effect. For example, Cohn and associates[57] administered sodium nitroprusside within the first 24 hours after onset of MI complicated by elevated left heart filling pressures. Despite improvement in hemodynamics, there was no effect on short- or long-term mortality. In fact, there appeared to be an adverse effect on mortality if the drug was initiated within the first 6 hours after the onset of chest pain. They speculated that worsening of ischemia and infarct extension may have been to blame for the adverse effect.

In contrast, Jugdutt and Warnica[58] reported a beneficial effect of nitroglycerin on early ventricular remodeling in a study in which hypotension was avoided by carefully titrating an intravenous infusion of the drug, which was initiated within 12 hours of the onset of infarction and continued for 2 days. Patients treated with active therapy had less infarct segment expansion; however, it is unclear whether the effect was due to a limitation of infarct size (the treatment group had lower peak creatinine kinase levels) or to a reduction in preload or afterload, all of which may be modified with intravenous nitroglycerin. Regardless of the mechanism, less of an unfavorable change in ventricular topography was seen in the treatment group as a whole and clinical outcome was substantially improved in the subset with anterior infarction.

On a much larger scale, the CONSENSUS II investigators randomized over 6,000 patients to enalapril or placebo within 24 hours of onset of symptoms of MI and followed the patients for 6 months.[59] That trial was prematurely terminated by the safety monitoring committee because of a lack of beneficial effect, with a trend towards increased mortality in the active therapy group. However, the recently completed ISIS-4 (captopril) and GISSI-3 (lisinopril) studies have now established in over 80,000 patients both the safety and efficacy of converting-enzyme inhibitors initiated within 24 hours of the onset of MI. In addition, several soon-to-be-reported studies have now confirmed the efficacy of converting-enzyme inhibitors initiated in the subacute phase of recovery, 2 to 16 days after MI. The Studies of LV Dysfunction (SOLVD) Prevention Arm randomized patients with asymptomatic LV dysfunction, predominantly ischemic in origin, to enalapril or placebo and demonstrated significant reductions in hospitalization for heart failure or recurrent MI.[60] By design, patients included in that study had not experienced a MI within at least a month preceding randomization, suggesting that even very late administration of converting-enzyme

inhibitor may favorably modify the remodeling process and reduce the rate of adverse cardiovascular events after MI.

SUMMARY

Transmural LV infarction initiates a complex cascade of ventricular healing and remodeling that continues months to years after the initial event. The occurrence of late ventricular remodeling, which may culminate in symptomatic congestive heart failure and death, appears to be closely related to changes in geometry within and remote from the infarct zone during the first hours to days after infarction. Efforts to limit the extent of the initial damage will undoubtedly be more effective than those aimed at controlling late ventricular remodeling, although both are critically important.

REFERENCES

1. Hutchins GM, Bulkley BH. Infarct expansion versus extension: Two different complications of acute myocardial infarction. *Am J Cardiol.* 1978;41:1127-1132.
2. Eaton LW, Weiss JL, Bulkley BH, et al. Regional cardiac dilatation after acute myocardial infarction. Recognition by two-dimensional echocardiography. *N Engl J Med.* 1979;300:57-62.
3. Erlebacher JA, Weiss JL, Weisfeldt ML, et al. Early dilation of the infarcted segment in acute transmural myocardial infarction: Role of infarct expansion in acute left ventricular enlargement. *J Am Coll Cardiol.* 1984;4:201-208.
4. Weisman HF, Bush DE, Mannisi JA, et al. Cellular mechanisms of myocardial infarct expansion. *Circulation* 1988;78:186-201.
5. Hochman JS, Bulkley BH. Pathogenesis of left ventricular aneurysms: an experimental study in the rat model. *Am J Cardiol.* 1982;50:83-88.
6. Meizlish JL, Berger HJ, Plankey M, et al. Functional left ventricular aneurysm formation after acute anterior transmural myocardial infarction: Incidence, natural history, and prognostic implications. *N Engl J Med.* 1984;311:1001-1006.
7. Schuster EH, Bulkley BH. Expansion of transmural myocardial infarction: A pathophysiologic factor in cardiac rupture. *Circulation.* 1979;60:1532-1538.
8. Pirolo JS, Hutchins GM, Moore GW. Infarct expansion: pathologic analysis of 204 patients with a single myocardial infarct. *J Am Coll Cardiol.* 1986;7:349-354.
9. Bulkley BH, Roberts WC. Steroid therapy during acute myocardial infarction: A cause of delayed healing and of ventricular aneurysm. *Am J Med.* 1974;56:244-250.

10. Brown EJ, Kloner RA, Schoen FJ, et al. Scar thinning due to ibuprofen administration after experimental myocardial infarction. *Am J Cardiol.* 1983;51:877-883.

11. Burton AC. The importance of the shape and size of the heart. *Am Heart J.* 1957;54:801-810.

12. Role L, Bogen D, McMahon TA, et al. Regional variations in calculated diastolic wall stress in rat left ventricle. *Am J Physiol.* 1978;235:H247-H250.

13. Weber KT, Janicki JS. The heart as a muscle-pump system and the concept of heart failure. *Am Heart J.* 1979;98:371-384.

14. Picard MH, Wilkins GT, Gillam LD, et al. Immediate regional endocardial surface expansion following coronary occlusion in the canine left ventricle: Disproportionate effects of anterior versus inferior ischemia. *Am Heart J.* 1991;121:753-762.

15. Mitchell GF, Lamas GA, Vaughan DE, et al. Left ventricular remodeling in the year following first anterior myocardial infarction: A quantitative analysis of contractile segment lengths and ventricular shape. *J Am Coll Cardiol.* 1991;19:1136-1144.

16. Lamas GA, Vaughan DE, Parisi AF, et al. Effects of left ventricular shape and captopril therapy on exercise capacity after anterior wall acute myocardial infarction. *Am J Cardiol.* 1989;63:1167-1173.

17. Weisman HF, Bush DE, Mannisi JA, et al. Global cardiac remodeling after myocardial infarction: A study in the rat model. *J Am Coll Cardiol.* 1985;5:1355-1362.

18. Bogen DK, Rabinowitz SA, Needleman A, et al. An analysis of the mechanical disadvantage of myocardial infarction in the canine left ventricle. *Circ Res.* 1980;47:728-741.

19. Janz RF. Estimation of local myocardial stress. *Am J Physiol.* 1982;242:H875-H881.

20. Lessick J, Sideman S, Azhari H, et al. Regional three-dimensional geometry and function of left ventricles with fibrous aneurysms. A cine-computed tomography study. *Circulation.* 1991;84:1072-1086.

21. Hutchins GM and Bulkley BH. Catenoid shape of the interventricular septum: possible cause of idiopathic hypertrophic subaortic stenosis. *Circulation.* 1978;58:392-397.

22. Cox DA, Vatner SF. Myocardial function in areas of heterogeneous perfusion after coronary artery occlusion in conscious dogs. *Circulation.* 1982;66:1154-1158.

23. Sheehan FH, Braunwald E, Canner P, et al. The effect of intravenous thrombolytic therapy on left ventricular function: a report on tissue-type plasminogen activator and streptokinase from the Thrombolysis in Myocardial Infarction (TIMI Phase 1) Trial. *Circulation.* 1987;75:817-829.

24. Anversa P, Olivetti G, Capasso JM. Cellular basis of ventricular remodeling after myocardial infarction. *Am J Cardiol.* 1991;68:7D-16D.

25. McKay RG, Pfeffer MA, Pasternak RC, et al. Left ventricular remodeling following myocardial infarction— a corollary to infarct expansion. *Circulation.* 1986; 74:693-702.

26. Mirsky I, Pfeffer JM, Pfeffer MA, et al. The contractile state as the major determinant in the evolution of left ventricular dysfunction in the spontaneously hypertensive rat. *Circ Res.* 1983,53:767-778.

27. Anversa P, Loud AV, Levicky V, et al. Left ventricular failure induced by myocardial infarction: 1. Myocyte hypertrophy. *Am J Physiol.* 1985;248:H876-H882.

28. Anversa P, Beghi C, Kikkawa Y, et al. Myocardial infarction in rats. Infarct size, myocyte hypertrophy, and capillary growth. *Circ Res.* 1986;58:26-37.

29. Olivetti G, Ricci R, Beghi C, et al. Response of the border zone to myocardial infarction in rats. *Am J Pathol.* 1986; 125:476-483.

30. Jeremy RW, Allman KC, Bautovitch G, et al. Patterns of left ventricular dilation during the six months after myocardial infarction. *J Am Coll Cardiol.* 1989;13:304-310.

31. Hammermeister KE, DeRouen TA, Dodge HT. Variables predictive of survival in patients with coronary disease: Selection by univariate and multivariate analyses from the clinical, electrocardiographic, exercise, arteriographic, and quantitative angiographic evaluations. *Circulation.* 1979; 59:421-430.

32. White HD, Norris RM, Brown MA, et al. Left ventricular end-systolic volume as the major determinant of survival after recovery from myocardial infarction. *Circulation.* 1987;76:44-51.

33. Erlebacher JA, Weiss JL, Eaton LW, et al. Late effects of acute infarct dilation on heart size: A two dimensional echocardiographic study. *Am J Cardiol.* 1982;49:1120-1126.

34. Mitchell GF, Lamas GA, Vaughan DE, et al. Infarct expansion does not contribute to late left ventricular enlargement. *Circulation.* 1989;80(suppl 2):589. Abstract.

35. Gaudron P, Eilles C, Kugler I, et al. Progressive left ventricular dysfunction and remodeling after myocardial infarction: Potential mechanisms and early predictors. *Am J Cardiol.* 1993;87:755-763.

36. Reimer KA, Jennings RB. The changing anatomic reference base of evolving myocardial infarction. Underestimation of myocardial collateral blood flow and overestimation of experimental anatomic infarct size due to tissue edema, hemorrhage and acute inflammation. *Circulation.* 1979;60:866-876.

37. Gibbons EF, Hogan RD, Franklin TD, et al. The natural history of regional dysfunction in a canine preparation of chronic infarction. *Circulation.* 1985;71:394-402.

38. Roberts CS, Maclean D, Maroko P, et al. Early and late remodeling of the left ventricle after acute myocardial infarction. *Am J Cardiol.* 1984:54:407-410.

39. Mitchell GF, Lamas GA, Vaughan DE, et al. Changes in local curvature accompany left ventricular enlargement following anterior myocardial infarction. *J Am Coll Cardiol.* 1990;15:15A. Abstract.

40. Braunwald E. Myocardial reperfusion, limitation of infarct size, reduction of left ventricular dysfunction, and improved survival. Should the paradigm be expanded? *Circulation.* 1989;79:441-444.

41. Scotti TM. Heart. In: Anderson WAD, Kissane JM (eds). *Pathology.* St. Louis, CV Mosby; 1977:737-855.

42. Hochman JS, Choo H. Limitation of myocardial infarct expansion by reperfusion independent of myocardial salvage. *Circulation.* 1987;75:299-306.

43. Hirai T, Fujita M, Nakajima H, et al. Importance of collateral circulation for prevention of left ventricular aneurysm formation in acute myocardial infarction. *Circulation.* 989;79:791-796.

44. Jeremy RW, Hackworthy RA, Bautovich G, et al. Infarct artery perfusion and changes in left ventricular volume in the month after acute myocardial infarction. *J Am Coll Cardiol.* 1987;9:989-995.

45. Pfeffer MA, Lamas GA, Vaughan DE, et al. Effect of captopril on progressive ventricular dilatation after anterior myocardial infarction. *N Engl J Med.* 1988; 319:80-86.

46. White HD, Norris RM, Brown MA, et al. Effect of intravenous streptokinase on left ventricular function and early survival after acute myocardial infarction. *N Engl J Med.* 1987;317:850-855.

47. Serruys PW, Simoons ML, Suryapranata H, et al. Preservation of global and regional left ventricular function after early thrombolysis in acute myocardial infarction. *J Am Coll Cardiol.* 1986;7:729-742.

48. Marino P, Zanolla L, Zardini P, et al. Effect of streptokinase on left ventricular modeling and function after myocardial infarction: The GISSI (Gruppo Italiano per lo Studio della Streptochinasi nell'Infarto Miocardico) Trial. *J Am Coll Cardiol.* 1989;14:1149-1158.

49. Cigarroa RG, Lange RA, Hillis LD. Prognosis after acute myocardial infarction in patients with and without residual anterograde coronary blood flow. *Am J Cardiol.* 1989;64:155-160.

50. Pfeffer JM, Pfeffer MA, Braunwald E. Influence of chronic captopril therapy on the infarcted left ventricle of the rat. *Circ Res* 1985;57:84-95.

51. Pfeffer MA, Pfeffer JM, Steinberg C, et al. Survival following an experimental myocardial infarction: Beneficial effects of chronic captopril therapy. *Circulation.* 1985;72:406-412.

52. Raya TE, Gay RG, Aguirre M, et al. Importance of venodilatation in prevention of left ventricular dilatation after chronic large myocardial infarction in rats: A comparison of captopril and hydralazine. *Circ Res.* 1989;64:330-337.

53. Sharpe N, Murphy J, Smith H, et al. Treatment of patients with symptomless left ventricular dysfunction after myocardial infarction. *Lancet.* 1988;1:255-259.

54. Bonaduce D, Petretta M, Paquale A, et al. Effects of captopril treatment on left ventricular remodeling and function after anterior myocardial infarction: comparison with digitalis. *J Am Coll Cardiol.* 1992;19:858-863.

55. Pfeffer MA, Braunwald E, Moye LA, et al. Effect of captopril on mortality and morbidity in patients with left ventricular dysfunction after myocardial infarction: Results of the Survival and Ventricular Enlargement Trial. *N Engl J Med.* 1992;327:669-677.

56. St. John Sutton M, Pfeffer MA, Plappert T, et al. Quantitative two dimensional echocardiographic measurements are major predictors of adverse cardiovascular events following acute myocardial infarction: The protective effects of captopril. *Circulation.* 1994;89:68-75.

57. Cohn J, Franciosa J, Francis G, et al. Effect of short-term infusion of sodium nitroprusside on mortality rate in acute myocardial infarction complicated by left ventricular failure. *N Engl J Med.* 1982;306:1129-1135.

58. Jugdutt BI, Warnica JW. Intravenous nitroglycerin therapy to limit myocardial infarct size, expansion, and complications. Effect of timing, dosage, and infarct location. *Circulation.* 1988;78:906-919.

59. Swedberg K, Held P, Kjekshus J, et al. Effects of the early administration of enalapril on mortality in patients with acute myocardial infarction: Results of the Cooperative New Scandinavian Enalapril Survival Study II (CONSENSUS II). *N Engl J Med.* 1992;327:678-684.

60. The SOLVD Investigators. Effect of enalapril on mortality and the development of heart failure in asymptomatic patients with reduced left ventricular ejection fractions. *N Engl J Med.* 1992;327:685-691.

17 Interventional Cardiology

Andrew C. Eisenhauer, MD
Stephen N. Oesterle, MD

PERCUTANEOUS TRANSLUMINAL CORONARY ANGIOPLASTY

Dramatic technological advances and unparalleled growth characterized the first 15 years of coronary angioplasty. Andreas Gruentzig first described the technique in the late 1970s.[1] In 1980, approximately 200 procedures were performed throughout the world. By the end of 1992, more than 300,000 procedures were performed annually in the United States alone.[2] This exponential growth in application, associated with broadened indications and vastly improved success rates, is largely attributable to technological improvements in angioplasty equipment.

Early dilatation devices, developed by Gruentzig in conjunction with Schneider-Medintag (Zurich), were neither steerable nor of low-profile. Guiding catheters were stiff and had very poor torque. Due to these technical shortcomings, percutaneous transluminal coronary angioplasty (PTCA) was initially limited to discrete proximal lesions. Furthermore, poor steerability precluded routine dilatation of distal stenoses, branch stenoses, and most lesions in the left circumflex coronary artery. These early procedures were often tedious and frequently prolonged; hence, multivessel angioplasty was rarely attempted.

The first PTCA registry, sponsored by the National Heart, Lung, and Blood Institute, was completed in 1982.[3] This registry reported an overall success rate for balloon angioplasty of just over 60%, with single vessel disease representing the large majority of cases. Around this time, Simpson introduced a "second generation" dilatation device (Advanced Cardiovascular Systems, Santa Clara, California), distinguished by an independently moveable guide wire.[4] Dilatation devices could be tracked over a wire, which was independently positioned across target stenoses. The first intracoronary guide wires were stiff and non-directional. Multiple advances in engineering and manufacturing have since produced a family of intracoronary guide wires with various degrees of flexibility and steerability. With the current generation of intracoronary guide wires, it is possible to position a wire in virtually every patent branch of the coronary tree.

Concurrent advances in balloon technology have led to further miniaturization of dilatation devices. New plastic materials, incorporated into the balloons and shaft, allow for lower crossing profiles and the ability to cross critical stenoses without significant "backup" support from guiding catheters. Some dilatation balloons attach directly to the guide wire, adding no more than 0.001-0.002 inches to the crossing profile of the bare wire. These low-profile devices have facilitated crossing of high-grade stenoses in the most distal aspects of the coronary anatomy. Different blends of plastic materials have allowed manufacturers to vary the compliance characteristics of balloon catheters. Noncompliant, high pressure balloons have been developed to treat inelastic lesions. Highly compliant balloons have facilitated the use of a single balloon for treating multiple lesions in arteries with varying luminal diameters.

Success rates for coronary angioplasty are now routinely better than 90% for single vessel disease.[5] Improved guide wire steerability and lower balloon profiles have expanded the indications for this procedure to include lesions that may be distal, heavily calcified, lengthy, eccentric, or involving branch vessels. Multi-lesion and multivessel dilatations now represent many of the successful cases.

Long-term benefits are clearly documented,

with follow-up extending beyond 10 years in selected groups of patients.[6-9] For most patients with symptomatic single-vessel coronary artery disease, angioplasty offers a very acceptable alternative to coronary artery bypass surgery and, for at least 70% of patients, results in significant improvement in symptoms and reduction in ischemia by objective criteria.[10] Therefore, PTCA has become the standard of care for patients with single vessel disease in need of revascularization. Whether patients with multivessel coronary disease are best treated by angioplasty or surgery remains controversial, and is the focus of several large randomized trials under way in both the United States and Europe.[11,12]

The first of these trials to publish preliminary findings originated from the United Kingdom: the Randomised Intervention Treatment of Angina (RITA) trial.[13] The primary trial endpoint was defined as the combined 5-year incidence of death and non-fatal myocardial infarction. The first report was for a mean 2.5 years of follow-up on 1,000 patients, randomized to either surgery or balloon angioplasty. This trial included patients with 1, 2, or 3 diseased coronary arteries in which equivalent revascularization was achievable by either procedure. Sixteen hospitals in England, Scotland and Ireland participated during 34 months of recruitment. More than 17,000 patients were referred for revascularization during this period; only 5% were randomized in the trial. At 2.5 years there was no significant difference in the risk of death or myocardial infarction between the 2 treatment groups; however, the bypass surgery group had less angina (31% vs 22%) and less frequent revascularization during the follow-up period. Repeat coronary arteriography was 4 times more common in PTCA than in surgery patients (31% vs 7%). Additional data are forthcoming that will highlight the relative costs of these treatment strategies over time.

INDICATIONS

With the multiple refinements in angioplasty equipment, the question is rarely, "Can it be done by balloon angioplasty," but, more frequently, "Should it be done?"

The American College of Cardiology and the American Heart Association have published guidelines for selecting patients for PTCA.[14]

The best candidates for PTCA generally have single-vessel disease with stenoses that are proximal, non-calcified, concentric, and do not involve major side branches. Patients considered for elective PTCA should be moderately to significantly symptomatic. Objective evidence of ischemia should be demonstrated by treadmill testing, nuclear scintigraphy, exercise echocardiography or exercise radionuclide ventriculography.

Many cardiologists offer patients angioplasty as an alternative to medical therapy, as a way to reduce or eliminate the need for taking medications. The efficacy and fiscal soundness of this approach has been validated by at least 1 well-designed trial, randomizing patients with single vessel disease between PTCA and medical therapy.[15]

Some patients undergoing PTCA are asymptomatic and have had their underlying coronary disease unmasked by surveillance treadmill testing or by the development of serious ventricular arrhythmias. Angioplasty is frequently offered to these patients with "silent ischemia," when they present with disease anatomically favorable for dilatation. This is particularly true when the silent disease involves segments of the coronary arteries that are proximal, and of large diameter. This strategy is currently under investigation in a multicenter trial sponsored by the National Heart, Lung, and Blood Institute.

Some patients with symptomatic multivessel CAD have several major stenoses, each of which have suitable location and morphology for treatment by PTCA. Others may have 1 or 2 vessels that are ideal for PTCA, while the remaining diseased vessels are poor targets because of lesion morphology. Incomplete revascularization, with dilatation limited to the putative "culprit lesion," is frequently advocated as an alternative to bypass surgery.[16,17] Although many of these patients can be relieved, or significantly improved, some physicians are critical of this incomplete treatment. The culprit angioplasty strategy can be defended on the basis of patient safety. Each additional vessel dilatation is associated with incremental risk to the patient.[18] For patients undergoing surgery, most of the risk is related to the thoracotomy and pump run; the incremental risk of additional bypasses is minimal. Hence, a plan for "complete" revascularization makes good sense in patients undergoing thoracotomy but may not be prudent in those receiving the less invasive percutaneous therapy.

Table 1. Relative Contraindications to PTCA

Chronic total occlusion (>3 months)
Long lesions (>2 cm)
Old vein grafts with diffuse disease
Ostial stenosis of the right coronary artery or
  vein grafts
Stenoses involving major side branches that
  cannot be protected
Stenoses with associated organized thrombus
Stenoses within *severely* angulated segments
Extensive calcification of the involved arterial
  segment
Coronary spasm as a predominant component of
  stenosis (lesion <70%)
Very recent reperfusion with tissue plasminogen
  activator
Presence of noncritical left main coronary artery
  disease when firm engagement of a left main
  guiding catheter is anticipated
Noncritical stenoses (<60%)

Table 2. Absolute Contraindications to PTCA

Unprotected left main coronary artery disease
Extensive myocardial jeopardy, i.e., where vessel
  occlusion following PTCA would result in loss of
  >60% of viable myocardium
Coronary stenoses in vessels uninvolved with
  acute myocardial infarction
Absence of timely surgical standby

Table 3. Type A Lesions

**Typically associated with high success and low
  complication rates**
Discrete (<10 mm length)
Concentric
Readily accessible
Nonangulated segment <45°
Smooth contour
Little or no calcification
Less than totally occlusive
Not ostial in location
No major branch involvement
Absence of thrombus

Table 4. Type B Lesions

**Typically associated with moderate success
  and complications**
Tubular (10-20 mm length)
Eccentric
Moderate tortuosity of proximal segment
Moderately angulated segment >45° <90°
Irregular contour
Moderate to heavy calcification
Total occlusion <3 months old
Ostial in location
Bifurcation lesions requiring double guidewires
Some thrombus present

Coronary bypass grafts, including autologous vein grafts and internal mammary artery grafts, usually can be dilated;[19,20,21] however, restenosis and embolization of vein graft debris are common problems following dilatation.

The role of PTCA in the setting of an acute myocardial infarction is controversial. Angioplasty can be effective either as direct therapy for recanalization or as an adjunct to thrombolytic therapy. These issues are discussed more extensively in a later section.

RELATIVE CONTRAINDICATIONS

Tables 1 and 2 present a synthesis of the conservative guidelines of the AHA/ACC Task force 14 coupled with our experience. Table 1 lists "relative" contraindications. Although skilled operators can expect initial success rates of more than 90% for ideal lesions, PTCA for lesions listed in Table 1 will be less successful. (Success for PTCA is generally defined as >20% improvement in luminal diameter with a residual stenosis <50%, and no major complications such as death or the need for coronary bypass surgery during the hospitalization.) Tables 3–5 list an ACC/AHA classification of lesion morphology which has predictive value for PTCA success.[22]

Chronic total occlusions (>3 months) are not likely to be recanalized by conventional balloon angioplasty. Although the risks are low, failure is frequent with the attendant financial loss from spent equipment and personnel time. These occlusions are thought to be associated with low risk; however, attempted dilatation of chronic total occlusions has been associated with myocardial infarction and death.[23]

Table 5. Type C Lesions

Typically associated with low success and/or high complication rates
Diffuse (>2 cm length)
Excessive tortuosity of proximal segment
Extremely angulated segments >90°
Total occlusion >3 months old
Inability to protect major side branches
Degenerated vein grafts with friable lesions

Lesions greater than 2 centimeters in length are associated with a higher rate of dissection, abrupt closure, and restenosis.[24,25] Ostial stenoses of the right coronary artery or of a bypass graft are associated with poor results because of inability to seat the guiding catheter. Additionally, recoil from elastic fibers in the aorta accounts for sub-optimal dilatation of ostial lesions and a higher rate of restenosis.

Most side branches can be protected during angioplasty of an adjacent vessel; however, anatomic variability may preclude protecting major side branches.[26] These unprotected side vessels will either be occluded during angioplasty of the adjacent vessel (20% incidence or left as a potential source of coronary insufficiency). Frequently, such complex lesions are best treated surgically.

Organized thrombus, at the site of dilatation, dramatically increases the complications during PTCA.[27] Plaque associated thrombus is frequently treated adjunctively with intracoronary thrombolytic agents.[28] Stenoses of <60% diameter narrowing should not routinely be dilated, as they are unlikely to cause coronary insufficiency. Dilatation of these lesions is associated with the same risks of vessel occlusion and restenosis.[29] A trivial stenosis can be converted to a high-grade critical stenosis through the proliferative process of restenosis.

ABSOLUTE CONTRAINDICATIONS

Table 2 lists circumstances whereby PTCA is generally considered contraindicated. Although dilatation of a high-grade left main coronary artery stenosis is technically straightforward, complications including abrupt closure can threaten life. Restenosis in this subset of patients is also associated with out-of-hospital sudden death. For the rare patient who requires revascularization, and for whom surgery cannot be performed, PTCA can be facilitated by the use of special dilatation catheters which perfuse the distal coronary bed while the balloon is inflated[30] or with the circulatory support of a percutaneous cardiopulmonary pump system.[31,32]

Left main disease can be safely treated by PTCA when "protection" exists by way of a patent bypass graft to the left anterior descending or circumflex coronary arteries. In these circumstances the left main disease has been reduced functionally to "single vessel" disease.

The jeopardy of a single dilatation should be assessed before subjecting a patient to PTCA.[33] Frequently, a target vessel for angioplasty is the source of collaterals to another major coronary artery. Abrupt closure after angioplasty can result in massive infarction from compromise of both the target artery and the collateral artery. An attempt should be made to open the collateral artery before dilating the target artery. If the collateral artery cannot be opened with PTCA, and the amount of jeopardized myocardium represents more than 60% of the remaining viable myocardium, surgery should be considered. Elective bypass surgery will generally be associated with lower risk for the patient in such a situation.

Angioplasty for myocardial infarction is extensively discussed in a later section. In the setting of a myocardial infarction, angioplasty of coronary vessels uninvolved with the acute event can lead to catastrophe and should be deferred until the reperfused "stunned" myocardium recovers.

Emergency bypass surgery will continue to be necessary for 1%-2% of patients, at the time of angioplasty, until a reliable percutaneous solution to abrupt vessel closure is developed. Although stents have mitigated the need for standby surgery, not all vessel disruptions can be successfully stented (see following section on intracoronary Stents). Therefore, angioplasty is contraindicated in settings where cardiac surgery is not readily available.

PATIENT MANAGEMENT

The management of patients before, during, and after coronary angioplasty is directed predominantly toward the anticipation of potential complications. Planning of the procedure, preparation of the patient, performance of the angioplasty and subsequent patient care all interact to determine the ultimate success of the procedure. Most elective coronary angioplasty is uncomplicated and elaborate precautions may therefore seem "unnecessary." However, many potentially unsuccessful procedures have been salvaged because of careful planning and anticipatory management.

SURGICAL SUPPORT

Coronary angioplasty and surgical myocardial revascularization are complementary and not competitive. The standby surgical team must be truly supportive and willing to perform cardiac surgery on patients with angioplasty complications under emergency conditions. Early in the development of coronary angioplasty, an operating room was held open for each patient. As angioplasty has improved, a designated, waiting operating room for all patients has become unnecessary. Accordingly, many centers have adopted a tiered approach to surgical standby. There are some patients for whom the potential need for emergency cardiac surgery during angioplasty approaches that associated with routine catheterization. Patients with chronic, well-collateralized occlusions of the right coronary artery, for example, are at low risk. Thus, dilatation of a chronically occluded vessel that supplies a moderate or small amount of myocardium and is well collateralized is very unlikely to require emergency surgical revascularization even if the procedure is unsuccessful. There are complications that may arise, such as guide wire perforation or proximal coronary dissection from the guiding catheter, that require urgent surgical intervention. For these "level O" angioplasties, an operating room need not be ready and there need be no greater surgical involvement than that for routine cardiac catheterization and angiography.

In the majority of other single-vessel coronary angioplasties, the surgical team simply needs to be aware that angioplasty is taking place and that a complication could arise requiring urgent surgery. In large centers with active cardiac surgical programs, no single operating room need be kept available; an available surgical team on site is sufficient. Single-vessel angioplasty involving the right or circumflex system, where the amount of jeopardized myocardium is relatively small, can fit into this group. With the

advent of coronary perfusion balloon catheters and stents for the control of acute reocclusions that do not respond to simple redilatation, many more patients may fall into this category requiring "level 1" backup.

If there is concern that significant hemodynamic compromise will result from uncontrollable coronary occlusion, and that immediate surgical revascularization may be necessary, a designated operating room and surgical team should be kept on standby until there is no longer a significant risk of occlusion. Angioplasties of arteries that supply a large myocardial segment—a proximal lesion in a very large circumflex system, left anterior descending lesions proximal to the first significant diagonal branch, or large arteries in patients with severely compromised left ventricular function—are best dealt with using this "level 2" backup. For some patients it is prudent to have an intra-aortic balloon pump console available with the electrocardiographic monitoring leads preconnected to the patient and both groins prepped for any easy second arterial access. An occasional patient is best supported on an intra-aortic balloon pump placed electively at the time of coronary intervention.

As increasingly complex and complicated angioplasties are performed, several additional support options have been developed. Angioplasty of the left main coronary artery or its hemodynamic equivalent has been carried out in a combined angiographic suite/operating room.[34] Other institutions keep equipment for open-chest cardiopulmonary bypass and surgery available in the catheterization laboratory. Percutaneous total cardiopulmonary bypass systems have been developed to support hemodynamically unstable patients during potentially dangerous angioplasty procedures.[35] In some cases patients thought to develop hemodynamic compromise or collapse during balloon inflation can have distal coronary perfusion maintained by a perfusion balloon[30] or perfusion with an oxygen-carrying fluorocarbon.[36] Retroperfusion of the coronary sinus has also been used to ameliorate ischemia in this setting.[37]

PRE-PROCEDURE PLANNING

All patients should be fully and openly informed about their interventional procedure and its potential risks. Written or videotaped educational materials are helpful adjuncts, as is the use of nurse-clinicians to provide further teaching and support. The concept of surgical standby should be discussed with the patient to ensure complete understanding. The patient's oral intake should be managed in preparation for possible intubation and general anesthesia. Consideration should be given to the presence of dentures or other oral appliances. Relative contraindications to intubation and surgery (such as critical obstructive lung disease) should be kept in mind. Although it is seldom needed, all information relative to the patient's tolerance of emergency intubation, anesthesia, and cardiac surgery should be sought in the preoperative period, as there will be little time to do so should emergency surgery be necessary. Hospital admission for elective coronary angioplasty need not occur until the day of the procedure in many cases. A stable and free-running intravenous line should be started in the forearm and the patient kept well hydrated (be mindful of the potential for fluid overload in patients with impaired renal or cardiac function). Many pre-procedure regimens for sedation exist and most are satisfactory. Patients should be started on low-dose soluble aspirin before their procedure. In consideration of the possibility of emergency "bailout" stent placement, dipyrimadole 75 mg t.i.d. should be begun before the procedure. If the lesion to be treated appears high risk for acute occlusion, a low molecular weight dextran infusion should either be started or be quickly available in the event that stent placement is needed. A blood sample should be sent to the blood bank for typing and screening for antibodies that would make crossmatching difficult in the event that blood is needed for surgery. Blood is not routinely reserved for patients undergoing angioplasty.

MANAGEMENT OF PATIENTS DURING PTCA

Control of Periodic and Unintended Coronary Occlusion

Successful coronary angioplasty creates controlled, periodic coronary occlusion. The most common problems that an operator must deal with during angioplasty are those arising when control of occlusion is lost. It is difficult to predict the response of an individual patient and

individual artery to the resulting ischemia, but prediction can be attempted by evaluating the amount of myocardium that will be ischemic during balloon inflation and estimating its contribution to cardiac performance and hemodynamic stability. Dilatation of a small distal right coronary artery is unlikely to render a large amount of myocardium ischemic during balloon inflation. Nevertheless, elective right coronary dilatation can result in hypotension that is vagally mediated or caused by the Bezold-Jarisch reflex. In a similar fashion, balloon deflation can result in paradoxical hypotension or bradycardia.[38] The judicious use of atropine and fluid therapy to correct reflex vasodilatation can help to mitigate this problem. On the other hand, the dilatation of certain vessels, such as the proximal left anterior descending coronary, may be associated with hemodynamic compromise simply because they supply a large amount of contracting muscle. The proper choice of inflation times, or the use of distal perfusion,[39-41] may help in situations where acute depression of left ventricular function occurs. In some patients, the prophylactic use of intra-aortic balloon counter pulsation or other cardiopulmonary support may be warranted.

The occurrence of unintended occlusion during coronary procedures is infrequent, and the ability to gain control over these occlusions has increased. Early in the history of coronary angioplasty it was feared that coronary emboli from plaque debris might be a significant problem. Plaque embolization is now known to be uncommon in native vessels but can occur in deteriorating, aging, saphenous vein bypass grafts. The distal embolization of thrombus occurs more frequently and is reason for caution in the dilatation of arteries containing large amounts of thrombus.[27] Some operators advocate prolonged pre-treatment with intravenous heparin, some use no adjuvant therapy, and others use local thrombolytic agents.[42] Particular caution should be exercised in vessels totally occluded with plaque and sub-acute thrombus—the notion that a patient with an occluded vessel cannot be "made worse" by an unsuccessful percutaneous transluminal coronary angioplasty of a totally occluded artery is untrue. Embolization can compromise collateral flow to the distal vessel and create or worsen ischemia. Unintended but controllable coronary ischemia can also occur from inappropriate or inept manipulation of equipment. The inadvertent injection of air or thrombus from improperly or inadequately flushed catheters can create profound ischemia and hemodynamic collapse, or simulate other forms of uncontrollable coronary occlusion. This is entirely preventable by careful attention to equipment setup and manipulation.

Ostial coronary occlusion can result from obstruction by the guiding catheter. This may occur when a minimal ostial narrowing is present or when a guide catheter is deeply seated to provide support for advance of the balloon catheter. The resulting persistent ischemia after balloon deflation is often misinterpreted by inexperienced operators as a more distal coronary occlusion due to spasm, dissection or embolus. Unseating the catheter, using a guiding catheter with a different configuration, or using a catheter with side holes for coronary perfusion, will usually alleviate this problem. Should "side hole" catheters be used, care must be taken to ensure that there is adequate coronary flow—the mere presence of an arterial pressure wave form at the catheter tip does not guarantee this.

All types of coronary instrumentation, including angioplasty, can produce coronary spasm. Spasm may occur at the site of coronary dilatation and can be associated with continuing ischemia following balloon deflation. Although there are some common angiographic features of spasm, there is no absolutely characteristic appearance—it is often indistinguishable from other forms of occlusion or near-occlusion at the angioplasty site. In such situations, the administration of intracoronary nitroglycerin can sometimes ameliorate ischemia and thus is diagnostic. If spasm at the site of dilatation is resistant to nitroglycerin, redilatation (often at higher pressures, with a larger balloon or of a longer duration) may resolve it.

Vasospasm can occur in the non-dilated portions of the instrumented artery or even in a contralateral coronary vessel. Guide catheter tips can produce ostial spasm and profound ischemia. A guide wire tip can cause mechanical irritation and spasm and impede distal flow in a fashion similar to an embolus. These kinds of spasm often respond to repositioning of the offending device and to the liberal use of intracoronary nitroglycerin. Intracoronary verapamil is also occasionally used. Rarely, intra-aortic balloon counter pulsation has been associated with the reversal of profound coronary spasm and amelioration of hemodynamic compromise.

Managing Coronary Dissection

Coronary dissection is probably the most feared management difficulty during coronary intervention. Unfortunately, it is also the most common. At times, the deep seating of a guiding catheter may cause ostial coronary dissection. Left main dissection with occlusion is rare but often fatal. Right coronary ostial dissection with occlusion, because of possible acute right ventricular failure and compromise of both the sinoatrial and atrioventricular nodal arteries, is also a dire complication. Ostial dissections are not always associated with complete occlusion and can simply create further reduction in the lumen. Dye staining or irregularities characterize their angiographic appearance. Their prompt recognition and management can prevent myocardial infarction and death. Though right coronary ostial dissections have been successfully managed without surgery, the consequences of abrupt closure of an unprotected left main coronary are so dire that the dissections of it are nearly always managed surgically. This applies even if they are initially successfully treated percutaneously. Non ostial dissections are now often managed with catheter-based techniques. Prompt balloon redilatation, the placement of a coronary perfusion "bailout,"[43] or perfusion balloon catheter,[30,44] directional atherectomy,[45] or stent placement, may salvage the situation. Finally, urgent coronary bypass surgery may be necessary. Figure 1 illustrates a proximal dissection precipitated by deep-seating a guiding catheter. More distal coronary dissection may also be instigated by passage of a guide wire tip through an area of disrupted or friable plaque. The guide wire tip or other coronary instrumentation can raise a "flap" and cause luminal compromise or occlusion at any point along the vessel. This accounts for the difficulty in separating guide wire-mediated distal coronary dissection from spasm. Most commonly however, coronary dissection occurs at the site of dilatation.

It might be argued that most successful angioplasties are associated with dissection simply because the predominant mechanism of angioplasty is to produce a controlled dissection

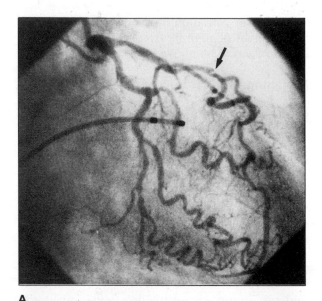

A

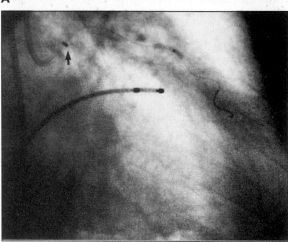

B

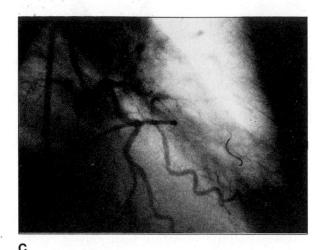

C

Figure 1. Proximal dissection in the left anterior descending coronary artery caused by deep seating of the guiding catheter. The pre-angioplasty angiogram (A) reveals both proximal left anterior descending plaquing and a distal shelf-like stenosis (arrow) in a tortuous vessel. Very forceful seating (B, arrow) of the guide was required to "force" the balloon across the stenosis. Though the distal lesion was dilated, the guide catheter caused disruption of the proximal LAD resulting in acute occlusion unresponsive to dilatation and necessitating emergency surgical revascularization (C).

over a limited area.[46–48] "Pathologic" dissection results when there is sufficient disruption of plaque to collapse the vessel lumen and compromise distal flow.[49,50] Multiple techniques have been proposed to reduce the incidence of pathologic dissections, including the under-sizing or over-sizing of balloons, the use of low pressure-long duration inflations, intraprocedural monitoring of balloon/vessel compliance, sequential dilatation with successively larger balloons, or limiting the rate of balloon inflations.[51–53] There is no proven "best" strategy—most dilators opt to increase the rate of pressure slowly during inflation and to avoid over dilatation. Interestingly, the presence of an angiographically visible dissection without luminal compromise has been correlated with undiminished or improved[54–56] long-term patency. Characteristics that suggest an increased risk of dissection may include calcification of the vessel, lesion location, and the angiographic appearance of the stenosis.[57,58]

The management of dissection consists primarily of its avoidance; and as PTCA equipment and operators have improved, the rate of uncontrollable dissections has decreased. Yet, there seem to be some arteries where dissection will occur no matter what technique is employed—an operator-independent variable. Under these circumstances, redilatation is the first-line therapy, in most cases using the same balloon inflated for a longer time, at a higher pressure, or both. Occasionally, the

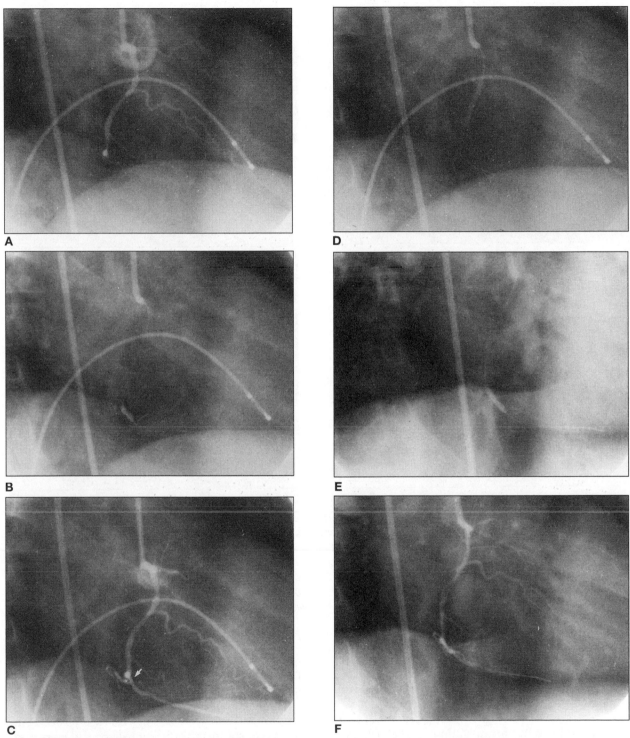

Figure 2. *Right coronary artery illustrating several pitfalls encountered by the inexperienced operator. In (A), the diagnostic angiogram of the right coronary artery shows a complete occlusion in the distal vessel. The occlusion is crossed with a wire and an appropriate inflation is made in (B). Distal flow is restored but a residual lesion is present in the distal vessel (C). A second dilatation is performed in the proximal portion of the vessel using a long balloon (D). However, in the subsequent angiogram, flow is compromised into the distal vessel. At this point, redilatation is appropriate. However, in this case, the balloon is inflated too proximally and fails to resolve the obstruction (E). The obstruction has migrated proximally because the operator has failed to identify the location of the distal dissection (F) and has incorrectly concluded that the origin of the obstruction is in the proximal vessel.*

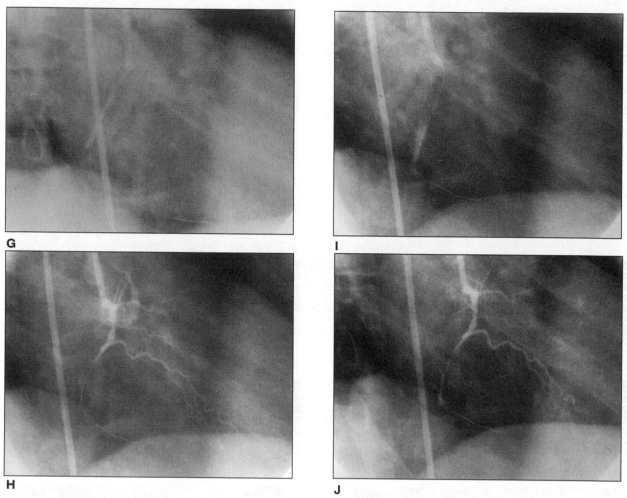

Figure 2 continued. *A second long-duration redilatation is also performed (G)—also too proximally. Flow is not restored (H) and a final attempt is made to "open" the dissected vessel (I); but once again the operator failed to appreciate that the distal vessel was occluded and that no amount of dilatation in the proximal vessel would restore outflow. The final result in (J) shows a more proximal occlusion in the right coronary than that with which the patient presented. Overall, this case illustrates the need to identify correctly the site of atherosclerotic obstruction—whether it is in an elective setting or in an emergency. Accurate balloon placement and an understanding of the responses of vessels to the trauma of dilatation are required for high quality and successful coronary intervention.*

substitution of a larger balloon will be required to "tack down" a recalcitrant flap. Empirical intra-coronary nitroglycerin, if permitted by the patient's blood pressure, may help to rule out or treat concomitant coronary spasm. The duration, number, and extent of redilatations that should be used in the management of dissection are functions of operator experience, the degree of ischemia, and the patient's hemodynamic status.

At times, redilatation and other interventions fail to control the dissection and urgent stent placement is considered. The operator must then not only be able to deliver the stent(s) successfully but also (and perhaps most importantly) he/she must balance the benefit of avoiding emergency surgery against the risks of vigorous anticoagulation, access site complications, and sub-acute closure. If surgery is chosen, the use of coronary perfusion balloon catheters may relieve or reduce ischemia while preparations for surgery are being made. When severe hypotension or hemodynamic compromise occurs, the prompt insertion of an intra-aortic balloon or other circulatory assist device may help to achieve hemodynamic stability in preparation for emergency surgery.

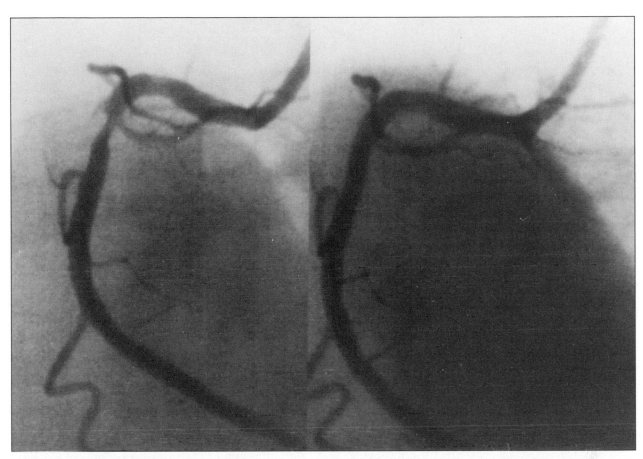

Figure 3. *Shown in the left panel is a focal dissection in the proximal portion of a large caliber right coronary artery after balloon angioplasty several hours earlier. "Salvage" directional coronary atherectomy was performed retrieving a "flap" of tissue and yielding the final result shown in the right panel. Directional atherectomy is a valuable technique for controlling focal dissections in large caliber coronaries.*

POSTPROCEDURE MANAGEMENT

The most important long-term management problem after coronary angioplasty is restenosis, discussed in detail in the next section of this chapter. However, the management of acute closure is of paramount concern in the immediate post angioplasty period.

Routinely following a successful angioplasty (if the procedure has been performed from the femoral approach), vascular access sheaths are left indwelling and the patient is continued on intravenous heparin. Should acute occlusion occur, vascular access is readily available for redilatation. Attempts have been made to predict acute closure from clinical and angiographic characteristics,[24] but in practice, the greatest

concern is raised by the continued presence of thrombus, semi-occlusive dissection, or incomplete dilatation at the termination of the procedure. The appropriate duration of systemic heparinization is not known. As a practical matter, most operators leave the vascular sheaths in place from 4 to 24 hours. Interruption of heparinization and the removal of the sheaths on the day after most interventions is therefore the rule. Special attention must be paid to anticoagulation following coronary stent placement. Under these circumstances, patients are continued on dextran, aspirin and dipyrimidole, and warfarin is begun. Heparin is interrupted for vascular sheath removal and then reinstituted after which the dextran is stopped. Heparin is continued for at least 3 days or until the INR on warfarin is 4 to 5. It is important to confirm the

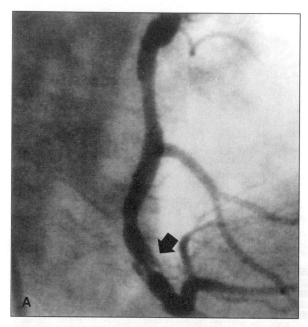
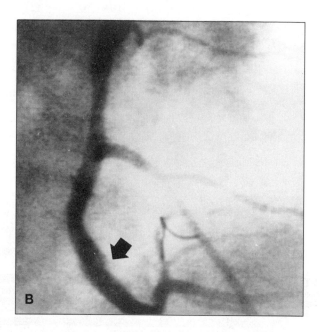

Figure 4. *In panel (A) an enlarged view of a distal right coronary circumferential dissection is shown. This had resulted in recurrent angina and electrocardiogram changes following balloon angioplasty and is pictured after both prolonged perfusion balloon dilatation and attempted atherectomy. A single Cook Flexstent results in a much improved angiographic appearance (B).*

stability of the INR off heparin. Hospital discharge can be accomplished if all else is in order. Post discharge, the coronary stent patient should remain in close contact for careful anticoagulation monitoring. The potential complications of stent thrombosis on the one hand, and significant hemorrhage on the other, can be life-threatening and it is vitally important that protocol orders, staff training, and patient education be put in place and periodically re-evaluated if this is to be a widely successful therapeutic option.[59]

In the past most post-intervention patients were monitored in intensive care units, as these were the only places in the hospital where arterial catheters could be maintained. Many institutions now have special areas where stable post-angioplasty patients can be followed overnight. This has reduced costs and increased patient comfort.

Under all circumstances, careful monitoring for the development of peri-access and retroperitoneal bleeding is appropriate. Femoral hematomas can be difficult to detect unless the clinician is alert for their presence. The development of hypotension, or a vasovagal reaction several hours after coronary angioplasty, should always prompt suspicion of hemorrhage. In most instances bleeding is minimal but it is uncomfortable and cosmetically unap-

pealing. In some cases, blood loss itself is ongoing and hemodynamically significant. As interventional procedures have become more complex, the amount of intra-procedural blood loss has increased and a hematocrit decline is often seen in the post-procedure period. This does not necessarily indicate ongoing blood loss. In contrast, "rescue" angioplasty in patients who have received systemic thrombolytics and the need for vigorous anticoagulation in stent placement, has increased the likelihood of major blood loss in these settings. These confounding forces must be appreciated and it is important that the rate of decline of the post-procedure hematocrit, the presence or absence of clinical correlates, and potential hemodilution be kept in mind when considering whether blood loss is ongoing. If blood loss occurs and bleeding cannot be "seen," retroperitoneal and (less likely) gastrointestinal hemorrhage must be considered. Anticoagulation should be interrupted or reversed, blood products readied and treatment of the source of bleeding begun.

In addition, patients have often undergone diagnostic catheterization before angioplasty and are then kept without their usual oral intake. The subsequent angioplasty procedure entails the use of radiographic contrast material and an ensuing osmotic diuresis. Following angioplasty, therefore, patients tend to be intravascularly volume-depleted and may require vigorous fluid replacement. Thus, the major differential diagnosis in post procedural hypotension is blood loss versus simple dehydration volume-depletion. Occasionally vasovagal reactions or medication-related bradycardias also account for hypotension. The development of pseudoaneurysm or arteriovenous fistula is possible and should be considered in the patient with groin hematoma or unusual groin tenderness in the post procedure period.

In the past, there was great concern over the late development of clinically important coronary spasm after angioplasty. Patients were thus routinely kept on nitrates and/or calcium channel blockers. The development of significant delayed coronary vasospasm is uncommon. Although some luminal narrowing may often occur,[60] its immediate clinical significance is doubtful. Since most patients are managed on calcium channel blockers before their procedure, many are continued on them afterwards. We generally discharge patients on a calcium channel blocker and continue it for at least 6 weeks. In this way, should the patient develop early restenosis, some protection against angina will be on board. We do not routinely perform pre-discharge exercise testing in patients with adequate angiographic results. Occasionally, following a very difficult procedure or those with uncertain angiographic results, the performance of a "second look" coronary angiogram is appropriate before sheath removal and hospital discharge. This is also appropriate in patients with recurrent symptoms after dilatation. It should be emphasized to nurses and other monitoring personnel that the development of recurrent ischemic symptoms after dilatation is a medical emergency that is often best dealt with by repeat angiography and angioplasty. It is not a situation in which the administration of nitrates and/or analgesics is sufficient. In most instances, the discharge of patients from the hospital can be accomplished within 24-36 hours after completion of a successful procedure. This is predicated on the patient being ambulatory and without complications after removal of the vascular access. Repeat exercise testing or other objective confirmation of the abolition of ischemia can be accomplished on an outpatient basis.

RESTENOSIS

Restenosis after successful balloon dilatation occurs in 20%-35% of patients and requires repeat angioplasty.[56,61-62] The majority of cases of restenosis occur in the first 2-3 months following PTCA and are generally heralded by either recurrent angina or a clearly positive exercise treadmill test.[63,64] Although both thallium scintigraphy and exercise echocardiography are more sensitive indicators of coronary insufficiency than is treadmill testing alone, their cost makes them less attractive for routine surveillance. Patients who have not developed restenosis at 6 months will generally have continued patency of the dilated coronary segment for years. Repeat angioplasty for restenosis is associated with favorable results and lower complication rates, but recurrent restenosis can occur.[65-67] Mini dilatations are performed,[68] but a patient is generally declared an angioplasty failure after 3 dilatations and should be considered for an alternate therapy.

Restenosis is rarely a simple re-accumulation of plaque. It is a sequela of "healing" at the site of dilatation.[69] Platelets adhere to the sites of endothelial trauma and may stimulate a complex cascade that leads to restenosis over the course of weeks to months.[70-72] The primary "culprit" appears to be smooth muscle cell proliferation which is stimulated by various growth mediators released from platelet aggregates, endothelial cells, and local macrophages in response to the local injury from balloon angioplasty. Molecular biology techniques such as in-situ hybridization and the use of the polymerase chain reaction (PCR) to detect genes that are active in the process of cell proliferation are under investigation.[73] It is hoped that once specific genes are implicated in restenosis, alternate or mutant genes can be delivered locally at the time of intervention to ablate or blunt the response.[74] Anti-platelet receptor antibodies have been tested. They are hoped to offer the potential of blocking platelet adherence.[75,76] Anti-sense oligonucleotides have prevented smooth muscle cell proliferation in an animal model of restenosis.[77] However, no conventional drug therapy has yet significantly altered the incidence of restenosis.[77-80] Fish oil has been proposed as a potential agent in the prevention of clinical restenosis; but, the data remain conflicting and the overall sense is that even the positive results are not dramatic.[81–83] Animal data exist that suggest that a modification in the level of serum cholesterol might reduce the development of a proliferative response following balloon dilatation.[84] There are some suggestive studies that this approach may be applicable to the human situation and some interventionalists use cholesterol-lowering medications in an attempt to modify restenosis.[85–86]

Mechanical solutions to the problem are also being sought and attempts have been made to understand the relationship of clinical parameters and procedural results to the development of restenosis.[87] The medium-term (6-month) results of balloon angioplasty and other interventional modalities are made up of the "acute gain" (the increase in luminal diameter owing to the procedure) and the "late loss" (recoil and restenosis). The relationship of acute gain to late loss may be device specific and predict, for a given post-procedure result, the likelihood of restenosis. The development of some "late loss" or restenosis seems to be a universal phenomenon and the incidence of clinical restenosis will depend upon whether this response has "room" to occur before compromising flow. Within a population of patients, the late luminal diameter is predicted by the immediate post-procedural luminal diameter. Though this does not permit the prediction of restenosis in an individual patient, it strongly suggests that the larger the post-procedure lumen the less likely the patient is to develop restenosis. Though there does seem to be a greater late loss produced by greater acute gain, this is less significant than the initial greater increase in lumen. Further, because late loss in luminal diameter is a universal phenomenon, there is a predictable limit beyond which mechanical devices will not reduce restenosis.[88–90]

The clinical implication of these notions are that the likelihood of restenosis can be reduced by obtaining the maximum possible luminal diameter at the time of the initial intervention. It was hoped that devices that allowed the achievement of a near-zero residual stenosis would lower the rate of clinical restenosis— small series of coronary stent placement and directional atherectomy support this concept.[90] The results of the randomized CAVEAT trial comparing balloon angioplasty with directional atherectomy suggest that directional atherectomy, when performed successfully, significantly

but mildly reduces the incidence of restenosis over balloon angioplasty.[91] Unfortunately, this may have been accomplished at the cost of more complications in the atherectomy cohort. Both this trial, and the CCAT trial of atherectomy[92] have been criticized because their participants did not routinely reduce the patients' residual stenosis beyond what some consider "balloon angioplasty" levels.[93] Following balloon angioplasty, many operators have previously accepted a 20%-30% residual stenosis either because recoil prevents further dilatation or because of the fear of causing a coronary dissection from over-dilatation.

At present, the best clinical strategy for the prevention of restenosis is likely the attempt to achieve the greatest post-procedure lumen possible while being mindful of the potential trade-off in increased acute and sub-acute complications to achieve potential long-term benefit. In addition, the continued modification of risk factors should not be forgotten in the complete care of the patient.

ANGIOPLASTY IN ACUTE MYOCARDIAL INFARCTION

In the early history of coronary angioplasty, the presence of intracoronary thrombus was considered a near absolute contraindication to the procedure. As operators became more comfortable with the technique, its indications expanded and cardiologists began to use angioplasty to restore patency of coronary arteries that remained severely obstructed after administration of intracoronary thrombolytic therapy.[94] It was quickly realized that angioplasty without thrombolytic agents could also be used as primary therapy to restore coronary patency.[95] Using currently available equipment, skilled operators can now successfully and stably recanalize approximately 90% of infarct related vessels in the setting of an acute myocardial infarction[96] (Fig. 5). At this time, effective, easily administered, intravenous thrombolytic agents have been developed that also effect successful and stable coronary reperfusion. Tissue plasminogen activator (t-PA), despite its high cost, has become the mainstay of coronary thrombolytic therapy in the United States and its relationship to, and interaction with, angioplasty have been studied extensively.[97–99]

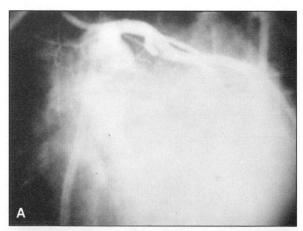

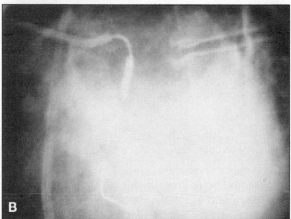

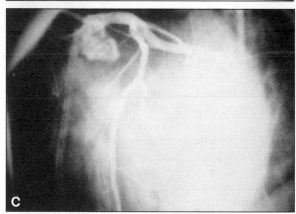

Figure 5. *Acute occlusion at the left anterior descending coronary for which the patient was referred for acute PTCA (A). The occlusion was crossed easily and dilatation performed (B). The result is a widely patent artery with amelioration in the patient's symptoms (C).*

Coronary angiography performed during myocardial infarction has shown clearly that when thrombolytic therapy is applied to an infarct-related vessel, there is often an underly-

ing residual stenosis after dissolution of the intracoronary thrombus.[94] The assumption had been that presence of this residual stenosis might be flow-limiting or that it could somehow become biologically active, engendering rethrombosis. Therefore, concern was raised that simple dissolution of thrombus would not be sufficient to prevent rethrombosis once the thrombolytic effect waned. A logical strategy evolved recommending intravenous thrombolytic therapy followed by emergent or urgent coronary angioplasty.

While thrombolytic therapy could be given easily in nearly every emergency room and hospital setting, the performance of emergency coronary angioplasty required appreciably greater organization, facilities, and personnel. Thus, coronary angioplasty was and is not always available for all patients. The cost of making it available was clearly substantial and the benefits uncertain. Fortunately, this dilemma prompted organized and large-scale scientific investigation. Randomized trials of t-PA, with and without routine coronary angioplasty, confirm that if thrombolytic therapy is the first line of intervention, routine angioplasty offers no benefit in short term survival or in improved ventricular function.[97–99] In fact, the vascular access required for the performance of PTCA may engender more short term complications.

Significant clinical issues in the relationship of PTCA to thrombolytic therapy were not addressed in these trials. For example, angioplasty without prior thrombolytic therapy was not compared to thrombolytic therapy in a large scale prospective trial. In centers where primary angioplasty had been used for acute MI patients, mortality has been as low as that reported in large scale thrombolysis trials.[100–102] In cardiogenic shock patients, direct coronary angioplasty has been shown to be the intervention of choice; it has achieved significant reductions in mortality compared with historic controls.[103,104] Data also indicate that in the setting of acute myocardial infarction, a patent infarct-related artery at the time of hospital discharge may confer an improved prognosis.[105,106] The improvement may be unrelated to the degree of myocardial salvage or ventricular function.[107,108] ISIS-2, a large-scale thrombolysis trial, indicated that reperfusion delayed for up to 24 hours after the onset of symptoms may confer a survival advantage.[109] Delayed direct angioplasty

Table 6. Studies of Direct Angioplasty in Acute MI

	PAMI[84]		NETHERLANDS[85]		MAYO[86]	
Number of Patients	395		142		108	
Hours eligible post onset	12		6 (24)		12	
PTCA success	97%		95%		93%	
	t-PA	PTCA	SK	PTCA	t-PA	PTCA
Death (%)	6.5	2.6	6	0	4	4
Death ("not low risk")**	10.4*	2.0				
Reinfarction	6.5	2.6	13*	0	1	0
Death + Reinfarction	12.0	5.1				
Post-Infarct Angina			19*	6		
Patency			68*	91		
Residual stenosis			76*	36		
Salvage					15	13
EF	53	53	45*	51	50	53
Late reinfarction + death	16.8*	8.5				
Need for additional revascularization	48	14	42	14	36	15
Bleeding	6	4	8	3		
Intracerebral hemorrhage	2*	0				

*$P < .05$ compared with PTCA group.
** "Not low risk"=age >70, anterior infarct or HR >100
Summary of the 3 recently published randomized trials of PTCA versus thrombolytic therapy for acute myocardial infarction. Though the study designs and endpoints differed somewhat among the studies, the salient points are that mortality and myocardial salvage are equivalent and that hemorrhagic complications and subsequent adverse events may be reduced in the PTCA groups.

may also be effective.[110,111] Recently, the results of 3 randomized trials comparing direct PTCA with thrombolytic therapy have become available. They indicate that primary balloon angioplasty offers equivalent mortality reduction benefits and ventricular salvage to thrombolytic therapy. It is also suggested by these trials that direct angioplasty may result in fewer intracerebral hemorrhages than thrombolytic therapy.[112–114] The results of these studies are summarized in Table 6. Many clinical and interventional cardiologists now believe that, when it can be applied as rapidly as thrombolytic therapy, direct angioplasty offers additional benefits in safety and efficacy.

At present, the patient successfully reperfused with thrombolytic therapy should not routinely be treated with balloon angioplasty. However, there is danger in assuming that the biologic activities of all lytic agents and all other non-balloon interventions will make this conservative approach universally appropriate. What should be the intervention strategy for those patients for whom direct angioplasty is available, who clinically fail chemical reperfusion, develop recurrent ischemia after chemical reperfusion, have a contraindication to thrombolytic therapy, or who simply cannot receive lytic therapy within 4-6 hours after the onset of infarction? In many institutions, patients in these groups are catheterized emergently and undergo PTCA. A flow chart used at The Lahey Clinic Medical Center and Stanford University Medical Center for the management of patients with myocardial infarction is shown in Figure 6. Although it is not necessary to transport every infarct patient to a catheterization laboratory for intervention, every infarct patient may need subsequent intervention. It is also clear that a significant percentage of patients who receive initial thrombolytic therapy will require such emergent angiography and intervention. Some will need "elective" procedures for symptoms that develop after hospital discharge, and a significant num-

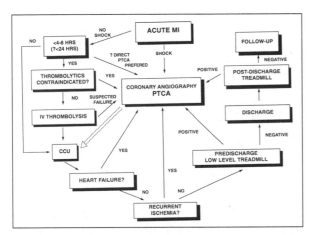

Figure 6. *Flow diagram for the management of acute myocardial infarction using interventional techniques. The central concept is that reperfusion should be achieved as quickly as possible. Definition of coronary anatomy is essential in complicated situations (shock, thrombolytic failure, or recurrent ischemia) to plan mechanical therapy. In instances where direct PTCA is available, it may be preferable. Arrows toward the center represent potential transfer from primary to tertiary center. In high-risk patients or those with a complicated clinical course or ongoing ischemia, definition of coronary anatomy and possible mechanical reperfusion are valuable adjuncts.*

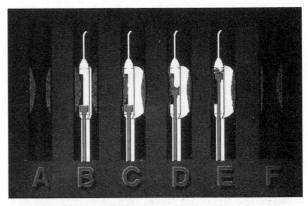

Figure 7. *Schematic representation of atherectomy using the Simpson AtheroCath. In plate B, the device is positioned across the stenosis with the aid of a guide wire. A stabilizing balloon is inflated at low pressures and the rotational cutting device is advanced at 2,000 rpm, "shaving" plaque into the metal housing (C-E). The device can be rotated to shave additional plaque, or withdrawn. (Courtesy of John Simpson, MD)*

ber will require emergency angiography and angioplasty to control recurrent or ongoing ischemia. And while it may not be cost effective to ensure instant local availability of coronary intervention for all patients, it is desirable to develop systems that give community hospitals direct access to the full range of emergency interventional cardiology services on a regionalized and cost effective basis.

The challenge for the future is not only to develop the best thrombolytic agent, but also to determine how best to combine interventional techniques with thrombolytic reperfusion, and to determine if and when direct intervention without thrombolysis is not only "equivalent" but preferable. In comparing techniques with drugs, one must remember that a drug can be given in essentially the same way from patient to patient. A technique, however, is operator dependent. Equally skilled operators at different institutions may develop subtly different techniques for the

management of patients with acute MI using interventional techniques. This fact makes it difficult to use the results of multicenter prospective trials to guide therapy for an individual patient; and it places a premium on clinical judgment of the interventional cardiologist.

NEWER INTRAVASCULAR DEVICES

ATHERECTOMY

The Simpson directional atherectomy device (Athero Cath,™ Devices for Vascular Intervention, Redwood City, California) was developed as an alternative to balloon angioplasty.[115] Figure 7 is a schematic representation of directional atherectomy with the Athero Cath.™ This percutaneous device has a rigid metal housing that facilitates cutting and extraction of intracoronary plaque, leaving a relatively smooth luminal surface. Simpson coined the word "atherectomy" in describing this "cut and retrieval" device. He postulated that the type of "controlled" intravascular injury it effected might lead to a reduction in the incidence of restenosis routinely seen following the barotrauma of balloon angioplasty. This device received approval from the FDA in 1988. Two randomized trials have since been completed, compar-

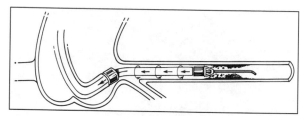

Figure 8. Schematic representation of the transluminal extraction catheter (TEC). The device consists of a motorized cutting head with triangular blades controlled by a steerable guidewire. The cutting head rotates at 750 rpm, and a suction apparatus removes excised plaque. From Stack. With permission.

ing the rates of restenosis following directional atherectomy (DCA) with PTCA.[91,92] Neither of these studies confirmed a reduction in restenosis with this new device. Directional atherectomy has nevertheless emerged with an effective niche: Its cutting mechanism is particularly well suited for treating eccentric lesions in large non-tortuous arteries. It has also been effective in treated ostial lesions where PTCA has frequently failed.

The transluminal extraction catheter (TEC) (Interventional Technologies, San Diego, California) is similar to the AtheroCath™ in that it is an "over the wire" system that cuts and removes plaque.[116] It is a cutting device with 2 blades that revolve in a conical fashion as the device advances. Continuous suction through a contiguous hypo-tube theoretically removes shaved debris (Fig. 8). Although this device has not mitigated restenosis rates, it has promise as a "niche device." Its design gives this device potential in treating diffusely diseased vein grafts and thrombus-laden coronary segments.

High speed rotational atherectomy is accomplished with the Auth-Rotablator device (Heart Technology, Bellevue, Washington). Atherectomy is a misnomer in that pulverization of plaque, without retrieval, occurs.[117,118] Various sizes of diamond coated, elliptical burrs (Fig. 9) can be advanced down the coronary artery, over a wire, at rotational speeds of 150,000-200,000 rpm. Like an orthopedic cast saw, the Rotablator™ works by the principal of differential cutting: rigid or inelastic plaque is ablated, while soft elastic tissue is pushed aside, unharmed.[119] Atherosclerotic plaque is pulverized into debris less than 10 microns in size. This particulate debris flows into the distal micro-circulation, without apparent infarction.[120] The Rotablator™ can easily track over a wire and offers flexibility for delivery into branched and distal vessels. Like the TEC device, fixed profiles of the rigid burr require large lumen guiding catheters for delivery of the device. High speed rotational atherectomy has not lessened the rate of restenosis seen with PTCA;[121] however, it has emerged as a preferred device for treating heavily calcified stenoses. The Rotablator™ appears to be the only percutaneous device that will reliably treat such lesions.

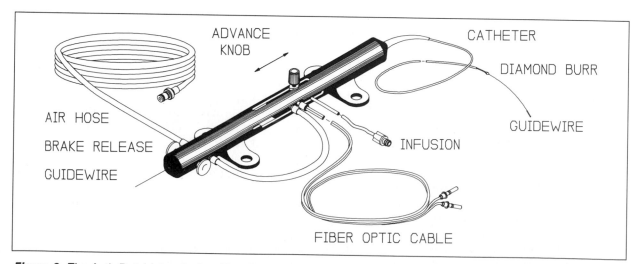

Figure 9. The Auth-Rotablator device. The diamond burr is rotated at high speed by an air-drive turbine. Rotational speed is monitored with the fiber optic cable. The burr is advanced over an independently moveable guide and "pulverizes" plaque. (Courtesy of David Auth, MD.)

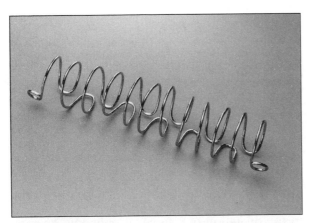

Figure 10. *Expanded Gianturco-Roublin Flexstent. Photography courtesy of Cook Cardiology, Cook Inc. Bloomington, IN.*

STENTS

The first use of intracoronary stents was described by Sigwart, while working in Lausanne, Switzerland, in 1987.[122] The idea of buttressing or stenting an artery with an expandable metal tube was quickly embraced by multiple companies in the United States and Europe. There are at least five intracoronary stents undergoing clinical trials in the United States under Investigational Device Exemptions. The designs include both balloon expandable and self-expanding stents, using a variety of metal alloys. The Gianturco-Roubin FlexStent™ (Cook, Inc., Bloomington, Indiana) was the first intracoronary stent to receive FDA approval (1993). Figure 10 depicts a typical balloon expandable FlexStent™. The device was approved for use in coronary arteries with abrupt closure or threatened closure, because of dissection. These stents can restore coronary flow in vessels compromised by dissection flaps.[123] The advent of coronary stents has lessened the need for emergency bypass surgery following failed angioplasty.

Although stents have obvious application in the setting of acute dissection and abrupt vessel closure, enthusiasm has spread for their potential to reduce the clinical incidence of restenosis following successful angioplasty. Elastic recoil of the dilated coronary segment has been implicated as one of the important factors in early restenosis. Rigid stenting of the dilated segment clearly limits this phenomenon. Stents also facil-

itate the development of larger residual lumens following angioplasty. The larger residual lumen permits the proliferative response of restenosis to occur with less clinical impact.[89,124] "Tacking" up dissections may also limit the exposure of damaged intima and media to circulating platelets and, theoretically, reduce the stimulation of smooth muscle cell proliferation and attendant restenosis.[125,126]

It is anticipated that stents might substantially reduce the incidence of embolization during balloon dilatation of friable vein grafts by entrapping the plaque debris as dilatation occurs with the expanding stent.[127]

Intracoronary stents have been associated with 2 serious complications: abrupt thrombotic closure and hemorrhage. These metallic devices are inherently thrombogenic. The first reports from Europe, with Sigwart's Wallstent™ (Medinvent, Lausanne), were associated with a high rate of both in-hospital and out-of-hospital thrombosis.[128] These abrupt closures were frequently associated with acute myocardial infarction and occasionally death. It appears that the incidence of thrombosis (and stent restenosis) is indirectly related to the size of the stent.[89,129] Larger diameter stents (≥ 3.0 mm) are significantly less prone to closure.

Clinical trials of coronary stenting in America have avoided a high incidence of thrombotic closure by use of an aggressive anticoagulation approach during and following stent implantation. Patients are pre-treated with aspirin. In the catheterization laboratory they receive intravenous heparin and dextran. Following stent deployment, patients are continued on heparin while they receive warfarin orally. Once an appropriate therapeutic level of anticoagulation is achieved (INR > 3-4) they are discharged on aspirin, dipyridamole and warfarin. While this anticoagulation approach has lessened the occurrence of stent thrombosis, it has led to an increase in bleeding complications, particularly at the site of vascular entry. Very recent investigative reports from Europe have questioned the need for anticoagulation.

LASER ANGIOPLASTY

The use of lasers in the treatment of coronary artery disease has appeal because of the potential to deliver a high energy source over a flexible optical fiber. Enthusiasm for the clinical development of laser angioplasty was held back several years by the premature application of continuous wave lasers and the so-called "hot tip" laser.[130] These devices caused massive thermal injury, resulting in high rates of restenosis.

The first laser system to realize the potential for effective treatment of coronary artery disease was a pulsed ultraviolet laser system: excimer[131] (Spectranetics, Colorado Springs, Colorado). Lasers interact with tissue, causing both thermal and acoustic trauma. The ultraviolet excimer laser putatively disrupts molecular bonds, effecting tissue ablation without attendant thermal injury.[132–133] Although the device has not had an impact on the incidence of restenosis,[134] the FDA has approved the excimer laser for clinical use. It has been a particularly effective tool for treating long (>20 mm) stenoses and ostial lesions.

A mid-infrared laser system is being evaluated (as an alternative to the excimer laser) under an Investigational Device Exemption.[135] The Holmium laser (Eclipse Surgical Technologies, Palo Alto, California) has the theoretical advantage of possessing high absorption characteristics in water, an important component of most plaques.

The direction and depth of ablation are poorly controlled with both laser systems. The inability to fully control the energy at the tip of the fiber has led to inadvertent vessel perforations. These fiber optic devices may eventually be coupled to a sensing mechanism (such as intracoronary ultrasound or angioscopy) to deliver the ablating power in a more effective and safe fashion.

With the possible exception of intracoronary stents, none of the new devices described have had a mitigating impact on the incidence of restenosis. They have, nevertheless, received FDA approval because of their potential "niche applications." Table 7 summarizes their role as adjuncts to conventional balloon angioplasty.

BALLOON VALVOTOMY

The successful development of coronary angioplasty gave rise to the possibility of dilatation of other stenotic cardiac lesions. Such an idea was also a probable outgrowth of interventional techniques such as balloon atrial septostomy[136] or blade septostomy[137] that have been applied in pediatric cardiology. Consideration was first given

Table 7. Niche Technology	
DCA	Proximal eccentric stenoses; ostial stenoses
Rotablator	Calcified/inelastic stenoses
TEC	Diffuse disease: Vein Grafts
LASER	Long (>20 mm) stenoses, ostial stenoses
DCA=Directional Coronary Atherectomy; TEC=Transluminal Extraction Catheter	

to the dilatation of congenital pulmonic stenosis in children through use of a moving, inflated balloon like that used for septostomy.[138] "Angioplasty-like" static balloon dilatation was first proposed by Kan.[139] The pathology of congenital valvular pulmonic stenosis involved fusion of valve leaflets or the development of a supravalvular membrane; balloon dilatation of these noncalcified valves might result in commissural splitting and a low incidence of distal embolization. In addition, it was believed that brief occlusions of the pulmonary artery might be well tolerated and that small distal embolizations would be less of a problem in the pulmonary circuit than in the left heart. These assumptions proved true. The first catheters used for pulmonic dilatation were modifications of those developed for peripheral angioplasty. The procedure has been successful and has become the treatment of choice for congenital valvular pulmonic stenosis.[140–142] Interest soon developed in the balloon dilatation, or valvotomy, of adult acquired stenotic valvular heart disease.[143] Rheumatic mitral and tricuspid stenoses were first attempted[143–145] with large balloons that permitted transvalvular passage, inflation, and dilatation, resulting in disruption of rheumatic commissural fusion. High-quality transthoracic and transesophageal echocardiography and color flow Doppler mapping have facilitated the pre-procedure risk stratification of patients with mitral stenosis and helped in evaluating the results of the balloon valvotomy procedure. As is the case for surgical commissurotomy, ideal valvotomy patients are those whose valvular stenosis is a result primarily of commissural fusion and not of chordal foreshortening and subchordal scarring, and whose valve leaflets are not calcified. Echocardiographic identification of left atrial thrombus, which increases the chance of systemic or cerebral embolization, can also be made before

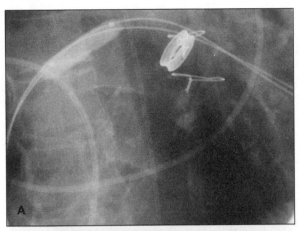

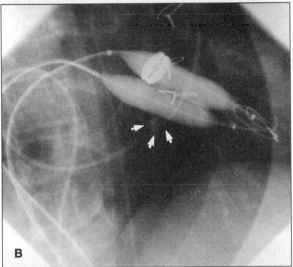

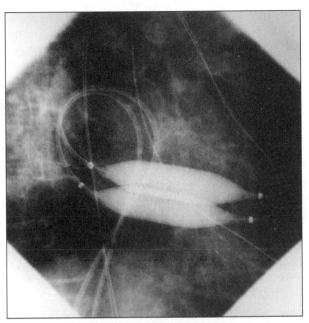

Figure 12. *An alternate method of valvotomy useful in some cases is to pass the guide wires into the aorta. If large (.035 in or .038 in) wires can be used, they are often sufficient to guide the balloons through the mitral annulus. At times, however, smaller diameter flexible guide wires must be snared and fixed in the descending aorta to permit the balloons to be pulled into place as shown in this anteroposterior view.*

Figure 11. *Transseptal mitral balloon dilatation. Dilatation of the intra-atrial septum with a small (8 mm) balloon shown in (A) is necessary to permit the passage of two large (15-20 mm) balloons into the mitral annulus (B). In this instance (seen in the right anterior oblique view) the relatively stiff .035 inch diameter guide wires are coiled and end in the left ventricle. Calcification in the mitral annulus is visible (arrow) and a waist is seen as the balloons inflate.*

the procedure. A quantitative scoring system has been developed to evaluate patients and to predict the results of balloon valvotomy.[146]

Mitral valvotomy is performed typically via the transseptal approach. Arterial and venous access is obtained from the right groin. Retrograde transseptal catheterization of the left heart is performed and a transmitral gradient measured. Following confirmation of mitral stenosis, a balloon flotation catheter is passed from the left atrium to the left ventricle through the mitral valve. A stiff guide wire or guide wires are then passed transseptally to the left ventricle or, in some cases, out into the aorta. The skin tract through the groin and into the femoral vein is enlarged and dilatation of the intra-atrial septum is performed with an 8-10 mm balloon. This accommodates the larger balloon catheters needed for effective dilatation. Both single- and double-balloon techniques are employed; several types of balloons have been developed that permit more stable seating within the mitral apparatus.[147,148] After dilatation and confirmation of a reduction in transvalvular gradient, the mitral valve area is measured using standard catheterization techniques. Figures 11 and 12 illustrate balloon dilatation of the interventricular septum and mitral valve. Contrast ventriculography or echocardiography is employed to assess the change in degree of mitral regurgitation, if any, and oximetry is used to assess the magnitude of the atrial-septal defect produced by dilatation of the intraventricular septum.

The short- and long-term results of mitral valvotomy are encouraging.[149] Reported restenosis rates at 9 months have been less than 5%.[150] Although the technique has been in use for far less time than surgical commissurotomy, the mechanism of balloon valvotomy is similar and the long term results are expected to be similar.[157,158] An additional benefit of balloon valvotomy is that it does not involve a sternotomy or a thoracotomy, and it is easily reapplied to appropriate patients. Today, balloon mitral valvotomy is considered by many cardiologists to be the most widely applicable first-line therapy in patients with rheumatic mitral stenosis.[153,154]

Although noncalcific congenital aortic stenosis is effectively treated with balloon valvotomy, balloon dilatation of acquired aortic stenosis has not fared as well. This experience parallels that of surgical valvotomy of rheumatic aortic valves. It results in part from the way aortic valvotomy has been applied in the United States—to degenerative calcific aortic stenosis, the most common type of adult aortic stenosis. Although it was feared initially that obstruction of the aortic valve orifice would be very dangerous and potentially fatal, this obstruction was quickly shown to be well tolerated if associated with subsequent reduction in aortic stenosis.

Retrograde aortic valvotomy requires crossing of the aortic valve with guide wires and the retrograde passage of a dilating balloon or balloons through the orifice (Fig. 13) or, alternatively, antegrade passage via the transseptal approach. A high degree of technical success has been achieved with the procedure. In degenerative calcific aortic stenosis however, the mechanism of reduction in stenosis is the cracking and deformation of areas of calcification in the valve leaflets; the disruption of commissural fusion is less apparent in these valves than in mitral valves.[155] For this reason, just as in surgical valvotomy, the long-term results of balloon valvotomy in calcific aortic stenosis have been relatively poor. Up to 50% of patients develop restenosis within 6 months[156] and the natural history of the patients who are dilated may be indistinguishable from those treated medically.[157] Outside the United States, where aortic stenosis is more likely to be rheumatic in origin, better long term success has been reported with balloon valvotomy.[158]

In the United States, valvotomy of the aortic valve should be reserved for patients who are too

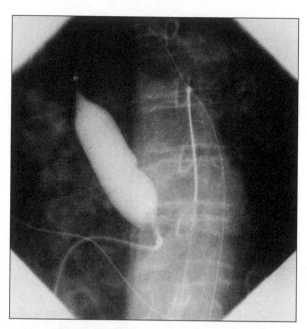

Figure 13. *Antegrade aortic balloon dilatation. A guide wire is passed into the aorta through a balloon flotation catheter that has been introduced transseptally into the left heart. A single balloon is guided into the area of the aortic valve and the dilatation performed. This approach, while technically more demanding than the retrograde passage of a balloon, avoids the necessity of a very large bore (12-14 Fr.) arterial access.*

ill to undergo aortic valve replacement or in patients whose expected survival because of intercurrent disease (malignancy, for example) is brief. In addition, balloon aortic valvotomy may be used as protective therapy should other major noncardiac surgery be required.[159] Another potential use is diagnostic: there exists a group of patients with extremely poor ventricular function and aortic stenosis in whom the clinician may question whether relief of aortic obstruction will improve ventricular function or symptoms. A trial balloon valvotomy may occasionally be appropriate to determine whether the patient will be a candidate for subsequent valve replacement. However, even in elderly patients, surgical valve replacement seems to be the preferred therapy.[160]

NONCORONARY INTERVENTIONS

In recent years, because of a large experience with the care of critically ill patients, interventional cardiologists have been increasingly called

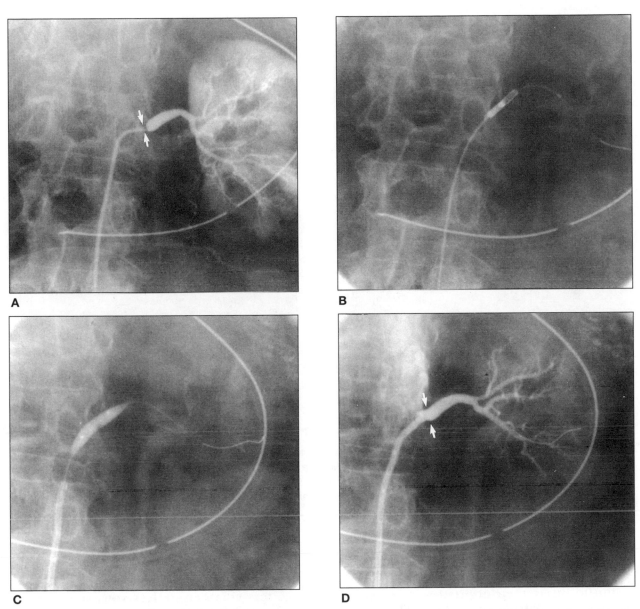

A

B

C

D

Figure 14. *Renal atherectomy. An aorto-ostial stenosis of the left renal artery is shown (A). This is less favorable for simple balloon dilatation than a lesion in the body of the artery. Directional atherectomy was chosen as an alternative. Using careful catheter placement and digital roadmapping, a .014" wire is passed into the renal artery and the angiographic catheter removed. A 7 Fr. G SCA-I catheter or "small vessel" peripheral atherotrack catheter is used to excise as much tissue as possible (B) and is followed by final balloon dilatation (C). The final result shows a smooth lumen with minimal residual stenosis (D). The use of directional atherectomy may facilitate the final balloon dilatation by providing stress relief to control both elastic recoil and the propagation of dissection.*

upon to develop, assist in, or perform other types of interventional procedures. Interventionalists who treat pediatric patients have led the way—the percutaneous closure of patent ductus arteriosus[161] or atrial septal defect[162] and the stenting of the ductus arteriosus[163] have all been reported.

The therapeutic embolization of congenital coronary arteriovenous malformations or the percutaneous closure of persistent side branches of the internal mammary artery (IMA) that cause coronary "steal" after bypass surgery are now the first-line therapies for those conditions.

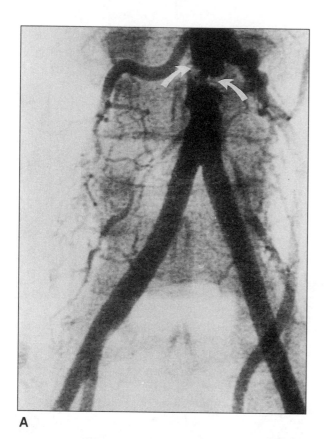
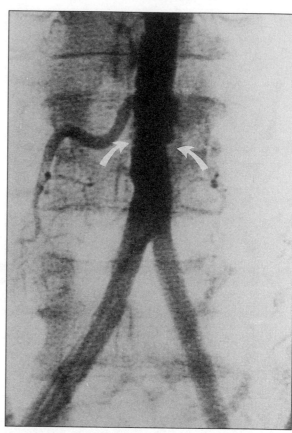

Figure 15. *Aortic stent placement. As interest develops among interventionalists in treating aortic disease, more creative uses of stents are found as shown here. (A) shows a distal aortic stenosis resulting in severe (<50 ft.) claudication in a young female smoker. Following stent placement, the pre-procedure translesional gradient of 60 mm Hg is abolished and there is wide patency of the aorta with an excellent angiographic result (B) and complete relief of symptoms.*

Increasingly, however, cardiologists have begun to direct their efforts toward common non-coronary vascular pathology. The evaluation of renovascular hypertension, renal arterial balloon angioplasty, atherectomy,[164] and stent placement,[165] are all performed by a growing group of cardiovascular interventionalists from cardiologic, radiologic and surgical subspecialties who are capable not only of performing procedures but also of providing clinical care to the severely ill patient. Similarly, the therapy of peripheral vascular disease with local thrombolytic therapy, balloon angioplasty, atherectomy and stent placement are increasingly a part of the complete therapy of the patient with cardiovascular disease.

Many of the conditions treated by the car-diovascular interventionalist are those that are less common or less stereotyped than coronary atherosclerosis but that occur primarily in patients who also have coronary artery disease. The mortality and morbidity suffered by patients with claudication is much more a function of their underlying (sometimes inapparent) coronary artery disease[166] than it is of their peripheral vascular obstruction. Thus, it is appropriate that catheter-based technology be studied which will permit therapy of underlying vascular conditions without compromise of the patient's cardiac status. For example, the percutaneous placement of stent-grafts to control aortic dissection or aneurysm is an active area of investigation[167] in the hope that a less morbid non-

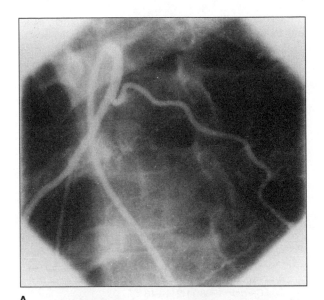

A

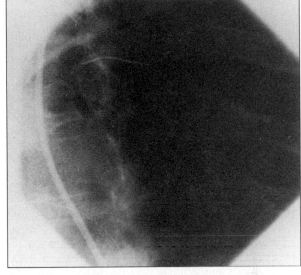

B

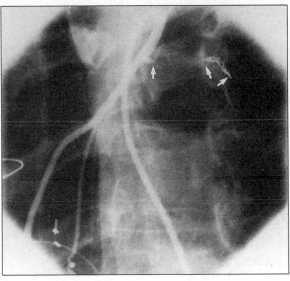

C

Figure 16. *Embolization therapy. This patient had prior coronary bypass surgery that included construction of a left internal mammary artery-LAD anastomosis. Shortly after surgery, the patient noted recurrent angina. Exercise testing with radionuclide imaging showed an area of anterior ischemia. Coronary angiography revealed patency of all grafts and the presence of a large intercostal that had not been ligated at the time of surgery (A). Coronary "steal" was suspected and several fibered coils were delivered to the side branch (B) resulting in its occlusion (C). The symptoms were abolished and a repeat exercise radionuclide exam was improved.*

surgical alternative can be found for these patients.

As technology improves and economic issues become more prominent, it remains important that centers of excellence continue to be developed and maintained where dedicated interventional clinicians can apply skills, creativity, and technology to improve the quality of life of patients with cardiovascular disease.

REFERENCES

1. Gruentzig AR, Senning A, Siegenthaler WE. Nonoperative dilatation of coronary-artery stenosis: Percutaneous transluminal coronary angioplasty. *N Engl J Med.* 1979;301:61-68.
2. Explosive growth of coronary angioplasty. Success story of a less than perfect procedure. *Circulation.* 1993;5:1489-1497. Editorial; comment.
3. Kent KM, Bentivoglio LG, Block PC, et al. Percutaneous transluminal coronary angioplasty: Report from the registry of the National Heart, Lung and Blood Institute. *Am J Cardiol.* 1982;49:2011-2020.
4. Simpson JB, Baim DS, Robert EW, et al. A new catheter system for coronary angioplasty. *Am J Cardiol.* 1982;49:1216-1222.
5. Tuzcu EM, Simpendorfer C, Badhwar K, et al. Determination of primary success in elective percutaneous transluminal coronary angioplasty for significant narrowing of a single major coronary artery. *Am J Cardiol.* 1988;62:873-875.

6. Gruentzig AR, King SB, Schlumpf M, et al. Long-term follow-up after percutaneous transluminal coronary angioplasty. The early Zurich experience. *N Engl J Med.* 1987;316:1127-1132.

7. Cowley MJ, Vetrovec GW, Disciascio G, et al. Coronary angioplasty of multiple vessels: Short term outcome; and long term results. *Circulation.* 1985;72:1314-1320.

8. Weintraub WS, Ghazzal ZM, Douglas JS Jr, et al. Long-term clinical follow-up in patients with angiographic restudy after successful angioplasty. *Circulation.* 1993;3:831-840.

9. King SB III, Schlumpf M. Ten-year completed follow-up of percutaneous transluminal coronary angioplasty: the early Zurich experience. *J Am Coll Cardiol.* 1993;2:353-360.

10. Talley JD, Hurst JW, King SB, et al. Clinical outcome 5 years after attempted percutaneous coronary angioplasty in 427 patients. *Circulation.* 1988;77:820-829.

11. Editorial. BARI, CABRI, EAST, GABI and RITA: Coronary angioplasty on trial. *Lancet.* 1990;335:1315-1316.

12. Anonymous. Protocol for the bypass angioplasty revascularization investigation, *Circulation.* 1991;84(suppl V):V1-V27.

13. Coronary angioplasty versus coronary artery bypass surgery: the Randomised Intervention Treatment of Angina (RITA) trial; RITA trial participant report; *Lancet.* 1993;341:573-600.

14. ACC/AHA Task Force Report. Guidelines for percutaneous transluminal coronary angioplasty. *J Am Coll Cardiol.* 1993;7:2033-2054.

15. Parisi AF, Folland ED, Hartigan P, on behalf of the Veterans Affairs ACME Investigators. A comparison of angioplasty with medical therapy in the treatment of single-vessel coronary artery disease. *N Engl J Med.* 1992;326:10-16.

16. Wohlgelernter D, Cleman M, Highman HA, et al. Percutaneous transluminal coronary angioplasty of the "culprit lesion" for management of unstable angina pectoris in patients with multivessel coronary artery disease. *Am J Cardiol.* 1986;6:460-464.

17. Bell MR, Bailey KR, Reeder GS, et al. Percutaneous transluminal angioplasty in patients with multivessel coronary disease: How important is complete revascularization for cardiac event-free survival? *J Am Coll Cardiol.* 1990;16:553-562.

18. Faxon DP, Ghalill K, Jacobs AK, et al. The degree of revascularization and outcome after multivessel coronary angioplasty. *Am Heart J.* 1992;123:854-859.

19. Cote G, Myler RK, Stertzer SH, et al. Percutaneous transluminal angioplasty of stenotic coronary artery grafts: 5 years experience. *J Am Coll Cardiol.* 1987;9:8-17.

20. Plaiko W, Holman J, Whitlow P, et al. Percutaneous transluminal angioplasty of saphenous vein graft stenoses: long-term follow-up. *J Am Coll Cardiol.* 1989;14:1645-1650.

21. de Feyter PJ, van Suylen RJ, de Jaegere PP, et al. Balloon angioplasty for the treatment of lesions in saphenous vein bypass grafts. *J Am Coll Cardiol.* 1993;7:1539-1549.

22. Ellis SG, Vandormael MG, Cowley MG, et al. Coronary morphologic and clinical determinants of procedural outcome with angioplasty for multi-vessel coronary disease; implications for patient selection. *Circulation.* 1990;82:1193-1202.

23. Stewart JT, Denne L, Bowker TJ, et al. Percutaneous transluminal coronary angioplasty in chronic coronary artery occlusion. *J Am Coll Cardiol.* 1993;6:1371-1376.

24. Ellis SG, Roubin GS, King SB, et al. Angiographic and clinical predictors of acute closure after native vessel coronary angioplasty. *Circulation.* 1988;77:372-379.

25. Ellis SG, Roubin GS, King SB, et al. In-hospital cardiac mortality after acute closure after coronary angioplasty: Analysis of risk factors from 8,207 procedures. *J Am Coll Cardiol.* 1988;11:211-216.

26. Oesterle SN. Angioplasty techniques for stenoses involving coronary artery bifurcations. *Am J Cardiol.* 1988;61:29G-32G.

27. Cameron J, Buchbinder M, Wexler L, et al. Thromboembolic complications of percutaneous transluminal coronary angioplasty for myocardial infarction. *Cathet Cardiovasc Diagn.* 1987;13:100-106.

28. Topol EJ. Integration of anticoagulation, thrombolysis and coronary angioplasty for unstable angina pectoris. *Am J Cardiol.* 1991;68:136B-141B.

29. Ischinger T, Gruentzig AR, Hollman J, et al. Should coronary arteries with less than 60% diameter stenosis be treated by angioplasty? *Circulation.* 1983;68:148-154.

30. Stack RS, Quigley PJ, Collins G, et al. Perfusion balloon catheter. *Am J Cardiol.* 1988;61:77G-80G.

31. Vogel RA, Shawl F, Tommaso C, et al. Initial report of the National Registry of Elective Cardiopulmonary Bypass Supported Coronary Angioplasty. *J Am Coll Cardiol.* 1990;15:23-29.

32. Ellis SG, Myler RK, King SB III, et al. Causes and correlates of death after unsupported coronary angioplasty: implications for use of angioplasty and advanced support techniques in high-risk settings. *Am J Cardiol.* 1991;68:1447-1451.

33. Califf RM, Phillips HR III, Hindman MC, et al. Prognostic value of a coronary artery jeopardy score. *J Am Coll Cardiol.* 1985;5:1055-1063.

34. McAuley BJ, Selmon M, Sheehan J, et al. Coronary angioplasty of high risk patients in a combined catheterization laboratory-operating room setting. *Circulation.* 1985;72(suppl III):217. Abstract.

35. Tommaso CL, Vogel JH, Vogel RA. Coronary angioplasty in high risk patients with left main coronary stenosis: results from the National Registry of Elective Supported Angioplasty. *Cathet Cardiovasc Diagn.* 1992;25:169-173.

36. Jaffe CC, Wohlgelerntner D, Cabin HS, et al. Preservation of left ventricular ejection fraction during percutaneous transluminal coronary angioplasty by distal transcatheter coronary perfusion of oxygenated Fluosol DA 20%. *Am Heart J.* 1988;115:1156-1164.

37. Incorvati RL, Tauberg SG, Pecora M, et al. Clinical applications of coronary sinus retroperfusion during high risk percutaneous transluminal coronary angioplasty. *J Am Coll Cardiol.* 1993;22:127-134.

38. Gacioch GM, Topol EJ. Sudden paradoxic clinical deterioration during angioplasty of the occluded right coronary artery in acute myocardial infarction. *J Am Coll Cardiol.* 1989;14:1202-1209.

39. Erbel R, Clas W, Busch U, et al. New balloon catheter for prolonged percutaneous transluminal coronary angioplasty and bypass flow in occluded vessels. *Cathet Cardiovasc Diagn.* 1986;12:116-123.

40. Turi ZG, Rezkalla S, Campbell CA, et al. Amelioration of ischemia during angioplasty of the left anterior descending coronary artery with an autoperfusion catheter. *Am J Cardiol.* 1988;62:513-517.

41. Turi ZG, Campbell CA, Gottimukkala MV, et al. Preservation of distal coronary perfusion during prolonged balloon inflation with an autoperfusion angioplasty catheter. *Circulation.* 1987;75:1273-1280.

42. Cohen BM, Buchbinder M, Kozina J, et al. Rethrombosis during angioplasty in myocardial infarction and unstable syndromes: Efficacy of intracoronary urokinase and redilation. *Circulation.* 1988;78(suppl): II-8. Abstract.

43. Ferguson TB Jr, Hinohara T, Simpson J, et al. Catheter reperfusion to allow optimal coronary bypass grafting following failed transluminal coronary angioplasty. *Ann Thorac Surg.* 1986;42:399-405.

44. Van der Linden LP, Bakx AL, Sedney MI, et al. Prolonged dilatation with an autoperfusion catheter for refractory acute occlusion related to percutaneous transluminal coronary angioplasty. *J Am Coll Cardiol.* 1993;22:1016-1023.

45. Mc Keever LS, Marek JC, Kerwin PM, et al. Bail-out directional atherectomy for abrupt coronary occlusion following conventional angioplasty. *Cathet Cardiovasc Diagn.* 1993;(suppl I):31-36.

46. Block PC, Myler RK, Stertzer S, et al. Morphology after transluminal angioplasty in human beings. *N Engl J Med.* 1981;305:382-384.

47. Soward AL, Essed CE, Serruys PW. Coronary arterial findings after accidental death immediately after successful percutaneous transluminal coronary angioplasty. *Am J Cardiol.* 1985; 56:794-795.

48. Mizuno K, Kurita A, Imazeki N. Pathologal findings after percutaneous transluminal coronary angioplasty. *Br Heart J.* 1984;52:588-590.

49. Waller BF, Gorfinkel HJ, Rogers FJ, et al. Early and late morphologic changes in major epicardial coronary arteries after percutaneous transluminal coronary angioplasty. *Am J Cardiol.* 1984;53:42C-47C.

50. Waller BF. "Crackers, breakers, stretchers, drillers, scrapers, shavers, burners, welders and melters." The future treatment of atherosclerotic coronary disease? A clinical-morphologic assessment. *J Am Coll Cardiol.* 1989;13:969-987.

51. Jain A, Demer LL, Raizner AE, et al. In vivo assessment of vascular dilatation during percutaneous transluminal coronary angioplasty. *Am J Cardiol.* 1987;60:988-992.

52. Levin DC, Boxt LM, Abben R, et al. Sequential balloon technique in angioplasty of severe coronary arterial obstructions. *Am J Cardiol.* 1985;56:789-791.

53. Simpfendorfer C, Belardi J, Bellamy G, et al. Frequency, management and follow-up of patients with acute coronary occlusions after percutaneous transluminal coronary angioplasty. *Am J Cardiol.* 1987;59:267-269.

54. Matthews BJ, Ewels CJ, Kent KM. Coronary dissection: A predictor of restenosis? *Am Heart J.* 1988;115:547-554.

55. Leimgruber PP, Roubin GS, Anderson HV, et al. Influence of intimal dissection on restenosis after successful coronary angioplasty. *Circulation.* 1985;72:530-535.

56. Leimgruber PP, Roubin GS, Hollman J, et al. Restenosis after successful coronary angioplasty in patients with single-vessel disease. *Circulation.* 1986;73:710-717.

57. Bredlau CE, Roubin GS, Leimgruber PP, et al. In-hospital morbidity and mortality in patients undergoing elective coronary angioplasty. *Circulation.* 1985;72:1044-1052.

58. Cowley MJ, Dorros G, Kelsey SF, et al. Emergency coronary bypass surgery after coronary angioplasty: The National Heart, Lung, and Blood Institute's Percutaneous Transluminal Coronary Angioplasty Registry experience. *Am J Cardiol.* 1984;53:22C-26C.

59. George BS, Voorhees WD, Roubin GS, et al. Multicenter Investigation of Coronary stenting to treat acute or threatened closure after percutaneous transluminal angioplasty: clinical and angiographic outcomes. *J Am Coll Cardiol.* 1993;22:135-143.

60. Fischell TA, Derby G, Tse TM, et al. Coronary artery vasoconstriction routinely occurs after percutaneous transluminal coronary angioplasty — a quantitative arteriographic analysis. *Circulation.* 1988;78:1323-1334.

61. Holmes DR Jr, Vlietstra RE, Smith HC, et al. Restenosis after percutaneous transluminal coronary angioplasty (PTCA): A report from the PTCA Registry of the National Heart, Lung, and Blood Institute. *Am J Cardiol.* 1984;53:77C-81C.

62. Meier B, King SB III, Gruentzig AR, et al. Repeat coronary angioplasty. *J Am Coll Cardiol.* 1984;4:463-466.

63. Serruys PW, Luitjen HE, Beatt KJ, et al. Incidence of restenosis after successful coronary angioplasty: A time-related phenomenon. A quantitative angiographic study in 342 consecutive patients at 1, 2, 3, and 4 months. *Circulation.* 1988;77:361-371.

64. Nobuyoshi M, Kimura T, Nosaka H, et al. Restenosis after successful percutaneous transluminal coronary

angioplasty: Serial angiographic follow-up of 229 patients. *J Am Coll Cardiol.* 1988;12:616-623.

65. Quigley PJ, Hlatky MA, Hinohara T, et al. Repeat percutaneous transluminal coronary angioplasty and predictors of recurrent restenosis. *Am J Cardiol.* 1989;63:409-413.

66. Glazier JJ, Varricchione TR, Ryan TJ, et al. Factors predicting recurrent restenosis after percutaneous transluminal coronary balloon angioplasty. *Am J Cardiol.* 1989;63:902-905.

67. Bonan R. Angioplasty and restenosis revisited: Diagnosis and management of restenosis. *J Invasive Cardiol.* 1989;1:69-75.

68. Teirstein PS, Hoover CA, Ligon RW, et al. Repeat coronary angioplasty: Efficacy of a third angioplasty for a second restenosis. *J Am Coll Cardiol.* 1989;13:291-296.

69. Faxon DP, Sanborn TA, Haudenschild CC. Mechanism of angioplasty and its relation to restenosis. *Am J Cardiol.* 1987;60:5B-9B.

70. Harker LA. Role of platelets and thrombosis in mechanisms of acute occlusion and restenosis after angioplasty. *Am J Cardiol.* 1987;60:20B-28B

71. Ross R. The pathogenesis of atherosclerosis—an update. *N Engl J Med.* 1986;314:488-500.

72. Fuster V, Badimon L, Cohen M, et al. Insights into the pathogenesis of acute ischemic syndromes. *Circulation.* 1988;77:1213-1220.

73. Simons M, Leclerc G, Satan RD, et al. Relation between activated smooth-muscle cells in coronary-artery lesions and restenosis after atherectomy. *N Engl J Med.* 1993;328:608-613.

74. Riessen R, Rahimizadeh H, Takeshita S, et al. Successful vascular gene transfer using a hydrogel-coated balloon angioplasty catheter. *J Am Coll Cardiol* 1993;21:74A. Abstract.

75. Coller BS, Scudder LE, Berger HJ. Inhibition of human platelet function in vivo with a monoclonal antibody with observation on the newly dead as experimental subjects. *Ann Intern Med.* 1988;109:635-638.

76. Gold HK, Coller BS, Yasuda T, et al. Rapid and sustained coronary artery recanalization with combined bolus injection of recombinant tissue-type plasminogen activator and monoclonal antiplatelet GIIb/IIIa antibody in a canine preparation. *Circulation.* 1988;77:670-677.

77. Simons M, Edelman ER, DeKeyser J, et al. Antisense c-myb oligonucleotides inhibit intimal arterial smooth muscle cell accumulation in vivo. *Nature.* 1992;359:67-70.

78. Harker LA, Fuster V. Pharmacology of platelet inhibitors. *J Am Coll Cardiol.* 1986;8(suppl):21B-32B.

79. Kyrle PA, Eichler HG, Jager U, et al. Inhibition of prostacyclin and thromboxane A_2 generation by low-dose aspirin at the site of plug formation in man in vivo. *Circulation.* 1987;75:1025-1029.

80. Blackshear JL, O'Callaghan WG, Califf RM. Medical approaches to prevention of restenosis after coronary angioplasty. *J Am Coll Cardiol.* 1987;9:834-848.

81. Dehmer GJ, Popma JJ, Van den Berg EK, et al. Reduction in the rate of early restenosis after coronary angioplasty by a diet supplemented with n-3 fatty acids. *N Engl J Med.* 1988;319:733-740.

82. Gapinski JP, VanRuiswyk JV, Heudebert GR, et al. Preventing restenosis with fish oils following coronary angioplasty. A meta-analysis. *Arch Intern Med.* 1993;153:1595-1601.

83. Grigg LE, Kay TWH, Valentine PA, et al. Determinants of restenosis and lack of effect of dietary supplementation with eicosapentaenoic acid on the incidence of coronary artery restenosis after angioplasty. *J Am Coll Cardiol.* 1989;13:665-672.

84. Bellows SD, Clugston RA, Kloner RA, et al. A porcine model of postangioplasty "restenosis": effects of cholesterol. *J Vasc Med Biol.* 1993;4:64-69.

85. Sahni R, Maniet AR, Voci G, et al. Prevention of restenosis by lovastatin after successful coronary angioplasty. *Am Heart J.* 1991;122:171-187.

86. Weintraub WS, Bocuzzi SJ, Brown CL, et al. Background and methods for the lovastatin restenosis trial after percutaneous transluminal coronary angioplasty. *Am J Cardiol.* 1992;70:293-299.

87. Weintraub WS, Kosinski AS, Brown CL, et al. Can restenosis after coronary angioplasty be predicted from clinical variables? *J Am Coll Cardiol.* 1993;21:6-14.

88. Kuntz RE, Safian RD, Schmidt DA, et al. Novel approach to the analysis of restenosis after the use of three new coronary devices. *J Am Coll Cardiol.* 1992;19:1493-1499.

89. Kuntz RE, Safian RD, Carrozza JP, et al. The importance of acute luminal diameter in determining restenosis after coronary atherectomy or stenting. *Circulation.* 1992;86:1827-1835.

90. Kuntz RE, Gibson CM, Nobuyoshi M, et al. A generalized model of restenosis following conventional balloon angioplasty, stenting, and directional atherectomy. *J Am Coll Cardiol.* 1993;21:15-25.

91. Topol EJ, Leya F, Pinkerton CA, et al. A comparison of directional atherectomy with coronary angioplasty in patients with coronary artery disease. *N Engl J Med.* 1993;329:223-227.

92. Adelman AG, Cohen EA, Kimball BP, et al. A comparison of directional atherectomy with balloon angioplasty for lesions of the left anterior descending coronary artery. *N Engl J Med.* 1993;329:228-233.

93. Safian RD. Coronary atherectomy versus angioplasty. *N Engl J Med.* 1993;329:1891. Letter.

94. Meyer J, Merx W, Schmitz H, et al. Percutaneous transluminal coronary angioplasty immediately after intracoronary streptolysis of transmural myocardial infarction. *Circulation.* 1982;66:905-913.

95. Hartzler GO, Rutherford BD, McConahay DR, et al. Percutaneous transluminal coronary angioplasty with and without thrombolytic therapy for treatment of acute myocardial infarction. *Am Heart J.* 1983;106:965-973.

96. O'Neill WW, Brodie B, Knopf W, et al. Initial report of the primary angioplasty revascularization (PAR) multicenter registry. *Circulation.* 1991;84(suppl 2):II-536. Abstract.

97. The TIMI Study Group. Comparison of invasive and conservative strategies after treatment with intravenous tissue plasminogen activator in acute myocardial infarction. Results of the thrombolysis in myocardial infarction (TIMI) phase II trial. *N Engl J Med.* 1989;320:618-627.

98. Guerci AD, Gerstenblith G, Brinker JA, et al. A randomized trial of intravenous tissue plasminogen activator for acute myocardial infarction with subsequent randomization to elective coronary angioplasty. *N Engl J Med.* 1987;317:1613-1618.

99. Topol EJ, Califf RM, George BS, et al. A randomized trial of immediate versus delayed elective angioplasty after intravenous tissue plasminogen activator in acute myocardial infarction. *N Engl J Med.* 1987;317:581-588.

100. Sinclair IN, McCabe CH, Sipperly ME, et al. Predictors, therapeutic options and long-term outcome of abrupt reclosure. *Am J Cardiol.* 1988;61:61G-66G.

101. Rutherford BD, Hartzler GO, McConahay R, et al. Direct balloon angioplasty in myocardial infarction: Long-term results. *Circulation.* 1988;78:II-502. Abstract.

102. Giorgi LV, Rutherford BD, Hartzler GO, et al. Direct PTCA for acute MI in patients commonly excluded from thrombolytic trials. *Circulation.* 1988;78(suppl II):377. Abstract.

103. Lee L, Bates ER, Pitt B, et al. Percutaneous transluminal coronary angioplasty improves survival in acute myocardial infarction complicated by cardiogenic shock. *Circulation.* 1988;78:1345-1351.

104. O'Neill WW. Primary percutaneous coronary angioplasty: A protagonist's view. *Am J Cardiol.* 1988;62:15K-20K.

105. Stack RS, Califf RM, Hinohara T, et al. Survival and cardiac event rates in the first year after emergency coronary angioplasty for acute myocardial infarction. *J Am Coll Cardiol.* 1988;11:1141-1149.

106. Topol EJ, Califf RM, George BS, et al. Coronary arterial thrombolysis with combined infusion of recombinant tissue-type plasminogen activator and urokinase in patients with acute myocardial infarction. *Circulation.* 1988;77:1100-1107.

107. Hochman JS, Choo H. Limitation of myocardial infarct expansion by reperfusion independent of myocardial salvage. *Circulation.* 1987;75:299-306.

108. Sager PT, Perlmutter RA, Rosenfeld LE, et al. Electrophysiologic effects of thrombolytic therapy in patients with a transmural anterior myocardial infarction complicated by left ventricular aneurysm formation. *J Am Coll Cardiol.* 1988;12:19-24.

109. ISIS-2 (Second International Study of Infarct Survival) Collaborative Group. Randomized trial of intravenous streptokinase, oral aspirin, both, or neither among 17,187 cases of suspected acute myocardial infarction: ISIS-2. *Lancet.* 1988;2:349-360.

110. Eisenhauer AC, Matthews RV, Moore L. Late direct angioplasty in patients with myocardial infarction and fluctuating chest pain. *Am Heart J.* 1992;123:553-559.

111. Ellis SG, O'Neill WW, Bates ER, et al. Coronary angioplasty as primary therapy for acute myocardial infarction 6 to 48 hours after symptom onset: Report of an initial experience. *J Am Coll Cardiol.* 1989;13:1122-1126.

112. Grines CL, Browne KF, Marco J, et al. Comparison of immediate angioplasty with thrombolytic therapy for acute myocardial infarction. *N Engl J Med* 1993;328:673-679.

113. Zijlstra F, de Boer MJ, Hoorntje JC, et al. A comparison of immediate coronary angioplasty with intravenous streptokinase in acute myocardial infarction. *N Engl J Med.* 1993;328:680-684.

114. Gibbons RJ, Holmes DR, Reeder GS, et al. Immediate angioplasty compared with the administration of a thrombolytic agent followed by conservative treatment for myocardial infarction. *N Engl J Med.* 1993;328:685-691.

115. Simpson JB, Selmon MR, Robertson GC, et al. Transluminal atherectomy for occlusive peripheral vascular disease. *Am J Cardiol.* 1988;61:96G-101G.

116. Stack R. New interventional technology. *Am J Cardiol.* 1988;62:3F-24F.

117. Auth DC. Angioplasty with high speed rotary ablation. In: Serruys PW (ed). *Restenosis After Intervention With New Mechanical Devices.* New York: Kluwer Academic Publishers; 1992:275-288.

118. Mintz GS, Potkin BN, Karen G, et al. Intravascular ultrasound evaluation of the effect of rotational atherectomy in obstructive atherosclerotic coronary artery disease. *Circulation.* 1992;5:1383-1393.

119. Hansen DD, Auth DC, Hall M, et al. Rotational endarterectomy in normal canine arteries: preliminary report. *J Am Coll Cardiol.* 1988;5:1073-1077.

120. Hansen DD, Auth DC, Vracko R, et al. Rotational atherectomy in atherosclerotic rabbit iliac arteries. *Am Heart J.* 1988;115:160-165.

121. Stertzer SH, Rosenblum J, Shaw RE, et al. Coronary rotational ablation: initial experience in 302 procedures. *J Am Coll Cardiol.* 1993;2:296-297.

122. Sigwart U, Puel J, Mirkovitch V, et al. Intravascular stents to prevent occlusion and restenosis after transluminal angioplasty. *N Engl J Med.* 1987;316:701-706.

123. Roubin GS, Cannon AD, Agrawal SK, et al. Intracoronary stenting for acute and threatened closure complicating percutaneous transluminal coronary angioplasty. *Circulation.* 1992;3:916-927.

124. Gibson CM, Kuntz RE, Nobuyoshi M, et al. Lesion-to-lesion independence of restenosis after treatment by conventional angioplasty, stenting, or directional atherectomy. Validation of lesion-based restenosis analysis. *Circulation.* 1993;4:1123-1129.

125. Haudenschild CC. Pathobiology of restenosis after angioplasty. *Am J Med.* 1993;94:40S-44S.

126. de Jaegere PP, de Feyter PJ, van der Giessen WJ, et al. Endovascular stents: preliminary clinical results and future developments. *Clin Cardiol.* 1993;16:369-378.

127. Urban P, Sigwart U, Golf S, et al. Intravascular stenting for stenosis of aortocoronary venous bypass grafts. *J Am Coll Cardiol.* 1989;13:1085-1097.

128. Serruys PW, Strauss BH, Beatt KJ, et al. Angiographic follow-up after placement of a self-expanding coronary-artery stent. *N Engl J Med.* 1991;324:1595-1598.

129. Carrozza JP Jr, Kuntz RE, Levine MJ, et al. Angiographic and clinical outcome of intracoronary stenting: Immediate and long-term results from a large single-center experience. *J Am Coll Cardiol.* 1992;20:328-337.

130. Sanborn TA, Faxon DP, Kellet MA. Percutaneous coronary laser thermal angioplasty. *J Am Coll Cardiol.* 1986;8:1437-1440.

131. Litvack F, Grundfest W, Hickey A, et al. Percutaneous coronary excimer laser angioplasty in animals and human. *J Am Coll Cardiol.* 1989;13:61A.

132. Grundfest WS, Litvack F, Forrester JS, et al. Laser ablation of human atherosclerotic plaque without adjacent tissue injury. *J Am Coll Cardiol.* 1985;5:929-932.

133. Litvack F, Grundfest WS, Papaloannou T, et al. Role of laser and thermal ablation devices in the treatment of vascular diseases. *Am J Cardiol.* 1988;61:81G.

134. Reeder GS, Bresnahan JF, Holmes DR Jr, et al. Excimer laser coronary angioplasty: results in restenosis versus de novo coronary lesions. *Cathet Cardiovasc Diagn.* 1992;3:195-199.

135. Heuser RR, Mehta SS. Holmium laser angioplasty after failed coronary balloon dilation: use of a new solid-state, infrared laser system. *Cathet Cardiovasc Diagn.* 1991;3:187-189.

136. Rashkind WJ, Miller WW. Creation of an atrial septal defect without thoracotomy: A Palliative approach to complete transposition of the great arteries. *JAMA.* 1966;196:991-992.

137. Park SC, Zuberbuhler JR, Neches WH, et al. A new atrial septostomy technique. *Cathet Cardiovasc Diagn.* 1975;1:195-201.

138. Semb BKH, Tjonneland S, Stake G, et al. "Balloon valvulotomy" of congenital pulmonary valve stenosis with tricuspid valve insufficiency. *Cardiovasc Radiol.* 1979;2:239-241.

139. Kan JS, White RI Jr, Mitchell SE, et al. Percutaneous balloon valvuloplasty: A new method for treating congenital pulmonary valve stenosis. *N Engl J Med.* 1982;307:540-542.

140. Kveselis DA, Rocchini AP, Snider AR, et al. Results of balloon valvuloplasty in the treatment of congenital valvar pulmonary stenosis in children. *Am J Cardiol.* 1985;56:527-532.

141. Ali Khan MA, Yousef SA, Mullins CE. Percutaneous transluminal balloon pulmonary valvuloplasty for the relief of pulmonary valve stenosis with special reference to dou-ble balloon technique. *Am Heart J.* 1986;112:158-166.

142. Radtke W, Keane JF, Fellows KE, et al. Percutaneous balloon valvotomy of congenital pulmonary stenosis using oversized balloons. *J Am Coll Cardiol.* 1986;8:909-915.

143. Lock JE, Khalilullah M, Shrivastava S, et al. Percutaneous catheter commissurotomy in rheumatic mitral stenosis. *N Engl J Med.* 1985;313:1515-1518.

144. McKay RG, Lock JE, Keane JF, et al. Percutaneous mitral valvuloplasty in an adult patient with calcific rheumatic mitral stenosis. *J Am Coll Cardiol.* 1986;7:1410-1415.

145. Palacios IF, Lock JE, Keane JF, et al. Percutaneous transvenous balloon valvotomy in a patient with severe calcific mitral stenosis. *J Am Coll Cardiol.* 1986;7:1416-1419.

146. Wilkins GT, Weyman AE, Abascal VM, et al. Percutaneous balloon dilatation of the mitral valve: An analysis of echocardiographic variables related to outcome and the mechanism of dilatation. *Br Heart J.* 1988;60:299-308.

147. Meier B, Friedli B, Oberhaenlsi I, et al. Trefoil balloon for percutaneous valvuloplasty. *Cathet Cardiovasc Diagn.* 1986;12:277-281.

148. Park, SJ, Kim JJ, Song JK, et al. Immediate and one year results of percutaneous mitral balloon valvuloplasty using the Inoue and double-balloon techniques. *Am J Cardiol.* 1993;71:938-943.

149. Palacios IF, Block PC, Brandi S, et al. Percutaneous balloon valvotomy for patients with severe mitral stenosis. *Circulation.* 1987;75:778-784.

150. Vahanian A, Michel PL, Cormier B, et al. Results of percutaneous mitral commissurotomy in 200 patients. *Am J Cardiol.* 1989;63:847-852.

151. McKay RG, Lock JE, Safian RD, et al. Balloon dilation of mitral stenosis in adult patients: Postmortem and percutaneous mitral valvuloplasty studies. *J Am Coll Cardiol.* 1987;9:723-731.

152. John S, Bashi VV, Jairaj PS, et al. Closed mitral valvotomy: Early results and long-term follow-up of 3,724 consecutive patients. *Circulation.* 1983;68:891-896.

153. Roberts WC. Good-bye to thoracotomy for cardiac valvulotomy. *Am J Cardiol.* 1987; 59:198-202. Editorial.

154. Cheng TO. Percutaneous balloon mitral valvuloplasty: are Chinese and Western experiences comparable? *Cathet Cardiovasc Diagn.* 1994;31:23-28.

155. McKay RG, Safian RD, Lock JE, et al. Balloon dilatation of calcific aortic stenosis in elderly patients: Postmortem, intraoperative, and percutaneous valvuloplasty studies. *Circulation.* 1986;74:119-125.

156. Block PC, Palacios IF. Clinical and hemodynamic follow-up after percutaneous aortic valvuloplasty in the elderly. *Am J Cardiol.* 1988;62:760-763.

157. Lieberman EB, Hermiller JB, Pieper KS, et al. Balloon aortic valvuloplasty: The final chapter. *Circulation.* 1992;86:I595. Abstract.

158. Letac B, Cribier A, Koning R, et al. Results of percuta-

neous transluminal valvuloplasty in 218 adults with valvular aortic stenosis. *Am J Cardiol.* 1988;62:598-605.

159. Roth RB, Palacios IF, Block PC. Percutaneous aortic balloon valvuloplasty: Its role in the management of patients with aortic stenosis requiring major noncardiac surgery. *J Am Coll Cardiol.* 1989;13:1039-1041.

160. Bernard Y, Etievent J, Mourand JL, et al. Long-term results of percutaneous aortic valvuloplasty compared with aortic valve replacement in patients more than 75 years old. *J Am Coll Cardiol.* 1992;20:796-801.

161. Gray DT, Fyler DC, Walker AM, et al. Clinical outcomes and costs of transcatheter as compared with surgical closure of patent ductus arteriosus. *N Engl J Med.* 1993;329:1517-1523.

162. Rome JJ, Keane JF, Perry SB, et al. Double umbrella closure of atrial defects. Initial clinical applications. *Circulation.* 1990;80:751-758.

163. Ruiz CE, Gamra H, Zhang HP, et al. Brief report: stenting of the ductus arteriosus as a bridge to cardiac transplantation in infants with the hypoplastic left heart syndrome. *N Engl J Med.* 1993;328:1605-1608.

164. Dake MD, Oesterle SN, Robertson GR, et al. Percutaneous directional atherectomy for treatment of rerenal artery stenosis. *Radiology.* 1991;181:295. Abstract.

165. Dorros G, Prince C, Mathiak. Stenting of a renal artery stenosis achieves better relief of the obstructive lesion than balloon angioplasty. *Cathet Cardiovasc Diagn.* 1993;29:191-198.

166. Hertzer NR. The natural history of peripheral vascular disease: implications for its management. *Circulation.* 1991;(suppl I)83:I12-I19.

167. Chuter T, Green RM, Ouriel K, et al. Transfemoral endovascular aortic graft placement. *J Vasc Surg.* 1993;18:185-197.

CHAPTER 18 Valvular Heart Disease

Sylvia A. Mamby, MD

Valvular heart disease continues to be a dominant factor in the spectrum of cardiovascular disease. While rheumatic fever is no longer the major etiologic consideration, documentation of several sporadic outbreaks of the disease indicates a clear resurgence.

Cardiovascular ultrasound remains the predominant method by which valvular heart pathology is characterized, quantified, and judged regarding the need for definitive intervention. The safety, facility, relative low cost, and reproducibility of echocardiography makes it the ideal tool. Invasive diagnostic studies to assess valvular pathology are performed far less frequently than in the past. However, the technique remains the standard, particularly in settings of limited noninvasive data. Most commonly, however, coronary angiography is performed to evaluate concomitant coronary artery disease.

Finally, the concept of timing for intervention has become increasingly important. Long-term investigations through either the continued pursuit of science and/or socioeconomic demand continue to emerge and elucidate our understanding of appropriate timing of intervention.

RHEUMATIC FEVER AND RHEUMATIC CARDITIS

Overall, the incidence of rheumatic fever has declined considerably in the United States over the past 100 years. Reasons for the decline are debatable; however, improved health care, including the emergence of antimicrobial agents (although the decline predated this era), diminished household overcrowding, and socioeconomic factors are all believed to have contributed.[1]

Despite this decline, several recent outbreaks of acute rheumatic fever have been reported in Utah, northeastern Ohio, western Pennsylvania, Tennessee, and at a naval training center in San Diego, California.[2-6] The explanation for this resurgence, which began in the mid-1980s, is unclear; however, theories relate primarily to 2 considerations. New strains of streptococci associated with outbreaks of rheumatic fever have recently been demonstrated.[7] Secondly, there has been an increase in the numbers of immigrants entering the United States from territories where rheumatic fever remains prevalent. There is some evidence that patients with rheumatic fever have a genetic predisposition, i.e., that the abnormal immune response is genetically programmed. Using a monoclonal antibody, a B-cell marker has been identified in 90% to 100% of all patients with rheumatic fever tested in 5 different geographical ethnic populations under study.[8]

Acute rheumatic fever is characterized by exudative and proliferative inflammatory lesions of the connective tissues, particularly the heart, joints, and subcutaneous tissues. Later in the course of the disease, circumvascular inflammatory lesions called Aschoff's nodules develop in the heart and are considered pathognomonic. These nodules consist of central areas of fibrosis within a zone of lymphocytes, plasma cells, and large basophilic cells.

Clinically, rheumatic fever presents itself as a generalized inflammatory disease complicating an upper respiratory infection. It tends to affect young people 5-15 years of age, and is generally uncommon in adults. Although the precise mechanism by which the bacterium triggers the inflammatory response is unknown, current belief favors the theory of autoimmunity, whereby tissue damage is created by the body's own immunologic response to the antecedent streptococcal infection. This indeed is supported by the relatively long latency between pharyngitis and acute rheumatic fever.

The Jones criteria, proposed to guide the diagnosis of acute rheumatic fever, were established in 1944.[9] Since this time, subcommittees of the American Heart Association have modified and revised these criteria.[10-12] A high probability of acute rheumatic fever is likely in the presence of 2 major or 1 major and 2 minor criteria, if supported by evidence of a preceding Group A streptococcal infection (Table 1). Symptoms include fever, chills, migratory polyarthritis, fatigue, weakness, irritability, and epistaxis. Though nonspecific, tachycardia out of proportion to fever which persists during sleep is often present. When carditis develops, it typically involves the pericardium, myocardium, and endocardium, and clinically a murmur of valvulitis is nearly always present. When a murmur is not present, one should diagnose isolated myocarditis or pericarditis due to cardiac rheumatic involvement with great reluctance.

The diagnosis of rheumatic fever may be made without firm adherence to the Jones criteria in 3 situations. Chorea may present itself as the only manifestation of rheumatic fever. Carditis may also present in this manner. Finally, in those with a history of rheumatic fever or rheumatic heart disease (typically at increased risk for recurrences), a high level of suspicion for the diagnosis should be present with any rheumatic complaint.[12]

On chest x-ray, an enlarged cardiac silhouette may be seen and is due to cardiac chamber enlargement or pericardial effusion. Signs of congestive heart failure may also be evident.

Electrocardiographic findings, primarily PR-interval prolongation, are frequently observed. Other abnormalities include sinus tachycardia, second-and third-degree heart block, diminished voltage of QRS complexes, and prolongation of the QT interval. With pericarditis, the ST segments are elevated; however, with myocarditis, ST-segment changes are often nonspecific.

Table 1. Guidelines for the Diagnosis of Initial Attack of Rheumatic Fever (Jones Criteria, Updated 1992)*

MAJOR MANIFESTATIONS	MINOR MANIFESTATIONS	SUPPORTING EVIDENCE OF ANTECEDENT GROUP A STREPTOCOCCAL INFECTION
Carditis	Clinical findings	Positive throat culture or rapid
Polyarthritis	Arthralgia	streptococcal antigen test
Chorea	Fever	Elevated or rising streptococcal
Erythema marginatum	Laboratory findings	antibody titer
Subcutaneous nodules	Elevated acute phase reactants	
	Erythrocyte sedimentation rate	
	C-reactive protein	
	Prolonged PR interval	

*If supported by evidence of preceding Group A streptococcal infection, the presence of 2 major manifestations or of 1 major and 2 minor manifestations indicates a high probability of acute rheumatic fever.

From the Special Writing Group of the Committee on Rheumatic Fever, Endocarditis, and Kawasaki Disease of the Council on Cardiovascular Disease in the Young of the American Heart Association. Guidelines for the Diagnosis of Rheumatic Fever. Jones Criteria, 1992 Update. *JAMA*. 1992;268:2069-2073.

Supraventricular and ventricular tachyarrhythmias also occur.

Therapy for acute rheumatic fever includes rest and sodium restriction. The arthritic component usually responds to salicylates. Although antibiotic therapy neither alters the course of rheumatic fever nor influences the development of carditis, antibiotics are indicated to eradicate the streptococcal infection. The following regimens are suggested: benzathine penicillin G 600,000 units IM for children <27 kg; benzathine penicillin G 1.2 million units for children >27 kg and adults; penicillin V 125-250 mg po qid for 10 days, or erythromycin 250 mg po qid for 10 days. Occasionally, prednisone 40-60 mg/day is given to patients with marked cardiac dysfunction. Prednisone will reduce the symptoms of rheumatic fever but does not shorten its course or prevent cardiac sequelae. Long-term rheumatic fever prophylaxis helps prevent recurrent attacks of rheumatic fever and subsequent cardiac damage. The most effective regimen appears to be 1.2 million units benzathine penicillin G monthly. The duration of the prophylaxis is debatable. Some clinicians suggest a lifelong regimen; others favor an individualized approach, since increasing age and disease-free interval from the previous attack are associated with a diminished likelihood of recurrence.

The development of valvular lesions is gradual, requiring 10-30 years to become manifest. In rheumatic heart disease, the mitral valve is involved in approximately 85% of cases, the aortic valve in 44%, and the tricuspid valve in 10% to 16%; the pulmonic valve is rarely involved.

MITRAL STENOSIS

By far the most common etiology of mitral stenosis is rheumatic heart disease. Congenital forms of mitral stenosis also occur, but rarely. Typically, rheumatic mitral stenosis is manifested by fusion of the valve leaflet cusps, and thickening and shortening of the chordae (Fig. 1). Subsequently, calcium deposition within the valve leaflets compounds the problem. The normal mitral valve area is 4–6 cm². The severity of symptoms depends primarily on the degree of stenosis. As the valve area decreases, a

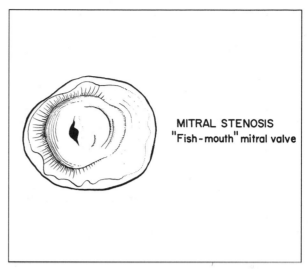

Figure 1. *Looking down into the left atrium at a stenotic mitral valve. The mitral valve leaflets are thickened with fusion of the commissures. The mitral valve orifice has a narrowed "fish-mouth" appearance.*

greater pressure gradient is required to generate flow from the left atrium to the left ventricle, resulting in substantial left atrial pressures. With increases in blood flow or reduction of mitral valve area, the gradient across the valve increases, thereby increasing both left atrial and pulmonary venous pressure (Fig. 2). Once pulmonary venous (capillary) pressure exceeds plasma oncotic pressure, transudation of fluid occurs (one of the mechanisms of hemoptysis in this disease). Subsequently, pulmonary arteriolar resistance increases and impedes right ventricular performance. The right ventricle hypertrophies, dilates, and ultimately fails. The left atrium, which also becomes severely dilated over time, may develop atrial fibrillation, losing its effective contraction. Rapid heart rates are poorly tolerated in mitral stenosis, allowing less time for already impaired ventricular filling to occur, and result in even higher left atrial pressures.

The progression of mitral stenosis is chronic and variable. Most commonly, symptoms begin in the patient's fourth decade of life. Mitral stenosis is far more common in women and may become evident with the onset of atrial fibrillation and pregnancy.

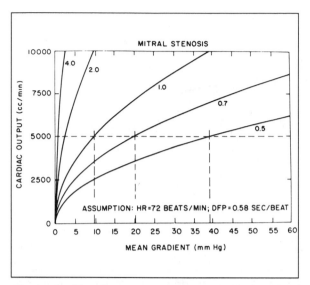

Figure 2. Cardiac output and mean transmitral pressure gradient for various mitral valve areas. The gradient increases for a variety of valve areas as cardiac output increases. From Carabello BA, Grossman W. Calculation of stenotic valve orifice area. In: Grossman W (ed). Cardiac Catheterization and Angiography, 4th ed. Philadelphia: Lea & Febiger; 1990. With permission.

DIAGNOSIS

Patients primarily complain of dyspnea, with progressive limitations on physical exertion as mitral stenosis worsens. Patients will also manifest orthopnea, paroxysmal nocturnal dyspnea, fatigue, weakness, and hemoptysis. When pulmonary vascular resistance increases, there may be a transient period during which left-sided symptoms diminish and right-sided symptoms increase. With advanced mitral stenosis, symptoms of right heart failure develop, including nausea, anorexia and right upper quadrant pain (secondary to hepatic congestion), ascites, hoarseness, and peripheral edema. Hoarseness, the primary manifestation of Ortner's syndrome, is created by compression of the left recurrent laryngeal nerve between the enlarged pulmonary artery, the aorta, and the ligamentum arteriosum, and not by the enlarged left atrium, as has often been assumed.[13] Chest pain can occur and is thought to be related to developing pulmonary hypertension. However, angina due to concomitant coronary artery disease may also be present. In 1 necropsy study of patients with mitral stenosis who were more than 30 years old, 50% had significant narrowing of at least 1 major epicardial coronary artery.[14]

Physical examination reveals characteristic ruddy cheeks (so-called mitral facies) and usually a normal arterial pulse unless atrial fibrillation is present. Rales may be present depending on the degree of interstitial and alveolar edema. With increased right-sided pressures, jugular venous distention is present, with a prominent a wave in patients in sinus rhythm. Palpitation reveals a normal or reduced left ventricular impulse, and often a right ventricular heave. Auscultation typically reveals a prominent S_1, a loud P_2 if pulmonary hypertension is present, and an opening snap occurring after the S_2. The murmur is a low-pitched diastolic rumble that begins with the opening snap and becomes loudest just before S_1 (presystolic accentuation). The opening snap is a high-pitched sound believed to be created by sudden tensing of the anterior mitral valve leaflet by the chordae tendineae after cuspal opening. Its presence implies valve mobility. The interval between A_2 and the opening snap has been used to estimate the severity of mitral stenosis. A shorter interval (<0.06–0.07 sec) suggests higher left atrial pressure, which supports more severe mitral stenosis. The reverse is not always true, however, since in elderly patients or those with systemic hypertension the decline in left ventricular systolic pressure may be prolonged. The diastolic rumble is best heard with the bell of the stethoscope at the apex, with the patient in the left lateral decubitus position. Its prolonged duration, more than its intensity, is the predictor of severe mitral stenosis. Associated murmurs include tricuspid regurgitation with severe right heart failure, and pulmonary regurgitation (Graham Steell murmur) with pulmonary hypertension. The tricuspid regurgitation murmur may be differentiated from mitral regurgitation (not uncommonly associated with mitral stenosis) by its enhancement during inspiration. Other signs of right ventricular failure also may be present, including a tender pulsatile liver, ascites, and

Table 2. Differential Diagnosis of Mitral Valve Stenosis	
DISEASE ENTITY	DIFFERENTIATING FEATURES
Left atrial myxoma (symptoms and signs especially diastolic murmur, mimic mitral stenosis)	Auscultatory findings change with body position, signs of systemic illness (weight loss, anemia, fever, emboli); usually no opening snap; tumor plop; characteristic echocardiographic findings
Atrial septal defect (increased flow across tricuspid valve causes diastolic flow murmur)	Fixed splitting of the S_2; absence of left atrial enlargement; abscence of Kerley B lines; echocardiography reveals normal mitral valve and large right ventricle; left-to-right shunt by catheterization study
High flow states, such as hyperthyroidism (diastolic flow rumbles across AV valves due to increased amount of blood traversing these valves)	Hyperactive cardiac state; signs of hyperthyroidism; echocardiogram shows normal mitral valve, hyperkinetic left ventricular motion
Mitral regurgitation (with large amounts of blood flowing across the mitral valve during diastole, a diastolic rumble may be present)	Holosystolic murmur of mitral regurgitation (although mitral regurgitation and mitral stenosis may coexist); concomitant S_3, signs of left ventricular enlargement
Cor triatriatum (uncommon congenital malformation consisting of a fibromuscular membrane that divides the left atrium and impedes flow from pulmonary veins to left ventricle)	Murmurs (both systolic and diastolic) are not typical of mitral stenosis; normal mitral valve by echocardiogram with characteristic echocardiogram in left atrium; left atrial angiography may visualize membrane
Congenital stenosis of pulmonary veins (unusual congenital entity resulting in signs of pulmonary hypertension, pulmonary venous congestion, and right ventricular failure)	No distinctive murmurs; mitral valve normal by echocardiogram
Primary pulmonary hypertension (signs of right ventricular failure; more common in women)	No opening snap or diastolic rumble; no left atrial enlargement or elevated pulmonary artery wedge pressure
Large mitral vegetations from endocarditis	Vegetations may be visualized by echocardiography
Ball-valve thrombus formation in the left atrium	Auscultatory findings change with body position; 2-dimensional echocardiography may be helpful

peripheral edema. Features of the differential of the cardiac examination are shown in Table 2.

Electrocardiographic findings, although not specific, may suggest mitral stenosis and include left atrial enlargement (p mitrale), right-axis deviation, and right ventricular hypertrophy.

Atrial fibrillation may be present, and represents a poor prognostic sign. The chest x-ray demonstrates signs of left atrial enlargement: an elevated left mainstem bronchus and double cardiac density, and prominent left heart border. A severely dilated left atrium suggests concomitant mitral regurgitation. Pulmonary vascular redistribution, interstitial edema, Kerley B lines, and prominence of the right ventricle and pulmonary artery also may be observed.

Echocardiography is the diagnostic tool of choice in mitral stenosis. The primary M-mode signs are reduction of the E to F slope (reduced left ventricular filling rate), thickening of the mitral valve leaflets, and concordant (rather than the normal discordant) motion of the posterior mitral valve leaflet with the anterior leaflet. Two-dimensional echocardiography reveals typical diastolic doming of the thickened mitral valve leaflets with restricted leaflet separation. An enlarged left atrium and rheumatic involvement of other valves may also be demonstrated. Doppler echocardiography reveals an increased velocity of transmitral flow. This technique allows an estimation of the severity of mitral stenosis by calculation of the mitral valve half-time, the time necessary for peak transmitral flow velocity to fall to half its value (Fig. 3). Doppler echocardiography can also provide an estimate of right heart pressure. A Doppler-derived mitral valve area can also be calculated using the continuity equation.[15] The calculation by this method provides a direct, easily obtainable estimation of mitral valve area; however, it cannot be applied in settings of significant concomitant mitral or aortic regurgitation.[16] Echocardiography is also helpful in ruling out other diagnoses in the differential of mitral stenosis, specifically, left atrial myxoma, atrial septal defect, cor

triatriatum, ball-valve thrombus in the left atrium, and large mitral valve vegetations. Transesophageal echocardiography may be useful for identifying thrombi in the left atrial appendage.

Cardiac catheterization, although not required for the diagnosis of mitral stenosis, is often performed before surgical intervention to evaluate concomitant coronary artery disease in older patients. Typical hemodynamic features are an elevated left atrial pressure and a significant left atrial-to-left ventricular diastolic gradient (Fig. 4). Cardiac catheterization derived mitral valve area can be calculated using the Gorlin formula:

$$MVA = \frac{CO/DFP \times HR}{0.85 \times 44.3 \sqrt{G}}$$

Where CO = cardiac output; DFP = diastolic filling period; HR = heart rate; and G = transmitral gradient. Elevated right heart pressures may also be observed, with associated tricuspid regurgitation manifested as tall, regurgitant systolic v waves on the atrial pressure tracing.

THERAPY

The management of mitral stenosis has changed considerably over the years. Medical management follows 5 general considerations: 1) prophylaxis against infective endocarditis; 2)

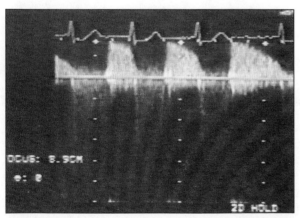

Figure 3. *Doppler echocardiographic profile of a stenotic mitral valve.*

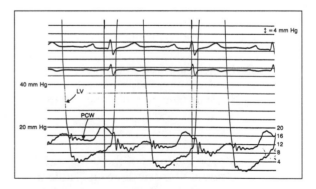

Figure 4. *Pressure wave forms in mitral stenosis. Pulmonary capillary wedge pressure (PCW) tracing shown against left ventricular (LV) pressure (off scale) and the significant diastolic gradient between them.*

efforts to limit elevations of left atrial pressure; 3) management of right heart failure; 4) management of atrial fibrillation; and 5) prophylaxis against systemic embolization.

Rapid atrial fibrillation is poorly tolerated. Digitalis is useful in slowing rapid ventricular response rates. Beta-blockers or diltiazem may be added to digitalis in patients with atrial fibrillation whose ventricular rate is not well controlled on digitalis alone. Antiarrhythmic therapy directed toward suppression of atrial fibrillation may help maintain sinus rhythm in those with recurrent paroxysms of atrial fibrillation. Diuretic therapy helps to reduce symptoms of pulmonary congestion and right heart failure. Oral anticoagulation is indicated in patients with atrial fibrillation.

Surgical therapy currently consists of either open commissurotomy or mitral valve replacement. Indications for surgical intervention include symptomatic patients (NYHA functional class II or higher) with moderate to severe mitral stenosis (mitral valve area <1.0 cm²).

An alternative to surgical correction of mitral stenosis is percutaneous balloon mitral valvuloplasty, during which a balloon catheter is advanced across the atrial septum and the stenotic mitral valve. With balloon inflation commissural separation occurs enhancing the mitral valve orifice. Application of echocardiographic scoring systems evaluating the level of valve deformity may help determine appro-

priate candidate selection for balloon valvuloplasty.[17,18] Good long-term results can be expected from those individuals with limited degrees of mitral valve deformity.[18]

MITRAL REGURGITATION

The integrity and preservation of normal mitral valve function requires the support of the components that make up the mitral valve apparatus. The mitral valve apparatus consists of anterior and posterior mitral valve leaflets, the chordae tendineae, the papillary muscles, and the mitral annulus. So-called primary mitral regurgitation results from pathology of any of these components. Secondary mitral regurgitation typically is created by left ventricular dysfunction and dilatation resulting in an incompetent mitral valve and implies normal mitral valve components. Various etiologies of mitral regurgitation are shown in Table 3.

Mitral regurgitation is manifested by significant systolic backflow of blood from the left ventricle into the left atrium across an incompetent mitral valve. This regurgitant load is returned to the left ventricle, resulting ultimately in dilation of both the left ventricle and left atrium. The presentation of acute mitral regurgitation is quite different from that of chronic mitral regurgitation; left atrial size is the mediator of these differences. In acute

Table 3. Etiologies of Mitral Valve Regurgitation

ACUTE	CHRONIC
Ruptured chordae tendineae	Rheumatic heart disease
Papillary muscle rupture	Papillary muscle dysfunction
Endocarditis	Mitral valve prolapse (click-murmur syndrome, Barlow's syndrome, floppy mitral valve)
Trauma	Endocarditis
	Calcification of the mitral valve annulus
	Accompanying hypertrophic obstructive cardiomyopathy
	Congenital endocardial cushion defect, corrected transposition
	Endocardial fibroelastosis
	Severe left ventricular dilatation

mitral regurgitation, initial left atrial size is small; sudden increased pressure in this noncompliant chamber results in pulmonary congestion. In chronic mitral regurgitation, the left atrium dilates over time and attempts to accommodate the regurgitant volume. The result is low left-atrial pressure and far less pulmonary congestion. Limited effective forward output, resulting from the failing dilated ventricle, appears to be the primary mechanism of symptoms in the chronic state.

DIAGNOSIS

In chronic mitral regurgitation, patients may be asymptomatic for 20-30 years, later presenting with dyspnea on exertion, orthopnea, weakness, and fatigue. A dilated left atrium may result in atrial fibrillation and the associated risk of systemic embolization, although not as often as in mitral stenosis. After long-standing severe mitral regurgitation, left ventricular failure inevitably results in right ventricular failure.

Because left ventricular ejection is actually hyperdynamic in the initial phases of regurgitation, the carotid pulse is brisk, as is the left ventricular impulse. The S_1 is generally soft and the S_2 widely split. An S_3 may also be present. The murmur of mitral regurgitation is characteristically high-pitched and holosystolic, and is most prominent at the apex with radiation to the axilla. Mild mitral regurgitation typically reveals a normal S_1 and a late systolic murmur. Table 4 lists features that help differentiate the murmur of mitral regurgitation.

The chest x-ray generally reveals enlargement of both the left atrium and ventricle, and occasionally, signs of pulmonary congestion. Calcification of the mitral valve annulus may be observed, which is a frequent cause of mitral regurgitation in the elderly. The most common electrocardiographic finding is left atrial enlargement. Atrial fibrillation and evidence of left ventricular hypertrophy may develop over

Table 4. Differential Diagnosis of Mitral Valve Regurgitation

DISEASE ENTITIES	DIFFERENTIATING FEATURES
Ventricular septal defect (murmur may be confused with mitral regurgitation)	Murmur localized over lower left sternal border. Radionuclide studies or Doppler confirm left-to-right shunt. Cardiac catheterization reveals O_2 step up from right atrium to ventricle.
Hypertrophic obstructive cardiomyopathy (or idiopathic hypertrophic subaortic stenosis [IHSS])	Associated mitral regurgitation murmur may be present. However, outflow murmur typical of hypertrophic obstructive cardiomyopathy (HOCM) is present as well, which increases with Valsalva maneuver and amyl nitrite and decreases with squatting, hand grip. Typical echocardiographic features of HOCM.
Aortic stenosis (murmur may be confused with mitral regurgitation)	The murmur is systolic ejection in quality. Confusion occurs when mitral regurgitation is due to prolapse of posterior papillary muscle or rupture of posterior chordae tendineae with radiation of the murmur to the aortic area. In some patients the murmur of aortic stenosis is loudest at the apex. With aortic stenosis, carotid upstroke is delayed, S_2 is soft, single or absent, echocardiographic features of aortic stenosis and calcification of the aortic valve are present.

time. In acute mitral regurgitation, as occurs with sudden papillary muscle rupture, signs of ischemia may be the only electrocardiographic finding.

Two-dimensional echocardiography with Doppler interrogation establishes the presence of mitral regurgitation and provides an assessment of its possible etiology by direct visualization of the mitral valve apparatus. A survey of structure and function may support a diagnosis of rheumatic valve involvement, prolapse, or vegetations as a possible culprit for regurgitation. One can also appreciate papillary muscle dysfunction or mitral annulus calcification in the differential of etiologies. Left ventricular function is typically hyperdynamic in the setting of acute mitral regurgitation. Chronic mitral regurgitation is manifested by left atrial and ventricular dilatation with a gradual decline of left ventricular performance. While Doppler echocardiography has become the cornerstone in making the diagnosis of mitral regurgitation, its interpretation of the severity of mitral regurgitation remains semi-quantitative. Despite this limitation, several recent investigations have provided supportive Doppler criteria to improve on the ability to quantitate mitral regurgitation. Specifically, calculation of the regurgitant fraction,[19] observation of proximal flow convergence[20,21] and pulmonary venous flow[22,23] have all emerged to provide a quantitation of mitral regurgitation.

Cardiac catheterization in acute mitral regurgitation demonstrates marked elevation of the pulmonary capillary wedge pressure and prominent systolic regurgitant v waves. Angiographically, regurgitant flow is observed in the left atrium during left ventriculography; if mitral regurgitation is severe, the flow may be tracked back into the pulmonary veins. Over time, as the left ventricle fails, end-diastolic pressure will rise and the ejection fraction falls. Left ventricular regurgitant fraction can be calculated by incorporating the formula:

$$\frac{\text{Angiographic cardiac output}-\text{FICK cardiac output}}{\text{Angiographic cardiac output}}$$

If the regurgitant fraction is greater than 60%, severe mitral regurgitation is present.

THERAPY

The primary goal of the medical management of mitral regurgitation is afterload reduction. Reduced impedance to left ventricular outflow serves to reduce regurgitation across the mitral valve. In acute mitral regurgitation, this is readily accomplished by use of intravenous sodium nitroprusside and/or intra-aortic balloon counterpulsation. Chronic afterload reduction can be achieved with hydralazine or angiotensin-converting enzyme (ACE) inhibitors. A low-sodium diet and aggressive diuretic therapy are also good supportive measures. Endocarditis prophylaxis is recommended in patients with mitral regurgitation associated with organic disease of the mitral leaflets.

Traditionally, parameters of left ventricular function have been used to guide the timing of intervention for mitral regurgitation. However, measurements of ejection fraction can be misleading, given that end-systolic volumes are smaller due to reduced impedance to left ventricular outflow. Appropriate timing of intervention is critical: premature intervention should be avoided, while delayed intervention can lead to irreversible left ventricular dysfunction. Once mitral regurgitation is corrected, the left ventricle confronts increased systolic wall stress, having lost the left atrial reservoir as an unloading chamber. Acute severe mitral regurgitation generally requires aggressive surgical intervention. Chronic mitral regurgitation with significant limiting symptoms also calls for intervention provided that left ventricular function is not severely depressed. Table 5 lists guidelines, described by Ross, for patient selection.

A strong prediction of surgical outcome in chronic mitral regurgitation is left atrial size as determined by 2-dimensional echocardiography. Reed and co-investigators found left atrial size to be equally important as a determinant of surgical outcome as left ventricular ejection fraction.[24] In patients with a left ventricular ejection fraction greater than 75%, left atrial size was the only predictor of cardiac death, while given a normal ejection fraction (i.e., 50% to 75%), left atrial size was

Table 5. Guidelines for Selecting Patients With Mitral Regurgitation for Operation

1. The downhill clinical course is relatively gradual in chronic mitral regurgitation once symptoms begin, and left ventricular dysfunction may develop insidiously.

2. With significant *limiting symptoms* and severe mitral regurgitation, operation is usually indicated provided left ventricular function is good or not severely depressed (ejection fraction <40%). Even when left ventricular function is sustained preoperatively, the ejection fraction will deteriorate to some degree after operation.

3. In patients with severe regurgitation who have *few or no symptoms*, operation should be considered to preserve left ventricular function provided serial noninvasive studies of the left ventricle show ejection fraction <55%, fractional shortening <30%, plus either A or B:

   A) End-diastolic diameter approaching 75 mm and end-systolic diameter approaching 50 mm or 26 mm/m² body surface area (end-systolic volume approaching 60 ml/m²).

   B) Both an end-systolic diameter approaching 26 mm/m² and a radius/wall thickness ratio at end-systole x systolic pressure approaching 195 mm Hg.

From Ross J.[64] With permission of the American College of Cardiology.

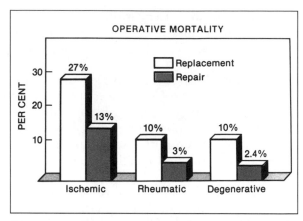

Figure 5. Operative mortality for mitral valve replacement exceeds that for mitral valve repair regardless of the etiology. From Cosgrove DM, Stewart WJ. *Mitral valvuloplasty.* Curr Probs Cardiol. 1989;14:359. With permission.

equally as important as left ventricular systolic function.

Surgical intervention takes 2 forms, i.e., either mitral valve replacement or valve repair. Whenever possible, mitral valve repair is favored over valve replacement, due to reduced infective endocarditis risk, reduced incidence of thromboembolism, and superior preservation of ventricular function.[25] Moreover, regardless of the etiology of mitral regurgitation the operative mortality is lower when the valve is repaired, as compared with mitral valve replacement (Fig. 5). Mitral valve repair of the posterior leaflet and chordae is generally easier than repair of the anterior mitral valve leaflet. Intra-operative transesophageal echocardiographic monitoring helps to evaluate the success of mitral valve repair.

When mitral valve replacement must be performed, chordae preservation has been shown to help maintain left ventricular geometry thus allowing better maintenance of left ventricular function.[26,27] The VA Cooperative Study established postoperative variables that predicted a poor surgical outcome following mitral valve replacement.[28] Patients with a postoperative left ventricular ejection fraction less than 50%, and an end-diastolic volume index greater than 101 ml/m², had significantly higher peri- and post-operative mortality, and tended to be NYHA functional class III or IV.

MITRAL VALVE PROLAPSE

Mitral valve prolapse represents an entity whereby 1 or both mitral valve leaflets exhibit exaggerated systolic bowing above the plane of the mitral valve annulus. Using echocardiographic criteria exclusively, the incidence of mitral valve prolapse is overestimated. Criteria that help to establish the diagnosis of mitral valve prolapse on clinical grounds, in

Table 6. Minor and Major Criteria for Establishing the Diagnosis of Mitral Valve Prolapse

MINOR CRITERIA	MAJOR CRITERIA

History
  Focal neurologic attacks or amaurosis fugax in the young patient
  First-degree relatives with major criteria
  Recurrent supraventricular tachycardia (documented)
Ausculatation
  Soft, inconsistent, or equivocal mid- to late-systolic sounds at the cardiac apex
Other physical signs
  Low body weight, asthenic habitus
  Low blood pressure
  Thoracic bony abnormalities
Two-dimensional/Doppler/color flow echocardiography
  Moderate superior systolic displacement of mitral leaflets with Doppler mitral regurgitation
Two-dimensionally targeted M-mode echocardiography
  Moderate (2 mm) late systolic buckling posterior to the line between points C and D
  Holosystolic displacement (3mm) posterior to the line between points C and D*
	Auscultation
	  Mid- to late-systolic clicks and a late systolic murmur at the cardiac apex
	  Mobile mid- to late-systolic clicks at the cardiac apex
	  Late systolic murmur at the cardiac apex in the young patient
	Auscultation plus echocardiography
	  Apical holosystolic murmur of mitral regurgitation plus echocardiographic criteria (below)
	Two-dimensional/Doppler echocardiocardiography
	  Marked systolic displacement of mitral leaflets with coaptation point at or on the left atrial side of the annulus
	  Moderate systolic displacement of the leaflets with at least moderate mitral regurgitation, chordal rupture, and annular dilatation
	Two-dimensionally targeted M-mode echocardiography
	  Marked ($\geq$ 3 mm) late systolic buckling posterior to the line between points C and D

* C represents complete closure of valve; D represents onset of valve opening. From Perloff JK et al.[29] With permission.

addition to echocardiographic features, were proposed by Perloff and truly yield a more appropriate incidence of the phenomenon (Table 6).[29]

Mitral valve prolapse may be structural, i.e., based on a specific structural abnormality of the valve or physiologic, in which concomitant physiologic circumstances are the dominant source of prolapse (Table 7).[30] Structurally mediated mitral valve prolapse is more likely to be associated with an increased morbidity than so-called physiologic prolapse.[31] The mechanism behind physiologic forms of mitral valve prolapse relate mainly to transient reduction in left ventricular cavity dimension. The classic structural form of mitral valve prolapse is due to myxomatous degeneration of the valve leaflets resulting in systolic bowing of the valve leaflets and subsequent loss of leaflet coaptation, ultimately producing mitral regurgitation. There appears to be some familial tendency for prolapse, as well as an association with disorders including various connective tissue diseases, e.g., systemic lupus erythematosus, polyarteritis nodosa, Wolff-Parkinson-White syndrome, neurocirculatory asthenia, anxiety neurosis, and straightback syndrome, to name just a few.

The vast majority of patients with mitral valve prolapse are asymptomatic. However, patients

Table 7. Causes of Mitral Valve Prolapse	
STRUCTURAL	PHYSIOLOGIC
Myxomatous degeneration	Valsalva maneuver
Ruptured chordae tendineae	Atrial septal defect
Papillary muscle rupture	Hyperthyroidism
Marfan's syndrome	Emphysema
Rheumatic fever	Hypertrophic cardiomyopathy
Infective endocarditis	
Collagen vascular disease	

From Carabello B.[25] With permission.

may complain of palpitations, chest pain, fatigue, dyspnea, lightheadedness, and syncope. Physical examination will generally reveal a midsystolic click (and sometimes multiple clicks). The click is often followed by the mid-to-late systolic murmur of mitral regurgitation. The murmur becomes more holosystolic with increasing severity of regurgitation. The electrocardiogram is usually normal, but may reveal nonspecific repolarization changes most often in the inferior leads.[32] Supraventricular tachycardia is the most frequent tachyrhythmia observed. An association of mitral valve prolapse with sudden death has been established, however, this complication is rare.

Two-dimensional echocardiography demonstrates the prolapsing motion of either/or both mitral valve leaflets into the left atrium during systole. Two-dimensional echocardiography may also reveal prolapse of the tricuspid and/or aortic valves. Doppler echocardiography may demonstrate associated mitral regurgitation.

Most patients with mitral valve prolapse have a benign course; however, a small number of individuals may experience 1 of the major complications of mitral valve prolapse, including infective endocarditis, development of severe mitral regurgitation, significant cardiac arrhythmias, or cerebrovascular events. In the Massachusetts General Hospital Study evaluating the course of patients with mitral valve prolapse, severe mitral regurgitation developed in 12% of patients with structurally abnormal valves versus prolapse alone.[31] Endocarditis occurred in 3.5% of patients with thickened

valve leaflets versus 0% in those with prolapse only. Surprisingly, the incidence of stroke was nearly comparable in both groups, i.e., those with and without thickened leaflets. Antibiotic prophylaxis against bacterial endocarditis is strongly recommended, particularly when valve leaflets are thickened and/or mitral regurgitation is present.

MITRAL ANNULAR CALCIFICATION

Calcification of the mitral annulus is frequently idiopathic and is a significant etiology of mitral regurgitation in the elderly. Although considered a degenerative change, it appears to be hastened by certain conditions, including hypertension, aortic stenosis, diabetes, Marfan's and Hurler's syndromes, and has been associated with hypertrophic obstructive cardiomyopathy.

There may be associated calcification of the aortic valve cusps as well. The chest x-ray may show a characteristic C-shaped calcification of the mitral valve annulus. The annular calcification can be assessed by echocardiography. If the calcium extends into the conduction system, atrioventricular or intraventricular conduction defects may develop. Functional mitral stenosis has also been reported in patients with massive annular calcification. The Framingham Heart Study has suggested an increased incidence of stroke independent of standard risk factors.[33] Moreover, there was a continuous relationship between the incidence of stroke and severity of mitral annular calcification (based on millimeter degrees of thickening) underscoring the impact of this entity on elderly populations.

AORTIC STENOSIS

There are 3 major varieties of adult valvular aortic stenosis: rheumatic, senile-calcific, or degenerative and congenital bicuspid aortic valve with secondary calcification (Fig. 6). In rheumatic aortic stenosis, the major pathologic feature is fusion of the commissures with

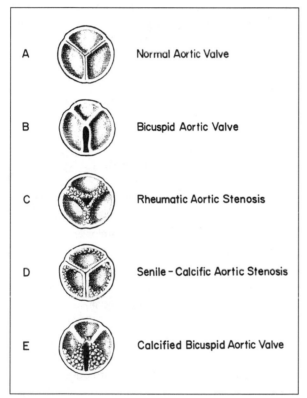

Figure 6. *Pathology of aortic stenosis. (A) Normal tricuspid aortic valve. (B) Bicuspid aortic valve. (C) Rheumatic aortic stenosis. The commissures are fused and the valve leaflets are thickened. (D) Senile-calcific aortic stenosis. Calcium deposits are present within the cusps of the aortic valve without primarily affecting the commissures. (E) Calcified bicuspid aortic valve. Adapted from Brandenburg RO, Fuster V, Giuliani E. Valvular heart disease. When should the patient be referred?* Pract Cardiol. *1979;5:50 and Fuster V, Brandenburg RO, Giuliani E, et al. Clinical approach and management of acquired valvular heart disease.* Cardiovasc Clin. *1980;10:126. With permission.*

thickening and fibrosis of the valve leaflets. Patients in their 20s and 30s may have a murmur, but symptoms might not occur until the sixth decade of life. In senile-calcific or degenerative aortic stenosis, calcium accumulates in the pockets of the aortic cusps with eventual fibrosis. Symptoms typically occur in the seventh decade of life. In congenital bicuspid aortic valve, calcific changes occur earlier in life, presumably secondary to increased turbulence. There is progressive narrowing of the valve orifice over time and symptoms develop in the fifth decade. Congenital aortic stenosis, in which the aortic valve is dome-shaped, causes symptoms early in life. Isolated aortic stenosis in the adult is unlikely to be secondary to rheumatic disease and more likely to be secondary to the congenital bicuspid or the senile-calcific variety.

Obstruction to flow between the left ventricle and aorta also may be due to hypertrophic obstructive cardiomyopathy, sub- or supra-valvular stenosis due to an abnormal membrane below or above the valve, or supravalvular stenosis due to a congenital narrowing of the ascending aorta. Supravalvular stenosis has been associated with hypercalcemia and mental retardation.

DIAGNOSIS

Aortic stenosis results in increased resistance to left ventricular outflow. The left ventricle compensates by developing hypertrophy in order to maintain an effective cardiac output. The hypertrophied muscle has diminished compliance, which results in a rise in left ventricular end-diastolic pressure. Left atrial contraction thus becomes more important for filling the left ventricle. Hence, patients with significant aortic stenosis often become more symptomatic when they develop atrial fibrillation and lose atrial contraction. Myocardial oxygen consumption is increased, largely due to increased left ventricular wall tension (due to increased left ventricular intracavitary pressure), while subendocardial coronary blood flow is compromised because of high subendocardial intramural pressure. Therefore, patients might exhibit symptoms and signs of ischemia without having coronary artery disease.

The traditional triad of symptoms in patients with aortic stenosis consists of angina, syncope, and heart failure. Lombard and Selzer evaluated the clinical and hemodynamic profiles of 397 patients with severe aortic stenosis, finding that 50.9% of patients had angina. Coexisting coronary disease was present in 60% of patients (mean age, 60 years); however, there was no difference regarding the incidence of angina in this group versus those without coronary disease.[34] These observations suggest that patients manifesting angina can have normal coronary arteries. Marcus and colleagues[35] demonstrated that reduced coronary reserve to the hypertrophied left ventricle can contribute to the mechanism of angina pectoris. In general, a 5-year life expectancy can be predicted once angina develops. Syncope is frequently exertional and can be secondary to exercise-triggered peripheral vasodilation with a fixed cardiac output; atrial or ventricular arrhythmias can also be a mechanism. Once syncope develops, mean survival is approximately 3 to 4 years. Signs of left ventricular failure may also develop, and are associated with a 2-year survival.[36] Occult aortic stenosis occasionally presents as intractable heart failure.[37]

Table 8. Differential Diagnosis of Aortic Valve Stenosis

DISEASE ENTITY	DIFFERENTIATING FEATURES
Aortic valve sclerosis of the elderly without stenosis (systolic murmur may mimic that of aortic stenosis)	Systolic murmur does not peak late. Carotids do not have delayed upstrokes. No left ventricular hypertrophy by ECG. Echocardiographic visualization of excursion of valve leaflets usually normal or mildly reduced, but valves may not be visualized. No hemodynamically significant aortic valve gradient by cardiac catheterization.
Hypertrophic obstructive cardiomyopathy (IHSS; systolic murmur may be confused with that of aortic stenosis)	Brisk bifid carotid upstrokes. Murmur usually does not radiate into neck. Characteristic change in murmur with various maneuvers. Pseudoinfarct pattern (large septal Q waves) on ECG. Characteristic echocardiographic features.
Mitral regurgitation (systolic murmur may be confused with that of aortic stenosis)	Murmur is holosystolic and radiates to axilla and not carotids. Carotid upstroke may be normal. Dilated left ventricle. Aortic valve normal on echocardiogram unless there is associated aortic valve disease.
Pulmonic stenosis (systolic murmur may be confused with that of aortic stenosis)	Murmur does not radiate into neck; loudest along the left sternal border. Physical exam, chest x-ray and ECG may reveal enlarged right ventricle. M-mode echocardiogram reveals right ventricular enlargement and hypertrophy and 2-dimensional echocardiography may visualize valve stenosis.

Sudden death occurs in 15% to 20% of patients with symptomatic aortic stenosis and is thought to be mediated through arrhythmias and myocardial ischemia.[38] It is in the rare instance that sudden death attributable to aortic stenosis occurs without some degree of antecedent symptomatology. Heyde's Syndrome, manifested by gastrointestinal bleeding due to angiodysplasias of the colon, has also been described.[39] Finally, although a rare presentation, abrupt partial or complete vision loss in 1 eye has been attributed to calcium emboli in individuals with calcific aortic stenosis.[40]

Physical examination reveals a delayed carotid upstroke with a prominent anacrotic notch at the time of peak turbulence across the valve. There is a prominent prolonged apical impulse, often with a palpable a wave. Auscultation reveals an ejection type systolic murmur beginning just after S_1. The murmur is harsh, crescendo-decrescendo and maximal at the second right intercostal space. The intensity and duration of the murmur bears a fair correlation with the severity of aortic stenosis. A high-frequency diastolic murmur of associated aortic regurgitation also can be present. The S_2 can be paradoxically split due to delayed left ventricular emptying. An S_4 is often heard in patients in sinus rhythm. A systolic ejection click can also be present, which suggests valve mobility and is heard frequently in congenitally bicuspid aortic valves. Differential diagnosis of the murmur of aortic stenosis is described in Table 8.

Since the left ventricle develops concentric hypertrophy in aortic stenosis, the cardiac silhouette may not change on early chest films. Eventually, the chest x-ray reveals a prominent left ventricle and a dilated ascending aorta (due to post-stenotic dilation). The aortic valve itself might be calcified. With decompensation, the left ventricle dilates and pulmonary venous congestion may appear. The electrocardiogram typically reveals left ventricular hypertrophy with secondary repolarization changes and left atrial enlargement. A left-axis deviation might be present and conduction defects (e.g., left bundle branch block, first-degree AV block, etc.) are frequently seen. With severe aortic stenosis, atrial fibrillation might be present.

Echocardiography has advanced considerably in establishing a diagnosis of aortic stenosis.

Two-dimensional imaging demonstrates thickened valve leaflets with limited excursion. Left atrial enlargement can be present, and while the presence of left ventricular hypertrophy can suggest significant aortic stenosis, the degree of left ventricular hypertrophy cannot be used to grade the severity of aortic stenosis.[41] Agreement between echo-Doppler and catheterization-derived aortic valve area is greater than 95%.[42] Doppler echocardiography provides a good estimate of systolic gradients and the aortic valve area using the continuity equation (Fig. 7).[43,44] In view of the occasional limitation of valve area calculation by the continuity equation in the setting of a reduced cardiac output, the peak velocity ratio has been described.[45,46] Using this method, a ratio of peak left ventricular outflow track velocity to peak transaortic velocity is calculated. A peak velocity ratio ≤ 0.26 has a sensitivity of 98%, specificity of 77%, and predictive value of 93% for identifying patients with severe aortic stenosis.[46]

Cardiac catheterization reveals a significant gradient between the left ventricle and aorta, as shown in Figure 8. A peak-to-peak gradient more than 50 mm Hg with a normal cardiac output has been considered severe. Left ventricular systolic and end-diastolic, and left atrial pressures are elevated. Critical aortic stenosis is present when the valve area is less than 0.75 cm² in an average-sized adult or 0.4 cm²/m² BSA (normal aortic valve area is 3.0–3.5 cm²).

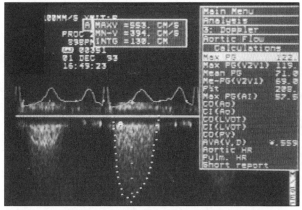

Figure 7. *Doppler echocardiographic profile of a stenotic aortic valve with the on-screen calculation of the valve area.*

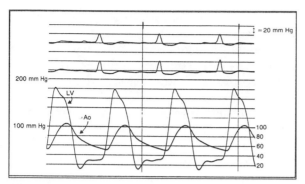

Figure 8. *A significant systolic pressure gradient is shown between the left ventricle (LV) and the central aorta (AO), in a patient with aortic stenosis.*

Coronary angiography is performed to determine if concomitant coronary artery disease is present, particularly in patients more than 40 years of age or those with significant risk factors for coronary artery disease. The incidence of concomitant coronary disease is approximately 35% in all patients with aortic stenosis, and 45% in those older than 60 years of age.[47]

THERAPY

Patients with truly asymptomatic significant aortic stenosis are at an increased risk for cardiac events within 2 years; however, during the time that they remain asymptomatic, the risk of sudden death is low.[48,49] These individuals are advised to be monitored closely with echo-Doppler examinations and symptom evaluation.

Once a patient becomes symptomatic with evidence of severe aortic valve stenosis, surgery generally is indicated. The patient's age per se is not a contraindication to aortic valve replacement. Unless the left ventricular ejection fraction is severely depressed, valve replacement should be strongly considered, since left ventricular function will improve in most instances. There is also evidence that left ventricular hypertrophy will regress over time.

Percutaneous balloon dilatation of stenotic aortic valves has been performed to treat nonsurgical candidates, although with less enthusiasm than in mitral stenosis. The technique has been largely limited to elderly populations with severe senile calcific degenerative aortic stenosis, in whom the risks of valve replacement are significant or other antecedent illness deems the patient not suitable for surgery. In-hospital morbidity and mortality, as well as long-term results have been poor.[50–52] The rate of restenosis is also considerable, with recurrence to prevalvotomy aortic valve area levels in as early as 8 days following the procedure.[53]

Medical management in aortic stenosis includes endocarditis prophylaxis for dental and surgical procedures and treatment of atrial fibrillation.

AORTIC REGURGITATION

Aortic regurgitation is caused by processes affecting either the valve leaflets or the aortic root. Primary diseases affecting the valve leaflets include rheumatic fever, infective endocarditis, congenital bicuspid valve, and ventricular septal defect (in which the aortic valve leaflet is pulled downward toward the ventricular cavity). Processes that dilate the ascending aorta can also create aortic regurgitation by preventing coaptation of the aortic valve leaflets. They include systemic hypertension, osteogenesis imperfecta, Reiter's syndrome, syphilitic aortitis, ankylosing spondylitis, Marfan's syndrome, cystic medial necrosis, and Ehlers-Danlos syndrome. Aortic regurgitation may be acute, as in acute bacterial endocarditis, aortic dissection, or trauma, or it may be chronic, as in systemic hypertension, rheumatic heart disease, or collagen vascular disease (Fig. 9).

DIAGNOSIS

In acute aortic regurgitation there is an abrupt increase in left ventricular end-diastolic volume, which results in marked elevations of left ventricular end-diastolic pressure. In chronic aortic regurgitation, the end-diastolic volume increases more slowly, allowing the left ventricle to compensate with gradual dilatation and hypertrophy. The left ventricle then ultimately fails. During diastole, the rapid runoff of blood volume back into the left ventricle yields a low peripheral diastolic pressure, which is the

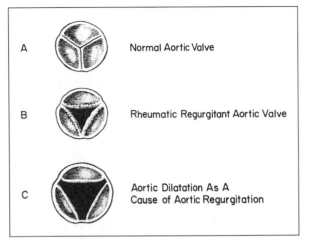

A — Normal Aortic Valve

B — Rheumatic Regurgitant Aortic Valve

C — Aortic Dilatation As A Cause of Aortic Regurgitation

Figure 9. (A) Normal aortic valve. (B) Rheumatic regurgitant aortic valve. The valve leaflets are fibrotic and shortened. (C) Aortic dilatation as a cause of aortic regurgitation. The valve leaflets are bowed and unable to coapt during diastole. There may be commissural separation.

mechanism behind many of the physical signs of aortic regurgitation. Low aortic diastolic pressures also reduce coronary perfusion pressure, making angina one of the features of this disease.

In acute aortic regurgitation, patients complain of weakness and severe dyspnea; hypotension may also be present. In chronic aortic regurgitation, patients are often asymptomatic for long periods. One of the first symptoms to develop includes an uncomfortable awareness of the heart beat due to an increased stroke volume. Other symptoms include exertional dyspnea, orthopnea, paroxysmal nocturnal dyspnea, and palpitations. Angina may also occur. Patients with acute aortic regurgitation are generally tachycardic with marked peripheral vasoconstriction and a normal pulse pressure. The patients appear ill and have signs of decompensated heart failure with pulmonary congestion and edema, S_3 and S_4. The S_1 may be diminished or absent because of premature mitral valve closure. The murmur of acute aortic regurgitation is a short, low-frequency diastolic murmur.

In patients with chronic aortic regurgitation, there is a wide pulse pressure due to elevated systolic pressure created by an enhanced stroke volume, and relatively low diastolic pressure created by the rapid runoff of blood volume. This situation creates a number of peripheral physical signs. The water-hammer (Corrigan's) pulse, described as a rapid upstroke and collapse, is noted on examination of peripheral pulses. De Musset's sign is head-bobbing with each systole. Palpation of the carotid pulse reveals a bisferiens or double-peaked quality. Duroziez' sign is the diastolic murmur auscultated when the stethoscope compresses the femoral artery, while Quincke's pulse refers to the visible capillary pulsations in the nailbed. Hill's sign, described as an increased popliteal systolic pressure over brachial systolic pressure of ≥ 40 mm Hg, is noted in severe aortic regurgitation. These peripheral signs may be absent if aortic regurgitation is acute or after development of severe left ventricular failure.

In chronic aortic regurgitation there is inferior and lateral displacement of the left ventricular impulse. The S_1 and A_2 can be diminished. In contrast to acute aortic regurgitation, the murmur is of high-frequency, blowing in quality, and decrescendo beginning just after S_2. The murmur also tends to be of longer duration. The more severe the aortic regurgitation, the longer the murmur persists in diastole. Auscultation can be facilitated with the patient sitting up and leaning forward, and with the use of the diaphragm of the stethoscope. When the murmur is heard best along the left sternal border, its cause is most likely to be damage to the valve leaflets; if the murmur is heard best along the right sternal border, the cause is most likely aortic root dilation. An Austin Flint murmur is often heard by the astute listener. This is a low-frequency, mid-diastolic apical rumble. The etiology of the murmur continues to be controversial (see chapter 2). Table 9 describes the differential features of aortic regurgitation.

The chest x-ray is far more helpful in chronic than in acute aortic regurgitation; it reveals an enlarged left ventricle with downward tilting of the apex. There can be calcification of the aortic valve, which is felt to be more suggestive of aortic regurgitation combined with stenosis, than of pure aortic regurgitation. Marked dilatation of the aorta can suggest aortic root

Table 9. Differential Diagnosis of Aortic Regurgitation

DISEASE ENTITY	DIFFERENTIATING FEATURES
Pulmonary regurgitation (diastolic murmur may be confused with aortic regurgitation)	Murmur of pulmonary insufficiency usually occurs in setting of pulmonary hypertension due to mitral stenosis or right-to-left cardiac shunt. Associated right ventricular enlargement. Absence of peripheral manifestations of aortic regurgitation.
Mitral stenosis (murmur may be confused with aortic regurgitation and Austin Flint murmur)	Murmur is low-pitched diastolic rumble with presystolic accentuation. Differentiated from Austin Flint murmur by using amyl nitrate. Austin Flint murmur diminishes with amyl nitrate; murmur of mitral stenosis remains unchanged or increases. Characteristic echocardiographic features of mitral stenosis.
Aortic stenosis (patients with aortic regurgitation typically have a prominent aortic systolic murmur due to the increased flow of blood volume across the aortic valve)	With aortic stenosis, there is a delayed carotid upstroke; the murmur tends to peak later in systole; and the echocardiographic features of aortic regurgitation (a hyperdynamic left ventricle and high-frequency vibrations of the anterior leaflet to the mitral valve during diastole) are absent.
Patent ductus arteriosus (murmurs may be confused with those of aortic insufficiency)	Murmur is continued throughout systole and diastole with peak of the murmur at S_2. Systolic ejection murmur accompanying aortic reguritation usually peaks in midsystole. Left-to-right shunt with radionuclide angiography and cardiac catheterization.

disease. Pulmonary venous congestion might also be present. The electrocardiogram generally reveals left ventricular hypertrophy and left atrial enlargement. A diastolic overload pattern might be noted on occasion, manifesting as left ventricular hypertrophy with Q waves anterolaterally.[54]

The M-mode echocardiogram can reveal fine diastolic fluttering of the mitral valve and ventricular septum and incomplete opening of the valve early in diastole. Early mitral valve closure can also be detected due to the marked elevation of left ventricular diastolic pressure. This finding is typical of acute severe aortic regurgitation. In time, left ventricular dilatation and inevitably a reduction in systolic performance

develop. Doppler echocardiography is the primary noninvasive method used to identify aortic regurgitation. Color-flow Doppler is particularly useful and can provide clues to the severity of regurgitation.

Diastolic mitral regurgitation is a phenomenon described by Downes and colleagues[55] that suggests acute aortic regurgitation. Premature mitral valve closure occurs due to the rapid rise of left ventricular diastolic pressure; this may be associated with the appearance of mitral regurgitation into the diastolic phase.[55]

Cardiac catheterization demonstrates a decreased diastolic systemic pressure and increased left ventricular end-diastolic pressure. There is a rapid diastolic fall on the aortic pressure tracing. Systolic arterial pressure is normal or increased and pulmonary capillary wedge pressure may be increased. Aortic root angiography is performed on occasion to quantitate the degree of the aortic regurgitation. Morphologic abnormalities of the aorta may also be seen, such as dissection, aortic root aneurysm, or calcification of the aortic valve.

THERAPY

Immediate surgical intervention is required for acute, hemodynamically unstable aortic regurgitation, since mortality is considerable without it. Intravenous pressors or sodium nitroprusside might be helpful while anticipating surgery.

The long-term prognosis for patients with chronic aortic regurgitation is primarily based on left ventricular systolic function and the severity of left ventricular dilatation. Asymptomatic patients with mild chronic aortic regurgitation generally need no treatment other than regular follow-up echocardiographic examinations to assess left ventricular cavity dimension and systolic performance. Antibiotic prophylaxis against bacterial endocarditis is also advisable. For symptomatic patients, diuresis and afterload reduction may be helpful.

Aortic regurgitation is generally tolerated for a significant duration before the development of heart failure; however, with the development of symptoms comes significant decline. Mean survival rates of under 2 years can be expected after the onset of congestive heart failure. Patients may survive 5 years after the development of angina, while 75% of patients overall with significant aortic regurgitation survive 5 years.[56]

The majority of patients who are asymptomatic with chronic severe aortic regurgitation and preserved left ventricular systolic function do well with a conservative nonoperative approach. Bonow and co-investigators note that 58% of patients in this category were alive and asymptomatic, with maintenance of normal left ventricular systolic function, at 11 years follow-up (representing an attrition rate of less than 5%/year).[57] A left ventricular end-systolic dimension of 50 mm or greater, however, predicted a 19% likelihood per year of symptom development or left ventricular dysfunction. Three indications for aortic valve replacement in chronic aortic regurgitation were proposed by the investigators: the development of symptoms, the development of left ventricular dysfunction at rest, or the development of marked left ventricular dilatation (end-diastolic diameter $\geq$ 80 mm or end-systolic dimension >55 mm). A recent study showed that vasodilator therapy with nifedipine could "reduce or delay" replacement of the aortic valve in patients with isolated, severe aortic regurgitation who were asymptomatic and had normal ventricular function.[57a]

TRICUSPID STENOSIS

The most common cause of tricuspid stenosis is rheumatic heart disease. Typically, tricuspid stenosis is present with concomitant mitral stenosis. Primary tricuspid stenosis can be present in carcinoid syndrome, systemic lupus erythematosus and endomyocardial fibrosis. Rarely, congenital tricuspid atresia and large tricuspid valve vegetations or right atrial tumors may obstruct right ventricular inflow, creating functional tricuspid stenosis. Symptoms are generally related to enhanced systemic venous pressure as well as reduced cardiac output owing to the obstruction between the right atrium and ventricle. Patients complain of generalized weakness and right upper quadrant discomfort due to hepatic venous congestion.

Physical examination is remarkable for jugular venous distention with a prominent a wave and slow y descent. There might be an opening snap on auscultation. The murmur is a high-frequency diastolic rumbling most prominent at the lower left sternal border. Both the opening snap and the murmur are intensified with inspiration. Additionally, in patients in sinus rhythm, there might be presystolic accentuation of the murmur. The liver is enlarged and tender, generally with hepatojugular reflux. Peripheral edema and ascites also might be present. The most common chest x-ray abnormality is right atrial enlargement typically without pulmonary arterial dilatation or other markers of pulmonary hypertension. The electrocardiogram characteristically demonstrates the prominent P waves of right atrial enlargement, and occasionally atrial fibrillation.

Two-dimensional echocardiography might demonstrate doming usually of the anterior tricuspid valve leaflet, with thickening and limited mobility of all leaflets. Doppler echocardiography demonstrates an increased transvalvular flow velocity during diastole.

Cardiac catheterization can be performed to confirm a significant gradient across the tricuspid valve elicited by Doppler electrocardiography. Simultaneous pressure measurements in the right atrium and ventricle must be performed. A normal gradient is less than 1 mm Hg. Significant tricuspid stenosis is usually present when the tricuspid valve area calculates to less than 1.5 cm^2.

If a patient fails intensive medical treatment consisting primarily of sodium restriction and diuresis, surgical intervention should be considered, particularly once the mean diastolic pressure gradient approaches 5 mm Hg. Either tricuspid valve replacement or surgical valvuloplasty can be considered. The state of other valve lesions, particularly mitral stenosis, may be the crucial factor in the timing of tricuspid valve intervention. Patients with tricuspid stenosis should receive antibiotic prophylaxis against infective endocarditis.

TRICUSPID REGURGITATION

Tricuspid regurgitation usually arises after the development of right ventricular and tricuspid annular dilatation. Any cause of right ventricular or pulmonary artery hypertension with subsequent right chamber dilatation can lead to tricuspid regurgitation. The most common etiology of primary tricuspid regurgitation is infectious endocarditis related to intravenous drug abuse. Other causes of tricuspid regurgitation include Ebstein's anomaly, carcinoid heart disease, rheumatic valvular involvement, prolapse due to myxomatous degeneration of the valve and trauma. Gayet and colleagues[58] reviewed 12 patients with traumatic tricuspid regurgitation, noting its occurrence with thoracic injuries. The investigators demonstrated the usefulness of echocardiography in making this diagnosis and emphasized the serious under-estimation of trauma as a possible etiology of tricuspid regurgitation.

Patients with tricuspid regurgitation complain of symptoms of right-sided heart failure, such as peripheral edema, right upper quadrant tenderness (due to hepatic venous congestion), nausea, and vomiting (due to splanchnic congestion). The physical examination reveals jugular venous distension with prominent regurgitant systolic v waves and a rapidly collapsing y descent. A palpable venous systolic thrill and murmur at the base of the neck, described by Amidi and coworkers,[59] might appear in severe tricuspid regurgitation. A right ventricular heave also may be present. If pulmonary hypertension is present, the P$_2$ will be accentuated. The murmur of tricuspid regurgitation typically is high-frequency, holosystolic, and most prominent along the lower left sternal border. Its enhancement during inspiration can help distinguish it from the murmur of mitral regurgitation. There also may be a right ventricular S$_3$. The liver might be enlarged and pulsatile, with hepatojugular reflux. Peripheral edema and ascites are often present.

The chest x-ray reveals enlargement of the right atrium and ventricle, often in association with prominence of the superior vena cava and azygous vein. The electrocardiogram displays right atrial enlargement with tall P waves, most clearly seen in the inferior leads. There may be right-axis deviation and prominent anterior forces as evidence of right ventricular hypertrophy. Atrial fibrillation might also be present.

Two-dimensional echocardiography reveals a dilated right ventricular chamber with paradoxical motion of the ventricular septum, implying right ventricular volume overload. The right atrium is also enlarged. If the tricuspid regurgitation is secondary to abnormalities of the valve itself, the echocardiogram might reveal tricuspid valvular vegetations, nonspecific thickening of the valve, prolapse, or evidence of Ebstein's anomaly. Doppler echocardiography is extremely sensitive in identifying tricuspid regurgitation. Using the continuous-wave mode, peak velocity of the regurgitant jet can be obtained and pulmonary artery systolic pressure estimated using the simplified Bernoulli equation. Color flow Doppler is also sensitive for diagnosing tricuspid regurgitation.

Cardiac catheterization typically reveals elevated right atrial and right ventricular end-diastolic pressures. A prominent regurgitant wave with a rapid y descent is observed in the right atrial pressure tracing. Although seldom required, right ventriculography demonstrates dilated right heart chambers with regurgitation of contrast into the right atrium.

Medical management consisting of sodium restriction, diuretics and digitalis can be sufficient for mild tricuspid regurgitation. Endocarditis prophylaxis should be administered for organic tricuspid valve disease. Surgical intervention is usually not employed unless there is evidence of severe tricuspid regurgitation. If tricuspid regurgitation is due to annular dilation, a technique developed by Carpentier and colleagues,[60] allowing suturing of the annulus to a prosthetic ring, has simplified surgical management considerably. If tricuspid regurgitation is due to primary valvular abnormalities, valve replacement is the usual treatment. However, there has been at least temporary success with excision of the valve in patients with tricuspid regurgitation due to recurrent infective endocarditis in the setting of intravenous drug abuse.[61]

PULMONIC STENOSIS

Pulmonic stenosis is generally congenital in origin and may be valvular, subvalvular, or supravalvular. On rare occasions, valvular pulmonic stenosis may be rheumatic in origin or secondary to plaque collection around the pulmonic valve (or the tricuspid valve) in malignant carcinoid syndrome. Extrinsic compression in the region of the pulmonic valve due to tumors or aneurysm of the sinus of Valsalva may occasionally lead to functional pulmonic stenosis. The normal pulmonic valve area is 2.0 cm^2/m^2.

Only moderate to severe pulmonic stenosis creates symptoms, which generally include fatigue, exertional dyspnea, lightheadedness, syncope, and, if severe, symptoms of right ventricular failure. The physical examination reveals a prominent jugular venous a wave with a right ventricular heave. The S_2 is widely split with a soft P_2 component. A right-sided S_3 and

S_4 also might be present. The murmur of pulmonic stenosis is a harsh systolic ejection murmur prominent at the upper left sternal border. Late peaking of the murmur implies increased severity of pulmonic stenosis. An ejection click preceding the murmur suggests that the stenosis is valvular rather than sub- or supravalvular. Cyanosis can be present with substantial reductions in cardiac output. With the development of right ventricular failure comes peripheral edema, ascites, and a tender enlarged liver.

The chest x-ray demonstrates post-stenotic dilatation of the main pulmonary artery, and ultimately dilatation of the right atrium and ventricle if pulmonic stenosis is severe. There might be generalized pulmonary oligemia as well. The electrocardiogram demonstrates right atrial enlargement and right ventricular hypertrophy in advanced pulmonic stenosis. Conduction disturbances, most commonly a right bundle branch block, are not infrequent.

Two-dimensional echocardiography is of limited usefulness in the diagnosis of pulmonic stenosis, as the pulmonic valve is the most difficult to demonstrate echocardiographically. A prominent a wave can be observed on the M-mode tracing of the pulmonic valve. A reasonably accurate transvalvular gradient can be obtained with Doppler echocardiography; the peak velocity is entered into the simplified Bernoulli equation to establish the transvalvular pressure gradient.

Cardiac catheterization may be used to assess the severity of the pulmonic stenosis. If the transvalvular gradient is >50 mm Hg, pulmonic stenosis is considered to be moderate; it is severe if the gradient is >80 mm Hg. Right ventricular end-diastolic pressure and right atrial systolic pressure (the a wave) may also be increased. Right ventriculography can display doming and thickening of the pulmonic valve leaflets. Cardiac catheterization is also useful in ruling out concomitant congenital lesions. Intervention, consisting of either surgical valve replacement or valvulotomy, is usually undertaken once the transvalvular gradient exceeds 50 mm Hg. Kan and coworkers[62] described success with percutaneous transluminal balloon valvuloplasty for pulmonic stenosis.

This lesion was among the first dilated by this technique. Patients with pulmonic stenosis should receive prophylaxis against infective endocarditis.

PULMONIC REGURGITATION

The most common cause of pulmonic valve regurgitation is physiologic, secondary to dilatation of the pulmonary valve ring, as in pulmonary hypertension, or to dilatation of the pulmonary artery. Infective endocarditis can also rarely cause pulmonic regurgitation. Pulmonic regurgitation may be congenital in origin occurring in association with tetralogy of Fallot, ventricular septal defect, or pulmonic valve stenosis.

Patients are generally asymptomatic unless severe pulmonic regurgitation develops with marked right ventricular dilatation and subsequent failure. In these cases, patients complain of generalized fatigue, exertional dyspnea, anorexia, nausea, vomiting, and right upper quadrant discomfort. There may be significant peripheral edema as well. Severe right heart failure may be particularly common in patients with pulmonic regurgitation due to infective endocarditis. These patients often develop septic pulmonary emboli with severe pulmonary hypertension.

The physical examination reveals a hyperdynamic right ventricular impulse and occasionally a palpable pulmonary artery impulse in the second left intercostal space. There is a widely split S$_2$, with prominence of the P$_2$ if pulmonary hypertension is present. The murmur of pulmonic regurgitation is a low-frequency, decrescendo diastolic murmur most prominent along the upper left sternal border, which is enhanced by inspiration. When the murmur is high-frequency and blowing in quality (Graham Steell murmur), pulmonic regurgitation is most likely secondary to pulmonary hypertension. Other physical findings relate to the development of right ventricular failure. The chest x-ray reveals enlargement of the main pulmonary artery as well as the right ventricle. The electrocardiogram displays evidence of right ventricular hypertrophy.

Two-dimensional echocardiography demonstrates the dilated right ventricle, with hyper-trophy if pulmonary hypertension is present. There is generally paradoxical interventricular septal wall motion typical of right ventricular overload states. Tricuspid valve leaflet fluttering during diastole can be observed (similar to that seen on the mitral valve in the setting of aortic regurgitation). Doppler echocardiography is fairly sensitive in identifying pulmonic regurgitation.

Pulmonary regurgitation alone, unless severe, rarely requires specific therapy. However, once evidence of right ventricular failure appears, valve replacement (or correction of the underlying lesion) should be undertaken. Infective endocarditis on the pulmonic valve will require appropriate antibiotic treatment and sometimes valve replacement. Patients with clinically significant pulmonic regurgitation due to structural abnormalities of the valve should have antibiotic prophylaxis against infective endocarditis.

PROSTHETIC HEART VALVES

The selection of a particular prosthetic valve should be done under the direction of the surgeon and cardiologist. There are 2 general categories of prosthetic valves—mechanical and bioprosthetic (Fig. 10).

MECHANICAL VALVES

The Starr-Edwards caged-ball valve with a cloth-covered sewing ring and silastic ball has the advantages of durability, a single orifice, reduced rate of thrombogenicity (as compared with others), and relative ease of insertion. In addition, the valve functions quietly and has a low incidence of endocarditis. Disadvantages include its large, bulky size, making it inappropriate for patients with a small left ventricle or aortic annulus. In addition, hemolysis occurs in a small percentage of patients. After undergoing modifications during 1960-1965, the Starr-Edwards valve has been unchanged since 1965.

To date, the Bjork-Shiley tilting disc family of valves has accounted for the majority of prosthetic valve implantations (more than

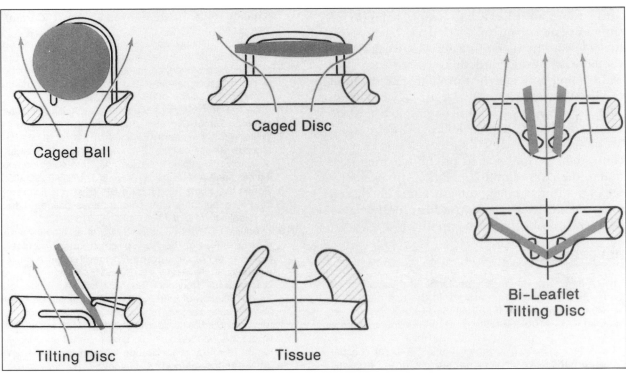

Figure 10. *Features and flow profiles of major categories of prosthetic heart valves. From Schoen FJ. Bioengineering aspects of heart valve replacement.* Ann Biomed Eng. *1982;10:97 and Schoen FJ.* Pathology of cardiac valve replacement. *In: Morse D, Steiner RM, Fernandez J (eds).* Guide to Prosthetic Cardiac Valves. *New York: Springer-Verlag; 1985:209. With permission.*

400,000).[63] The convexo-concave form of the valve, now discontinued owing to widely publicized failure caused by fracture of the welded outflow strut, has been replaced by the Bjork-Shiley monostent valve.[63] Although experiencing early favorable results in Europe, this prosthesis awaits FDA approval for usage in the United States at the present time.

The St. Jude valve consists of two semicircular leaflets which pivot open but do not rotate. The valve is coated with pyrolitic carbon and has excellent flow characteristics.

All mechanical valves require chronic anticoagulation therapy; usually this is instituted a few days into the postoperative course.

BIOPROSTHETIC VALVES

Bioprosthetic valves (Hancock, Carpentier-Edwards, Ionescu- Shiley, etc.), made of either porcine aortic valves or bovine pericardium, were developed primarily in an effort to avoid the need for anticoagulation that exists with mechanical valves. However, the bioprosthetic valves might be less durable; approximately 20% to 30% of patients need a second valve by 10 years after the first implantation. In patients younger than 30 to 35 years, the risk of bioprosthetic valve failure is far higher than in patients greater than 50 years. Calcification of bioprosthetic valves is also a frequent problem. For this reason, patients with chronic renal failure, secondary hyperparathyroidism, or abnormal calcium metabolism, and children who have active calcium metabolism, should receive mechanical prosthetic valves.

Even when bioprosthetic valves are used, anticoagulation might be desirable during the first three months of valve replacement. After three months, anticoagulation usually is not needed for bioprosthetic valves in the aortic or the mitral position if patients are in sinus rhythm and there is no evidence of atrial thrombi. However, in patients with atrial fibrillation and a large left atrium, a history of thromboembolism, or evidence of left atrial thrombus at the time of surgery, anticoagulation should be continued indefinitely.

In young patients, the durability and duration of effectiveness of the valve must be considered. The risk of long-term anticoagulation must be balanced against the probability of reoperation. Mechanical prosthetic valves are relatively contraindicated in women of child-bearing age, due to the risks of anticoagulation. In an elderly patient, a bioprosthetic valve is generally chosen to avoid anticoagulation; additionally, valve longevity may be less of an issue.

REFERENCES

1. Gordis L. The virtual disappearance of rheumatic fever in the United States. Lessons in the rise and fall of disease. *Circulation*. 1985;72:1155-1162.
2. Bisno A. Group A streptococcal infections and acute rheumatic fever. N Engl J Med. 1991;325:783-793.
3. Congeni B, Rizzo C, Congeni J, et al. Outbreak of acute rheumatic fever in Northeastern Ohio. *J Pediatr*. 1987;111:176-197.
4. Veasy L, Wiedmeier SE, Orsmond GS, et al. Resurgence of acute rheumatic fever in the intermountain area of the United States. *N Engl J Med*. 1987;316:421-427.
5. Wallace MR, Garst PD, Papadimes TJ, et al. The return of acute rheumatic fever in young adults. *JAMA*. 1989;262(18):2557-2561.
6. Westlake RM, Graham TP, Edwards KM, et al. An outbreak of acute rheumatic fever in Tennessee. *Pediat Infect Dis J*. 1990;9:97-100.
7. Stollerman GH. Rheumatogenic group A streptococci and the return of rheumatic fever. *Adv Intern Med*. 1990;35:1-25.
8. Gibofsky A, Khanna A, Suh E, et al. The genetics of rheumatic fever: Relationship to streptococcal infection and autoimmune disease. *J Rheumatol*. 1991;18(suppl 30):1-5.
9. Jones TD. Diagnosis of rheumatic fever. *JAMA*. 1944;126:481-484.
10. Committee on Standards and Criteria for Programs of Care. Jones criteria (modified) for guidance in the diagnosis of rheumatic fever. *Mod Concepts Cardiovasc Dis*. 1955;24:291-293.
11. Jones Criteria (revised) for guidance in the diagnosis of rheumatic fever. *Circulation*. 1984;69:204A-208A.
12. Dajani AS, Ayoub E, Bierman FZ, et al. Guidelines for the diagnosis of rheumatic fever. Jones Criteria, updated 1992. *Circulation*. 1993;87:302-307.
13. Case Records of the Massachusetts General Hospital. Case 19-1989. *N Engl J Med*. 1989;320:1260-1268.
14. Reis R, Roberts W. Amounts of coronary arterial narrowing by atherosclerotic plaques in clinically isolated mitral valve stenosis: Analysis of 76 necropsy patients older than 30 years. *Am J Cardiol*. 1986;57:1117-1123.
15. Nakatani S, Masuyama T, Kodama K, et al. Value and limitations of Doppler echocardiography in the quantification of stenotic mitral valve area: comparison of the pressure half-time and the continuity equation methods. *Circulation*. 1988;77:78-85.
16. Hatle L. Doppler echocardiographic evaluation of mitral stenosis. *Cardiol Clin*. 1990;8(2):233-247.
17. Wilkens GT, Weyman AE, Abascal VM, et al. Percutaneous balloon dilation of the mitral valve: An analysis of echocardiographic variables related to outcome and the mechanism of dilatation. *Br Heart J*. 1988;60:299-306.
18. Cohen DJ, Kuntz RE, Gordon SP, et al. Predictors of long-term outcome after percutaneous balloon mitral valvuloplasty. *N Engl J Med*. 1992;327:1329-1335.
19. Tribouilloy C, Wei FS, Slama MA, et al. Non-invasive measurement of the regurgitant fraction in pulsed Doppler echocardiography in isolated pure mitral regurgitation. *Br Heart J*. 1991;66:290-294.
20. Bargiggia GS, Tronconi L, Sahn DJ, et al. A new method for quantitation of mitral regurgitation based on color from Doppler imaging of flow convergence proximal to regurgitant orifice. *Circulation*. 1991;84:1481-1489.
21. Rivera JM, Vandervoort PM, Levine RA, et al. Quantification of mitral regurgitation with the proximal flow convergence method: A clinical study. *Am Heart J*. 1992;124:1289-1296.
22. Kamp O, Huitink H, Roos JP, et al. Value of pulmonary venous flow characteristics in the assessment of severity of native mitral valve regurgitation: An angiographic correlated study. *J Am Soc Echocardiogr*. 1992;5:239-246.
23. Appleton CP, Hartle LK, Nellessen U, et al. Flow velocity acceleration in the left ventricle: A useful Doppler echocardiographic sign of hemodynamically significant mitral regurgitation. *J Am Soc Echocardiogr*. 1990;3:35-45.
24. Reed D, Abbott RD, Smucker ML, et al. Prediction of outcome after survival valve replacement in patients with symptomatic chronic mitral regurgitation. *Circulation*. 1991;84:23-24.
25. Carabello B. Mitral valve disease. *Curr Probs Cardiol*. 1993;18:421-480.
26. Rozich JD, Carabello BA, Usher BW, et al. Mitral valve replacement with and without chordal preservation in patients with chronic mitral regurgitation. Mechanisms for differences in postoperation ejection performance. *Circulation*. 1992;86:1718-1726.
27. Hennein HA, Swain JA, Clark RE, et al. Comparative assessment of chordal preservation versus chordal resection during mitral valve replacement. *J Thorac Cardiovasc Surg*. 1990;99:828-837.
28. Crawford MH, Souchek J, Oprian CA, et al. Determinants of survival and left ventricular performance after mitral valve replacement. *Circulation*. 1990;83:1173-1181.
29. Perloff J, Child J. Clinical and epidemiologic issues in mitral valve prolapse: overview and perspective. *Am Heart J*. 1987;113:1324-1332.
30. Carabello BA. Mitral valve disease. *Curr Probs Cardiol*. 1993;18:421-480.

31. Marks AR, Choong CY, Sanfilippo AJ, et al. Identification of high-risk and low-risk subgroups of patients with mitral valve prolapse. N Engl J Med. 1989; 320:1031-1036.

32. Lobstein HP, Horwitz LD, Curry CC, et al. Electrocardiographic abnormalities and coronary angiograms in the mitral click-murmur syndrome. *N Engl J Med*. 1973;289:127-131.

33. Benjamin EJ, Plehn JF, D'Agostino RB, et al. Mitral annular calcification and the risk of stroke in an elderly cohort. *N Engl J Med*. 1992;327:374-379.

34. Lombard J, Selzer A. Valvular aortic stenosis: A clinical and hemodynamic profile of patients. *Ann Intern Med*. 1987;106:292-298.

35. Marcus M, Doty D, Hiratzka L, et al. Decreased coronary reserve. A mechanism for angina pectoris in patients with aortic stenosis and normal coronary arteries. *N Engl J Med*. 1982;307:1362-1366.

36. Ross J, Braunwald E. Aortic stenosis. *Circulation*. 1968;38(suppl 5):61-67.

37. Morgan D, Hall R. Occult aortic stenosis as a cause of intractable heart failure. *Br Med J*. 1979;1:784-787.

38. Frank S, Johnson A, Ross J, et al. Natural history of valvular aortic stenosis. *Br Heart J*. 1973;35:41-46.

39. Heyde EC. Gastrointestinal bleeding in aortic stenosis. *N Engl J Med*. 1958;259:196. Letter.

40. Brochmeier L, Adolph R, Gustin B, et al. Calcium emboli to the retinal artery in calcific aortic stenosis. *Am Heart J*. 1981;101:32-37.

41. Griffith MJ, Carey CM, Byrne JC, et al. Echocardiographic left ventricular wall thickness: A poor predictor of the severity of aortic valve stenosis. *Clin Cardiol*. 1991;14:227-231.

42. Shah PM, Graham BM. Management of aortic stenosis: Is cardiac catheterization necessary? *Am J Cardiol*. 1991;67:1031-1032.

43. Yeager M, Yock PG, Popp R, et al. Comparison of Doppler-derived pressure gradient to that determined at cardiac catheterization in adults with aortic valve stenosis: Implications for management. *Am J Cardiol*. 1986;57:644-648.

44. Skjaerpe T, Hatle L. Noninvasive estimation of valve area in patients with aortic stenosis by Doppler ultrasound and two-dimensional echocardiography. *Circulation*. 1985;72:810-818.

45. Oh JK, Taliercio CP, Holmes DR, et al. Prediction of the severity of aortic stenosis by Doppler aortic valve area determination: prospective Doppler-catheterization correlation in 100 patients. *J Am Coll Cardiol*. 1988;11:1227-1234.

46. Berger M, Hecht SR. Doppler echocardiographic assessment of aortic stenosis using the peak velocity ratio. *Am J Cardiol*. 1992;70:536-537.

47. Rahimtoola SH. Perspective on valvular heart disease: An update. *J Am Coll Cardiol*. 1989;14:1-23.

48. Pellikka PA, Nishimura RA, Tajik AJ, et al. The natural history of adults with asymptomatic, hemodynamically significant aortic stenosis. *J Am Coll Cardiol*. 1990;15:1013-1017.

49. Braunwald E. On the natural history of severe aortic stenosis. *J Am Coll Cardiol*. 1990;15:1018-1020. Editorial.

50. Lewin RF, Dorros G, King JF, et al. Percutaneous transluminal aortic valvuloplasty: Acute outcome and follow-up of 125 patients. *J Am Coll Cardiol*. 1989;14:1210-1217.

51. Dorros G, Lewin RF, Stertzer SH, et al. Percutaneous transluminal aortic valvuloplasty—the acute outcome and follow-up of 149 patients who under-went the double balloon technique. *Eur Heart J*. 1990;11:429-440.

52. Safian RD, Kuntz RE. Aortic valvuloplasty. *Cardiol Clin*. 1991;9:289-299.

53. Grollier G, Commeau P, Sesboue B, et al. Short-term clinical and hemodynamic assessment of balloon aortic valvuloplasty in 30 elderly patients. Discrepancy between immediate and eighth-day haemodynamic valves. *Eur Heart J*. 1988;9:155-162.

54. Cabrera E, Baxiola A. A critical re-evaluation of systolic and diastolic overload patterns. *Prog Cardiovasc Dis*. 1959;2:219-222.

55. Downes T, Nomeir A, Hackshaw B, et al. Diastolic mitral regurgitation in acute but not chronic aortic regurgitation: implications regarding the mechanism of mitral closure. *Am Heart J*. 1989;117:1106-1112.

56. Rapaport E. Natural history of aortic and mitral valve disease. *Am J Cardiol*. 1975;35:221-227.

57. Bonow RO, Lakatos E, Epstein SE, et al. Serial long-term assessment of the natural history of asymptomatic patients with chronic aortic regurgitation and normal left ventricular systolic function. *Circulation*. 1991;84:1625-1635.

57a. Scognamiglio R, Rahimtoola SH, Fasoli G, et al. Nifedipine in asymptomatic patients with severe aortic regurgitation and normal left ventricular function. *N Engl J Med*. 1994;331:689-694.

58. Gaynet C, Pierre B, Delahaye JP, et al. Traumatic tricuspid insufficiency—an underdiagnosed disease. *Chest*. 1987;92:429-432.

59. Amidi M, Irwin J, Salerni R, et al. Venous systolic thrill and murmur in the neck: A consequence of severe tricuspid insufficiency. *J Am Coll Cardiol*. 1986;7:942-945.

60. Carpentier A, Deloche A, Hanania G, et al. Surgical management of acquired tricuspid valve disease. *J Thorac Cardiovasc Surg*. 1974;67:53-65.

61. Arbulu A, Asfaw I. Tricuspid vulvulectomy without prosthetic replacement. Ten years of clinical experience. *J Thorac Cardiovasc Surg*. 1981;82:684-691.

62. Kan J, White R, Mitchell S, et al. Percutaneous transluminal balloon valvuloplasty for pulmonary valve stenosis. *Circulation*. 1984;69:554-560.

63. Grunkemeier GL, Rahimtoola SH, Starr A, et al. Prosthetic heart valve performance: Long-term follow-up. *Curr Probs Cardiol*. 1992;17(6):335-406.

64. Ross J. Afterload mismatch in aortic and mitral valve disease: Implications for surgical therapy. *J Am Coll Cardiol*. 1985;5:811-817.

19 Myocarditis and Cardiomyopathy

Shereif Rezkalla, MD
Robert A. Kloner, MD, PhD

MYOCARDITIS

Myocarditis is an inflammatory process involving the heart. There are many causes, including infectious agents, physical agents, chemicals, drugs, and radiation (Table 1).

INCIDENCE

Incidence varies widely in various reports, partly because of the difficulty in establishing the diagnosis, and the lack of uniform diagnostic criteria. An analysis of 12,747 consecutive autopsies performed at Malmö General Hospital (Sweden) revealed an incidence of about 1%.[1]

GENERAL CLINICAL MANIFESTATIONS

Clinical manifestations of myocarditis range from electrocardiographic abnormalities in an asymptomatic patient to severe congestive heart failure (CHF). Symptoms consist of fatigue, dyspnea, palpitations, chest pain suggestive of pericarditis or myocardial ischemia, and fever. Sinus tachycardia is usually present, and is out of proportion to the degree of fever. The S_1 is soft. Ventricular gallops, a transient apical systolic murmur, and a pericardial friction rub may be heard. In cases presenting with CHF, pulmonary rales and pulsus alternans may be present. Systemic or pulmonary emboli are complications of myocarditis. Physical findings related to the underlying cause of myocarditis should be sought (e.g., the suppurative pharyngeal membrane of diphtheria or skin rashes associated with rickettsial infection).

LABORATORY FINDINGS

Chest x-ray film is either normal or reveals cardiac enlargement, with or without signs of pulmonary congestion. Electrocardiogram reveals atrioventricular (AV) block, repolarization abnormalities during the acute phase of the disease, atrial abnormalities, left ventricular hypertrophy (LVH), and interventricular conduction delay during the chronic phase. Occasionally, patients may present with an electrocardiographic picture that is indistinguishable from acute myocardial infarction (MI).[2,3]

Echocardiography may demonstrate pericardial effusion and generalized uniform reduction in wall motion; however, regional wall motion abnormalities are not uncommon.[4] Transient ventricular aneurysm has also been observed.[5] Repeat echocardiograms may be the best means to follow up disease progression. Radionuclide ventriculography may detect reduced left ventricular function. Gallium scan[6] and Tc 99m WBC imaging,[7] while nonspecific, may suggest the presence of active inflammation. Electromagnetic resonance imaging may show the myocardium with higher signal intensity than does the skeletal muscle.[8]

TREATMENT

Although spontaneous recovery from acute myocarditis is common, a certain percentage of patients develop a fulminant illness and progress to severe, end-stage heart failure. Right ventricular function at the time of presentation is an important predictor of survival. If spontaneous recovery is to occur, it usually is seen within the first few months from the onset of infection. In general, therapy is supportive. Adequate rest and oxygenation are important as exercise and hypoxemia may increase myocardial damage. Congestive heart failure is treated with salt restriction, diuretics, and afterload reducers. Patients with myocarditis tend to be sensitive to digitalis; hence, it must be used with

---

Table 1. Etiologies of Myocarditis

Infectious Agents
Viral: coxsackievirus, echovirus, poliovirus, influenza, mumps, Epstein-Barr virus, viral hepatitis, rabies, rubella, rubeola, varicella, retrovirus
Bacterial: diphtheria, tuberculosis, salmonella (typhoid fever), streptococcus (rheumatic fever or direct streptococcal myocarditis), meningococcus, clostridia (gas gangrene or tetanus), brucellosis
Spirochetal myocarditis; syphilis, leptospirosis (Weil's disease), relapsing fever, Lyme disease
Rickettsial myocarditis: typhus, Rocky Mountain spotted fever, Q fever
Chlamydial: psittacosis
Primary atypical pneumonia (mycoplasma)
Fungal: candidiasis, aspergillosis, histoplasmosis, actinomycosis, blastomycosis
Protozoal myocarditis: Trypanosoma cruzi (Chagas' disease), African trypanosomiasis (sleeping sickness), malaria, toxoplasmosis, amebiasis
Metazoal myocarditis: schistosomiasis, trichinosis, ascariasis, cysticercosis, echinococcus

Myocardial Damage due to Chemicals, Drugs, Toxins
Antineoplastic agents: anthracyclines, cyclophosphamide, 5-fluorouracil
Metal poisoning: lead, mercury, arsenic
Antiparasitic agents: emetine, chloroquine, antimony compounds
Catecholamines (e.g., pheochromocytoma)
Psychotropic drugs: phenothiazines, lithium
Animal toxins: snake bite, wasp, spider, scorpion stings
Carbon monoxide, phosphorus

Physical Agents
Radiation, hypothermia, heat stroke

Hypersensitivity Reactions
Methyldopa, penicillin, sulfonamides, tetracycline, phenylbutazone, serum sickness, rejection of cardiac transplant, collagen vascular diseases

---

caution. Patients should be monitored for the development of conduction disturbances and arrhythmias. The use of steroids in the acute phase of the disease is controversial and should probably be avoided, particularly in the infectious myocarditides. Antibiotics are used in myocarditis secondary to bacterial, rickettsial, or mycoplasmal infections. Antitoxin is used for diphtheria myocarditis. If myocarditis is due to chemicals, drugs, or physical agents, the offending substance or agent must be withdrawn.

SELECTED SPECIFIC MYOCARDITIDES

Viral Myocarditis

Coxsackievirus A and B, echovirus, and influenza virus are the most common viruses causing myocarditis. The disease consists of 2 phases: the acute phase, characterized by viral replica-tion, during which the virus may be isolated from the myocardium, and usually represents the first 10 days of the illness. The late phase is characterized by slow deterioration of myocardial function or spontaneous recovery. It is believed that many cases of idiopathic dilated cardiomyopathy are due to antecedent viral myocarditis.[9] Endomyocardial biopsy in patients with dilated myopathy reveals a high incidence of myocarditis. Matoba et al[10] reported a case of biopsy proven myocarditis that progressed to dilated myopathy. Gwathmey et al[11] were able to show that acute viral myocarditis may progress to dilated cardiomyopathy in a swine model.

Helpful laboratory tests include isolation of virus from blood, throat, or rectal swabs, and determination of antibody titer during the acute and convalescent phases of the disease. A rise in the titers is more suggestive of the disease than the absolute value. Isolation of virus from the heart, although quite uncommon, is diagnostic for myocarditis. Recently, antimyosin antibody imaging has emerged as a new technique for detection of myocyte necrosis.[12,13] Animal as well as human studies show that it may be a useful technique in the evaluation of acute myocarditis. It is of particular use in patients with myocarditis presenting as acute myocardial infarction. In myocarditis the uptake is diffuse and extends beyond specific coronary territories. Endomyocardial biopsy supports a definite diagnosis when positive, but does not rule out the disease if negative. Its routine use is probably not warranted and should be reserved for those patients who show progressive deterioration in their symptoms and a definitive diagnosis must be established. Rest is indicated.[14] Nonsteroidal anti-inflammatory drugs should be avoided during the acute phase of myocarditis, since they may exacerbate the extent of cardiac pathology, and their use should be restricted to symptomatic treatment during the later phase of illness.[15,16] Beta-blockers should probably be avoided during the acute phase as well.[17] Alpha-adrenergic blockers were not beneficial when administered after the disease had been established.[18]

Several clinical reports suggest either a beneficial or a deleterious effect of immunosuppressive therapy on myocarditis. O'Connell and colleagues studied 35 patients with idiopathic myopathy presumed to be secondary to myocarditis. Twenty patients had a negative gallium scan and were treated with conventional therapy, and 15 with positive scans were treated with prednisone and azathioprine. Among the treated patients, 6 showed improvement while 9 did not.[19] Due to the lack of control groups in this study, the claimed benefit cannot be distinguished from spontaneous improvement. A randomized study failed to show any benefit of immunosuppressive therapy in patients with myocarditis. Further testing is currently underway to see if certain subgroups of patients may benefit from immunosuppressive therapy (personal communication).

A report on the use of intravenous ribavirin in influenza virus-associated acute myocarditis in 3 patients revealed that while viral-shedding abruptly terminated with therapy, 2 patients died shortly after treatment, and the third died 8 months later.[20] At present ribavirin does not appear to be of clear benefit in management of human myocarditis. Recently, captopril was beneficial during both the acute[21] and late phases[22] of the disease in a murine model of myocarditis.

Rezkalla, Kloner, and colleagues randomized 90 mice with coxsackie-myocarditis to captopril or saline during early and late phases of illness. Captopril was beneficial when administered early, with a reduction in left ventricular mass and myonecrosis, and a reduction in left ventricular mass when administered late. This was confirmed by further studies and the captopril benefit was dose-dependent. Other angiotensin-converting enzyme (ACE) inhibitors did not significantly affect myonecrosis. It does seem that the beneficial effect of captopril is, at least in part, due to its oxygen radical scavenging properties.[23] Controlled human studies are not yet available. Preliminary data suggest that high-dose gamma-globulin treatment may be beneficial in the pediatric population. However, this needs to be confirmed by controlled prospective studies.[24] Most patients recover from viral myocarditis within weeks, although electrocardiographic abnormalities often persist for months. Viral myocarditis is only occasionally fatal in adults; neonates tend to have a more malignant course than adults, and if improvement is lacking after a few weeks of captopril therapy, then cardiac transplantation should be considered for those with end-stage heart failure.

Diphtheria

Myocardial involvement occurs in approximately 25% of cases of diphtheria and may lead to severe cardiac dysfunction and, in some cases, sudden cardiovascular collapse and death. The myocarditis is due to a toxin produced by the diphtheria bacillus. Clinical manifestations of myocarditis typically appear at the end of the first week of illness and include CHF, arrhythmias, and conduction defects. Treatment includes administration of antitoxins, antibiotics (penicillin G or erythromycin), and respiratory support. Digitalis should be administered cautiously as it may increase atrioventricular block. Transvenous pacemaker therapy is instituted for complete AV block. Ramos et al reported that the addition of carnitine at 100 mg/kg/day results in a lower incidence of heart failure and improved survival.[25] Corticosteroid therapy is of no benefit.

Chagas' Disease (Trypanosomiasis)

Chagas' disease is the most common form of heart disease in Central and South America and is caused by the protozoan *Trypanosoma cruzi*. The protozoan is transmitted to humans through an insect bite. In the acute phase of the illness, patients may be asymptomatic or may experience constitutional symptoms of fever, sweating, muscle pains, vomiting, diarrhea, palpitations, and dyspnea. Tachycardia, signs of CHF, and hepatomegaly may be present. After a latent phase, 30% of patients progress to the chronic phase of the disease.

Chronic Chagas' disease may be due to autoimmune or neurogenic factors. Abnormalities in microcirculation could also contribute to it.[26] The disease is characterized by mononuclear cellular infiltration, fibrosis in the myocardium and its conduction systems, and often mural thrombi. Clinical manifestations include symptoms of CHF.[27] Chest pain is common and syncope may be reported. Thromboembolic events can occur which may be related to mural thrombi and increased platelet aggregability noted in this disease. Physical examination reveals a widely split S_2 due to right bundle branch block and a loud P_2 due to pulmonary hypertension. The murmur of mitral and tricuspid regurgitation may be present. Ventricular ectopic activity is a frequent finding and usually indicates a worsened prognosis. Laboratory evidence of Chagas' disease includes a complement-fixation test (Machado-Guerreiro test), a positive monoclonal antibody test, or a detection of the parasite in the blood of patients during the acute phase of illness. Electrocardiography is a good screening test in areas with a high prevalence of the disease.[28] Electrocardiographic abnormalities include AV and bundle branch block, low QRS voltage, prolonged QT interval, and various repolarization abnormalities. Echocardiography reveals systolic and diastolic dysfunction with or without regional wall motion abnormalities. Thallium perfusion abnormalities are common, particularly in patients with chest pain, and it is usually associated with normal epicardial coronary arteries as shown by coronary angiograms. Electrophysiologic testing reveals HV prolongation and may show inducible ventricular tachycardia in patients presenting with syncope. Endomyocardial biopsy reveals cellular infiltration myocardial necrosis and myocyte hypertrophy.

Prevention includes control of the insect vector. Patients with high-degree AV block may require pacemaker placement. Digoxin and amiodarone should be used with caution if indi-

cated. Two agents for treating acute Chagas' disease (benznidazole and nifurtimox) have shown promise in decreasing the length of illness and in reducing parasitemia. Verapamil may be a useful adjunct therapy. Captopril may also be beneficial. Roberti et al[29] conducted a single-blind, crossover trial of prolonged treatment with captopril or placebo. Captopril therapy led to a reduction in heart rate, urinary catecholamine levels, as well as frequency of premature ventricular contractions. Further studies are warranted to confirm these findings. Amiodarone may be beneficial in treating malignant ventricular arrhythmias often seen with this disease.

Prognosis depends on ventricular function and frequency of premature ventricular contractions. Although rare, Chagas' disease has been reported in the continental United States, and the disease may mimic coronary artery disease (CAD) or idiopathic cardiomyopathy in presentation.

Trichinosis

Trichinosis is an illness due to infestation with Trichinella spiralis. The larva invade skeletal muscle, the tongue, heart, lungs, and other organs, and the most serious complication of the disease is myocarditis. Cardiac damage may be due to inflammation or a hypersensitivity reaction mounted in response to the parasite. The initial clinical manifestations include muscle tenderness, periorbital edema, and eosinophilia. Cardiac symptoms include dyspnea, palpitation, and chest pain. These typically occur approximately 3 weeks after the initial onset of illness. Arrhythmias and CHF may be present. Electrocardiographic abnormalities are common and include low QRS voltage, prolonged PR interval, nonspecific interventricular conduction delay, and nonspecific ST- and T-wave abnormality. Echocardiography may show pericardial effusion, dilated cardiomyopathy, and regional wall motion abnormality. The diagnosis is established by demonstration of larval forms in muscle biopsy. Eosinophilia and a positive skin test provide supportive evidence of the diagnosis. Thiabendazole and corticosteroids may be beneficial.

AIDS Heart Disease

The acquired immune deficiency syndrome (AIDS) is probably one of the worst epidemics in

Table 2. Cardiac Involvement in AIDS

PERICARDIUM	MYOCARDIUM	ENDOCARDIUM
Pericardial effusion	Myocarditis	Infective endocarditis
Pericardial tamponade	Dilated myopathy	Nonbacterial thrombotic
Constrictive pericarditis	Kaposi's sarcoma	endocarditis
Infectious pericarditis	Malignant lymphoma	Mitral valve prolapse
Kaposi's sarcoma	Cor pulmonale	
Lymphoma		

history. In addition to an increasing number of symptomatic AIDS patients, it is estimated that about 2 million asymptomatic human immunodeficiency virus (HIV-1) patients exist in the United States and 5 million world-wide.

The disease carries a very poor prognosis. Among AIDS patients in San Francisco, the 1-year survival is 51% and 3-year survival is 3%. The cardiac involvement in AIDS patients is responsible for 5%-10% of morbidity and 1%-5% of disease mortality. The cardiac involvement was first reported in 1983 by Autran et al[30] who described a Kaposi's sarcoma found in the heart at autopsy. Since then, a variety of cardiac manifestations have been reported (Table 2). The incidence of cardiac involvement in patients with AIDS is about 50%.[31] Patients with cardiac manifestations tend to be older, with a mean age in 1 study of about 38 years compared with 29 years in those who have apparently normal hearts.[32] It also tends to be more common with severe disease, particularly when the CD_4 cell count drops to below 100 cells/ml[3]. Common cardiac abnormalities are pericarditis, myocarditis, dilated cardiomyopathy, Kaposi's sarcoma, and thrombotic nonbacterial endocarditis.[33,34]

Pericarditis and pericardial effusion are usually present in over 20% of patients presenting with cardiac abnormality. The nature of effusion is usually serosanguineous, yet it may be serofibrinous. The majority of patients will have small or moderate effusions, yet few may present with cardiac tamponade. In most cases, no pathogen can be identified. There is no specific treatment for small effusions, while pericardiocentesis is indicated for tamponade. Dilated cardiomyopathy is a common finding. In about one-half of the cases of cardiomyopathy at autopsy, foci of myocarditis are identified. Other less common etiologies for myopathy are pulmonary hypertension and selenium deficiency. In one case,

the HIV virus was isolated from an endomyocardial biopsy in the absence of histologic evidence for myocarditis.

Kaposi's sarcoma is present in about 18% of autopsy series and may be present in the pericardium or myocardium. Malignant lymphomas may also be seen infiltrating the myocardium. Both tumors can be suspected during echocardiographic examination, yet it is usually an autopsy finding. Routine screening with electrocardiogram and 2D echocardiogram is not recommended and should be reserved for symptomatic patients. When electrocardiograms are done, repolarization abnormalities, bundle branch block, and premature ectopic beats may be present. Almost all changes are nonspecific and are of limited clinical value. Perhaps the electrocardiogram is most important during Pentamidine therapy. Few patients will have prolongation of QT interval and may develop *torsades de pointes*. QT interval will revert to normal at the end of treatment. Treatment for AIDS heart disease is supportive and the prognosis depends on the disease progression.

Lyme Disease

Lyme disease is caused by the spirochete *Borrelia burgdorferi*, transmitted by the bite of the *Ixodes dammini* tick. Originally described in Lyme, Connecticut, the disease is endemic to Wisconsin, Minnesota, and the Northeastern United States. It usually manifests initially with a characteristic skin lesion (erythema chronicum migrans) and flu-like symptoms. If left untreated, it may progress with neurologic, arthritic, and cardiac manifestations. Cardiac involvement is usually a late manifestation, and it may manifest as various degrees of atrioventricular block, myopericarditis and myocardial dysfunction.[35]

Atrioventricular block is the most common

Table 3. Etiologies of Dilated (Congestive) Cardiomyopathy

Idiopathic
Peripartum
Post-myocarditis due to infectious agents (viral, parasitic, mycobacterial, Rickettsiae)
Alcoholic
Neuromuscular (muscular dystrophy, myotonic dystrophy)
Connective tissue disorders (systemic lupus erythematosus, rheumatoid disease, polyarteritis)
Beriberi
Glycogen storage disease
Toxins (cobalt, lead, arsenic)
Doxorubicin hydrochloride, cyclophosphamide, vincristine
Infiltrative: amyloid, hemochromatosis, sarcoid (may have congestive or restrictive features)
Inherited disorders: Fabry's disease, Gaucher's disease
Metabolic: chronic hypophosphatemia, hypokalemia, hypocalcemia, uremia

manifestation, usually requiring temporary pacemaker placement; however, the long-term prognosis with treatment is usually good. Gallium scanning may reveal diffuse myocardial uptake. Myocardial biopsy may show areas of lymphocyte infiltration and myocytic necrosis. Serologic testing is useful in establishing the diagnosis, particularly in the late phase of the disease. Antibiotic therapy with tetracyclines (250 mg 4 times/day for 10 days), or erythromycin in the same dose, is recommended to all patients. Despite scattered reports of possible benefit from corticosteroids or salicylates, their therapeutic role has not been well established.

CARDIOMYOPATHY

Cardiomyopathy is a disorder in which the prominent feature is a primary involvement of the cardiac muscle. Myocardial dysfunction due to systemic or pulmonary vascular disease (e.g., hypertensive heart disease), or structural abnormalities (e.g., valvular or congenital heart disease) is not included in this category.

The annual incidence of cardiomyopathy ranges from 0.7-7.5 cases per 100,000 population, and the prevalence has been reported by William and Olsen as 8,317 cases per 100,000.[1] Mortality due to cardiomyopathy constitutes about 0.7% of cardiac deaths in the United States, with higher rates among men and blacks.[2]

Cardiomyopathy may be classified on a functional basis as dilated (or congestive), hypertrophic, or restrictive. Alternatively, it may be classified on an etiologic basis (i.e., viral myocarditis, ischemic cardiomyopathy, alcoholic

cardiomyopathy). Kasper et al reviewed 673 consecutive patients with dilated cardiomyopathy. The most common cause was idiopathic cardiomyopathy, which was reported in 47% of patients. Myocarditis was found in 12% of patients, and coronary artery disease was the culprit in 11%.[2a]

DILATED CARDIOMYOPATHY

Dilated or congestive cardiomyopathy is characterized by a large, dilated heart with reduced systolic and abnormal diastolic function, frequently associated with the clinical features of CHF. There are numerous causes (Table 3), but the most common form is idiopathic cardiomyopathy. Although still controversial, considerable evidence suggests that at least some of the cases of dilated cardiomyopathy are a late sequelae of viral myocarditis. All 4 chambers of the heart are dilated. The degree of hypertrophy of the ventricular wall is disproportionately small in relation to the extent of ventricular dilatation. The clinical manifestations are those of CHF. They include dyspnea on exertion, orthopnea, fatigue, and paroxysmal nocturnal dyspnea. Peripheral edema, ascites, and hepatomegaly occur later, resulting from right-sided cardiac dysfunction. Systemic and pulmonary emboli may be present.

Diagnosis

Depending on the severity of cardiac dysfunction, physical examination may reveal a narrow pulse pressure, pulsus alternans, cold clammy

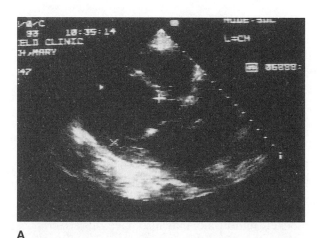 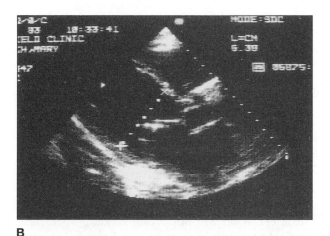

A   **B**

Figure 1. *Two-dimensional echocardiogram of a patient with dilated cardiomyopathy during systole (Fig. 1A) and diastole (Fig. 1B). Note global hypokinesia and dilation of left ventricular cavity. Courtesy of Bill Nugent and Jan Claringbole, Marshfield Clinic.*

skin, and jugular venous distention with prominent a waves. If tricuspid regurgitation is present, as is frequently the case, prominent regurgitant systolic v waves are present. The cardiac apical impulse is typically displaced leftward with a left ventricular heave and, in some cases, right ventricular heave. A palpable precordial a wave may be present. Auscultation may reveal paradoxical splitting of S_2, an S_3 gallop, and, in some cases, an S_4 gallop. The murmurs of mitral and tricuspid regurgitation may be heard. Other signs of left heart failure are common, including pulmonary rales or dullness at the lung bases due to pleural effusion; when right ventricular failure ensues, peripheral edema, ascites, and hepatomegaly are present as well.

Chest x-ray demonstrates diffuse cardiac enlargement, and when hemodynamic deterioration occurs, signs of CHF are seen, including pulmonary vascular redistribution, interstitial and alveolar edema, and pleural effusions. When right-sided heart failure is present, the azygous vein and superior vena cava are dilated; the right-sided cardiac chambers are dilated as well.

The ECG shows a variety of abnormalities. Supraventricular and ventricular ectopy and various conduction disturbances are common. Left atrial abnormality and either left ventricular hypertrophy or low-voltage QRS may be present. In the absence of a discrete infarction, the ECG may reveal pathologic Q waves and nonspecific ST-T-wave abnormalities. Wilensky and colleagues[3] showed that when serial ECGs from patients with cardiomyopathies were analyzed,

progressive prolongation of PR interval and QRS duration were noted. The presence of abnormal Q waves, left bundle branch block, and nonspecific interventricular conduction delay are associated with a worse prognosis.

Two-dimensional echocardiography is virtually diagnostic of cardiomyopathy (Figs. 1A, 1B). Dilated cardiac chambers with generalized poor ventricular function are observed. Mitral valve closure may be delayed and aortic valve closure may occur earlier than normal. Two-dimensional echocardiography is especially useful for detecting a left ventricular thrombus. Doppler echocardiography usually reveals multiple valvular regurgitation. Keren and colleagues studied 17 patients with dilated cardiomyopathy and no evidence of primary valvular disease. Mitral regurgitation was present in all but 1 patient, with regurgitant fraction ranging between 5% and 53%; regurgitant fraction was >20% in two-thirds of the patients.[4] Pulmonary hypertension may be detected by continuous-wave Doppler and is associated with a worse prognosis.[5]

Radionuclide ventriculography demonstrates increased ventricular volumes and reduced ejection fraction. There is controversy concerning the role of endomyocardial biopsy in patients with idiopathic dilated cardiomyopathy. Apart from its value in detecting early transplant rejection and cardiac involvement in systemic disease, other indications for biopsy are less clear. Even though it may yield a specific diagnosis on a few occasions, it rarely alters therapeutic decisions.

Cardiac catheterization reveals an elevated

left ventricular end-diastolic pressure (EDP) and left atrial pressure, and modest elevation in the pulmonary artery pressure. When right ventricular failure occurs, the right ventricular and right atrial pressures rise as well. The left ventricular EDP may be higher than that in the right ventricle, and the cardiac index is reduced. Diffuse hypokinetic wall motion, elevated systolic and diastolic volumes, and a reduced ejection fraction are observed during left ventriculography. Mitral regurgitation is frequently detected and, occasionally, mural thrombi are observed. Coronary angiography and cardiac catheterization are important in diagnosis, particularly to rule out other conditions that may mimic dilated myopathy.[6]

Therapy

Therapy for patients with dilated cardiomyopathy includes treatment for the underlying disease, if known. The basic therapy for cardiomyopathy is similar to treatment of heart failure including vasodilator therapy, preferably with angiotensin-converting enzyme inhibitors, diuretics, digitalis, and salt restriction. Inotropic drugs that bypass the cAMP system, such as cardiac glycosides, increase isometric tension in cardiomyopathic muscle, whereas agents that increase cAMP, such as phosphodiesterase inhibitors, have a less profound effect. Phosphodiesterase inhibitors have both inotropic and vasodilator effects; amrinone and milrinone may provide short-term improvement in left ventricular function, but chronic use of these drugs has been disappointing. In a study by Packer et al,[7] 1,088 patients with severe CHF were randomized to oral milrinone therapy or placebo. As compared to placebo, milrinone therapy was associated with 28% increase in mortality, more hospitalization, and more serious adverse cardiovascular reactions.[7] Infusions of inotropes such as dobutamine for a few days may provide clinical improvement lasting months, possibly by reconditioning the heart. However, this requires careful monitoring of the patient, and has not been shown to improve survival.

Although calcium-channel blockers may be beneficial in some cases of dilated cardiomyopathy, especially if patients have concomitant hypertension or coronary artery disease, their ultimate role in therapy is not yet clear, and they may occasionally cause significant left ventricular dysfunction, particularly when combined with β-blocker therapy. In 1 study by Figulla et al,[8] 47 patients with dilated cardiomyopathy were assigned to either conventional therapy alone or conventional therapy plus diltiazem in doses ranging from 180-270 mg/day. Patients in the diltiazem group had a significant improvement in both New York Heart Association functional class and mortality.[8] In preliminary trials, the newer calcium channel blocker, amlodipine, has been shown to improve symptoms of heart failure and exercise tolerance.[9] The dihydropyridine calcium-channel blocker, felodipine, may also have this effect.

Despite favorable reports about the efficacy of β-blockers in dilated cardiomyopathy, their role is still controversial. Waagstein et al[10] reported improved functional class, increased ejection fraction, and reduction of left ventricular dilatation, pulmonary wedge pressure, and mitral and tricuspid regurgitation during long-term therapy with metoprolol. The beneficial effect may have been related to an up-regulation of ventricular β-adrenergic receptors.

Perhaps the mainstay of therapy is vasodilators because they improve cardiac performance, relieve signs and symptoms of CHF, and improve survival. The Captopril Multicenter Research Group enrolled 92 patients with chronic CHF refractory to digitalis and diuretic therapy into a randomized, double-blind trial with either the ACE inhibitor, captopril, or placebo. The main cause of CHF was ischemic heart disease. Captopril therapy was well-tolerated, and was associated with better exercise tolerance, higher ejection fraction, and better clinical improvement. Hydralazine plus isosorbide dinitrate, enalapril, and captopril have been shown to improve survival in patients with heart failure.

Symptomatic, high-grade arrhythmias may be treated with antiarrhythmic agents, but because many of these agents have negative inotropic effects and may even have proarrhythmic effects, dosages must be carefully titrated and patients monitored frequently during administration of these drugs. Amiodarone, however, has a favorable therapeutic profile compared to other agents and has less tendency to worsen heart failure.[11] Patients who present with atrial fibrillation should have an attempt at cardioversion to sinus rhythm since this may improve their ejection fraction.[12] There is no clear role for electrophysiologic testing in guiding antiarrhythmic therapy in patients with dilated cardiomyopathy, except perhaps in preparation for implementation of an automatic implantable cardioverter-defibrillator (AICD), which may prove to be the most effective therapy for preventing sudden death in this group of patients.[13] Anticoagulant therapy probably should be administered if there are no contraindications.

In suitable candidates, cardiac transplantation may be considered for better quality of life and improved survival. With current immunosuppressive regimens, the 5-year survival rate is 75%, a substantial improvement from medical therapy alone in patients with end-stage dilated cardiomyopathy.[14]

Prognosis

Fuster et al[15] followed 104 patients with a diagnosis of idiopathic dilated cardiomyopathy for up to 20 years. Seventy-seven percent of patients in this study had an accelerated course, with the majority of patients dying within the first 2 years of diagnosis. Three factors were highly predictive of a poor prognosis: age over 50 years, a cardiothoracic ratio >0.55, and a cardiac index of <3 l/min/m^2. Hofmann et al[16] prospectively followed 110 patients with idiopathic dilated cardiomyopathy for 53 months. Two-year mortality was 34%, and poor left ventricular function was the major predictor of mortality.[16] Furthermore, patients with a low frequency of ventricular pairs/24 h on ambulatory ECG monitoring were more likely to die from CHF, while those with a high frequency of pairs were more susceptible to sudden cardiac death.

HYPERTROPHIC CARDIOMYOPATHY

Hypertrophic cardiomyopathy (HCM) refers to inappropriate hypertrophy of the left ventricle and often involves the interventricular system (asymmetric septal hypertrophy, ASH). If it is associated with a left ventricular outflow gradient, it is known as hypertrophic obstructive cardiomyopathy (HOCM), formerly referred to as idiopathic hypertrophic subaortic stenosis (IHSS).

Hypertrophic cardiomyopathy is characterized by a diastolic dysfunction with abnormal relaxation of the left ventricle. This feature impairs left ventricular filling, while systolic left ventricular function may actually demonstrate hypercontractility. While disproportionate ventricular wall thickness usually involves the septum in cases of HCM, it can be limited to the apex or to the upper part of the septum. With HOCM, the anterior mitral leaflet moves forward during systole (systolic anterior motion), and together with septal hypertrophy, may cause obstruction to blood flow. The obstruction may occur at rest or after provocative maneuvers that reduce blood volume.

Hypertrophic cardiomyopathy is an autosomal dominant disease with variable penetrance. A gene for hypertrophic cardiomyopathy has been identified and appears to be more prevalent than indicated by echocardiographic studies. Gene mutation may result in a variety of clinical expressions[17] and the clinical course of a specific gene mutation may be different in various ethnic backgrounds.[18] Genetic and nongenetic factors appear to determine the clinical course of the disease. The incidence of HCM ranges between 0.1%-1% in the population and represents 2%-6% of cases of cardiomyopathy, and is more common in males than females, and in blacks than whites. Occasionally patients with Pompe's disease, Friedreich's ataxia, or Noonan's syndrome present with cardiac findings indistinguishable from HCM.

Symptoms of HCM include dyspnea on exertion, orthopnea, paroxysmal nocturnal dyspnea, palpitations, angina, and syncope. Angina in the absence of concomitant coronary artery disease is probably due to small vessel disease, and to reduced coronary reserve in the setting of a hypertrophied ventricle. Thallium images frequently reveal perfusion defects that are reversed with dipyridamole.[19] Syncope may be due to decreased cerebral perfusion, emboli from mitral vegetations or ventricular thrombi, or arrhythmias. Stroke and transient ischemic attack may be a manifestation of the disease. In a study of 119 patients with HCM who were followed for 6.5 years, cerebrovascular events were observed in 26 patients.[20] Cardiac embolic events were common in patients with atrial fibrillation and a large left atrium, while carotid disease was the culprit in patients with significant hypertension. Increased risk of stroke was noted in females, in patients with mitral annular calcification, and/or hypertension. The average patient age at presentation was in the mid-20s; however, it is not uncommon to first recognize the condition at an older age. It should be pointed out that there is considerable variation from patient to patient in

Table 4. Effect of Various Maneuvers on Systolic Murmurs

	VALSALVA	PHENYLEPHRINE HANDGRIP	SQUATTING	AMYL NITRITE	LEG RAISING
Aortic stenosis	Decrease	Decrease	Increase or Decrease	Increase	Increase
Hypertrophic obstructive cardiomyopathy	Increase	Decrease	Decrease	Increase	Decrease
Ventricular septal defect	Decrease	Increase	No change	Decrease	Increase
Mitral regurgitation	Slight decrease	Increase	No change	Decrease	Increase

the degree of symptomatology, from totally asymptomatic to severely symptomatic patients presenting with end-stage heart failure. Relatives of patients with documented HCM may have echocardiographic evidence of the disease, but are often asymptomatic.

Diagnosis

There are several prominent physical findings in patients with HCM. The carotid pulse rises rapidly and typically has a double peak; the jugular venous pulse may reveal a prominent a wave. The apical impulse may be displaced leftward, is forceful, and typically consists of a presystolic impulse followed by a double systolic impulse. A systolic thrill may be palpable. Auscultation reveals an S_4 gallop and an S_2 that is normally split. An S_3 may be heard in some patients. The systolic murmur of HOCM is a harsh crescendo-decrescendo murmur heard best between the left lower sternal border and the apex. The murmur radiates toward the base of the heart and clavicle, but in general, not into the carotid artery. The severity of outflow obstruction and the loudness of the murmur are increased by factors which reduce ventricular volume, increase inotropy, or reduce afterload. Conversely, the severity of obstruction and the loudness of the murmur are reduced by maneuvers which increase ventricular volume, reduce inotropy, or increase afterload. The murmur increases with Valsalva maneuver, standing, and administration of amyl nitrite or isoproterenol. It decreases with squatting, handgrip, and administration of phenylephrine. The murmur of mitral regurgitation is commonly heard. The effects of various maneuvers on systolic murmurs are shown on Table 4.

Chest x-ray reveals various degrees of cardiomegaly. Unlike valvular aortic stenosis, poststenotic aortic dilatation and calcification of the aortic valve are absent, but calcification of the mitral annulus may be present. Electrocardiogram reveals left ventricular hypertrophy with repolarization abnormalities. Deeply inverted T waves may be present in the anterior leads, particularly in apical hypertrophy. Deep, narrow Q waves may be seen in up to 50% of patients, and are typically present in inferolateral leads. Left atrial abnormality and prolonged QTc may also be present. The echocardiogram is extremely useful in establishing the diagnosis. The left ventricular walls are hypertrophied with disproportionate septal thickness (Figs. 2A, 2B). Systolic anterior motion of the mitral valve may be seen (Fig. 3). The aortic valve leaflets may appear to partially close or flutter in systole due to the Venturi effect produced by the subvalvular stenosis. Doppler echocardiography may reveal a systolic gradient in the left ventricular outflow tract. While most patients will have normal systolic function, some will have a low ejection fraction, and occasionally a regional wall-motion abnormality in the absence of myocardial infarction. Thallium-201 may reveal an asymmetrically thickened septum. Perfusion abnormalities, in the absence of coronary artery disease, are not uncommon and may normalize following treatment with dipyridamole. Recently, magnetic resonance imaging has been utilized in the diagnosis of HCM.[21] While not routinely recommended, it is helpful in patients with apical hypertrophy and in those with a technically difficult echocardiographic study. Holter monitoring has been recommended for patients with HCM, because some studies have shown that patients with high-grade ventricular

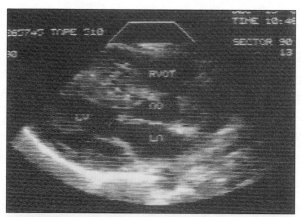

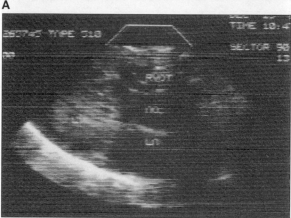

Figure 2. *Parasternal long-axis echocardiogram of a patient with hypertrophic cardiomyopathy during diastole (Fig. 2A) and systole (Fig. 2B). RVOT=Right ventricular outflow tract; Ao=Aorta; LA=Left atrium; LV=Left ventricle. Note virtual cavity obliteration during systole. Courtesy of Bruce Fye, MD, Marshfield Clinic.*

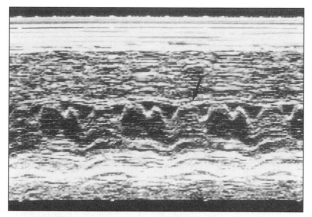

Figure 3. *M mode echocardiogram at the level of the mitral valve in a patient with hypertrophic cardiomyopathy. Note systolic anterior motion of the mitral valve (arrow). Courtesy of Bruce Fye, MD, Marshfield Clinic.*

ectopy are at high-risk of sudden death. Supraventricular arrhythmias are common; atrial fibrillation leads to a loss of atrial contraction with reduced left ventricular filling and clinical deterioration.[22]

Signal-averaged electrocardiograms may be abnormal. An abnormal test is common in patients with frequent nonsustained ventricular tachycardia and is useful in the prediction of sudden death in young patients with HCM.[23] Cardiac catheterization studies demonstrate elevated left ventricular EDP, and systolic pressure gradient between the body of the left ventricular cavity and the area below the aortic valve (in HOCM). The gradient can be provoked by Valsalva maneuver, amyl nitrite, nipride and isoproterenol (Fig. 4). Following a premature

beat, the gradient increases with a concomitant fall in aortic pulse pressure (Brockenborough's sign, Fig. 5). The systolic arterial wave-form may reveal a spike and dome configuration. There is usually a prominent a wave in the left atrial and left ventricular wave-forms due to diminished left ventricular compliance. Mild pulmonary hypertension is present in 25% of cases. Left ventricular angiography allows visualization of the obstruction, estimation of the degree of hypertrophy and visualization of the systolic anterior motion of the mitral valve. Concomitant coronary artery disease is not uncommon in patients over 50 years of age.

Therapy

The main therapies for HCM are β-blockers and calcium-channel blockers. Beta-blockers improve ventricular compliance and reduce myocardial oxygen demand, thus decreasing the frequency of angina.[24] Beta-blockers have some effect on decreasing resting gradient; however, their main benefit is in preventing the increase in gradient that occurs with exercise. Verapamil has been shown to reduce the left ventricular outflow gradient, improve exercise capacity, and improve peak left ventricular filling rate.[25] One study showed electrocardiographic evidence of regression of hypertrophy following long-term verapamil therapy. Nifedipine has also been shown to be effective in these patients with its

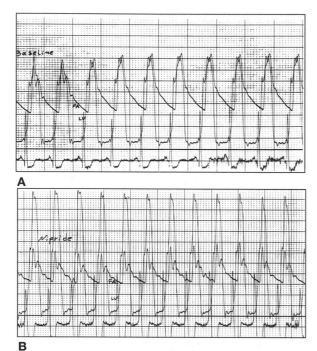

Figure 4. *Simultaneous left ventricular (LV) and femoral arterial (FA) pressures in a patient with hypertrophic cardiomyopathy at baseline recording (Fig. 4A), and following nipride infusion (Fig. 4B). A significant gradient is noted following nipride infusion. Courtesy of John Hayes, MD and Scott Neises, Marshfield Clinic.*

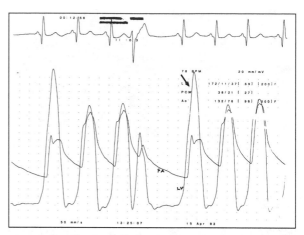

Figure 5. *Simultaneous left ventricular (LV) and femoral arterial (FA) pressures in a patient with hypertrophic cardiomyopathy. The contraction following a premature ventricular beat reveals accentuation of ventricular gradient, and concomitant reduction in arterial pulse pressure. Courtesy of Charles McCauley and Bonnie L Rogney, Marshfield Clinic.*

main action in improving left ventricular diastolic function. Other drugs that are beneficial in the medical therapy of HCM also include disopyramide and amiodarone. [26] Amiodarone may be particularly helpful in patients with symptomatic nonsustained ventricular tachycardia and/or atrial fibrillation. In patients who do not respond to medical therapy, surgical intervention in the form of septal myotomy-myomectomy, with or without mitral valve replacement may be considered.[27] In patients with significant mitral regurgitation and septal thickness less than 18 mm, mitral valve replacement alone may be beneficial. Surgical intervention improves symptomatology and alleviates significant interventricular gradient with operative mortality about 5% and 1.6% annual postoperative mortality in experienced centers. Dual-chamber pacing may be an effective alternative to surgical intervention. In a study of 44 consecutive patients with obstructive cardiomyopathy who failed medical therapy, dual-chamber pacing resulted in improvement in symptoms and in exercise tolerance. It is theorized that preex-

citation of the interventricular septum may cause the septum to move away from left ventricular free wall during systole, resulting in an increase in left ventricular outflow tract dimension.[28] An algorithm for management of patients with HCM is depicted in Figure 6.

Pregnant women with HCM may give birth by vaginal delivery unless there is a history of syncope or a severe gradient is documented. Spinal anesthesia should be avoided. General anesthesia with intravenous esmolol has been used to allow a reduced inotropic state with less obstruction.[29] Patients with HCM should avoid strenuous exercise if they have marked ventricular hypertrophy, significant gradient, history of ventricular tachycardia, atrial fibrillation, and family history of sudden death. Anticoagulation with warfarin should be considered in patients with atrial fibrillation to decrease the risk of systemic embolization. All patients should receive prophylactic antibiotics before dental or surgical procedures because of the risk of endocarditis. Sudden death was associated with a history of syncope, young age at initial diagnosis, and family history of hypertrophic myopathy or sudden death.[30] Although supraventricular and ventricular arrhythmias play an important role in the genesis of sudden death, they probably are not the only explanation. Amiodarone may be beneficial in decreasing the incidence of sudden death in

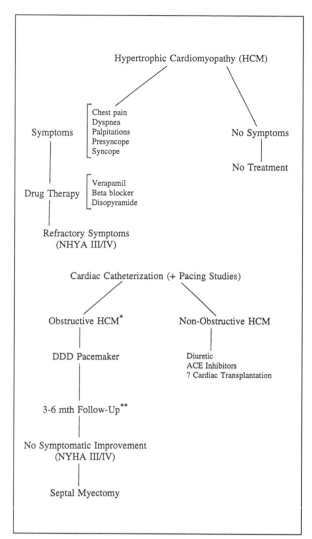

Figure 6. *An algorithm for management of patients with hypertrophic cardiomyopathy. (*) Left ventricular outflow tract gradient off all drugs more than 30 mm Hg at rest or more than 50 mm Hg after provocative maneuvers. (**) Repeat treadmill exercise tests to assess symptomatic improvement. Echocardiogram to establish a reduction in severity of anterior systolic motion and left ventricular outflow tract velocities. NYHA=New York Heart Association functional class; DDD=Dual chamber pacing; mth=Month. Modified after Fananapazir L, et al.[28]*

patients with HCM and nonsustained ventricular tachycardia. The prognosis of HCM is variable. Two-thirds of patients with obstructive symptoms may improve or remain stable; the remaining one-third have a worsening of symptoms. Sudden death may develop in patients, regardless of symptoms. Asymptomatic nonsustained

ventricular tachycardia on a Holter monitor is of benign prognostic significance. A sustained inducible ventricular tachycardia during electrophysiologic testing is associated with an increased risk for subsequent cardiac events.[31]

RESTRICTIVE CARDIOMYOPATHY

Restrictive cardiomyopathy is characterized by a restriction of ventricular filling during diastole due to reduced ventricular compliance. Systolic function is relatively intact. In the World Health Organization classification, 2 conditions of unknown cause are listed under restrictive cardiomyopathy; endomyocardial fibrosis and Löffler's endocarditis. The latter starts with eosinophilic infiltration of the heart muscle and passes through 3 stages: the necrotic stage, the thrombotic stage, and the fibrotic stage. The fibrotic stage is characterized by endomyocardial fibrosis, with the endocardium showing fibrotic plaques of various sizes and thickness; this condition is indistinguishable from endomyocardial fibrosis. The 2 conditions however, are now believed to represent 2 spectra of the same disease. A familial form of idiopathic cardiomyopathy has been described. It usually manifests in the third or fourth decade with atrioventricular block and is associated with skeletal myopathy. A variety of specific cardiac muscle diseases may present clinically with a picture similar to restrictive cardiomyopathy, and are listed in Table 5.

The clinical symptoms reflect the inability of the ventricle to fill during diastole and to provide an increase in cardiac output when needed. Fatigue, weakness, and poor exercise tolerance with dyspnea on exertion are common. Symptoms of reduced filling of the right ventricle include edema, ascites, right upper quadrant discomfort, and anorexia. Chest pain similar in quality to that caused by myocardial ischemia may be present in a small number of patients.

Diagnosis

Physical examination reveals signs of venous congestion and includes distended neck veins, Kussmaul's sign, edema, ascites, and an enlarged, tender liver. Peripheral arterial pulse pressure is typically narrow; the jugular venous pulse reveals a prominent a wave with a rapid x and y descent. The cardiac apex may be dis-

---

Table 5. Etiologies of Restrictive Cardiomyopathy

Infiltrative
  Sarcoidosis; Amyloidosis
  Hemochromatosis
  Neoplasia
Endocardial fibroelastosis
  Cardiac dilatation with diffuse endocardial hyperplasia. Thickened aortic and mitral valve; distorted papillary muscle; primary form affects infants
Endomyocardial fibrosis
  Fibrous endocardial lesions of the inflow portion of the ventricles; may involve AV valves and cause regurgitation. Occurs in tropical and subtropical Africa.
Löffler's endocarditis
  Dense endocardial fibrosis with overlying thrombosis; occurs following an arteritis and eosinophilic infiltrate of the myocardium. May be related to endomyocardial fibrosis.
Scleroderma
Adipositas cordis (fatty infiltration)
Radiation
Postmyocarditis
Glycogen storage disease
Becker's disease
  Cardiac dilatation with fibrosis of the papillary muscles and subendocardium associated with necrosis and mural thrombosis. Occurs in South Africa.

---

placed laterally, and in general, cardiomegaly is absent or mild. Sinus tachycardia and atrial and ventricular arrhythmias may be noted. The heart sounds are often soft and an S_3 and S_4 are common. Murmurs of tricuspid and/or mitral regurgitation are usually present. On a chest x-ray, the heart is normal in size or demonstrates mild cardiomegaly. Signs of pulmonary congestion may be present as well, and absence of pericardial calcification may differentiate the condition from constrictive pericardial disease, which has some similarity to restrictive heart disease.

Electrocardiographic features include diffuse low QRS voltage, nonspecific ST-T-wave abnormalities, conduction disturbances, and atrial and ventricular arrhythmias. Echocardiography reveals normal ventricular volumes and increased wall thickness, with preserved normal systolic function. Doppler echocardiography reveals shortened deceleration times across atrioventricular valves, which represent the abrupt premature cessation of ventricular filling, as well as abnormal central venous flow velocity reversals with inspiration. Mitral and tricuspid regurgitation are also frequently observed.

Technetium-99m pyrophosphate scans may show intense diffuse cardiac uptake, particularly in patients with amyloid disease. In patients with metastatic neoplasms or sarcoid granulomas, thallium-201 studies reveal defects in the myocardial walls. Magnetic resonance imaging reveals enlargement of the atria and inferior vena cava; a prominent signal within the atria in all phases of the cardiac cycle, suggesting impaired ventricular filling, and possibly mitral and/or tricuspid regurgitation.

Jugular venous pulse tracings reveal a prominent a wave, with rapid x and y descents resulting in a characteristic M-shaped tracing. Apexcardiography also reveals a prominent a wave. There are a number of ancillary tests and findings that aid in the diagnosis of the underlying disorder. These include high serum iron levels with hemochromatosis; hypercalcemia, which occurs in approximately 9% of patients with sarcoidosis; and rectal biopsy for diagnosing amyloidosis.

Cardiac catheterization is currently the gold standard in diagnosing restrictive cardiomyopathy. There is elevated ventricular EDP, with left ventricular EDP usually greater than right ventricular EDP. The diastolic portion of the ventricular pressure pulse reveals a dip and plateau

Table 6. Differentiating Features of Restrictive Cardiomyopathy Versus Constrictive Pericarditis

	RESTRICTIVE CARDIOMYOPATHY	CONSTRICTIVE PERICARDITIS
Pulmonary capillary wedge pressure (PCW)	PCW > right atrial pressure	PCW = right atrial pressure
Pulmonary artery systolic pressure	Usually >40-50 mm Hg	Usually <40-50 mm Hg
Right vs left ventricular end-diastolic pressures	Left ventricular > right ventricular end-diastolic pressure	Left ventricular usually = right ventricular end-diastolic pressure
Right ventricular end-diastolic pressure	Usually less than 1/3 of right ventricular systolic pressure	Usually about 1/3 of right ventricular systolic pressure
Cardiac output	Depressed	Often normal or only slightly depressed
Square-root sign in ventricular pressure tracings	More prominent in left ventricular tracing. May diminish with therapy	Sign is equally prominent in right and left ventricular pressure tracing
Right atrial pressure	<15 mm Hg if PCW not markedly elevated	Usually >15 mm Hg

configuration, resembling a square-root sign. The right atrial pressures are elevated and have an "M" or "W" shape due to rapid x and y descents. Table 6 reviews features that help to differentiate restrictive cardiomyopathy from constrictive pericarditis. Endomyocardial biopsy may be helpful in differentiating restrictive from constrictive disease and in finding a cause for restrictive disease[32] (such as amyloidosis, hemochromatosis, or sarcoidosis).

Therapy

Therapy for symptomatic cardiomyopathy includes a low-salt diet and diuretics. While vasodilator therapy is beneficial in dilated myopathy, its role in restrictive myopathy is less clear. In 1 study of children with restrictive cardiomyopathy, acute administration of captopril did not improve hemodynamics and was associated with significant hypotension.[33] Digitalis may be beneficial in some patients, but should be used with caution, since patients with restrictive cardiomyopathy may be prone to digitalis toxicity. If patients

develop complete heart block, AV sequential pacing is superior to ventricular pacing to allow atrial contraction and enhance ventricular filling. Antiarrhythmic agents are sometimes required, and anticoagulation is indicated to prevent thromboembolic complications. Specific treatment, if available, may be used: sarcoidosis may be treated with steroids, neoplasms with chemotherapy or radiation, and hemochromatosis with repeated phlebotomy and deferoxamine.

SPECIFIC MYOCARDIAL DISEASES

In the following section, we will discuss certain causes of cardiomyopathy that have specific clinical significance.

Ischemic Cardiomyopathies

Ischemic cardiomyopathy refers to severe systolic dysfunction with or without diastolic dysfunction of the myocardium due to severe diffuse coronary artery disease. Dysfunction due to loss of critical mass of the myocardium as a result of a massive infarction, or due to structural complications of myocardial infarction (i.e., ventricular septal defect, mitral regurgitation, or ventricular aneurysm), are not included in this syndrome. Inclusion of this entity under cardiomyopathies is not universally accepted. The pathogenesis of the disease is not well understood. Postmortem studies reveal that severe diffuse coronary disease with multiple sites of scarring might be responsible for ischemic cardiomyopathy. Alternatively, zones of hibernating or stunned myocardium may contribute. Some preliminary data suggest that it might be linked to HLA-DRW6 antigen.[34] In addition, remodeling of the left ventricle, which can occur after infarction, may contribute to this entity.

The clinical picture is that of dilated cardiomyopathy, but a restrictive picture is not uncommon. While noninvasive tests (thallium scans, positron emission tomography) may document ongoing ischemia, the presence of significant diffuse coronary disease on angiography helps confirm the diagnosis. Afterload reducers, captopril in particular, are beneficial in the management of such patients. Despite high operative mortality, coronary artery bypass surgery increases long-term survival in selected patients.

Cardiomyopathy Induced by Chemotherapeutic Drugs

Cyclophosphamide, vincristine, vinblastine, cisplatinum, and a variety of other chemotherapeutic agents have been implicated in toxic cardiac effects. The agents most commonly associated with cardiotoxicity are anthracyclines (e.g., doxorubicin) and 5-fluorouracil.

The incidence of anthracycline cardiotoxicity ranges from 5.3% to 28% in different series. The common clinical presentation is that of dilated cardiomyopathy, but it may present as restrictive disease, angina pectoris, acute myocardial infarction, or ventricular arrhythmia. The toxicity is dose related, and adoption of a once-a-week, low-dose regimen appears to lower the incidence of the disease. Echocardiography and radionuclide ventriculography support the diagnosis. For a reliable method of early diagnosis, however, exercise radionuclide ventriculography or ventricular biopsy is superior. Several therapeutic options have been suggested to decrease the possibility of cardiac toxicity, including use of free radical scavengers, calcium channel antago-

nists, and cardiac glycosides. No controlled prospective studies are available yet. Supportive therapy is indicated; in some cases, cardiac function may revert to normal. Calcium-channel blockers, especially those with significant negative inotropic effects, should be avoided because they have deleterious effects in animals models.

5-fluorouracil (5-FU) cardiotoxicity may present as congestive heart failure, Prinzmetal's angina, or myocardial infarction. In a prospective study of 25 patients receiving 5-FU infusion, patients had a significant increase in the incidence of ST-segment changes suggestive of ischemia during infusion (as compared to baseline recordings).[35] These changes were more common in patients with underlying coronary disease. The underlying mechanism of cardiotoxicity is not known, and no specific therapy for this condition is established.

Effect of Cocaine on the Heart

Cocaine use has been linked to the development of cardiomyopathy, myocarditis, endocarditis, and various ventricular arrhythmias.[36] The most common clinical presentation is acute myocardial infarction. The link between cocaine and development of cardiomyopathy is supported by the drug's depressant effect on cardiac function in animal models. A depressant effect was also shown in isolated myocyte preparations. Cocaine use in humans in small doses does not seem to have a consistent depressant effect on cardiac function. It is possible that in some subjects the negative inotropic effect is balanced by the drug's reflex sympathomimetic activity. Arrhythmogenic effects might be related to cocaine's cardiac ischemic effects, or to a direct effect on electrophysiologic properties of cardiac muscle. The mechanism of inducing myocardial ischemia is probably multifactorial. Cocaine has been shown to cause coronary spasm, increase intimal proliferation, and increase platelet aggregation. No specific therapy is universally accepted to control cardiac manifestations of cocaine, and various drugs may be individualized depending on the presentation. In patients presenting with hypertension and tachycardia but no evidence of coronary artery disease, use of β-blockers may be helpful. Patients presenting with myocardial ischemia may benefit from nitroglycerin and calcium-channel blockers. Aspirin and thrombolytic therapy should be considered in those presenting with acute myocardial infarction, provided there is no contraindication to their use. Caution in using these drugs is important since cocaine use may be associated with hypertension or cerebrovascular accidents, presentations in which thrombolytic therapy should be avoided. Those who present with acute onset of heart failure should be supported with inotropic drugs since cardiac dysfunction may be reversible.

Alcoholic Cardiomyopathy

Excessive alcohol consumption may lead to progressive myocardial dysfunction and dilated cardiomyopathy in susceptible individuals. Other cardiac effects of alcohol include exacerbation of conduction abnormalities, atrial and ventricular arrhythmias, increased risk of hypertension, and possibly increase in fetal cardiac abnormalities. The mechanism of alcohol-induced cardiac dysfunction is not fully understood, but is believed to be due to direct toxic effects on the myocytes, associated thiamine deficiency, and, occasionally, additives used in the alcohol manufacturing process. The heart increases in weight, with biventricular hypertrophy and dilatation and widespread focal myocardial fibrosis. Sudden death has been reported in alcoholic cardiomyopathy. Another manifestation of alcohol-induced heart disease is an increased propensity for atrial and ventricular arrhythmias. "Holiday heart" syndrome refers to the occurrence of arrhythmias (especially supraventricular tachyarrhythmias) after alcohol consumption, in the absence of overt cardiomyopathy. Acute alcohol ingestion in otherwise normal individuals may depress myocardial contractility. Cessation of alcohol intake is the only treatment available for alcoholic cardiomyopathy. Following abstinence, patients have shown normalization of chamber dimensions and ventricular function as determined by echocardiography.[37]

REFERENCES: MYOCARDITIS

1. Gravanis MB, Sternby NH. Incidence of myocarditis: A 10-year autopsy study from Malmö, Sweden. *Arch Pathol Lab Med.* 1991;115:390-392.
2. Dec GW Jr, Waldman L, Southern J, et al. Viral myocarditis mimicking acute myocardial infarction. *J Am Coll Cardiol.* 1992;20:85-89.
3. Narula J, Khaw BA, Dec GW Jr, et al. Recognition of acute myocarditis masquerading as acute myocardial infarction. *N Engl J Med.* 1993;328:100-104.
4. Joy J, Rao YY, Raveendranath M, et al. Coxsackie viral myocarditis: A clinical and echocardiographic study. *Indian Heart J.* 1990;42:441-444.
5. Fisher DZ, DiSalvo TG, Dec GW, et al. Transient left ventricular aneurysm in a patient with hypertrophic cardiomyopathy and myocarditis. *Clin Cardiol.* 1993;16:253-256.
6. Veluvolu P, Kamrani F, Horton DP, et al. Acute transient myocarditis evaluation by gallium imaging. *Clin Nuclear Med.* 1992;17:411-413.
7. Kao C, Wang S, Yeh S. Detection of myocarditis in dilated cardiomyopathy by Tc-99m HMPAO WBC myocardial imaging in a child. *Clin Nuclear Med.* 1992;17:678-679.
8. Gagliardi MG, Bevilacqua M, DiRenzi P, et al. Usefulness of magnetic resonance imaging for diagnosis of acute myocarditis in infants and children and comparison with endomyocardial biopsy. *Am J Cardiol.* 1991;68:1089-1091.
9. Maehashi N, Yokota Y, Takarada A, et al. The role of myocarditis and myocardial fibrosis in dilated cardiomyopathy: Analysis of 28 necropsy cases. *Jap Heart J.* 1991;32:1-15.
10. Matoba Y, Matsumori A, Ohtani H, et al. A case of biopsy-proven myocarditis progressing to autopsy-proven dilated cardiomyopathy. *Clin Cardiol.* 1990;13:732-737.
11. Gwathmey JK, Nakao S, Come PC, et al. An experimental model of acute and subacute viral myocarditis in the pig. *J Am Coll Cardiol.* 1992;19:864-869.
12. Rezkalla S, Kloner RA, Khaw BA, et al. Detection of experimental myocarditis by monoclonal antimyosin antibody, Fab fragment. *Am Heart J.* 1989;117:391-395.
13. Matsumori A, Ohkusa T, Matoba Y, et al. Myocardial uptake of antimyosin monoclonal antibody in a murine model of viral myocarditis. *Circulation.* 1989;79:400-405.
14. Rezkalla S, Kloner RA. Management strategies in viral myocarditis. *Am Heart J.* 1989;117:706-708.
15. Rezkalla S, Khatib G, Khatib R. Coxsackievirus B3 murine myocarditis: Deleterious effects of anti-inflammatory drugs. *J Lab Clin Med.* 1986;107:393-395.
16. Rezkalla S, Khatib R, Khatib G, et al. Effect of indomethacin in the late phase of coxsackievirus myocarditis in a murine model. *J Lab Clin Med.* 1988;112:118-121.
17. Rezkalla S, Kloner RA, Khatib R, et al. Effect of metoprolol in acute coxsackievirus B3 murine myocarditis. *J Am Coll Cardiol.* 1988;12:412-414.
18. Yamada T, Matsumori A, Okada I, et al. The effect of α1-blocker, bunazosin on a murine model of congestive heart failure induced by viral myocarditis. *Jpn Circ J.* 1992;56:1138-1145.
19. O'Connell JB, Robinson JA, Henkin RE. Immunosuppressive therapy in patients with congestive cardiomyopathy and myocardial uptake of gallium-67. *Circulation.* 1981;64:780-786.
20. Ray CG, Icenogle TB, Minnich LL, et al. The use of intravenous ribavirin to treat influenza virus-associated acute myocarditis. *J Infect Dis.* 1989;159:829-836.
21. Rezkalla S, Kloner RA, Khatib G, et al. Beneficial effect of captopril in coxsackievirus B_3 murine myocarditis.

Circulation. 1990;81:1039-1046.

22. Rezkalla S, Kloner RA, Khatib G, et al. Effect of delayed captopril therapy on left ventricular mass and myonecrosis during acute coxsackievirus murine myocarditis. *Am Heart J.* 1990;120:1377-1381.

23. Hiraoka Y, Kishimoto C, Kurokawa M, et al. Effects of polyethylene glycol conjugated superoxide dismutase on coxsackievirus B_3 myocarditis in mice. *Cardiovasc Res.* 1992;26:956-961.

24. Drucker NA, Colan SD, Lewis AB, et al. Gamma globulin treatment of acute myocarditis in the pediatric populations. *Circulation.* 1994;89:252-257.

25. Ramos AC, Elias PR, Barrucand L, et al. The protective effect of carnitine in human diphtheric myocarditis. *Pediatr Res.* 1984;18:815-819.

26. Marin-Neto JA, Marzullo P, Marrassa C, et al. Myocardial perfusion abnormalities in chronic Chagas disease as detected by thallium-201 scintigraphy. *Am J Cardiol.* 1992;69:780-784.

27. Hagar JM, Rahimatoola SH. Chagas heart disease in the United States. *N Engl J Med.* 1991;325:763-768.

28. Pless M, Juranek D, Kozarsky P, et al. The epidemiology of Chagas disease in a hyperendemic area of Cochabamba Bolivia: A clinical study including electrocardiography, seroreactivity to Trypanosoma cruzi, xenodiagnosis, and domiciliary triatomine distribution. *Am J Trop Med Hygiene.* 1992;47:539-546.

29. Roberti RR, Martinez EE, Andrade JL, et al. Chagas cardiomyopathy and captopril. *Eur Heart J.* 1992;13:966-970.

30. Autran BR, Gorin I, Leibowitch M, et al. AIDS in a Haitian woman with cardiac Kaposi's sarcoma and Whipple's disease. *Lancet.* 1983;1:767-768.

31. Levy WS, Simon GL, Rios JC. Prevalence of cardiac abnormalities in human immunodeficiency virus infection. *Am J Cardiol.* 1989;63:86-89.

32. Lewis W. AIDS: Cardiac findings from 115 autopsies. *Prog Cardiovasc Dis.* 1989;32:207-215.

33. Kaul S, Fishbein M, Siegel RJ. Cardiac manifestations of acquired immune deficiency syndrome: A 1991 update. *Am Heart J.* 1991;122:535-544.

34. Acierno L. Cardiac complications in acquired immunodeficiency syndrome (AIDS): A review. *J Am Coll Cardiol.* 1989;13:1144-1154.

35. Cox J, Krajden M. Cardiovascular manifestations of Lyme disease. *Am Heart J.* 1991;122:1449-1455.

REFERENCES: CARDIOMYOPATHY

1. William DG, Olsen EGL. Prevalence of overt dilated cardiomyopathy in two regions of *England. Br Heart J.* 1985;54:153-155.

2. Coughlin SS, Labenberg TR, Tefft MC. Black-white differences in idiopathic dilated cardiomyopathy: The Washington DC dilated cardiomyopathy study. *Epidemiology.* 1993;4:165-172.

2a. Kasper EK, Agema WP, Hutchins G, et al. The causes of dilated cardiomyopathy: A clinicopathologic review of 673 consecutive patients. *J Am Coll Cardiol.* 1994;23:566-590.

3. Wilensky KL, Yudelman P, Cohen AI, et al. Serial electro-cardiographic changes in idiopathic dilated cardiomyopathy confirmed at necropsy. *Am J Cardiol.* 1988;62:276-283.

4. Keren G, Katz S, Strom J, et al. Non-invasive quantification of mitral regurgitation in dilated cardiomyopathy: Correlation of two Doppler echocardiographic methods. *Am Heart J.* 1988;116:758-764.

5. Abramson SV, Burk JF, Kelly JJ Jr, et al. Pulmonary hypertension predicts mortality and morbidity in patients with dilated cardiomyopathy. *Ann Intern Med.* 1992;116:888-895.

6. Figulla HR, Kellermann AB, Stille-Siegener M, et al. Significance of coronary angiography, left heart catheterization, and endomyocardial biopsy for the diagnosis of idiopathic dilated cardiomyopathy. *Am Heart J.* 1992;124:1251-1257.

7. Packer M, Carver JR, Rodeheffer RJ, et al. Effect of oral milrinone on mortality in severe chronic heart failure. *N Engl J Med.* 1991;325:1468-1475.

8. Figulla HR, Rechenberg JV, Wiegand V, et al. Beneficial effects of long-term diltiazem treatment in dilated cardiomyopathy. *J Am Coll Cardiol.* 1989;13:653-658.

9. Packer M, Nicod P, Khandheria BK, et al. Randomized, multicenter, double-blind placebo controlled evaluation of amlodipine in patients with mild to moderate heart failure. *J Am Coll Cardiol.* 1991;17:274A.

10. Waagstein F, Caidahl K, Wallentin I, et al. Long-term ß-blockade in dilated cardiomyopathy. Effects of short-and long-term metoprolol treatment followed by withdrawal and readministration of metroprolol. *Circulation.* 1989;80:551-563.

11. Antiarrhythmic Drug Evaluation Group. A multicenter randomized trial on the benefit/risk profile of amiodarone, flecainide, and propafenone in patients with cardiac disease and complex ventricular arrhythmias. *Eur Heart J.* 1992;13:1251-1258.

12. Kieny JR, Sacrez A, Facello A, et al. Increase in radionuclide left ventricular ejection fraction after cardioversion of chronic atrial fibrillation in idiopathic dilated cardiomyopathy. *Eur Heart J.* 1992;13:1290-1295.

13. Tamburro P, Wilber D. Sudden death in idiopathic dilated cardiomyopathy. *Am Heart J.* 1992;124:1035-1045.

14. Kriett JM, Kaye MP. The registry of the international society for heart transplantation: Seventh official report — 1990. *J Heart Transplant.* 1990;9:323.

15. Fuster V, Gersh BJ, Giuliani ER, et al. The natural history of idiopathic dilated cardiomyopathy. *Am J Cardiol.* 1981;47:525-531.

16. Hofmann T, Meinertz T, Kasper W, et al. Mode of death in idiopathic dilated cardiomyopathy: A multivariate analysis of prognostic determinants. *Am Heart J.* 1988;116:1455-1463.

17. Epstein ND, Cohn GM, Cyran F, et al. Differences in clinical expression of hypertrophic cardiomyopathy associated with two distinct mutations in the ß-myosin heavy chain gene. *Circulation.* 1992;86:345-352.

18. Fananapazir L, Epstein ND. Genotype-phenotype correlations in hypertrophic cardiomyopathy. *Circulation.* 1994;89:22-32.

19. Koga Y, Kihara K, Yamaguchi R, et al. Therapeutic effect of oral dipyridamole on myocardial perfusion and car-

diac performance in patients with hypertrophic cardiomyopathy. *Am Heart J.* 1992;123:433-438.

20. Russell JW, Biller J, Hajduczok ZD, et al. Ischemic cerebrovascular complications and risk factors in idiopathic hypertrophic subaortic stenosis. *Stroke.* 1991;22:1143-1147.

21. Gaudio C, Pelliccia F, Tanzilli G, et al. Magnetic resonance imaging for assessment of apical hypertrophy in hypertrophic cardiomyopathy. *Clin Cardiol.* 1992;15:164-168.

22. Greenspan AM. Hypertrophic cardiomyopathy and atrial fibrillation: A change of perspective. *J Am Coll Cardiol.* 1990;6:1286-1287.

23. Cripps TR, Counihan PJ, Frenneaux MP, et al. Signal averaged electrocardiography in hypertrophic cardiomyopathy. *J Am Coll Cardiol.* 1990;15:956-961.

24. Hartmann A, Kuhn J, Hopf R, et al. Effect of propranolol and disopyramide on left ventricular function at rest and during exercise in hypertrophic cardiomyopathy. *Cardiology.* 1992;80:81-88.

25. Bonow RO, Rosing DR, Bacharach SL, et al. Effects of verapamil on left ventricular systolic function and diastolic filling in patients with hypertrophic cardiomyopathy. *Circulation.* 1981;64:787-796.

26. Hopf R, Kaltenbach M. Management of hypertrophic cardiomyopathy. *Annu Rev Med.* 1990;41:75-83.

27. Fritzsche D, Krakor R, Goos H, et al. Comparison of myectomy alone or in combination with mitral valve repair for hypertrophic obstructive cardiomyopathy. *Thorac Cardiovasc Surg.* 1992;40:65-69.

28. Fananapazir L, Cannon RO, Tripodi D, et al. Impact of dual-chamber permanent pacing in patients with obstructive hypertrophic cardiomyopathy with symptoms refractory to verapamil and ß-adrenergic blocker therapy. *Circulation.* 1992;85:2149-2161.

29. Doi LG, O'Shea PJ, Wood AJ. Use of esmolol in the post bypass management of hypertrophic obstructive cardiomyopathy. *Br J Anaesth.* 1993;70:104-106.

30. Maron BJ, Fananapazir L. Sudden cardiac death in hypertrophic cardiomyopathy. *Circulation.* 1992; 85(suppl 1):I-57–1-63.

31. Fananapazir L, Chang AC, Epstein SE. Prognostic determinants in hypertrophic cardiomyopathy. *Circulation.* 1992;86:730-740.

32. Vaitkus PT, Kussmaul WG. Constrictive pericarditis versus restrictive cardiomyopathy: A reappraisal and update of diagnostic criteria. *Am Heart J.* 1991; 122:1431-1441.

33. Bengur AR, Beekman RH, Rocchini AP, et al. Acute hemodynamic effects of captopril in children with a congestive or restrictive cardiomyopathy. *Circulation.* 1991; 83:523-527.

34. Limas CJ, Limas C. HLA-DRW6 antigen linkage in chronic congestive heart failure secondary to coronary artery disease (ischemic cardiomyopathy). *Am J Cardiol.* 1988;62:816-818.

35. Rezkalla S, Kloner RA, Ensley J, et al. Continuous ambulatory electrocardiographic monitoring during 5-fluorouracil therapy. *J Clin Oncol.* 1989;7:509-514.

36. Kloner RA, Hale S, Alker K, et al. The effects of acute and chronic cocaine use on the heart. *Circulation.* 1992;85:407-419.

37. Hicks RJ, Low RD, Arkles LB. Marked improvement in left ventricular systolic function 3 months after cessation of excess alcohol intake. *Clin Nucl Med.* 1993;18:101-103.

CHAPTER 20

Heart Failure

Robert A. Kloner, MD, PhD
Michael B. Fowler, MB, MRCP
Victor Dzau, MD

DEFINITION AND MECHANISMS OF HEART FAILURE

Heart failure (HF) affects approximately 1 million to 2 million Americans,[1] developing in about 400,000 each year. It is especially common in the elderly.[2] This clinical syndrome results from an abnormality of cardiac function such that the heart cannot pump blood at a volume adequate to meet the metabolic needs of the tissues of the body (forward failure), or it cannot distend sufficiently during diastole, leading to congestion (backward failure).[3] The syndrome is associated with an increase in atrial pressures, reduced exercise tolerance, ventricular arrhythmias, and shortened life expectancy.[4,5] The abnormality in cardiac function may be the result of an abnormality in the myocardial cells themselves (myocardial failure) or to some other structural abnormality, such as valvular stenosis, impairing ventricular ejection.

Myocardial failure may be attributable to a quantitative loss of functioning myofibers, as in HF associated with a large myocardial infarction (MI) or to a generalized qualitative abnormality in myocyte function, as occurs with congestive cardiomyopathy. The precise mechanism of abnormal myocyte function in myocardial failure is controversial. One possible mechanism is a reduction in myofibrillar ATPase, seen in the hearts of patients and experimental animals with congestive heart failure (CHF). Reduced myocardial contractility is associated with a change in myosin isozyme from myosin V_1 (a myosin with increased ATPase activity) to myosin V_3 (which has reduced ATPase activity).[6]

Another possible mechanism is suggested by animal and human studies, indicating that sarcoplasmic reticulum is defective in its ability to pump calcium owing to reduced activity of the enzyme calcium-activated ATPase in the sarcoplasmic reticulum.[7,8] Normally, the sarcoplasmic reticulum takes up intracellular calcium during the relaxation phase of the cardiac cycle. During electrical depolarization, extracellular calcium enters the cell, and intracellular calcium is released from the sarcoplasmic reticulum. The calcium interacts with the contractile apparatus, resulting in a contraction. Experimental studies suggest that in myocardial failure, the sarcoplasmic reticulum is defective in its ability to take up calcium during relaxation. As a result, little calcium is available for release to the contractile apparatus during systole. In myocardial failure, the mitochondria may become the main site of uptake of calcium and source of calcium for contraction. Because release of calcium from the mitochondria is a slow process, only limited amounts of calcium may be available to activate the contractile mechanism. Cardiac tissue from patients with heart failure who were undergoing cardiac transplantation also show reduced rates of calcium uptake by the sarcoplasmic reticulum, as well as reduced rates of release.

Other possible explanations for myocardial failure include reduced coronary blood flow and myocardial oxygen consumption per unit of tissue and alterations of mitochondrial function. Depletion of myocardial norepinephrine stores and decline in norepinephrine production have been observed in myocardial failure.[6] Although regional norepinephrine stores do not play a role in the intrinsic contractile state of the myocardium, the adrenergic nervous system is an important compensatory mechanism for the failing heart. The depleted norepinephrine levels may impede this compensatory mechanism. Decreased ß-receptors have been described in HF, although their importance remains controversial. Myocardial

407

hypertrophy with excess collagen deposition may also contribute to HF and has been implicated as a cause of diastolic dysfunction.

ASSOCIATED PATHOPHYSIOLOGY

There are several recently recognized pathophysiologic features that are associated with HF, including skeletal muscle abnormalities; alterations of sympathetic and parasympathetic nervous system, including altered baroreflex control; and abnormalities in endothelial function.

Patients with HF have been reported to have skeletal muscle deconditioning, atrophy, and abnormalities in skeletal muscle oxidative metabolism.[9–13] Some studies have suggested that diminished blood flow with reduced oxygen delivery to muscle may be in part responsible for this abnormality.[11,14] These alterations may contribute to the symptom of fatigue and may be reversible in part with supervised physical training.[15] Diaphragmatic work is increased in patients with HF and may contribute to the sensation of dyspnea.[12]

Patients with CHF have an increase in sympathetic nerve activity but a decrease in parasympathetic activity with a reduction in heart rate variability.[16–20] There is a decrease in the circadian fluctuations in heart rate and blood pressure in patients with HF.[21] Increased sympathetic activity, with stimulation of the α-receptors may stimulate left ventricular hypertrophy.[22]

Patients with CHF have abnormal baroreflex control of sympathetic neural activity. Administration of phentolamine to increase blood pressure does not result in the normal baroreflex decrease in heart rate; conversely, decreasing the blood pressure by administering nitroprusside does not result in the normal increase in heart rate.[23–25] Impaired baroreceptor mechanisms also may affect vascular resistance, capillary filtration, and contribute to the development of edema.[26,27]

Recent studies have shown that patients with CHF have elevated levels of endothelin,[28,29] which correlate with the degree of pulmonary hypertension.[30] Impaired endothelial-dependent vasodilator response to intravascular infusions of acetylcholine and methacholine have been reported in patients with HF, as have endothelium-independent vasodilator response to nitroglycerin.[31,32]

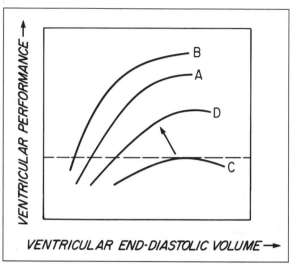

Figure 1. *Starling curves showing ventricular end-diastolic volume plotted on the horizontal axis and ventricular performance on the vertical axis. The horizontal axis could also be ventricular end diastolic pressure, and the vertical axis could be stroke volume or stroke work. Curve A represents the normal curve; curve B a curve of increased contractile state; curve C that of reduced contractile state; and curve D the curve of a failing heart after digitalis treatment.*

COMPENSATORY MECHANISMS IN HEART FAILURE

The heart relies on several compensatory mechanisms for maintenance of its pumping ability in the setting of myocardial failure or an excessive hemodynamic burden (such as systemic hypertension, aortic regurgitation, or stenosis). The first is the Frank–Starling mechanism, in which the force of contraction or extent of shortening depends on the initial muscle length. When the muscle and, therefore, sarcomere length is increased by an increase in preload to provide optimal overlap between the actin (thin) and myosin (thick) filaments, cardiac performance is enhanced.

Figure 1 shows a typical Frank–Starling curve. As ventricular end-diastolic volume or preload increases, so does ventricular performance. Braunwald[6] described factors that result in changes along a given curve (changes in preload resulting in different degrees of stretching of the myocardium) and changes that shift the curve (alterations of the contractile state of the myocardium). Factors that alter ventricular end-diastolic volume and, hence, result in movement along a given Frank–Starling curve include total blood volume, body position, intrathoracic and intrapericardial pressure, venous tone, the pumping action of skeletal muscle that returns blood to the heart, and the atrial contribution to ventricular filling. Factors that shift the Frank–Starling curve upward and to the left (increase in the contractile state of the myocardium as shown in curve B) include sympathetic nerve stimulation, circulating catecholamines, positive inotropic agents such as digitalis, and the force–frequency relationship (an increase in heart rate resulting in an increase in contractility). Factors that shift the Frank–Starling curve down and to the right (depressed contractile state of the myocardium [curve C]) include anoxia, hypercapnia, acidosis, pharmacologic depressants (such as quinidine and local anesthetic agents), loss of myocardium, and intrinsic myocardial depression.

Patients with myocardial failure function along this depressed (curve C) Frank–Starling curve. To maintain the same ventricular performance as in a normal heart, they must have a higher ventricular end-diastolic volume. If the metabolic demands of the body increase, requiring increased cardiac performance, this occurs in such patients at the expense of a higher ventricular end-diastolic volume (and increased left ventricular filling pressure), which may in turn result in the symptoms of dyspnea or even pulmonary edema (Fig. 2).

Neurohumoral systems are activated in HF. The effects include activation of the sympathetic nervous system with increased plasma catecholamine levels, activation of the renin–angiotensin–aldosterone system, and increased production of arginine vasopressin (antidiuretic hormone). Although the changes in these systems are meant to be compensatory to defend against traumatic loss of blood volume and dehydration—and are capable of restoring blood pressure—they may have adverse effects in patients with HF (Fig. 2). Sympathetic stimulation, renin release, and arginine vasopressin act to increase systemic vascular resistance and promote salt and water retention. The increase in cardiac afterload can ultimately depress cardiac performance, and the increase in volume may worsen congestive symptoms. Increase in heart rate attributable to sympathetic stimulation may precipitate arrhythmias as well as ischemia.

Levels of atrial natriuretic peptide (ANP) are

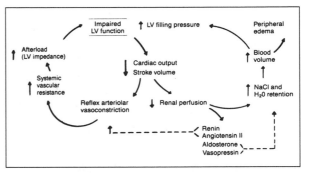

Figure 2. *Two interrelated vicious cycles in congestive heart failure. Left: Impairment of left ventricular (LV) function leads to a decrease in cardiac output. This leads to a reflex increase in systemic vascular resistance by the neurohumoral mechanisms. This increases the effective afterload of the left ventricle and further reduces stroke volume. Right: A reduction in cardiac output and arterial pressure leads to a decrease in renal perfusion. This activates the renin-angiotensin-aldosterone system. Overall, there is retention of salt (NaCl) and water (H₂O), leading to a further increase in filling pressure and to peripheral edema. These cycles, therefore, can feed back on each other to worsen the heart failure state. Reprinted from McCall et al.[41] With permission of the American Heart Association.*

elevated in patients with HF. Atrial natriuretic peptides are located within secretory granules within the atria and are released upon increased atrial pressure or volume. In animal and human studies, infusion of atrial extracts has been shown to induce natriuresis, diuresis, and vasodilation. Saito et al[33] showed that infusion of ANP in patients with congestive HF reduced pulmonary capillary wedge pressure, improved stroke volume, and reduced systemic vascular resistance. The effect of ANP on diuresis was blunted compared with that in healthy patients. Presumably, release of ANP is a compensatory mechanism in HF; whether exogenous administration of ANP in patients with HF will have an important therapeutic role remains to be determined.

Recent studies suggest that the form of neuroendocrine activation may depend on the degree of HF. Patients with left ventricular ejection fractions of less than or equal to 35% but with no or mild HF symptoms have increased plasma norepinephrine, ANP, and arginine vasopressin levels but normal plasma renin activity. Once clinical signs of congestive HF are present, plasma renin activity is increased as well.[34,35]

Long-term compensatory mechanisms of the heart with valvular or myocardial abnormalities include myocardial hypertrophy and dilatation. In the initial stages of HF, the compensatory mechanisms may sustain the circulatory needs of the body. Eventually, however, as myocardial failure progresses, the compensatory mechanisms can no longer maintain the pump function of the heart and the clinical syndrome of HF emerges.

THE CLINICAL SYNDROME OF HEART FAILURE

FORWARD VERSUS BACKWARD HEART FAILURE

The clinical syndrome of HF has been hypothesized to arise from backward, forward cardiac failure, or both. *Backward failure* refers to blood damming up behind 1 or both ventricles, because the ventricle cannot discharge its contents. Symptoms result from an increase in systemic venous pressure with right ventricular failure, resulting in transudation of fluid into the interstitium of the liver, mesentery, and subcutaneous tissue; or from an increase in pulmonary venous pressure with left ventricular failure, resulting in transudation of fluid into the interstitium of the lung. The *forward failure* hypothesis refers to inability of the heart to pump an adequate amount of blood into the arterial tree, resulting in symptoms of underperfusion of the vital organs. Reduced perfusion to the kidneys results in increased sodium and water retention, leading to an increase in extracellular fluid level and tissue congestion. The renal mechanisms for increased water retention are complex; they include reduced renal water excretion caused by decreased renal blood flow with reduced glomerular filtration rate, enhancement of the renin–angiotensin–aldosterone system, and enhanced antidiuretic hormone release. Reduced forward output to the brain results in mental confusion; reduced output to the skeletal muscles results in exercise intolerance and weakness.

In most patients with chronic HF, both backward and forward failure result in symptoms.[3]

RIGHT- VERSUS LEFT-SIDED HEART FAILURE

Right ventricular failure, associated with blood "damming up" in the systemic venous circuit, includes symptoms and signs of edema, congestive hepatomegaly, ascites, and, eventually, signs of low forward output, including weakness and mental confusion. Symptoms and signs of left ventricular failure are attributable to blood damming up behind the left ventricle and to pulmonary congestion. Long-standing left ventricular failure may eventually result in signs of right ventricular failure, with generalized accumulation of fluid. Experimental studies show that failure of 1 ventricle induced by a hemodynamic stress eventually results in biochemical changes (depletion of norepinephrine and abnormalities in the activity of actin-myosin ATPase) of the other ventricle. This may be secondary to the fact that muscle bundles composing 1 ventricle are in continuity with those of the other ventricle.

LOW- VERSUS HIGH-OUTPUT CARDIAC FAILURE

Heart failure causing low cardiac output is the most common form of HF and is usually traceable to an ischemic, valvular, hypertensive, congenital, or cardiomyopathic process. Heart failure also may result from several high-output states such as beriberi, Paget's disease, thyrotoxicosis, arteriovenous fistula, and anemia.[3] Low-output failure is characterized by reduced stroke volume, peripheral vasoconstriction with cold and pale extremities, reduced pulse pressure, and widened arteriovenous oxygen difference. High-output failure is characterized by a widened pulse pressure and peripheral vasodilatation, with warm and flushed extremities. High-output states are associated with reduced arteriovenous oxygen difference. Arteriovenous oxygen difference does not decrease much in patients with high-output states once CHF develops.

CAUSES OF HEART FAILURE

The general underlying causes of HF are outlined in Table I. It is important to realize that 50% of episodes of clinical HF are secondary to a precipitating cause. Thus, in treating HF, both the underlying and precipitating causes must be recognized. The most common underlying causes of HF (in the United States) are coronary artery disease, hypertension, cardiomyopathy, and valvular heart disease.

Table 1. Causes of Heart Failure

Primary abnormality of myocardial cells
- Cardiomyopathy and myocarditis

Secondary abnormality of myocardial cells
- Due to prolonged exposure to a hemodynamic burden (i.e., aortic regurgitation, hypertensive heart disease, primary or secondary pulmonary hypertension)
- Due to reduced O_2 delivery (ischemia)

Structural abnormalities
- Valvular heart disease
- Congenital heart disease
- Pericardial disease
- Coronary artery disease (ischemia, myocardial infarction, left ventricular aneurysm)
- Intracavity outflow obstruction

High-output states

Precipitating causes
- Increased salt intake
- Inappropriate reduction of a drug regimen
- Excess exertion or emotion
- Arrhythmias
- Systemic infection
- Onset of high-output states: anemia, hyperthyroidism, pregnancy
- Pulmonary embolism
- Increased fluid load
- Renal failure
- Myocardial ischemia
- Cardiac depressants (e.g., disopyramide)

THE CONCEPT OF DIASTOLIC HEART FAILURE

Heart failure is usually associated with an abnormality of systolic function (reduced ability to expel blood from the ventricular cavities); it also may occur with an abnormality of diastolic function despite normal systolic function (reduced ability of the left ventricle to accept or fill with blood).[36,37] In fact, approximately 30% of patients with classic symptoms and signs of HF have normal systolic function; that is, their HF is caused by diastolic dysfunction. Heart failure attributable to diastolic dysfunction is especially common in hypertensive heart disease, coronary artery disease, hypertrophic cardiomyopathy, and restrictive cardiomyopathy. The pathophysiology of diastolic dysfunction may involve abnormal calcium handling by myocytes as well as myocardial fibrosis.[38,39] When the ventricles fail to relax adequately to accept blood, ventricular diastolic pressures increase, causing atrial pressures to increase and leading to systemic or pulmonary congestion. Transient diastolic HF may be seen in patients with coronary artery disease who, during ischemia, have a reduction in left ventricular compliance, an increase in left ventricular filling pressures, and subsequent dyspnea.

One study suggested that a combination of diastolic blood pressure of 105 mm Hg or more and an absence of jugular venous distension was predictive of HF in patients with normal systolic function.[40] Patients with HF and primarily diastolic rather than systolic dysfunction may respond to angiotensin-converting enzyme inhibitor, calcium blocker, or ß-blocker therapy.

SYMPTOMS OF LEFT-SIDED HEART FAILURE

The major clinical symptoms of left ventricular HF include exertional dyspnea, orthopnea, paroxysmal nocturnal dyspnea, dyspnea at rest, exercise intolerance, weakness, fatigue, nocturia, and mental confusion.[3]

Dyspnea is the sensation of breathlessness, difficulty in breathing, or increased awareness of breathing that occurs with elevation in left atrial pressure resulting from pulmonary capillary hypertension. It is associated with a restrictive ventilatory defect caused by the replacement of air with fluid or blood in the lungs. The work of breathing is increased in order to distend the stiffened lungs. In the early phases of left ventricular HF, the dyspnea occurs only with exertion; with increasing HF, the level of exertion resulting in dyspnea diminishes until, in severe HF, dyspnea occurs at rest. Orthopnea is dyspnea that occurs while the patient is recumbent and is relieved by standing or sitting. It is caused by redistribution of fluid from the dependent parts of the circulation to the thorax, where the depressed left ventricle cannot pump the additional volume of delivered blood. Orthopnea results from pulmonary venous and capillary congestion. The severity of the orthopnea can often be determined by asking the patient how many pillows he or she uses when sleeping.

Paroxysmal nocturnal dyspnea, an extreme form of orthopnea, occurs when a patient wakes from sleep with a sense of severe breathlessness and suffocation. It is often associated with bron-

Table 2. Noncardiac Causes of Pulmonary Edema

Decreased plasma oncotic pressure: hypoalbuminemia due to renal, hepatic disease, nutritional cause, or protein-losing enteropathy
Altered alveolar-capillary membrane permeability (often referred to as adult respiratory distress syndrome [ARDS])
    Pneumonia: viral, bacterial, parasite, aspiration
    Inhaled toxins: smoke, nitrogen dioxide, phosgene
    Circulating toxins: bacterial endotoxins, snake venom
    Radiation pneumonitis
    Endogenous vasoactive substances: kinins, histamines
    Disseminated intravascular coagulation
    Uremia
    Immunologic reactions: hypersensitivity pneumonitis
    Associated with drowning
Lymphatic insufficiency: carcinomatosis, fibrosing lymphangitis
Unknown or not well understood
    Narcotic overdose: heroin
    High altitude pulmonary edema
    Neurogenic: subarachnoid hemorrhage, central nervous system trauma
    Eclampsia
    Post-cardiopulmonary bypass
    Post-cardioversion
    Post-anesthesia

chospasm and hence has been called "cardiac asthma." Paroxysmal nocturnal dyspnea usually occurs at night and often is unrelieved by sitting upright. A pathophysiologic feature of this condition is interstitial pulmonary edema.

Pulmonary edema associated with HF occurs when left atrial pressure is markedly elevated, with subsequent transudation of fluid into the alveoli. It is the severest form of breathlessness associated with HF. In acute pulmonary edema, patients are severely short of breath at rest, with associated agitation or dizziness. Pulmonary edema, which is considered a medical emergency, can be caused by any etiology of HF (Table 1). Several noncardiac causes of pulmonary edema (increased capillary "leakage" without elevation of atrial pressures) should be considered (Table 2).

Differentiating between dyspnea associated with cardiac disease and dyspnea due to pulmonary disease may be difficult, especially when they coexist. Table 3 presents some differentiating features.

Other symptoms of left-sided HF reflecting reduced forward output include fatigue, weakness, and, in severe cases, mental confusion.

The New York Heart Association (NYHA) devised a functional classification of heart disease that grades the severity of HF according to the amount of exertion required to cause symptoms. Although the classification is based on subjective findings, it is useful in following the course of patients during their disease, assessing results of therapy, and comparing groups of patients. The following is a summary of the classifications:

- Class I—no limitation of physical activity. No dyspnea, fatigue, or palpitations with ordinary physical activity
- Class II—slight limitation of physical activity. These patients have fatigue, palpitations, and dyspnea with ordinary physical activity, but are comfortable at rest
- Class III—marked limitation of activity. Less than ordinary physical activity results in symptoms, but patients are comfortable at rest
- Class IV—symptoms are present at rest, and any physical exertion exacerbates the symptoms

SYMPTOMS OF RIGHT-SIDED HEART FAILURE

The common specific etiologies of right-sided HF are listed in Table 4. A rare form of cardiomyopathy affects primarily the right ventricle and is called arrhythmogenic right ventricular dysplasia. This entity is associated with arrhyth-

---

Table 3. Differentiation of Cardiac Versus Pulmonary Dyspnea

CARDIAC DYSPNEA	PULMONARY DYSPNEA
Onset of dyspnea more sudden	Dyspnea tends to occur more gradually (except with infectious bronchitis, pneumonitis, pneumothorax, asthma)
Dyspnea usually not associated with sputum production	Dyspnea at night often associated with sputum production and relieved by coughing up sputum
No history of pulmonary disease	History of chronic obstructive lung disease; smoking history; noxious inhalants
No history of smoking	
No evidence of lung disease on chest x-ray film	Chest x-ray evidence of lung disease
Restrictive ventilatory defect by pulmonary function tests	Obstructive or restrictive ventilatory defect by pulmonary function tests
Arm-to-tongue circulation time usually increased (> 16 sec)*	Arm-to-tongue circulation time more likely to be normal

*The circulation time may be a useful test to perform when trying to distinguish pulmonary from cardiac dyspnea and low-output from high-output heart failure. 3–5 mL of Decholin is injected intravenously, and the time until the patient senses a bitter taste is measured. Normal values are 9–16 seconds. In patients with low-output heart failure, values are > 16 sec; in patients with high-output failure, circulation time is normal or reduced; in patients without heart failure, values are normal.

Table 4. Specific Causes of Right-Sided Heart Failure

Mitral stenosis with pulmonary hypertension
Cor pulmonale caused by chronic obstructive lung disease
Pulmonary valve stenosis
Pulmonary hypertension due to other causes
  • Congenital heart disease
  • Primary pulmonary hypertension
  • Collagen vascular disease
Tricuspid valve regurgitation (causes right ventricular [RV] failure)
Tricuspid valve stenosis (obstruction of flow into RV without RV myocardial failure)
Right ventricular myocardial infarction
Chronic left-sided congestive heart failure attributable to valvular or ischemic disease
Arrhythmogenic RV dysplasia

---

mias, right-sided HF, and sudden death in young patients.

Symptoms of predominantly right-sided HF are those of systemic venous congestion, including dependent edema; right upper quadrant pain resulting from stretching of the hepatic capsule from liver engorgement; anorexia, nausea, and bloating attributable to congestion of the mesentery and liver; and fatigue as forward output diminishes. Pulmonary symptoms are uncommon unless concomitant left-sided HF is present.

SIGNS OF HEART FAILURE

The general appearance of patients in left-sided HF depends on the severity of the HF. With mild failure, patients may appear entirely comfortable sitting at rest and do not appear breathless or in any distress until they undertake physical activity or lie flat. With severe failure, patients at rest may appear to be in severe distress, tachypneic, pale, and with cool extremities. They may be cyanotic.

Examination of the lungs in patients with mild left HF reveals moist rales at the bases; with severe failure and pulmonary edema, rales may be heard over the entire lung fields and may be associated with blood-tinged sputum. Dullness on percussion at the lung bases may reflect a pleural effusion.

If HF is secondary to left ventricular failure, evidence of dilatation and/or hypertrophy of that chamber may be present, including displacement of the apical impulse downward and toward the axilla (dilatation) and a left ventricular heave, which is a localized sustained outward motion of the ventricle during systole (left ventricular hypertrophy). With right ventricular enlargement, the right heart border may be percussed to the right of the sternum and a right ventricular heave may be felt as a diffuse lift over the lower portion of the sternum.

The S_1 is often normal; the P_2 may be accentuated with the development of left ventricular failure and pulmonary hypertension. A protodiastolic, or S_3 gallop, heard 0.13 to 0.16 second after the S_2, is a common sign of CHF.[42] This sound occurs in association with increased ventricular volumes and is caused by a rapid deceleration of ventricular inflow occurring just after the early filling phase of the ventricle. Reduced ventricular distensibility may contribute to the gallop sound.

A fourth heart sound (presystolic gallop) may be heard when CHF is associated with conditions in which the atrium contracts forcibly into a noncompliant ventricle and occurs with ventricular hypertrophy. Gallops emanating from the left ventricle are best heard at the apex with the patient in the left lateral decubitus position; gallops emanating from the right ventricle are best heard at the lower left sternal border and, typically, increase with inspiration. Gallops are best heard using the bell of the stethoscope. Murmurs caused by mitral regurgitation or tricuspid regurgitation secondary to ventricular dilatation are not uncommon in HF.

Tachycardia is another common manifestation of HF and is a compensatory mechanism whereby the heart attempts to maintain cardiac output in the setting of reduced stroke volume. Pulsus alternans is characterized by a regular rhythm in which there is an alternation of strong and weak contractions as detected by palpation of the pulse or by sphygmomanometry. This phenomenon occurs secondary to alternating stroke volume due to incomplete recovery of contractile cells on every other beat. Ventricular arrhythmias are a frequent complication of CHF. Cheyne–Stokes respiration occurs in patients with advanced cardiac failure and is characterized by alternating periods of apnea and hyperpnea. This condition is caused by a reduced sensitivity of the respiratory center to CO_2 and prolonged circulation time from lung to brain associated with left ventricular failure. When congestive failure is severe and longstanding, cardiac cachexia may occur with anorexia and weight loss.

Signs of right ventricular failure include jugular venous distention, hepatojugular reflux, hepatomegaly, right upper quadrant tenderness, edema, and ascites. When severe congestion of the viscera occurs, a protein-losing enteropathy may exacerbate development of ascites by a reduction in plasma oncotic pressure. With development of tricuspid regurgitation, a systolic regurgitant V wave may be seen and palpated in the jugular veins.

LABORATORY EXAMINATION IN CONGESTIVE HEART FAILURE

A typical chest x-ray feature of congestive HF includes cardiomegaly with a cardiothoracic ratio of more than 0.5. The appearance of the lung fields serves as an estimate of the pulmonary capillary pressure. Normally, the apices of the lung are less well perfused than the bases. With pulmonary capillary pressures of 15 to 20 mm Hg, apical and basal perfusions equalize; with pulmonary capillary pressures of 20 to 25 mm Hg, upper lobe pulmonary veins become more prominent than those in the lower lobe. With pulmonary capillary pressures greater than 25 mm Hg, interstitial pulmonary edema and Kerley B lines (interlobular edema) occur, and with pressures greater than 25 mm Hg, alveolar edema and pleural effusions may be seen (see Chapter 4).

The electrocardiogram (ECG) may help define the underlying etiology (especially ischemia) of the HF and confirm the presence of ventricular hypertrophy (see Chapter 3). Ventricular arrhythmias may be detected. Runs of nonsustained ventricular tachycardia in patients with HF associated with dilated cardiomyopathy are associated with an increased risk of sudden death.[43]

Echocardiography is useful in assessing the severity and etiology of HF and may aid in serial evaluation of the effect of therapy. Surgically correctable valvular disease must first be excluded. Global or diffuse left ventricular dysfunction suggests a cardiomyopathic process. Regional wall motion abnormalities are suggestive of coronary artery disease. Doppler echocardiography may be useful for assessing diastolic dysfunction. Typically, a tall a wave of mitral inflow velocity and prolonged isovolumic relaxation time are suggestive of abnormal diastolic function. Radionuclide ventriculography is another useful noninvasive technique for assessing both ventricular systolic and diastolic function. Serial ejection fractions may be followed and areas of abnormal ventricular wall motion detected. Serial exercise testing and exercise radionuclide ventriculography may be used to follow the response of patients with chronic HF to treatment regimens. Coronary angiography may be undertaken to diagnose significant coronary artery disease, which may be treated with angioplasty or surgical therapy. Cardiac catheterization is also useful in identifying other underlying causes of HF but is rarely needed to make the diagnosis of HF. Catheterization may be helpful in assessing the effect of pharmacologic interventions such as vasodilators or experimental inotropic agents in patients whose HF is refractory to other forms of medical therapy.

Several blood chemistry tests may be abnormal in patients with CHF, including elevated liver enzyme levels (SGOT, SGPT) and bilirubin secondary to hepatic congestion. Urinalysis may reveal proteinuria and high urine specific gravity. With reduced renal flow, the blood urea nitrogen concentration becomes elevated. With chronic cor pulmonale, polycythemia may occur. Serum electrolyte levels are usually normal in patients with mild-to-moderate CHF before treatment. With severe HF, diuretic therapy, salt restriction, and reduced ability to excrete free water result in dilutional hyponatremia.

Hypokalemia may result from thiazide or loop diuretics. Hyperkalemia may result from spironolactone administration, especially in the presence of a nonsteroidal anti-inflammatory drug or an angiotensin-converting-enzyme (ACE) inhibitor. It may occur in severe HF with markedly reduced renal blood flow or underlying diabetic nephropathy.

PROGNOSIS

The 5-year mortality rate for HF is generally high: 60% for men and 45% for women. Patients with class IV HF have worse prognoses, with a 1-year survival rate of only 50%. Other markers of a worse prognosis include coronary artery disease as the etiology of HF; reduced exercise capacity; poor hemodynamic function of the heart, especially reduced ejection fraction; low serum sodium concentration; low serum potassium level; high plasma renin, norepinephrine, vasopressin, and ANP concentrations; and presence of ventricular arrhythmias.[3] Sudden death accounts for 33% to 47% of deaths in patients with severe HF. Only recently have certain vasodilator agents been shown to improve survival in patients with HF (see below).

THERAPY FOR CONGESTIVE HEART FAILURE

Therapy for CHF is directed at reversing the pathophysiological processes described in the first section of this chapter. The treatable conditions among the causes listed in Table 1 should be corrected. Treatment of HF can then be separated into 2 clinical syndromes: 1) acute HF, often requiring management in the hospital and 2) chronic HF, where therapy is effective at reducing symptoms, improving functional capacity, and prolonging survival.

ACUTE HEART FAILURE

Acute pulmonary edema is a common presentation of acute HF. Any cause of left-sided HF may cause acute pulmonary edema; conditions with a major mechanical component, such as mitral regurgitation from chordal or papillary muscle rupture, or aortic stenosis will usually require urgent surgical intervention. More frequently, acute pulmonary edema is seen as an initial or recurrent presentation in patients with left ventricular failure. Therapy is directed toward reducing the symptoms of terrified breathlessness by reducing left ventricular end-diastolic pressure and improving oxygenation. The management strategy depends on the precipitating factor or factors (which have to be recognized and corrected) and the severity of the patient's

---

Table 5. Intravenous Agents Used to Treat Acute Heart Failure

Epinephrine: Full ß-adrenoceptor agonist. Also, α- and β_2-agonist actions. Heart rate response frequently excessive. Proarrhythmic. Sometimes combined with calcium in cardiogenic shock ("Epical")

Dopamine: β_1, α- and dopaminergic-receptor stimulation. At doses above 7.5 μg/kg/min, α adrenergic vasoconstriction becomes more pronounced and may compromise cardiac output and tissue perfusion through an excessive increase in systemic vascular resistance. Often used in combination with intravenous vasodilators such as sodium nitroprusside to control systemic vascular resistance. Dopaminergic receptor stimulation may augment renal blood flow—seen at low doses, <5 μg/kg/min. Relies partly on release of norepinephrine stores for inotropic properties.

Dobutamine: Racemic mixture with β_1, β_2, and α-adrenergic agonist activity. Countering effects of peripheral β_2 (vasodilator) and α (vasoconstrictor) actions on the peripheral circulation result in an agent with a relatively pure β_1 inotropic effect on the myocardium. Tends to have less effect on heart rate than epinephrine. Widely prescribed in acute heart failure with compromised systemic blood pressure and/or cardiac output.

Amrinone, Milrinone: Phosphodiasterase inhibition limits breakdown of 3,5-cyclic AMP. May circumvent ß-adrenergic receptor down regulation. Synergistic effects with ß-adrenoceptor agonists. Produces vasodilation coupled with inotropic and chronotropic effects. Thrombocytopenia seen especially with prolonged amrinone infusions—use now largely superseded by milrinone.

Nitroprusside: "Balanced" arteriolar and venous vascular smooth muscle relaxation through cyclic GMP. Very effective agent with predictable titratable dose response. Often combined with inotropic support in hypotensive patients.

Nitroglycerin: Probably more effect on the venous capacitance system. Vascular smooth muscle relaxation through cyclic GMP. May be the preferred agent in patients following acute myocardial infarction or evidence of ischemia.

---

condition. Patients with only early changes on the chest x-ray, pulmonary venous congestion, or interstitial edema with a well-preserved blood pressure will often respond promptly to intravenous direct therapy. A loop diuretic such as furosemide or bumetanide will cause a rapid reduction in the pulmonary capillary pressure and usually alleviate symptoms. The dramatic clinical response often appears to precede the diuresis and is consistent with an early reduction of pulmonary artery pressure. An initial report[44] suggesting a direct decrease in pulmonary artery pressures is not supported by later studies, where an increase in pulmonary capillary wedge pressure and an increase in systemic vascular resistance can be related to renin release and vascular effects through angiotensin II.[45] Patients with more severe forms of acute pulmonary edema require additional agents to reduce the pulmonary capillary pressure. Intravenous nitroprusside or nitroglycerin are most commonly used. Nitroprusside is particularly effective for the treatment of acute pulmonary edema in patients with preserved or increased blood pressure.[46–48] Appropriate and optimal infusion rate can be determined by monitoring right heart pressures using a pulmonary artery monitoring catheter (Swan–Ganz catheter). In patients with hypotension and acute pulmonary edema, such monitoring becomes almost mandatory in order to optimally reduce left ventricular end-diastolic pressure and augment cardiac output without further compromising systemic blood pressure.[49]

Patients with hypotension in acute pulmonary edema are at high risk of developing cardiogenic shock and aggressive therapy should be initiated promptly.[49] Intravenous inotropic agents are required (Table 5). Dobutamine and dopamine are the agents most commonly employed. Dobutamine has the advantage of not increasing systemic vascular resistance, which is seen with higher doses of dopamine.[49–53] The increase in cardiac output and blood pressure after therapy with dobutamine and dopamine may provide the hemodynamic support required for intravenous vasodilator therapy.

Intravenous ANP and more recently brain

natriuretic peptide (BNP) have also been shown to reduce filling pressure and systemic vascular resistance, and augment cardiac output in HF. These agents also possess natriuretic and diuretic properties that provide an attractive pharmacological profile for acute HF. The agents, however, are still investigational, and extensive clinical trials in acute HF are still needed.[54]

Patients with acute HF will also respond to general measures. Intravenous morphine will alleviate anxiety and dyspnea. Acute hemodynamic studies have shown that these agents also reduce pulmonary artery pressure, probably through a reduction in sympathetic induced vasoconstriction.[55] Morphine is safe in the majority of patients who have acute pulmonary edema, although the drug should be used with caution in patients with hypotension and not be used in patients with chronic obstructive airways disease. Aminophylline, rotating tourniquets, and therapeutic phlebotomy have no place in the hospital management of HF in the Northern Hemisphere.

Attention should be paid to arterial pH and oxygenation, and any electrolyte imbalance aggressively corrected. Critically ill patients with severe hypoxia may require urgent intubation and assisted ventilation. Almost all patients will benefit from supplemental oxygen.

Acute HF may also present as hypotension without overt pulmonary edema. This is more common in patients already receiving diuretics and may be related to over-diuresis. The acute presentation of HF may masquerade as primary disease in other organ systems. Hepatic dysfunction, ascites, or recurrent thrombotic events are not uncommonly caused by HF. These patients will usually respond to judicious use of diuretics, with or without low-dose dopamine inotropic support to enhance renal perfusion. As the patient responds to these measures to treat acute HF, the therapeutic goals shift toward the management of chronic HF.

CHRONIC HEART FAILURE

As patients respond to the measures to treat acute HF, the therapy required for chronic management should be instituted. Intravenous diuretics will be switched to oral therapy. Most patients who have had an episode of acute HF will require long-term oral diuretics (except where the underlying cause is correctable). The

dose of diuretic agents will depend on the severity of the underlying condition, the intensity of earlier diuretic response, and importantly, the degree of patient compliance to a low salt diet. Dose of concomitant angiotensin-converting enzyme (ACE) inhibitor drugs also affects the final diuretic requirements.

Clinical stability, disease progression, and survival appear to be dependent on the neuroendocrine activation that accompanies chronic HF. Diuretics and ACE inhibitor drugs should be considered together in the management of HF because of their profound and interrelated effects on the clinical manifestations and neuroendocrine status in patients with HF.

Table 6 lists the principal diuretics used to control the clinical manifestations of HF. Patients with mild HF or patients who are highly compliant to a less than 2 g/day sodium diet will only require a modest diuretic regimen. Some patients will remain free of clinical evidence of right- or left-sided HF with only thiazide diuretics. The combination of hydrochlorothiazide with triamterine may be particularly useful in this setting. In patients with more advanced HF, loop diuretics, such as furosemide or bumetanide, are usually required to prevent symptoms and signs from excess fluid retention. Even patients with advanced HF can usually be diuresed in an inpatient setting to the point where there is no clinical evidence of pulmonary edema. Some patients, particularly those with tricuspid regurgitation, will continue to have raised neck veins, but overt right HF with ascites, abdominal organ congestion, and severe peripheral edema can usually be controlled with loop diuretics or a combination of loop diuretics with thiazide or triamterine/thiazide combinations. Patients who readily respond to inpatient diuretic therapy but who are readmitted with redevelopment of pulmonary or peripheral edema usually have dietary or drug noncompliance to explain their recurrent episodes of "decompensated" HF.[56]

Diet

Patients have to be instructed as how to adhere to a diet of less than 2 g/day of sodium. In practice, this means virtually no preserved foods or strict attention to the labeled sodium control of such food. Most restaurant or fast food has to be avoided. Some patients will present to emergency rooms in acute HF, or experience parox-

Table 6. Commonly Used Diuretics in Heart Failure

DRUG	SITE OF ACTION	TOTAL DAILY DOSE IN CHF	FREQUENCY	COMPLICATIONS
Acetazolamide	Proximal tubule	250-375 mg	qod or qd x 2 days, skip day 3	Metabolic acidosis
Thiazides Hydrochlorothiazide Chlorothiazide	Distal tubule	50-200 mg 500-1,500 mg	qd to bid qd to bid	Hyponatremia, hypokalemia, metabolic alkalosis, hyperuricemia, glucose intolerance, lipid abnormalities, hypercalcemia, reduced GFR, allergy, thrombocytopenia, agranulocytosis, leukopenia, anemia, sexual dysfunction
Indapamide	Distal tubule (Direct vasodilator)	2.5-5 mg	qd	As above, but hypokalemia and lipid abnormalities less common
Phthalimidine derivatives Chlorothalidone Metolazone*	Distal tubule	50-200 mg 2.5-10 mg	qd qd	Similar to thiazides, but hypokalemia may be profound
Loop diuretics Furosemide	Loop of Henle	40-320 mg	qd to bid	Hyponatremia, hypokalemia, metabolic alkalosis, hyperuricemia, glucose intolerance, interstitial nephritis, ototoxicity, thrombocytopenia, agranulocytosis, leukopenia, anemia
Ethacrynic acid		50-400 mg	qd to bid	
Bumetanide		0.5-10 mg	qd, bid-tid qod	
Potassium-sparing Diuretics Spironolactone	Distal tubule	25-200 mg	qd to tid	Hyperkalemia, mental confusion, nausea, and gynecomastia (spironolactone only)
Triamterene Amiloride		100-300 mg 5-20 mg	qd to bid qd	

* Not recommended for maintenance therapy.

ysmal nocturnal dyspnea (having been previously clinically stable) after eating pizza, Chinese food, or other foods that are high in sodium. A low sodium diet is the foundation on which successful pharmacologic management of the patient with chronic HF is based.

ACE-Inhibitor Drugs

Captopril, enalapril, lisinopril, and quinapril have FDA labeling approval for the management of HF. The benefits of ACE inhibition is probably a shared "class" benefit of all ACE-inhibitor drugs, but differing pharmacology and a paucity of information regarding the optimal dose argues against the routine use of nonapproved agents. Moreover, there is mounting evidence that the effects of ACE inhibitors on disease progression, especially their influence on the processes of myocardial and vascular remodeling, may be dependent on the ability of each specific agent to affect the local or tissue angiotensin–aldosterone system.[57]

Large-scale randomized trials have demonstrated that the ACE inhibitor enalapril prolongs survival and reduces hospitalization in patients with NYHA classes II to IV HF. The CONSENSUS trial,[58] which compared enalapril with placebo in class IV HF, showed a 40% reduction in mortality. As the placebo mortality in this class of patients is high, the number of patients needed to be treated for 1 year to "save 1 life" is particularly low. Although the survival benefit demonstrated in the SOLVD treatment trial[59] in patients with mainly symptomatic NYHA class II-III HF was lower (the overall mortality reduction was 16%), the effect on the larger number of patients with class II HF was great. In the same study, a 26% reduction in the combined endpoint of hospitalization and mortality was reported. In clinical practice, all patients with symptomatic HF receiving therapy with a diuretic should also be treated with ACE inhibitors. The exception may be patients at high risk for vasodilation. Such patients would include those with significant aortic stenosis or obstructive cardiomyopathy. Patients with renal artery stenosis, a fixed obstruction to afferent glomerular arteriolar perfusion pressure, become dependent on the resultant high levels of angiotensin II for efferent arteriolar vasoconstriction to maintain an adequate glomerular filtration pressure. Such patients will experience an acute and possibly progressive rise in creatinine and blood urea nitrogen (BUN) levels after institution of ACE-inhibitor therapy. It is also possible that the effect of these drugs to inhibit the breakdown of vasodilating bradykinins contribute to this adverse effect in the setting of obstructive renal artery disease (Fig. 3).

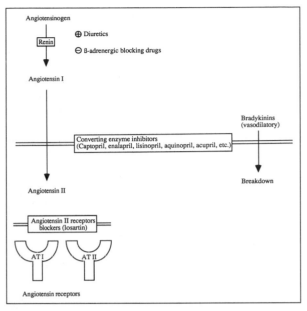

Figure 3. *Drugs and the renin–angiotensin system.*

A similar adverse rise in BUN or creatinine concentrations and/or an excessive symptomatic fall in systemic blood pressure may occur when the intravascular compartment is depleted from overdiuresis. Hyponatremia demonstrated in patients with HF correlates indirectly to circulating renin levels and is a clinical indicator for patients at risk for these complications during initiation of ACE-inhibitor therapy. Paradoxically, such patients probably achieve the most benefit from ACE inhibition.[60] The drugs are effective in reducing hyponatremia,[61] presumably as they break the vicious cycle of thirst and excess fluid ingestion in the setting of diuretic therapy. Unfortunately, many patients who experience renal dysfunction or symptomatic hypotension with ACE inhibitors have the therapy permanently withdrawn or reduced to a very low, possibly ineffective dose. If therapy with these agents is temporarily discontinued and reintroduced after the diuretic dose has been reduced, ACE inhibitors will frequently be tolerated. Stable elevations in BUN and creatinine levels are frequently an acceptable price to pay for the symptomatic and clinical benefit that accompanies ACE inhibition. After ACE-inhibitor therapy has been initiated, it is often possible to slowly titrate the daily dose to higher levels.

The daily dose of ACE inhibitors in the large-scale clinical trials is frequently higher than the

Table 7. Dose of ACE-Inhibitor Drugs in Major Heart Failure Trials

TRIAL	DRUG	ENDPOINT	MEAN DAILY DOSE
Consensus (I)	Enalapril	40% reduction in 6 mo. mortality	18.4 mg
V-Heft (II)	Enalapril	Greater survival benefit than hydralazine/nitrates*	15 mg
SOLVD	Enalapril	16% reduction in mortality risk	16.6 mg
AIRE	Ramipril	27% mortality reduction	5 mg bid. (77% of patients)

* Mortality at 2 yr 18% vs 25% with hydralazine/isosorbide dinitrate.

dose used in clinical practice. Table 7 shows the dose used in various major clinical trials of ACE inhibitors in HF.

Preliminary randomized dosage studies have suggested that the higher doses, which can usually be achieved by gradual dose titration, and appropriate reduction of diuretic dose may confer greater benefit than the low dose frequently prescribed in clinical practice. Large-scale randomized trial with lisinopril (double-blind, randomized; survival endpoint) and quinapril (open, randomized; morbidity endpoint) are underway to directly address this important point.

Oral Vasodilators

In addition to, or in patients intolerant of ACE inhibitors, various medications with vasodilating properties are beneficial to patients with HF.[61,62] The combination of hydralazine and nitrates were shown by Cohn et al[63,64] in V-HEFT studies I and II to improve survival, ejection fraction, and exercise capacity compared with placebo. V-HEFT II, which compared the survival benefit between enalapril and the hydralazine/nitrate combination demonstrated a greater survival benefit with the ACE-inhibitor drug, although subgroup analysis showed this effect to be limited to those patients with the highest circulating norepinephrine levels. Other orally active vasodilators have not been subjected to survival studies in HF. Prazosin use, which causes marked acute hemodynamic improvement, is associated with the rapid development of tachyphylaxis and does not improve survival. It is interesting that, despite problems with tolerance during chronic nitrate use, that isosorbide dinitrate was effective when combined with the arteriolar vasodilator hydralazine in the V-HEFT tri-

als. Hydralazine itself has some phosphodiesterase properties and can increase heart rate. It is not yet clear whether newer vasodilator agents or the mononitrates in their various release preparations will prove to be superior to the hydralazine/isosorbide dinitrate combination used for survival benefit in the V-HEFT trials.

Vasodilating Calcium-Channel Blockers

The dihydropyridine calcium-channel blockers combine the negative inotropic and other central effects of inhibition of the slow inward calcium channel with vascular smooth muscle relaxation. Nifedipine, the original dihydropyridine approved for clinical use, has not been shown to be useful for the management of patients with HF.[65] Worsened heart failure, the principle adverse effect, may have been in part a result of its original pharmacology, where the onset of action was rapid and associated with a presumably reflex increase in heart rates through sympathetic stimulation.[65] Recently, the second-generation dihydropyridines have been developed with a greater degree of vasodilation for any unit of negative inotropism. In vitro experiments with papillary muscle and vascular smooth muscle have shown those agents to have 10- to 100-fold increase in vascular effects relative to negative inotropic effects compared with nifedipine. Preliminary studies have demonstrated improved tolerability and short-term benefits on hemodynamics, exercise capacity, and quality of life in patients with mild to moderate HF. The second-generation dihydropyridines approved in the U.S. for hypertension are nicardipine, isradipine, felodipine, and amlodipine. The later 2 have been most extensively tested in HF. Their effect on mortality is currently being evaluated (V-HEFT III and PRAISE trials). A preliminary report by Packer et al[65a] for the PRAISE investigators suggested that amlodipine given to patients with severe heart failure was safe; in patients with nonischemic dilated cardiomyopathy, amlodipine resulted in a 45% reduction in the risk of death. Generally, however, calcium-channel blockers—certainly those without vasodilator properties—should be avoided or used with caution in the routine treatment of chronic HF. The adverse effects of diltiazem were demonstrated in patients with pulmonary congestion or a left ventricular ejection fraction of less that 40% in the MDPIT trial of diltiazem versus placebo following acute myocardial infarction.[66]

Digoxin

Digitalis glycosides[67,68] have been used to treat patients with HF for at least 200 years, when Withering first described their use in patients with "dropsy." Recent randomized withdrawal trials did show that approximately one-third of patients developed worsening HF within 3 months of stopping digoxin regardless of the use of ACE inhibitors.[69,70] Despite this convincing evidence for beneficial effects, even in patients with sinus rhythm, there are many unresolved issues regarding dose and the effect of the agents on arrhythmic sudden death and/or disease progression.[67] Recent experience with the oral agent flosequinan, briefly approved in the United States for the treatment of HF, has shown that an agent can have demonstrable benefit in symptoms and exercise capacity in relatively short-term trials[71] but an adverse effect on survival and probably disease progression [unpublished survival trial data, PRO-FILE trial]. Probably because of the adverse effect on disease progression, the "randomized withdrawal" of flosequinan (which was effected when the randomized survival trials of flosequinan were terminated) resulted in further clinical deterioration in those patients withdrawn from active treatment with flosequinan. The large-scale, prospective randomized trial of digoxin therapy currently being undertaken in patients with HF should help resolve many of these issues, which have caused controversy regarding its role in patients with HF in sinus rhythm.

Digoxin acts as an inotropic agent through sodium/potassium ATPase inhibition. Although this action can be demonstrated in acute inter-vention studies of left ventricular function, the hemodynamic effect is modest.[67] It is of interest that digoxin has also been recently demonstrated to have an antisympathetic effect on the heart by resetting the reduced sympathetic inhibitory input to the heart that accompanies chronic HF.[72] This antisympathetic influence of digoxin in HF is consistent with other beneficial agents in HF, which ameliorate or reduce the neuroendocrine response described in the first section of this chapter.

Oral Inotropic Agents

Digoxin remains the only oral inotropic agent widely prescribed in HF. Inotropic effects can be achieved with other approved drugs used in patients with HF, but the clinical trials that support their use have been small or inconclusive. Thus L-dopa will be partially converted to dopamine and has been prescribed in chronic HF. Salbutomol and other orally active β_2-agonists have also been evaluated, but the results of survival trials with agents designed to treat HF through any augmented sympathetic stimulation have shown an adverse effect on survival. The phosphodiesterase inhibitors were initially thought to have an attractive pharmacological profile for HF treatment.[73] Amrinone, milrinone, and enoximone caused inotropic effects combined with vasodilation as a result of the myocardial and vascular effects of enhanced levels of 3,5 cyclic AMP, the second messenger for adrenergic stimulation. Although the acute hemodynamic effects appeared beneficial, it was hard to show benefit during chronic therapy. Subsequent large-scale, randomized, survival trials with milrinone (PROMISE) and enoximone were discontinued after an increased mortality was observed in the active treatment group.[74] No class of patients was spared this increase in mortality, which was greatest in patients with class IV HF (56% increase in mortality). It seems probable that attempts to circumvent the downregulation in β-adrenergic receptors through phosphodiesterase inhibition has an adverse effect on disease progression. Cautious attention should be given to the results of these trials and the randomized trials of outpatient intravenous dobutamine therapy, which were also stopped early because of increased mortality in the dobutamine group, before patients are prescribed outpatient sympathomimetic intravenous or oral therapy.[75]

Table 8. Potential Harm From Excess Sympathetic Stimulation in Heart Failure

Excessive Heart Rate
Increased Ischemia
Promotion of Arrhythmias
Direct Toxicity
• Intracellular Calcium Excess
• Free Radical Formation
• ß-Receptor Downregulation
Increased Renin Formation
Effect of Remodeling (Hypertrophy)

Pimobendan is another investigational inotropic agent that has been evaluated in patients with chronic HF.[76] The agent appears to produce inotropic effects that are at least in part caused by enhanced calcium sensitivity. The effect of this agent on mortality in patients with HF is still unknown.

Vesnarinone is an interesting new investigational inotropic agent under evaluation in patients with HF. This quininolone derivative has phosphodiesterase properties at higher doses. It also affects the slow inward rectifying potassium and outward potassium currents that produces an inotropic effect. Higher doses improve central hemodynamics and tend to increase exercise capacity. However, in a recently published survival and morbidity trial, the higher dose (120 mg/day) limb of the study was discontinued on the advice of an independent safety board because of increased mortality. The 60-mg dose on the other hand reduced mortality by 60% compared with placebo.[77] Neutropenia has been observed in association with this agent as well as torsades de points ventricular arrhythmias.

ß-Adrenergic Blocking Drugs

ß-Adrenergic blocking drugs have traditionally been considered contraindicated in patients with HF. There is little doubt that this class of drugs can have adverse effects—especially in the setting of acute HF, where the beneficial influence of sympathetic activation may predominate. For chronic HF, the adverse effects of chronic sympathetic activation (a pathophysiological state) seem to predominate.

Table 8 lists the potential adverse effects of chronic sympathetic activation in patients with HF. Small clinical trials, initiated by the group from Gothenburg, Sweden, and first reported in 1975, resulted in a reconsideration of the role of ß-adrenergic blocking drugs in HF, particularly in patients with idiopathic dilated cardiomyopathy.[78–83]

In 1979, the Swedish group published survival data for a group of patients with dilated cardiomyopathy treated with metoprolol.[78] Survival was better in the treatment group than in historical controls. Subsequently, other small trials in patients with dilated cardiomyopathy or ischemic HF showed beneficial responses. In the largest trial to date, 383 patients with dilated cardiomyopathy were randomized between placebo and metoprolol.[84] A *P* value of .056 was reported on the decreased need for heart transplantation and mortality, the primary endpoints of the trial.

Bucindolol and Carvedilol

ß-Adrenergic blocking drugs with vasodilator properties, either through α-blockade (carvedilol) or direct vasodilator properties (bucindolol), are currently being tested in clinical trials in patients with HF.[85,86] The addition of vasodilator properties appears to result in improved tolerance to initiation of drug therapy associated with the acute hemodynamic benefit of vasodilation.[85] Chronic randomized studies with bucindolol and carvedilol have shown improved hemodynamics, left ventricular ejection fraction, and quality of life scores. In contrast with metoprolol, which has been shown to upregulate ß-receptors and the contractile response to exogenous sympathetic stimulation, carvedilol and bucindolol do not upregulate myocardial ß-receptor density and have not been shown to improve maximum exercise capacity. Submaximal exercise is improved with carvedilol.[86]

Xamoterol

Xamoterol is a sympathomimetic agent with ß-agonist and antagonist properties. It occupies ß-adrenergic receptors but with 40% of the sympathetic agonist activity of isoproterenol. In patients largely with ischemic heart disease and mild HF, the agent improved symptoms and exercise capacity. In severe HF, mortality was increased.[87] It is not clear whether the harm was from the ß-blocking or ß-adrenergic properties of the drug. Heart rates with xamoterol were higher during the nighttime (presumably because of low intrinsic sympathetic tone and the ß-agonist effects of the drug) but lower during the daytime hours.

DIASTOLIC DYSFUNCTION

Increasing attention is being focused on the importance of relaxation abnormalities, diastolic dysfunction, in the pathogenesis of acute or chronic HF. In its pure form, patients with this abnormality will have HF in the setting of normal left ventricular systolic function. More commonly, mild-to-severe relaxation abnormalities will accompany patients with systolic dysfunction. This group of patients can appropriately be treated as other patients with systolic dysfunction and will usually require digoxin, diuretics, and ACE-inhibitors as already discussed. In patients with more pure forms of diastolic dysfunction, perhaps the largest group being the "hypertensive hypertrophic cardiomyopathy of the elderly,"[88] it is not clear to what extent the conventional therapy for HF can be prescribed.[89] Most of these patients will require chronic diuretic therapy coupled with general measures, such as a low salt diet. The important role of the circulating renin–angiotensin–aldosterone system in salt and water homeostasis; and perhaps more importantly the role of the tissue components of this system in the vascular and myocardial structural changes (principally hypertrophy and collagen formation) argue strongly for including ACE-inhibitor drugs in the treatment of patients with this condition.[90] Here, the agents are not being used strictly as vasodilators, but the majority of these patients will have an increased systemic vascular resistance and probably have a common pathophysiology route in hypertension where the ACE-inhibitor drugs appear to have the greatest influence on reversing hypertrophy.[91] For similar reasons, ß-adrenergic blockade may have long-term benefits in patients with HF from diastolic dysfunction, particularly when there is a history or clinical evidence of hypertrophy. Patients with diastolic dysfunction may be critically dependent on diastolic filling time. Any drug that controls excessive heart rate may thus be beneficial.

Based on largely theoretical considerations, the calcium-channel blockers have developed a reputation, particularly in the United States, as being the drugs of choice in patients with diastolic dysfunction.[89] Very limited data are available to support these views. What studies do exist, have largely been carried out in highly selected patients, often with familial hypertrophic *obstructive* cardiomyopathy. Here, the beneficial effects of the drugs demonstrated in some studies may be attributable to negative inotropism in patients with obstructive cardiomyopathy. Much of the confusion stems from the absence of studies specifically in patients with HF and "pure" nonobstructive diastolic dysfunction. It is also virtually impossible in humans to measure independently the interrelated effects of loading, heart rate, and elasticity in determining alterations of diastolic function. It is sometimes forgotten that systolic function and diastolic function are inexorably linked within the energy-consuming process of the cardiac cycle of contraction and relaxation.

Based on our current understanding, it is probably appropriate to avoid potent vasodilators in patients with diastolic dysfunction, but it is interesting to note that the largest patient group with HF and diastolic dysfunction who were subjected to a long-term randomized trial can be found within the V-HEFT populations. Here, these patients were found to have a better prognosis than the cohort with systolic dysfunction but to respond similarly to vasodilator therapy!

OTHER THERAPIES

Heart Transplant (See Chapter 36)

Anticoagulation

Long-term therapy with warfarin is controversial. Benefit has been shown in patients with atrial fibrillation, particularly in the elderly and those with left ventricular dysfunction.[92] It is highly unlikely that selected patients, who are compliant and under close supervision, would not benefit from low-dose (INR, 1.5–2.0) warfarin therapy with a reduction in pulmonary and systemic embolic events.

Antiarrhythmic Therapy

Drug treatment has not been shown to improve survival in placebo controlled trials. Selective

Table 9. Precipitating Factors in Chronic Heart Failure	
	% OF PATIENTS
Lack of compliance	64
With diet	22
With drugs	6
With both (diet and drugs)	37
Uncontrolled hypertension	44
Cardiac arrhythmias	29
Atrial fibrillation	20
Atrial flutter	7
Multifocal atrial tachycardia	1
Ventricular tachycardia	1
Environmental factors	19
Inadequate therapy	17
Pulmonary infection	12
Emotional stress	7
Administration of inappropriate medications or fluid overload	4
Myocardial infarction	6
Endocrine disorders (thyrotoxicosis)	1
Adapted from Ghali JK et al.[56]	

patients may benefit from automated implantable tachycardia terminating devices with defibrillation capability. In patients with advanced left ventricular failure and severe HF, it is not clear that long-term benefit results. Some studies have shown 2-year survival to be similar to those patients not implanted with an automatic implantable cardioverter-defibrillator.[93,94]

Other Drugs

The comorbidity of patients with advanced HF frequently complicates their therapy and adversely affects the prognosis. Nonsteroidal anti-inflammatory drugs should be avoided where possible. These drugs have adverse effects on sodium balance and mitigate the actions of some thiazide diuretics and ACE inhibitors. Their use can be associated with renal failure in patients taking ACE inhibitors. Acute gout can be treated with colchicine and allopurinol, which can reduce the incidence of recurrent attacks. Aspirin may also diminish the benefits of ACE inhibition, although this largely theoretic interaction is almost certainly outweighed by the benefits to patients with atherosclerosis.

Finally, it is critical that precipitating causes of HF be diagnosed and treated. These are listed in Table 9.

DRUG TOLERANCE/ALLERGIES

Cough is frequently encountered in patients with HF and may be attributable to ACE inhibition. Therapeutic trials should be undertaken to ensure that the cough is drug related before the agent is abandoned in favor of other vasodilator agents. In the future, angiotensin-II–receptor blocking agents may become a therapeutic option.

Drug allergies causing a rash or skin irritation are frequently encountered. Some patients will require treatment with drugs without a sulphydryl group. Furosemide or bumetamide can be switched to ethracrynic acid, captopril to one of the newer ACE inhibitors, and thiazide diuretics (frequently the culprit agent) avoided.

SUMMARY

Heart failure is a very common condition that will be encountered across all ages and by family practitioners, internists, and specialists. Patients are frequently aware of the poor prognosis of this condition and will need a high level of support and monitoring if they are to receive the full benefits of our current understanding of the condition, and optimal therapy is to be prescribed. A surprising number of patients will respond to aggressive and diligent management of this condition with improved quality and duration of life.

REFERENCES

1. Schocken DD, Arrieta MI, Leaverton PE, et al. Prevalence and mortality rate of congestive heart failure in the United States. *J Am Coll Cardiology.* 1992;20:301-306.
2. Tighe D, Brest, AN. Congestive heart failure in the elderly. *Cardiovasc Clin.* 1992;22:127-138.
3. Braunwald E, Grossman W. Clinical aspects of heart failure. In Braunwald E (ed): *Heart Disease: A Textbook of Cardiovascular Medicine.* 4th Ed. Philadelphia: W.B. Saunders; 1992:444-463.
4. Cohn JN. Current therapy of the failing heart. *Circulation.* 1988;78:1099-1107.
5. Parmley WW. Pathophysiology and current therapy of congestive heart failures. *J Am Coll Cardiol.* 1989;13:771-785.
6. Braunwald E. Pathophysiology of heart failure. In Braunwald E (ed): *Heart Disease. A Textbook of Cardiovascular Medicine,* 4th Ed. Philadelphia: W.B. Saunders; 1992:393-418.
7. de la Bastie D, Levitsky D, Rappaport L, et al. Function of the sarcoplasmic reticulum and expression of its Ca^{++} - ATPase gene in pressure overload-induced cardiac hypertrophy in the rat. *Circ Res.* 1990;66:554-564.
8. Mercadier JJ, Lompre AM, Duc P et al. Altered sarcoplasmic reticulum Ca^{++}-ATPase gene expression in the human ventricle during end-stage heart failure. *J Clin Invest* 1990;85:305-309.
9. Mancini DM, Walter G, Reichek N, et al. Contribution of skeletal muscle atrophy to exercise intolerance and altered muscle metabolism in heart failure. *Circulation.* 1992;85:1364-1373.
10. Minotti JR, Christoph I, Massie BM. Skeletal muscle function, morphology, and metabolism in patients with congestive heart failure. *Chest.* 1992;101(suppl 5):333S-339S.
11. Poole-Wilson RA, Buller NP, Lindsay DC. Blood flow and skeletal muscle in patients with heart failure. *Chest.* 1992;101(suppl 5):330S-332S.
12. Mancini DM, Henson D, LaManca J, et al. Respiratory muscle function and dyspnea in patients with chronic congestive heart failure. *Circulation.* 1992;86:909-918.
13. Drexler H, Riede V, Munzel T, et al. Alterations of skeletal muscle in chronic heart failure. *Circulation.* 1992;85:1751-1759.
14. Mancini DM, Ferraro N, Nazzaro D, et al. Respiratory muscle deoxygenation during exercise in patients with heart failure demonstrated with near-infrared spectroscopy. *J Am Coll Cardiol.* 1991:18:492-498.
15. Coats AJ, Adamopoulos S, Radaelli A, et. al. Controlled trial of physical training in chronic heart failure: Exercise performance, hemodynamics, ventilation, and autonomic function. *Circulation.* 1992;85:2119-2131.
16. Casola G, Balli E, Taddei T, et al. Decreased spontaneous heart-rate variability in congestive heart failure. *Am J Cardiol.* 1989;64:1162-1167.
17. Ferguson DW, Berg WJ, Sanders JS. Clinical and hemodynamic correlates of sympathetic nerve activity in normal humans and patients with heart failure: Evidence from direct microneurogenic recordings. *J Am Coll Cardiol.* 1990;16:1125-1134.
18. Nolan J, Flapan AD, Capewell S, et al. Decreased cardiac parasympathetic activity in chronic heart failure and its relation to left ventricular function. *Br Heart J.* 1992;67:482-485.
19. Woo MA, Stevenson WG, Moser DK, et al. Patterns of beat to beat heart rate variability in advanced heart failure. *Am Heart J.* 1992;123:704-710.
20. Kienzle MG, Ferguson DW, Birkett CL, et al. Clinical, hemodynamic and sympathetic neural correlates of heart rate variability in congestive heart failure. *Am J Cardiol.* 1992;67:761-767.
21. Van de Borne P, Abramowicz M, Degre S, et al. Effects of chronic congestive heart failure on 24-hour blood pressure and heart rate patterns: A hemodynamic approach. *Am Heart J.* 1992;123:998-1004.
22. Leier CV, Binkley PF, Cody RJ. Alpha-adrenergic component of the sympathetic nervous system in congestive heart failure. *Circulation.* 1990;82(suppl 2):68-76.
23. Ferguson DW, Berg WJ, Roach PJ, et al. Effects of heart failure on baroreflex control of sympathetic neural activity. *Am J Cardiol.* 1992;69:523-531.
24. Mancia G, Seravalle G, Giannattasio C, et al. Reflex cardiovascular control in congestive heart failure. *Am J Cardiol.* 1992;69:17G-23G.
25. Creager MA. Baroreceptor reflex function in congestive heart failure. *Am J Cardiol.* 1992;69:10G-15G.
26. Jacobson TN, Kassis E, Amtorp O. Effects of orthostatic stress on peripheral capillary filtration in mild congestive heart failure after healing of myocardial infarction. *Am J Cardiol.* 1993;72:418-422.
27. Wroblewski H, Kastrup J, Mortensen SA, et al. Abnormal baroreceptor-mediated vasodilation of the peripheral circulation in congestive heart failure secondary to idiopathic dilated cardiomyopathy. *Circulation.* 1993;87:849-856.
28. Lerman A, Kubo SH, Tschumperlin LK, Burnett Jr JC. Plasma endothelin concentrations in humans with end-stage heart failure and after heart transplantation. *J Am Coll Cardiol.* 1992;20:849-853.
29. Cody RJ. The potential role of endothelin as a vasoconstrictor substance in congestive heart failure. *Eur Heart J.* 1992;13:1573-1578.
30. Cody RJ, Haas GJ, Binkley PF, et al. Plasma endothelin correlates with the extent of pulmonary hypertension in patients with chronic congestive heart failure. *Circulation.* 1992;85:504-509.
31. Katz SD, Schwarz M, Yuen J, et al. Impaired acetyl choline-mediated vasodilation in patients with conges-

tive heart failure. Role of endothelium-derived vasodilating and vasoconstricting factors. *Circulation.* 1993;88:55-61.

32. Kubo SH, Rector TS, Bank AJ, et al. Endothelium-dependent vasodilation is attenuated in patients with heart failure. *Circulation.* 1991;84:1589-1596.

33. Saita Y, Nakao K, Nishimura K, et al. Clinical application of atrial natriuretic polypeptide in patients with congestive heart failure: Beneficial effects on left ventricular function. *Circulation.* 1987;76:115-124.

34. Francis GS. Neuroendocrine activity in congestive heart failure. *Am J Cardiol.* 1990;66:33D-39D.

35. Francis GS, Benedict C, Johnstone DE, et al. Comparison of neuroendocrine activation in patients with left ventricular dysfunction with and without congestive heart failure. A substudy of the Studies of Left Ventricular Dysfunction (SOLVD). *Circulation.* 1990;82:1724-1729.

36. Brutsaert DL, Sys SU, Gillebert TC. Diastolic failure pathophysiology and therapeutic implications. *J Am Coll Cardiol.* 1993;22:318-325.

37. Bonow RO, Udelson JE. Left ventricular diastolic dysfunction as a cause of congestive heart failure: Mechanisms and management. *Ann Intern Med.* 1992;117:502-510.

38. Klug D, Robert V, Swynghedauw B. Role of mechanical and hormonal factors in cardiac remodeling and the biologic limits of myocardial adaptation. *Am J Cardiol.* 1993;71:46A-54A.

39. Grossman W. Diastolic dysfunction and congestive heart failure. *Circulation.* 1990;81(suppl 2):1-7.

40. Ghali JK, Kadakia S, Cooper RS, et al. Bedside diagnosis of preserved versus impaired left ventricular systolic function in heart failure. *Am J Cardiol.* 1991;67:1002-1006.

41. McCall D, O'Rourke R. Congestive heart failure. *Mod Concepts Cardiovasc Dis.* 1985;52:55.

42. Patel R, Bushnell DL, Sobotka PA. Implications of an audible third heart sound in evaluating cardiac function. *West J Med.* 1993;158:606-609.

43. Podrid PJ, Fogel RI, Fuchs TT. Ventricular arrhythmia in congestive heart failure. *Am J Cardiol.* 1992;69:82G-96G.

44. Dikshit, K, Vyden JK, Forrester JS, et al.: Renal and extrarenal hemodynamic effects of furosemide in congestive heart failure after acute myocardial infarction. *N Engl J Med.* 1973;288:1087-1090.

45. Larsen FF: Hemodynamic effects of high vs low dose furosemide in acute myocardial infarction. *Eur Heart J.* 1988;9:125-131.

46. Leier CV, Bambach D, Thompson MJ, et al. Central and regional hemodynamic effects of intravenous isosorbide dinitrate, nitroglycerin, and nitroprusside in patients with congestive heart failure. *Am J Cardiol.* 1981;48:1115-1123.

47. Franciosa JA, Guiha NH, Limas CL, et al. Improved left ventricular function during nitroprusside infusion in acute myocardial infarction. *Lancet.* 1972;1:650-654.

48. Miller RR, Vismara LA, Zelis R, et al. Clinical use of sodium nitroprusside in chronic ischemic heart disease. *Circulation.* 1975;51:328-336.

49. Leier CV. Acute inotropic support: intravenously administered positive inotropic drugs. In: Leier CV (ed). *Cardiotonic Drugs*, 2nd Ed. New York: Marcel Dekker; 1991:63-106.

50. Francis GS, Sharma B, Hodges M. Comparative hemodynamic effects of dopamine and dobutamine in patients with acute cardiogenic circulatory collapse. *Am Heart J.* 1982;103:995-1000.

51. Leier CV, Heban PT, Huss P, et al. Comparative systemic and regional hemodynamic effects of dopamine and dobutamine in patients with heart failure. *Circulation.* 1978;58:466-475.

52. Loeb HS, Winslow EBJ, Rahimtoola SH, et al. Acute hemodynamic effects of dopamine in patients with shock. *Circulation.* 1971;44:163-173.

53. Holzer J, Karliner JS, O'Rourke RA, et al. Effectiveness of dopamine in patients with cardiogenic shock. *Am J Cardiol.* 1973;32:79-84.

54. Wei CM, Heublein DM, Perrella MA, et al. Natriuretic peptide system in human heart failure. *Circulation.* 1993;88:1004-1009.

55. Vismara LA, Leaman DM, Zeliv R. The effects of morphine on venous tone in patients with acute pulmonary edema. *Circulation.* 1976;54:335-337.

56. Ghali JK, Kadakia S, Cooper R, et al. Precipitating factors leading to decompensation of heart failure. Traits among urban blacks. *Arch Intern Med.* 1988;148:2013-2016.

57. Hirsch AT, Talsness CE, Schunkert H, et al. Tissue-specific activation of cardiac angiotensin converting enzyme in experimental heart failure. *Circ Res.* 1991;69:475-482.

58. CONSENSUS Trial Study Group. Effects of enalapril on mortality in severe congestive heart failure: Results of the Cooperative New Scandinavian Enalapril Survival Study. *N Engl J Med.* 1987;316:1429-35.

59. The SOLVD Investigators. Effect of enalapril on survival in patients with reduced left ventricular ejection fractions and congestive heart failure. *N Engl J Med.* 1991;325:293-302.

60. Lee WH, Packer M. Prognostic importance of serum sodium concentration and its modification by converting enzyme inhibition in patients with severe chronic heart failure. *Circulation.* 1986;73:257-267.

61. Cohn JN. Efficacy of vasodilators in the treatment of heart failure. *J Am Coll Cardiol.* 1993;22(suppl A):135A-138A.

62. Massie B, Ports T, Chatterjee K, et al. Long-term vasodilator therapy for heart failure: Clinical response and its relationship to hemodynamic measurements. *Circulation.* 1981;63:269-278.

63. Cohn JN, Archibald DG, Phil M, et al. Effect of vasodilator therapy on mortality in chronic congestive heart failure. Results of a veterans administration cooperative study. *N Engl J Med.* 1986;314:1547-1552.

64. Cohn JN, Johnson G, Ziesche S, et al. A comparison of enalapril with hydralazine-isosorbide dinitrate in the treatment of chronic congestive heart failure (V-HEFT II). *N Engl J Med.* 1991;325:303-310.

65. Elkayam U, Amin J, Mehra A, et al. A prospective, randomized, double-blind, crossover study to compare the efficacy and safty of chronic nifedipine therapy with that of isosorbide dinitrate and their combination

in the treatment of chronic congestive heart failure. *Circulation.* 1990;82:1954-1961.

65a. Packer M, for PRAISE investigators. The PRAISE Trial (Prospective Randomized Amlodipine Survival evaluation): Background and Main Results. Presented at the 44th annual American College of Cardiology Meeting. New Orleans. March, 1995

66. Multicenter Diltiazem Postinfarction Trial Research Group. The effect of diltiazem on mortality and reinfarction after myocardial infarction. *N Engl J Med.* 1988;319:385-392.

67. Smith TW. Digoxin in heart failure (editorial). *N Engl J Med.* 1993;329:51-53.

68. Jaeschke R, Oxman AD, Guyatt GH. To what extent do congestive heart failure patients in sinus rhythm benefit from digoxin therapy? A systematic overview and meta-analysis. *Am J Med.* 1990;88:279-86.

69. Packer M, Gheorghiade M, Young JB, et al. Withdrawal of digoxin from patients with chronic heart failure treated with angiotensin-converting enzyme inhibitors: RADIANCE Study Group. *N Engl J Med.* 1993;329:1-7.

70. Massie BM, Berk MR, Brozena SC, et al. Can further benefit be achieved by adding flosequinan to patients with congestive heart failure who remain symptomatic on diuretic, digoxin, and an angiotensin converting enzyme inhibitor? Results of the flosequinan-ACE inhibitor trial (FACET). *Circulation.* 1993;88:492-501.

71. Packer M, Narahara KA, Elkayam U, et al. Double-blind, placebo-controlled study of the efficacy of flosequinan in patients with chronic heart failure. *J Am Coll Cardiol.* 1993;22:65-72.

72. Ferguson DW, Berg WJ, Sanders JS, et al. Sympathoinhibitory responses to digitalis glycosides in heart failure patients: Direct evidence from sympathetic neural recordings. *Circulation.* 1989;80:65-77.

73. Packer M. Effects of phosphodiasterase inhibitors on survival of patients with chronic congestive heart failure. *Am J Cardiol.* 1989;63:41A-45A.

74. Packer M, Carver JR, Rodeheffer RJ, et al. Effect of oral milrinone on mortality in severe chronic congestive heart failure. *N Engl J Med.* 1991;325:1468-1475.

75. Curfman GD. Inotropic therapy for heart failure: An unfulfilled promise. *N Engl J Med.* 1991;325:1509-1510.

76. Kubo SH, Gollub S, Bourge R, et al. Beneficial effects of pimobendan on exercise tolerance and quality of life in patients with heart failure: Results of a multicenter trial: the Pimobendan Multicenter Research Group. *Circulation.* 1992;85:942-949.

77. Feldman AM, Bristow MR, Parmley WW, et al. Effects of vesnarinone on morbidity and mortality in patients with heart failure: Vesnarinone Study Group. *N Engl J Med.* 1993;329:149-155.

78. Swedberg K, Hjalmarson Å, Waagstein F, et al. Prolongation of survival in congestive cardiomyopathy by beta-receptor blockade. *Lancet.* 1979;1:1374-1376.

79. Engelmeier RS, O'Connell JB, Walsh R, et al. Improvement in symptoms and exercise tolerance by

metoprolol in patients with dilated cardiomyopathy: A double-blind, randomized, placebo-controlled trial. *Circulation.* 1985;72:536-546.

80. Currie PJ, Kelly MJ, McKenzie A, et al. Oral beta-adrenergic blockade with metoprolol in chronic severe dilated cardiomyopathy. *J Am Coll Cardiol.* 1984;3:203-209.

81. Anderson JL, Gilbert EM, O'Connell JB, et al. Long-term (2 year) beneficial effects of beta-adrenergic blockade with bucindolol in patients with idiopathic dilated cardiomyopathy. *J Am Coll Cardiol.* 1991;17:1373-1381.

82. Woodley SL, Gilbert EM, Anderson JL, et al. ß-blockade with bucindolol in heart failure caused by ischemic versus idiopathic dilated cardiomyopathy. *Circulation.* 1991;84:2426-2441.

83. Heilbrunn SM, Shah P, Bristow MR, et al: Increased ß-receptor density and improved hemodynamic response to catecholamine stimulation during long-term metoprolol therapy in heart failure from dilated cardiomyopathy. *Circulation.* 1989;79:483-490.

84. Waagstein F, Bristow MR, Swedbert K, et al, Beneficial effects of metoprolol in idiopathic dilated cardiomyopathy. *Lancet.* 1993;342:1441-1446.

85. Fowler MB (ed). Beta-adrenergic blockade In the management of chronic heart failure. *Am J Cardiol.* 1993;71:9:1C-70C.

86. Olsen SL, Gilbert EM, Renlund DG, et al. Carvedilol improves symptoms and left ventricular function in patients with congestive heart failure due to ischemic or idiopthic dilated cardiomyopathy. *J Am Coll Cardiol.* 1993;21:114A:725-732.

87. The Xamoterol in Severe Heart Failure Study Group: Xamoterol in severe heart failure. *Lancet.* 1990;336:1-6.

88. Topol EJ, Traill TA, Fortuin NJ. Hypertensive hypertrophic cardiomyopathy of the elderly. *N Engl J Med.* 1985;312:277-283.

89. Bonow RO, Udelson JE. Left ventricular diastolic dysfunction as a cause of congestive heart failure: Mechanisms and management. *Ann Intern Med.* 1992;117:502-510.

90. Schunkert H, Dzau VJ, Tang SS, et al. Increased rat cardiac angiotensin converting enzyme activity and mRNA expression in pressure overload left ventricular hypertrophy: effects on coronary resistance, contractility, and relaxation. *J Clin Invest.* 1990;86:1913-1920.

91. Hill LS, Monoghan M, Richardson PJ. Regression of left ventricular hypertrophy during treatment with antihypertensive agents. *Br J Clin Pharmacol.* 1979;7(suppl 2):225s-260s.

92. The Boston Area Anticoagulation Trial for Atrial Fibrillation Investigators. The effect of low-dose warfarin on the risk of stroke in patients with nonrheumatic atrial fibrillation. *N Engl J Med.* 1990;323:1505-1511.

93. Stevenson WG, Stevenson LW, Middlekauff HR, et al. Sudden death prevention in patients with advanced ventricular dysfunction. *Circulation.* 1993;88:2953-2961.

94. Bardy GH, Hofer B, Johnson G, et al. Implantable transvenous cardioverter-defibrillators. *Circulation.* 1993;87:1152-1168.

CHAPTER 21

Diagnosis and Management of Cardiac Arrhythmias

Thomas B. Graboys, MD

Management of patients presenting with rhythm disorders requires judgment, experience, and integration of the electrocardiographic (ECG) abnormality within the context of each patient's clinical status.

This chapter presents a unified, concise approach to diagnosis and management of arrhythmias.

DIFFERENTIAL DIAGNOSIS OF TACHYARRHYTHMIAS

The differential diagnosis of cardiac arrhythmias is facilitated by a classification based on the width of the QRS interval and the regularity or irregularity of the RR cycle. Thus, when a tachycardia is seen, a logical progression in the differentiation of the rhythm is to determine if the QRS is wide or narrow and the cycling regular or irregular (Table 1). The major differential diagnosis of any wide regular tachycardia would be ventricular tachycardia (VT), supraventricular tachycardia (SVT) with aberration, or preexcita-

tion with antegrade accessory tract conduction.

Wide irregular tachyarrhythmia is probably atrial fibrillation with either aberrancy or fixed or rate-related bundle branch block. Narrow QRS regular tachycardias are classified as sinus, SVT, junctional tachycardia, or atrial flutter. Irregular, narrow complex tachycardias are classified as atrial fibrillation or multifocal atrial tachycardia (MAT).

WIDE, REGULAR TACHYCARDIA

VENTRICULAR TACHYCARDIA

By standard definition, 3 or more consecutive rapid ventricular beats constitute a salvo of VT. The QRS is wide and, at times, bizarre, particularly if the origin of the tachycardia is far enough from the normal specialized conduction system. Ventricular activity is independent of that within the atrium, resulting in atrioventricular (AV) dissociation (Fig. 1). The hallmark on the ECG is

Table 1. Classification of Tachycardias

QRS COMPLEX			
WIDE (≥ 0.12 SEC)		NARROW (≤ 0.12 SEC)	
Regular	Irregular	Regular	Irregular
VT	AF	ST	AF
SVT (aberration)	(aberration or bundle branch block)	PSVT	MAT
		NPJT	
WPW		AFL	

AF=Atrial fibrillation; AFL=Atrial flutter; MAT=Multifocal atrial tachycardia; NPJT=Nonparoxysmal junctional tachycardia; PSVT=Paroxysmal supraventricular tachycardia; SVT=Supraventricular tachycardia; VT=Ventricular tachycardia; ST= Sinus tachycardia; WPW=Wolff-Parkinson-White syndrome.

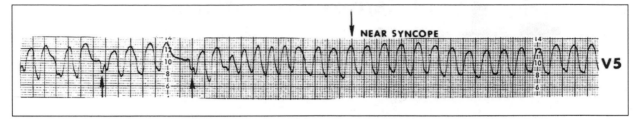

Figure 1. *Ventricular tachycardia with atrioventricular dissociation (arrows).*

partial capture if the sinus mechanism coincides with ventricular depolarization from the VT focus, resulting in a fusion beat. A full 12-lead ECG should be obtained, so as not to base the diagnosis of a tachyarrhythmia on a single lead in which the QRS may be spuriously narrow.

The rate of VT is variable and depends on the clinical circumstances. The form of VT occurring within the setting of an acute myocardial infarction (so-called VT of the vulnerable period) is typically rapid and accelerating, and deteriorates to ventricular fibrillation (VF), often within 30-60 seconds. Paroxysmal VT in the nonischemic setting may have a constant rate of 150 beats/min. Typically, VT salvos have a rate of 150-200 beats/min. Therapy with antiarrhythmic drugs may result in slower nonsustained salvos, with rates of 100-150 beats/min. The rate of VT may exceed 200 beats/min; SVT with aberration should be suspected if the rate exceeds 250 beats/min and the ORS is 120-140 msec.

Slow ventricular loci may represent an idioventricular escape mechanism (60-100 beats/min), VT with 2:1 exit block from the site of tachycardia, or the electrophysiologic effect of antiarrhythmic drugs producing periods of "slow VT." At times, it may be difficult to differentiate electrocardiographically an accelerated idioventricular focus from VT in which the rate has been slowed.

SUPRAVENTRICULAR TACHYCARDIA WITH ABERRANCY

In SVT with aberrancy (Table 2), the rate of the tachycardia is usually 160-220 beats/min, although frequently it exceeds 250 beats/min in the presence of concealed bypass tracts or

Table 2. Factors in the Electrocardiographic Diagnosis of Ventricular Tachycardia or Supraventricular Tachycardia With Aberration

	VT	SVT WITH ABERRATION
AV dissociation	+	—
Fusion beats	+	—
QRS width	>140 msec	<140 msec
QRS morphology		
RBBB	Monophasic, LAD	Triphasic, normal axis
LBBB	Wide R in lead V_1	—
	RAD	—
Regularity	80%	95%
Onset	VBP	APB with ↑ QRS
CSP	−(<2%)	+(30%)
Rate (beats/min)	150-200	>200

APB=Atrial premature beat; CSP=Carotid Sinus pressure; LAD=Left axis deviation; LBBB=Left bundle branch block; RAD= Right axis deviation; RBBB=Right bundle branch block; SVT=Supraventricular tachycardia; VPB=Ventricular premature beat; VT=Ventricular tachycardia.

known preexcitation. The QRS is between 0.11 and 0.13 second. A right bundle branch block pattern is more common, although left ventricular tachycardia may also appear as right-sided intraventricular conduction disturbance. One helpful distinguishing characteristic is that SVT with aberration usually does not result in a QRS duration >0.13 sec. The presence of P waves preceding each QRS should be sought, utilizing special leads if necessary (Lewis, esophageal, or right atrial). Differentiation from VT may be facilitated if onset of the tachycardia is recorded. The initial premature beat is noted to be narrow, followed by progressive widening of the QRS as rate-related aberrancy ensues.

Carotid sinus massage (CSM) often assists in differentiating SVT with aberration from VT. Carotid sinus massage may interrupt the reentrant mechanism by inducing vagotonia and terminating the tachycardia. If the mechanism is atrial flutter, CSM may slow conduction, converting a 2:1 or 1:1 response transiently to 2:1 or 4:1, resulting in normalization of conduction and confirming the presence of aberration. Rarely, CSM may terminate an episode of VT.

Certain physical findings are helpful in differentiating an aberrant rhythm from VT. Heart sounds are constant in SVT, as opposed to the variable intensity and splitting of both S_1 and S_2 during VT. The presence of cannon a waves observed in the jugular pulse indicates AV dissociation and a ventricular origin of the tachycardia.

PREEXCITATION SYNDROMES

Preexcitation syndromes are discussed in detail in a later section. Among patients with Wolff-Parkinson-White syndrome (WPW) whose atrial mechanism is fibrillation or flutter, the refractory period of the anomalous pathway may be so short that rapid conduction with rates in excess of 300 beats/min ensues (Fig. 2).

WIDE, IRREGULAR TACHYCARDIA

TORSADES DE POINTES

Torsades de pointes (Fig. 3) represents chaotic, nonsustained ventricular activity that is invariably associated with serious symptoms. The ECG hallmark is rapid, bizarre QRS complexes with recurrent alteration of the QRS axis. Mechanisms include antiarrhythmic drugs (the

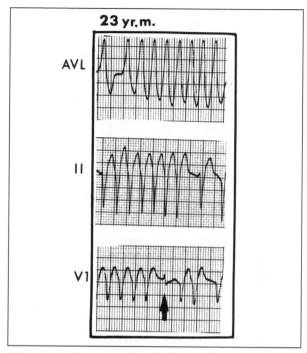

Figure 2. *Atrial fibrillation with rapid ventricular response in a patient with Wolff-Parkinson-White syndrome, indicating antegrade accessory tract conduction.*

most common being quinidine), phenothiazines, electrolyte disturbances (particularly hypokalemia), hereditary and acquired QT prolongation, AV block, and coronary vasospasm.

ATRIAL FIBRILLATION WITH ABERRANCY OR BUNDLE BRANCH BLOCK

Occasionally, patients with acute onset of atrial fibrillation, particularly in the setting of left ventricular failure, present with a wide-QRS, slightly irregular tachycardia that may be confused with VT. Close scrutiny of the cycle lengths and carotid sinus pressure (CSP) that slows the ventricular response invariably secure the diagnosis.

NARROW, REGULAR TACHYARRHYTHMIAS

SINUS TACHYCARDIA

Sinus tachycardia is defined as acceleration of the normal sinus mechanism beyond 105 beats/min. P waves with the same general morphology as the normal sinus P wave precede each QRS. As the rate increases, the P wave may appear somewhat peaked, and the PR interval may shorten, indicating facilitation of AV conduction. Rates rarely exceed 160 beats/min in the adult. However, under unusual circumstances (e.g., thyrotoxicosis), sinus tachycardia may range from 150-200 beats/min. The rhythm is typically regular, and the response to CSM is gradual slowing, with prompt resumption of the tachycardia. Carotid sinus massage is particularly helpful if there is either rate-related or underlying bundle branch block. In this circumstance, particularly if the PR interval is somewhat prolonged, the P wave becomes fused with the preceding T wave at rapid rates and the rhythm may appear to be VT. With CSM, slowing unveils the P waves and confirms the presence of a sinus mechanism.

SUPRAVENTRICULAR TACHYCARDIA

When there is a rapid atrial mechanism (150-200 beats/ min), the diagnosis of paroxysmal SVT (PSVT) should be considered (Figs. 4 and 5). Recent developments in the techniques of intracardiac recordings have led to better understanding of the pathophysiologic mechanisms of PSVT. The 2 basic mechanisms are *reentry* and *enhanced automaticity*. Reentrant rhythms involve a complex mechanism, the substrate of which is electrophysiologic inhomogeneity of adjacent cardiac tissue. Reentry accounts for some 90% of episodes of PSVT.

Sixty percent of PSVTs are AV nodal reentrant tachycardia. In about three-fourths of patients with AV nodal (junctional) reentrant tachycardia, dual AV nodal pathways are identified in the electrophysiology laboratory. The AV node contains 2 functionally different pathways, designated α and ß. The α pathway is slower conducting, but its refractory period is shorter than the faster conducting ß pathway. Atrial premature beats (APBs) that are sufficiently early block the ß pathway and conduct slowly in the antegrade direction down the α pathway. The ß pathway is then available for retrograde conduction, and the appropriate substrate for reentrant tachycardias is established. As with most forms of reentrant SVT, either an APB or ventricular premature beat (VPB) can initiate AV nodal reentrant tachycardias.

If the mechanism of atrial tachycardia is enhanced automaticity, a P wave precedes each QRS. The P wave will be morphologically different from the sinus P wave and it will fire at a constant rate of 160-250 beats/min.

The response to vagal maneuvers such as CSM is variable. If the mechanism is reentry, the reentrant tachycardia may be slowed or terminated. If the mechanism of arrhythmia is based on automaticity, such maneuvers may have no effect or only briefly return the rhythm to sinus.

ATRIAL FLUTTER

Atrial flutter is characterized by coarse, regular, "sawtooth" undulations of the baseline, referred to as F waves. These F waves appear at a rate of approximately 300 beats/min (Fig. 6). Atrial flutter is usually associated with 2:1 AV block and a resultant ventricular response of 150 beats/min. Indeed, any regular narrow tachycardia at 150

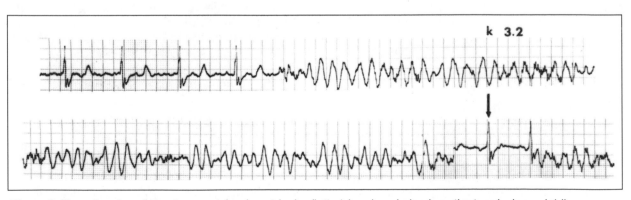

Figure 3. Torsades de pointes (nonsustained ventricular flutter) in a hypokalemic patient recieving quinidine.

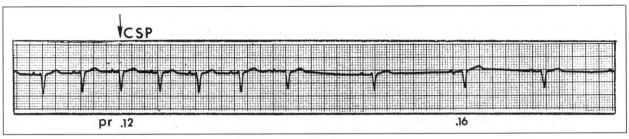

Figure 4. *Slow paroxysmal supraventricular tachycardia (PSVT) at 100 beats/min, which reverted to sinus rhythm with carotid sinus pressure (CS).*

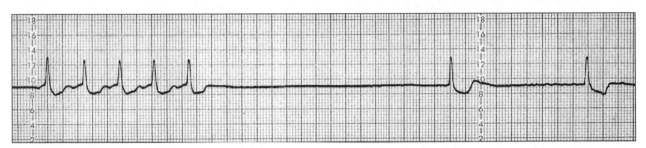

Figure 5. *Spontaneous termination of paroxysmal supraventricular tachycardia with asymptomatic offset pause and junctional escape beat.*

beats/min should be considered atrial flutter until proved otherwise. Carotid sinus massage is, as noted earlier, most helpful in diagnosis because it induces an increase in AV block, slowing of the ventricular response, and disclosure of the flutter waves. The bulk of data suggests that atrial flutter is due to a reentrant mechanism involving pathways in the atrium. This reentrant mechanism results in a predominantly negative deflection of the flutter waves in the inferior leads. A less common type of atrial flutter involves an oppositely directed reentrant circuit, such that the flutter waves are predominantly positive in the inferior leads.

When the frequency of the atrial rate is as low as 250 beats/min, it must be differentiated from SVT; at higher frequencies — 400 beats/min — atrial flutter must be differentiated from atrial fibrillation. Pharmacological interventions may alter the rate of the flutter mechanism. Thus, drugs that prolong the effective refractory period, such as quinidine, procainamide, and disopyramide (class IA drugs), will reduce the flutter rate from 300 to 200-250 beats/min. If the flutter rate is sufficiently slowed, it is possible to inter-

mittently conduct 1:1. Hence, in some patients, administration of class IA agents without concomitant use of drugs to block the AV junction may result in acceleration of heart rate. Drugs that shorten repolarization, such as digitalis, may enhance the flutter rate, as is often seen during digitalis treatment. About half of patients in atrial flutter convert to atrial fibrillation.

NONPAROXYSMAL JUNCTIONAL TACHYCARDIA (NPJT)

Nonparoxysmal junctional tachycardia, also termed accelerated junctional rhythm, is a manifestation of enhanced automaticity of the AV junction. The average rate is 70-130 beats/min. This arrhythmia may be a manifestation of digitalis toxicity or it may be associated with inferior myocardial infarction. It may be seen in the postoperative cardiac patient or in patients with severe mitral valvular disease. Patients with acute rheumatic fever and rare patients who have no other significant heart disease may manifest NPJT. Antiarrhythmics such as procainamide and quinidine may induce NPJT.

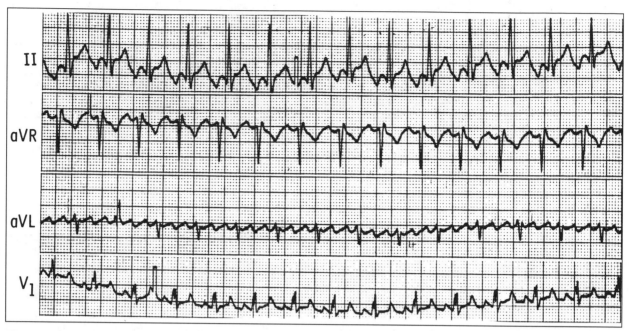

Figure 6. *Atrial flutter with atrial rate of 315 beats/min and 3:1 atrioventricular response.*

NARROW, IRREGULAR TACHYCARDIAS

ATRIAL FIBRILLATION

It has been suggested that both atrial flutter and fibrillation are part of a spectrum of intra-atrial reentry. A shift of atrial flutter to fibrillation can be seen when the flutter waves break down into multiple smaller reentrant wavelets. The creation of such wavelets depends on the circulating impulses encountering areas of inhomogeneous refractoriness, resulting in secondary wavelets in multiple areas of reentry. This produces the chaotic, small-amplitude fibrillatory waves seen in atrial fibrillation. Borderline cases are seen and may be described as impure flutter or flutter-fibrillation. Because of the extremely high rate of discharge of the fibrillating atrium (500-600 cycles/min), impulses arriving in the AV junction present a disorganized wave front with insufficient potency to be consistently conducted to the ventricular specialized conduction system.

Although atrial fibrillation may be paroxysmal, it is often a chronic stable rhythm. The critical determinant of the clinical response to atrial fibrillation is the rapidity of the ventricular rate. The average ventricular response to atrial fibrillation among patients not receiving ß-blockers or digitalis drugs is 160 beats/min. More rapid ventricular responses are noted in certain clinical conditions. Thus, patients with thyrotoxicosis, preexcitation, or serious myocardial or valvular disease; patients receiving sympathomimetic agents, such as those used to treat chronic obstructive pulmonary disease; patients with alcoholic cardiomyopathy; and patients with certain electrolyte disorders, such as hypokalemia and hypomagnesemia, may exhibit a ventricular rate >160 beats/min (Fig. 2). Patients with an intrinsic AV junctional conduction abnormality may exhibit slower ventricular responses. Thus, the patient who is not receiving medication and presents with a ventricular response to atrial fibrillation between 60 and 100 beats/min should be considered to have an intrinsic AV junctional conduction disorder. Occasionally, athletes with extreme vagotonia may present with atrial fibrillation and a slow ventricular response.

MULTIFOCAL ATRIAL TACHYCARDIA

Multifocal atrial tachycardia is defined as a tachyarrhythmia in which the atrial rate is >100 beats/min (Fig. 7). There are well-organized discrete P waves of at least 3 separate morphologies, and there is an irregular variation in the P-P interval. An isoelectric baseline is noted between P waves. This tachycardia is associated with a high mortality rate, primarily due to its association with severe decompensated pulmonary disease, although MAT is often seen among patients receiving bronchodilators. The mechanism must be distinguished from that of other supraventricular rhythm disturbances. Although sinus tachycardia with multifocal APBs usually has a rate greater than 100 beats/min, it can be differentiated from MAT by the predominantly uniform P-P intervals and P-wave morphology except for isolated APBs. The most important differentiation is atrial fibrillation versus MAT. The indistinct morphology of atrial activity and undulating baseline of atrial fibrillation contrast with the discrete P waves and isoelectric baseline seen in MAT. Carotid sinus pressure may transiently decrease the rate of atrial activity in MAT, but this quickly returns to control levels after release of CSP. At times, patients with MAT also have atrial fibrillation, complicating a unified diagnosis of the dysrhythmia.[1]

THERAPY FOR CARDIAC ARRHYTHMIAS (TABLES 3 AND 4)

VENTRICULAR TACHYCARDIA

Ventricular tachycardia in the acute stage of myocardial infarction (MI) must be treated immediately. Clinical circumstances dictate the acute management. Patients whose condition is hemodynamically unstable during VT and who exhibit a change in mental status should be promptly cardioverted. If the patient loses consciousness, a precordial blow may be successful in reverting VT to sinus rhythm. The small amount of energy delivered by a precordial thump (1 watt-second) is frequently sufficient to depolarize enough myocardium and initiate a propagated response by electromechanical transduction. If VT degenerates to VF, the steep rise in energy requirement for termination of VF

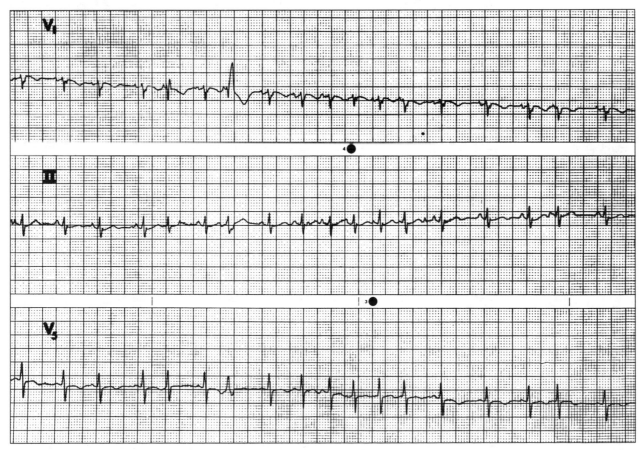

Figure 7. *Multifocal atrial tachycardia (MAT). Note variable rate and P-wave morphology.*

Table 3. Clinical Pharmacology of Antiarrhythmic Drugs

DRUG	INDICATIONS	EFFECT ON ECG	DOSE	ADVERSE EFFECTS	THERAPEUTIC PLASMA LEVELS
Bretylium	VT-VF		5 mg/kg IV; 5-10 mg/kg q6h	Hypotension; GI (Nausea, vomiting); possible aggravation of arrhythmia	
Disopyramide	VEA AEA	QRS, QT, PR prolongation	100-200 mg q6h	Anticholinergic effects; hypotension; heart failure; heart block; tachyarrhythmia	2-8 µg/ml
Lidocaine	VEA	± QT shortening	Loading: 200-300 mg given as 50-100 mg every 5 min with rebolus after 20-40 min prn. Maintenance: 2-4 mg/min	CNS (drowsiness, agitation, seizures); rarely CHF or heart block	1-5 µg/ml
Phenytoin	VEA	± QT shortening	100-300 mg IV given as 50 mg every 5 min (ineffective as oral agent)	CNS (ataxia, nystagmus, drowsiness); hypotension and heart block with rapid IV injection	5-20 µg/ml
Procainamide	VEA AEA	QRS, QT prolongation	500-1,000 mg q4-6h (po); 1 g IV load as 100 mg every 3-5 min Maintenance: 2-6 mg/min	Lupus-like syndrome; GI; insomnia; rash; hypotension; aggravation of arrhythmia; blood dyscrasias	3-8 µg/ml
Quinidine	VEA AEA	QRS, QT prolongation	200-600 mg q4-6 h (po) (average oral dose 300 mg q6h)	Aggravation of arrhythmias ("quinidine syncope"); Thrombocytopenia; fever; rash; cinchonism; GI symptoms; digoxin-quinidine interaction (elevation of digoxin levels)	2-7 µg/ml
β-adrenergic blockers	AEA VEA	PR prolonged	Propranolol (80-160 mg/day); atenolol (50-100 mg/day; nadolol (40-100 mg 1-2x/day); metoprolol (50-100 mg 2-3 x/day)	Cardiac (heart block, hypotension, heart failure); asthma; hypoglycemia; lethargy; impotence	
Verapamil	AEA	—	5-15 mg IV; 40-160 mg po q8h	CHF, asystole, constipation	

AEA=Atrial ectopic activity; CHF=Congestive heart failure; CNS=Central nervous system; GI=Gastrointestinal; VEA=Ventricular ectopic activity.

Table 4. Clinical Pharmacology of Newer Antiarrhythmic Drugs

DRUG	INDICATIONS	IV DOSE	ORAL DOSE	ADVERSE EFFECTS	COMMENTS
Mexiletine	VEA	Loading: 1200 mg/12 h Maintenance: 250-500 mg mg/12h	Loading: 400-600 mg Maintenance: 200-300 mg q8h	GI; neurologic	Lidocaine-like drug Local anesthetic; half-life, 8-14 h
Tocainide	VEA	Loading: 0.5-0.75 mg/kg/min for 15 min	Loading: 400-600mg Maintenance: 400-800 mg q8h	GI; neurologic	Lidocaine-like drug Half-life, 11 h in normals;14-16 h in patients with high-grade VEA
Amiodarone	AEA (especially in patients with WPW) VEA	IV loading: 300 mg Maintenance: 50 mg/h	Loading: 400-1,200 mg/day x 5 d Maintenance: 200-800 mg/day	Constipation; skin rash; may uncover hypo- or hyperthyroid-ism; nausea; headache; corneal deposits; pulmonary infiltrates	Very long half-life (20-40days). May increase digoxin level. May worsen existing cardiac conduction disturbances. May prolong Coumadin effect.
Sotalol	VT SVT AFib.	—	80-160 mg bid (gradual dose adjustments every 2-3 days)	Cardiac (CHF); bronchospasm	Proarrhythmia: Dose related and parallels QT prolongation
Flecainide	VT SVT WPW	—	100-200 mg bid	GI; CNS; cardiac (incessant VT)	+++Negative inotropism, QRS, PR prolongation
Propafenone	VT AF	—	150-300 mg tid	GI; CNS; cardiac	++ Negative inotropism

AEA=Atrial ectopic activity; VEA=Ventricular ectopic activity; VT=Ventricular tachycardia; SVT=Supraventricular tachycardia; WPW=Wolff-Parkinson-White; CNS=Central nervous system; GI=Gastrointestinal; AF=Atrial fibrillation.

renders chest thumping ineffective. The current recommendation is that chest thump be reserved for monitored patients only, the concern being that a thump delivered during the ventricular vulnerable period may result in VF. However, the risk of this event is less than 5%. Lidocaine is the drug of choice for complex forms of VPBs (repetitive, early cycle) and VPBs occurring during acute MI, and is the initial agent used for paroxysmal VT. Second-line agents include intravenous procainamide and bretylium.[2–4]

Therapy for torsades de pointes requires special mention. Ordinarily, traditional agents are ineffective for this arrhythmia, although lido-caine or phenytoin should certainly be tried. Prevention of torsades de pointes requires shortening of the refractory period. This can be accomplished either by isoproterenol infusion or pacing at rates sufficient to overdrive ectopic activity. Administration of magnesium sulfate has also been useful therapy. The inciting agent (i.e., quinidine) or contributing factors (hypokalemia, hypomagnesemia) should be eliminated.[5]

SUPRAVENTRICULAR TACHYCARDIA

Management of acute SVT is generally directed toward increasing vagal tone with methods such as CSM or the Valsalva maneuver, or evoking the dive reflex by applying ice water to the forehead. If the basis of the arrhythmia is a reentry circuit involving the AV junction, digitalis, ß-adrenergic blocking agents, or verapamil may be effective in restoring normal rhythm. Cardioversion is rarely necessary in PSVT.

Administration of either intravenous calcium-channel drug or adenosine will convert the majority of episodes of SVT. In a study by Hood and Smith comparing adenosine versus verapamil for the treatment of acute supraventricular tachycardia, adenosine converted 100% of the patients randomized to that agent, versus 73% for those receiving intravenous verapamil.[6] Adenosine interrupts reentrant circuits by direct action on the AV node. The advantage of the agent is that its half life is less than 10 seconds as it is rapidly eliminated by vascular endothelial cells and erythrocytes. It is administered by a rapid intravenous bolus of 6 mg, waiting 1 to 2 minutes, and then repeating with a 12 mg bolus which may be repeated after several minutes if the tachycardia has not reverted. The mean time for reversion with adenosine intravenously is 31 seconds. The drug is antagonized by methylxanthines, caffeine, and theophylline. Side effects are brief and include facial flushing, a sense of breathlessness or chest pressure, occasional lightheadedness, headache, nausea or dizziness. These side effects last but a few seconds.

Long-term management of patients with recurrent supraventricular tachycardia is dependent upon the patients' age, frequency of the event, duration of the episode and whether it is associated with significant hemodynamic compromise and resultant symptoms.

Over the past several years transcatheter ablation of cardiac tissue for the management of various types of arrhythmias has emerged as an effective and safe approach. The use or radiofrequency ablating is now associated with approximately a 95% success rate among patients who can be mapped and are inducible at the time of electrophysiologic study.[7] It has been our practice to offer antiarrhythmic therapy for patients with infrequent episodes that are not associated with significant symptoms, particularly if the dysrhythmia is occurring in an older patient. However, for younger patients, particularly those with pre-excitation syndromes (Wolf-Parkinson-White syndrome), radiofrequency ablation may be the "therapy of choice."

ATRIAL FLUTTER

Atrial flutter is more difficult to treat pharmacologically. Cardioversion is the treatment of choice. Rapid atrial pacing has also been used to revert flutter. Digitalis glycosides may reduce the ventricular response to atrial flutter, but the response is variable. At times, large doses of digoxin are necessary, presenting a risk of development of digitalis toxicity, including paroxysmal atrial tachycardia (PAT) with block. If the patient is receiving quinidine concomitantly, differentiation of atrial flutter with a slow flutter mechanism and PAT with block may be difficult. Diminutive atrial complexes in the inferior leads with an isoelectric baseline favors PAT with block. In about half of patients, digitalis converts the rhythm to atrial fibrillation, and in the remainder, sinus rhythm is restored after a brief period of atrial fibrillation. Verapamil rapidly slows the ventricular response while the patient is being readied for cardioversion. Once sinus rhythm is restored, maintenance with quinidine, procainamide, or disopyramide may decrease the risk of recurrence.

ATRIAL FIBRILLATION

Treatment of atrial fibrillation depends on whether the rhythm disturbance is a paroxysmal event in the absence of congestive heart failure, or whether it is a manifestation of decreased left ventricular function. In the former, membrane-stabilizing drugs (quinidine, disopyramide, or procainamide) or cardioversion are effective in reverting atrial fibrillation to sinus rhythm. In the latter, digitalis with other measures to improve left ventricular function restores sinus rhythm.

Management of the patient with paroxysmal (lone) atrial fibrillation may present a complex problem. Typically, the patient has no overt heart disease, normal left atrial size, and fine (~2 mm) fibrillatory waves on the ECG. Many such patients are sensitive to changes in vagal tone; if they are, digitalis may be profibrillatory because of the heterogeneity of cholinergic fibers within the atria. Quindine and disopyramide are useful agents for treating this condition. Procainamide is effective for short-term oral or IV use, but few patients can remain on chronic therapy for longer than 3 months. Several drugs approved for ventricular arrhyth-

Table 5. Comparison of 5 Randomized Trials of Warfarin for Atrial Fibrillation

	AFASAK	SPAF	BAATAF	CAFA	SPINAF
Mean age (yr)	74	67	68	68	67
Chronic (%)/ paroxysmal (%)	100/0	66/34	83/17	94/6	100/0
Aspirin (mg/day)	75	325	—	—	—
Aspirin effective	No	Yes<75yr No>75yr	—	—	—
Risk of major bleeding (%)	<1	1.5	<1	2.5	1.3
Warfarin therapeutic level (INR)	2.8-4.2	2.0-3.5	1.5-2.7	2.0-3.0	1.4-2.8
Warfarin effect on mortality	No	No	Yes	No	Yes
Reduction in risk of stroke (%)	60	67	86	44	79

AFASAK=Atrial Fibrillation, Aspirin, Anticoagulation; BAATAF=Boston Area Anticoagulation Trial for Atrial Fibrillation; CAFA=Canadian Atrial Fibrillation Anticoagulation Study; SPAF=Stroke Prevention in Atrial Fibrillation; SPINAF=Stroke Prevention in Nonrheumatic Atrial Fibrillation.[8-14] Reprinted from Cheng TO, et al.[11] With permission.

mia are also effective for atrial fibrillation, particularly amiodarone and propafenone.

Verapamil administered either orally or intravenously slows the response to both atrial fibrillation and flutter. Use of this agent for prevention of atrial fibrillation has not yielded impressive results. However, for the patient in whom atrial fibrillation is a fixed rhythm, verapamil may be helpful in maintaining rate control.

The most common cause of atrial fibrillation, particularly in the acute phase of MI, is elevated left ventricular filling pressure. Thus, slowing of the ventricular response is mandatory before sinus rhythm can be established and maintained. Cardioversion offers little advantage in the patient with decompensated cardiac function and atrial fibrillation. Once optimal ventricular function and control of the ventricular response is effected, electrical reversion may be undertaken if necessary. In our experience, oral quinidine or IV procainamide is helpful in stabilizing the atrium before cardioversion and will result in a 10% to 15% chance of pharmacologic reversion.

A number of recent studies have documented the benefit of anticoagulation with warfarin for patients with both recurrent and fixed atrial fibrillation (Table 5).[8-14] A review of the prospective anticoagulation trials suggests that there is a relative risk reduction in stroke of approximately 60% for the patients with nonvalvular atrial fibrillation placed on chronic warfarin therapy.[8,9] The optimal degree of anticoagulation is an international normalized ratio (INR) of approximately 2.0-3.0. We are no longer using the prothrombin time ratio, abandoned in favor of the INR because of the wide range of sensitivities of commercial thromboplastins. This may result in variability of the prothrombin ratios among patients at the same level of anticoagulation.[10]

MULTIFOCAL ATRIAL TACHYCARDIA

The treatment of MAT is primarily the treatment of the underlying pulmonary disease. Modification of bronchodilator therapy may also reduce the density of MAT. Some success has been reported with verapamil, which may reduce automaticity within the atrium.

"COCKTAIL" THERAPY FOR PAROXYSMAL ARRHYTHMIAS

If the patient's dysrhythmia occurs infrequently — once or twice yearly — and if the patient tolerates the arrhythmia, then the physician might use a therapeutic "cocktail" to revert the arrhythmia.[15] In these situations, the patient does not require chronic antiarrhythmic therapy. Use of a single agent or group of drugs only at the time of the cardiac arrhythmia is the treatment of choice. Thus, for the patient experiencing PSVT, use of verapamil or a ß-adrenergic blocking agent and mild sedatives may be effective in controlling infrequent episodes of tachycardia. Paroxysmal atrial fibrillation may be treated with a "cocktail" of quinidine, a ß-adrenergic blocking agent, and sedative. Atrial flutter usually does not respond to this approach.

PREEXCITATION SYNDROMES AND THERAPY

Preexcitation syndromes (PES) include ECG and clinical conditions resulting from accelerated transmission of impulses from atrium to ventricle via accessory tracts which bypass the normal physiologic delay in the AV junction. Electrocardiographic findings reflect the pathoanatomic tracts. Classic syndromes include Wolff-Parkinson-White (WPW) and Lown-Ganong-Levine (LGL) syndromes, although a number of variations may be encountered. In patients with WPW, a short or normal PR interval is inscribed; the "slurring" of the QRS is a result of fusion of early ventricular depolarization via the accessory Kent bundle and that which occurs over the normal His-Purkinje system. In LGL syndrome, the ECG hallmark is a short PR interval with normal QRS complex. Conceptually, an anomalous connection circumvents a portion of the AV junction. This tract, described by James, is believed to explain the short PR interval (<0.12 second) and normal QRS in the LGL syndrome.[16-18]

A rare form of preexcitation involves the fibers of Mahaim. Accessory pathways from either the lower AV junction or His bundle pass directly to the ventricular myocardium. Thus, the PR interval is normal because there is no bypass of the AV junction. The QRS complex exhibits a delta wave that is due to premature depolarization of the ventricle as in the WPW syndrome.

Preexcitation syndromes are common entities. Slightly more men are affected, and about two-thirds of patients have no associated evidence of organic heart disease. An array of congenital heart defects is associated with preexcitation syndromes, the most common of which is Ebstein's anomaly of the tricuspid valve.

Most patients with symptomatic preexcitation have SVT. The mechanism is a reciprocating, or reentrant, tachycardia. Usually there is antegrade conduction down the AV node with retrograde conduction from ventricle to atrium by the anomalous pathway. The QRS morphology is regular. In a small proportion of WPW patients, antegrade conduction down the anomalous pathway with retrograde conduction through the AV node or a second accessory pathway occurs. This results in a regular tachycardia, but with a wide and aberrant QRS complex. This tachyarrhythmia is clinically significant in the acute setting because of its ECG similarity to VT.

Atrial fibrillation, which may be seen more often in older WPW patients, can result in rapid depolarization of the ventricle, leading to VF and sudden death. Atrial flutter can be a significant problem when 1:1 conduction occurs over the accessory tract.

Therapy is guided by the clinical circumstances: the patient's symptoms, the rate of the tachyarrhythmia, and the nature of the atrial mechanism (fibrillation, flutter, or reciprocating tachycardia). In an emergency setting, when a patient presents with a bizarre, extremely rapid tachycardia (rates in excess of 250 beats/min), expedient treatment is mandatory.

Intravenous procainamide or lidocaine often block the accessory pathway, reducing the ventricular response and allowing for more definitive therapy. Cardioversion is the therapy of choice if the atrial mechanism is flutter or fibrillation. Quinidine and disopyramide also impede conduction through accessory pathways and are alternatives to IV lidocaine. Digitalis drugs, verapamil, and ß-adrenergic blocking agents are useful if the arrhythmia is a regular reciprocating tachycardia (rates 200 beats/min) with antegrade conduction through the His-Purkinje system. Digitalis drugs and verapamil are contraindicated if the tachyarrhythmia is atrial fibrillation, the concern being that digitalis or verapamil will shorten the refractory period of the accessory pathway in a few patients, promoting enhanced conduction with potential deterioration to ventricular fibrillation. One cannot predict by ECG analysis which patients are susceptible to this problem. It has been suggested that patients with an effective refractory period of the bypass tract of approximately 200 msec (corresponding to a ventricular rate of 300 beats/min) are at highest risk.

Beyond the acute management of patients with dysrhythmias in the setting of pre-excitation as mentioned, electrophysiologic study carried out to map accessory pathways followed by radio frequency ablation is an increasingly attractive option for patients with pre-excitation.

SICK SINUS SYNDROME AND THERAPY

Sick sinus syndrome is a heterogeneous entity, both in terms of definition and underlying pathophysiologic mechanisms. The term, coined by Lown in reference to the condition in patients after cardioversion who exhibited bradycardia, sinoatrial arrest, and escape junctional mechanisms, now refers to evidence of sinus node dysfunction producing clinical symptoms; it is also used to describe an asymptomatic patient who has evidence of failure of proper sinoatrial pacemaker function. In effect, sick sinus syndrome represents a generalized disorder of the conduction system of the heart, sinus node dysfunction being only one aspect. Evidence of sinus node dysfunction is observed in diverse populations of patients. The spectrum may range from extreme vagotonia and minor sclerodegenerative changes in the conduction system to bradycardia-tachycardia syndromes, in which the patient experiences ventricular or atrial tachyarrhythmias and becomes symptomatic during prolonged offset pauses.[19] Therapy must be individualized, and insertion of pacemakers should be confined to patients who experience documented symptomatic bradyarrhythmias. One should not assume apriori that patients with asymptomatic offset pauses of as long as 3 seconds after a bout of tachyarrhythmia require permanent pacing. Antiarrhythmic drugs that suppress the tachyarrhythmia may eliminate offset pauses and may not provoke sinoatrial or AV conduction problems in and of themselves. Patients should undergo careful monitoring to establish their response to antiarrhythmic therapy.

CARDIOVERSION AND DEFIBRILLATION

Use of electrical energy for reverting cardiac tachyarrhythmias has become standard practice in the last 25 years because of its safety and reliability. The term *defibrillation* generally applies to depolarization during VF of the entire heart, or a major portion of it, by an unsynchronized electrical discharge. The ensuing cardiac asystole is then terminated by emergence of the cardiac pacemaker with the highest automaticity (usually the sinoatrial node).

Cardioversion is the use of electrical energy to revert specific cardiac arrhythmias. It differs from defibrillation in that the electrical discharge is synchronized with the R wave to avoid triggering VF by accidental discharge during the vulnerable period of the ventricle. The vulnerable period is a span of approximately 30 msec just before inscription of the apex of the T wave on the surface ECG, but may be considerably longer under conditions of ischemia. Discharge of a low-intensity shock will produce VF only when delivered during a vulnerable period. For the sake of simplicity, the R wave has been selected for triggering the electrical discharge. The physiologic basis for cardioversion is that an electrical discharge depolarizes a part of the reentrant pathway that is nonrefractory and interrupts the circus movement.[2,20]

METHOD OF DEFIBRILLATION

Almost all cardiac arrests are a result of VF. Defibrillation constitutes definitive treatment for this condition, and success is assured only if prompt defibrillation is accomplished. Initial defibrillation of adults should be conducted with a setting between 100-300 watt-seconds. There is no evidence that energies in excess of 400 watt-seconds are needed in humans for defibrillation, provided proper technique is used. Higher energies may result in prolonged periods of asystole or complete heart block, resulting in resumption of VF.

Paddle position for defibrillation and cardioversion is the same. Both anteroposterior and anterolateral electrode positions are used. The anterior electrode is held firmly along the right sternal border at the level of the second and third intercostal spaces while the posterior electrode is placed at the angle of the left scapula. If a lateral paddle is used, it should be placed between the apex and anterior axillary line. The electrodes must be completely covered with conductive gel, particularly along the edges, to reduce the likelihood of skin burns.

METHOD OF CARDIOVERSION

Cardioversion may be done under both elective and nonelective circumstances. The conscious patient with VT who is hemodynamically compromised should be promptly cardioverted after receiving small amounts of IV diazepam or short-acting barbiturates. Alternatively, the patient with atrial fibrillation who is to be electively cardioverted should have the procedure fully explained to allay as much anxiety as possible. Digitalis drugs need not be withheld. Serum levels of digoxin and electrolytes should be determined before the procedure; and, if the patient has had anticoagulation therapy, a recent prothrombin time determination is necessary. Cardioversion may be done at the patient's bedside or in a room equipped for cardiopulmonary resuscitation. There should be a minimum of personnel and activity. A short-acting barbiturate should be administered 1-2 hours before the procedure. This sedation reduces the amount of diazepam given subsequently. At the time of cardioversion, an initial IV dose of 5 mg of diazepam is administered, followed by 2.5-mg increments every 2-3 minutes. Both blood pressure and respiratory rates are monitored before each dose. An average of 15 mg of diazepam is required to achieve adequate sedation, although the range is variable.

The main danger in transthoracic electric discharge is provocation of VF. The current generation of cardioverters incorporates a display that indicates the portion of the QRS to which the circuit is synchronized. The lead that displays the highest R-wave amplitude should be selected for discharge synchronization. Improper synchronization may result when the ECG signal contains artifactual spikes, when there are extremely prominent T waves, and in bundle branch block when the R' wave is taller than the R wave. The energy levels required to terminate specific arrhythmias are listed in Table 6. During elective cardioversion, energy titration should be used. Low energies may

disclose rhythm disturbances in patients with subclinical digitalis toxicity or electrolyte disturbance, and they also reduce myocardial damage.

INDICATIONS FOR PACEMAKER INSERTION

Table 7 lists indications for temporary and permanent pacemaker implantation. During acute MI, indications for temporary pacing are the occurrence of complete heart block or advanced AV block in the setting of anterior wall MI. Progressive first- and second-degree AV block in the setting of acute bundle branch block is another indication for temporary pacing. Controversy remains as to the absolute need for pacing in the patient with acute bundle branch block and no evidence of AV conduction disorder whose condition is otherwise stable.[21-23]

A permanent pacemaker should be placed only in patients with symptomatic bradyarrhythmia, brady-tachy syndromes, and evidence of Stokes-Adams syncope. Use of pacemaker technology for management of recurrent atrial and ventricular tachyarrhythmias is reserved for only a minority of patients with drug-refractory tachycardia.

Because of the rapidly increasing complexity of types of pacemakers, a code for pacemaker identification[24] was developed to describe essential features of each type. The code consists of 5 letters. The first letter represents the chamber (or chambers) paced (A, atrium; V, ventricle; D, double chamber); the second letter represents the chamber(s) sensed (A, V, D, or 0 [none]); the third letter represents the mode of response (I, inhibited; T, triggered; D, double [atrial triggered and ventricular inhibited]; O, not applicable). The fourth and fifth letters indicate more sophisticated pacing features, such as programmability or special tachyarrhythmia functions. The bulk of current pacemaker therapy involves the standard ventricular demand pacemaker. The first 3 letters of the code used to describe this type of device are VVI (ventricular pace, ventricular sensed, and inhibited by natural electrical activity in the ventricular chamber).

In some patients, if there is no competing atrial rhythm, synchronization of atrial and ventricular contraction may improve cardiac performance. Devices capable of this can sense or pace the atrium, and then perform sequential ventricular pacing (VAT, DVI, DDD). If AV conduction is intact, atrial demand pacing may be used (AAI).

Table 6. Average Energy Level Required for Cardioversion

RHYTHM	ENERGY (WATT-SEC)
VT	10
Atrial flutter	20
Atrial fibrillation	100
SVT	150

SVT=Supraventricular tachycardia; VT=Ventricular tachycardia.

Table 7. Indications for Pacing

Temporary
Occurrence of the following events during an acute myocardial infarction:
  Complete heart block
  Mobitz II atrioventricular block (anterior wall infarct)
  Atrioventricular block and acute bifascicular block
  Overdrive suppression of ventricular arrhythmia
Permanent
  Complete heart block
  Bradycardia-tachycardia syndrome
  Symptomatic bradyarrhythmia
  Proven efficacy of overdrive suppression

STRATEGIES IN THE APPROACH TO SUDDEN CARDIAC DEATH AND INDICATIONS FOR TREATMENT OF VENTRICULAR ARRHYTHMIA

Sudden death from heart disease is the leading cause of death in developed countries. In the past 2 decades, many advances have been made in the management of the patient with malignant ventricular arrhythmia, as well as in the use of antiarrhythmic drugs for long-term survival.[25] The concept of antiarrhythmic drug aggravation of arrhythmia is now accepted, and accordingly, indications for therapy have been modified.[26-28]

PROARRHYTHMIA

In addition to the syndrome of torsade de pointes, substantial data underscore the observation that every antiarrhythmic drug has the potential to aggravate the arrhythmia we hope to suppress. This concept of proarrhythmia is manifest either by a significant increase in the density of single ectopic beats; emergence of nonsustained VT when the clinical arrhythmia had only been VPBs; conversion of nonsustained VT to sustained VT; or provocation of cardiac arrest in a patient who had not experienced that event. Proarrhythmia is more likely to occur in the setting of left ventricular dysfunction and if the clinical arrhythmia is either noninfarction VF or sustained VT. As with provocation of torsade de pointes, concomitant diuretic and digitalis therapy enhances the risk of proarrhythmia.

INDICATIONS FOR TREATMENT OF VENTRICULAR ECTOPIC ACTIVITY

The recognition of proarrhythmia as a real entity has reduced the enthusiasm for initiating chronic antiarrhythmic therapy. Although VPBs are associated with an enhanced risk for sudden cardiac death, this finding lacks specificity. The finding of advanced forms of ectopic activity in an asymptomatic, otherwise healthy person is cause for neither alarm nor treatment. Table 8 details indications for treatment of VPBs. Only a few persons with VPBs require chronic antiarrhythmic therapy. For patients who have so-called malignant ventricular arrhythmia, i.e., noninfarction VF or sustained VT, there is no debate as to the need for aggressive therapy. Except for patients who have unusual cardiac conditions such as hypertrophic obstructive cardiomyopathy, hereditary long QT syndrome, or nonsustained VT categorically correlated with symptoms, antiarrhythmic therapy is not associated with an improved survival rate. The Cardiac Arrhythmia Suppression Trial (CAST) showed a 2.5-fold higher incidence of cardiac death or nonfatal cardiac arrest among patients

Table 8. Indications for the Chronic Treatment of Ventricular Arrhythmias

Primary (noninfarction-related) VF
Sustained symptomatic VT
Mitral valve prolapse in patient with family history of sudden cardiac death and with paroxysms of symptomatic VT
Long QT syndrome with syncope or family history of sudden death
Obstructive cardiomyopathies, particularly with a family history of sudden death
Symptomatic VPBs

VF=Ventricular fibrillation; VPBs=Ventricular premature beats; VT=Ventricular tachycardia.

receiving one of the IC drugs (encainide or flecainide), underscoring the concern as to the appropriate use of these agents.[29,30]

For patients with malignant ventricular arrhythmia, defined as noninfarction-related VF or hemodynamically compromising VT, a systematic approach using electrophysiologic study or noninvasive assessment to antiarrhythmic drug testing and therapy is mandatory because of the risk of recurrence and high annual mortality rate among such patients. Many of these patients can be successfully treated with a combination of antiarrhythmic drugs, significantly improving long-term survival.[25,31]

The past 2 decades have seen tremendous advances in the technology available for terminating sustained ventricular tachycardia and reversion of ventricular fibrillation. While Amiodarone continues to represent a significant option for many patients with malignant arrhythmia,[25,31] increasingly, patients are undergoing electrophysiologic study as to suitabllity for an implantable cardioverter-defibrillator. The ability to implant non-thoracotomy lead systems is associated with a significant reduction in operative mortality. Patients with sustained ventricular tachycardia may undergo burst pacing, cardioversion, or defibrillation with these newer devices. The new generation of devices allows for a tiered therapy in which the device "determines" the appropriate method for tachycardia termination.[32–34]

As is the situation with supraventricular reentrant tachycardia, patients with intact ventricular function who have right ventricular outflow tachycardia may be suitable for mapping and ablation procedures.

REFERENCES

1. Shine KI, Kastor JA, Yurchak PM. Multifocal atrial tachycardia: Clinical and electrocardiographic features. *N Engl J Med.* 1968;179:344.
2. Lown B. Electrical reversion of cardiac arrhythmias. *Br Heart J.* 1967;29:469-489.
3. Lown B, Podrid PJ, DeSilva RA, et al. *Sudden Cardiac Death: Management of the Patient at Risk.* Chicago: Year Book Medical Publishers; 1980;4-62.
4. Lown B, Graboys TB. Ventricular premature beats and sudden cardiac death. In: McIntosh H (ed). *Baylor Cardiology Series.* 1980;3:1-24.
5. Fisch C. Relation of electrolyte disturbances to cardiac arrhythmias. *Circulation.* 1973;47:408-420.
6. Hood MA, Smith WM. Adenosine versus verapamil in the treatment of supraventricular tachycardia. A randomized double crossover trial. *Am Heart J.* 1962;123:1543-1549.
7. Kay GN, Epstein AE, Dailey SM, et al. Selective radiofrequency ablation of the slow pathway for the treatment of atrial ventricular nodal reentrant tachycardia. Evidence for involvement of perinodal myocardium within the reentrant circuit. *Circulation.* 1992;85: 1675-1688.
8. Boston Area Anticoagulation Trial for Atrial Fibrillation (BAATAF) Investigators. The effect of low-dose warfarin on the risk of stroke in patients with non-rheumatic atrial fibrillation. *N Engl J Med.* 1990;323:1505-1511.
9. Stroke Prevention in Atrial Fibrillation (SPAF) Investigators. Stroke prevention in atrial fibrillation. Final Results. *Circulation.* 1991;84:527-539.
10. Hirsch J, Potter L, Deykin D, et al. Optimal therapeutic range for oral anticoagulants. *Chest.* 1989;95:5S-11S.
11. Cheng TO. Atrial fibrillation, stroke, and antithrombotic treatment. *Am Heart J.* 1994;127:961-968.
12. Petersen P, Boysen G, Godtfredsen J, et al. Placebo-controlled, randomized trial of warfarin and aspirin for prevention of thromboembolic complications in chronic atrial fibrillation: the Copenhagen AFASAK Study. *Lancet.* 1989;I:175-179.
13. Connolly SJ, Laupacis A, Gent M, et al. Canadian Atrial Fibrillation Anticoagulation (CAFA) Study. *J Am Coll Cardiol.* 1991;18:349-355.
14. Ezekowitz MD, Bridgers SL, James KE, et al. Warfarin in the prevention of stroke associated with nonrheumatic atrial fibrillation. *N Engl J Med.* 1992;327:1406-1412.
15. Margolis B, DeSilva RA, Lown B. Episodic drug treatment in the management of paroxysmal arrhythmias. *Am J Cardiol.* 1980;45:621-626.
16. Lown B, Ganong WF, Levine SA. The syndrome of short RR interval, normal QRS complexes and paroxysmal rapid heart action. *Circulation.* 1952;5:693-698.
17. Rigby WFC, Graboys TB. Current concepts and management of the preexcitation syndromes. *J Cardiovasc Med.* 1981;6:277-293.
18. Wolff L, Parkinson J, White PD. Bundle branch block with short PR interval in healthy young people prone to paroxysmal tachycardia. *Am Heart J.* 1930;5:685-691.
19. Moss AF, Davis RJ. Brady-tachy syndrome. *Prog Cardiovasc Dis.* 1974;16:439-458.
20. DeSilva RA, Graboys TB, Podrid PJ, et al. Cardioversion and defibrillation. *Am Heart J.* 1980;100:881-885.
21. Goodman MJ, Lassers BW, Julian DG. Complete bundle branch block complicating acute myocardial infarction. *N Engl J Med.* 1970;282:237.
22. Hindman MC Wagner GS, Jaro M, et al. The clinical significance of bundle branch block complicating acute myocardial infarction. *Circulation.* 1978;58:689-699.
23. McAnulty JH, Rahimtoola S, Murphy ES. A prospective study of sudden death in "high risk" bundle branch block. *N Engl J Med.* 1978;299:209-216.
24. Parsonnet V, Furman S, Smyth NPD. A revised code for pacemaker identification. *PACE.* 1981;4:400-408.

25. Graboys TB, Lown B, Podrid PJ, et al. Long term survival in patients with malignant ventricular arrhythmia treated with antiarrhythmic drugs. *Am J Cardiol.* 1982;50:437-443.
26. Velebit V, Podrid PJ, Lown B, et al. Aggravation and provocation of ventricular arrhythmias by antiarrhythmic drugs. *Circulation.* 1982;65:886-894.
27. Minardo JD, Heger JJ, Miles WM, et al. Clinical characteristics of patients with ventricular fibrillation during antiarrhythmic drug therapy. *N Engl J Med.* 1988;319:257.
28. Podrid P, Lampert S, Graboys TB, et al. Aggravation of arrhythmias by antiarrhythmic drugs-incidence and predictors of occurrence. *Am J Cardiol.* 1987;59:38E-44E.
29. Cardiac Arrhythmia Suppression Trial (CAST) Investigators. Preliminary report: Effect of encainide and flecainide on mortality in a randomized trial of arrhythmia suppression after myocardial infarction. *N Engl J Med.* 1989;321:406-411.
30. Ravid S, Graboys TB. Undesirable cardiovascular antiarrhythmic drug effects: Incidence, mechanisms and practical considerations. In: Fisch C, Surawicz B (eds). *Advances in Cardiac Electrophysiology and Arrhythmias.* New York: Elsevier; 1991:314-322.
31. Pfisterer M, Kiowski W, Burckhardt D, et al. Beneficial effects of amiodarone on cardiac mortality in patients with asymptomatic complex ventricular arrhythmias after acute myocardial infarction and preserved but not impaired left ventricular function. *Am J Cardiol.* 1992;69:1399-1402.
32. Rosenthal ME, Josephson ME. Current status of antitachycardia devices. *Circulation.* 1990;82:1889-1899.
33. ACC/AHA Task Force Report. Guidelines for Implantation of Cardiac Pacemakers and Antiarrhythmia Devices. *J Am Coll Cardiol.* 1991; 18:1-13.
34. Manolis AS. Transvenous endocardial cardioverter defibrillator systems. Is the future here? *Arch Intern Med.* 1994;154:617-622.

22 Atrioventricular Conduction Disorders

Dusan Z. Kocovic, MD
Peter L. Friedman, MD, PhD

PHYSIOLOGY OF ATRIOVENTRICULAR CONDUCTION

In normal hearts the cardiac impulse is initiated in the pacemaker or P cells of the sinoatrial node, situated in the high lateral right atrium near the orifice of the superior vena cava. Depolarization spreads from this region through the right atrium, probably over discrete anatomic pathways, eventually reaching the atrioventricular (A-V) node. Transmembrane action potentials recorded from A-V nodal cells are characterized by a relatively low level of resting membrane potential of approximately -60 mV and a very slow rate of rise of phase 0. Such action potentials, know as "slow responses," are generated by an inward slow current, Isi, which is believed to be carried predominately by Ca^{2+} ions. The membrane channels through which Isi flows open and close slowly as compared to the channel through which the fast inward Na^+ current flows. They also remain inactivated for a time even after the cell has repolarized to its full maximum diastolic potential, thereby giving A-V nodal cells the property of time-dependent as well as voltage-dependent refractoriness.[1-3] Because of all these features of A-V nodal action potentials, conduction velocity through the A-V node is quite slow and decremental. This slow decremental conduction is further contributed to by the fact that the A-V node is composed of relatively small fibers that are sparsely distributed and interconnected in a complex network. This anatomic arrangement favors fragmentation of wave fronts of depolarization, predisposing to conduction block.

After traversing the A-V node, the impulse then travels over the bundle of His. The His bundle in the normal human heart originates near the central fibrous body at a point where fibers from the distal end of the A-V node coalesce into large, longitudinally oriented Purkinje fibers. Anatomically, it forms a discrete bundle that usually courses down the left side of the membranous interventricular septum to the crest of the muscular septum, where it bifurcates into the right and left bundle branches. The right bundle branch is itself a discrete bundle that continues down the right side of the muscular septum to the right ventricular apex, at which point it arborizes into the septal and right ventricular free wall myocardium. In contrast, the left bundle branch fans out broadly over the left septal surface shortly after its origin. The left bundle branch functions electrophysiologically as though it were composed of 2 separate divisions, the anterior and posterior fascicles. This is based on commonly observed electrocardiographic patterns of left ventricular conduction defects (see below). Unlike A-V nodal cells, Purkinje fibers in the His bundles and bundle branches are large cable-like cells with resting membrane potentials that normally exceed -90 mV and with action potentials that are characterized by a rapid phase 0, carried largely by Na^+ ions. Because of these characteristics, conduction velocity in the His-Purkinje system is quite rapid.

The P-R interval in the surface electrocardiogram (ECG) represents the total time required for transmission of the cardiac impulse from its point of origin in the sinus node to the ventricular myocardium. This interval is the sum of conduction times over each different segment of the A-V conducting system; namely, conduction time between the sinus and A-V nodes, conduction time through the A-V node itself, and conduction time from the His bundle to ventricular myocardium. Although specific information about conduction over each of these segments is not apparent from the surface

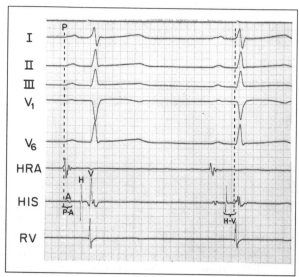

Figure 1. *Simultaneous recordings of surface electrocardiographic leads I, II, III, V₁ and V₆ along with bipolar intracardiac electrograms from the high right atrium (HRA), His bundle region (HIS), and right ventricular apex (RV). One-second time lines are shown in top trace. See text for discussion.*

ECG, it is available from simultaneous recordings of the surface ECG and a His bundle electrogram.

The interval between the onset of a normal sinus P wave in the surface ECG and depolarization of the right atrial myocardium (A in the His bundle electrogram) represents intra-atrial conduction time from the sinus node to the A-V node (Fig. 1). This time is referred to as the PA interval, normally requiring between 10 and 55 msec, and is determined by conduction velocity over the specialized internodal tracts and through atrial myocardium. Because intra-atrial conduction normally is quite rapid, the PA interval accounts for only a small part of the PR interval. Most of the normal delay during A-V transition occurs within the A-V node, where cells generate slowly rising low amplitude action potentials, and conduction velocity is accordingly slow. Atrioventricular nodal conduction time, therefore, accounts for the majority of the PR interval. Since the atrial deflection recorded by a His bundle electrode catheter represents depolarization of atrial muscle near the cranial border of the A-V node, the AH interval provides an accurate measure of A-V nodal conduction time (Fig. 1). A-V nodal

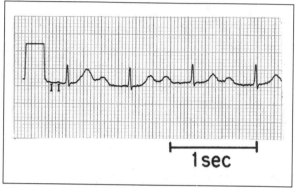

Figure 2. *Marked first-degree atrioventricular (A-V) block. The normal QRS suggests that the site of block is in the A-V node.*

conduction times in normal persons span a wide range, usually between 50 and 140 msec, due largely to variations in sympathetic and parasympathetic tone within the richly innervated A-V node. The terminal portion of the PR in the surface ECG represents conduction through all segments of the A-V conduction system distal to the A-V node. This includes conduction over the His bundle, down to right and left bundle branches and through the subendocardial ramifications of the Purkinje network to ventricular myocardium. Total conduction time in this subnodal portion of the A-V conduction system is reflected in the HV interval, measured from the H spike in the His bundle electrogram to the earliest point of ventricular depolarization in any intracardiac or surface lead (Fig. 1). Since conduction velocity in the His-Purkinje system is so rapid, the HV interval is normally quite short, ranging between 35 and 55 msec.

ELECTROCARDIOGRAPHIC MANIFESTATIONS OF ABNORMAL ATRIOVENTRICULAR CONDUCTION

ATRIOVENTRICULAR BLOCK

Atrioventricular block, simply defined, is the delay in transmission of the cardiac impulse from atrium to ventricle or the actual failure of transmission of 1 or more such impulses. Traditionally, A-V block is divided into 3 categories, based on electrocardiographic characteristics of the block. First-degree A-V

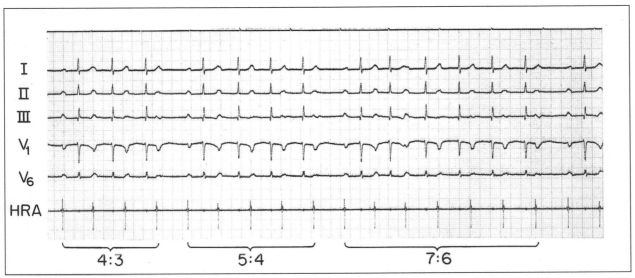

Figure 3. *Multiple surface electrocardiographic leads recorded simultaneously with a high right atrial electrogram (HRA) during type I second-degree atrioventricular block. The HRA electrograms are coincident with regularly occurring P waves. During the cycle labeled "5:4," there is typical Wenckebach periodicity, the RR intervals progressively decreasing with a progressively increasing PR interval. The cycle labeled "7:6" is atypical.*

block refers to simple delay of the A-V transmission. Second-degree block refers to actual failure of 1 or more P waves but not all P waves to be conducted. Third-degree A-V block is complete absence of A-V conduction.

The ECG manifestations of first-degree A-V nodal block are a 1:1 relationship between P waves and QRS complexes but with a PR interval of greater than .20 seconds (Fig. 2). The magnitude of PR prolongation seen in different patients spans a wide range; although A-V conduction can occur with a PR interval of 1.0 seconds or greater, it is much more common to see PR interval prolongation in the range of 0.2 to 0.6 seconds. Even in the same patient the PR interval may vary over a wide range, depending on the interplay among such factors as heart rate, autonomic tone, drug levels, and metabolic state.

The cardinal ECG manifestation of second-degree A-V block is the failure of some but not all P waves to be conducted to the ventricles. Three stereotypical patterns of second-degree A-V block are recognized. Type I second-degree A-V block is characterized by Wenckebach periodicity, in which the PR interval gradually prolongs until a P wave fails to conduct to the ventricles. After the blocked P wave conduction then resumes, the PR interval of this next

conducted beat is the shortest during the Wenckebach cycle (Fig. 3). In its "typical" form the largest increment in PR interval occurs between the first and second beat of the Wenckebach cycle (Fig. 3). Although the PR interval continues to lengthen during subsequent beats, it does so by progressively smaller increments. Thus, during such "typical Wenckebach" cycles the RR intervals actually decrease progressively, even though the PR intervals are progressively increasing. The term "typical Wenckebach periodicity" is actually a misnomer, since it is seen in fewer than 50% of cases showing Wenckebach periodicity. Changing sinus rates, as would occur with sinus arrhythmia, and moment-to-moment fluctuations of autonomic tone are probably the most common factors that upset "typical" Wenckebach periodicity. Thus, it is quite common to observe RR intervals that do not decrease progressively or PR intervals that may actually stabilize or shorten for several beats during the Wenckebach cycle (Fig. 3).

Type II second-degree A-V block is characterized by sudden failure of 1 or several consecutive P waves to conduct to the ventricles without progressive lengthening of the PR interval prior to the blocked P wave (Figs. 4, 5). In some patients apparent type II second-

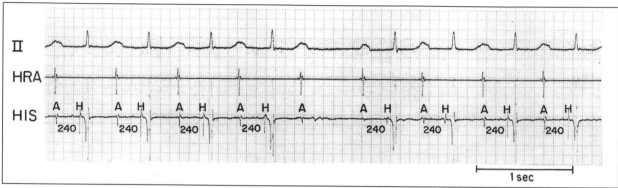

Figure 4. *Surface electrocardiographic (ECG) lead II recorded simultaneously with high right atrial (HRA) and His bundle (HIS) bipolar electrograms. The ECG shows type II second-degree atrioventricular (A-V) block. The fifth P wave fails to conduct through the A-V node despite constant PR and AH intervals before and after the blocked P wave. This may reflect momentary increase in vagal tone.*

degree block may actually be the same electrophysiologic phenomenon as type I block, but with increments in the PR interval too small (i.e., <50 msec) to be detected at the usual ECG recording paper speed of 25 mm/sec. Another explanation for apparent type II A-V nodal block is the sporadic occurrence of concealed junctional extrasystoles.[4] The third ECG pattern of second-degree A-V block is characterized by a fixed ratio of P waves to QRS complexes, e.g., 2:1, 3:1, 4:1, etc. This type of block cannot be classified as type I or type II and instead is usually referred to as "advanced" or "high-grade" second-degree block.

Third-degree, or complete, A-V block is the total absence of conduction between atria and ventricles. In the presence of sinus rhythm or some other organized atrial rhythm, such as atrial tachycardia, there is A-V dissociation, the ventricular rate being slower than the atrial rate and being governed by a subsidiary sub-A-V nodal pacemaker (Fig. 6). Complete A-V block in the presence of atrial fibrillation may be easily overlooked with only casual inspection of the ECG. A regular ventricular rate in the presence of atrial fibrillation should heighten one's suspicion of complete A-V block.

Atrioventricular block can result from delay or blockade of impulse transmission between the sinoatrial and A-V nodes, i.e., intra-atrial block. It can be the result of delay or blockade of impulse transmission within the A-V node

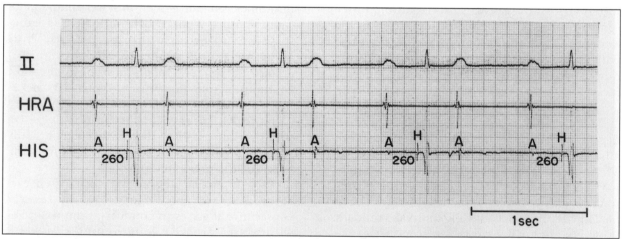

Figure 5. *Two to one (2:1) atrioventricular (A-V) nodal block. Note absence of His depolarization following the blocked P waves. This localizes the site of block to the A-V node.*

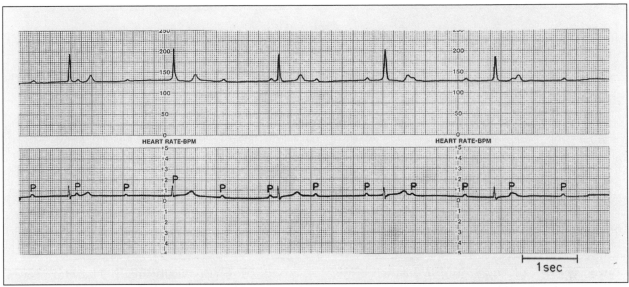

Figure 6. *Complete atrioventricular block. The P waves and QRS complexes are dissociated with regular RR intervals that are slower than the PP intervals. Note that PP intervals that span a QRS complex (sixth and seventh P waves, eighth and ninth P waves) are shorter than other PP intervals (fifth and sixth P waves). This is referred to as ventriculo-phasic sinus arrhythmia.*

itself, i.e., A-V nodal block. Alternatively, it can be the result of delay or blockade of impulse transmission in the distal conducting system, i.e., intra-His or infra-His block. Certain patterns of A-V block more commonly reflect impaired conduction in 1 particular segment of the A-V conducting system as compared to others. For example, type I second-degree A-V block with a normal QRS complex is almost always due to A-V nodal block. In contrast, the site of block in an individual with complete A-V block and a wide QRS is usually within or below the His bundle. However, sufficient overlap occurs so that it often is not possible to determine with certainty which part of the conduction system is responsible for A-V block based on the ECG pattern of block alone.

INTRAVENTRICULAR CONDUCTION DEFECTS

When conduction delay or block occurs in the anterior fascicle of the left bundle branch, the result is delayed activation of the upper anterior wall of the left ventricle. This pattern of intraventricular conduction is referred to as left anterior hemiblock. The electrocardiographic hallmarks of left anterior hemiblock include a QRS axis in the frontal plane equal to or more

negative than -45°, small initial R waves in the inferior leads, and then large S waves inferiorly, with dominant R waves in leads I and aVL. Conduction delay or block in the posterior fascicle of the left bundle branch results in a different electrocardiographic pattern, referred to as left posterior hemiblock. The salient electrocardiographic features of left posterior hemiblock include a QRS axis in the frontal plane greater than or equal to +110°, a small initial R wave in lead I, small inferior Q waves, and an initial R wave in lead V_1. This electrocardiographic diagnosis, however, can be made only in the absence of clinical evidence for right ventricular hypertrophy or pulmonary disease. Left posterior hemiblock is less common than left anterior hemiblock, in all likelihood because the posterior fascicle usually has a dual blood supply from both the left anterior descending and posterior descending coronary arteries. The ECG characteristics of complete left bundle branch block (LBBB) include QRS interval prolongation to 120 msec or longer; delayed intrinsic deflection in lead V_6; absent Q waves and slurred broad R waves in leads I, aVL, and V_6; Rs or QS deflection in leads V_1 and V_2; and an ST- and T-wave vector 180° discordant to the QRS vector. The ECG

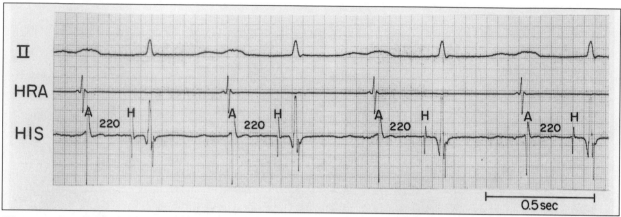

Figure 7. *Same organization of tracings as in Figure 4. The prolonged PR interval is due to prolongation of the AH interval. This localizes the site of atrioventricular (A-V) conduction delay to the A-V node.*

characteristics of right bundle branch block (RBBB) are QRS interval prolongation to 120 msec or longer with normal activation during the first half (60 msec) of the QRS complex, delayed intrinsic deflection in lead V_1, and abnormal anterior and rightward forces during the terminal portion of the QRS complex.

CLINICAL ELECTROPHYSIOLOGY OF ATRIOVENTRICULAR BLOCK

In patients with manifest ECG evidence of A-V block the site of block can be localized with certainty during electrophysiologic study. First-degree A-V block occurring in the A-V node, for example, is characterized by a prolonged AH interval, whereas first-degree A-V block occurring below the A-V node is characterized by a prolonged HV interval (Figs. 7, 8). Individuals with type I second-degree A-V nodal block typically have progressive lengthening of the AH interval with eventual block between the atrial and His deflections in the His bundle recording lead. During type II or high degree second-degree A-V nodal block, the blocked P waves fail to conduct through the A-V node, whereas conducted P waves have a normal or prolonged AH interval that is constant. Third-degree, or complete, A-V nodal block would appear as AH dissociation.

Prolonged intra-His conduction is present if the total duration of the His bundle deflection is more than 30 msec. In contrast to A-V nodal conduction, the range of values of intra-His

conduction is typically small. Therefore, even marked delays of intra-His conduction are not usually reflected by prolongation of the PR interval on the surface ECG. A rare expression of intra-His conduction delay is the recording of distinct proximal and distal His bundle deflections, referred to as a "split-His" potential. Second-degree A-V block (typically type II) or complete A-V block rarely can be due to intra-His block occurring between the proximal and

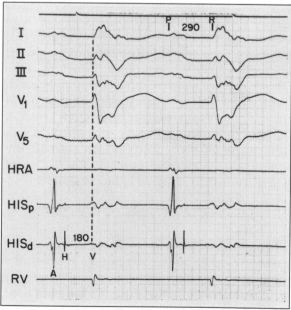

Figure 8. *Same organization of tracings as in Figure 1. Two His bundle recording sites are shown: HIS_p = proximal His; HIS_d = distal His. The prolonged PR interval is due to prolongation of the HV interval.*

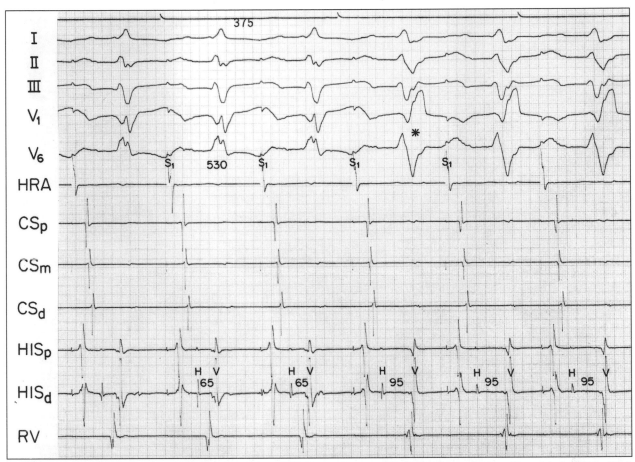

Figure 9. *Multiple surface electrocardiographic (ECG) leads recorded simultaneously with a high right atrial electrogram (HRA), proximal, mid- and distal coronary sinus electrograms (CS_p, CS_m, and CS_d, respectively), proximal and distal His bundle electrograms (HIS_p and HIS_d) and a right ventricular electrogram (RV) during atrial pacing at a CL of 530 msec. Initially, the HV interval is only slightly prolonged (65 msec), associated with an incomplete left bundle branch block pattern in the surface ECG leads. The HV interval then prolongs to 95 msec, associated with the appearance of right bundle branch block (*).*

distal deflections of the "split-His" potential. Usually, however, first-, second-, or third-degree A-V block due to abnormal His-Purkinje conduction is caused by delay or block of impulses between the His bundle and ventricular muscle, i.e., infra-His block. The degree of infra-His delay can be variable, typically ranging from 60–100 msec, although an HV interval of 345 msec has been reported.[5] Such marked delay is very uncommon, probably because it progresses quickly to higher degrees of block. Second-degree block with type I or type II characteristics can result from abnormal infra-His conduction. In type I second-degree infra-His block, a gradual prolongation of the HV intervals occurs until a His deflection is not followed by ventricular depolarization. Type II second-degree infra-His block occurs in the absence of HV prolongation, and it is typically sudden and unexpected. Third-degree infra-His block is the most common cause of chronic complete heart block in adults over 30 years old. It accounts for approximately 60% of patients with complete heart block and is characterized by AH association plus HV dissociation with an underlying idioventricular rhythm. Of interest, retrograde ventriculo-atrial conduction may still be present in 20% of these patients.[6]

Electrophysiologic studies can be useful for demonstrating latent A-V conduction distur-

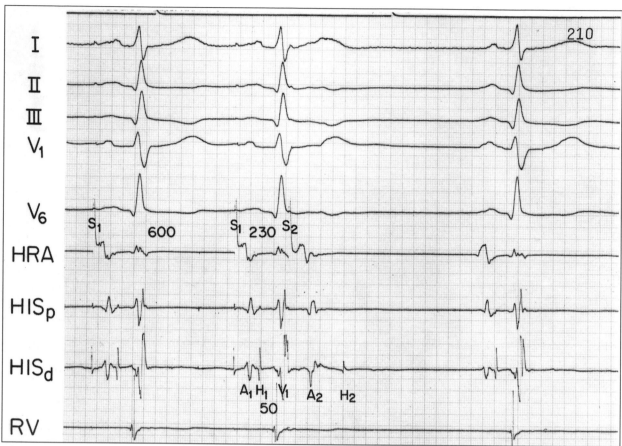

Figure 10. *Same organization of tracings as in Figure 8. A single atrial premature stimulus (S₂) is delivered during fixed-rate atrial pacing at a cycle length of 600. The HV interval during the basic drive (H_1V_1) is normal. However, the atrial premature impulse (A_2) fails to conduct to the ventricles, the site of block being localized to the distal His-Purkinje system.*

bances that may not be apparent from inspection of the surface ECG. Atrial pacing, for example, may precipitate the occurrence of type I second-degree A-V nodal block at much slower paced atrial rates than in normal individuals or may even provoke intra-His or infra-His block (Fig. 9). Similarly, atrial extrastimulus testing may reveal abnormally prolonged A-V nodal or His-Purkinje refractory periods (Fig. 10). Provocative maneuvers, such as carotid sinus massage, may be employed to demonstrate hypersensitive responses to vagal stimulation. Finally, one may use electrophysiologic testing after acute intravenous administration of drugs, such as cardiac glycosides, ß-blockers, calcium antagonists, and type I antiarrhythmic drugs, to uncover possible adverse effects of A-V

conduction that might be encountered during long-term oral therapy with such agents.

ETIOLOGY OF ATRIOVENTRICULAR BLOCK AND INTRAVENTRICULAR CONDUCTION DEFECTS

A variety of conditions or disease processes may lead to impaired A-V conduction, and the degree of impairment of A-V conduction in each of these circumstances may range in severity from first-degree A-V block to third-degree or complete A-V block (Table 1). In general the prognosis in such situations is determined by the nature of the condition or disease process leading to A-V block rather than the severity of the A-V block itself.

Table 1. Causes of A-V Block

1. Congenital block
   Associated with other anomalies (ostium primum defect, corrected transposition of great arteries)
   Not associated with other congenital anomalies
2. Primary causes
   Cardiomyopathy
   Lev's disease
   Lenegre's disease
3. Secondary causes
   Atherosclerotic heart disease
      Acute myocardial infarction
         Anterior
         Inferoposterior
      Myocardial infarction, healed
   Calcific interruption of A-V conduction system
      Calcified mitral or aortic valve or combination
   Inflammatory diseases
      Acute infective endocarditis ("ring abscess")
      Myocarditis
         Bacterial
            Acute rheumatic fever
            Diphtheria, syphilis, pertussis, Lyme disease, tuberculosis
         Parasitic
            Chagas disease
         Viral
            Mumps, measles
   Drugs
   Collagen disease
      Dermatomyositis, scleroderma, SLE, rheumatoid arthritis, ankylosing spondylitis, Wegener's granulomatosis
   Infiltrative diseases
      Hemochromatosis, primary oxalosis, sarcoidosis
   Trauma
      Surgical trauma, radiation therapy, catheter ablation
   Tumors
      Rhabdomyoma, rhabdomyosarcoma, mesothelioma
4. Functional block
   Vagally induced

A-V=Atrioventricular; SLE=Systemic lupus erythematosus.

Since the A-V node is exquisitely sensitive to the influence of the autonomic nervous system, any condition that leads to an increase in vagal tone may result in varying degrees of A-V nodal block. Vagal tone is heightened during sleep and may cause A-V nodal block that disappears during waking hours with resumption of normal daily activities. Similarly, Valsalva maneuver or carotid sinus massage can cause transient A-V nodal block in the absence of any intrinsic abnormality of A-V nodal conduction. Abnormally elevated vagal tone associated with conditions such as carotid sinus hypersensitivity or neurally mediated syncope may also lead to transient A-V nodal block.[7]

Drugs are a very common cause of impaired A-V conduction. Therapeutic levels of digitalis glycosides slow conduction and prolong the refractory period of the A-V node. At therapeutic levels such effects can be largely attributed to the parasympathetic effects of these agents.[8] Quinidine and disopyramide shorten the AH interval, an effect that is likely attributable to the vagolytic action of these drugs.[8-11] The direct effects of disopyramide and procainamide on A-V node are prolongation of the functional refractory period and slowing of conduction.[12,13] Quinidine, procainamide, and disopyramide modestly increase HV interval and QRS duration and significantly increase the effective refractory period of ventricular muscle.[14] Propafenone depresses A-V nodal conduction directly and also indirectly by virtue of its weak ß-blocking and weak calcium-channel blocking activity.[15] Flecainide and encainide increase markedly the HV interval and prolong QRS duration. Beta-blockers increase conduction time through the A-V node and prolong refractoriness. This effect is largely indirect, although in very high concentrations the ß-blockers may directly depress A-V nodal conduction. Calcium antagonists inhibit conduction through the A-V node. Upon exposure to verapamil, action potentials of the upper and middle sections of the A-V node develop diminished amplitude and upstroke velocity, the refractory period of the A-V node is prolonged, and conduction velocity is suppressed. Verapamil and diltiazem slow conduction through the A-V node and prolong the A-V nodal effective and functional refractory periods. Nifedipine, in contrast, has no detectable effect on A-V conduction.[9] Amiodarone also slows A-V conduction, although the mechanism of this action of amiodarone is not completely known.[16] Adenosine, an A_1-receptor agonist, activates an outward potassium current in all supraventricular tissues (sinus node, atrium, and A-V node) that causes membrane hyperpolarization and an abbreviation of the action potential. In addition, an inward calcium current is attenuated. This latter effect in the A-V node may be the principal mechanism by which adenosine exerts its negative chronotropic effects on A-V nodal conduction.[17]

Atrioventricular block and intraventricular conduction defects may occur as a result of changes in the A-V conduction system itself or in nearby structures, such as the central fibrous body, mitral or tricuspid annulus, membranous septum, aortic valve, or crest of the ventricular septum. Such pathologic changes may be primary (idiopathic), secondary to other underlying diseases, such as hypertension or coronary artery disease, or congenital. The most common pathological process underlying permanent A-V block is termed idiopathic bilateral bundle branch fibrosis. The process is characterized by a slow and progressive loss of conduction fibers and is described in 2 distinct forms: Lev's disease and Lenegre's disease. Lev's disease is characterized by a loss of fibers predominantly in the proximal left bundle and portions of the branching A-V bundle. With advancing age, the crest of the ventricular septum, membranous septum, central fibrous body, aortic annulus, and mitral annulus undergo degenerative changes, including fibrosis and calcification. This process may start as early as 40 years of age, progressing from left axis deviation to LBBB and then to complete A-V block by the eighth decade of life. Lenegre's disease is a more diffuse conduction system disease affecting the middle and distal portions of both bundle branches.[18,19]

Diseases or conditions that cause inflammation in the A-V node or in the atrial approaches to the A-V node, His-Purkinje system, and the bundle branches may be causes of transient or chronic A-V block. Inflammation in these regions can be the result of bacterial or viral illnesses, such as diphtheria, infectious mononucleosis, acquired immunodeficiency syndrome (AIDS), or *Borrelia burgdorferi* infection. Acute myocarditis of any cause, whether viral, rheumatic or idiopathic, can cause A-V block. In general, the A-V conduction disturbances seen in such transient inflammatory conditions resolve as the underlying illness subsides. Myocardial ischemia is another common cause of A-V block, as is trauma such as that seen after mitral or aortic valve surgery. Conditions or diseases that lead to necrosis, disruption, or replacement of A-V nodal cells and the fibers surrounding the A-V node typically cause fixed or progressive A-V nodal block rather than transient conduction abnormalities. Infarction of the A-V node or surgical disruption of the A-V node fall into this category. Infectious endocarditis, particularly with virulent organisms involving the aortic valve, may extend into and disrupt the A-V node, leading to permanent A-V block. Irreversible A-V block may also result from infiltrative diseases such as tumors, sarcoid, amyloidosis, and hemochromatosis; neuromuscular diseases such as progressive muscular dystrophy; or connective tissue disorders, such as systemic lupus erythematosus, progressive systemic sclerosis, dermatomyositis, rheumatoid arthritis, and ankylosing spondylitis. Finally, it must be remembered that A-V nodal block may be congenital.[18–21]

PREVALENCE AND PROGNOSIS OF ATRIOVENTRICULAR BLOCK AND INTRAVENTRICULAR CONDUCTION DEFECTS

Many conditions or disease states that affect A-V nodal conduction also affect conduction in other segments of the conduction system. Since the sites of block usually cannot be determined precisely from electrocardiographic criteria alone and since most clinical studies of A-V block are based on electrocardiographic criteria alone, it is virtually impossible to describe accurately the prevalence or significance of A-V block occurring in any single component of the conducting system. Nevertheless, some general statements are possible.

Table 2. A-V Block in Acute Myocardial Infarction

	ANTERIOR MI	INFEROPOSTERIOR MI
Pathology	Extensive infarction Injury to His-Purkinje system, infranodal block	Less extensive infarction Nodal block
Hemodynamic compromise	Often present	Often absent
QRS width	Wide	Narrow
Treatment	Pacing	No therapy Atropine Infrequent pacing
Prognosis	80% mortality	30% mortality

Several large studies have indicated that the incidence of unexplained PR prolongation of greater than 0.2 seconds in a healthy population ranges between 0.5% and 1.5%.[22-24] Importantly, the morbidity and mortality in the group of individuals with first-degree A-V block are generally the same as expected in a normal population without first degree A-V block. First-degree A-V block occurring in a young, otherwise healthy individual with no obvious cause for impairment of A-V conduction usually is simply a manifestation of enhanced vagal tone with resultant slowing of conduction in the A-V node and is of no prognostic significance. Such a finding is particularly likely in well-trained endurance athletes, who may even have periods of type I (Wenckebach) second-degree A-V block. The only important exception to this generalization is patients with familial heart block. This condition is inherited in an autosomal dominant pattern with incomplete penetrance and is characterized by progressive A-V nodal block that usually first appears during adulthood.[25,26] The site of block in these patients typically is in the A-V node, although there may be associated bundle branch block. Early recognition of these patients is important because they have a high incidence of syncope and sudden death.[25-27]

Unlike first-degree A-V nodal block and second-degree type I A-V nodal block, which are usually asymptomatic and of no prognostic significance in otherwise healthy young individuals, complete A-V block is rarely asymptomatic and may affect prognosis adversely. The most common cause of acquired complete A-V block is acute myocardial infarction (MI) (Table 2). In the setting of acute inferior MI due to occlusion of a dominant right or dominant left circumflex coronary artery, the A-V nodal blood supply via the A-V nodal artery is interrupted. Complete A-V nodal block may be encountered in 10%–15% of such patients.[28] Complete A-V block in this setting is rarely sudden in onset and usually is preceded by a period of second-degree type I block. The site of A-V block in such patients is typically the A-V node and is due to a combination of factors, including ischemia of the A-V node, local release of adenosine, and activation of autonomic reflexes.[29,30] This type of A-V block often responds readily to treatment with atropine or isoproterenol and seems not to have an adverse impact on the overall prognosis of affected patients. In some patients the atrial rate may be relatively slow due to reflex mechanisms or as a result of ischemic involvement of the sinoatrial node. Furthermore, ischemia and edema in the region of the A-V junction may cause subsidiary pacemakers in this region to fire at faster than normal rates. This combination of a relatively slow atrial rate and an accelerated junctional escape rate (45–70 beats/min) often results in A-V dissociation, which can give the appearance of A-V block when none exists. This is a transient rhythm disturbance lasting from 1–3 days usually and responds to the same treatment measures as A-V block associated with inferoposterior MI. Complete A-V block in the setting of acute anterior MI is less common, occurring in only 5% of patients.[18,29,30] The site of block in such patients is usually the bundle of His rather than the A-V node.[18,29,31] Although such patients have a much more grave prognosis than do individuals with complete A-V block in the setting of inferior infarction, this is probably due to the greater extent of necrosis usually seen in anterior infarction rather than the accompanying A-V block per se.

In rare patients complete A-V block is congenital; the site of block in such patients is typically the A-V node.[32] Congenital complete A-V block may occur as an isolated abnormality or it may be seen in association with other cardiac defects, such as corrected transposition, Ebstein's anomaly, and ventricular septal defect. The existence of systemic lupus erythematosus or Rh incompatibility in the mother appears to be related to the occurrence of complete A-V block in some infants, perhaps because anti-tissue antibodies cross the placenta and produce conduction system disease in the infant heart.[33] The prognosis of patients with congenital complete A-V block is good and is largely determined by the nature and severity of accompanying anatomic lesions, if any are present. The majority of infants with complete A-V block as their sole cardiac abnormality will develop and grow normally. Studies and case reports in children and young adults with congenital complete A-V block indicate that the heart rate in such patients, which is usually determined by automaticity in the His bundle, responds well to a variety of hemodynamic and pharmacologic stimuli.[34] The patients can engage in active sports and can even carry normal pregnancies to term. However, this benign prognosis has been questioned recently.[35] Patients with resting heart rates of less than 50 beats/min may be prone to syncope and may require permanent pacing to relieve symptoms,

particularly as they grow older.[18,32] Sudden death has also been reported to occur in this group of patients.[26,32] The mechanism of sudden death in such patients has not been clarified, but fatal bradyarrhythmia and pause-dependent torsades de pointes ventricular tachycardia are likely possibilities. Both of these lethal outcomes should be preventable with permanent pacemaker therapy.

The incidence of RBBB has been estimated to be 0.15% case per 1,000 in an asymptomatic population below the age of 40 years, and 0.29% in an asymptomatic population over 40 years of age. Estimates of the incidence of LBBB in patients younger and older than 40 years of age are 0.009% and 0.036%, respectively.[36,37] The right bundle branch is a relatively thin structure throughout its course and could be more vulnerable to disruption which may, in part, explain the higher incidence of RBBB. In hospitalized patients, the incidence of RBBB with left anterior hemiblock (LAHB) and RBBB with right posterior hemiblock (RPHB) are approximately 1% and 0.1%, respectively. The natural history of patients with such evidence of chronic bifascicular block is still unclear. Early retrospective studies suggested that up to 60% of these individuals eventually developed complete A-V block during follow-up intervals ranging up to 10 years. More recently, several prospective studies have been undertaken in an attempt to determine the percentage of patients with bifascicular block who have prolonged HV intervals and to determine whether such a finding is predictive of subsequent development of complete A-V block. For patients with RBBB + LAHB, a prolonged HV interval has been found in 50% to 70% of individuals. For patients with RBBB + RPHB, the incidence of a prolonged HV interval approaches 100%. Rosen and coworkers reported several series of patients with chronic bifascicular block. In each of these groups the incidence of eventual development of complete A-V block during follow-up was approximately 6% and could not be predicted by the length of the HV interval, even when it was markedly prolonged (>80 msec). Furthermore, AV nodal block, not intra-His or infra-His block, was the underlying mechanism of complete heart block in more than 50% of such patients. Furthermore, 20% of patients with chronic bifascicular block did not exhibit clinical evidence of coexisting organic heart disease.[36,37] Second-degree or complete A-V block developed at a rate of less than 1% per year in patients without underlying organic heart disease as compared to 2% per year in patients with organic heart disease. In contrast, studies of Scheinman and coworkers indicated a strong association between the finding of a markedly prolonged HV interval (>80 msec) and the subsequent development of complete A-V block during a 2-year follow-up period. A more recent study found that a prolonged HV interval (>70 msec) was an independent risk factor for sudden death, particularly in patients with an HV interval greater than 100 msec. Of interest was the observation that although permanent pacing effectively relieved symptoms related to A-V block, it did not reduce the risk of sudden death. This observation suggests that sudden death in patients at risk for developing complete A-V block is due to causes other than the A-V block per se.[5,6,36,37]

GUIDELINES FOR TREATMENT

Decisions about treatment of A-V nodal block are influenced by whether the block is related to some transient active problem or occurs as a chronic condition. Acute A-V nodal block, such as that encountered in the setting of digitalis toxicity or acute inferior MI, usually subsides with resolution of the underlying problem. The need for intervention in such patients should be determined by the symptomatic state of the patient. First-degree A-V nodal block is not an indication for treatment. However, acute second- and third-degree block that results in symptomatic bradycardia is an indication for therapy. Intravenous atropine 0.5 mg to 1.0 mg administered as a bolus is often helpful at reducing the degree of block or eliminating block altogether in patients with acute block. Intravenous infusion of isoproterenol may also be used in emergency situations, but is not recommended in patients with digitalis intoxication or acute MI because of the likelihood of precipitating ventricular arrhythmias or exacerbating myocardial ischemia. If symp-

tomatic bradycardia persists despite atropine, a temporary pacemaker should be utilized. Atrioventricular block occurring below the level of the A-V node is usually not the result of a transient, active problem but rather reflects chronic and often progressive disease in the His-Purkinje system. Atropine does not effectively reverse block occurring below the level of the A-V node and may actually increase the degree of block by virtue of the increased sinus rate that results from administration of the drug. In acute situations, isoproterenol may improve His-Purkinje conduction and, thereby, help to avoid the need for temporary pacing.

In chronic A-V block, prognosis is determined predominantly by the nature and severity of the associated underlying heart disease. The major contribution of permanent pacemaker implantation is relief of symptoms related to bradycardia rather than a marked impact on prognosis. Guidelines have been published by the joint American Heart Association/American College of Cardiology task force for implantation of permanent pacemakers.[38] The guidelines have been divided into 3 categories. Category I includes situations in which permanent pacemaker implantation is definitely recommended. This category applies to patients with complete A-V block, whether the site of block is in or below the A-V node, provided that it occurs in association with any of the following: 1) symptomatic bradycardia; 2) congestive heart failure; 3) confusional state that clears with temporary pacing; 4) ectopic rhythms or other conditions that require the use of drugs that would suppress the automaticity of subsidiary pacemakers; 5) documented periods of asystole greater than 3 seconds in duration or escape heart rate less than 40 beats/min; 6) following intentional A-V nodal ablation; and 7) myotonic dystrophy.

Category I also applies to patients with second-degree A-V block, whether in or below the A-V node, if it is associated with symptomatic bradycardia. Category II includes situations in which there is divergence of opinion whether permanent pacemaker implantation should be recommended. This category applies to patients with asymptomatic complete A-V block, whether in or below the A-V node, with ventricular rates greater than or equal to 40 beats/min. Category III includes situations in which a permanent pacemaker is not recommended. This category applies to patients with asymptomatic second-degree A-V nodal block or first-degree A-V block.

REFERENCES

1. Watanabe Y, Dreifus LS. Factors controlling impulse transmission, with special reference to A V conduction. *Am Heart J.* 1975;89:790-793.
2. Hoffman BF, Cranefield PF. *Electrophysiology of the Heart.* New York: McGraw-Hill; 1960:132-174.
3. Janse MJ, van Capelle FJL, Anderson RH, et al. Electrophysiology and structure of the atrioventricular node of the isolated rabbit heart. In: Wellens HJJ, Lie KI, Janse MJ (eds). *Conduction System of the Heart.* Leiden: Stefert Kroese; 1976:296-315.
4. Moore EN, Knoebel SB, Spear JF. Concealed conduction. *Am J Cardiol.* 1971;28:406-413.
5. Josephson ME. *Clinical Cardiac Electrophysiology. Techniques and Interpretations*, 2nd Ed. Philadelphia: Lea & Febiger; 1993:96-149.
6. Puech P, Wainwright RJ. Clinical electrophysiology of AV block. *Cardiol Clin.* 1983;1:209-224.
7. Hutchinson EC, Stock JTT. Carotid sinus syndrome. *Lancet.* 1960;2:445.
8. Watanabe Y, Dreifus LS. Electrophysiologic effects of digitalis on A-V transmission. *Am J Physiol.* 1966; 211:1461-1466.
9. Antman EM, Stone PH, Muller JE, et al. Calcium channel blocking agents in the treatment of cardiovascular disorders. Part I. Basic and clinical electrophysiologic effects. *Ann Intern Med.* 1980;93:875-885.
10. Alboni P, Cappato R, Paparella N, et al. Electrophysiological effects and mechanism of action of oral quinidine in patients with sinus bradycardia and first degree A-V nodal block. *Eur Heart J.* 1987;8:1080-1089.
11. Mason JW, Winkel RA, Rider AK, et al. The electrophysiologic effects of quinidine in the transplanted human heart. *J Clin Invest.* 1977;59:480-489.
12. Birkhead JS, Vaughan Williams WM. Dual effect of disopyramide on atrial and atrioventricular conduction and refractory periods. *Br Heart J.* 1977;39:657-660.
13. Josephson ME, Caracta AR, Ricciutti MA, et al. Electrophsyiologic properties of procainamide in man. *Am J Cardiol.* 1974;33:596-603.
14. Ogunkelu JB, Damato AN, Akhatar M, et al. Electrophysiologic effects of procainamide in sub-therapeutic to therapeutic doses on human atrioventricular conduction system. *Am J Cardiol.* 1976;37:724-731.
15. Seipel L, Breithardt B. Propafenone—a new anti-arrhythmic drug. *Eur Heart J.* 1980;1:309-313.
16. Zipes DP, Prystowsky EN, Heger JJ. Amiodarone: Electrophysiologic actions, pharmacokinetics, and clinical effects. *J Am Coll Cardiol.* 1984;3:1059-1071.
17. Pelly A, Miyagawa A, Michelson EL, et al. On the mechanisms of cardiac electrophysiologic actions of adenosine and adenosine triphosphate. In Mazgalev T,

Dreifus LS, Michelson EL. *Electrophysiology of the Sinoatrial and Atrioventricular Nodes.* New York, NY: Alan R. Liss; 1988:133-155.
18. Lev M, Bharati S. Atrioventricular and intraventricular conduction disease. *Arch Intern Med.* 1975;135:405-416.
19. Lev M. The pathology of atrioventricular block. *Cardiovascular Clin.* 1972;4:159-168.
20. Davies MJ. *Pathology of Conducting Tissue of the Heart.* New York: Appleton-Century-Crofts; 1971:60-114.
21. Jones ME, Terry G, Kenmure ACF. Frequency and significance of conduction defects in acute myocardial infarction. *Am Heart J.* 1977;94:163-169.
22. Bures AR. First degree AV block: Anatomy and physiology as illustrated by a twenty year follow-up. *Aerospace Med.* 1965;36:780-784.
23. Calleja HB, Guerrero MX. Prolonged PR interval and coronary artery disease. *Br Heart J.* 1973;35:372-376.
24. Johnson RL, Averill KH, Lamb LE. Electrocardiographic findings in 67,375 asymptomatic subjects. VII. Atrioventricular block. *Am J Cardiol.* 1960;6:153-164.
25. Waxman MB, Catching JD, Felderhof CH, et al. Familial atrioventricular heart block: An autosomal dominant trait. *Circulation.* 1975;51:226-231.
26. Reid JM, Coleman EN, Doig W. Complete congenital heart block: Report of 35 cases. *Br Heart J.* 1982; 48:236-241.
27. Sarachek NS, Leonard JJ. Familial heart block and sinus bradycardia: Classification and natural history. *Am J Cardiol.* 1972;29:451-460.
28. Rotman M, Wagner GS, Wallace AG. Bradyarrhythmias in acute myocardial infarction. *Circulation.* 1973;45:703-710.
29. Rosen KM, Loeb HS, Chuquimia R, et al. Site of heart block in acute myocardial infarction. *Circulation.* 1970;42:925-936.
30. Brown RW, Hunt D, Sloman JG. The natural history of atrioventricular conduction defects in acute myocardial infarction. *Am Heart J* 1969;78:460-467.
31. Lie KI, Wellens HJ, Schuilenberg RM, et al. Factors influencing prognosis of bundle branch block complicating acute antero-septal infarction: The value of His bundle recordings. *Circulation.* 1974;50:935-941.
32. Nakamura FF, Nadas AS. Complete heart block in infants and children. *N Engl J Med.* 1964;270:1261-1268.
33. Kenmure ACF, Cameron AJV. Congenital complete heart block in pregnancy. *Br Heart J.* 1967;29:910-912.
34. Corne RA, Mathewson FAL. Congenital complete atrioventricular heart block: A 25-year follow-up study. *Am J Cardiol.* 1972;29:412-415.
35. Mymin D, Mathewson FAL, Tate RB, et al. The natural history of primary first-degree atrioventricular heart block. *N Engl J Med.* 1986;315:1183-1187.
36. Narula OS. Current concepts of atrioventricular block. In: Narula OS (ed). *His Bundle Electrocardiography.* Philadelphia: FA Davis; 1975:32-40.
37. Narula OS. Atrioventricular block. In: Marula OS (ed). *Cardiac Arrhythmias.* Baltimore: Williams & Wilkins; 1979:85-140.
38. Dreifus LS, Fisch C, Griffin JC, et al. Guidelines for implantation of cardiac pacemakers and antiarrhythmia devices. *J Am Coll Cardiol.* 1991;18:1-13.

23 Pacemaker Therapy

David T. Martin, MBBS
Andrew C. Eisenhauer, MD

BACKGROUND

When the first pacing system was implanted in 1958 by Senning, artificial cardiac pacing was largely viewed as a therapy to prevent recurrent syncope and death due to complete AV block.[1] At that time pacemaker implantation required thoracic surgery and committing a patient to a lifetime of cardiac pacing was done with trepidation on the part of the clinician. Over the last 30 years it has become clear that pacemaker therapy for the treatment of heart block is life saving.[2-5] Today, transvenous cardiac pacing has become routine therapy not only for treating manifest syncope but also for controlling near syncope and other non–life-threatening symptoms of bradycardia.

This chapter will discuss both traditional and innovative indications for pacemaker implantation as well as the evolution of lead and pulse generator technology. In addition we will address common problems in electrocardiographic (ECG) interpretation and troubleshooting of pacing systems, as well as some of the frequent sources of interference with pacing system function.

INDICATIONS

Indications for the implantation of a permanent pacing system have been evaluated and a consensus developed by a combined committee of the American Heart Association (AHA), American College of Cardiology (ACC), and North American Society of Pacing and Electrophysiology (NASPE).[6,7] In addition, the United States Health Care Finance Administration (HCFA) has published guidelines for reimbursement for pacemaker procedures.

Adherence to the guidelines is important since major discrepancies in pacemaker utilization between countries with comparable medical resources have been demonstrated.[8,9] Allowing for diagnostic differences, it remains of great interest why the proportion of pacemakers implanted for complete heart block far outweigh the number for sinus node disease in European countries and Canada compared with the United States where these proportions are reversed and overall utilization is much greater. This apparent over-utilization has led to close scrutiny, by peer review organizations in some states, of the indications for implantation, but studies of such interventions have demonstrated no reduction in implantation rates.[10] There is good reason to believe Wyse's argument that appropriate and parsimonious use of this expensive technology, as well as attainment of the highest standards of practice is optimized by centralizing pacemaker implantation in high volume referral centers.[11]

The clinician contemplating the recommendation of permanent pacing should understand that the notion of a pacemaker is often very distressing to the patient and misunderstood by him or her. Patients often place their hopes for resolution of nonbradycardia-related symptoms, such as fatigue or confusion, on permanent pacing. The clinician must clearly define for the patient and his or her family what symptoms can reasonably be expected to improve after pacing and what symptoms can not. This can prevent disappointment from unmet expectations following pacemaker implantation.

Clinically, the reason for implanting a permanent pacing system is generally to treat and prevent symptoms from an inappropriately slow heart rate. As a result, a central requirement for bradycardia pacing support is the presence of a

Table 1. Indications for Pacing in Sinus Node Dysfunction	
Class I	**General Agreement Favors Pacing** Documented symptomatic bradycardia
Class II	**Divergence of Opinion** Bradycardia <40 beats/min without clearly associated symptoms
Class III	**Pacing not Indicated** Asymptomatic sinus bradycardia <40 beats/min due to drug therapy Symptoms suggestive of sinus bradycardia shown by monitoring not to be associated with slow heart rate
Modified from Dreifus LS, et al.[7]	

Table 2. Indications for Pacing in Chronic Acquired AV Block	
Class I	**General Agreement Favors Pacing** A. Complete heart block (fixed or intermittent) accompanied by: Symptomatic bradycardia Congestive heart failure Ventricular ectopy Escape rate <40 beats/min or asystole >3 sec Confusional state that clears with temporary pacing B. Second degree heart block with symptomatic bradycardia C. Atrial fibrillation/flutter with conditions under A (above)
Class II	**Divergence of Opinion** A. Asymptomatic third degree AV block with escape rate >40 beats/min B. Asymptomatic type II second degree AV block C. Asymptomatic type I second degree AV block at the intra-His or infra-His level
Class III	**Pacing not Indicated** A. Asymptomatic type I second degree AV block at the supra-His (AV node) level B. First degree AV block
Modified from Dreifus LS, et al.[7]	

documented symptomatic bradyarrhythmia (Tables 1–4). When such an event occurs and is not due to a temporary, remediable or otherwise treatable cause (such as drug toxicity, Lyme disease,[12] or neurally mediated syncope[13] [Fig. 1]), permanent pacing is generally indicated. A symptomatic bradycardia may be operationally defined as a pause in cardiac rhythm of 3 or more seconds accompanied by subjective experience of syncope or presyncope. Although the mechanism underlying such a pause is generally of no importance in deciding whether pacemaker implantation is indicated, it is relevant, along with other clinical data, in the choice of pacing mode to be employed.

Occasionally, despite an extensive evaluation, the clinician is faced with the inability to document bradyarrhythmias as the cause of recurrent syncope, near syncope, or light-headedness. Under these circumstances it may be appropriate to implant a pacing system based solely on clinical judgment. This is an uncommon situation, but well within the range of acceptable clinical practice. By distinction, sinus pauses and periods of sinus bradycardia are very common, particularly in elderly patients and in young physically active patients. The mere presence of these findings without correlation with associated symptoms should not result in the implantation of a pacing system (Table 1). Outside of the placebo effect, such an implant does not improve the patient's overall sense of well-being.

"Prophylactic" permanent pacing is not usually required except in very specific instances such as the witnessed development of permanent bundle branch block in the face of an acute myocardial infarction. However, implantation of a pacemaker in such circumstances has been shown to have no influence upon mortality (in contrast with the effects of pacing in sclerodegenerative disease of the cardiac conduction system) since mortality is predominantly determined by the size of the infarct, of which the development of bundle branch block is a powerful clinical indicator. Pacemaker implantation in the "asymptomatic" patient is only very rarely warranted; examples of such indications include development of acquired complete AV block (a potentially lethal condition) or the gradual slowing in junctional escape rate that occurs with increased age in patients with congenital heart block. These patients frequently realize in retrospect that prior to pacemaker implantation they were not truly asymptomatic. Implantation of a

Table 3. Indications for Pacing in Chronic Bifascicular or Trifascicular Block	
Class I	**General Agreement Favors Pacing** Bifascicular block with intermittent complete heart block associated with symptoms of bradycardia Bifascicular or trifascicular block with asymptomatic intermittent type II second degree heart block
Class II	**Divergence of Opinion** Bifascicular or trifascicular block with syncope that is not proved to be due to heart block but no other causes are apparent Markedly prolonged HV interval (>100 ms) Pacing induced infra-His block
Class III	**Pacing Not Indicated** Fascicular block without AV block or symptoms Asymptomatic fascicular block with first degree AV block
Modified from Dreifus LS, et al.[7]	

Table 4. Clinical Factors That May Influence Pacemaker Implantation Decisions

Absence of other life-threatening comorbidity
Associated cardiac condition aggravated by bradycardia
Motor vehicle operator
Remote or inaccessible medical attention
Need for medication that suppresses cardiac conduction/automaticity
Slow basic escape mechanism
Cerebrovascular disease exacerbated by bradycardia
Desires of patient and family

pacemaker in a patient with the tachycardia-bradycardia variant of sinus node disease is frequently justified on the grounds that it is needed prior to the necessary use of anti-tachycardia drugs which are likely to further depress intrinsic cardiac automaticity and conduction. This management strategy has never been subjected to a randomized trial, and there is theoretic support for the counter-argument that effective drug suppression of tachycardia will lead to effective abolishment of bradycardia since offset pauses will no longer occur.

In vasodepressor or neurally-mediated syncope, episodic bradyarrhythmias may only be part of a complex disturbance in consciousness (Fig. 1). Here, correcting the bradyarrhythmia, although sometimes appropriate, may, at best, only partially relieve symptoms. Generally, the initial therapy of this usually benign condition should be with trials of ß-blocking or anticholinergic agents in an attempt to block the vagal reflex that leads to profound vasodilatation.[13]

Recent studies have led to the emergence of new indications for permanent pacemaker implantation: hemodynamic improvement of patients with hypertrophic or dilated cardiomyopathy.[14–16] There are multiple potential mechanisms for the benefit of pacing in these conditions, and these are the subject of ongoing research. Patients with obstructive hypertrophic cardiomyopathy have been shown to have substantial hemodynamic and symptomatic improvement with dual-chamber pacing provided the pulse generator is programmed such that the AV delay is very short (typically less than 100 msec). It is suggested that the short AV interval combined with the altered sequence of ventricular activation during pacing abolishes the dynamic obstruction that develops during normally conducted left ventricular systole. There remains no evidence of survival benefit, but it is clear that pacing in this condition offers a major improvement in quality of life and, in many patients, obviates the requirement for septal myomyectomy. Many questions remain unanswered about this new indication for pacing:[15] If benefit is due to the altered sequence of ventricular activation, why do patients with intrinsic left bundle branch block not benefit to the same extent? Why do some patients evidence no apparent hemodynamic benefit when studied acutely in the catheterization laboratory, but later seem to be much improved by pacing?

TECHNICAL CONSIDERATIONS

Organizationally, a pacing system can be conceptualized as performing 2 general medical functions—diagnosis and treatment. Diagnostically, a pacemaker must determine the

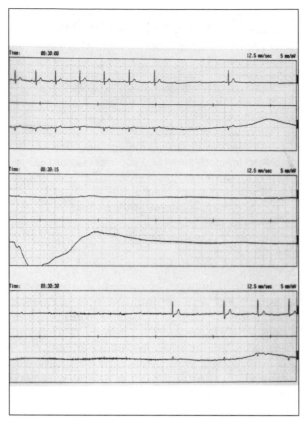

Figure 1. *Holter monitor recording of a syncopal spell in a young patient with reflex ("vasovagal") syncope. The pathophysiology is complex and not well understood, but entails profound vasodepression as well as bradycardia. Enhanced vagal tone is suggested by the appearance of both AV block with depressed junctional escape mechanism and sinus bradycardia leading to sinus arrest. Note that paper speed in 12.5 mm/S. This patient did not require pacemaker implantation.*

presence or absence of appropriate cardiac activity. Therapeutically, the device supplies electrical stimuli to trigger cardiac activity that is lacking. From a logical or "software" perspective, the 3 areas of pacemaker function are sensing, analysis (logic), and stimulation. Sensing and stimulation involve not only the basic electronic system, but its interface with the patient.

The components of the "hardware" that make up a modern pacing system consist of: 1) the electrode/lead system, and 2) the pulse generator. The pulse generator itself is comprised of an energy source (battery) and electronic circuitry enclosed by a housing which shields the energy

supply and circuit from contact with body fluids. In addition, since all modern pacemakers are externally adjustable with a specific radio frequency programming device, the programmer and its associated software should be considered an integral part of the pacing system. Most currently used programmers are sophisticated computers with bi-directional telemetry capabilities allowing medical personnel to obtain detailed diagnostic data relating to the patient and the device, and the delivery of both programming instructions and software upgrades to the implanted pulse generator. Unfortunately each manufacturer's programming system uses proprietary radiofrequency telemetric technology and there is little prospect of the development of a "universal" programmer.

The performance and reliability of a pacing system is determined by the performance and reliability of its weakest component. Thirty years ago unexpected and unintended pulse generator component failures were common; today these are rare. Most pacing system anomalies seen in current clinical practice are not component failures but a complex interaction of pacemaker programming, and the patient's intrinsic cardiac electrophysiology.

POWER SUPPLY

A reliable pacemaker obviously requires a reliable power source. Power is usually supplied by an electrolytic cell or cells arranged in a battery. An electrolytic cell consists of a positive and negative electrode separated by an electrolytic medium. The connection between these 2 electrodes will cause current to flow outside of the cell from the electrochemical reaction. Normal cells contain a certain calculated maximum energy that can be provided over their useful lifetime. The theoretical maximum however, is greater than that actually realized because of internal losses. Further, the amount of energy contained in the cell in proportion to its size (energy density) is critical in developing compact pacing devices.[17]

In the early days of pacing, mercury zinc cells were used. They were relatively low in energy density and their internal losses subjected them to unpredictable and sudden failure. Subsequently, a number of cells have been developed using lithium as the anode. In general, these have been very successful and have provided high-energy densities which, in combination with decreasing pacemaker power requirements, have resulted in very long-lived devices.[18] During the search for a reliable long-lived power source, rechargeable cells, biogalvanic power sources, and nuclear energy sources have also been used. Interestingly, nuclear sources were technically quite successful, but their usefulness has been limited by concern (both real and imagined) over radiation exposure and component disposal. The availability of good electrolytic power supplies and failure of other associated components as a limit on pacer longevity have also served to discourage the use of nuclear power sources.

ELECTRONIC CIRCUIT

Early electronic circuits of the first implanted devices were made possible by the invention of the transistor. The circuit consisted of little more than a crystal oscillator to provide rhythmic outputs of the stimulating signals. These devices were "fixed-rate devices" and did not incorporate the ability to sense intrinsic cardiac activity. It quickly became apparent that it was desirable to develop miniature sense amplifiers so that intrinsic cardiac activity could be sensed through the exploring electrode at times when stimulation was not occurring. A device's output could then be suppressed or triggered depending on the needs of the patient. Unfortunately, the manufacturing, connection, and soldering of the transistors in these devices was a major source of reliability difficulties. With the advent of microcircuitry in the late 1970s, solid-state devices could be coupled with these chips in which transistor equivalent components number in the several thousand. This offered greater reliability and the possibility of incorporating more functions into a smaller space. Modern devices now employ large-scale integrated circuit technology and microprocessors to provide the equivalent of several hundred thousand solid-state components. These components drain far less current from the power source than did the early simple transistor devices. Current pacemakers can be thought of as small programmable computers that are called upon to modulate cardiac sensing and stimulation.[19–22]

HOUSING

The function of the medium enclosing the components of the pulse generator is simple in concept but quite difficult to achieve in practice. It must be inert chemically and biologically, and yet confer protection from the hostile environment of the human body. It also must protect the patient from the outward leak of hazardous electrolytes. Early devices utilized silicone or epoxy coatings and were subject to expansion following the encroachment of moisture. Modern devices are hermetically sealed in 3 layers with the electronic circuit and power supply individually isolated in a final sealed "can" constructed of titanium or stainless steel.

LEADS AND ELECTRODES

Early pacing systems stimulated the heart through surgically applied epicardial electrodes which were frequently unreliable due to development of conductor fractures and high pacing thresholds over time. In 1958, the development of temporary transvenous pacing and subsequent refinement of the surgical techniques has led to its primacy in modern cardiac pacing. A transvenous pacing lead consists of a conductor and insulator, and also of an exposed electrode(s) to provide the bioelectric interface.[23] Insulation material may be manufactured from silicone rubber or polyurethane; the former is bulkier and creates more friction between leads during the implantation of a dual-chamber system but is historically more durable than the latter. The tip of the lead may be fixed in the heart passively (by fins or tines that snag trabeculae in the right atrium or ventricle) or actively (usually by a screw mechanism that may itself be electrically active or passive). In addition, the tip of the lead may incorporate a small pellet of steroid material that acts locally in the myocardium during the 2 years after implantation to prevent the rise in pacing and sensing thresholds commonly seen due to local inflammation.[24]

In unipolar systems, a single electrode at the tip of the lead serves as the cathode and a metallic pacemaker "can" is an electrically active anode in contact with the tissue fluid. In contrast, bipolar leads are made up of 2 internal conductors that are insulated one from the

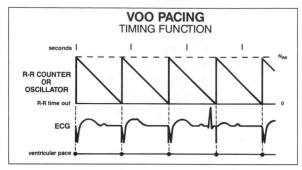

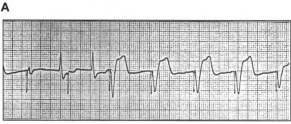

B

Figure 2. *(A) Timing "ladder" diagram for VOO pacing. The pacemaker events are listed on the left. Time is along the horizontal axis from left to right. In this figure, following a ventricular paced event (the first QRS on the left), the RR counter resets and begins "counting down" a prescribed length of time. At the end of this RR interval or "RR timeout," a second stimulus artifact is placed in the oscillator which is then reset. Rhythmic stimulus artifacts are produced throughout the remainder of this figure. A native QRS occurs and, appropriately, is not sensed. (B) Accompanying EKG strips of a patient with a VOO pacemaker, showing appropriate capture but a complete lack of sensing of ventricular events (All Ladder Diagrams courtesy J.W. Harthorne, MD).*

other and from the external environment. Each is connected to a separate electrode. The cathode is formed by an electrode at the tip of the lead and the anode by a ring electrode mounted 1-2 cm more proximally. Unipolar leads can generally be manufactured with a smaller diameter and are easier to handle during implantation. The stimulus artifact produced by the output of a unipolar system is large and easily visible electrocardiographically. However, the "antenna effect" created by the wide separation of anode and cathode, subjects these systems to clinically relevant external interference (see below).[25] Bipolar systems in comparison tend to be larger and provide smaller stimulus artifacts, but are far more resistant to external interference at high programmed sensitivities.[26]

MODES OF CARDIAC PACING

In order to clarify the rationale for the plethora of available pacing modes when current practice essentially restricts use to the VVI and DDD modes, this discussion will use a historical approach illustrating that evolution of pacing modes was determined by evolving engineering capabilities. The first implanted artificial cardiac pacemakers were simply devices to rhythmically stimulate the heart (Fig. 2). Generally, the patients in whom they were implanted had little or no intrinsic ventricular activity without cardiac pacing. The sensing of patients' native QRS complexes to avoid potential competition was not a serious problem. In fact, even when patients did have intrinsic cardiac activity, competition between it and artificial pacemaker activity did not usually result in adverse reactions. The insertion of a stimulus into the vulnerable portion of the T-wave only rarely resulted in the generation of a ventricular tachyarrhythmia. This difficulty was initially resolved by developing sensing amplifiers which would trigger a pacemaker output immediately upon sensing a QRS complex. This triggering also provided direct ECG evidence of appropriate sensing and stimulation by "marking" each of these events with a stimulus artifact. Additional impulses would be triggered if no intrinsic activity was sensed during a time corresponding to the escape rate of the pacemaker (Fig. 3). This mode of pacing worked very well, but it failed to achieve the potential advantage of the ability to sense intrinsic cardiac activity—the reduction in the frequency of stimulus outputs and the resulting conservation in energy. As a result, other sensing circuitry was developed to inhibit pulse generator output except following periods of cardiac electrical "silence" (Fig. 4). These devices, that either sensed or triggered pacemaker output could also, under certain circumstances, be applied to atrial pacing. It soon became necessary to develop a nomenclature for the description of pacemaker function. The Intersociety Commission on Heart Disease Resources (ICHD) developed the first 3-position pacemaker code; the first position refers to the chamber(s) paced, the second position to the chamber whose activity is sensed, and the third position to the mode of response (Table 5). The pacemaker that paced and sensed the ventricle and responded to intrinsic cardiac activity by

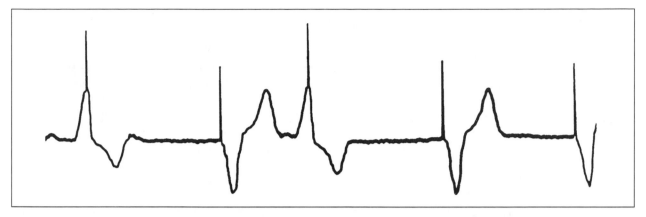

Figure 3. *VVT EKG strip. Every QRS is marked by a stimulus artifact. In this fashion, appropriate sensing is easily demonstrated.*

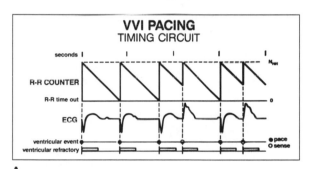

A

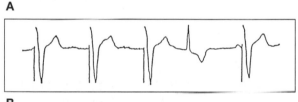

B

Figure 4. *VVI timing diagram (A) and accompanying EKG (B). In the timing diagram, the sensing function is apparent. In the rhythm strip (B), the fourth QRS from the left is above the pacing rate and resets the RR counter.*

triggering a stimulus output functioned in the VVT mode. In a similar fashion, a ventricular pacemaker whose output was suppressed by a native QRS complex was a device in the VVI mode. The earliest fixed-rate, non-sensing devices were VOO pacemakers. Devices with their single leads placed in the atrium are AOO, AAT and AAI devices. The ICHD code was subsequently revised by a joint commission of NASPE and the British Pacing and Electrophysiology Group ("NBG") which expanded the mode designations to 5 positions. The fourth position outlines programmable and rate-modu-

lated functions and the last indicates antitachycardia features (Table 5). These later additions have not been widely incorporated into routine clinical practice.

Even before the first permanent implant in 1958, some investigators realized that ventricular pacing was not a good physiologic solution to the problem of complete or episodic atrioventricular block. The normal cardiac impulse arises in the SA node and after the appropriate AV nodal delay (corresponding to the PR interval on surface ECG) travels to the ventricles producing a QRS complex and subsequent mechanical ventricular systole. Simple ventricular pacing did not mimic normal cardiac activation and did not seem to be the ideal solution to the problem of AV block, the most common indication for implantation at that time. In 1954, Folkman developed an apparatus for replacing AV conduction in the canine model of heart block.[27] The apparatus consisted of a sense amplifier that would identify intrinsic atrial activity and, after an appropriate delay, stimulate the ventricle. This was the forerunner of the VAT pacemaker in which ventricular pacing is induced by atrial activity (Fig. 5). Though this mode is not used today, it is an essential component of the DDD mode, and understanding how it was developed and how it behaves is important in the understanding of modern dual chamber mode.

VAT PACING

With the development of the VAT mode of atrial-triggered ventricular pacing, came the

Table 5. The 5-Position NBG Pacemaker Code

Position	I	II	III	IV	V
Category	Chamber(s) paced	Chamber(s) sensed	Mode of response(s)	Programmable functions	Special tachyarrhythmia functions
Letters used	V-Ventricle	V-Ventricle	T-Triggered	P-Simple programmable (rate and/or output)	B-Bursts
	A-Atrium	A-Atrium	I-Inhibited	M-Multi-programmable	N-Normal rate competition
	D-Double	D-Double	D-Double*	C-Multi-programmable with telemetry	S-Scanning
				R-Rate-modulated	
			O-None		
		O-None	R-Reverse†	O-None	E-External
Manufacturer's designation only	S-Single chamber‡	S-Single chamber‡			

*Atrial triggered and ventricular inhibited
†Activated by tachycardia and (usually) bradycardia
‡Can be used for atrial or ventricular pacing (manufacturer's designation)

need to develop an electronic analogy of conduction system refractoriness. Just as 1:1 AV conduction at the onset of atrial flutter could be deleterious to a non-paced patient, so too could rapid ventricular pacing triggered by atrial tachyarrhythmias in a patient with a VAT device (Fig. 6). Thus, sensing circuitry is required to be "deaf" (or refractory) to intrinsic atrial activity that occurs above a selected rate to prevent inappropriate rapid ventricular pacing from the sensing of atrial tachyarrhythmias or extracardiac signals.

An additional technical problem was created by sensing and pacing in multiple chambers. The voltage required to stimulate is 3 orders of magnitude greater than that produced by intrinsic cardiac activity. Thus, the stimulus outputs produced in 1 chamber could be sensed by an alert sense amplifier connected to another chamber. For example, a theoretical VAT device could sense atrial activity and produce a stimulus output in the ventricle and then sense that remote or "far-field" stimulus as another atrial

event. This would trigger a ventricular stimulus output which would be sensed by the atrial channel inducing a third stimulus output and continuing indefinitely with rapid paced rates. A potential solution to this problem is to render the sense amplifiers completely refractory during a stimulus output and its associated polarization artifact. This property, referred to as "blanking," serves to prevent self-inhibition or self-triggering known as "crosstalk."

Early VAT pacing was fraught with difficulties. Devices were bulky and the passive fixation atrial leads were large and difficult to position reliably. Intrinsic ventricular activity was not sensed so there was often competition with ventricular extrasystoles, junctional beats, or, if heart block was not continual and complete, normally conducted beats. In addition, blanking periods and refractoriness of the atrial channel were sufficiently long to prevent the appropriate tracking of even modest degrees of sinus tachycardia.

Even with the poor reliability of early atrial sensing leads, technical problems with pro-

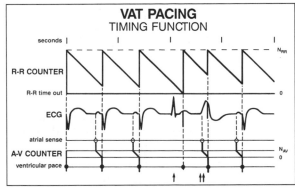

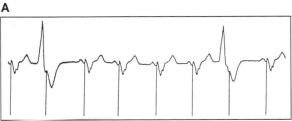

B

Figure 5. VAT timing diagram (A) and accompanying EKG (B). Following the first paced QRS in this diagram, the RR counter is reset (there is no ventricular sensing). A P wave occurs which initiates another timing cycle (the AV counter), represented at the bottom of the diagram. Following this AV delay, a ventricular stimulus is produced that resets the RR counter. This series of events is repeated. Following the third QRS, the RR counter is reset again and begins counting down. A premature ventricular complex (PVC) occurs (first arrow) and it is appropriately not sensed. A ventricular stimulus is produced on the T wave of this PVC and the RR counter is reset. A hidden P wave occurs (second 2 arrows) triggering another ventricular stimulus artifact this time in the middle of a PVC. The RR counter is reset once again. Note the atrial refractory period during which atrial sensing cannot occur. (Courtesy J.W. Harthorne) The EKG illustrates VAT pacing.

longed atrial refractory periods, blanking and ventricular competition, it became clear some patients *required* this early dual-chamber pacing. In these patients, simple ventricular pacing was intolerable. Some became hypotensive, sensed cannon "A" waves in the neck and noted very poor exercise tolerance; a few developed congestive heart failure. These patients were suffering from what has become known as the "pacemaker syndrome" and are now known to have had ventriculo-atrial conduction with retrograde activation of the atria during ventricular pacing.

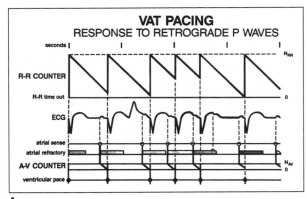

A

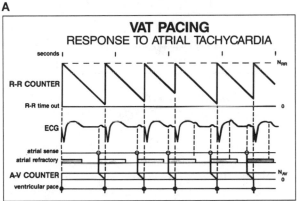

B

Figure 6. VAT pacing response to retrograde P waves (A) and to atrial tachycardia (B). Note in (A) the development of a pacemaker-mediated tachycardia (the fourth, fifth, and sixth QRS complexes from the left). The retrograde P wave, after the sixth QRS falls within the atrial refractory period and is therefore not sensed. The next event is therefore lower rate ventricular pacing. In (B) the atrial rate has accelerated so that only every other P wave falls outside the refractory period resulting in tracking this fast rate in a 2:1 fashion.(Courtesy J. W. Harthorne.)

While not all patients with VA conduction have the pacemaker syndrome, all patients with the syndrome have VA conduction.

DVI PACING

A potential electronic solution to the problem of the need to maintain AV synchrony but to avoid the difficulties of VAT pacing was to couple an atrial stimulus output with a ventricular pacemaker. In this mode, both chambers are paced but only ventricular activity inhibits pacemaker output. This "DVI" mode maintains atrioventricular synchrony, but at the expense of being

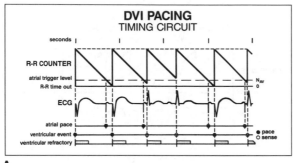

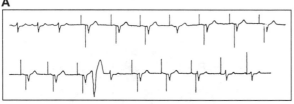

B

Figure 7. *DVI timing diagram (A) and EKG (B). Note, on the EKG, the appropriate lack of atrial sensing.*

unable to track intrinsic atrial activity (Fig. 7). Unlike VAT pacing, it is not an arrangement that produces "replacement" of AV nodal function. It was, however, a good solution for maintaining AV synchrony at least in patients who had chronically slow sinus rates. However, just as VAT pacing provides potential competition between ventricular stimulus outputs and intrinsic ventricular activity, DVI pacing can compete with intrinsic atrial activity and may promote the development of atrial fibrillation.

An additional electronic problem became evident as DVI pacing developed. The earliest DVI pulse generators were "noncommitted" and could not distinguish between appropriate AV conduction, a PVC, or extracardiac electronic noise occasionally leading to crosstalk inhibition of ventricular output. To solve this problem, later DVI devices became "committed" that is, a ventricular stimulus output was committed to occur following the preceding atrial stimulus regardless of what happened during the AV delay; this prevented crosstalk inhibition but caused frequent competition between native conduction and ventricular pacing. The final generation of DVI devices were "partially committed:" everything in the early part of the AV delay (the crosstalk-sensing window) was ignored and the pulse generator would emit a ventricular spike after the AV delay ended (so-called "safety pacing"); ventricular output was appropriately inhibited should a ventricular event be sensed in the later part of the AV interval.

HYSTERESIS

It quickly became apparent that not only was it desirable to maintain AV synchrony in patients with the pacemaker syndrome, but a number of individuals clearly required AV synchrony to maintain ventricular filling and optimum cardiac output. In some patients sinus bradycardia at 35 beats/min was hemodynamically preferable to ventricular pacing at 60 beats/min with the associated loss of AV synchrony. For this reason, "hysteresis" was added as a programmable option to some VVI pacemakers. Hysteresis allowed the pacing rate to be programmed to exceed the escape rate by a selected amount. For example, a VVI device with a programmed rate of 70 and 20 beats/min of hysteresis would require the heart rate to fall to ≤ 50 beats/min before it initiated pacing at a rate of 70 beats/min. While theoretically helpful, the EKG consequences were often confusing to the uninitiated. Further, frequent ineffective premature ventricular contractions (especially in a bigeminal pattern) could reduce the effective pacing heart rate to below the hysteresis level and produce symptoms from unsupported bradycardia. While hysteresis was designed for the patient with intermittent bradycardia as a simple energy saving mechanism permitting normal conduction and intrinsic heart rates for most of the time, its use without thoughtful programming of rate frequently leads to 100% pacing since many patients are unable to develop a heart rate high enough to inhibit the pulse generator once it has been triggered.

DDD PACING

The benefits of the maintenance of AV synchrony became particularly apparent in patients postoperatively following cardiac surgery. Improved blood pressure and cardiac output could often be related to the maintenance of AV synchrony. However, neither VAT nor DVI devices could track atrial activity, provide AV nodal replacement, and maintain AV synchrony under all conditions. Technical developments in hybrid and microcircuit design made possible the development of devices that function in the DDD mode with sensing and pacing in both chambers. A device that can be programmed to the DDD mode is, in effect, 2 separate pacing devices interconnected with logic circuitry.

The DDD mode's prime "objective" is to prohibit an RR interval from being longer than that corresponding to the programmed lower rate of the pacemaker. In the DDD mode the cardiac cycle is divided into 2 periods: the AV interval and the VA interval. Electrocardiographic interpretation is greatly facilitated by thinking of these 2 basic intervals in DDD timing. Thus, following a sensed or paced ventricular event and the appropriate refractory periods, both atrial and ventricular channels are alert. The next "expected event" would be the appearance of a P wave. This is expected with an interval corresponding to that of the lower rate minus the programmed AV delay. For example, if the device is programmed to a lower rate of 60 beats/min, the corresponding RR interval is 1,000 msec. If the device's AV delay is programmed to 200 msec, then a P wave would be expected within the 800 msec following a ventricular event. If a P wave does not occur during this VA interval, the device stimulates the atrium and remains alert for the expected occurrence of a QRS complex within the programmed AV delay. If a QRS does not occur, a ventricular stimulus is emitted. During the AV delay, with the exception of the blanking period, the ventricular channel remains alert for the occurrence of premature ventricular contractions and may pace asynchronously if such an event occurs in the crosstalk sensing window. In this fashion, the device senses and paces in both chambers (Figs. 8, 9). Thus, the DDD mode was conceived to be the universal (ideal) or physiologic pacing mode.

However, there were a number of problems with early DDD devices that have required software-based engineering solutions. These problems were related to preserved VA conduction and upper rate response, and are discussed below.

PACEMAKER-MEDIATED TACHYCARDIA

Approximately 25% of patients with complete anterograde AV block have preserved VA conduction. In addition, many patients with sinus node disease have intact retrograde conduc-

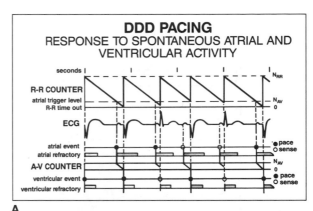

A

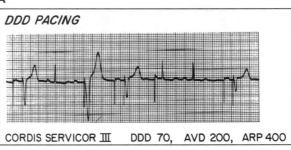

CORDIS SERVICOR III   DDD 70,   AVD 200,   ARP 400

B

Figure 8. *DDD timing diagram (A) and EKG (B). In the EKG the first complex illustrates atrioventricular pacing with fusion between pacemaker stimulus artifact and QRS. The second complex shows spontaneous atrial activity with normal AV conduction. The third complex is P-triggered ventricular pacing. The fourth complex again shows AV pacing with ventricular fusion and the fifth, atrial pacing with normal AV conduction and suppression of ventricular output. Although at first glance, this strip appears confusing, it outlines all the appropriate and normal responses of a system programmed to the DDD mode. (Panel A courtesy J. W. Harthorne.)*

tion.[28,29] Retrograde conduction is most frequently seen after a premature ventricular contraction, (PVC), but may also occur in dual-chamber systems when there is atrial undersensing or loss of atrial capture.[30] The retrograde P wave seen by the sense amplifier of current pulse generators is electronically indistinguishable from a sinus P wave; however, theoretic studies indicate that it may, in the future, be possible to separate the 2 entities.[31-33] If a current dual-chamber device's atrial channel is not refractory when a retrograde P wave occurs, it senses this as another P wave and initiates an AV delay; assuming that no intrinsic ventricular event occurs, there would next be a ventricular paced event followed by another retrograde P wave. This endless loop, in which macro-reentry

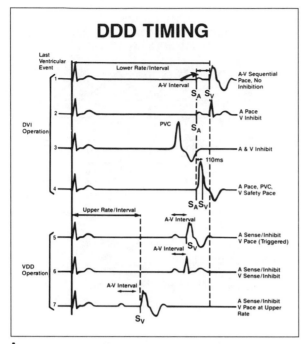

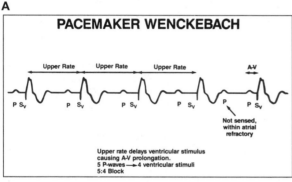

Figure 9. *(A) The variety of responses possible for a dual-chamber pacemaker programmed to the DDD mode. (B) Pacemaker Wenkebach. (Courtesy J. W. Harthorne.)*

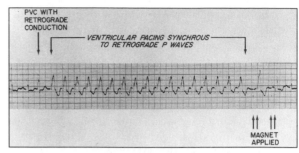

Figure 10. *Pacemaker-mediated tachycardia. Note the initiation by a premature ventricular contraction with retrograde conduction and its termination by applying a magnet to the pacemaker (disabling its sensing functions) and interrupting the "endless" feedback loop.*

occurs utilizing the pacemaker as the antegrade limb and the native conduction system as the retrograde limb could continue indefinitely as long as VA conduction is maintained, producing a "pacemaker-mediated" tachycardia (Fig. 10). Characteristically the tachycardia rate is exactly at, or a little below, the upper-rate limit programmed in the pulse generator. Since the pacemaker cannot violate the upper-rate limit, paced tachycardias of any mechanism can never be faster than this programmed value.

These pacemaker-mediated or "endless loop" tachycardias (PMT) were common early in DDD experience and engendered a number of inge-

nious programmable and automatic software features to prevent or treat the arrhythmia.[34] The initiation of the tachycardia could be partially avoided by rendering the atrial channel refractory during and immediately following a ventricular event. This period, known as the post ventricular atrial refractory period (PVARP), was a fixed interval of approximately 250 msec in early devices. It quickly became clear that ventriculo-atrial conduction was a dynamic phenomenon at times occurring at relatively long intervals and producing P waves outside these short refractory periods. Pacemaker mediated tachycardia often occurred and presented formidable problems when a wide range of physiologic heart rates were required. In order to prevent the initiation of PMT, the PVARP had to be prolonged, thereby significantly limiting upper-rate limit programmability since the atrial channel alert period for each cardiac cycle was curtailed. At present, the PVARP is programmable on all currently available devices and must be adjusted to prevent sensing of retrograde P waves in patients with VA conduction. A large number of engineering and pharmacologic solutions to the problem of PMT, some ingenious, some clinically unattractive, have been suggested.[35-41]

In newer devices a number of PVARP extension options are available after the pulse generator recognizes a PVC (defined as a ventricular event not preceded by an atrial event). This enables the use of a shorter PVARP permitting higher upper rates for most of the time, with PVARP extension occurring only after an event

---

Table 6. Management Strategies for Pacemaker-Mediated Tachycardia

Manual Termination
    Apply Magnet: This disables atrial sensing by converting pacemaker to DOO mode.
    Vagal maneuver (e.g., Carotid massage or Valsalva): This blocks retrograde VA conduction.

Automatic Termination
    Atrial insensitivity for a single event if the pacemaker operates at the upper rate limit for a specific number of paced ventricular events.
    Mode switch to DVI or VVI at a preselected (fallback) rate prior to resumption of atrial sensing.

Prevention
    Program the PVARP beyond the measured retrograde conduction time.
    Automatic PVARP extension (typically to 400 msec) after a PVC. This does not prevent PMT initiation by other less common mechanisms.

---

likely to trigger PMT. Table 6 illustrates other methods of PMT management.

UPPER-RATE RESPONSES

The DDD mode of pacing was originally thought to be "universal" or "physiologic" because of the ability to pace the heart at physiologic rates as determined by the sinus node. P-triggered ventricular pacing is permitted for the range of heart rates between the lower-rate and upper-rate limits, retaining for the patient (if sinus node function is normal), the ability to increase ventricular rate with increasing sinus rates up to the upper-rate limit. The absolute upper-rate limit at which 2:1 AV block occurs is a function of the 2 periods of atrial refractoriness: the AV delay, and the PVARP; these values (in msec) added together produce the total atrial refractory period (TARP). The atrial rate at which 2:1 block occurs (in bpm) can be calculated by dividing 60,000 by the TARP. The development of 2:1 AV block is usually highly symptomatic and should be avoided by judicious programming.

In all modern dual-chamber pulse generators the upper-rate limit and the components of the TARP are separately programmable thereby permitting a number of possible upper-rate behaviors. For example, if the TARP is 500 msec (corresponding to a 2:1 AV block rate of 120 bpm), and the upper-rate limit is programmed to 130 bpm, the pacemaker will respond to an increased atrial rate by abruptly developing 2:1 AV block at 120 beats/min and will not ever reach the programmed upper-rate limit; in this scenario the de facto upper-rate limit is determined by the TARP. If the programmed upper-rate limit is now set below the TARP (100 bpm, for example), the pacing system behaves differently with increased atrial rates. Figure 9B illustrates such a scenario: once the ventricular rate reaches the programmed upper-rate limit, lengthening of the AV interval occurs with further increases in the atrial rate until a P wave falls in the PVARP and block of a single beat occurs. This is known as pacemaker Wenckebach behavior, and is a function of continued atrial sensing during a tachycardia that has reached the programmed upper-rate limit.

It will be seen from the foregoing discussion that enabling a wide range of physiologic heart rates in the context of preserved VA conduction is a challenge to the physician's evaluation and programming skills in order to prevent both PMT and inappropriately low upper-rate limits. Recently, a number of manufacturers have helped in this task by producing pulse generators with rate adaptive AV delay.[42] This programmable feature gradually shortens the AV interval with increasing sinus node rates as occurs in normal physiology. Shortening the AV delay also allows higher upper-rates to be achieved prior to the development of 2:1 AV block. Management options for the patient with intermittent atrial arrhythmias leading to nonphysiologic upper-rate pacing are outlined in Table 7.

Table 7. Indications for Rate-Modulated Pacemakers and Programmed Pacing Modes

Single-Chamber
    AAIR: Chronotropic incompetence with normal AV conduction (rare).
    VVIR: Fixed atrial arrhythmias with slow ventricular response.

Dual-Chamber
    DDDR: Chronotropic incompetence with abnormal AV conduction (unusual).
    DDDR: Requirement for high-paced rates when retrograde conduction is preserved (frequent in young patients).
    DDDR with automatic mode switching to VVIR: Predominant sinus rhythm with intermittent atrial tachyarrhythmias (common).
    DDIR: Predominant sinus rhythm with intermittent atrial tachyarrhythmias (common).

RATE-MODULATED PACING

The ideal candidate for a dual-chamber pacemaker programmed to the DDD mode is a patient with AV block and normal sinus node function. The dual-chamber device will restore the patient's AV integrity by replacing the AV node, and the heart rate will be determined by the efficient integration of neurologic, hemodynamic, and hormonal influences upon sinus node behavior. The normal heart rate response to exercise will occur with P wave-triggered ventricular pacing as the patient's sinus rate increases. However, many candidates for cardiac pacing may not present with such ideal circumstances. Often the patient with a documented symptomatic bradyarrhythmia has sclerodegenerative conduction system disease, affecting the entire conduction pathway in the heart from the SA node through the His Purkinje system. In addition, these patients may have episodic atrial tachyarrhythmias, and/or sinus bradycardia with inappropriate sinus node responses to exercise. In the case of those with established atrial tachyarrhythmias, AV synchrony can not and should not be maintained. In those patients with atrial fibrillation, effective atrial contraction is lost and the maintenance of AV synchrony with pacing is no longer possible.

In the quest to normalize AV conduction and exercise response, engineers and clinicians have attempted to duplicate the sinus node response to exercise.[43] The first of these attempts to become applicable in clinical cardiac pacing was the development of a piezoelectric sensor that reflected body motion/vibration. Body motion and motion of the large muscle groups corre-

lates well with exercise. Exercise in turn, is associated with an increased sinus rate in healthy individuals. The incorporation of such a sensor into a cardiac pacemaker allows the development of a device responsive not only to intrinsic cardiac electrical events, but to body motion as well. Such devices have become widely used in patients with fixed, established atrial fibrillation or flutter and have been shown to be effective in increasing objective exercise performance over single-chamber non-rate modulated pacing.[44,45] Although body motion correlates well with physiologic demand to exercise, it may poorly reflect body demands under certain conditions, such as walking down stairs, in which the sensor indicated rate is consistently higher than walking upstairs. Also, helicopter travel has been shown to drive up the sensor rate in these vibration-sensitive pacemakers. Clearly this sensor cannot respond to mental stress, a problem with most putative biosensors. Minute ventilation derived by integration of transthoracic impedance measurements between pacing lead anode and pacemaker has recently gained wide acceptance as a valid biosensor closely reflective of physiologic demand during many types of exertion.[46] This sensor is incorporated in single- and dual-chamber pacemakers released in the United States and performs well, although there have been concerns about device longevity since the sensor requires the emission of a constant low-energy pulse of current in order to measure impedance. In addition, this sensor performs inappropriately in artificially ventilated patients and should be disabled under such circumstances.

Recently, sensors (predominantly those based upon body movement or minute ventilation)

Table 8. Options for the Prevention of Rapid Ventricular Rates During Intermittent Atrial Arrhythmias in Patients With Dual-Chamber Pacemakers

IN DDD PACEMAKERS WITHOUT RATE MODULATION

1. Reduce upper rate limit in DDD mode.
   Disadvantage: Inability to track physiologically normal rapid sinus rates.
2. Program to DVI or DDI mode.
   Disadvantage: Inability to track atrial rate during normal sinus activity; DVI pacing may cause atrial fibrillation by asynchronous atrial pacing.
3. Retriggering of TARP by intrinsic atrial event occurring within TARP ("dual demand"); pacemaker therefore functions in DVI mode during atrial arrhythmias with asynchronous atrial pacing at the lower-rate limit.
   Disadvantage: May facilitate atrial fibrillation.
4. Program to VVI mode.
   Disadvantage: Loss of atrioventricular synchrony during sinus rhythm.

IN DDDR (RATE-MODULATED) PACEMAKERS

1. Program to DDIR mode.
   Disadvantage: Inability to track atrial rates above the lower rate is controlled only by the sensor.
2. Automatic mode switch to VVIR when atrial events are sensed within the TARP with automatic reversion to DDDR mode when the atrial arrhythmia terminates.
   Disadvantage: Frequent atrial premature beats can lead to long periods of VVIR pacing with associated loss of atrioventricular synchrony.
3. Conditional ventricular tracking limit which limits tracking of rapid atrial rates when the sensor indicates no activity is being performed.
   Disadvantage: Prevents tracking of appropriate sinus tachycardias not associated with biosensor triggering (e.g., fever, anxiety); this may lead to 2:1 block.
4. Program to VVIR mode.
   Disadvantage: Loss of atrioventricular synchrony during sinus rhythm.

have been added to dual-chamber devices for use in a rate-modulated DDD mode. These "DDDR" devices are gaining wider popularity for use in patients for whom the maintenance of rate response and AV synchrony seem clinically important. The main indication for rate responsive dual-chamber pacemaker implantation is the presence of "chronotropic incompetence," a condition that has been historically difficult to define but which describes an inadequate elevation in sinus node rate to exercise or other stress. A number of operational definitions and standardized exercise tests for the assessment of chronotropic incompetence have been developed,[47] and indications for sensor-based systems are suggested in Table 7.

There are, however a number of other important indications for the use of a rate-responsive dual-chamber mode of pacing. Patients with frequent episodes of atrial arrhythmias (either atrial flutter/fibrillation, or atrial tachycardias in association with tachycardia/bradycardia syndrome) may benefit from a change in pacing mode at the onset of such a tachycardia. This so-called "mode switching" (usually to VVIR mode) prevents tracking of high atrial rates and permits physiologic pacing for the duration of the arrhythmia. When the episode terminates, the pacemaker automatically reverts to the dual-chamber mode. This automatic mode switching feature permits physiologic pacing in patients with paroxysmal atrial arrhythmias who are in sinus rhythm for most of the time. In pacemakers that do not possess this automatic mode switching feature it may be helpful to use the DDIR mode in patients with frequent atrial tachyarrhythmias.[48] This mode prevents tracking of atrial activity at any rate but permits the sensor to determine the heart rate with preserved AV synchrony when the patient is in sinus rhythm. Other strategies for managing atrial arrhythmias in patients with pacemakers are outlined in Table 8.

A third emerging indication for the use of DDDR pulse generators is in young patients with preserved VA conduction who require rapid rates with exercise; using the DDDR mode to drive the pacemaker during exercise may allow development of very rapid rates since the sensor derived rate may be programmed higher than the TARP-derived rate at which 2:1 block develops.

Other potential biosensors including those that measure central venous temperature, oxygen saturation or pH, QT interval, and pre-ejection period have been developed and are at various stages of preclinical and clinical evaluation for use in pacemakers in the United States.[49-51] The latter 2 sensors offer the possibility of rate-response to mental as well as physical stress since their outputs are significantly determined by neural and catecholamine influences. A potential disadvantage of devices utilizing central venous blood measurements is that they all require a special lead with a sensor (such as a thermistor or light source for saturation measurements) incorporated in the lead body. These sensors add bulk and complexity to the lead and have a history of unreliability in long-term implants. A challenge for the future is to evaluate the relationship between the improved objective measurements of exercise tolerance and an improved subjective feeling of well-being. Further, all rate-modulated devices currently require careful and individualized programming and follow-up to achieve maximum benefit.[52] This requires more careful postimplant evaluation and follow-up than has generally been the practice in the past for non-rate-modulated systems. Future devices may incorporate sensors that permit autocalibration of sensor to patient, as well as other automated programmability. A number of manufacturers are currently developing dual sensor-based pacemaker systems. It is hoped that such devices will permit more appropriate heart rate determinations for the patient's level of activity by use of sensor "cross-checking" and other software-based algorithms.[53,54]

CLINICAL PACEMAKER SELECTION

A large variety of pacemakers are in clinical use. Each system has a limited number of programmable modes and other features. It is therefore important that careful thought be given each patient's current and likely future requirements at the time of implantation. An important and still unresolved debate in the pacemaker literature is the importance of atrial-based pacing modes in patients who are mostly or always in sinus rhythm. There is consistent and compelling data from a number of large studies indicating that such patients who are paced in the VVI mode more frequently develop atrial fibrillation, heart failure, stroke, and death than do patients who are paced in the DDD or other atrial-based mode.[55-60] These studies are all retrospective, however, and a number of prospective randomized trials are currently underway in order to examine these important issues. In addition, there is considerable debate as to the frequency with which patients paced in the AAI mode later develop distal conduction system disease requiring "upgrade" to a dual-chamber system.[62-66]

INTERFERENCE WITH PACEMAKER FUNCTION

Extraneous signals may interfere with normal pacemaker function.[67] While there is reason to recommend that pacemaker patients do not enter close proximity to arc welding, running automobile engines, powerful radio transmitters or magnets, these exposures are uncommon in both home and occupational environments. Paradoxically, the environment that poses most risk to the pacing system is the hospital. Powerful magnets (MRI), and x-ray sources (radiotherapy) as well as ultrasound beams (lithotripsy) may all transiently or permanently impair pacing and/or sensing functions.[68,69]

Consultation from a pacemaker specialist should be routinely requested for all patients admitted for general surgery and other potentially damaging procedures. Because of the potential for intraoperative damage, it is the consultant's responsibility to ensure that the pacemaker is functioning satisfactorily prior to the operation. This usually entails interrogating the unit and evaluating the sensing and pacing thresholds as well as routine clinical examination and electrocardiography. It is essential at this time to determine if the patient is pacemaker-dependent; for these purposes pacemaker dependency is inferred if sudden inhibition of the pacemaker would lead to hemodynamic embarrassment due to an inadequate escape rate.

Table 9. Perioperative Care of the Pacemaker Patient

General Advice
Use bipolar cautery only.
If cautery has to be unipolar, the indifferent electrode should be as far away from the pacemaker as possible.
Never use cautery within 12 inches of the pacemaker.
Use the shortest bursts of cautery possible.

For the Pacemaker-Dependent Patient (see text)
For older nonprogrammable units, a magnet should be taped over the pulse generator for the duration of the procedure, thus rendering it insensitive.
For all other devices the asynchronous mode (VOO or DOO) should be programmed in the holding area prior to anesthesia induction, and the original mode restored in the recovery room.

SURGERY

The hazards of surgery are largely and most commonly a consequence of the use of electrocautery. The radiofrequency energy used by this technique may be sensed by the pacemaker which is then temporarily inhibited. More worrisome, the circuitry of the pacemaker can also be permanently damaged by cautery. This occurs most frequently in cardiac or open chest surgery where the cautery output is physically close to the pulse generator or electrode, but damage may also occur in any operation if a unipolar pacing system is implanted. Cautery in the chest cavity has also been reported to damage the electrode-tissue interface at the endocardial level and cause dramatic and acute elevations in pacing and sensing thresholds. Occasionally, this endocardial damage has provoked ventricular fibrillation.

In the past, the inappropriate inhibition of the pacemaker by the cautery was overcome by the prior application of a magnet to convert the pacemaker to the asynchronous (insensitive) mode. Currently, this is only recommended for older nonprogrammable devices since most modern pulse generators rely upon magnet application in order to open the telemetry circuit for receipt of new programming instructions. Radiofrequency interference in close proximity to a programmable pacemaker that has a magnet applied is potentially dangerous because reversion to "backup" or "reset" mode may occur. The reset mode is idiosyncratic for each model, but is usually VVI or VOO (even for dual-chamber devices). It usually simulates end-of-life behavior and may require a special pro-

grammer from the manufacturer to restore normal function. Recommended perioperative procedures for the pacemaker patient are outlined in Table 9.

CARDIOVERSION

Patients with pacemakers frequently develop atrial fibrillation requiring direct current (DC) cardioversion. In addition, this procedure may be indicated emergently for other arrhythmias in such patients. The high-voltage pulse delivered during cardioversion and defibrillation may damage pacing systems in a number of ways.[70]

All presently implanted devices are, in theory, protected from the sudden current surge seen during the delivery of an external DC shock. However the "Zener diode" located at the input of the device may protect the sensitive sensing circuitry of the unit at the expense of the lead system. Shunting of current down the pacemaker lead can damage the electrode-tissue interface leading to both acute and, if shocks are repeated, chronic loss of sensing and capture. Older pacemakers and modern units may all be damaged by external defibrillation. Reprogramming, as with electrocautery, and permanent damage to the pulse generator have been reported for a wide range of pacemakers. An unusual but serious complication of external DC shocks in the patient with a programmable-polarity pacemaker as well as an implanted defibrillator is reversion of the pacemaker to the unipolar backup mode causing inappropriate internal shocks due to double or triple counting of both the pacemaker artifact and the evoked electrogram. Table

Table 10. Care of the Pacemaker Patient Undergoing External Cardioversion/Defibrillation

Keep paddles as far from pulse generator as possible.

Use AP paddle orientation if possible.

Titrate dose of electrical energy used.

If procedure is elective, evaluate pacing and sensing prior to and after cardioversion.

If patient is pacemaker-dependent program to asynchronous mode (VOO or DOO) prior to cardioversion.

---

10 provides general advice for the care of patients undergoing cardioversion.

TROUBLESHOOTING

Successful implantation of a pacing system is not a panacea against the development of other symptoms. Thus, when patients with pacemakers develop other illnesses or associated symptoms, one is often asked, "Is the pacemaker working?" When faced with this question, it is first appropriate to ask if there has been any evidence of pacemaker dysfunction and if there is electrocardiographic documentation of it. In addition, the identity of the pacing system must be known or determined from records, the patient's pacemaker identification card, from chest radiography, or other information. Finally, a diagnostic session with the patient, the programmer, and an ECG machine is necessary.

In modern pulse generators, an isolated electronic malfunction is very rare and should never be assumed to be the cause of an apparent malfunction without an exhaustive search for other problems. Most electronic "abnormalities" are in fact an explicable and normal reaction of the pacing system to changing patient conditions, or are the misinterpretation of normal and appropriate function. For example, the failure to sense atrial activity in a device programmed to the DVI mode is normal — not a "failure" of atrial sensing. An exception to this rule is that the loss of atrial sensing in dual-chamber devices programmed to the DDD mode is relatively common (especially if the atrial signal was poor at the time of implant).[71] Devices nearing

battery depletion, and pulse generators and leads known to be subject to catastrophic premature failure, may produce unusual electronic manifestations. Only rarely is it necessary to explore a modern pacing system surgically to confirm a diagnosis of pacing system failure. Before surgical exploration is undertaken, the system should be evaluated by a pacemaker specialist to help ensure that unnecessary generator or lead replacement is not performed.

It is always embarrassing for the physician when a patient with a pacemaker returns with recurrent syncope. It is important during the analysis of a potential pacing system malfunction, that a witnessed ECG anomaly is shown to be causative of the symptoms noted. For example, myopotential triggering or inhibition is very easily and commonly provoked in unipolar pacing systems programmed to high sensitivities.[25] However, this phenomenon is often only of electrocardiographic significance — the triggering or inhibition may not be causing any clinical symptoms. Its mere electrocardiographic presence does not necessarily indicate a "malfunction." Thus, the correlation of clinical symptoms with pacemaker performance is of utmost importance before deciding that an anomaly is of clinical significance.

True pacing system malfunction should always be considered in patients in whom symptoms for which the pacing system was implanted recur, particularly if this occurs long after the system has been in place. Recurrent syncope, dizziness, or light-headedness are potential manifestations. The report of such symptoms merits a full and complete pacemaker evaluation. This, of course, begins with obtaining a complete history. Careful attention should be paid to the analysis of activities that may elicit symptoms. In particular, for unipolar systems, the use of the upper extremity on the side of the pacemaker implant may cause myopotential inhibition of pacemaker output. This can lead to the recurrence of symptoms of dizziness, light-headedness, or syncope associated with activity such as combing the hair.[25] Postural dizziness, on the other hand, is a frequent symptom in elderly individuals and may not represent a recurrent bradyarrhythmia or pacing failure. The occurrence of episodic symptoms immediately after pacemaker implantation, may indicate that the pacing system, despite normal operation, has not relieved the symptom for which it was placed. Symptoms from carotid sinus hypersensitivity, for example, may be blunted by rate support from a pacemaker, but the vasodepressor component of the condition may not be controlled even by a properly functioning dual-chamber system.[13]

Physical examination in a symptomatic patient with a pacemaker should concentrate first on potential nonpacemaker-related problems that may induce symptoms. For example, aortic stenosis, carotid bruits, carotid sinus vasodepressor effects, atrial myxoma, hypertrophic cardiomyopathy, and other central nervous system disorders should be checked. Postural vital signs should be recorded with the pacing system programmed to allow the patients underlying rhythm, if any, be dominant and recorded again with pacing. At times, the onset of ventricular pacing while standing, results in sufficient hypotension to cause light-headedness or syncope, whereas the onset of pacing with the patient in the supine position does not induce symptoms. The search for myopotential inhibition or triggering with the patient in various positions is also important. In addition, careful inspection of the pulse generator site, tugging on the pulse generator, and pressing on the underlying lead can bring out potential component malfunction such as a loose setscrew or lead fracture. With the exception of device or lead failures, much inappropriate pacemaker function such as the presence of pacemaker-mediated tachycardia, myopotential inhibition, or triggering can be remedied with reprogramming after such a diagnostic session.

In some instances, even after a careful history, physical examination and pacemaker evaluation, the relationship of the pacing system to a symptom remains obscure. Under these conditions, it becomes important to obtain an ECG recording during a symptom. This can be accomplished if symptoms are frequent (daily) with continuous ambulatory ECG (Holter) monitoring. If symptoms are less frequent, loop-type event recording should be undertaken until a symptomatic ECG is recorded. Real-time transtelephonic transmission alone is inadequate because by the time communication is established, symptoms have usually abated.

Examination of a putatively dysfunctional pacemaker ECG record should be performed systematically with all information about the device and its programmed characteristics available. Evidence of loss of capture is usually readily apparent from a pacemaker artifact that does not result in an atrial or ventricular event. Evidence of inappropriate sensing (either oversensing or undersensing) often has to be deduced from knowledge of the programmed timing cycles in the device. Oversensing is apparent when no pacemaker output is seen at a point on the ECG recording where such output is expected from knowledge of the programmed settings in the device. Undersensing is observed when an intrinsic cardiac event fails to inhibit subsequent pacemaker output.

Every implanted pulse generator, given sufficient time, will develop power source depletion. Each manufacturer has adopted its own indicators for battery depletion. In modern telemetric pacemakers, there are usually multiple indicators including direct information on battery voltage and impedance. Most commonly, a rate decrease and/or a pacing pulse width increase (with, or without magnet application) accompany battery depletion. In general, the slope of this decrease is sufficiently shallow to offer 6 months to 1 year of reliable pacing even after the manifestations of battery depletion have occurred. Each manufacturer has designated an elective replacement time (ERT) that reflects the time at which the pulse generator should be replaced. In the vast majority of devices, battery depletion is a predictable slowly-occurring phenomenon. It is this need for timely identification of power source depletion that is the fundamental rationale for pacemaker follow-up; much of this surveillance can now be done from the patient's home by telephone transmission of the patient's rhythm with and without magnet application over the pulse generator.

Pacemaker leads, though much more reliable than in the past, are still the weak link in the chain of pacemaker performance. Lead components can fail either because of insulation failure or because of conductor break. Broken conductors can make intermittent contact and the lead can appear to function perfectly normally at times. When traction is applied and the broken conductor and the ends no longer touch, failure of both sensing and pacing can occur. Most often, conduction fracture results in complete sensing and pacing failure. Careful evaluation of the chest x-ray may reveal the problem. However, a more accurate test is fluoroscopy of the pacing system under conditions which allow the observer to place traction on the pacemaker and/or the lead.

Insulation failure is sometimes more difficult to detect. Lead impedance, where it can be obtained by telemetry, may decrease if the failure is incomplete and current is lost to extracardiac sources. This can also result in extracardiac stimulation or myopotential sensing. In the case of lead or insulation failure, pacing system function is unreliable and the lead should be replaced.

Most lead "failures" are actually a failure of the electrode-tissue interface. Following implantation, as edema develops around the stimulating electrode, endocardial potentials fall and pacing thresholds rise. In the ventricle, these return to approximately 80% of baseline within about 8 weeks. Because of the large size of ventricular electrograms, the failure of ventricular sensing is uncommon. However, during this period of "acute threshold rise," atrial-sensing failure is more common. In the acute phase, should atrial-sensing failure occur, fluoroscopy should be performed to rule out gross lead dislodgment. If the lead is not dislodged, it is usually best to wait several weeks and re-evaluate the performance periodically to determine if sensing function has returned before repositioning the lead.

The best protection against an unanticipated and untreated pacemaker failure is for patients to be followed by a pacemaker clinic that can perform and interpret periodic transtelephonic monitoring and conduct "in-person" testing. Though malfunction of a modern well-implanted system is uncommon, periodic evaluation of the pacing system in an organized way by an expert physician, nurse, or technician will often prevent the rare catastrophe.

SUMMARY

Cardiac pacing has evolved from the simple implantation of fixed-rate devices into the prescription, implantation, and follow-up of sophisticated computer-based rhythm control systems. However, the basic principles of thorough patient evaluation and follow-up have changed little. This short review can only begin to point out some of the more important issues in cardiac pacing. The clinician confronted with a pacemaker problem must approach it logically

and with knowledge of both the electronic and clinical factors involved. He or she must demonstrate integrity in the prescription of pacing devices, pay meticulous attention to detail in performing the implantation procedure and, provide methodical assessment during follow-up. No clinician can remember all the nuances of pacemaker function and it is perhaps more important to recognize when one's knowledge is incomplete than it is to forge ahead with unquestioning self-assurance.

REFERENCES

1. Elmqvist R, Senning. An implantable pacemaker for the heart. In: *Proceedings of the Second International Conference on Medical Electronics*. London: Iliffe; 1960:253.
2. Friedberg CK, Donoso E, Stein WB. Nonsurgical acquired heart block. *Ann N Y Acad Sci.*. 1964;111:833-847.
3. Gadboys HL, Wisoff BG, Litwak RS. Surgical treatment of complete heart block: an analysis of 36 cases. *JAMA.* 1964;189:97-102.
4. Donmoyer TL, DeSanctis RW, Austen WG. Experience with implantable pacemakers using myocardial electrodes in the management of heart block. *Ann Thorac Surg.* 1967;3:213-227.
5. Edhag O, Swahn A. Prognosis of patients with complete heart block or arrhythmic syncope who were not treated with artificial pacemakers: a long term follow up study of 101 patients. *Acta Med Scand.* 1976;200:457-463.
6. Parsonnet V, Furman S, Smyth NP, et al. Optimal resources for implantable cardiac pacemakers. Pacemaker Study Group. *Circulation.* 1983;68:226A-244A.
7. Dreifus LS, Fisch C, Griffin JC, et al. Guidelines for implantation of cardiac pacemakers and antiarrhythmia devices. A report of the American College of Cardiology/ American Heart Association Task Force on Assessment of Diagnostic and Therapeutic Cardiovascular Procedures (Committee on Pacemaker Implantation). *J Am Coll Cardiol.* 1991;18:1-13.
8. Bernstein AD, Parsonnet V. Survey of cardiac pacing in the United States in 1989. *Am J Cardiol.* 1992;69:331-338.
9. Goldman BS, Fraser JD, Morgan CD. Survey of cardiac pacing in Canada. *Can J Cardiol.* 1991;7:391-398.
10. Falk RH. Impact of prospective peer review on pacemaker implantation rates in Massachusetts [see comments]. *J Am Coll Cardiol.* 1990;15:1087-1092.
11. Wyse DG, Gillis AM. Funding for cardiac pacing and defibrillators in Calgary: The Robin Hood philosophy. *PACE Pacing Clin Electrophysiol.* 1993;16:2305-2309.
12. McAlister HF, Klementowicz PT, Andrews C, et al. Lyme carditis: an important cause of reversible heart block [see comments]. *Ann Intern Med.* 1989;110:339-345.
13. Sra JS, Jazayeri MR, Avitall B, et al. Comparison of cardiac pacing with drug therapy in the treatment of neurocardiogenic (vasovagal) syncope with bradycardia or asystole [see comments]. *N Engl J Med.* 1993;328:

1085-1090.

14. Hochleitner M, Hortnagl H, Fridrich L, et al. Long-term efficacy of physiologic dual-chamber pacing in the treatment of end-stage idiopathic dilated cardiomyopathy. *Am J Cardiol.* 1992;70:1320-1325.

15. McAreavey D, Fananapazir L. Altered cardiac hemodynamic and electrical state in normal sinus rhythm after chronic dual-chamber pacing for relief of left ventricular outflow obstruction in hypertrophic cardiomyopathy. *Am J Cardiol.* 1992;70:651-656.

16. Fananapazir L, Cannon RO, Tripodi D, et al. Impact of dual-chamber permanent pacing in patients with obstructive hypertrophic cardiomyopathy with symptoms refractory to verapamil and beta-adrenergic blocker therapy. *Circulation.* 1992;85:2149-2161.

17. Greatbatch W. Pacemaker technology: energy sources. *Cardiovasc Clin.* 1983;14:239-246.

18. Hauser RG, Wimer EA, Timmis GC, et al. Twelve years of clinical experience with lithium pulse generators. *PACE Pacing Clin Electrophysiol.* 1986;9:1277-1281.

19. Wittkampf FH, Candelon B, van Arragon GW. The importance of software programmable pacemakers: in vivo programming of a prototype device. *PACE Pacing Clin Electrophysiol.* 1984;7:1207-1212.

20. Benedek ZM, Furman S. The role of the computer in cardiac pacemaker technology. *PACE Pacing Clin Electrophysiol.* 1984;7:1217-1227.

21. Ripart A, Fontaine G, Mugica J. How should the software pacemaker be programmed during manufacturing and after implantation? *PACE Pacing Clin Electrophysiol.* 1984;7:1202-1206.

22. Segerstad CH, Lekholm A, Elmqvist H. Pacemaker architecture: a pacemaker with an attached computer or a computer with an attached pacemaker. *PACE Pacing Clin Electrophysiol.* 1984;7:1213-1216.

23. Harthorne JW. Pacemaker leads. *Int J Cardiol.* 1984;6:423-429.

24. Mond HG, Stokes KB. The electrode-tissue interface: the revolutionary role of steroid elution. *PACE Pacing Clin Electrophysiol.* 1992;5:95-107.

25. Gross JN, Platt S, Ritacco R, et al. The clinical relevance of electromyopotential oversensing in current unipolar devices. *PACE Pacing Clin Electrophysiol.* 1992;15:2023-2027.

26. Mond HG. Unipolar versus bipolar pacing — poles apart. *PACE Pacing Clin Electrophysiol.* 1991;14:1411-1424.

27. Folkman MJ, Watkins E. An artificial conduction system for the management of experimental complete heart block. *Surg Forum.* 1958;8:331.

28. Klementowicz P, Ausubel K, Furman S. The dynamic nature of ventriculoatrial conduction. *PACE Pacing Clin Electrophysiol.* 1986;9:1050-1054.

29. Hayes DL, Furman S. Atrioventricular and ventriculo-atrial conduction times in patients undergoing pacemaker implant. *PACE Pacing Clin Electrophysiol.* 1983;6:38-46.

30. Frumin H, Furman S. Endless loop tachycardia started by an atrial premature complex in a patient with a dual chamber pacemaker. *J Am Coll Cardiol.* 1985;5:707-710.

31. McAlister HF, Klementowicz PT, Calderon EM, et al. Atrial electrogram analysis: antegrade versus retrograde. *PACE Pacing Clin Electrophysiol.* 1988;11:1703-1707.

32. Pannizzo F, Amikam S, Bagwell P, et al. Discrimination of antegrade and retrograde atrial depolarization by electrogram analysis. *Am Heart J.* 1986;112:780-786.

33. Throne RD, Jenkins JM, Winston SA, et al. Discrimination of retrograde from anterograde atrial activation using intracardiac electrogram waveform analysis. *PACE Pacing Clin Electrophysiol.* 1989;12:1622-1630.

34. Harthorne JW, Eisenhauer AC, Steinhaus DM. Pacemaker-mediated tachycardias: an unresolved problem. *PACE Pacing Clin Electrophysiol.* 1984;7:1140-1147.

35. Calfee RV. Pacemaker-mediated tachycardia: engineering solutions. *PACE Pacing Clin Electrophysiol.* 1988;11:1917-1928.

36. Greenspon AJ, Greenberg RM. Noninvasive evaluation of retrograde conduction times to avoid pacemaker-mediated tachycardia. *J Am Coll Cardiol.* 1985;5:1403-1406.

37. Duncan JL, Clark MF. Prevention and termination of pacemaker-mediated tachycardia in a new DDD pacing system (Siemens-Pacesetter model 2010T). *PACE Pacing Clin Electrophysiol.* 1988;11:1679-1683.

38. Pitney M, Davis M. Catheter ablation of ventriculoatrial conduction in the treatment of pacemaker-mediated tachycardia [see comments]. *PACE Pacing Clin Electrophysiol.* 1991;14:1013-1017.

39. Lamaison D, Girodo S, Limousin M. A new algorithm for a high level of protection against pacemaker-mediated tachycardia. *PACE Pacing Clin Electrophysiol.* 1988;11:1715-1721.

40. Nitzsche R, Gueunoun M, Lamaison D, et al. Endless-loop tachycardias: description and first clinical results of a new fully automatic protection algorithm. *PACE Pacing Clin Electrophysiol.* 1990;13:1711-1718.

41. Barold SS, Falkoff MD, Ong LS, et al. Pacemaker endless loop tachycardia: termination by simple techniques other than magnet application. *Am J Med.* 1988;85:817-822.

42. Mehta D, Gilmour S, Ward DE, et al. Optimal atrioventricular delay at rest and during exercise in patients with dual chamber pacemakers: a non-invasive assessment by continuous wave Doppler. *Br Heart J.* 1989;61:161-166.

43. Furman S. Rate-modulated pacing. *Circulation.* 1990;82:1081-1094.

44. Abrahamsen AM, Barvik S, Aarsland T, et al. Rate responsive cardiac pacing using a minute ventilation sensor. *PACE Pacing Clin Electrophysiol.* 1993;16:1650-1655.

45. Pollak A, Falk RH. Pacemaker therapy in patients with atrial fibrillation. *Am Heart J.* 1993;125:824-830.

46. Lau CP, Antoniou A, Ward DE, et al. Reliability of minute ventilation as a parameter for rate responsive pacing. *PACE Pacing Clin Electrophysiol.* 1989;12:321-330.

47. Wilkoff BL, Miller RE. Exercise testing for chronotropic assessment. *Cardiol Clin.* 1992;10:705-717.

48. Vanerio G, Maloney JD, Pinski SL, et al. DDIR versus VVIR pacing in patients with paroxysmal atrial tachyarrhythmias. *PACE Pacing Clin Electrophysiol.* 1991;14:1630-1638.

49. Lau CP, Butrous GS, Ward DE, et al. Comparison of exercise performance of six rate-adaptive right ventricular cardiac pacemakers. *Am J Cardiol.* 1989;63:833-838.

50. Lau CP, Ward DE, Camm AJ. Single-chamber cardiac pacing with two forms of respiration-controlled rate-responsive pacemaker. *Chest.* 1989;95:352-358.

51. Lau CP, Stott JR, Toff WD, et al. Selective vibration sens-

ing: a new concept for activity-sensing rate-responsive pacing. *PACE Pacing Clin Electrophysiol.* 1988;11:1299-1309.

52. McAlister HF, Soberman J, Klementowicz P, et al. Treadmill assessment of an activity-modulated pacemaker: the importance of individual programming. *PACE Pacing Clin Electrophysiol.* 1989;12:486-501.

53. Paul V, Garratt C, Camm AJ. Combination of sensors to provide optimal pacing rate response. *Clin Cardiol.* 1989;12:400-404.

54. Cowell R, Morris-Thurgood J, Paul V, et al. Are we being driven to two sensors?: clinical benefits of sensor cross-checking. *PACE Pacing Clin Electrophysiol.* 1993; 16:1441-1444.

55. Sgarbossa EB, Pinski SL, Maloney JD, et al. Chronic atrial fibrillation and stroke in paced patients with sick sinus syndrome. Relevance of clinical characteristics and pacing modalities. *Circulation.* 1993;88:1045-1053.

56. Hesselson AB, Parsonnet V, Bernstein AD, et al. Deleterious effects of long-term single-chamber ventricular pacing in patients with sick sinus syndrome: the hidden benefits of dual-chamber pacing. *J Am Coll Cardiol.* l992;19:1542-1549.

57. Zanini R, Facchinetti Al, Gallo G, et al. Morbidity and mortality of patients with sinus node disease: comparative effects of atrial and ventricular pacing. *PACE Pacing Clin Electrophysiol.* 1990;13:2076-2079.

58. Santini M, Alexidou G, Ansalone G, et al. Relation of prognosis in sick sinus syndrome to age, conduction defects and modes of permanent cardiac pacing. *Am J Cardiol.* 1990;65:729-735.

59. Sgarbossa EB, Pinski SL, Maloney JD. The role of pacing modality in determining long-term survival in the sick sinus syndrome. *Ann Intern Med.* 1993;119:359-365.

60. Camm AJ, Katritsis D. Ventricular pacing for sick sinus syndrome — a risky business? *PACE Pacing Clin Electrophysiol.* 1990;13:695-699.

61. Katritsis D, Camm AJ. AAI pacing mode: when is it indicated and how should it be achieved? *Clin Cardiol.*

1993;16:339-343.

62. Elshot SR, el Gamal MI, Tielen KH, et al. Incidence of atrioventricular block and chronic atrial flutter/fibrillation after implantation of atrial pacemakers; follow-up of more than ten years. *Int J Cardiol.* 1993;38:303-308.

63. Haywood GA, Ward J, Ward DE, et al. Atrioventricular Wenckebach point and progression to atrioventricular block in sinoatrial disease. *PACE Pacing Clin Electrophysiol.* 1990;13:2054-2058.

64. Sneddon JF, Camm AJ. Sinus node disease. Current concepts in diagnosis and therapy. *Drugs.* 1992;44: 728-737.

65. Brandt J, Anderson H, Fahraeus T, et al. Natural history of sinus node disease treated with atrial pacing in 213 patients: implications for selection of stimulation mode. *J Am Coll Cardiol.* 1992;20:633-639.

66. Rosenqvist M. Atrial pacing for sick sinus syndrome. *Clin Cardiol.* 1990;13:43-47.

67. Kaye GC, Butrous GS, Allen A, et al. The effect of 50 Hz external electrical interference on implanted cardiac pacemakers. *PACE Pacing Clin Electrophysiol.* 1988;11:999-1008.

68. Sager DP. Current facts on pacemaker electromagnetic interference and their application to clinical care. *Heart Lung.* 1987;16:211-221.

69. Cooper DJ, Wilkoff BL, Masterson M, et al. Effects of extracorporeal shock wave lithotripsy on cardiac pacemakers and its safety in patients with implanted cardiac pacemakers. *PACE Pacing Clin Electrophysiol.* l988;11:1607-1616.

70. Levine PA, Barold SS, Fletcher RD, et al. Adverse acute and chronic effects of electrical defibrillation and cardioversion on implanted unipolar cardiac pacing systems. *J Am Coll Cardiol.* 1983;1:1413-1422.

71. Hummel J, Fazio G, Lawrence J, et al. The natural history of dual chamber pacing. *PACE Pacing Clin Electrophysiol.* 1991;14:1745-1747.

CHAPTER **24** The Implantable Cardioverter-Defibrillator: Technology and Clinical Applications

David S. Cannom, MD

HISTORY OF IMPLANTABLE CARDIOVERTER-DEFIBRILLATOR INDICATIONS

The first defibrillator was implanted at The Johns Hopkins Hospital in Baltimore, Maryland, in 1980 in a patient who had had 2 cardiac arrests while receiving medication. The initial investigational protocol restricted the defibrillator to patients with at least 2 prior cardiac arrests incurred while being treated with antiarrhythmic drugs. To qualify for the Intec device between 1980 and 1982, a patient needed the following: 1) a clinical event with electrocardiographic (ECG) documentation of ventricular tachycardia (VT) or ventricular fibrillation (VF) at a time the patient was unconscious; 2) a history of recurrent VT/VF while on antiarrhythmic medications; 3) an electrophysiologic study during which VT or VF was induced and the patient lost consciousness; 4) a life expectancy of 6 months; and 5) emotional maturity and availability for long-term follow-up.[1]

It is probably fortunate that the initial indications for the device were so narrowly defined. Only patients with documented cardiac arrest were eligible for implantation. The initial insistence on an inducible arrhythmia at electrophysiologic study meant that reversible causes of cardiac arrest were excluded. Complete clinical follow-up data were a requisite for implantation. By restricting the device to a population with a known high recurrence rate, the efficacy of the device was tested in the sickest clinical population. Until 1982 the automatic implantable defibillator (AID) device was initially limited to experimental centers, which implanted 54 devices over 20 months.

The indications for the AID device in the clinical trial were relaxed somewhat in 1982 and came to reflect more closely what was finally approved by the Food and Drug Administration (FDA) in 1985. Device availability was expanded to 40 centers during the remainder of the clinical trial. On October 4, 1985, the FDA published approved indications for the automatic implantable cardioverter-defibrillator (AICD) and required that electrophysiologic evaluation be part of the patient's diagnostic work-up.[2] These indications, slightly reworded, include: 1) A patient who has survived at least 1 episode of cardiac arrest presumably due to hemo-dynamically unstable VT/VF and not associated with (i.e., at the time of) acute infarction; and/or 2) A patient who has not had an arrest but has had recurrent ventricular tachyarrhythmias and is inducible into VT and/or VF despite conventional antiarrhythmic drugs.

In 1994, these 2 FDA-approved indications still serve as the standards for defibrillator implantation, although they have since been reworked slightly by 2 expert panels (see below). Beginning in 1985, a documented cardiac arrest was not the sole requisite as it was initially in 1980, and the patient with syncope due to sustained VT was included as an implantable cardioverter-defibrillator (ICD) candidate. The FDA indications also establish electro-physiologic (EP) testing as the cornerstone for evaluating potential patients for the device. During an EP study the induction of the causative ventricular arrhythmia is not required if the patient is the survivor of an episode of cardiac arrest.

The FDA indications assume the implanting physician and hospital will have access to an

483

electrophysiology laboratory. Beyond this, no certification process or documented training is required by the FDA. The manufacturer will sell the device to any licensed physician who states that he or she is trained as an electrophysiologist.

INDICATIONS FOR DEVICE THERAPY: AHA/ACC/NASPE

Two expert panels recently released a summary of indications for the ICD. One was formulated by a combined group from the American College of Cardiology (ACC) and the American Heart Association (AHA) and the other from the North American Society of Pacing and Electrophysiology (NASPE).[3,4] The reports do not differ greatly in substance, nor do they significantly alter the original FDA guidelines (Table 1).

Each divides the possible indications into 3 classes:
- Class I: ICD is indicated by general consensus.
- Class II: ICD is an option but there is not consensus.
- Class III: ICD therapy is generally not justified.

The indications for ICD therapy by class, then, include:

CLASS I INDICATIONS

1) A patient with VT or VF in whom EP testing or Holter monitoring cannot be used to predict efficacy of therapy. This indication is intended to include the patient who is noninducible at EP testing.

2) A patient with recurrent VT or VF despite drug therapy as guided by EP testing or Holter monitoring. This indication covers the patient

---

Table 1. Indications for the ICD (AHA/ACC/NASPE)

Indications for the 1980s
- Survivor of a cardiac arrest (Class I)
- Sustained VT in a patient who at EPS is either (Class I)
  - Noninducible
  - Nonsuppressed with antiarrhythmic drugs
  - Nonsuppressed after ablative surgery or catheter ablation
  - Noncompliant or intolerant of drugs
- Syncope due to sustained VT at EPS (Class II)

Possible new indications for the 1990s (not yet approved)
- Sustained VT without syncope that is pace-terminable (third-generation device candidate)
- CAD patient with EF <40% and nonsustained VT (as defined by CABG-PATCH, MADIT, and MUSTT trials)

ICD Not Indicated (Class III)
- Cardiac arrest or sustained VT associated with
  - Acute myocardial infarction
  - Drugs (type I)
  - Electrolyte imbalance
- Incessant VT or frequent long runs of nonsustained VT
- Syncope not due to sustained VT
- Psychologically unstable patient
- Significant comorbidity

ICD=Implantable cardioverter-defibrillator; AHA=American Heart Association; ACC=American College of Cardiology; NASPE=North American Society of Pacing and Electrophysiology; VT=Ventricular tachycardia; EPS=Electrophysiologic study; CAD=Coronary artery disease; EF=Ejection fraction; CABG-PATCH=Coronary artery bypass grafting surgery plus implantable cardioverter-defibrillator; MADIT=Multicenter Automatic Defibrillator Implantation Trial; MUSTT=Multicenter Unsustained Tachycardia Trial.

who is a clinical failure on antiarrhythmic drugs that were predicted to be effective at initial EP testing.

3) A patient with spontaneous VT or VF in whom drugs are not tolerated or not taken.

4) A patient with VT or VF who remains persistently inducible despite the best drug therapy, surgical therapy, or catheter ablation. This category covers the persistently inducible patient without qualification in terms of the number of drug trials or rate of the tachycardia on drugs.

The indications do not go beyond the original 1985 FDA guidelines. The ACC guidelines mention that the VT must be hemodynamically significant, but NASPE does not.

CLASS II INDICATIONS

1) A patient with syncope of uncertain cause and with sustained VT or VF induced at EP-testing in whom drugs are not tolerated, ineffective, or not taken.

This indication was not clearly specified in the 1985 guidelines, although it was not excluded either.

CLASS III INDICATIONS (CONTRAINDICATIONS)

1) A patient with sustained VT or VF due to acute ischemia, recent infarction, or reversible metabolic/toxic etiologies.

2) A patient with recurrent syncope of uncertain cause who is noninducible.

3) A patient with incessant VT or VF.

4) A patient with VF secondary to the Wolff-Parkinson-White syndrome.

5) A patient with medical, surgical, or psychiatric contraindications.

CONTRAINDICATIONS TO ICD IMPLANTATION

There is no change in contraindications from the 1985 guidelines. The contraindications to device implantation are clearly spelled out in the FDA guidelines and are well substantiated in

clinical practice. It is critical that these contraindications be considered before recommending an ICD for a particular patient.

An episode of VF or VT caused by electrolyte imbalance, usually hypokalemia, is a relatively rare event. The potassium level is often reduced acutely in the cardiac arrest survivor, and it is often difficult to sort out the role of hypokalemia in causing the arrest. More often the patient is hypokalemic and taking an antiarrhythmic drug when cardiac arrest occurs. The approach to such patients is to perform electrophysiologic study when the patient is no longer receiving antiarrhythmics and the potassium level is normal. If the patient is then entirely noninducible, the clinician can consider treating the patient without a device. Such decisions are difficult and often depend on the magnitude of hypokalemia.

It is obvious that a patient with incessant VT is not suitable for surgery until the tachycardia is controlled. Frequent episodes of nonsustained tachycardia also must be controlled with antiarrhythmic medication before a device is implanted. In either case, a patient will receive an unacceptable number of shocks unless preoperative VT is controlled. The flexible programming features and antitachycardia pacing (ATP) function of third-generation devices make these decisions easier.

CURRENT GUIDELINE IMPLEMENTATION IN THE LITERATURE

A review of the early, large, published series of ICD patients discloses a strict adherence to the published FDA guidelines. In the earliest series, all patients had experienced a cardiac arrest,[5] but a sizable percentage (20%–40%) presented with syncope and turned out to have inducible VT at EP study. There is also a sizable proportion of patients (10%–20%) in these series who are noninducible at EP study.[5,6]

In the Cardiac Pacemakers Inc. (CPI) data registry (which records the clinical history of 38,000 ICD patients), a declining percentage of patients who present with cardiac arrest is also noted. This figure now represents only 50% of the total. The remaining 50% have sustained VT but without cardiac arrest at presentation.

ADDITIONAL IMPACT OF THE CURRENT PROSPECTIVE CLINICAL TRIALS

Nearly all the ICDs implanted to date have been in patients who have experienced cardiac arrest or sustained VT. A number of clinical trials are currently under way to assess the role of the ICD in patients who are at a high risk for future cardiac arrest but have not yet had a serious cardiac arrhythmia.

There are many similarities among these trials, which are called coronary artery bypass graft surgery plus implantable cardioverter-defibrillator (CABG-PATCH), the Multicenter Automatic Defibrillator Implantation Trial (MADIT), and the multicenter unsustained tachycardia trial (MUSTT). All 3 trials are large, are multicenter, and have a prospective and randomized design. All deal with high-risk patients as defined by known coronary artery disease, the presence of a low ejection fraction (at least less than 40%), and some marker of electrical instability (either a positive signal averaged ECG and/or inducibility at EP testing). Although the study protocols vary, a proportion of the study population in each will be assigned to ICD therapy. In the CABG-PATCH trial each group also receives coronary artery bypass surgery. All 3 studies have total cardiac mortality as a primary end point and sudden cardiac death (SCD) as a secondary end point.[7]

The important results of these trials will probably not be available until at least 1997-98. While most investigators believe such patients to be at high risk, both the exact risk and the role of the ICD therapy in these populations are unknown. Very few physicians currently implant the ICD in such high-risk patients, although the benefit of this strategy has not been proven in a prospective clinical trial. At present there is no indication to implant an ICD in a high-risk, "pre-event" patient unless he or she is enrolled in one of the major clinical trials.

If such trials prove the device to be of use in these patient categories, we will need a "pre-event" ICD. Ideally, this device will have a single transvenous lead attached to a generator small enough to be placed below the clavicle. It will need only the capacity to deliver a few shocks and will have limited memory.

We are at a critical crossroads in the indications for ICD therapy. The indications identified in the 1985 FDA guidelines were used during the 1980s, and the device had a remarkably beneficial effect on survival from sudden death. In the mid-1990s we will likely witness further expansion of ICD indications due to the efficacy of third-generation devices, which will extend ICD therapy to hemo-dynamically stable VT patients. A further extension of the indications for the ICD will occur if any or all of the clinical trials under way show the device to have a favorable impact on survival in high-risk groups. These data are not yet available. We must be sure that new data regarding the benefit of the ICD are clear in well-done clinical studies and are articulated both by the FDA and by cardiology specialty societies. We cannot afford to assume clinical benefit until proven by such trials as CABG-PATCH, MADIT, and MUSTT.[8]

THE FIRST-GENERATION DEVICE

The first-generation device, the automatic implantable defibrillator (AID®), was first implanted in February 1980 after years of development in the animal laboratory by its inventors, Michel Mirowski and Morton Mower.[9] It sensed arrhythmias using a transcardiac (superior vena caval spring electrode to left ventricular apical epicardial patch) modified bipolar electrocardiographic signal. It weighed 250 grams, delivered shocks of 25J and 30J, and had a total discharge capability of 100 shocks (Table 2).

The first device employed a relatively crude detection algorithm called the probability detection function (PDF) for arrhythmia sensing. It had no cardioverting capability and no heart rate detection criteria. The PDF, which is a histogram of the time spent by the ventricular electrogram signal on the isoelectric line, was good at detecting VF but not VT.

Despite these limitations in arrhythmia sensing, the initial clinical results with the AID device were very positive. Of the first 52 patients receiving the AID between 1980 and 1982, 33% received successful defibrillating shocks.[10] There was an actual 1-year SCD mortality of 8.5% and all-cause mortality of 22.9%. The expected (i.e., calculated by assuming those patients who received a shock would have died without an AID) 1-year SCD rate was 48%. Although these statistical assumptions have been challenged, the remarkable clinical efficacy of the AID device was apparent from the outset.

A radical new therapy for sudden death survivors had been introduced. Between 1980 and 1985, ICD implantation was restricted by the FDA to 25 centers. Some 400 defibrillators were implanted during the initial clinical trial before the FDA approved the device for expanded clinical use in October 1985.

FEATURES OF SECOND-GENERATION ICDs

The second-generation devices were until very recently the only market-released ICDs; they are manufactured by Cardiac Pacemaker Inc., St. Paul, Minnesota. Between October 1985 and the present, 38,000 second-generation devices have been implanted in 25,000 patients. They are relatively simple devices (Fig. 1). The energy output is fixed at 28J to 37J. There is limited programmability. The detection rate for VT can be programmed between 110 and 200 beats/min. The delay between sensing a tachycardia and charging the capacitors can also be programmed from 2.5–10 sec. This extended delay is a useful feature in patients having runs of nonsustained VT.

The second-generation devices provide accurate rate sensing and do not under-detect VT or VF. However, second-generation devices store very little information about device function or charging history for use in clinical follow-up. Retrievable data in this device include only the number of shocks, capacitor charge time, and lead impedance of the shocking leads.

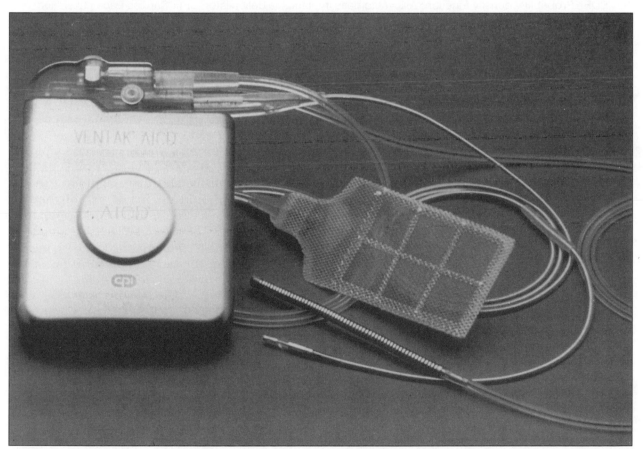

Figure 1. *The CPI second-generation automatic implantable cardioverter-defibrillator. Shown is the generator, a right ventricular rate sensing lead, a right atrial spring lead, and a small epicardial patch.*

Table 2. Differences in Generations

	FIRST	SECOND	THIRD
Sense (detect)	PDF	PDF, rate	Rate and enhancements
Energy (output)	25J–30J	28J–37J	Programmable to 0.1J–40J
Lead system	Spring-patch or patch-patch	Spring-patch, patch-patch or transvenous system alone	Patch-patch or transvenous system alone
Size	250 g	230 g	230 g
Committed	Yes	Yes	No
Programmable features	No	Rate Cutoff Delay (sense)	Extensive (Table 4)
Models	AID	AIDB AIDBR Ventak 1500 Ventak 1555 Ventak 1600 Ventak P	CPI PRx 1, PRx 2, P2, Medtronic 7217, 7219C, 7219D, Ventritex Cadence, Intermedics RESQ, Siemens Siecure, Teletronics 4210 ATP

PDF=Probability density function; AID=Automatic implantable defibrillator; CPI=Cardiac Pacemakers Inc.

Both device features and programmability are severely limited (Table 2).

LEAD SYSTEMS FOR SECOND-GENERATION ICDs

The early lead systems used in first-generation ICDs employed a transvenous superior vena caval spring electrode as the anode and a flat epicardial patch as the cathode. In the mid-1980s, a 2 patch system implanted directly on the epicardium became popular as it was shown that this configuration required less energy to defibrillate the heart (Fig. 2).[11] The currently used patches are composed of titanium mesh and come in 2 sizes, a 13.9 cm² ("small patch") and a 27.9 cm² ("large patch").

Rate sensing was first accomplished in 1982 via a bipolar electrode pair that was screwed directly onto the surface of the heart. Alternatively, a transvenous bipolar endocardial sensing lead in the right ventricle apex could be used. Either system is reliable and continues in use today.

Intraoperative testing of the implanted lead system was first done in 1982 with the development of the external cardioverter defibrillator (ECD) testing device. Guidelines were quickly established as to what value constitutes adequate defibrillation energy at acute testing (usually ≤ 20J) and what R wave amplitude constitutes an adequate signal for rate sensing (>5mV).[12]

The lead systems that have been employed for the past 10 years in clinical practice have been very reliable and their method of testing during implantation firmly established. If proper procedures are followed at operation, the patient can be assured of reliable long-term function of the lead system. Little change is anticipated in the design and function of the traditional transthoracic lead system.

WEAKNESSES OF THE SECOND-GENERATION ICD

The clinical utility of the ICD over the past 10 years, established during the era of the second-generation ICD, cannot be overemphasized. Experts in the field do not think that patient survival rates can be improved on no matter what changes are made in device design (Table 3).

Yet the second-generation ICD is a relatively crude clinical instrument with inflexible and

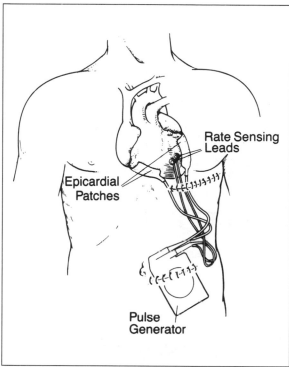

Figure 2. *Standard transthoracic (open chest) lead system including 2 patches for defibrillation, 2 screw-in electrodes for rate sensing, and the generator in the left upper quadrant of the abdomen.*

nondiscriminating tachycardia detection, limited and fixed therapies, virtually no memory, and limited programmability. It is a reliable but simple rate counter that delivers a fixed energy shock when a threshold rate is exceeded.

The weaknesses of the second-generation device include (Table 3):

GENERATOR-DEPENDENT WEAKNESSES

1) There is no antitachycardia pacing (ATP) or low energy cardioversion (LEC). This is unfortunate as the majority of sustained VT episodes that are induced in the EP laboratory are pace terminable, especially if the rate is under 200 beats/min.

2) There is no backup bradycardia pacing. Patients receiving the ICD have a significant incidence of clinically symptomatic bradycardia, and nearly 10% ultimately require a permanent pacemaker. Equally significant numbers develop

a post-ICD shock asystolic pause of greater than 2.5 seconds and require short-term bradycardia pacing.

3) The first and second generations of ICDs are "committed" devices. After detecting VT/VF, the second generation does not reconfirm that the arrhythmia persists before delivering therapy. Episodes of nonsustained VT that quickly convert to sinus rhythm can cause an inappropriate ICD discharge into sinus rhythm. Spurious shocks are prevented if the device reconfirms VT or VF before delivering a shock.

4) There is no device telemetry. A variety of device-related diagnostic information is desirable. This includes pacing lead impedance, measured battery voltage, capacitor charge times, and the ability to test pacing thresholds.

5) There is no way to distinguish supraventricular tachycardia (SVT) from VT. The second-generation ICDs record only whether the device has discharged. The clinician must depend on clinical criteria (i.e., did the patient have palpitations or syncope before the shock?) to categorize shocks as either true or spurious.

6) The generator size is large. Current ICD generators are large and weigh 197 to 280 grams. The large size of the device is due chiefly to its capacitor function and requires that it be implanted in the abdomen. Patients complain about the large size and the square shape of the device.

7) Second-generation ICDs do not permit noninvasive programmed stimulation. The

---

Table 3. Weaknesses of Second-Generation Devices

No antitachycardia pacing or low-energy cardioversion
No backup bradycardia pacing
Is a committed device
No device telemetry
No way to distinguish SVT from VT
Generator size is large
No way to perform noninvasive programmed stimulation

SVT=Supraventricular tachycardia;
VT=Ventricular tachycardia.

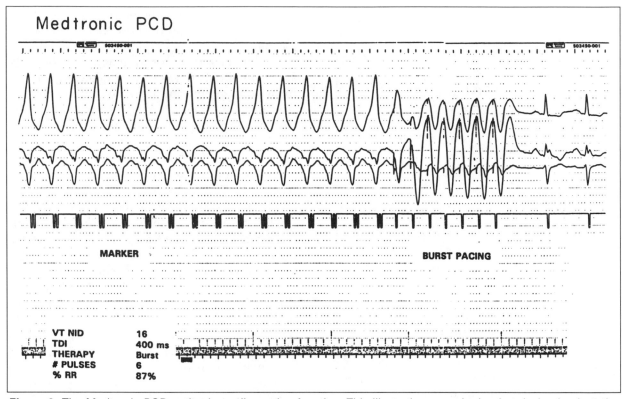

Figure 3. *The Medtronic PCD antitachycardia pacing function. This illustration was obtained at device implantation and both a 3-lead electrocardiogram and marker channels are shown. A 6 beat train of burst pacing is delivered at 87% of the ventricular tachycardia (VT) cycle length. The result is sinus rhythm. The device programmed values are shown at the lower left-hand corner. NID refers to the number of intervals for detection of VT (16) and TDI refers to tachycardia detection interval (or lower rate cutoff) (400 msec).*

capability to test device function noninvasively (especially the efficacy of ATP algorithms) improves both patient safety and acceptance.

8) A small number of patients have high defibrillation thresholds (DFTs). The second-generation ICD generator uses a monophasic waveform to defibrillate the heart. In a small number of cases adequate defibrillation thresholds cannot be achieved with this waveform. Approximately 5% of all trans-thoracic ICD implantations using an epicardial lead system have DFTs over 25J.[13] When a transvenous lead system is used with a monophasic energy source, the resulting DFTs are over 25J in one-quarter of patients. Clearly, a more efficient energy source is a necessity if all patients are to have an adequate safety margin at device implantation (see below).

IMPROVEMENTS IN TECHNOLOGY MAKING POSSIBLE THIRD-GENERATION ICDs

1) There have been significant improvements in tachycardia detection. First- and second-generation ICDs rely on ventricular rate alone to determine the presence of tachycardia (Table 2). It is desirable to distinguish VF from VT. It is also important to separate sinus tachycardia, which typically has a gradual onset, from VT, which usually has an abrupt onset. The third-generation devices employ features to help distinguish VT from SVT. These include sudden onset, rate stability, and rate duration. If properly programmed, these features allow most episodes of tachycardia due to a sinus mechanism or atrial fibrillation (AF) to be distinguished from VT.

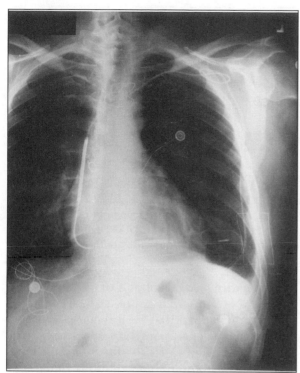

Figure 4. *Chest x-ray of a patient with a CPI ENDOTAK C 0060 lead. The right atrial and right ventricular coils are seen. The catheter tip is higher than usual and may not be at the true right ventricular (RV) apex. Defibrillation thresholds were 20J. In this case a subcutaneous patch was also employed.*

2) Improvements in tachycardia termination have been developed. A variety of pacing schemes to terminate VT have been studied, and each may have a role in terminating reentrant VT. The most useful algorithms employ simple burst pacing usually in combination with either adaptive or scanning methods.[14,15] The adaptive mode introduces burst pacing as a percentage of the basic VT cycle length (usually 80%–90% of cycle length). Use of this mode diminishes the significance of any changes or variability in spontaneous VT cycle length and is superior to fixed burst pacing. Another useful feature is scanning, which introduces each successive pacing train with increasing prematurity until the tachycardia is terminated. Other modes are described but are much less useful clinically (Fig. 3).

3) Improved lead systems are already in use. Endocardial (transvenous) sensing and defibrillation lead systems have been under development since the early canine work of Mirowski and Mower. In 1988 the first use of the CPI ENDOTAK transvenous lead in man was reported.[16] However, the early experience was plagued by lead complications in 6 of 10 patients, including lead fracture in either the transvenous lead or subcutaneous patch. The result was either spurious shocks or inadequate sensing and device function.[17] The transvenous lead systems are undergoing rapid development. There are many similarities but some important differences between the lead systems, which are in clinical trials from CPI and Medtronic. Both the CPI ENDOTAK and Medtronic Transvene leads are implanted via the left subclavian vein. The CPI lead is a single 9.6F lead that incorporates a proximal (right atrial) and distal (right ventricular) coil for delivery of defibrillating shocks and a porous tip and distal spring electrode (separated by 6 mm) for bipolar sensing. The Medtronic lead is 11F, and it is a 2-catheter system that includes a right ventricular lead and a second lead, which is placed in the SVC or coronary sinus. Sensing is accomplished between a distal helical tip and a distal ring electrode. Both systems incorporate a third component—a subcutaneous patch—that is placed in the left lateral or anterior pectoral region for patients having high (>24J) DFTs with a lead-only configuration (Fig. 4). Early clinical experience with both lead systems suggests that the ENDOTAK lead has superior handling characteristics, lower DFTs (less need for a patch), and a lower dislodgement rate. Either system, however, represents an enormous advantage over traditional epicardial systems.

4) All first- and second-generation defibrillators employ a truncated waveform with a fixed tilt (angle of the monophasic pulse) of 60%.[18] This waveform results in adequate DFTs in approximately 95% of patients receiving a standard epicardial system and 72%–88% of patients receiving a transvenous system.[19,20] A variety of different waveforms are under investigation in third-generation devices to improve defibrillation efficacy. A sequential waveform differs from the standard monophasic

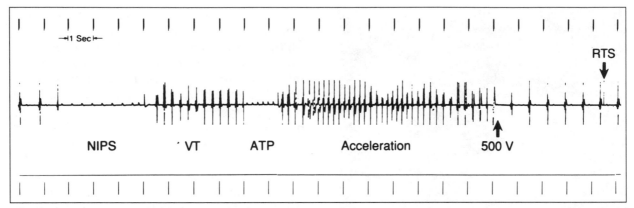

Figure 5. *Stored electrogram from a Ventritex Cadence. In this example, ventricular tachycardia is induced via noninvasive programmed stimulation (NIPS). An attempt at antitachycardia pacing (ATP) accelerates the tachycardia, and a 500-volt shock restores sinus rhythm. Such interval clinical information is helpful in reprogramming therapy at follow-up visits. VT=Ventricular tachycardia.*

waveform as a separate second monophasic pulse is delivered across a second pathway at the end of the first pulse. A biphasic waveform is different. At the end of phase 1, the defibrillation shock polarity is completely reversed and delivery continues along the same pathway but in the opposite direction. The published clinical data has shown that biphasic pulses are superior to either monophasic or sequential pulses. Bardy compared monophasic and biphasic waveform pulses in 22 patients undergoing epicardial lead system implantation. He found the DFTs were 8.5J for a monophasic pulse and 6.3J for a biphasic pulse.[21] Saksena made a similar comparison in 33 patients undergoing implantation of a transvenous system using a triple electrode configuration and bidirectional shocks. Again, simultaneous biphasic shocks resulted in lower DFTs than simultaneous monophasic pulses (15J vs 9J) for all arrhythmias tested.[22] In 2 recent series using the ENDOTAK lead and a biphasic pulse, the DFTs were less than 20J in 25 consecutive patients in 1 series and in 17 consecutive patients in another. In each series the superiority of a biphasic or monophasic pulse was shown.[23,24] The biphasic pulse will allow the transvenous lead to be employed in nearly all patients. There is still debate about which type of biphasic waveform shape is best. The issues are those of whether the capacitor should be single or dual, what the pulse width of the 2 phases should be, and the relationship of the

initial leading edge voltage of the 2 phases. Despite these unsolved issues, the early clinical utility of the biphasic has been remarkable.

5) Second-generation ICDs store only data about battery and capacitor function and have limited information about device discharges. Enormous progress has been made in this area. The third-generation ICDs provide information about number and type of events, therapy delivered and clinical success. The data that is retrieved by interrogating the ICD is printed in tabular form. One device (Ventritex) is able to store electrograms from the last 1 to 7 therapies, which encompass 120 seconds of data. This information can be of great help in diagnosing the cause of shocks, including lead fracture as a cause of spurious shocks.[25] Other devices (CPI and Medtronic) store arrhythmia events as R-R intervals before and after therapy so no analysis of morphology is possible (Fig. 5). Stored electrograms are promised in all future manufacturers' products. They will be features of the CPI PRx2 and the Medtronic 7219; both of these devices are undergoing evaluation clinical trials. Real time electrograms are available in all of the third-generation devices. However, the signals displayed vary considerably in their fidelity due to differences in the way that they are processed by each of the devices. Only the Cadence gives real time data about R wave morphology and T wave amplitude that helps sort out sensing problems (especially due to T wave oversensing) and helps

diagnose lead fracture or lead adaptor problems. Other valuable stored information in third-generation devices includes data about electrode status (lead resistance and pacing threshold), battery life (indicating the need for generator replacement), and pacing thresholds.

6) Key to the development of the third-generation ICDs is the concept of a hierarchical approach to ventricular arrhythmia treatment.[26] This critical concept proposes treating ventricular arrhythmias first with a safe and painless therapy (antitachycardia pacing) and then moving on to cardioversion and defibrillation. To carry out such therapy, a device must be extremely flexible and easy to program, have reliable tachycardia detection criteria, and the capacity to easily test and validate therapies through noninvasive programmed stimulation.

The clinical goals driving these improvements are those of patient comfort and safety. Patient comfort is maximized by attempts at antitachycardia pacing before cardioversion or defibrillation. Patient safety is ensured by limiting the duration of potentially ineffective therapy (ATP) and by moving toward established effective therapy (namely defibrillation). The design and specifications of the third-generation ICD generators are quite similar (Table 4). The device features that clinicians desire in the next generation of ICDs are widely agreed upon among device manufacturers. The third-generation ICDs are similar in concept but are proving to be very different in their application. A number of the differences between ICDs are minor and relate to the ease of programming the software; most of these shortcomings can be redesigned as future generations are introduced. Other shortcomings have been of great importance and relate to errors in sensing arrhythmias that have forced cancellation of clinical trials in progress.

PREOPERATIVE EVALUATION

Patients who are being considered for ICD therapy must undergo a comprehensive anatomic and electrophysiologic evaluation. A standard work-up can be accomplished in just a few days and an appropriate therapy recommended (Table 5).

Most device candidates have survived a recent episode of out-of-hospital SCD or sustained VT and must be clinically stable before any work-up is done. In the early phase of the hospitalization, a careful search for potentially reversible causes of the clinical arrhythmia should be sought and are frequently found. The most important causes include electrolyte abnormalities, the proarrhythmic effect of certain antiarrhythmic drugs (especially quinidine, flecainide, and moricizine), and transient ischemia. Approximately 25% of cardiac arrest survivors are receiving an antiarrhythmic drug when they arrest, which makes this an important part of the work-up.

When the patient is clinically stable, a cardiac catheterization and thorough hemodynamic evaluation is mandatory. The underlying abnormal substrate is thereby quickly determined, and the role of coronary artery disease and its contribution to the clinical event is better understood. At this juncture, the patients with cardiomyopathies can be differentiated from the patients with coronary artery disease and further work-up planned. An occasional patient will suffer cardiac arrest due to coronary artery spasm, and ergonovine testing should be done if suspected. Such patients are usually younger, smoke cigarettes, and have minimal coronary artery disease on routine angiography; often rapid nonsustained VT is a clue to the diagnosis.

In an occasional patient without obvious anatomic abnormalities, further testing is done to look for an occult cardiomyopathy. Such testing includes on occasion a magnetic resonance imaging scan to diagnose right ventricular dysplasia or an endocardial biopsy to find an infiltrative or infective myocardial process. Such testing requires expertise in interpreting the often confusing results that are inherent in such techniques.

In the coronary patient, a stress test of some kind is necessary to evaluate the role of ischemia and the need for revascularization. Each center has its favorite way of doing this, and a thallium treadmill stress test, an exercise echocardiogram, or dobutamine echocardiogram is sufficient. This test also gives an idea of the

Table 4. Characteristics of Third-Generation Devices

	VENTRITEX CADENCE	MEDTRONIC PCD (7216A/7217B)	CPI PRX1	TELECTRONICS 4210 ATP	INTERMEDICS RESQ 101-01	SIEMENS SIECURE
Weight (g)	237	197	224	280	240	225
Tachycardia detection						
rate	yes	yes	yes	yes	yes	yes
duration	yes	yes	yes	ye	yes	yes
Antitachycardia pacing						
fixed	yes	yes	yes	yes	yes	yes
adaptive	yes	yes	yes	yes	yes	no
scan	yes	no	yes	yes	yes	yes
autodecremental	yes	yes	yes	yes	yes	yes
Tiered therapy	yes	yes	yes	yes	yes	yes
Detection algorithms	RT, SO RS	RT, SO RS, TPM	RT, SO,	RT RS	RT, SO RS	RT, SO
Shocking Energy (stored)	0.1J–42J	0.2J–34J	0.1J–37J	0.1J–30J	0.2J–40J	0.5J–40J
Waveform	Bi	Mono	Mono	Mono	Bi	Mono
Committed	no	no VT/ yes VF	no	no	yes	no
Bradycardia pacing	yes	yes	yes	yes	yes	yes
Holter						
Total episodes	yes	yes	yes	yes	yes	yes
Last R-R intervals	no	yes	yes	yes	no	yes
EGM						
Real time	yes	yes	yes	yes	yes	yes
Stored	yes	no	no	no	no	no
Noninvasive EPS	yes	yes	yes	no	yes	yes
Life span (nonshocking)	5	5	4-5	4-5	2+	5
Number implanted	1,500	3,500	1,000	700	50	70

CPI=Cardiac Pacemakers Inc.; RT=Rate; RS=Rate Stability; SO=Sudden Onset; TPM=Turning point morphology; EGM=Electrogram; EPS=Electrophysiologic study.

maximally attained sinus rate, which is later useful for device programming. If there is definite evidence of ischemia in a SCD patient with a preserved ejection fraction, the work-up is truncated and the patient referred for revascularization.

Most patients will next be referred for a comprehensive EP study. It is important to define carefully atrioventricular (AV) nodal conduction and to determine if AV nodal reentry is present. Bypass tracts must be excluded as a possible cause of syncope or even sudden death. The most important aspect of the study is a complete ventricular induction study. Any and all VTs must be characterized as to rate, morphology, pace terminability, and associated clinical symptoms. Such data are critical to device selection and subsequent programming. It is also helpful to determine the response to intravenous procainamide both in terms of tachycardia suppression and rate slowing. Such data are important in making the initial decision as to whether a patient can be controlled with antiarrhythmic drugs alone or will need an implantable device. Furthermore, the response to procainamide is a useful guide to what, if any, drug will be useful later if a drug is needed after device implantation.

Over the past few years, there has been less and less use of serial drug testing in the EP

Table 5. Preoperative Evaluation

Rule out reversible causes of cardiac arrest or VT
Define right and left ventricular anatomy by
    Echocardiography
    MRI
    Catheterization
Define coronary anatomy by arteriography
Establish the presence or absence of ischemia by
    Treadmill or
    Thallium or
    Exercise echocardiography
Comprehensive electrophysiologic test
Holter monitor or extended telemetry
Assess psychological stability and family support
Preoperative teaching

VT = Ventricular tachycardia; MRI = Magnetic resonance imaging.

laboratory. There are many studies that show that the chance of finding an antiarrhythmic drug that suppresses VT is low (less than 20%) and that if intravenous procainamide is not effective, then the chance of another drug working is very unlikely. In the patient with suspected occult long QT syndrome, we administer isoproterenol to look for paradoxical QT lengthening.

These scientific data are added to the increasing economic pressures to keep the preoperative work-up to an absolute minimum. We will perform the cardiac catheterization on day 1 and the EP study with procainamide on day 2; at that point we make a clinical decision for a specific therapy, which is undertaken on day 3.

There are other important aspects to the preoperative work-up that need to be carefully carried out. If the patient has congestive heart failure, this must be maximally treated with diuretics and angiotensin-converting enzyme inhibitors; this reduces operative risk and morbidity. Chronic lung disease must be treated as completely as possible if an operation is contemplated. Any potential source of infection must be completely eliminated if a device is planned. Common problems include infected intravenous sites, skin infections, or infected teeth; the latter must be removed before a

device is implanted. Diabetes must be carefully managed if present.

It is important to know how much, if any, nonsustained VT is present. This can be accomplished either by Holter monitoring or by careful attention to the telemetry on the typical cardiology ward. We make an effort to suppress any significant nonsustained VT before ICD implantation. Also, atrial fibrillation must be controlled as its presence greatly complicates postoperative care. The patient with a low ejection fraction (<30%) should receive prophylactic digitalis preoperatively.

The final aspect of the preoperative evaluation is an understanding of the patient's psychologic stability and family support system. Patients with a strong family structure seem to do better both through the implantation period and during follow-up. An occasional patient is not referred for an ICD because of psychosocial instability.

CONSIDERATION OF ALTERNATIVE THERAPIES

The ICD has quickly emerged as the treatment of choice in the patient with aborted SCD or sustained VT who has failed a trial of antiarrhythmic drugs in the EP laboratory. A great deal of clinical judgment affects just which and how many antiarrhythmic drugs are used before a failure is declared (Tables 6 and 7). In the older patient or the poor operative candidate, more drugs might be tried. In the noninducible patient, there is, of course, no role for serial drug testing, and other therapies (ICD or bypass surgery) must be used.

The benefit of coronary artery bypass surgery either as primary or adjunctive therapy for this patient group cannot be overemphasized. The patient with ischemia as the cause of a VF arrest should receive coronary artery bypass surgery as the principal therapy. If, in addition, the patient has a normal or near normal ejection fraction, it is debatable whether a preoperative EP study is needed. In the past, such patients received a prophylactic epicardial ICD lead system in case they had inducible VT postoperatively. This is such an unusual event that we have abandoned it; if an ICD is needed, a transvenous lead

Table 6. Best Candidates for Antiarrhythmic Drugs
Hemodynamically stable VT Preserved ejection fraction Respond to IV procainamide at EPS "Older and sicker"
VT=Ventricular tachycardia; IV=Intravenous; EPS=Electrophysiologic study.

Table 7. Best Candidates for ICD
Hemodynamically unstable VT Pace terminable or noninducible Poor response to IV procainamide at EPS Survivors of SCD Low ejection fraction Concomitant cardiac surgery
ICD=Implantable cardioverter-defibrillator; VT=Ventricular tachycardia; IV=Intravenous; EPS=Electrophysiologic study; SCD=Sudden cardiac death.

system can be used postoperatively.

In patients with a reduced ejection fraction (<40%) and significant coronary disease, revascularization is also important, but prophylactic patches are warranted as many such patients will still have inducible VT postoperatively. If inducible, then a device can be implanted as a second-stage procedure.

There is still a role for direct arrhythmia surgery, but its role is limited and confined to centers with a special interest and expertise in such procedures. The ideal patient for a map-directed myocardial resection will have a large anterior or anterior-apical aneurysm with a relatively preserved (>40%) ejection fraction. Aneurysms located inferiorly can also be resected but run the risk of disrupting the mitral valve. In the proper setting, such surgery offers the chance of a cure as late sudden death rates in the large surgical series are comparable to survival rates with the ICD. Only a very few experienced surgical centers have been able to do this difficult surgery with an operative risk of less than 10%. As the operative risk with the transvenous ICD is under 1%, this procedure is difficult to justify except for the unusual patient.

Patients who do not need revascularization as part of their therapy for their arrhythmia constitute most of the VT/VF clinical population. Most of these patients have a reduced ejection fraction on either an ischemic or idiopathic basis. The choice often comes down to that of an ICD or empiric amiodarone. A number of large series of VT/VF patients show that subsequent arrhythmic death is less with the ICD than with amiodarone but that amiodarone is better than any other drug. There is a large cohort of patients who are not good ICD candidates because of age or concomitant disease in whom amiodarone is the best alternative therapy. A final disagreeable but clear reality is the increasing reluctance of some insurers to pay for the more expensive ICD, and thus amiodarone in some cases becomes the preferred therapy because of price.

The patients with an idiopathic dilated cardiomyopathy are often the best ICD candidates because of their very high risk of subsequent arrhythmic death (50% at 2 years in most series) and the frequent continued decline in their ejection fraction. Electrophysiologic testing is much less predictive in this group as well.

The central role of ejection fraction in determining any patient's long-term prognosis is the key to clinical decision making at this time. Patients with a relatively preserved ejection fraction (>40%) tend to do well over time irrespective of whether they are inducible or whether an effective antiarrhythmic drug is found. However, if the ejection fraction is low, then the long-term prognosis as defined by subsequent total mortality or sudden death is dramatically worse than in the near normal ejection fraction group. The ICD virtually eliminates subsequent sudden death in this low ejection fraction group and is more important the lower the ejection fraction. Whether the ICD in reducing subsequent SCD rates will also reduce subsequent total mortality is a hotly debated topic and the subject of the NIH-sponsored AVID (Antiarrhythmic Versus Implantable Defibrillator) trial.

The sudden death survivor who is non-inducible in the EP laboratory runs a high risk

(30%) of a subsequent arrhythmic event and needs special attention. If revascularization is possible, then this alone is adequate therapy. If the patient is not an operative candidate, then an ICD is usually recommended.

ICD IMPLANTATION

Implantable defibrillators can be implanted quickly and safely if certain guidelines are followed. Over the past 10 years, ICDs have nearly always been implanted in the operating room using a transthoracic approach to place an epicardial lead system directly on the heart. However, as transvenous lead systems are now the industry standard and as generators become smaller, the site for device implantation in many centers is becoming the EP laboratory. No matter where the device is implanted, certain guidelines must be followed.

The personnel needed for transthoracic ICD implantation include an anesthesiologist, cardiac electrophysiologist, cardiac surgeon, electrophysiology nurse, and support staff from the device company itself. An experienced team is important for some implantations will be difficult and demand both technical skill and good judgment. The operating room should be large and preferably one dedicated to heart surgery. We try to use the same room each time to allow the same setup and avoid electrical noise. The most important element is that each member of the implanting group know his or her role and work well together as a team. Implantations should be scheduled early in the day if possible and not at the end of a busy day as some of these procedures will be very tedious and time-consuming.

The patient is given anesthesia. The typical approach used in 1995 is a transvenous one. Nonetheless, we briefly review the transthoracic approach which was the chief way ICDs were implanted in the late 1980s until the ENDOTAK lead was approved. In the transthoracic approach 2 large patches are placed on the heart usually in an anterior-posterior position with as much of the septum as possible between the patches. Two epicardial sensing leads are screwed into the heart away from the patches and in what appears to be

viable muscle. Usually the high lateral surface of the left ventricle is used.

Regardless of whether the system is epicardial or transvenous, a careful set of measurements is then made by the electrophysiologist. The amplitude of the signal provided by the rate sensing lead must be greater than 5 mV and the pacing threshold less than 2.0 volts. Other measurements including lead impedance and rate sensing duration are made. Strict adherence to minimal standards is critical if the device is to sense and pace normally in the future life of the generator.

Next, a measurement of the energy needed to defibrillate the heart is made. A variety of protocols for performing this procedure have evolved. The critical concept is that the energy needed to defibrillate the heart must be at least 10J less than the maximal output of the defibrillator generator to allow a safety margin. Most protocols call for beginning the testing at 20J and stepping down by 5J per test until the pulse fails to defibrillate and a rescue shock is needed.

The defibrillation threshold (DFT) is the least amount of energy that reproducibly reverts VF to sinus rhythm. The technique used is important. First, VF must be induced and not VT. Also, a delay of 8–10 seconds between VF induction and delivery of the shock is recommended because if longer delays are used the DFT will be higher. If the first patch position used does not give DFTs less than 20J (or at most 24J for a 34J output device), then other patch positions should be tested. On occasion with high (>30J) DFTs, ingenious hybrid 3-patch systems will be required. In an occasional patient, the DFTs are consistently over 35J and a device cannot be implanted.

The factors causing high DFTs are not completely understood. The antiarrhythmic drug amiodarone is associated with high DFTs, but this is the only drug having this effect. The dilated end-stage left ventricle at times seems more likely to have high DFTs, but so-called normal hearts will, on occasion, have high DFTs.

We favor limiting DFT testing to as few tests as will convince the implanting team that an adequate safety margin has been achieved. This is important for patient safety. Protracted DFT testing can cause hemodynamic instability and make DFT results less reproducible. In the most straightforward case, a success at 20J then at 15J with a failure at 10J (a successful rescue shock of 30J) constitutes adequate albeit minimal DFT testing.

Irrespective of whether the lead is epicardial or transvenous, the surgeon next tunnels the leads and creates the pocket for the generator in the left upper quadrant of the abdomen. The leads are attached to the generator, and the device function is checked one further time. Again, VF is induced and the device itself allowed to terminate the arrhythmia. We limit testing of the device in the operating room and do all programming of pacing algorithms in subsequent sessions in the EP laboratory.

If coronary artery bypass surgery is part of the same procedure, then it is completed before the ICD is implanted. The same procedure is followed except the patches are placed epicardially. Again, DFT testing is kept to a minimum and usually done on partial circulatory bypass.

The era of transvenous lead systems has simplified the implantation procedure and made it a safer one. The same general principles and procedures are used, but the lead system is placed via the left subclavian vein in the operating room or EP laboratory. The same meticulous measurement of pacing and sensing parameters is required. A similar protocol for DFT testing is used.

In the early experience with transvenous lead systems that used generators that had a monophasic waveform, adequate DFTs could be achieved in approximately 75% of patients. The remaining 25% had to have an epicardial system. At the present time, 1 of the market-released devices (Ventritex) has a biphasic waveform, and the other manufacturers have devices in clinical trials (CPI PRx2, Medtronic 7219C and D) that have biphasic waveforms. Using these devices with a transvenous lead system, a DFT of less than 24J is possible in nearly 100% of patients. This new era will virtually eliminate the need for an open chest procedure and in turn will make device implantation both safer and associated with a shorter hospital stay.

One of the major complications of device implantation is infection with an incidence of from 2%–3%. Most of these episodes result from wound contamination at implantation and tend to occur more frequently in diabetics. The strictest attention to sterile technique will help reduce this serious complication, which demands device explantation. The risk of infection is another reason to keep intra-operative testing to a minimum.

The postoperative treatment of the ICD patient is not complicated if simple routines are followed. Any hospital that has developed care patterns for the routine coronary artery bypass and valve patients will have no difficulty caring for the ICD patient. However, if carefully planned routines are not carefully followed, the result can be unnecessary patient morbidity or even excessive operative mortality.[12]

POSTOPERATIVE ROUTINE

Our routine, and that of most implanting centers, is to begin the immediate postoperative care of the ICD patient in the same cardiac surgical unit in which other open heart surgery patients recover. This approach seems clinically logical as one-third of patients receiving an ICD will have concomitant heart surgery of some type as well. It is advantageous to have a nursing unit dedicated to the care of cardiovascular cases only. By concentrating ICD patients in 1 unit, nurses have the opportunity to care for large numbers of ICD patients which in turn lessens the chance for human error.

Patients in our center leave the operating room with the ICD turned off. This allows the surgeons to use cautery freely in the operating room at the conclusion of the case without affecting device function. Patients are not routinely treated with antiarrhythmic drugs in the early hours and days postoperatively. Once in the cardiac surgical unit, 1 of the EP nursing staff carefully documents the device status in the chart. We have used brightly colored stickers ("ICD on"/"ICD off") on the front of the chart and in the progress notes to alert the nursing staff as to the device status.

The care of ICD patients does not differ from the routine postoperative care of the coronary artery bypass graft or valve patient. Meticulous management of hemodynamic status is especially important because the typical ICD patient has a reduced ejection fraction (mean, 33%) and is therefore very sensitive to changes in preload. We routinely use a Swan-Ganz catheter to monitor filling pressures and cardiac output. The use of pressors does not differ from that used in other postoperative patients.

It is our routine to extubate the patient the evening of surgery if hemodynamics are stable. We think that this minimizes pulmonary complications and shortens the stay in the cardiac surgical unit. By the second day, most patients are ready for transfer to the cardiac telemetry unit. By then the patient has been extubated for nearly 24 hours, and the chest tubes and the Swan-Ganz catheter have been removed.

On the telemetry floor, the patient is progressively ambulated until ready for the predischarge EP study and home. Predischarge teaching begins as soon as the patient arrives on the telemetry floor. The patient who suffers complications will, of course, stay in the cardiac intensive care unit until stable for transfer.

The second-generation devices (defibrillator only) are usually activated when the patient moves from the cardiac surgical unit to the telemetry unit. If the patient has survived a known VF arrest, we turn the ICD on with as high a rate cutoff as possible (190–200 beats/min) in order to avoid spurious discharges if the patient develops postoperative AF. If the patient has VT rather than VF, we activate the rate cutoff at 10 beats below the clinical VT rate. In patients with multiple VT rates, clinical judgment is required; usually the device rate cutoff that is chosen is below the slowest clinically relevant VT.

The postoperative use of antiarrhythmic drugs is highly variable and subject to physician choice. Some centers soon after surgery give ICD patients an antiarrhythmic drug predicted to be effective at the preoperative EP study, while others wait until the postoperative EP study or until the patient first receives a shock. We withhold antiarrhythmic drug treatment unless it seems likely from the postoperative telemetry (which may show high density ectopy or frequent runs of nonsustained VT) that the patient will receive frequent shocks in the future. If antiarrhythmic drugs are used, they should be started before the postoperative EP test because of their effects on pacing algorithms and DFTs. The antiarrhythmic drugs employed are those that were judged to be most effective in preoperative EP studies. If no drugs were effective in EP studies and an antiarrhythmic is still judged to be needed, amiodarone is usually started in low dose.

It is critical that each center establish its own formula for the safe care of postoperative ICD patients. The principles that ensure success include the following:

1) Thorough in-service training on ICD function for all the intensive care specialists, surgeons, fellows (both EP and surgical), and nurses who will be caring for ICD patients. The night shift personnel especially must be trained.

2) A system for letting all care providers know whether the ICD is programmed on or off.

3) An established and unwavering clinical care algorithm for all patients. This is critical to minimize mistakes.

4) A physician, usually the attending electrophysiologist, is designated as "in charge" of postoperative antiarrhythmic drug treatment and device status. Confusion results if the nurses are receiving mixed signals from many sources.

POSTOPERATIVE SUPRAVENTRICULAR TACHYCARDIA

Supraventricular tachycardia occurring within the first week after ICD implantation is a relatively common occurrence and is reported to occur in approximately 35% of patients undergoing the open chest procedure.[27] The most common arrhythmia is atrial fibrillation (30%), although atrial flutter (4%) and paroxysmal atrial tachycardia (1%) less commonly occur. Other series have reported a postoperative incidence of atrial fibrillation varying from 9%–20%.

If the device is activated and atrial fibrillation develops, the device inappropriately discharges, which can have serious medical and psychologic consequences. This is especially true if the staff is unable to deactivate the device quickly and multiple shocks result.

The frequent incidence of postoperative atrial fibrillation is a strong argument for setting the rate cutoff of the activated device to a high cutoff (greater than 180 beats/min or so) if this will not render VT treatment ineffective. Also, the nursing staff must know how to deactivate the device with a magnet if atrial fibrillation results in device discharge. The practice of taping a donut magnet to the end of the bed for use in emergency device deactivation is a sound one.

A strong case can be made for the prophylactic use of digitalis in patients who are at high-risk for the development of atrial fibrillation. This high risk group includes patients with low ejection fraction (<35%), an enlarged left atrium, or a concomitant coronary bypass operation. A calcium channel blocker can be added if there is a history of rapid ventricular response to atrial fibrillation.

POSTOPERATIVE VENTRICULAR ARRHYTHMIAS

A significant percentage of patients will develop serious, sustained VT in the early days after ICD implantation. The incidence of this complication is relatively constant in the literature and has varied from 10%[28] to 17%.[29] The rhythm that develops is typically VT rather than VF. In a small percentage of patients, the VT becomes incessant and of hemodynamic importance.

Serious postoperative ventricular arrhythmias usually develop within the first week after surgery. No published series details the development of VT after postoperative day 9. The complication is extremely important clinically, as in all series it conveys a small but real increase in perioperative mortality due to incessant VT.

The development of postoperative VT is a serious complication that demands very intensive therapy with antiarrhythmic drugs. The ICD must be turned off and the patient treated in a critical care environment. The full spectrum of antiarrhythmic drugs is often necessary; lidocaine, bretylium, and at times intravenous amiodarone are necessary. It is also important to give enough magnesium and potassium by vein to keep serum levels in the high-normal range. In rare clinical settings, if intravenous medications fail, the clinician may resort to the intra-aortic balloon pump to terminate the VT.

The commonly seen postoperative pulmonary problems include left lower lobe collapse, pneumonia, and left pleural effusion. These complications occurred in 29% of the patients in 1 series[30] and were nearly exclusively related to the use of an anterolateral thoracotomy approach for patch placement. The use of a midline sternotomy or subxiphoid approach helps to avoid these problems.

Such problems resolve with the aggressive use of chest physiotherapy, although antibiotics and bronchoscopy are often needed. The clinical course of such patients is often protracted; this in itself can cause other complications (e.g., deep vein thrombophlebitis) in addition to patient discomfort and added cost.

A syndrome of postoperative adult respiratory distress syndrome has been reported in patients receiving amiodarone who undergo aortocoronary bypass surgery.[31] Similar postoperative complications have been described in postoperative ICD patients on amiodarone. We attempt to stop amiodarone preoperatively for days or even weeks before operation if possible. If a patient does undergo surgery while receiving amiodarone, we keep intraoperative testing (DFT determination) and systemic hypotension to an absolute minimum, although we cannot prove this to be of benefit.

Some fluctuation is noted in the pulse generator pocket postoperatively in the majority of patients, but in only a small percentage (2%) is the accumulation of fluid tense or painful enough to require drainage. The patients in whom this must be done have marked discomfort at the generator site due to the mechanical compression caused by the effusion; virtually all sterile effusions will spontaneously resolve if left alone. If the generator pocket must be tapped for clinical indications, it is done with meticulous sterile technique to avoid infection.

Many patients develop pericardial friction rubs postoperatively, but in only a small percentage (3%) does a clinical syndrome of fever, pleuritic chest pain, and echocardiographic evidence of pericardial effusion develop.[30] Such patients respond to a short course of anti-inflammatory drugs.

Deep venous thrombophlebitis occurs infrequently (2%)[30] and is usually seen in patients placed on bed rest for protracted periods of time. The usual preventive measures of early ambulation and prophylactic low-dose heparin can prevent this complication. We have not seen it since we stopped using anterior thoracotomies, which on occasion required long periods of bed rest.

The transvenous lead system will expand the number of patients receiving ICDs and will greatly simplify and shorten their postoperative care. Most of the complications we now see will become historic curiosities. Postoperative pulmonary complications, postoperative atrial fibrillation or VT storm, and complications of prolonged bed rest will no longer occur.

PATIENT CARE ISSUES

Patients with ICDs and their families are particularly vulnerable to psychologic setbacks in the early postoperative period. Often the ICD is placed after a long illness with many studies in the catheterization and EP laboratory, which leaves the patient and family vulnerable and insecure.

For these reasons, it is critical that patients and family be well prepared for what is to occur during the postoperative period. Every center develops its own method of teaching patients and family. We assign a nurse coordinator to each patient to teach and answer questions, but this function could be done by an electrophysiologist, fellow, or EP nurse. Contact with each patient and family twice daily is important to ease anxieties and ensure the patient goes home on time with all questions answered.

POSTOPERATIVE FOLLOW-UP

A set routine is necessary to ensure satisfactory follow-up of ICD patients. Most implanting physicians prefer to follow patients implanted at their center, but this is not mandatory if careful protocols are developed at smaller centers.

Most ICD manufacturers recommend that their devices be checked every 2 months. The visit is usually conducted in an outpatient setting and performed by an EP nurse and physician. It must be a setting where the programmers are located and resuscitation equipment is available. It should be a comfortable and relaxed environment as some of the interrogations and treatment can be time-consuming.

At each visit an interval history is taken and the device interrogated. Of particular importance is the patient's awareness of any device discharges or any symptoms, such as presyncope, palpitations, or syncope, that might suggest a ventricular arrhythmia. Also important are any changes in the underlying cardiac status or changes in medication.

Therapy from the second-generation defibrillators is shock only, and good data exist on how frequently these occur. At 1 year approximately 40% of patients will have received a shock, and this figure rises to 80% at 5 years. It was long thought that asymptomatic shocks usually represented a spurious shock due not to VT but to sinus tachycardia or atrial fibrillation. However, recent data from third-generation devices demonstrate that fully 20% of asymptomatic shocks are due to a ventricular arrhythmia.

The second-generation devices gave information only about battery function and the number of shocks. The third-generation devices take more time to interrogate but give much more complete diagnostic information. At each visit the interrogation discloses the number of events and therapy for each, data about battery life, and some more precise information about the rate and stability of the last arrhythmic episode or episodes. The devices vary widely on what is available and how it is presented. The Ventritex device has extensive stored electrograms, and other devices in clinical trials (CPI PRx2 and Medtronic 7219) will have similar data. The Ventritex device also gives R wave amplitude and the resistance of the sensing leads as well as real time electrograms, which are useful for detecting lead fracture.

The follow-up visit gives precise information on the extent and nature of ICD activity. If the device has not been used or there have been few but successful therapies, then nothing more is usually needed. If the device delivered frequent but successful therapies, a change in anti-arrhythmic drugs might be necessary. If therapies have been unsuccessful or have made the arrhythmias more difficult to treat, then an inpatient reprogramming session may be necessary. At such a session, the use of different ATP algorithms or the addition of low-energy cardioversion might be tested. If antiarrhythmic drugs are changed, then a retesting of therapies on the new regimen is required. Often in patients with frequent VT episodes, the addition of low-dose amiodarone is very effective in decreasing the number of episodes of VT; however, both DFTs and ATP must then be rechecked.

The transvenous lead systems should be routinely checked by chest x-ray for lead migration. The Medtronic Transvene lead system has had a higher dislodgment rate (5%–10%) than the CPI ENDOTAK and needs careful follow-up.

The outpatient monitoring of ICD activity is simplified if a transtelephonic monitoring system is developed. If a patient receives a shock or has symptoms that warrant concern, this 24-hour number is called and the patient's ECG transmitted. We locate this service in our CCU, and our nurses are trained to take a history, identify the rhythm, and then contact the attending physician. A decision about next steps can quickly be made, and unnecessary trips to the emergency room department can be avoided. We do not routinely see a patient after a single shock if the rhythm is stable. However, with multiple or clustered shocks, we will usually ask the patient to come for a device interrogation.

We also have developed a very active support group, which meets quarterly with patients and families. Each center will develop its own format. We have found that the success of such a group depends on having steady participation by the electrophysiologists and nurses as well as having psychiatric support at each meeting.

DRIVING

There is no more problematic area for patients with ICDs and their physicians than what to recommend regarding resumption of driving. A recent NASPE conference addressed the issue. We usually recommend that patients do not drive for 6 months or until they have received a shock during which they were nonsyncopal. Patients who receive syncopal shocks probably should not drive. Despite these recommendations, many patients drive anyway.

GENERATOR REPLACEMENT

Each generator has indices of battery life that tell the physician when generator replacement is necessary. Generator longevity is now anywhere from 24 to 40 months depending on the specific manufacturer as well as how much bradycardia pacing and defibrillation therapy is used. It is important to replace a generator even if no ATP or defibrillating events have occurred as there is a linear increase in first-time device activity over the initial 5 years after implantation.

The routine for generator change is simple. The previously placed device is removed. The lead system is tested as at initial implantation. If R wave signals are not adequate (<5 mV), then a new sensing system is placed; this is usually done via an RV sensing lead placed via the left subclavian. Defibrillation thresholds are again checked and if adequate, the new device is implanted and checked once. The total hospital stay is 1 day.

SURVIVAL DATA

The results of the widespread clinical application of the ICD have been extensively published and are uniformly impressive. A summary of the 11 largest clinical series published in the United States is summarized in Table 8.[30,32–41] All of these series are retrospective, yet deal with comparable patient groups in terms of presenting arrhythmia and ejection fraction. All series show that the recurrent sudden death rate has been lowered to 2%–3% or less per year with the ICD. The total cardiac mortality, more a reflection of severe left ventricular dysfunction, is high in this population and reaches 40% at 10 years.[32]

There is some disagreement among various investigators about the true impact of the ICD on patient survival. While the ICD has reduced the SCD rate dramatically, it has not lowered the total cardiac death rate in a proportional fashion.[42,43] Enthusiasts of the ICD state that it is enough to reduce sudden death mortality alone. Its detractors think that to be of clinical utility the ICD should so favorably impact sudden death mortality that total cardiac mortality will also be reduced in the ICD population.

These issues are complicated and arise for a variety of reasons. First, in the literature there is no agreed-upon set of definitions of commonly used terms, such as sudden death, operative mortality, cardiac death, and total mortality. A NASPE conference to standardize ICD outcome reporting held in February 1993 helped to correct this deficiency. Second, all of the published clinical ICD series are retrospective and uncontrolled; some data sets are small, which opens their interpretation to bias. A National Heart, Lung, and Blood Institute study, the AVID trial, began enrolling patients in June 1993. It uses a prospective, randomized design to compare survival between sudden death survivors receiving the ICD and those receiving sotalol or amiodarone. It may help define the true role of the ICD in this patient population, but there are serious design flaws in the trial that concern many electrophysiologists. Many electrophysiologists believe that the AVID investigators will not enroll their sickest (either in terms of clinical presentation or low ejection fraction) patients in the trial. If a less sick group of patients is randomized, it will be difficult for the ICD to have any benefit. Also, the absence of any EP criteria used in patient selection puts this protocol at odds with standard EP practice at most centers. Thus, potential drug responders are lumped together with nonresponders, which may dilute any measure of device efficacy.

What do these data above have to do with technologic advances in the ICD? It is remarkable that after only 9 years of widespread clinical use, the ICD has become the cornerstone of treatment for the high-risk patient with ventricular arrhythmias in the United States. There is remarkable consistency among published clinical ICD series as to indications, operative mortality and morbidity, frequency of shocks, sudden death rates, and total mortality.

In contrast, published reports on the efficacy of map-directed arrhythmia surgery or of electrophysiology-guided drug therapy in similar patients have been neither as uniformly favorable as to outcome or uniformly consistent among series as is true of the ICD literature.[44]

FUTURE ICD DEVELOPMENT

The next 5 to 10 years will likely see continuation of the progress of the past 12 years. Although patient survival figures will likely not improve any further, there will continue to be significant engineering improvements in third-generation defibrillators.

1) Tachycardia sensing will improve. There are many unsolved problems in tachycardia sensing. One of the most vexing clinical problems is that of spurious shocks due to supraventricular tachycardia. Sensing enhancements, such as sudden onset and rate stability, are 1 way to deal with this problem. Another way to diagnose atrial fibrillation is to employ an atrial sensing lead that will detect atrial fibrillation and inhibit spurious device discharges caused by this mechanism.

2) The superior efficacy of biphasic waveforms for defibrillation has been demonstrated. Biphasic waveforms are now the industry norm and will be incorporated into the next generation of devices from all the manufacturers. A number of devices entering clinical trials within the next year will have biphasic shocks available. These include the CPI PRx2, the Medtronic 7219, the Intermedics RES-Q 101-01, and the Telectronics Guardian ATP2 model 4211.

3) Transvenous leads are now used routinely. The transvenous lead has proven to be both extremely safe and cost-effective. Further improvements in transvenous leads are anticipated. They will be both smaller (11F rather than 14F) and have improved handling characteristics. They will come in 2 lengths (70 cm or 100 cm) depending on whether the generator is to be placed in a pectoral or abdominal position. The leads will have either active or passive fixation. Atrial leads will be employed for sensing atrial fibrillation and will by necessity employ active fixation.

Table 8. United States Experience With the ICD

	WINKLE	VELTRI	EDEL	FOGOROS	PALATIANOS	PAULL	KELLY	OLINGER	MANOLIS	HARGROV	TCHOU	TOTAL
No pts	555	163	322	118	111	192	84	77	77	77	70	1,767
Mean EF (%)	33	36	33	36	33	32	33	38	36	32	37	34.5
Presenting arrhythmia												
Arrest	48	61	41	51	72	56	54	62	64	91	77	
VT	47	39	55	49	28	44	39	38	36	—	23	
Operative mortality	1.7	4.9	4.0	—	1.0	3.0	3.0	—	2.5	3.0	1.2	2.2
Follow-up (yrs)	10	2	2	2	3	1	3	3	3	2		
Survival (%)	59.1	77	86	88	82	89	95	88	75	60	93	
Freedom from SCD	89.7	96	96	97	98	100	99	97	92	90	99	

ICD=Implantable cardioverter-defibrillator; EF=Ejection fraction; VT=Ventricular tachycardia; SCD=Sudden cardiac death.

4) Dual-chamber pacing will be available. A small percentage of patients with ICDs require dual chamber pacing sometime in their clinical course. This figure is estimated at between 5% and 10%. A dual-chamber pacing function increases the size of the device, and it is unlikely that devices small enough to be implanted in the pectoral region will also have dual-chamber pacing.

5) Diagnostics and stored electrograms will improve. Stored electrograms are extremely helpful in refining device programming as the Ventritex Cadence device has proven. Stored electrograms are available in the CPI PRx2 and Medtronic 7219 devices, which are in clinical trials. More complete memory will be available with extended electrogram storage. Complete information about each arrhythmia episode will be notated, including the time of the event, rate of the tachycardia, applied therapy, and resultant rhythm. Also available will be intracardiac electrograms from each episode with lead impedance if a shock is used. These data should be ample for making therapeutic decisions until an atrial sensing lead is employed, in which case there will be another set of electrograms to analyze.

6) Implantable cardioverter-defibrillator generators will be miniaturized for pectoral implantation. There is a stampede in the device industry to reduce the size of the generator so that it can be implanted in the pectoral region. Most clinicians agree that when device size

reaches approximately 100 cc in volume, pectoral implantation of a generator is possible. Both CPI and Medtronic have devices, which are soon to start clinical trials, that are small enough to employ a pectoral implantation site. The CPI PRx3 is 102 cc and 197 grams, and the Medtronic 7219D (Jewel) is 83 cc and 136 grams. The initial experience with the Medtronic Jewel (7219D) has been extremely favorable. This device is only 83 cc in size and has a biphasic waveform. In the first 140 patients worldwide, a DFT <24J was achieved in 95% and a pectoral implantation site was possible in 63%. The time of implantation was reduced to roughly 100 minutes. Such devices herald both a new and simpler era in the history of ICD technology. Both will have a 34J output (biphasic), antitachycardia pacing, stored electrograms, and noninvasive programmed stimulation. However, memory will be limited, and there will be no hemodynamic sensor or dual-chamber pacing. It is possible that generator size will decrease to as small as 70 cc when the CPI Mini series enters clinical trials in 1996. However, to miniaturize the device to this size, it is likely that generator output will be limited to 20J–25J. The reasons for reducing device size need to be examined carefully by the EP community. Patients complain about the size of the current device and its square corners when implanted in the abdomen. However, even a modest decrease in the size of the current device with some rounding of its shape will likely diminish patient complaints about device bulkiness.

7) Transtelephonic monitoring and programming of ICDs will allow easier follow-up. Third generation devices are time-consuming to follow because of the complexity of the device interrogation that is completed at each patient visit. Also, only a few centers currently have third-generation devices. Long travel distances are necessary for some patients even for routine interrogation. Although the technology exists for routine device follow-up over the telephone, little clinical experience has been gathered.

8) New patch arrays will further lower DFTs. A new subcutaneous array developed by CPI has advantages over the standard subcutaneous patch in use with a transvenous lead system. Preliminary data from European clinical trials have shown a 30% reduction in DFTs and a 17% reduction in lead system impedance using this array. These reductions in DFTs are similar to those provided by biphasic waveforms alone and show the critical importance of subcutaneous patch design and placement. Such innovative technology will help ensure the near 100% success of transvenous lead systems.

We are at a critical crossroads in the development of device therapy. The goals of the patient have been realized and include the established utility and safety of the device and the feasibility of transvenous lead system implantations. The next era (which will incorporate the changes cited above) will further enhance the function of the ICD. However, future changes will not be nearly as important to the patient as what has gone on in the previous 12 years. Lead systems will be improved, the size of the device will continue to be reduced, and the patient follow-up will be easier. Further down the road, there will be use of an atrial sensing lead that will make the diagnosis of atrial fibrillation easier and permit dual-chamber pacing.

The development of the ICD is a tribute to the creativity and determination of Drs. Michel Mirowski and Morton Mower. The ICD is now reaching middle age and has become a clinical tool of remarkable efficacy and flexibility that its inventors hoped for but hardly imagined possible.

American industry has been responsible for these amazing technologic improvements. A development of equal surprise, however, is the reaction of the EP community. In a short period of time, really between 1985 and 1990, arrhythmia specialists understood the enormous efficacy of the ICD for individual patients. It is now the gold standard of therapy for high-risk patients, and its further technologic improvements will only further enhance its clinical utility.

ACKNOWLEDGMENT

Portions of this chapter were written by the author in 3 previously published textbooks: Naccarelli GV, Veltri EP (eds). *Implantable Cardioverter Defibrillators.* Cambridge, MA: Blackwell Scientific Publications: 1992; Estes NA, Manolis A, Wang P (eds). *Indications for the Implantable Cardioverter Defibrillator.* New York: Marcel Dekker:1993; and Podrid PJ, Kowey PR (eds). *Cardiac Arrhythmia: Mechanism, Diagnosis and Management.* Philadelphia: William & Wilkins:1994.

REFERENCES

1. Intec Systems Inc. Protocol for the Clinical Investigation of the Automatic Implantable Defibrillator (AID). July 1980.
2. US Food and Drug Administration. 50 Federal Register 47276. 1985.
3. Dreifus LS, Fisch C, Griffin JC, et al. Guidelines for implantation of cardiac pacemakers and antiarrhythmic devices: A report of the American College of Cardiology/American Heart Association Task Force on Assessment of Diagnostic and Therapeutic Cardiovascular Procedures (Committee on Pacemaker Implantation). *J Am Coll Cardiol.* 1991;18:1-13.
4. Lehman MH, Saksena S. Implantable cardioverter defibrillators in cardiovascular practice: Report of the Policy Conference of the North American Society of Pacing and Electrophysiology. NASPE Policy Conference Committee. *PACE.* 1991;14:969-979.
5. Reid PR, Griffith LS, Platia EV, et al. The automatic implantable cardioverter-defibrillator: Five-year clinical results. In: Breithardt G, Borggrefe M, Zipes DP (eds). *Nonpharmacological Therapy of Tachyarrhythmias,* New York: Futura Publishing; 1987:477-486.
6. Myerburg RJ, Kessler KM, Estes, D, et al. Long-term survival after prehospital cardiac arrest: Analysis of outcome during an 8 year study. *Circulation.* 1984;70:538-546.

7. Bigger JT Jr. Future studies with the implantable cardioverter defibrillator. *PACE.* 1991;14:883-889.

8. Cannom DS. Implantable cardioverter defibrillator: The promise and perils of an evolving technology. *PACE.* 1992;15:1-4.

9. Mirwoski M, Mower MM, Langer A, et al. A chronically implanted system for automatic defibrillation in active conscious dogs: Experimental model for treatment of sudden death from ventricular fibrillation. *Circulation.* 1978;58:90-94.

10. Mirowski M. The implantable cardioverter-defibrillator: An update. *J Cardiovasc Medicine.* 1984;9:191-199.

11. Troup PJ, Chapman PD, Olinger GN, et al. The implanted defibrillator: Relation of defibrillating lead configuration and clinical variables to defibrillation threshold. *J Am Coll Cardiol.* 1985;6:1315-1321.

12. Cannom DS, Winkle RA. Implantation of the automatic implantable cardioverter defibrillator (AICD): Practical aspects. *PACE.* 1986;9:793-809.

13. Epstein AE, Ellenbogen KA, Kirk KA, et al. Clinical characteristics and outcome of patients with high defibrillation thresholds: A multicenter study. *Circulation.* 1992;86:1206-1216.

14. Fisher JD, Johnston DR, Kim SG, et al. Implantable pacers for tachycardia termination: Stimulation techniques and long-term efficacy. *PACE.* 1986; 9:1325-1333.

15. denKulk K, Kersschot IE, Brugada P, et al. Is there a universal antitachycardia pacing mode? *Am J Cardiol.* 1986;57:950-955.

16. Saksena S, Parsonnet V. Implantation of a cardioverter-defibrillator without thoracotomy using a triple electrode system. *JAMA.* 1988;259:69-72.

17. Tullo NG, Saksena S, Krol RB, et al. Management of complications associated with a first-generation endocardial defibrillation lead system for implantable cardioverter-defibrillators. *Am J Cardiol.* 1990; 66:411-415.

18. Troup PJ, O'Rourke RA, Crawford MH (eds). *Current Problems in Cardiology.* Chicago: Medical Publishers; 1989:675-815.

19. Ehrlich S, for The ENDOTAK Investigator Group. Early survival and follow-up characteristics of 151 patients undergoing transvenous cardioverter defibrillator lead system implantation. *J Am Coll Cardiol.* 1992;19:208A.

20. Block M, Hammel D, Isbruch F, et al. Three year experience with nonthoracotomy (NTL) defibrillation leads in 120 patients. *Circulation.* 1992;86:I-58.

21. Bardy GH, Ivey TD, Allen MD, et al. A prospective randomized evaluation of biphasic versus monophasic waveform pulses on defibrillation efficacy in humans. *J Am Coll Cardiol.* 1989;14:728-733.

22. Saksena S, An A, Mehra R, et al. Prospective comparison of biphasic and monophasic shocks for implantable cardioverter-defibrillators using endocardial leads. *Am J Cardiol.* 1992;70:304-310.

23. Ruppel R, Siebels J, Schneider MA, et al. The single endocardial lead configuration for ICD implantation: Biphasic versus monophasic waveform. *J Am Coll Cardiol.* 1993;21:128A.

24. Trappe HJ, Conrad-Weber O, Fieguth HG, et al. First experience with a new biphasic cardioverter defibrillator system. *J Am Coll Cardiol.* 1993;21:308A.

25. Hook BG, Marchlinski FE. Value of ventricular electrogram recordings in the diagnosis of arrhythmias precipitating electrical device shock therapy. *J Am Coll Cardiol.* 1991;17:985-990.

26. Haluska EA, Whistler SJ, Calfee RJ. A hierarchical approach to the treatment of ventricular tachycardias. *PACE.* 1986;9:1320-1324.

27. Paulowski JJ, Joye JD, Fogoros RN, et al. Incidence of supraventricular tachycardia after defibrillator implantation. *J Am Coll Cardiol.* 1992;19:123A.

28. Gartman DM, Bardy GH, Allen MD, et al. Short-term morbidity and mortality of implantation of automatic implantable cardioverter-defibrillator. *J Thorac Cardiovasc Surg.* 1990;100:353-359.

29. Kim SG, Fisher JD, Furman S, et al. Exacerbation of ventricular arrhythmias during the postoperative period after implantation of an automatic defibrillator. *J Am Coll Cardiol.* 1991;18:1200-1206.

30. Kelly PA, Cannom D, Garan H, et al. The automatic implantable cardioverter-defibrillator: Efficacy, complications and survival in patients with malignant ventricular arrhythmias. *J Am Coll Cardiol.* 1988; 11:1278-1286.

31. Nalos PC, Kass RM, Gang ES, et al. Life-threatening postoperative pulmonary complications in patients with previous amiodarone pulmonary toxicity undergoing cardiothoracic operations. *J Thorac Cardiovasc Surg.* 1987;93:904-912.

32. Winkle RA, Mead RH, Ruder MA, et al. Ten-year experience with implantable defibrillators. *Circulation.* 1991;84(suppl I):II-426.

33. Veltri EP, Mower MM, Mirowski M, et al. Follow-up of patients with ventricular tachyarrhythmia treated with the automatic implantable cardioverter-defibrillator: Programmed electrical stimulation results do not predict clinical outcome. *J Electrophysiol.* 1989; 3:467-476.

34. Edel TB, Maloney JD, Moore S, et al. Six-year clinical experience with the automatic implantable cardioverter defibrillator. *PACE.* 1991;14:1850-1854.

35. Fogoros RN, Elson JJ, Bonnet CA, et al. Efficacy of the automatic implantable cardioverter-defibrillator in prolonging survival in patients with severe underlying cardiac disease. *J Am Coll Cardiol.* 1990;16:381-386.

36. Palatianos GM, Thurer RJ, Cooper DK, et al. The implantable cardioverter-defibrillator clinical results. *PACE.* 1991;14:297-301.

37. Paull DL, Fellows CL, Guyton SW, et al. Continuing experience with the automatic implantable cardioverter defibrillator. *Am J Surg.* 1992;163:502-504.

38. Olinger GN, Chapman PD, Troup PJ, et al. Stratified application of the automatic implantable cardioverter defibrillator. *J Thorac Cardiovasc Surg.* 1988;96:141-149.

39. Manolis AS, Tan-DeGuzman W, Lee MA, et al. Clinical experience in seventy-seven patients with the automatic implantable cardioverter defibrillator. *Am Heart J.* 1989;118:445-450.

40. Hargrove WC III, Josephson ME, Marchlinski FE, et al. Surgical decisions in the management of sudden cardiac death and malignant ventricular arrhythmias. Subendocardial resection, the automatic internal defibrillator, or both. *J Thorac Cardiovasc Surg.* 1989;97:923-928.

41. Tchou PJ, Kadri N, Anderson J, et al. Automatic implantable cardioverter defibrillators and survival of patients with left ventricular dysfunction and malignant ventricular arrhythmias. *Ann Intern Med.* 1988;109:529-534.

42. Kim SG. Implantable defibrillator therapy. Does it really prolong life? How can we prove it? *Am J Cardiol.* 1993;71:1213-1218.

43. Saksena S. Survival of implantable cardioverter-defibrillator recipients. Can the iceberg remain submerged? *Circulation.* 1992;85:1616-1618.

44. Akhtar M, Avitall B, Jazayeri M, et al. Role of implantable cardioverter defibrillator therapy in the management of high-risk patients. *Circulation.* 1992;85(suppl I):I131-139.

CHAPTER 25

Congenital Heart Disease in the Adult

Richard R. Liberthson, MD

The past half century has witnessed a profound alteration in the fate of patients with congenital heart disease. Advances in clinical detection, diagnostic precision, and medical and surgical therapy have bequeathed today's adult cardiologist a diverse, challenging and often intimidating patient population. Some of these individuals present with lesions that allow natural survival, some have had previous palliative procedures, and some have had more definitive anatomic or physiologic revision. Both operated and unoperated adults often have acquired complications such as pulmonary vascular obstruction, heart failure and arrhythmia, and those who had previous palliative or reparative surgical procedures may suffer complications attributable to technical inadequacy and prosthetic material failure.

This review is an abbreviated synopsis intended to highlight the most frequent issues facing the practitioner caring for adults with congenital heart disease. It is neither all encompassing nor definitive, and for further details, readers are referred to more dedicated texts.[1-3] For each of the most commonly encountered lesions the pathophysiology, clinical presentation, physical findings, noninvasive and invasive assessment will be discussed, as well as the major palliative and more definitive surgical interventions and their postoperative course and pitfalls.

ATRIAL SEPTAL DEFECT

Atrial septal defect (ASD) accounts for approximately 25% of congenital heart lesions seen in the adult. Patients who have eluded earlier diagnosis as well as those who have undergone earlier correction of the defect may present to the cardiologist. Women with this disorder outnumber men by 3 to 1.

ANATOMY

Size and contour of the defect are variable. Defects are classified as secundum (70%), primum or partial atrioventricular (AV) canal (15%), and sinus venosus types (15%). These classifications are based on the location of the defect within the septum: in the region of the fossa ovalis, the AV junction, or the posterior septum, respectively. This classification system is useful because each type has different associated anomalies: one-third of secundum defects have associated mitral valve prolapse, two-thirds of primum defects have a cleft anterior mitral valve leaflet, and one-half of sinus venosus defects have anomalous drainage of the right pulmonary veins.

PHYSIOLOGY

Regardless of ASD type, the physiology of uncomplicated defects (those with normal pulmonary arteriolar resistance) is the same. Shunting from the left to the right atrium occurs during diastole and is determined by the relative right and left ventricular compliance (the former being greater in the patient with an uncomplicated defect) and by defect size. Pulmonary blood flow is increased. When the defect is small, the shunted volume is small and hemodynamic sequelae are minimal. In larger defects, chronic "left-to-right" shunting causes right atrial and right ventricular volume overload (Fig. 1A). In the patient with an uncomplicated course, the left heart is conspicuously spared and left atrial, left ventricular, and aortic size are normal.

CLINICAL COURSE

Symptoms and complications, except for an increased incidence of respiratory tract infec-

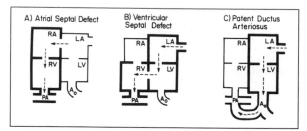

Figure 1. *(A) The pathophysiologic consequences in an uncomplicated ASD revealing right atrial (RA), right ventricular (RV), and pulmonary artery (PA) dilation and preservation of normal left atrial (LA), left ventricular (LV), and aortic (A_o) size. (B) Uncomplicated VSD showing LA, LV, RV, and PA enlargement, with preservation of normal RA and A_o size. (C) Uncomplicated patent ductus arteriosus, including LA and LV enlargement, dilation of both the A_o and PA, and preservation of normal RA and RV size.*

tions, are uncommon in the infant and small child, and early findings are subtle even in patients with large defects. Adolescents and young adults also have few symptoms. When present, symptoms include fatigue, palpitations, and mild dyspnea. Often, ASD is neither suspected nor diagnosed until adult life. Pregnancy is well tolerated. By the fifth decade, however, exercise intolerance, fatigue, and dyspnea are increasingly common and are nearly universal after age 50 years. By this time, the right atrium and ventricle are dilated and contractility is decreased. After the sixth decade, atrial fibrillation is present in 50% of patients; its onset often heralds progressive symptoms and findings of heart failure. Both primum and secundum ASD may have mitral regurgitation. In the former, this manifests early in life and is secondary to the associated cleft mitral valve. With secundum defects, mitral incompetence is rare until age 50 years but thereafter occurs in up to 20% of patients, and is secondary to myxomatous and fibrotic degeneration of the mitral valve. Severe pulmonary vascular obstruction with Eisenmenger's physiology is uncommon, occurring in approximately 5% of cases. It is rare before adolescence and rare after age 50 years. Severe irreversible pulmonary vascular obstruction causes reversal of shunt flow through the ASD from left-to-right to right-to-left. Progressive right heart failure, systemic desaturation, erythrocytosis, and paradoxical embolus

occur; the patient usually dies within 15 years of diagnosis of severe pulmonary vascular obstruction. Both pulmonary and paradoxical systemic embolization occur in the older patient with ASD, particularly in those with atrial arrhythmia and heart failure. Infective endocarditis is rare; when it occurs, it usually involves an associated mitral valve lesion. Endocarditis chemoprophylaxis is prudent regardless of earlier surgical repair. Lutembacher's syndrome (associated mitral stenosis) is rare. The average age of death of patients with uncorrected ASD secundum is 55 years; for primum ASD, it is 35 years.

CLINICAL FINDINGS

Body habitus is usually normal. Patients with Holt-Oram syndrome (congenital hypoplasia of the thumb and radial bones) often have associated ASD. In the absence of severe pulmonary vascular obstruction, patients are acyanotic. The salient clinical findings include an enlarged hyperdynamic right ventricle and a widely and nearly fixed split second heart sound (S_2). Even with the patient standing, the S_2 does not become single. A grade II/VI basal systolic ejection murmur secondary to increased blood flow across the pulmonic valve is present and increases with inspiration. Thrills are unusual. In older patients, heart failure and atrial fibrillation are common, and an apical holosystolic murmur secondary to mitral incompetence may be present. With severe pulmonary vascular obstruction and shunt reversal, the right ventricle hypertrophies, the pulmonic closure sound becomes loud, splitting narrows, and the pulmonic flow murmur becomes soft. A high-pitched diastolic decrescendo murmur of pulmonary incompetence, a pulmonic ejection sound, a right-sided S_4, cyanosis, and clubbing are late findings of this complication.

The electrocardiogram (ECG) reveals right ventricular volume overload, showing incomplete right bundle branch block in younger patients and often a complete right bundle block after middle age. Secundum and sinus venosus defects typically have right-axis deviation, although one-fourth have a normal frontal-plane QRS axis. Left-axis deviation is rare and suggests associated coronary, myocardial, or mitral valve disease. In contrast, in primum type defects, marked left-axis deviation is the rule. It is secondary to congenital hypoplasia and attenuation of the anterior radiations of the left bundle branch. Atrial fibrillation is common in the elderly patient.

The chest x-ray film shows right atrial and ventricular enlargement, dilation of the main and proximal pulmonary arteries, and increased pulmonary vascular markings (Fig. 2). The aorta appears to be small, and with uncomplicated ASD, the left heart is normal sized (Fig. 1). If left atrial enlargement is present, mitral incompetence should be suspected.

The 2-dimensional echocardiogram delineates the presence, size, and location of the ASD (Fig. 3A); the existence of associated cardiac anomalies; and the extent of secondary findings such as right atrial and right ventricular enlargement. Doppler study estimates the right ventricular and pulmonary artery pressures as well as the interatrial pressure gradient. Paradoxical interventricular septal motion correlates with significant right ventricular volume overload. Use of color Doppler or an agitated saline intravenous bolus document the presence of interatrial shunt flow and the diameter of the defect (Figs. 3B, C).

CARDIAC CATHETERIZATION

Catheterization may not be required in children with typical noninvasive findings. In older patients and in those with any questionable findings, catheterization is advisable before surgical repair. Confirmation of the defect is accomplished by catheter passage from the right to the left atrium. Essential data include assessment of right heart and pulmonary artery pressures, pulmonary arteriolar resistance, and the ratio of pulmonic to systemic blood flow. Table 1 lists formulas used to calculate the magnitude of the shunt.[4] After the fourth decade, coronary angiography and left ventriculography are advisable to identify acquired heart disease. For suspected primum defects (patients with left-axis deviation on the ECG), biplane left ventriculography is necessary to evaluate an associated cleft mitral valve or interventricular septal defect. Patients with pulmonary hypertension should receive a trial of pulmonary vasodilation while in the laboratory with either 100% oxygen inhalation for 10 minutes, priscoline or inhaled nitric oxide[5] and then repeat assessment of

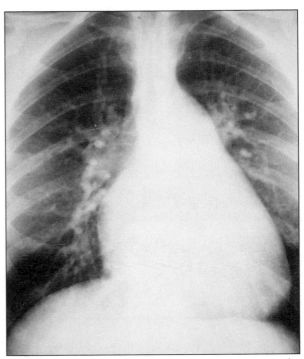

Figure 2. *Posteroanterior chest roentgenogram of a 22-year-old woman with a large secundum atrial septal defect. There is a large right atrium and right ventricle, a dilated pulmonic trunk, and increased pulmonary blood flow. Reprinted with permission from Liberthson RR. Congenital heart disease in the child, adolescent and adult. In: Johnson RA, Haber E, Austen WG (eds).* Practice of Cardiology. *Boston: Little, Brown; 1980.*

shunt size and pulmonary resistance to assess reversibility of pulmonary vascular obstruction. Patients with net right-to-left shunting—Eisenmenger's physiology—are inoperable. In contrast, patients with net left-to-right shunting are usually surgical candidates, regardless of the presence of pulmonary hypertension, systemic desaturation, or moderately elevated pulmonary vascular resistance. In these latter patients, the larger the net left-to-right shunt is, the more favorable will be the postoperative result. Transcatheter closure of secundum-type ASDs is possible using a variety of devices.[6] However, at present, these are still partially restricted from general availability owing in part to technical difficulties related to device frailties. It is my belief that these problems will be overcome and that transcatheter ASD closure will play a major role in secundum ASD management. At present,

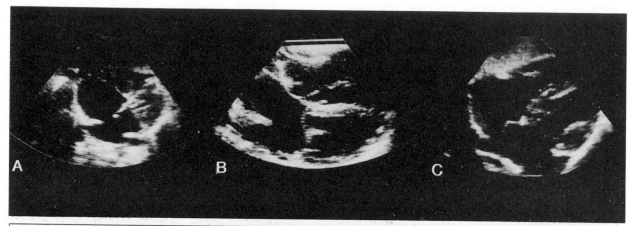

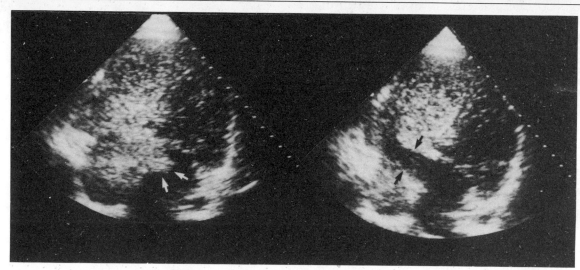

Figure 3. (Top:) Two-dimensional echocardiograms in the subcostal view illustrating (A) secundum-type, (B) primum-type, and (C) sinus venosus-type ASDs. (Bottom:) Saline contrast images in the apical 4-chamber views from a 16-year-old girl who has a large primum-type ASD. (Left:) positive contrast appears in the atrium (arrows), (Right:) Negative contrast is created by unopacified left atrial blood streaming left-to-right across the septal defect (arrows). (C) Color flow imaging of left-to-right shunt flow through an iatrogenic ASD created by a transseptal catheter that provided access to the left heart to permit mitral balloon valvuloplasty (see color plate in front of book). Reprinted with permission from Liberthson RR. Congenital Heart Disease: Diagnosis and Management in Children and Adults. Boston: Little, Brown; 1989.

surgical closure remains the recommendation for most who have larger defects.

SURGICAL INTERVENTION

Surgery consists of either suture closure (usually possible in the young patient) or patch closure in older patients, those with large defects, and in those with primum or sinus venosus defects. For best results, surgery should be performed before school age. Thereafter, ASD closure is indicated when the diagnosis is confirmed. The ASD population is predominantly female. The defect should be repaired before marriage and childbearing to avoid the tendency for further delay while raising a young family. Repair before the fourth decade usually results in return of normal heart size and function.[7] Thereafter, although both size and function of the right heart chambers improve, they rarely become normal. Safe repair may be performed through the seventh decade. Clinical improvement, even in older patients, is marked,

---

Table 1. Calculations of Shunts by Oximetric Analysis

1. Shunts are expressed as:
   Q_P/Q_S: The ratio of pulmonary blood flow (Q_P) to systemic blood flow(Q_S)
   and
   Q_P–Q_S: The value is positive if there is a net left-to-right (L→R) shunt, and negative if there is a net right-to-left (R→L) shunt.

2. Calculation of pulmonary blood flow (Q_P) in L/min:

$$Q_P = \frac{O_2 \text{ consumption (ml/min)}}{PVO_2 \text{ content (ml/L)} - PAO_2 \text{ content (ml/L)}}$$

   where PV=pulmonary venous blood and PA=pulmonary arterial blood.

   If a pulmonary vein has not been entered, systemic arterial O_2 content may be used for PVO_2 if systemic arterial O_2 saturation is 95% or more. If it is <95%, a determination must be made as to whether a R→L shunt is present. If a R→L shunt is present, an assumed value for PVO_2 content is determined as 98% x O_2 capacity. If systemic arterial saturation is <95% and no R→L shunt is present, the observed systemic arterial content is used.

3. Systemic blood flow (Q_S) in L/min:

$$Q_S = \frac{O_2 \text{ consumption (ml/min)}}{\text{Systemic arterial } O_2 \text{ content (ml/L)} - \text{mixed venous } O_2 \text{ content (ml/L)}}$$

   where mixed venous O_2 content is average O_2 content of blood in chamber immediately proximal to the shunt. If the shunt is at the level of the right atrium, one commonly used method for estimating mixed venous O_2 content is calculated as: $\frac{3 \text{ SVC } O_2 \text{ content} + 1 \text{ IVC } O_2 \text{ content}}{4}$

   where SVC=superior vena cava and IVC = inferior vena cava.
   Some institutions use the SVC O_2 content as the mixed venous sample, as the sample gives the maximal shunt size.

4. If bidirectional shunting is present, a more complex formula is used.*

*Adapted from Grossman W et al.[4]

---

particularly when associated mitral valve incompetence is relieved. In older patients, chronic anticoagulation therapy is advisable, particularly if heart failure, pulmonary hypertension, or atrial fibrillation is present. The use of anticoagulation therapy for young patients or those undergoing primary suture closure is generally not advised. In patients with ASD primum, mitral valve clefts may require plasty revision at the time of ASD closure; with rare exception, these mitral valve reconstructions have been remarkably durable over 2 and 3 decades follow-up. Older adults with secundum defects should have intraoperative assessment of the severity of

mitral valve insufficiency.[8]

The postoperative course in patients who undergo repair before the fourth decade is typically benign and lifestyle is normal. No restriction is indicated. The course of pregnancy and delivery is normal. Chemoprophylaxis for bacterial endocarditis should be a lifetime commitment, regardless of surgical repair, because of the frequent association with mitral valve prolapse. With pregnancy, prophylaxis for vaginal organisms should be started with the onset of labor and continued for several days after delivery. In the absence of surgical damage to the sinus node or its vascular supply, young patients retain normal rhythm. For those with supraventricular ectopy or atrial fibrillation, digitalis administration is indicated. Patients who have new atrial fibrillation after surgery warrant a trial of electrocardioversion after 6 weeks; anticoagulation and digitalis treatment should precede this, and additional antiarrhythmic drugs may be needed to maintain sinus rhythm. After the sixth decade, postoperative arrhythmia is typical in spite of medical management. Routine postoperative clinical evaluation is indicated for all patients, particularly for those who undergo repair past middle age. Longevity in those repaired before that time is normal. Thereafter, residual (but improved) heart failure may be present, and pulmonary or systemic embolization may occur. In the older patient, late progressive mitral insufficiency may occur despite ASD closure.[8] In the young patient undergoing repair, the postoperative examination, chest x-ray film, and ECG become normal except for a residual right ventricular conduction defect. In older patients with preoperative heart failure, pulmonary hypertension, and arrhythmia, some right heart enlargement may persist.[7]

DIFFERENTIAL DIAGNOSIS

Entities sometimes confused with ASD include persistent patency of the foramen ovale, which occurs in 10% to 20% of normal autopsies; this finding is of no hemodynamic consequence and has no clinical sequelae unless the pulmonary pressure is elevated and paradoxical embolization then becomes a risk. Partial anomalous pulmonary venous drainage with intact atrial septum is associated with similar clinical findings but rarely causes symptoms or requires correction. Mitral valve stenosis, pectus abnormalities, and pulmonic stenosis may all have similar clinical findings; however, both ultrasound and radionuclide scanning are usually sufficient to differentiate them from ASD.

VENTRICULAR SEPTAL DEFECT

Although VSD occurs in 1 in 500 normal births, nearly 50% close spontaneously during childhood; thus, in adults it is less common and accounts for approximately 12% of congenital heart abnormalities. Adult patients presenting

to the physician include those with small, inconsequential defects, those who have undergone earlier palliative or corrective surgical procedures and those with acquired complications. If a patient survives unimpaired to adult age and does not have Eisenmenger's physiology, the VSD is probably small.

ANATOMY

Ventricular septal defects are classified according to location within the interventricular septum. Seventy percent are membranous defects and involve the pars membranacea. They are variably sized and shaped and often close spontaneously. Muscular defects occur within the muscular portion of the septum and may involve the apex as well as the mid and peripheral muscular regions; defects may be multiple and spontaneous closure occurs. Atrioventricular canal type defects involve the posterobasal inlet septum, are usually large and are associated with mitral and tricuspid valve clefts, as well as a primum type ASD. These are common in patients with Down's syndrome.

Supracristal (juxta-arterial) defects are uncommon (5%) although more frequent in Oriental populations. They are usually small; however, their strategic location beneath the aortic annulus may undermine aortic leaflet support and may cause progressive aortic incompetence. In some of these patients the connective tissue of the aortic valve itself may be abnormal[10] and contribute to progressive aortic insufficiency.

PHYSIOLOGY

The hemodynamic consequences of VSD vary with defect size. When small, they are minimal. With uncomplicated VSD (those with normal right ventricular pressure and normal pulmonary artery resistance), shunting occurs from the left ventricle to the right ventricle. If the defect is large, both ventricles enlarge and pulmonary blood flow increases. Left atrial return is increased, causing left atrial enlargement. When left-to-right shunt flow is very large, heart failure occurs. The right atrium is normal sized in uncomplicated VSD (Fig. 1B). With large defects, pulmonary hypertension and pulmonary vascular obstruction may develop early in life, which

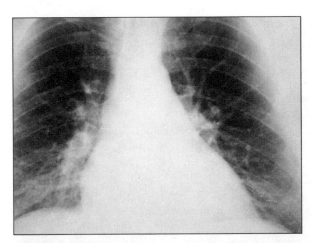

Figure 4. *Posteroanterior chest roentgenogram of a 30-year-old man with a large ventricular septal defect. There is biventricular and left atrial enlargement, a dilated pulmonic trunk, and increased pulmonary blood flow.*

thereafter leads to pulmonary artery and right ventricular hypertension, decreased left-to-right shunting, and eventually right-to-left shunting (Eisenmenger's syndrome).

CLINICAL COURSE

The clinical course of patients with VSD is variable depending on defect size, the common occurrence of spontaneous defect closure, development of complications in the unoperated patient, and the now common practice of early surgical intervention for those with large defects.

Patients with small defects have a history of a loud murmur present from early infancy but typically not at birth. They are asymptomatic, and complications are rare, except for bacterial endocarditis.

Overt clinical heart failure occurs in the infant with large VSD and may be fatal. Chronic left-heart volume overload may cause dyspnea and both symptoms and findings of heart failure may be late sequelae in adult life.

In patients who had large shunts, often with heart failure during infancy, pulmonary vascular obstruction and Eisenmenger's syndrome occur. In these patients, the chronic effects of increased pulmonary artery pressure include right ventricular hypertension, and reversal of interventricular shunt flow from the previous left-to-right direction to right-to-left. Systemic desaturation,

cyanosis (which is often increased with exertion), and erythrocytosis develop. Late right-heart failure, hemoptysis, and systemic embolization may occur. Because of right-to-left shunting, iatrogenic systemic embolization may occur secondary to careless intravenous technique. Bacterial endocarditis occurs regardless of VSD size or earlier repair and often involves the right ventricular outflow tract. In approximately 5% of patients with VSD, progressive hypertrophy of the right ventricular infundibulum develops and obstructs pulmonary blood flow, causing right ventricular hypertension and hypertrophy, with right-to-left interventricular shunting (see "pink tetralogy"), (Tetralogy of Fallot section). Patients with supracristal defects may have aortic insufficiency, which is progressive and may become severe. Patients with AV canal defects often have heart failure during infancy, and Eisenmenger's syndrome is typical. These patients commonly have Down's syndrome.

CLINICAL FINDINGS

Body habitus in VSD is normal except in patients with Down's syndrome, who have characteristic features. The patient with uncomplicated VSD has a systolic thrill at the left sternal border, an enlarged hyperdynamic left ventricle, and a loud holosystolic murmur heard best at the left sternal border on expiration and with isometric maneuvers. In general, the louder the murmur, the smaller the defect. This murmur begins with the S_1 and ends with S_2. With muscular defects, the murmur may end before the S_2 if the defect closes with ventricular contraction. Progressive pulmonary vascular obstruction causes this murmur to diminish in intensity. In these patients, right ventricular hypertrophy, a loud pulmonic closure sound, an ejection sound, and late cyanosis develop. With late right ventricular failure, pulmonary and tricuspid incompetence occur. Patients with aortic incompetence have a high-pitched diastolic decrescendo murmur. With canal defects, mitral or tricuspid incompetence murmurs may be present.

The ECG is helpful in diagnosing the type of defect and the presence of complications. With small defects, the ECG is normal. Larger defects cause a right ventricular conduction defect and both left atrial and left ventricular enlargement. Uncomplicated defects have a normal frontal-

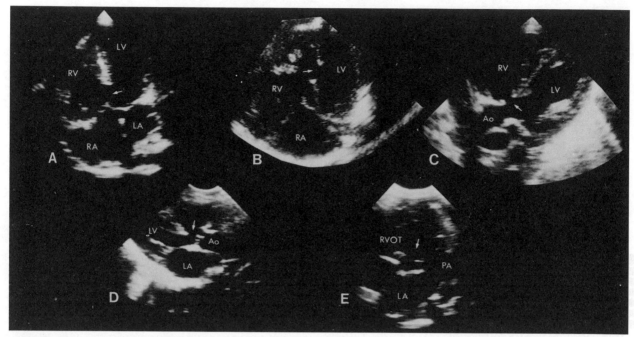

Figure 5. *Two-dimensional echocardiograms illustrating typical apical 4-chamber views in patients with (A) a complete atrioventricular canal-type VSD, (B) a muscular VSD, (C) a membranous defect (in the subcostal 5-chamber view), (D) a malalignment-type VSD viewed from the parasternal long-axis position, and (E) a supracristal VSD viewed from the short-axis parasternal view of the aorta. Arrows point to the defect. An infracristal VSD (not shown) would lie just leftward of the supracristal defect (E) from 10 to 12 o'clock on the aortic circumference. RVOT=Right ventricular outflow tract; LV=Left ventricle; RV=Right ventricle; LA=Left atrium; RA=Right atrium; Ao=Aorta; PA=Pulmonary artery. Reprinted with permission from Liberthson RR.* Congenital Heart Disease: Diagnosis and Management in Children and Adults. *Boston: Little, Brown; 1989.*

plane QRS axis. The QRS axis is an accurate indicator of right ventricular pressure in older children and adults. A normal axis (between –30° and +90°) usually rules out severe right ventricular hypertension, thus making pulmonary vascular obstruction or right ventricular infundibular obstruction unlikely; right-axis deviation suggests their presence. As with primum-type ASD, patients with canal-type VSD have marked left-axis deviation (more negative than –30°) regardless of pulmonary artery pressure or previous surgical correction.

In the patient with a small, uncomplicated VSD, the chest x-ray film is normal. With larger defects, characteristic findings (Fig. 4) include increased pulmonary vascular markings, left atrial and left ventricular enlargement, a small aortic shadow and, sometimes, right ventricular enlargement. The right atrium is normal-sized (Fig. 1B).

Two-dimensional echocardiography and Doppler examination are diagnostic; they delineate the presence, size, and location of VSDs (Fig. 5), and the presence of associated cardiac lesions

and secondary problems including right ventricular and pulmonary artery hypertension. Continuous-wave Doppler sampling of a tricuspid regurgitant flow jet allows estimation of right ventricular pressure (Fig. 6). Color flow Doppler is particularly useful in delineating shunt flow, especially for small residual communications after surgery or for small muscular defects associated with larger VSDs. Ultrasound study permits identification of associated great artery abnormalities such as transposition, double outlet right ventricle, and truncus arteriosus, and differentiation of the defect from single ventricle.

CARDIAC CATHETERIZATION

In general, asymptomatic patients with small defects, normal-sized hearts, normal ECGs (including a normal axis), and no evidence for associated valvular abnormalities do not require catheterization. For the remainder, catheterization is necessary before surgical intervention. Its

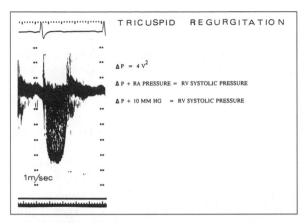

TRICUSPID REGURGITATION

$\Delta P = 4 V^2$

$\Delta P + RA\ PRESSURE = RV\ SYSTOLIC\ PRESSURE$

$\Delta P + 10\ MM\ HG = RV\ SYSTOLIC\ PRESSURE$

1m/sec

Figure 6. *Continuous-wave Doppler sampling of a tricuspid regurgitant flow jet in a patient with a large VSD, illustrating the presence of right ventricular systolic hypertension. The magnitude of the tricuspid regurgitant jet estimates a pressure gradient of 64 mm Hg. When this is added to the estimated right atrial pressure of 10 mm Hg (assuming absence of right heart failure), the patient has an estimated right ventricular pressure of 74 mm Hg. P=Pressure; V=Volume; RA=Right atrium; RV=Right ventricle. Reprinted with permission from Liberthson RR.* Congenital Heart Disease: Diagnosis and Management in Children and Adults. *Boston: Little, Brown; 1989.*

objectives include assessment of left-to-right shunt size, pulmonary artery pressure and resistance, and right ventricular pressure. Angiographic delineation of the defect and any associated lesions is necessary. Transcatheter device closure for selected muscular type VSDs is possible (although not yet widely available) and may have future application. Eisenmenger's syndrome (net right-to-left shunting) must be identified because affected patients are not standard surgical candidates. Because catheterization in these latter patients carries increased risk, it should be undertaken cautiously and only after careful noninvasive assessment, and should be performed only by those experienced with this problem.[11] Patients with pulmonary hypertension should receive a trial of pulmonary vasodilator therapy during catheterization to determine whether obstruction is reversible.[5]

SURGICAL INTERVENTION

Asymptomatic patients with small defects, normal heart size, normal ECG, and no associated valvular defects do not require surgery. Endocarditis chemoprophylaxis, including coverage for vaginal delivery, is recommended in all patients with VSD. Palliative banding of the pulmonary artery is infrequently performed today but was common in earlier years. This procedure protects the pulmonary circulation from increased flow and pressure, however, it produces right ventricular hypertension, often with right-to-left shunting through the VSD. The late sequelae of pulmonary banding include cyanosis, erythrocytosis, and systemic embolization. Pulmonary bands sometimes distort the pulmonary arteries as well. Patients who have undergone previous banding require catheterization to delineate the pulmonary artery pressure and anatomy as well as the VSD before VSD closure and band removal.

Corrective VSD surgery consists of either suture or prosthetic patch closure of the defect. It is indicated for patients who have symptoms, cardiomegaly, elevated pulmonary pressure (including elevated pulmonary resistance, provided there is still net left-to-right shunting), and for those with significant left-to-right shunting (>2:1). Patients with associated infundibular stenosis should undergo VSD closure and often also require infundibulectomy. Young patients with supracristal VSD who do not have aortic incompetence or who have only mild incompetence often benefit from VSD closure, to buttress the aortic annulus, thus preventing progressive insufficiency. This sometimes, but not always, obviates the need for later aortic valve replacement. Surgery is indicated for infants with medically refractory heart failure. Patients with severe pulmonary vascular obstruction and net right-to-left shunts are not surgical candidates.

After successful VSD closure, postoperative problems are minimal and a normal lifestyle is usual. Patients may have a residual VSD that was not appreciated at the time of repair or may have incomplete patch closure, but only when left-to-right shunting is large do these require reoperation. The late course of patients with a buttressed aortic valve in supracristal defects or of the palliated AV valvular incompetence in canal defects is variable, and these patients require closer follow-up. The latter sometimes suffer AV block

Patients with Eisenmenger's syndrome usually die within 15 years from the time of this diagnosis.[12] They are not candidates for VSD closure. They are at increased risk for death when subjected to any form of surgery or to general anesthesia. These patients are also at increased risk with strenuous physical exertion and may suffer incremental symptoms with exposure to high altitude. Pregnancy carries an increased risk of death and fetal wastage and must be prevented.[13] Birth control pills hasten the progression of the pulmonary vascular obstruction and are contraindicated. Intrauterine devices carry a risk of bacterial endocarditis and should not be used. The procedure of tubal ligation itself is a risk because of associated vasovagal reflexes. Bacterial endocarditis chemoprophylaxis is essential. Cautious phlebotomy with replacement of excessive volume loss with volume expanders may be helpful for those with severe erythrocytosis and hematocrit level greater than 65%. In patients with heart failure, medical treatment may improve symptoms. Heart and lung transplantation, or for appropriate candidates, lung transplantation with VSD closure, will play an increasing future role in the care of these patients.

DIFFERENTIAL DIAGNOSIS

The differential diagnosis of VSD includes single ventricle with small outlet chamber and VSD associated with abnormality of the great artery position including complete transposition, double outlet right ventricle, and truncus arteriosus. Although similar clinically to patients with large VSD, patients with these abnormalities also often have cyanosis. Ultrasound examination differentiates these patients from those with simple VSD.

PATENT DUCTUS ARTERIOSUS

Patent ductus arteriosus (PDA) is an obligatory component of the normal fetal circulation; however, persistent patency beyond early infancy is abnormal. Patent ductus arteriosus is present in 10% of adults with congenital heart abnormalities. Both unoperated patients and those with previously corrected PDA may present to the physician. Patent ductus arteriosus is particularly common in infants whose mothers had rubella infection during their first trimester of pregnancy, in premature infants, in infants with lung disease, and in infants born at high altitude. It is more common in women than in men.

PATHOPHYSIOLOGY

The anatomic spectrum of PDA includes a wide range of duct caliber, length, and shape. The ligamentum arteriosus is the fibrotic remnant of the obliterated ductus. The physiologic consequences vary, depending on the cross-sectional area of the ductus lumen. In patients with uncomplicated ductus (those with normal pulmonary arteriolar resistance), flow of blood is from the aorta to the pulmonary circulation (left to right). Large ducts allow large volume pulmonary blood flow, which causes increased pulmonary artery pressure, increased left atrial return, left ventricular enlargement, and enlargement of the aorta proximal to the ductus (Fig. 1C). The right atrium and ventricle are normal in size.

CLINICAL COURSE

The natural history depends on ductus size. Many ducts close spontaneously during early infancy. Thereafter, until age 40 years, an annual spontaneous closure rate of 0.6% has been reported.[14] Patients with a small ductus are asymptomatic. Heart failure occurs in infants with large ductus and may be fatal. Adults with large ductus have both symptoms and findings of heart failure. In patients with large ductus, pulmonary vascular obstruction may develop early in life. In these patients, the late sequelae of Eisenmenger's physiology (right-to-left shunting) include cyanosis and right-sided heart failure. Regardless of ductus size, infective endocarditis may occur. It typically involves the pulmonary side of the ductus. There may be infected pulmonary embolization. Rarely, ductal calcification, aneurysmal dilation, and dissection develop in elderly patients. These may be preceded by hoarseness secondary to left vocal cord paralysis attributable to left recurrent laryngeal nerve compression.

CLINICAL FINDINGS

Facies and body habitus are normal except in those with congenital rubella syndrome, who have cataracts and are deaf and retarded. In patients with congenital rubella syndrome, search for associated branch pulmonic stenosis is mandated. Patients with uncomplicated ducts of large size have hyperdynamic arterial pulses, wide pulse pressure, and an enlarged hyperdynamic left ventricle. These findings are absent in those with small ductus. Regardless of ductus size, a loud continuous machinery-like murmur is typically present, and heard best in the left infraclavicular area. It may obliterate the heart sounds in this region. With severe pulmonary vascular obstruction, the diastolic murmur shortens and becomes softer and pulmonic closure intensity increases. When reversal of shunt direction occurs in patients with PDA, the lower extremities receive the desaturated pulmonary artery blood flow, and cyanosis and clubbing of the toes develop. In contrast, the upper extremities still receive fully oxygenated blood from the ascending aorta; therefore, the fingers (particularly of the right hand) are pink and are not clubbed. This differential cyanotic distribution is diagnostic of PDA with Eisenmenger's physiology.

The ECG reveals left ventricular and left atrial enlargement when shunt flow is large. It is normal with a small ductus. If the ductus is small, the chest x-ray film appears normal; if the ductus is large, the x-ray may be diagnostic (Fig. 7). Pulmonary plethora, dilation of the proximal pulmonary artery and of the ascending aorta, a prominent aortic knob (in contrast with patients with intracardiac shunts, who have a small aortic knob), and left atrial and left ventricular enlargement are seen. The right heart is conspicuously normal-sized in uncomplicated PDA (Fig. 1C). In older adults the ductus may calcify.

Two-dimensional echocardiography and Doppler study allow direct imaging of the ductus. Doppler study allows assessment of shunt magnitude and color Doppler mapping is useful for delineation of the small and tortuous ductus. Associated cardiac lesions and secondary findings are readily identified. Magnetic resonance imaging can also accurately delineate the presence and size of a PDA.

Catheterization confirms the presence of a PDA and is generally performed in patients being assessed for correction. Its objectives include assessment of shunt size and pulmonary pressure and resistance. The catheter should be passed through the ductus to confirm its existence and to differentiate ductus from other great artery shunts, such as aorticopulmonary window, and from coronary arteriovenous fistula. Angiographic delineation of the ductal

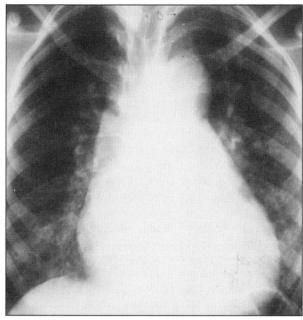

Figure 7. *Posteroanterior chest roentgenogram of a 19-year-old woman with a large patent ductus arteriosus and pulmonary artery hypertension. There is cardiomegaly with left atrial and left ventricular enlargement, and enlarged pulmonic trunk and aortic knob, and increased blood flow. Reprinted with permission from Liberthson RR. Congenital heart disease in the child, adolescent and adult. In: Johnson RA, Haber E, Austen WG (eds).* Practice of Cardiology. *Boston: Little, Brown; 1980.*

anatomy is useful in the adult to alert the surgeon to aneurysms or atypical anatomy. Patients with elevated pulmonary artery pressure should have a trial of pulmonary vasodilation to identify reversible pulmonary vascular obstruction. Patients with net left-to-right shunting should have ductus closure; those with net right-to-left shunting are not closure candidates.

Transcatheter methods for closing a PDA with a Teflon plug have been performed since 1967, and more recently, a double-umbrella device and coil implantation are employed.[15] Transcatheter techniques will clearly play an increasing role in future management of selected PDA patients.

SURGICAL INTERVENTION

Surgical intervention for PDA consists of double ligation of the ductus with or without division to insure obliteration. It does not require heart–lung bypass. It is performed through a left posterior thoracotomy. In children, all ducts should be closed. The optimal age for elective ligation is 1 year. Emergency surgery is indicated for infants with medically refractory heart failure. Elective ligation is indicated thereafter at the time of confirmed diagnosis. Older adults with aneurysmal dilation or calcification of the ductus warrant appropriate surgical precautions, including the availability of cardiac bypass, as dissection and rupture may occur.

Postoperatively, the patient typically has no further difficulties. Very rarely, recanalization of an improperly ligated and undivided ductus occurs. Patients with a large ductus and those who undergo repair after early childhood should receive postoperative bacterial endocarditis chemoprophylaxis because of the presence of residual endothelial irregularity, which may be a nidus for infection.

It is not established whether the asymptomatic young adult with small PDA and normal heart size, normal pulmonary artery pressure, and normal pulmonary resistance must have duct closure. Aneurysmal dilation and dissection are rare. We generally advise elective closure; however, close interim observation for the short term may be an acceptable alternative as transcatheter closure becomes increasingly available.

Indomethacin may stimulate "medical" closure of PDA in the newborn but is of no value in older children or adults. It acts by inhibition of prostaglandin activity, which functions to sustain ductal patency.

DIFFERENTIAL DIAGNOSIS

An innocent venous hum is often confused with PDA. Appropriate clinical maneuvers, including auscultation with the patient lying flat or cervical venous compression readily differentiate these conditions. More critical is identification of patients with aorticopulmonary window, because this condition requires heart–lung bypass surgery and median sternotomy. Patients with VSD and aortic incompetence have some similar clinical findings but can usually be differentiated both clinically and noninvasively. Sinus of Valsalva and coronary arteriovenous fistulas may resemble PDA clinically; but in both, the murmur is typically louder over the heart than beneath the left clavicle. Angiography is the confirmatory differentiating procedure for both. Angiography is also required to differentiate patients with pulmonary or systemic arteriovenous fistulas, in whom findings on physical examination may closely resemble those of PDA.

COARCTATION OF THE AORTA

Coarctation accounts for 15% of congenital heart abnormalities in adults. Increasing numbers of patients with coarctation are being identified by hypertension screening programs. Often patients with coarctation who have not undergone previous repair are seen. Men with this condition outnumber women by 2 to 1. This discussion concerns adult type, or periductal coarctation.

PATHOPHYSIOLOGY

Coarctation is a fibrotic narrowing of the aortic lumen in the region of the insertion of the ductus or ligamentum arteriosus. The caliber, configuration, and extent of narrowing varies, as does its relationship to the origin of the left subclavian artery and insertion of the ductus or ligamentum. In some patients, the left subclavian artery arises distal to the coarctation. At least one-third of patients have an associated bicuspid aortic valve. Infants who have early symptoms often have associated VSD, PDA, or aortic and or mitral stenosis.

Physiologically, coarctation causes obstruction to left ventricular outflow. The left ventricle and the proximal aorta and its proximally arising branches (the carotid and the subclavian arteries) have elevated blood pressure and strong pulses relative to the distal aorta and lower limbs, which have lower blood pressure and delayed arterial pulse. Concentric left ventricular hypertrophy occurs, although in late adult life there may be heart failure and left ventricular dilation. With significant coarctation, blood flow to the lower body derives in large part from collateral arterial circulation, which arises predominantly from the subclavian arteries. The internal mammary and posterior intercostal arteries become enlarged; these latter cause characteristic erosions along the posterior inferior rims of the mid zone ribs (rib notching). The more severe the coarctation, the more extensive the collateral development.

CLINICAL COURSE

Symptoms are minimal or absent in the young patient and, when present, are secondary to hypertension, which occurs in nearly all patients regardless of age. Headache, epistaxis, forceful carotid pulsations, and lower extremity claudication with exertion occur. Infants who have significant associated defects may have heart failure, which may be fatal, but with isolated coarctation this is uncommon. Heart failure is rare after infancy and before the fourth decade, but thereafter occurs in two-thirds of patients. About 8% of patients have a cerebral vascular accident; it is rare in infants and uncommon in children, but occurs in 20% of older adults.[16] It is attributed to both chronic hypertension and to the increased incidence of congenital berry aneurysm of the circle of Willis associated with coarctation. Cerebral vascular accident is less common after correction but may still occur notably in those with residual hypertension. Infective endocarditis occurs in 5% of patients, including some who have had repair. It may involve the coarctation or the surgical resection site, or associated lesions, notably a congenitally bicuspid aortic valve. Significant stenosis of the bicuspid aortic valve is uncommon until late in life, when calcification and fibrosis develop. Significant aortic valve stenosis or insufficiency may develop regardless of earlier coarctation repair, and late aortic valve replacement may be necessary. Aortic dissection at or near the site of the coarctation is rare. Coarctation may complicate pregnancy. Both severe hypertension and toxemia are more common in these pregnant women, and aortic dissection is a risk. In the absence of earlier repair, survival beyond age 50 years is unusual.

CLINICAL FINDINGS

Body habitus is usually normal, although some patients have underdeveloped lower extremities and hypertrophy of their arms and upper body. With Turner's syndrome, coarctation is common and these patients have a typical Turner's appearance. The clinical findings in patients with coarctation are diagnostic. Upper extremity hypertension is nearly always present. The upper extremity pulses are more forceful than those in the lower extremities; which are typical-

ly weak and delayed or absent. All pulses should be checked, as aberrant subclavian artery origin distal to the coarctation occurs. In patients with extensive collaterals, femoral pulses may be surprisingly strong, but careful comparison with the carotid or brachial pulses reveals a relative difference. Extensive collaterals are evident by both palpation and auscultation over the chest wall. Unlike the normal person, whose blood pressures in the legs are slightly higher than in their upper extremities, in the patient with coarctation, the leg pressures are lower than those in the arms. Left ventricular hypertrophy is present. An ejection sound, which derives from an associated bicuspid aortic valve or from the dilated ascending aorta, may be present. A soft systolic ejection murmur, secondary to a bicuspid valve, may also be present; and a systolic murmur over the left upper back, originating from the coarctation, is typical. Findings of heart failure are common in older patients.

Electrocardiographic findings are nonspecific. The left ventricle is the dominant chamber; however, frank left ventricular hypertrophy and strain are often absent until the third or fourth decade. In younger patients, a right ventricular conduction abnormality is common.

The chest x-ray film is often diagnostic (Fig. 8). The coarctation itself is demarcated by an indentation bordered proximally by the dilated left subclavian artery and distally by poststenotic aortic dilation "figure 3" sign. The ascending aorta is dilated. Rib notching develops by adolescence and increases with age. Notching sometimes resolves after correction. Heart size is normal, except in those with heart failure who have left ventricular and left atrial enlargement. Calcification of an associated bicuspid valve may be a late finding.

Two-dimensional echocardiography and Doppler study provide diagnostic confirmation and often nearly complete preoperative assessment of coarctation. The morphology, location and severity of obstruction are readily determined in infants and children but are somewhat more difficult to evaluate in adults. Doppler ultrasound helps to localize the site and severity of the coarctation, although those with a large PDA or very extensive collaterals may have a minimal pressure gradient. Ultrasound is particularly useful for those with residual or recurrent postoperative coarctation. Magnetic resonance imaging is also of value in delineating the anato-

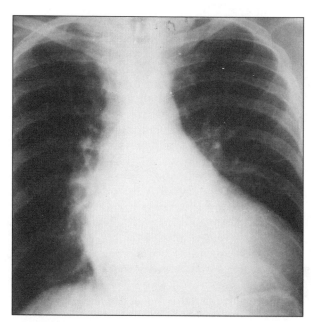

Figure 8. *A posteroanterior chest roentgenogram of a 64-year-old woman with coarctation of the aorta. The heart is enlarged owing to left ventricular enlargement and heart failure. The left subclavian artery is enlarged, and there is postcoarctation dilation, caus-* ing a "figure 3" sign. There is prominent rib notching. Reprinted with permission from Liberthson RR. Congenital heart disease in the child, adolescent and adult. In: Johnson RA, Haber E, Austen WG (eds). *Practice of Cardiology. Boston: Little, Brown; 1980.*

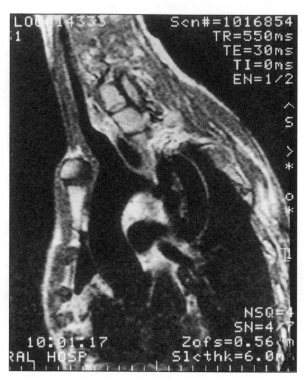

Figure 9. *Magnetic resonance image in a lateral projection from a 32-year-old man with aortic coarctation and a functioning dacron tubular shunt that bypasses the obstruction.*

my of coarctation particularly in patients who have atypical residual or recurrent postoperative stenosis (Fig. 9).

CARDIAC CATHETERIZATION

For most adults, cardiac catheterization and aortic arch angiography is recommended before repair. Its objectives are delineation of the specific coarctation anatomy and the anatomy of the arch vessels; assessment of the presence of adequate collateral circulation to permit safe aortic cross-clamping, without risk of spinal cord ischemia; and identification of associated cardiac lesions, particularly aortic and mitral stenosis, VSD, and PDA.

In older patients, evaluation to rule out acquired coronary and myocardial disease is advisable. Determination of the pressure gradi-

ent across the coarctation has limited value because the severity of the coarctation varies directly with the extent of collateral development, which in turn decreases the transcoarctation gradient.

Percutaneous balloon angioplasty to dilate residual stenosis or restenosis after earlier surgical repair is currently a preferred alternative to surgical revision for many patients.[17] For previously unoperated coarctation, dilation carries some risk of late aneurysm development; thus, its role for these patients remains controversial. It should be avoided for women who may subsequently become pregnant.

SURGICAL INTERVENTION

Surgery consists of coarctectomy and either primary aortic reanastomosis tubular bypass grafting or patch reconstruction. For infants, the left subclavian is often used as an overlay flap to enlarge the coarctation site; in these patients, the distal left subclavian artery is ligated. Hence, as adults, there is no left arm pulse or blood pressure [Waldenhausen procedure]. Optimally, elective repair should be performed before school age to avoid residual hypertension. Thereafter, surgery is still indicated at the time of diagnosis regardless of age. Even older adults who have long-standing hypertension should undergo correction, because 50% still become normotensive postoperatively and the remainder have more manageable pressures.[16] Older patients with heart failure also benefit from correction with improvement in or loss of heart failure postoperatively.[16]

Postoperative problems include residual coarctation, which is rare except in those who undergo correction during infancy. Residual hypertension with a blood pressure gradient of more than 20 mm Hg systolic between the arms and legs is an indication for recatheterization and reoperation or balloon dilation. Children who undergo aortic repair before school age rarely have postoperative hypertension and have a normal lifestyle free of restriction. Thirty percent to 50% of those who undergo surgical repair after childhood do have hypertension, although it is usually mild and often does not require antihypertensive medication.[16] In those with an associated bicuspid aortic valve, it is important to watch for late stenosis. Chemoprophylaxis for infective endocarditis should be a lifetime commitment regardless of previous repair.

DIFFERENTIAL DIAGNOSIS

The clinical findings in acquired aortic obstruction secondary to arteritis, notably Takayasu's disease, may resemble those of coarctation, although the 2 are readily differentiated noninvasively or by angiography. Patients with aortic dissection and traumatic para-aortic hematoma or tumor may also have similar findings. Preoperative differentiation of the above greatly alters management. Pseudocoarctation is associated with radiologic features similar to those of coarctation but does not have its clinical sequelae because there is neither aortic obstruction nor hypertension. It does not warrant correction. So-called "fetal coarctation" is sometimes confused semantically with adult-type coarctation. The difference is great, however, in that the former is a

variant of the hypoplastic left-heart syndrome and has associated hypoplastic left ventricle and ascending aorta, and often aortic and mitral stenosis or atresia. The right heart perfuses the systemic circulation via a large patent ductus. Affected infants usually die within weeks of birth, although extensive staged surgical revision (Norwood procedure) or cardiac transplantation currently offer "guarded" hope.

PULMONIC STENOSIS

Pulmonic stenosis accounts for approximately 10% of congenital heart abnormalities in adults. Both unoperated and postoperative patients are commonly seen in general cardiology practice.

PATHOPHYSIOLOGY

In most cases, pulmonic stenosis is valvular and secondary to partially fused bicuspid or tricuspid valve leaflets. These valves have a domed, "fish-mouth" appearance. Because of the chronic pressure load imposed on the right ventricle, that chamber hypertrophies. Sometimes there is selective hypertrophy of the infundibulum beneath the pulmonic valve, which contributes to the overall right ventricular outflow tract obstruction. This may selectively progress with duration of valvular obstruction.

Pulmonary branch stenosis is rare and occurs in patients with congenital rubella syndrome, Williams' syndrome, Takayasu's disease, and as an isolated lesion. It also exists as an iatrogenic complication in patients who had previous Waterston shunts (ascending aorta to right pulmonary artery) and in those who had prior surgical pulmonary artery banding. Many such pulmonary artery branch stenoses are now manageable with transcatheter balloon dilation, as are most with valvular stenosis.

The physiologic consequences of pulmonic stenosis vary with its severity. When severe, there is right ventricular hypertension with decreased right ventricular compliance and elevation of end-diastolic pressure. Pulmonic stenosis is classified as mild, moderate, and severe, according to the pressure gradient between the right ventricle and the pulmonary artery. These gradients are less than 40 mm Hg in patients with mild stenosis, between 40 mm

Hg and 70 mm Hg in moderate stenosis, and greater than 70 mm Hg in severe stenosis.

CLINICAL COURSE

Patients with mild-and-moderate pulmonic stenosis have few or no symptoms, and their lifestyle is generally unaffected. The condition may not be diagnosed until adult life, but often the patient has a long-standing history of a loud, asymptomatic murmur. Complications, even late in life, are few. Some patients with moderate stenosis have progressive fatigue and dyspnea late in life. Severe stenosis may cause heart failure and cyanosis during infancy owing to right-to-left shunting through a patent foramen ovale. Fatigue and dyspnea occur in children and adults with severe stenosis, but overt clinical heart failure is uncommon. With severe stenosis, chest pain can mimic angina pectoris. It is attributed to the excessive demand placed on coronary flow by the hypertrophied right ventricle. Right ventricular ischemia and infarction occur but are rare. Infective endocarditis is also rare. With severe stenosis and chronic heart failure, "cardiac" cirrhosis of the liver may develop secondary to passive congestion. Paroxysmal dyspnea is uncommon but is an ominous finding that sometimes heralds sudden death with severe stenosis.

CLINICAL FINDINGS

Body habitus is normal except for patients who have branch stenosis and manifest findings of their associated syndromes along with retardation in some. Patients are acyanotic unless they have an associated patent foramen ovale or ASD, which permits right-to-left shunting and, therefore, systemic desaturation. With valvular stenosis, there is an ejection sound. Its position relative to the S_1 correlates inversely with the severity of stenosis. When very close or merged with the S_1, stenosis is severe. The ejection sound is louder during expiration than inspiration, unlike other right heart auscultatory phenomena. Patients have a systolic ejection murmur heard best at the upper left sternum that is loudest with inspiration. Its intensity and duration correlate directly with the severity of stenosis. Very loud and long murmurs that reach to the S_2 indicate

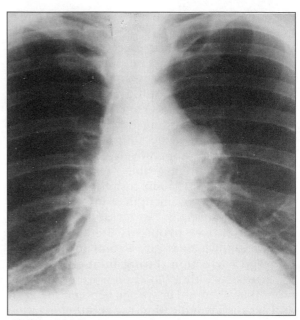

Figure 10. *Posteroanterior chest roentgenogram from a 48-year-old man with valvular pulmonic stenosis. There is prominent poststenotic dilation of the main and left pulmonary artery. Reprinted with permission from Liberthson RR. Congenital heart disease in the child, adolescent and adult. In: Johnson RA, Haber E, Austen WG (eds).* Practice of Cardiology. *Boston: Little, Brown; 1980.*

severe stenosis. The later the peaking of the murmur, the more severe the stenosis. Pulmonic valve closure intensity correlates inversely with the severity of stenosis. The more severe the stenosis, the softer the pulmonic closure intensity. In addition, the more stenotic the valve, the more delayed the pulmonic closure sound from aortic closure. Patients with moderate or severe stenosis have palpable right ventricular hypertrophy and, typically, a systolic thrill at the upper left sternal border. A prominent jugular venous a wave and a right ventricular S_4 are present with severe stenosis.

The ECG shows right atrial and right ventricular hypertrophy and right-axis deviation in moderate and severe stenosis; the ECG is normal in patients with mild gradients.

The chest x-ray film is often diagnostic. Patients with moderate or severe stenosis have right ventricular and right atrial enlargement. Patients with valvular stenosis have characteristic poststenotic dilation of the main and left pulmonary arteries (Fig. 10). Poststenotic dilation does not correlate with severity of stenosis. Pulmonary blood flow is normal.

Cardiac ultrasound examination delineates the location and severity of pulmonic stenosis and the presence and significance of associated anomalies and secondary complications. It also permits estimation of the size of the stenotic valve annulus, which is helpful in those undergoing percutaneous balloon angioplasty.

CARDIAC CATHETERIZATION

Patients with mild stenosis and no symptoms do not require catheterization, in contrast with those with cardiomegaly or symptoms or clinical findings suggesting moderate or severe stenosis. In adults, catheterization is always indicated before surgical intervention. Its objectives include assessment of right ventricular pressure, both absolute and relative to systemic pressure, and determination of the right ventricular outflow tract gradient. Detailed angiographic delineation of the

right ventricular outflow tract is essential.

For both children and adults with moderate or severe valvular stenosis, percutaneous balloon pulmonic valvuloplasty offers results comparable with those achieved surgically and has increasingly become the therapeutic intervention of choice in most centers (Fig. 11).

SURGICAL INTERVENTION

Patients with mild stenosis do not require intervention. Those with cardiomegaly, symptoms, and severe stenosis should have surgical or transcatheter relief.

Pulmonic valve surgery consists of plasty revision to open the valvular commissures and relieve obstruction. Pulmonic valve replacement is rarely necessary. Some patients require resection of hypertrophied and obstructing infundibular muscle, and some require an outflow tract patch if the pulmonary annulus is hypoplastic. Varying degrees of postoperative pulmonic insufficiency occur.

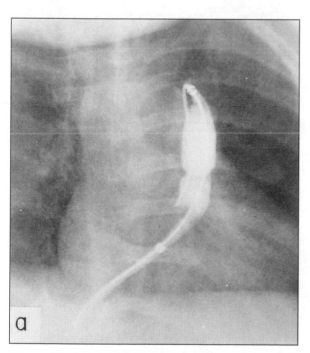 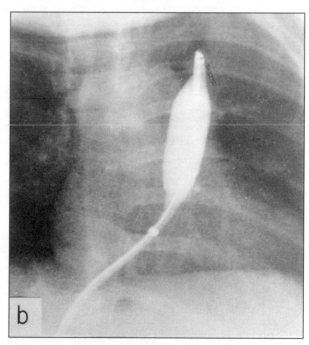

Figure 11. Anterior-posterior (A and B), and lateral (C and D) pre (A and C) and post (B and D) percutaneous pulmonary valvuloplasty. In A and C, there is a waist seen indenting the contrast-filled balloon that is formed by the stenotic valve. This waist is no longer seen after dilation (B and D). Prevalvuloplasty (E) and postvalvuloplasty (F), right ventricular outflow tract gradients in pressure taken on pullback of the catheter from the pulmonary artery (PA) to the right ventricular (RV) illustrate postprocedure absence of significant stenosis (F). Reprinted with permission from Liberthson RR. Congenital Heart Disease: Diagnosis and Management in Children and Adults. Boston: Little, Brown; 1989.

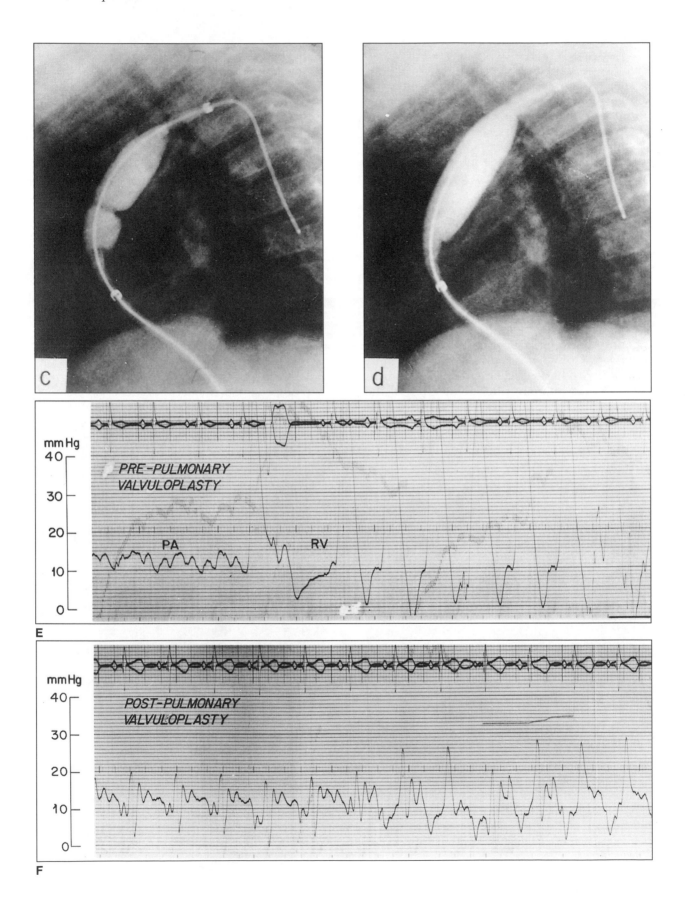

The postoperative and postvalvuloplasty course after successful relief of obstruction is excellent, and patients become asymptomatic. A soft residual systolic murmur and sometimes a low-pitched pulmonic diastolic murmur may be present. Residual stenosis occurs but usually is limited to those with unicuspid valves or annular stenosis. It may necessitate reoperation or valvuloplasty if severe. Pulmonary valve incompetence is generally well tolerated, although when significant over long duration, atrial tachyarrhythmias occur. In the older adult who has fibrosis secondary to chronic right ventricular hypertrophy, right ventricular dysfunction with fatigue, dyspnea, and, sometimes, ventricular arrhythmia may be present.

DIFFERENTIAL DIAGNOSIS

Patients with the "straight back syndrome," pectus deformity of the sternum, small ASD, and idiopathic dilation of the pulmonic artery have some findings on physical examination that resemble those of mild pulmonic stenosis. These conditions are rarely confused with more significant stenosis, however. They can be differentiated noninvasively.

DISCRETE SUBAORTIC STENOSIS

Discrete subaortic stenosis is the etiology of left ventricular outflow tract obstruction in 15% of young patients (<40 yr).[19] It is rare in infants and rare in the elderly. Patients are generally subdivided into those with discrete membranous or fibromuscular obstruction, and those less frequent patients who have more extensive tunnel-like narrowings that diffusely obstruct the left ventricular outflow tract. These latter entities are found mostly during early infancy; they are formidable surgical challenges, and few patients survive. Hence, the focus here will be on the more discrete and more common former entity. Hypertrophic cardiomyopathy with obstruction is covered elsewhere in this text.

Discrete subaortic obstructions occur at variable distances below the aortic valve. Rarely, there is adherence to an aortic leaflet or the annulus, but most occur from several millimeters to a centimeter below the valve. Obstructions are of variable thickness from fibrous membranes to fibromuscular bars. They involve varying degrees of the circumference beneath the aortic valve, some being circumferential, some hemicircular, and some "ridge-like." The rightward membranous attachment is to the upper interventricular septum near the region of the left bundle branch, and the leftward attachment is typically to the proximal portion of the anterior mitral valve leaflet near the annulus. The severity of obstruction varies from mild to critical. It is pertinent that these are not static magnitudes of obstruction and rapid progression does occur. Discrete subaortic stenosis also can be complicated (about 15% of patients) by development of submembranous fibromuscular hypertrophy adding to the overall left ventricular outflow tract obstruction.[19] Commonly, the aortic valve is thickened and fibrotic after the first few decades of life, owing at least in part to the hemodynamic jet created by the membrane, which strikes the valve. This valvular deformity produces degrees of aortic insufficiency, which may be progressive, and often become significant by the fourth decade.

Clinical sequelae in discreet subaortic stenosis vary with the severity of overall obstruction. When mild, patients are typically asymptomatic. Severe obstruction causes presyncope, syncope, chest pain, heart failure, and often exertion-related sudden death. Bacterial endocarditis occurs in 15% of patients.[19] Familial occurrence is common (15%), hence, screening relatives is necessary.

Clinical findings include typically normal body habitus. When obstruction is significant, peripheral pulses are weakened and delayed as in valvular aortic stenosis; left ventricular hypertrophy, systolic thrills, and transmitted carotid bruits occur. The second heart sound is typically preserved in these patients, and an ejection sound is notably absent in contrast with young patients with valvular aortic stenosis. As many as 50% of patients have an aortic incompetence murmur.

The ECG is similar to that in patients with valvular aortic stenosis. The chest x-ray is also similar, although there is a notable absence of poststenotic dilation of the ascending aorta in patients with discrete subaortic obstruction in contrast with those with valvular aortic stenosis. The echocardiogram is diagnostic for the presence, morphology, severity of obstruction, and concurrence of associated lesions (Fig. 12). Cardiac catheterization is helpful for these patients to confirm the noninvasive findings.

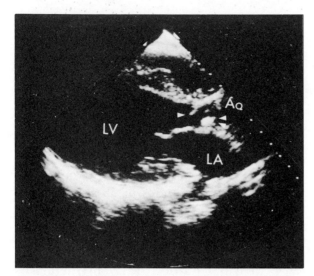

Figure 12. *Two-dimensional echocardiogram in the parasternal long-axis view of the left ventricular outflow tract showing a discrete subaortic membrane (single arrow) in a 17-year-old girl. There is a small aortic annulus and an abnormal aortic valve with a discrete vegetation (double arrows) on 1 leaflet. LV=Left ventricle; LA=Left atrium; Ao=Aorta. Reprinted with permission from Liberthson RR.* Congenital Heart Disease: Diagnosis and Management in Children and Adults. *Boston: Little, Brown; 1989.*

Using an end-hole catheter, a continuous pressure recording from the left ventricular apex across the subaortic membrane and then across the aortic valve provides a classical hemodynamic assessment (Fig. 13).

Management of patients with discrete subaortic stenosis varies with the severity of obstruction, but even those with mild obstruction require close follow-up, as these lesions may rapidly progress. Although still controversial, it has been the general experience that transcatheter dilation for most patients with discreet subaortic stenosis is suboptimal, although occasional, totally circumferential lesions that allow for splitting of the circumferential membrane might be acceptable lesions for dilation. More often, patients with subaortic stenosis require surgical resection when the obstruction is severe. Careful preservation of the integrity of the mitral valve as well as the left bundle branch is important. Patients in their 40s and beyond should have careful consideration of aortic valve replacement at the time of resection of the membrane, as these valves are often deformed and incompe-

tent. Patients with subaortic stenosis need close postoperative follow-up as nearly 15% have either residual or recurrent left ventricular outflow tract obstruction.[19] Women with subaortic stenosis contemplating pregnancy should be carefully apprised of both the familial tendency (15%) as well as the possibility that pregnancy may worsen their overall cardiac function.

TETRALOGY OF FALLOT

Ten percent of adults with congenital heart disease have tetralogy of Fallot. It is the most common cyanotic cardiac lesion seen after infancy and accounts for more than 50% of cyanotic heart disease in adults. Internists infrequently see a patient with tetralogy of Fallot who has not undergone surgery, but more often see patients who have had either previous palliative surgery or definitive corrective procedures.

ANATOMY

By definition, tetralogy has 4 anatomic components: 1) Right ventricular obstruction is secondary to both infundibular and pulmonic valvular stenosis. Both are of variable severity. Some patients have complete atresia of the right ventricular outflow tract. The pulmonary arteries themselves may also be small and sometimes hypoplastic, which may prevent surgical correction. 2) The VSD is membranous and large and approximates the size of the aortic annulus. 3) Aortic overriding across the ventricular defect is of variable degree and may approach 50% in those with severe pulmonic stenosis. 4) The right ventricle is hypertrophied secondary to its chronic pressure load; patchy interstitial right ventricular fibrosis occurs in older adults.

PHYSIOLOGY

Tetralogy has 2 essential physiologic components: 1) the right ventricular outflow tract obstruction causes decreased pulmonary blood flow, and 2) the large VSD allows blood to flow from the right ventricle to the systemic circulation (right-to-left shunting). Systemic desaturation is variable, depending on the severity of right ventricular obstruction. When severe,

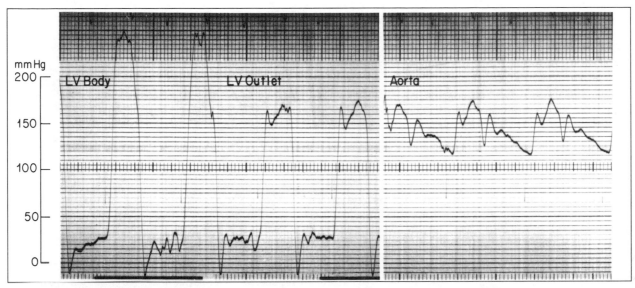

Figure 13. *Catheter withdrawal from the apex of the left ventricle (LV) across a discrete subaortic stenosis with moderate obstruction, into the subvalvular LV outlet chamber, then across the aortic valve into the aorta in a 12-year-old boy who has discrete membranous subaortic stenosis. Note the presence of equal ventricular end-diastolic pressures above and below the membrane and equal systolic pressures above the membrane. Reprinted with permission from Liberthson RR.* Congenital Heart Disease: Diagnosis and Management in Children and Adults. *Boston: Little, Brown; 1989.*

desaturation is marked. In order to survive without surgical intervention, patients with severe pulmonic stenosis or atresia must develop collateral blood flow from the systemic to the pulmonary circulation. In older patients, these natural collateral channels are extensive. When right ventricular obstruction is mild, right-to-left shunting is minimal, and patients may be acyanotic ("pink tetralogy").

CLINICAL COURSE

Cyanosis is typically present from early infancy and is progressive and worsened by exertion. A history of "tet spells" during the first years of life is sometimes offered by the patients. Spells typically occur in hot weather, follow exertion or feeding, and are characterized by irritability, dyspnea, hyperventilation, cyanosis, and, sometimes, syncope, seizure and death. Some patients have late residua of these spells, including seizure disorders and cerebral vascular accident. Spells are rare after age 2 years. Squatting is learned from infancy and is often incorporated into a child's activities. Squatting is nearly exclusive to patients with tetralogy. More socially acceptable squatting postures, such as crossing the legs when sitting, are sometimes adopted by

adults. Squatting increases systemic resistance and, therefore, decreases right-to-left blood flow across the ventricular defect and forces more blood to the lungs. Patients with chronic right-to-left shunting and systemic desaturation compensate by increased erythropoietin secretion, and erythrocytosis develops. When the erythrocytosis becomes excessive (hematocrit level >65%), however, dyspnea, fatigue and in situ thrombosis may occur. Patients who have not undergone surgical intervention may have a history of repeated phlebotomy. With long-standing erythrocytosis, uric acid elevation and symptomatic gout may be present. Abnormalities of factors V, VII, and IX as well as decreased and abnormal platelets result in increased perioperative bleeding, which can be ameliorated by preoperative phlebotomy.

Chronic right-to-left shunting subjects both unoperated patients and those who have had only palliative surgical procedures to the risk of systemic embolization. This may occur with careless intravenous technique. Cerebral abscess is another sequela of chronic right-to-left shunting, and must be suspected in patients with neurologic symptoms or findings. Bacterial endocarditis occurs in patients with uncorrected tetralogy and in those with palliated and corrected tetralogy. It usually involves the right ventricular outflow tract, the

VSD, or the overriding aortic valve, but it may occur at the site of palliative shunt insertion. Chemoprophylaxis is, therefore, a lifetime obligation. In the adult, ventricular tachyarrhythmia is an ominous finding and may herald sudden death. The risk of mortality is increased in pregnant women with uncorrected tetralogy, and the incidence of fetal death is also greatly increased.

CLINICAL FINDINGS

The salient findings in unoperated patients include generalized cyanosis and digital clubbing. Body habitus is normal, although kyphoscoliosis occurs in 20%. Those who have had a previous palliative procedure have a thoracotomy scar. Corrective procedures are performed via a median sternotomy. In the adult who has not had earlier surgery, continuous collateral bruits are heard throughout the chest. Those with a functioning palliative shunt will have a continuous bruit beneath their thoracotomy scar.

The cardiac examination in patients with palliative shunts and those who have not had prior surgery is the same because both still have the anatomic components of tetralogy. Successfully palliated patients differ only in having less cyanosis, because their pulmonary blood flow has been augmented: They may have no digital clubbing. However, patients with previous palliated shunts may outgrow or close their shunts and develop progressive cyanosis. In both patients with uncorrected or palliated shunts, there is palpable right ventricular hypertrophy and a palpable systolic thrill secondary to pulmonic stenosis. The S_1 is normal; the S_2 is single and often loud—it corresponds to aortic closure. Patients with very mild tetralogy ("pink tet") may have an audible pulmonic closure sound, which is otherwise atypical in tetralogy of Fallot. An ejection sound is common and arises from the overriding aortic valve and is best heard on expiration. A systolic ejection murmur secondary to right ventricular outflow tract obstruction is typical. The length, intensity, and contour of this murmur help the clinician to assess the severity of pulmonic stenosis. Long, loud, late-peaking murmurs indicate less severe right ventricular obstruction than do short, soft, early-peaking murmurs. With pulmonary atresia, an outflow tract murmur is not present, although collateral continuous bruits may be striking throughout the thorax.

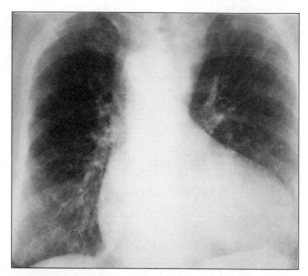

Figure 14. *Posteroanterior chest roentgenogram from a 59-year-old woman with tetralogy of Fallot and extensive systemic-to-pulmonary collateral vasculature with secondary rib notching. The cardiac silhouette has a distinctive "boot" shape secondary to the upturned apex, right ventricular hypertrophy, and the concave pulmonary artery segment. There is a right aortic arch. Reprinted with permission from Liberthson RR. Congenital heart disease in the child, adolescent and adult. In: Johnson RA, Haber E, Austen WG (eds).* Practice of Cardiology. *Boston: Little, Brown; 1980.*

The ECG reveals right ventricular hypertrophy and right-axis deviation in patients with either uncorrected or palliated tetralogy. Atrial flutter sometimes with one-to-one conduction are common beyond the third decade.

The chest x-ray film is often diagnostic. In the young patient, pulmonary vascular markings are diminished. However, with age and proliferation of collateral circulation, pulmonary vascular markings may actually be increased (Fig. 14). Functioning palliative shunts also cause increased pulmonary markings and enlargement of the pulmonary branch into which they enter. In unoperated patients and in those with palliative shunts, the cardiac silhouette is typical. There is an upturned apex, secondary to right ventricular enlargement, and a concave left basal region caused by the small main pulmonary artery. This combination gives the heart a boot shape. Approximately 25% of patients with tetralogy of Fallot have a right-sided aortic arch.

Ultrasound examination (Fig. 15) delineates the morphology of the right ventricular obstruc-

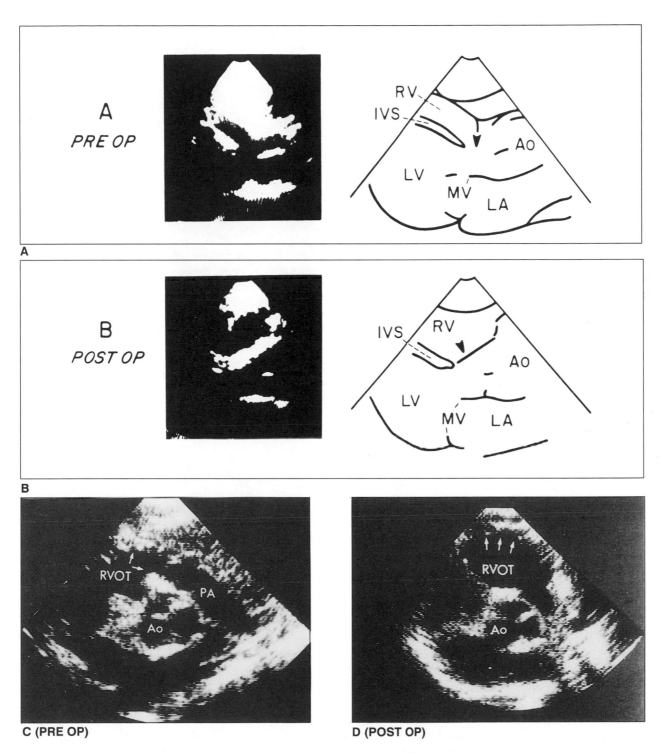

Figure 15. *Preoperative (A and C), and postoperative (B and D) 2-dimensional echocardiograms from 2 patients with tetralogy of Fallot in the parasternal long-axis projection (A and B), and the parasternal short axis (C and D) projection illustrating the VSD and overriding aorta (Ao) before and after patch revision (arrow) (A and B), and the right ventricular outflow tract (RVOT) obstruction (C and D) before and after resection and outflow patch enlargement (arrows). RV=Right ventricle; IVS=Ventricular septum; LV=Left ventricle; MV=Mitral valve; LA=Left atrium; PA=Pulmonary artery. Reprinted with permission from Liberthson RR.* Congenital Heart Disease: Diagnosis and Management in Children and Adults. *Boston: Little, Brown; 1989.*

tion, the VSD, the overriding aorta, and the hypertrophied right ventricle. It also differentiates tetralogy of Fallot from more complex entities, including single ventricle and variants of transposition of the great arteries. It is particularly helpful in accessing postoperative patients who have residual defects such as VSD or pulmonic stenosis.

CARDIAC CATHETERIZATION

Catheterization is required before surgical intervention. The objectives of the catheterization include detailed angiographic study of the right ventricular obstruction, including assessment of the caliber of the pulmonary arteries; assessment of the VSD and exclusion of multiple or atypical septal defects; and evaluation of the coronary arteries to identify the approximately 5% of patients who have anomalous origin of major left coronary branches from the right coronary. These branches cross the anterior right ventricle and can be damaged at the time of right ventriculotomy if not identified. In patients who have had previous palliative shunts, pulmonary artery anatomy, pressure, and resistance must be assessed because long-standing shunts may cause severe pulmonary vascular obstruction as well as kinking and hypoplasia of a pulmonary branch. Angiographic identification of these surgical shunts is also important before surgical revision (Fig. 16). Catheterization must also exclude more complex entities; notably, variants of double outlet right ventricle.

SURGICAL INTERVENTION

Surgery for tetralogy of Fallot began with the palliative procedures involving creation of a shunt between the systemic and pulmonary circulations to increase pulmonary blood flow and to alleviate systemic desaturation. The Blalock–Taussig shunt involves ligation of the distal subclavian artery and insertion of its proximal end into the ipsilateral pulmonary artery (Fig. 16). Complications with this procedure when performed before school age are rare, and

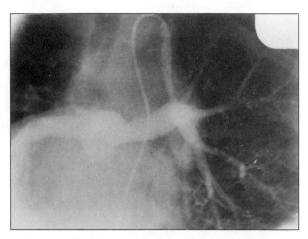

Figure 16. *Selective angiogram with the catheter in a patent Blalock–Taussig shunt, in the anterior–posterior projection illustrating contrast filling the pulmonary artery in a 49-year-old woman with tetralogy of Fallot. The catheter was passed retrogradely up the aorta. Reprinted with permission from Liberthson RR. Congenital Heart Disease: Diagnosis and Management in Children and Adults. Boston: Little, Brown; 1989.*

excellent long-term alleviation of desaturation is typical. Both pulse and blood pressure in the ipsilateral arm are sacrificed, but arm function and development are usually normal. Modified Blalock–Taussig shunts employing prosthetic tube grafts may be performed at any age and do not compromise the subclavian circulation. The Potts shunt involves creation of a surgical window between the left pulmonary artery and the descending aorta. It also achieves excellent long-term palliation of desaturation. However, in about one-fourth of patients, early heart failure owing to excessive pulmonary flow or late pulmonary vascular obstruction develops. Patients with these shunts require assessment of pulmonary artery pressure and resistance at the time of catheterization. When the latter is high, corrective surgery may be precluded. The Waterston shunt is a surgical window between the ascending aorta and the right pulmonary artery. It also provides excellent palliation. However, its complications include hypoplasia and stenosis of the right pulmonary artery secondary to kinking; early heart failure if the shunt is too large; and, occasionally, pulmonary vascular obstruction. Regardless of shunt type, patients may outgrow them or they may kink or close, and recurrent and progressive cyanosis occurs. If so, catheterization and further surgery are indicated. Despite their success in relieving cyanosis, shunts do not alter the intracardiac pathology of the tetralogy; therefore, the chronic sequelae of right-to-left shunting and right ventricular hypertension remain. For these reasons, most patients with palliative shunts should still have definitive surgical repair and shunt closure.

Correction of tetralogy of Fallot consists of surgical relief of right ventricular obstruction (which may require patch augmentation of the outflow tract) and patch closure of the VSD such that left ventricular outflow is directed to the overriding aorta. When the outflow tract requires a patch to enlarge it, patients have residual pulmonic incompetence that manifests as a low-pitched diastolic decrescendo murmur. Most centers perform elective total correction during infancy or early childhood. Infants who have tet spells require either emergency palliation or definitive repair. In all other cases, surgery should be performed when the diagnosis is confirmed. After the fifth decade of life, risks of total correction increase because of right ventricular dysfunction secondary to chronic hypertrophy and fibrosis.

After successful tetralogy repair, patients become acyanotic, clubbing resolves over a period of years, exercise tolerance markedly improves, and lifestyle becomes normal. Some patients have residual problems and all require continued surveillance. Problems include an incompletely closed VSD and residual right ventricular obstruction, which, when severe (gradient >50 mm Hg), requires reoperation. In the former, when shunt size exceeds 2:1, repeat operation is appropriate. Patients with right ventricular outflow tract patches have pulmonic incompetence, but this is usually well tolerated. If an anomalous left coronary artery branch was damaged at the time of repair, patients may have anterior wall myocardial infarction. Ventricular ectopy usually arises from the right ventricle and may be secondary to fibrosis owing to chronic right ventricular pressure overload or to aneurysm or infarction in those patients with a damaged anomalous coronary artery. It is an ominous finding and requires intensive antiarrhythmic treatment; invasive electrophysiologic study may help in the selection of an antiarrhythmic regimen but is far less predictive than in patients with coronary artery disease. When ventricular ectopy is associated with significant residual right ventricular obstruction, residual VSD, or severe pulmonic incompetence, patients may require reoperation. Right bundle branch block and left anterior hemiblock occur in 10% of patients after repair, but rarely lead to more advanced degrees of heart block. Syncope in these patients is uncommon.

DIFFERENTIAL DIAGNOSIS

Patients with pulmonic stenosis and VSD who also have variants of transposition of the great arteries, as well as those who have single ventricle rather than a VSD alone, may be impossible to differentiate clinically from those with tetralogy of Fallot. Both ultrasound and angiography are important in identifying these patients. The latter is essential because in some, reparative surgery is precluded and in others its risk may be increased.

EBSTEIN'S ANOMALY OF THE TRICUSPID VALVE

Although uncommon, Ebstein's anomaly is particularly pertinent to the adult cardiologist as it often allows prolonged survival, hence knowledge of both its diagnosis and management are essential. Ebstein's births have been observed more commonly among mothers who have taken Lithium during pregnancy.

The morphologic spectrum of Ebstein's anomaly varies from mild to severe. It should be thought of as an abnormality involving the entire right heart rather than merely the tricuspid valve.[20] In these patients, displacement downward into the right ventricle of the tricuspid valve elements occurs to a variable degree. Typically, the anterior leaflet maintains an attachment to the annulus at its leftward aspect. The anterior leaflet is generally large and "sail-like." It may be thickened and quite billous. The inferior and septal leaflets are often small fibrotic and dysplastic with fused chordal attachments that at times appear as mere excrescences on the ventricular wall. To the extent that the tricuspid apparatus is displaced downward into the ventricle, the functional right atrium is enlarged, and the functional contractile right ventricle is diminished in size. In addition to being small, the functional right ventricle is usually fibrotic, and the endocardial surface may be fibroelastic. In addition, the majority of patients have an interatrial communication that may also vary in size and may be either a patent foramen ovale or an actual septal defect. These patients have variably severe right ventricular inflow obstruction owing to the small and abnormal "true" right ventricle, have varying degrees of tricuspid insufficiency, and have variable degrees of right atrial enlargement depending on the presence and size of an interatrial communication, which allows right-to-left decompression, and the severity of tricuspid valve displacement and insufficiency. When an interatrial communication is absent, the right atrial enlargement may be profound, as there is no decompression and arrhythmias and early death are common. In the presence of interatrial communication, right-to-left shunting occurs and varying degrees of systemic desaturation along with other complications, notably systemic abscess or paradoxical embolus occur.

The body habitus with Ebstein's anomaly is typically normal, save for cyanosis and clubbing when present. With heart failure, jugular venous distension and tricuspid insufficiency may exist, depending on the dampening effect of the enlarged right atrium and the right-to-left egress provided by the interatrial communication, which allows "blow-off" for the regurgitant tricuspid volume. The right ventricular impulse is notably diminished or absent, although the right atrium may be evidenced by an "undulating-like" movement caused by contraction of the "atrialized" portion of the right ventricle. In addition, at the left sternal border, the right ventricular infundibulum may be palpable. The first heart sound is widely split as is the second sound. Extrasystolic sounds along the right sternum as well as a scratchy mid-systolic murmur at this site occur. Patients often also have a mid-diastolic tricuspid filling sound.

The ECG shows right atrial enlargement, decreased right ventricular voltage, a rightward axis, prolongation of the PR interval and typi-

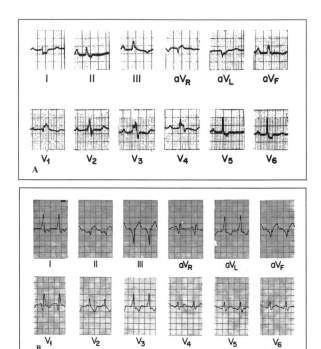

Figure 17. *(A) Twelve-lead ECG of a 52-year-old woman with Ebstein's anomaly of the tricuspid valve. There is right-axis deviation, first-degree atrioventricular block, and complete right bundle branch block with marked splintering of the R' deflection. (B) ECG in a 6-year-old girl who has Ebstein's anomaly and associated Wolff-Parkinson-White syndrome with a posterior bypass tract. Reprinted with permission from Liberthson RR.* Congenital Heart Disease: Diagnosis and Management in Children and Adults. *Boston: Little, Brown; 1989.*

cally a right bundle branch block pattern with marked splintering of the R prime wave, evidenced in the right precordial leads (Fig. 17A). In addition, supraventricular tachycardia is common, as is a "type B" Wolff–Parkinson–White pattern, which is seen in up to 15% of patients with Ebstein's anomaly (Fig. 17B). The chest x-ray film reveals a globular and often markedly enlarged cardiac silhouette owing to right atrial enlargement as well as leftward displacement of the right ventricular outflow tract (Fig. 18) which may give the heart a box-like appearance. Depending on the presence and magnitude of cyanosis, pulmonary vascular markings vary from normal to diminished.

The echocardiogram allows definitive diagnosis as well as assessment of the structural and functional aspects of Ebstein's anomaly. The anatomy and function of the tricuspid valve itself, the

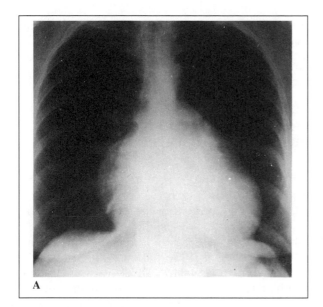

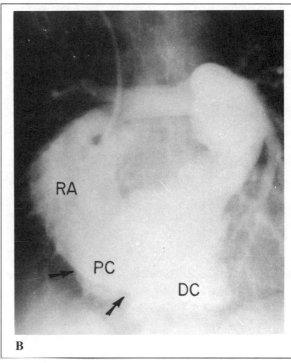

Figure 18. *(A) Posteroanterior chest roentgenogram of a 52-year-old woman with Ebstein's anomaly of the tricuspid valve. The right atrium is enlarged and the right ventricular outflow tract is displaced leftward. (B) Right atrial angiogram in the posteroanterior projection opacifying the enlarged right atrium (RA). The small distal right ventricular chamber (DC) and the leftward displaced right ventricular outflow tract are shown. Arrows indicate the junctions between the atrialized portion of the right ventricle (PC) and the right atrium and the distal right ventricular chamber.* Reprinted with permission from Liberthson RR. Congenital Heart Disease: Diagnosis and Management in Children and Adults. *Boston: Little, Brown; 1989.*

degree of displacement into the right ventricle, the size and contractility of the functional right ventricle, the size of the right atrium, the presence of an interatrial communication, the magnitude of tricuspid incompetence, and any associated cardiac abnormalities can all be assessed sufficiently well by ultrasound (Fig. 19); hence, cardiac catheterization is not often needed for these patients, and in fact carries some increased risk.

The clinical course and management are intimately entwined. Ebstein's anomaly may be minimal and go undetected for decades. Alternatively, when severe, death occurs during infancy. Classical presentation for adults with Ebstein's anomaly include persistent supraventricular tachyarrhythmia often associated with "type-B" Wolff–Parkinson–White syndrome, cyanosis and complications of right-to-left shunting including paradoxical embolus, systemic abscesses, right heart failure manifestations (dyspnea and fatigue), ventricular tachyarrhythmia with occasional sudden cardiac

death, and bacterial endocarditis. Management of Ebstein's anomaly depends on the severity of the deformity and the occurrence of symptoms and complications. Electrophysiology assessment before surgical intervention, aimed at identifying and ablating any preexcitation pathways present as well as assessing these patients for inducible ventricular tachyarrhythmia that may require postoperative management is recommended. For patients with marked cardiomegaly and those with significant systemic desaturation or right-to-left shunting complications or those with heart failure, attempts at surgical plasty revision of the tricuspid valve are warranted and have been accomplished with increasing success in recent years.[21] These are particularly appropriate for women who may still desire pregnancy, and hence need to avoid anticoagulation with warfarin if tricuspid reconstruction fails and prosthetic valve replacement is needed. It is not yet known whether these surgical plasty attempts will be as long lived as tri-

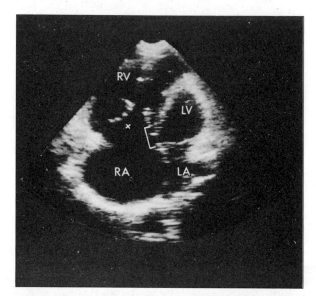

Figure 19. Two-dimensional echocardiogram in the apical 4-chamber view of a 19-year-old man with Ebstein's anomaly. Bracket shows the distance between the septal insertion of the tricuspid septal leaflet and the anterior mitral valve leaflet. There is a moderate degree of displacement of the tricuspid apparatus into the right ventricle (RV), creating the atrialized portion of the right ventricle (x). An atrial septal defect is present. RA=Right atrium; LA=Left atrium; LV=Left ventricle. Reprinted with permission from Liberthson RR. Congenital Heart Disease: Diagnosis and Management in Children and Adults. Boston: Little, Brown; 1989.

cuspid valve prostheses, although when possible, the plasty repairs are desirable. Ultrasound assessment can help identify the likelihood of achieving surgical valvuloplasty. Patients with a large mobile and nonadherent anterior tricuspid valve leaflet are more favorable candidates for valvuloplasty. When plasty is not possible, tricuspid valve replacement is necessary, and in all patients, repair of the interatrial communication when present is performed. When appropriate, reduction in the size of the right atrium should be considered.

After surgical repair, patients with Ebstein's anomaly generally experience marked improvement in symptoms. The risks of systemic embolization as well as cyanosis are eliminated. Some patients continue to suffer atrial tachyarrhythmia, and many require medication. All require chemoprophylaxis for bacterial endocarditis, and those with smaller and more dysfunctional "true" right ventricles may have persisting degrees of right heart failure. Although

surgery is not yet a truly elective procedure for patients with the anomaly, my personal threshold to recommend repair for selected individuals continues to decline.

ECTOPIC ORIGIN OF A CORONARY ARTERY FROM THE AORTA WITH ABERRANT PROXIMAL COURSE

Although uncommon, patients with ectopic origin of a coronary artery from the aorta are increasingly identified, owing to the many invasive and noninvasive cardiac procedures performed as well as to the not uncommon presentation of some of these patients with exertion-related ventricular tachyarrhythmia and sudden death. The clinical significance and management of these patients have only recently been delineated.[22] The most common clinically important entities are illustrated in Figure 20. As shown, aberrant origin may involve either the right or the left coronary artery and less often an isolated left coronary artery branch. The aberrant right or left coronary artery usually arise separately or from a common orifice adjacent to the normally arising artery. The ostium is often "slit-like," and the artery traverses the aortic wall in an oblique fashion in the region between the aorta and the right ventricular outflow tract. In patients clinically affected, the origin of the aberrant artery is commonly hypoplastic to varying degrees, hence obstructed proximally. The distal portion of the artery is either normal or relatively small. Less often, there is focal intraluminal obstruction of the aberrant artery in the region where it passes between the aorta and the outflow tract of the right ventricle. Proximal coronary obstruction is augmented during strenuous physical exertion by torsion of the great vessels caused by increased output as well as dilation of the aorta and right ventricular outflow tracts. In clinically affected patients, the aberrantly arising coronary arteries are large and perfuse major areas of myocardium and hence are dominant vessels. Although aberrant left coronary arteries more commonly have clinical sequelae, large aberrant right coronary arteries can also be clinically significant. It is important to emphasize that aberrant coronary arteries that are small and those that are not proximally obstructed do not have clinical sequelae and may go undetected throughout life.

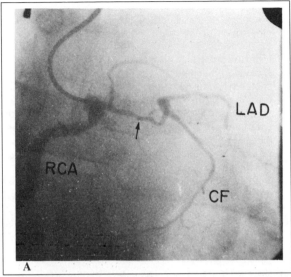 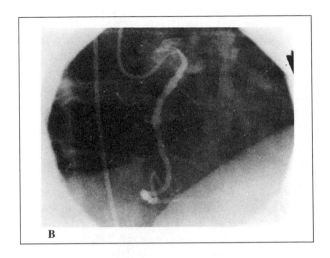

Figure 20. *(A) Selective right coronary arteriogram in the right anterior oblique projection of a 36-year-old man with anomalous origin of the left coronary artery (arrow) from the right coronary artery (RCA). The left coronary artery is small and passes posteriorly and leftward between the aorta and the right ventricular outflow tract; it then gives rise to small left anterior descending (LAD) and circumflex (CF) arteries. The right coronary artery is large and extends around the apex to the anterior left ventricular wall. (B) Selective right coronary angiogram in a 48-year-old man with aberrant origin of the right coronary artery form the left sinus of Valsalva. There is marked narrowing of this artery at its origin. Reprinted with permission from the American Heart Association from Liberthson RR et al.[22] and Liberthson RR. Congenital Heart Disease: Diagnosis and Management in Children and Adults. Boston: Little, Brown; 1989.*

In patients with significant proximal obstruction of a dominant artery, whether the right or the left coronary artery, the presentation is commonly that of exertion-induced ventricular tachycardia, exertional angina or sudden death. Clinically affected patients are generally young adults or teenagers. In contrast, patients who have an aberrant origin and proximal course of a coronary artery but who do not have proximal obstruction, or who have an aberrantly arising, but only small artery are not infrequently identified beyond mid-life as part of evaluation for unrelated acquired coronary artery disease. In these patients, symptoms are not related to the proximal compromise and aberrant origin itself. Noteworthy in these patients is the fact that their longer survival itself (particularly when the patient is older than 50 yr) bears testimony to the fact that proximal coronary artery obstruction is not severe enough to have lethal arrhythmic consequences; hence, specific management of the aberrancy is rarely indicated.

There are no specific clinical identifying criteria for these patients with aberrant coronary origins other than the fact that all young individuals presenting with exertional ventricular arrhythmia or angina in the absence of standard coronary risk factors should be screened for this anatomy. In the absence of myocardial ischemia or infarction, the resting ECG is either normal or shows mild nonspecific ST-wave changes. With exercise, it may or may not show ischemia in the area of aberrant coronary artery distribution, or ventricular tachyarrhythmia. Stress thallium imaging often reveals ischemia when there is significant proximal obstruction. Transthoracic cardiac ultrasound in the short-axis or parasternal or aortic views when performed by a "dedicated technician," illustrates the presence of an aberrantly arising right or left coronary artery and its proximal size and course relative to the right ventricular outflow tract. Doppler assessment of proximal coronary artery flow is also obtainable. Coronary angiography (Fig. 20), is required to delineate definitively the anatomy in these patients. It is often challenging for the physician performing the catheterization to engage the small, aberrantly arising coronary ostia. Both lateral and right anterior oblique projections ideally with a pulmonary artery catheter in place to help clarify the relationship of the aberrantly arising artery to the pulmonary artery are helpful. Functional assessment by atrial pacing with ECG recording from the anterolateral or inferior leads depending on the vessel involved and coronary sinus lactate levels provide useful functional information.

Optimal management of these patients may be difficult to determine. Patients who present with ventricular tachyarrhythmia and documented myocardial ischemia related to aberrancy of the proximally arising coronary artery should undergo a bypass surgical procedure. Because of the young age of these patients an arterial bypassing vessel should be used whenever possible. Patients identified after age 50 years, particularly by evaluations for other issues, have generally already demonstrated by their longevity that the proximal artery aberrancy is not their culprit lesion; particularly when the aberrant artery is small, the proximal portion of the aberrant artery seems unobstructed, and distal ischemia has not been confirmed. Middle-aged patients who have lesser degrees of proximal coronary compromise or small involved vessels must be carefully assessed and individualized to determine optimal management, particularly if their clinical presentation was suspicious.

The above sections have reviewed the pertinent clinical aspects of some of the more common forms of congenital heart disease which manifest in the adult. These patients present a continued challenge to the managing physician as they acquire the burdens of cardiac aging superimposed on their underlying lesions and earlier repairs.

REFERENCES

1. Liberthson RR. *Congenital Heart Disease: Diagnosis and Management in Children and Adults.* Boston: Little, Brown; 1989.
2. Kirklin JW, Barrett-Boyes BC. *Cardiac Surgery: Morphology, Diagnostic Criteria, Natural History, Techniques, Results and Indications.* New York: Churchill-Livingston; 1993.
3. Perloff JK, Child JS. *Congenital Heart Disease in Adults.* Philadelphia: WB Saunders; 1991.
4. Grossman W, Barry MM. Cardiac catheterization. In: Braunwald E (ed). *Heart Disease.* Philadelphia: WB Saunders; 1988:242-267.
5. Roberts JD, Lang P, Bigatello LM, et al. Inhaled nitric oxide in congenital heart disease. *Circulation.* 1993;87:447-453.
6. Rome JJ, Keane JF, Perry SB, et al. Double umbrella closure of atrial septal defects. *Circulation.* 1990; 82:751-758.
7. Liberthson RR, Boucher CA, Dinsmore RE, et al. Evaluation of the right heart function in adults with atrial septal defect using gated cardiac blood pool scanning. Presented at the American College of Cardiology 29th Annual Scientific Session, Houston, Texas, March 1980.
8. Liberthson RR, Boucher CA, Fallon JT, et al. Severe mitral regurgitation: a common occurrence in the aging patient with secundum atrial septal defect. *Clin Cardiol.* 1981;4(suppl):229-232.
9. Soto B, Ceballos R, Kirklin JW. Ventricular septal defects: A surgical viewpoint. *J Am Coll Cardiol.* 1989;14:1291-1297.
10. Kawashima Y, Danno M, Shimuzu Y. Ventricular septal defect associated with aortic insufficiency: Anatomic classification and method of operation. *Circulation.* 1973;47:1057-1064.
11. Neutze JM, Ishikawa T, Clarkson PM, et al. Assessment and follow-up of patients with ventricular septal defect and elevated pulmonary vascular resistance. *Am J Cardiol.* 1989; 63:327-331.
12. Wood P. The Eisenmenger syndrome. *Br Med J.* 1958;2:755-762.
13. Spinnato JA, Kraynack BJ, Cooper MW. Eisenmenger's syndrome in pregnancy: Epidural anesthesia for elective cesarean section. *N Engl J Med.* 1981;304:1215-1217.
14. Campbell M. Natural history of persistent patent ductus arteriosus. *Br Heart J.* 1968;30:4-13.
15. Mullins CE. Pediatric and congenital therapeutic cardiac catheterization. *Circulation.* 1989;79:1153-1159.
16. Liberthson RR, Pennington DG, Jacobs M, et al. Coarctation of the aorta: Review of 234 patients and clarification of management problems. *Am J Cardiol.* 1979;43:835-840.
17. Hellenbrand W, Allen H, Golinko R, et al. Balloon angioplasty for aortic recoarctation: Results of Valvuloplasty and Angioplasty of Congenital Anomalies Registry. *Am J Cardiol.* 1990;65:793-797.
18. Stanger P, Cassidy SC, Girod DA, et al. Balloon pulmonary valvuloplasty: Results of the Valvuloplasty and Angioplasty of the Congenital Anomalies Registry. *Am J Cardiol.* 1990;65:775-783.
19. Katz N, Buckley MJ, Liberthson RR. Discrete membranous subaortic stenosis: Report of 31 patients, review of the literature, and delineation of management. *Circulation.* 1977;56:1034-1038.
20. Lev M, Liberthson RR, Joseph RH, et al. The pathologic anatomy of Ebstein's disease. *Arch Pathol.* 1970; 90:334-343.
21. Danielson GK, Maloney JD, Devloo RAE. Surgical repair of Ebstein's anomaly. *Mayo Clinic Proc.* 1979;54:185-192.
22. Liberthson RR, Dinsmore RE, Fallon JT. Aberrant coronary artery origin from the aorta: Report of 18 patients, review of the literature and delineation of natural history and management. *Circulation.* 1979;59:748-754.

26 Pericardial Diseases

Haim Hammerman, MD
Robert A. Kloner, MD, PhD

PERICARDIAL DISEASES

The mode of presentation of pericardial disease depends on both the etiology and the type or stage of pericardial inflammatory reaction. Thus, pericardial diseases are classified by etiology and according to stage. The etiologies of pericardial disease are classified as infectious, neoplastic, metabolic, autoimmune-related, traumatic, and idiopathic (Table 1). The stages of inflammatory reactions include acute, subacute, and chronic, with or without effusion and constriction (Table 2).

Clinically, pericardial involvement may manifest as an acute disease, with or without evidence of pericardial effusion or tamponade. Sometimes it presents as a subacute constrictive disease, or effusive constrictive process. Chronic pericarditis can manifest as 1) relapses of acute attack, 2) chronic pericardial effusion, or 3) chronic constrictive pericarditis.[1,2]

ACUTE PERICARDITIS

Common etiologies of acute pericarditis include viral, post-myocardial infarction (MI), uremic, idiopathic, and autoimmune-related diseases. In immunologically competent patients, most of the cases of primary pericardial disease are idiopathic. Acute pericarditis is a clinical entity characterized by 3 major features: chest pain, friction rub, and fever. The pain of pericarditis characteristically is sharp or stabbing, variable in intensity, persistent, and aggravated by respiration, coughing, and movement. The pain is usually precordial, sometimes substernal, and occasionally radiates to the neck, arms, and back. It may be relieved by leaning forward or sitting and exacerbated by lying down. Some patients have acute pericarditis without pain; in others, the pain mimics that of ischemic disease.

The most characteristic physical sign is a precordial friction rub. This is a scratchy noise, caused by friction between the pericardial layers, and may have 3 components: presystolic, systolic, and protodiastolic. All 3 components are not always heard in any 1 patient. The quality of the rub typically changes with patient position and often is transitory. The rub is best heard during expiration, with the patient leaning forward. Although a pericardial friction rub is pathognomonic for pericarditis, it is found in only 60%-70% of patients with acute pericarditis. It may be difficult to distinguish the rub from a murmur when only 1 component of the rub is heard. Therefore, every attempt must be made to repeat the auscultatory examination in order to detect other components or a change in the friction rub. Absence of a friction rub does not rule out pericardial effusion. Other common signs of acute pericarditis are fever and tachycardia. Associated symptoms and signs of systemic disease should be sought. Patients should be evaluated for clinical signs of cardiac compression (e.g., tamponade).[1-3]

Laboratory findings depend on the etiology of the disease. In cases of viral, immune-related, infectious, or idiopathic pericarditis, sedimentation rate and leukocyte count may be elevated. The electrocardiogram (ECG) shows sinus tachycardia and diffuse ST-segment elevation in multiple leads in the early stages. This ST elevation is different from that in acute myocardial infarction (MI), in which it is localized and accompanied by Q-wave formation. Sometimes only T-wave changes are detected. A decrease in QRS amplitude is seen in patients with pericardial effusion, and atrial arrhythmias occasionally are detected. Chest x-ray film may be normal or, with pericardial effusion, the heart shadow may be enlarged (see Chapter 4).

Table 1. Etiologic Classification of Pericardial Disease

Infectious
    Viral (Coxsackie B, A; echo; influenza; infectious mononucleosis)
    Bacterial (pneumococci, staphylococci, meningococci, gonococci)
    Tuberculous
    Fungal (histoplasmosis, aspergillosis)
    Parasitic
    Acquired immunodeficiency syndrome (AIDS)
Pericarditis associated with acute myocardial infarction
    Neoplastic
    Primary (meosthelioma)
    Secondary (lung, breast, melanoma, lymphoma, leukemia)
Metabolic
    Uremia
    Myxedema
    Cholesterol
Autoimmune related
    Connective tissue diseases (systemis lupus erythematosus, rheumatoid arthritis, scleroderma,
        polyarteritis nodosa, Takayasu's disease, Wegener's granulomatosis)
    Post-cardiac injury (late postmyocardial infarction syndrome–Dressler's syndrome, postcardiotomy
        syndrome, post-trauma syndrome)
    Drug induced (procainamide, hydralazine, penicillin, isonicotinic acid hydrazide, phenylbutazone,
        minoxidil, high-dose cyclophosphamide in children)
Trauma
    Penetrating chest injury
    Closed chest injury
    After throacic surgical procedures
    After cardiac catheterization and pacemaker insertion
    Rupture of heart or great vessels
Aortic dissection and rupture of heart
Radiation
Miscellaneous
    Sarcoidosis
    Amyloidosis
    Acute pancreatitis
    Chylopericardium
    Familial Mediterranean fever
    Familial pericarditis
Idiopathic

Management of acute pericarditis includes: 1) observation for development of pericardial effusion and signs of tamponade (monitor heart rate, arterial and venous pressure); 2) determining and treating the underlying etiology; and 3) analgesics and anti-inflammatory agents for viral or idiopathic pericarditis. Most patients with viral or idiopathic pericarditis recover rapidly with the help of symptomatic therapy, such as aspirin, for a few days. Indomethacin is often used, but probably has little advantage over aspirin. Glucocorticosteroids are more potent but should be used only in severe cases that do not respond to nonsteroidal anti-inflammatory agents. Chronic recurrent or relapsing pericarditis may follow acute pericarditis. This syndrome often develops in patients who have been treated with glucocorticosteroids and later had the dose reduced. Management of this relapsing syndrome includes very slow reduction of the glucocorticosteroid dose. Pericardiectomy should be

Table 2. Stages of Inflammatory Reaction in Pericarditis

Acute pericarditis
    Noneffusive (fibrinous)
    Effusive
Subacute pericarditis
    Effusive constrictive
    Constrictive
Chronic pericarditis
    Effusive
    Constrictive
    Adhesive

considered in relapsing cases that require long periods (more than a year) of steroid therapy.[1–6]

ACUTE PERICARDITIS WITH PERICARDIAL EFFUSION

Pericardial effusion (accumulation of fluid in the pericardial space) can occur in the acute phase of pericarditis and develop either rapidly or slowly and insidiously. Pericardial effusion can be associated with compression of the heart. If fluid has accumulated to a point of causing increased intrapericardial pressure, compression of the heart can develop. The rate at which the fluid accumulates is important, because slow accumulation allows the pericardium to stretch over time; with rapid accumulation this compensatory mechanism does not have time to develop. The primary effect of accumulation of fluid in the pericardial space is eventual restriction of diastolic filling. The influence on systolic contraction is negligible. Systemic arteriolar contraction, salt and water retention, and increased venous tone act initially as compensatory mechanisms to preserve cardiac output (see section on cardiac tamponade). Thus, the clinical picture of compensated pericardial effusion with compression is increased systemic venous pressure. In cases of cardiac tamponade, there is failure of the compensatory mechanisms with a drop in cardiac output. Pericardial effusion can present as a wide range of clinical syndromes,

from an asymptomatic undetected effusion without hemodynamic compromise to dramatic life-threatening tamponade. The 2 main factors governing presentation are the amount of fluid and rate of accumulation. Extent of prior inflammation or thickening of the pericardium affects its capability to stretch and, hence, the amount of fluid required for tamponade.

Clinical findings of pericardial effusion include the pain of associated pericarditis (sometimes the pain may become less sharp in quality once fluid accumulates), shortness of breath, orthopnea, cough, tachycardia, elevated central venous pressure, hepatic enlargement, a weak apical cardiac impulse, and faint heart sounds. The friction rub of pericarditis may disappear. In large effusions there may be an area of dullness to percussion and bronchial breathing at the angle of the left scapula, probably caused by lung compression (Ewart's sign).

Electrocardiographic findings are similar to those noted above. In large effusions, typically, QRS amplitude is decreased.

The chest x-ray film reveals an enlarged cardiac silhouette (Chapter 4) with clear lungs. Epicardial fat lines may be seen within the cardiac shadow. Fluoroscopy shows diminished cardiac pulsations. Echocardiography is an accurate and convenient noninvasive tool for diagnosing pericardial effusion (see Chapter 7). Both M-mode and 2-dimensional echocardiograms show fluid accumulation and pericardial thickening. In general, the amount of fluid can be semiquantitated by M-mode echocardiography. In small to moderate effusions, fluid appears as an echo-free space posterior to the left ventricle. In the absence of adhesions, fluid also appears anteriorly in moderate to large effusions. Very large effusions often extend behind the lower left atrium. Exaggerated heart movements ("swinging heart") are seen with large effusions and are often associated with an echocardiographic appearance simulating mitral and tricuspid prolapse ("pseudoprolapse"). Two-dimensional echocardiography provides a better idea as to the quantitation of fluid, especially if a large volume has accumulated or if the fluid is loculated (Figs. 1, 2). Serial echocardiography is valuable in following the course of pericardial

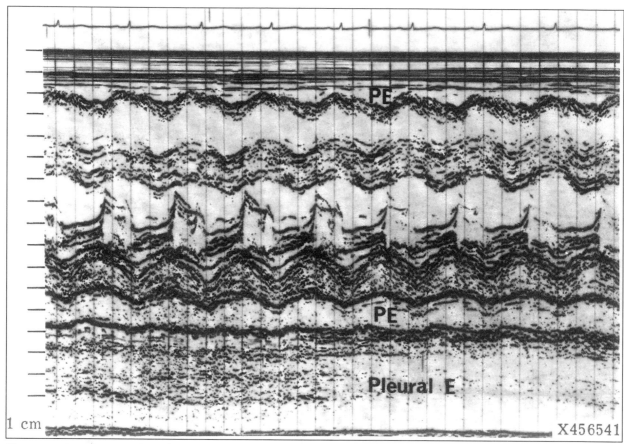

Figure 1. *M-mode echocardiogram from a patient with pericardial and pleural effusions (E). The pericardial effusion (PE) can be seen both anteriorly and posteriorly. From Feigenbaum H.[7] With permission.*

effusions. Radionuclide scans and intravenous injection of CO with contrast angiocardiography may be used to detect effusion in cases in which echocardiography is unsatisfactory.[1,2,7]

CARDIAC TAMPONADE

Cardiac tamponade is an accumulation of fluid in the pericardium in an amount sufficient to cause serious restriction of diastolic filling, with failure of compensatory mechanisms. Development of tamponade is related to distensibility of the pericardium and the speed of fluid accumulation. It is not proportional to the amount of fluid present, since massive effusions may be present without tamponade, and relatively small amounts of fluid collecting quickly may produce severe compression and tamponade. Circulation cannot be sustained for

long, once pericardial pressure exceeds venous pressure. Any cause of pericardial effusion can induce cardiac tamponade. Frequent causes are neoplasms, radiation, trauma, bleeding after cardiac surgery, pyogenic infections, tuberculosis, and uremia (Table 3). Tamponade occasionally occurs during acute viral or idiopathic pericarditis and in patients treated with anticoagulants during the course of acute pericarditis.[1,2,8]

The clinical manifestations are the result of a fall in cardiac output and elevated venous pressure. Patients complain of lightheadedness and dizziness as forward output decreases, as well as other symptoms of pericardial effusion discussed above. Physical examination reveals jugular venous distention, tachycardia, systemic hypotension, narrow pulse pressure, paradoxical pulse and, in some cases, tender and enlarged liver. When tamponade is severe, there is

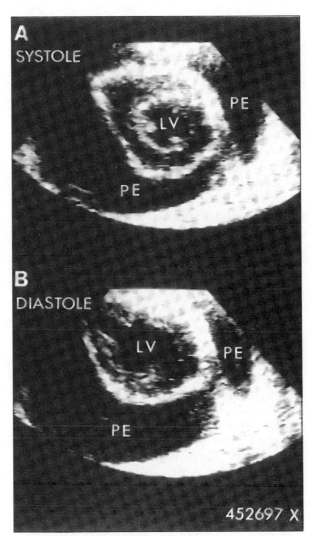

Figure 2. *Short-axis 2-dimensional echocardiogram from a patient with a large pericardial effusion (PE) demonstrating the shift in cardiac position from systole to diastole. LV=Left ventricle. From Feigenbaum H.[7] With permission.*

evidence of a shock state with signs of organ hypoperfusion.

Paradoxical pulse, defined as an abnormally large (>10 mm Hg) drop in arterial systolic pressure with inspiration, is a valuable sign of cardiac tamponade. This physical sign can be detected by palpation of the pulse. During inspiration the amplitude of the pulse drops markedly. The degree of paradoxical pulse can be estimated by measuring blood pressure during the respiratory cycle. It should be measured during normal respiration, since deep breathing as well as artificial respiration exaggerate paradoxical pulse. In cases of severe hypotension, this sign is difficult to appreciate. Paradoxical pulse can be accurately determined by means of direct arterial pressure measurements. In patients with chronic constrictive pericarditis, paradoxical pulse is often minimal or absent. Although this finding is consistently found in tamponade, it is not pathognomonic of it; it is seen in acute and chronic obstructive lung diseases, severe myocardial failure, hemorrhagic shock, and in some forms of restrictive cardiomyopathies. Kussmaul's sign (rise in central venous pressure with inspiration) occasionally occurs in cardiac tamponade, but it is more common in patients with constrictive pericarditis; it also occurs in some patients with tricuspid valve disease. Typically, the x and y descents of the jugular venous pulse are approximately equal, or the x descent is predominant. Auscultation typically reveals tachycardia; the heart sounds may be faint with or without a pericardial friction rub.[1,2,8,9]

The ECG shows features similar to those described for effusion. Electrical alternans (alternation of the QRS amplitude on every other beat) appears in severe cases of tamponade.

The chest x-ray film may show either a normal or large heart shadow, with clear lung fields. Symmetric enlargement of the heart shadow occurs when more than 200-300 ml of fluid accumulates. Fluoroscopy reveals diminished cardiac pulsations.

Table 3. Common Causes of Tamponade

Neoplastic disease
Idiopathic pericarditis
Uremia
Trauma
Infection (tuberculous, pyogenic)
Rupture of heart or great vessels
Anticoagulant therapy (during pericardial disease)
Iatrogenic (after thoracic surgery, catheterization, pacemaker)
Radiation

Echocardiography establishes the presence of pericardial fluid and allows a reasonably accurate estimation of the size of the effusion (Figs. 1, 2). Detection of abnormal diastolic right ventricular wall motion may be a sensitive indicator of a hemodynamically significant pericardial effusion. There is posterior motion of the anterior right ventricular wall that represents true collapse of the right ventricle in early diastole. Echocardiographic findings of a pericardial effusion—an inspiratory increase in right ventricular dimensions and right atrial and ventricular diastolic collapse—strongly suggest cardiac tamponade. In various studies, the sensitivity and specificity of right ventricular collapse for tamponade are 79%-92% and 90%-100%, respectively. Patients with pulsus paradoxus and severe cardiac tamponade have a marked increase in respiratory variation in transvalvular flow velocities, flow velocity integrals and left ventricular ejection and isovolumic relaxation times. These changes were seen also in some patients with pericardial effusion but without overt hemodynamic compromise.

However, tamponade is diagnosed primarily on the basis of clinical findings and characteristic hemodynamic features rather than echocardiography. In cases of life-threatening tamponade, echocardiography should not be performed if it will delay the decision to perform pericardiocentesis. The clinical features of right ventricular infarction sometimes mimic tamponade. Detection of fluid by echocardiography with no evidence of right ventricular enlargement or abnormal right ventricular contractility favor the latter diagnosis.[1,2,6,10,11]

Cardiac catheterization is not required when the diagnosis is certain, but it is important in equivocal cases or when an element of pericardial constriction is suspected. Characteristically, venous pressure is elevated with normal inspiratory decline (Kussmaul's sign usually absent). Prominent y descent, which is characteristic of constrictive pericarditis (described later), is absent in tamponade. Paradoxical pulse can be recorded from a systemic artery or from left ventricular pressures, and, in extreme cases, pulsus alternans (alternation of systolic pressure amplitude every other beat) can be recorded. Typically, both right and left ventricular diastolic pressures equal intrapericardial pressure. Right atrial pressure is elevated above normal, and right atrial pressure, right ventricular end-diastolic pressure, pulmonary artery diastolic pressure, and pulmonary capillary wedge pressure are within 5 mm Hg of each other. After pericardial aspiration, pericardial and right atrial pressures fall, right ventricular diastolic pressure comes down to a normal level, and cardiac output increases.

Patients with acute pericarditis should be observed carefully for development of pericardial effusion with tamponade. In the presence of pericardial effusion, heart rate and arterial and central venous pressures should be monitored continuously and serial echocardiograms recorded to detect any change in the amount of pericardial fluid. In case of cardiac tamponade, the definitive emergency treatment is removal of pericardial fluid by pericardiocentesis or surgical drainage. Medical support is often necessary to stabilize the patient's condition while preparations are made for the definitive procedures. Intravenous fluids are administered in order to help restore left ventricular filling volumes. Despite venous congestion, significant volumes should be administered (up to 300-500 ml/15 min). Inotropic support may be beneficial in improving cardiac output. Isoproterenol is infused initially at a rate of 2-4 μg/min and the rate is increased up to 20 μg/min until improvement or appearance of arrhythmias. Dobutamine may be infused starting at a rate of 1-2 μg/kg/min and the rate is increased to 15 μg/kg/min. Expansion of blood volume combined with nitroprusside has been shown to increase cardiac output and improve blood pressure in numerous studies of animals with tamponade. However, in humans, the hemodynamic benefits of volume expansion alone or combined with nitroprusside are very limited. Medical support is not an alternative mode of treatment and should not cause a delay in performing pericardiocentesis or surgical drainage.[1–8,10,11]

PERICARDIOCENTESIS

Pericardiocentesis—needle aspiration of the pericardial sac—has been used successfully in the management of pericardial effusion and tamponade. Pericardiocentesis is performed for 2 major reasons: therapeutically, for relief of tamponade as an emergency procedure or, in cases of large effusion, for relief of symptoms; and to obtain fluid for diagnostic purposes. Pericardiocentesis is associated with potentially dangerous complications (e.g., ventricular laceration or puncture, coronary artery laceration, ventricular arrhythmias, MI, and even cardiac arrest), and should be performed by those experienced in this procedure. Some believe that pericardiocentesis should be performed only for emergency relief of cardiac tamponade, and recommend surgical drainage in elective cases.

Optimally, pericardiocentesis is performed in the cardiac catheterization laboratory under ECG and fluoroscopic control. However, it can be performed at the bedside with proper monitoring. In general, a needle is inserted 2-4 cm below the junction of the subxiphoid process and the left costal margin at an angle of 20-30 degrees, so that it passes underneath the sternum into the pericardial sac. A chest lead of the ECG is connected to the needle and monitored throughout the insertion. When the needle touches the myocardium, ST elevation is detected. The location of the needle can also be determined by fluoroscopy (sometimes with the aid of a contrast agent injection), by echocardiography, by measuring pressure contour from the needle, or by identifying the type of fluid aspirated. Aspirated bloody fluid should be compared to venous blood for its hemoglobin content in order to determine whether a cardiac chamber was punctured. Bloody pericardial fluid tends not to clot, in contrast to blood aspirated accidentally from a cardiac chamber. The pericardiocentesis tends to be low risk when there is a large anterior pericardial effusion, determined by echocardiography. Intrapericardial pressures should be measured before and after aspiration of fluid. In tamponade, this pressure exceeds or equals central venous pressure, and in some cases it may exceed 20 mm Hg. Intrapericardial pressure drops after removal of fluid. Some pericardial needles have a plastic cannula over them; after successful entry into the pericardial space, the needle is removed, leaving the cannula for drainage. Most cardiologists prefer to exchange the needle for a catheter, and this is performed by passing a soft floppy tip guide-wire through the needle and then passing a 6 or 7 French multihole catheter over the guide-wire into the pericardial sac. This catheter can be left for continuous drainage or for intrapericardial drug administration (e.g., cytotoxic or sclerosing agent) in large recurrent or malignant effusions.

Open surgical drainage is an alternative treatment for cardiac tamponade. Subxiphoid pericardiotomy under local anesthesia can be performed in acutely ill patients for relief of tamponade. Surgical drainage is indicated in cases of repeated accumulation of pericardial effusion.

The pericardial fluid should be analyzed for color, turbidity, cell counts, cultures, chemistries, and cytology. However, in a number of diseases (viral pericarditis, collagen-vascular diseases, uremia) the pericardial fluid has no pathognomonic features. The quality of fluid inspected visually may be of some diagnostic yield. Serosanguineous or sanguineous effusion is found after cardiac surgery, trauma, pericarditis after acute MI treated with anticoagulants, neoplastic pericarditis, and rupture of the heart and great vessels. Serous effusion is commonly found in viral pericarditis, radiation pericarditis, heart failure, tuberculous pericarditis, collagen diseases, and hypoalbuminemia. Chylous effusion may follow cardiac surgery with injury to lymph vessels or when neoplasm interferes with lymph drainage. Cholesterol effusion is found in cases of myxedema.

The fluid should be characterized as a transudate (protein <3 g/100 ml) or an exudate (protein >3g/100 ml). Transudates occur in heart failure, hypoalbuminemia, Dressler's syndrome, postpericardiotomy syndrome, drug-induced pericarditis, cases of collagen diseases, and radiation pericarditis. Exudates are more likely to occur in infection, neoplasms, uremia, chylous pericarditis, and collagen diseases.

Cholesterol content is elevated in cases of myxedema. Glucose content of the fluid is low in bacterial pericarditis.

Other tests that should be performed include blood cell count and differential; gram stain; Ziehl-Neelsen stain; cultures for aerobic and anaerobic bacteria; cultures for tuberculosis; and, when suspected, fungal cultures. Positive cytologic findings have been reported in 50%-75% of patients with neoplastic involvement of the pericardium, depending on the number of samples examined. Pericardiocentesis can provide positive culture diagnosis in 15% of cases of tuberculosis and in almost all cases of pyogenic pericarditis.

As mentioned previously, pericardiocentesis is not without hazards; therefore, it, as well as surgical exploration, should be performed only when indicated, namely, in tamponade or high pressure pericardial effusion, suspicion of pyogenic pericarditis, and the need to obtain fluid for diagnosis.[1,2,8,12]

CHRONIC PERICARDITIS

Chronic pericarditis may be associated with relapses of acute pericarditis, chronic pericardial effusion or constriction, or adhesion to surrounding structures. Chronic pericardial effusion can follow any cause of pericarditis, presenting as a wide variety of clinical pictures depending on the degree of compression of the heart and the manifestations of the underlying disease. In some patients chronic asymptomatic pericardial effusion develops that does not progress to compression or cardiac constriction.

CHRONIC CONSTRICTIVE PERICARDITIS

This condition occurs when the healing of acute pericarditis is followed by formation of scar tissue surrounding the heart, compressing its chambers and restricting diastolic filling. Constrictive pericarditis may follow idiopathic pericarditis, tuberculosis, pyogenic infection, radiation, uremia, neoplasm, trauma, viral and connective tissue diseases. Often the etiology of pericarditis cannot be determined in late stages of constrictive pericarditis. The fundamental pathophysiologic abnormality characteristic of

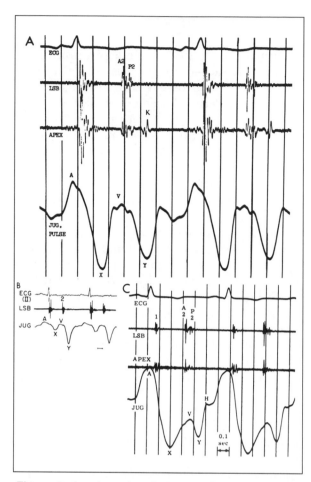

Figure 3. *Jugular pulses in 3 examples of pericardial constriction. In example A, both x and y descents are deep. A pericardial "knock" (K) coincides with the y trough. Example B shows a deep y descent but a shallow x descent. A few sound vibrations are located in early diastole at the expected time of the knock. Example C displays a deep x descent with a relatively short y descent. All 3 examples display early v-wave peaking (around the time of S2), an early y trough (less than 0.2 second after A2), and an early, prominent H wave. These features are characteristic of pericardial constriction. From Tavel ME.[13] With permission from Year Book Medical Publishers.*

constrictive pericarditis is restriction of diastolic filling due to limitation imposed by the fibrous scarred pericardium. Stroke volume is diminished and ventricular end-diastolic pressures as well as mean atrial pressure and systemic and pulmonary vein pressures are equally elevated. Sometimes pericardial fibrosis is associated with myocardial fibrosis, which leads to ventricular contraction abnormality.

Clinical manifestations include shortness of breath, orthopnea, and fatigue due to limited cardiac output reserve, and elevated systemic jugular venous pressure. Kussmaul's sign may be present. The jugular venous pulse has a characteristic wave form. The peak of the v wave is early, and there is a deep y descent. This is followed by an early diastolic rise, terminating in an early H wave and a plateau (Fig. 3).[3] Paradoxical pulse is observed in some cases. Signs of congestive hepatomegaly, spleno-megaly, and ascites may be found; dependent edema is less common than ascites. Constrictive pericarditis is a frequently missed diagnosis. Patients with chronic constrictive pericarditis may be erroneously diagnosed as having cirrhosis of the liver; others are suspected of having gastrointestinal malignancy and undergo a lengthy clinical workup. These diagnostic errors can be avoided simply by careful examination of the venous pressure, which is elevated in constrictive pericarditis. The precordial pulse is either imperceptible or appears to retract during systole. Heart sounds typically are faint. A diastolic pericardial knock, which is an early, high pitched sound (0.06-0.12 sec after aortic closure), may be heard and is related to the phase of early diastolic filling of the heart. It coincides with the y trough described for the venous pulse. Studies have related this sound to the sudden halt of ventricular filling in constrictive pericarditis. This sound, like Kussmaul's sign, occurs frequently in constrictive pericarditis but rarely in cardiac tamponade.

Hancock[14] suggested that there are 2 forms of constriction, 1 elastic and the other more rigid. These 2 forms are believed to cause different patterns of diagnostic signs. The elastic form is similar to cardiac tamponade and is associated with prominent paradoxical pulse and systolic descent in venous tracings. The rigid type has a less prominent paradoxical pulse and a more conspicuous diastolic descent in the venous pressure tracing, often associated with a pericardial knock.[14]

Electrocardiographic abnormalities in about 25% of patients include low QRS amplitude, T-wave changes, notched P waves, and atrial fibrillation. Chest x-ray shows a normal or slightly enlarged cardiac shadow, with clear lung fields. Pericardial calcification may be seen (see Chapter 4). Computed tomography as well as magnetic resonance imaging are valuable in identifying pericardial thickening and other findings consistent with constrictive pericarditis, including dilatation of large systemic veins and narrowing of the right ventricle. Pericardial thickening on echocardiography in the absence of effusion is a nonspecific finding and is not diagnostic of constriction. Abnormal left ventricular filling, as reflected by a sharp posterior motion of the posterior wall in early diastole followed by a flat segment, can be seen in constriction, with prominent early diastolic anterior motion of the ventricular septum. Two-dimensional echocardiography may show small ventricles with enlarged atria, dilatation of the inferior vena cava, and bulging of the interventricular and interatrial septa into the left side of the heart on inspiration. Patients with constrictive pericarditis can be differentiated from those with restrictive cardiomyopathy by comparing respiratory changes in transvalvular flow velocities. Patients with constrictive pericarditis show respiratory variation in left ventricular isovolumic relaxation time and in peak mitral flow velocity in early diastole. These changes disappear after surgery and are not present in patients with restrictive cardiomyopathy or in normal subjects. The relatively larger pulmonary venous systolic/diastolic and greater respiratory variation in pulmonary venous systolic, and especially diastolic flow velocities by trans-esophageal echocardiography can be useful signs in distinguishing constrictive pericarditis from restrictive cardiomyopathy.[1,3,15–17]

Cardiac catheterization reveals that ventricular end-diastolic pressures are elevated. Right ventricular pressure shows a consistent steep early diastolic dip, followed by a plateau ("square-root sign"). The end-diastolic pressure of the right ventricle is higher or equal to one-third of its systolic pressure. The wave form and amplitude of left ventricular diastolic pressure is identical to that of the right ventricle. Pulmonary arterial diastolic pressure is equal to end-diastolic pressure in the ventricles. Severe

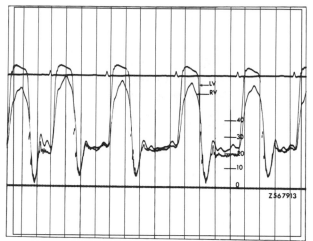

Figure 4. *Simultaneous left ventricular and right ventricular pressure recordings from a patient with constrictive pericarditis. The classic "square root" sign of the ventricular pressures during diastole can be noted. From Feigenbaum H.[7] With permission.*

constriction is associated with filling pressures of 20-25 mm Hg (Fig. 4). The right atrial pressure pulse has an M-shaped pattern. The typical venous M-shaped pattern and ventricular square-root sign are characteristic of constriction and differentiate it from tamponade. Cardiac catheterization helps differentiate constrictive pericarditis from restrictive cardiomyopathy. Transvenous endomyocardial biopsy may be of value when differential diagnosis between restrictive myocardial or constrictive pericardial disease is necessary.

Pericardial resection is the treatment of choice in symptomatic cases. Operative mortality is about 5%. Long-term results are satisfactory, especially in radical resection of the pericardium; however, hemodynamic improvement may be gradual. In cases with no improvement, one should look for either myocardial involvement or inadequate pericardial resection. Recurrence of constriction is rare.[1-3,18]

SUBACUTE EFFUSIVE-CONSTRICTIVE PERICARDITIS

In this condition, constrictive pericarditis coexists with pericardial effusion and tamponade. The constriction is by the visceral pericardium rather than by the parietal pericardium. Causes of effusive-constrictive pericarditis include tuberculosis, recurrent relapses of idiopathic pericarditis, trauma, radiation effects, uremia, and connective tissue diseases. Physical findings include paradoxical pulse and elevated venous pressure with prominent x descent. An S_3 or diastolic knock may be present. The ECG reveals low or borderline QRS amplitude with T-wave changes. Chest x-ray film reveals a large heart and echocardiography often reveals effusion and pericardial thickening. After removal of fluid by pericardiocentesis, venous pressure typically remains elevated due to remaining constriction. The intracavitary pressure tracings shift from those typical of tamponade before pericardiocentesis (x = y descent or x > y descent, no square-root sign) to those typical of constriction after pericardiocentesis (y > x descent, square-root sign). This condition may progress to chronic constrictive pericarditis. Surgical excision of the pericardium is indicated in severe cases.[19]

ADHESIVE PERICARDITIS

In this condition, there are adhesions between pericardium and structures in the mediastinum. Adhesive pericarditis usually does not interfere with cardiac function.

FEATURES OF SPECIFIC FORMS OF PERICARDIAL DISEASE

VIRAL OR ACUTE BENIGN FORM OF PERICARDITIS

Viral pericarditis is common and can be caused by a wide range of viruses (Coxsackie B or A, influenza, echo, herpes simplex, mumps, chicken pox, and adenovirus). It can cause a variety of inflammatory reactions (serous, fibrinous, hemorrhagic, or suppurative), probably depending on the virus. Sometimes acute pericarditis is related to or associated with a viral infection by history. Viral cultures are not always helpful; 4-fold or greater increases in convalescent serum titer are usual, but because most infections are benign, this variable is not tested. When viral etiology cannot be established but is presumed, the illness is referred to by some physicians as acute benign pericarditis. This condition is more frequent in young adults.

Pain is usually accompanied by fever; pneumonitis and pleuritis are common. There is evidence of pericardial effusion, but tamponade is unusual. The acute disease lasts for 10-14 days and relapses of the acute disease occur in 20% of cases. No specific therapy is available. Analgesic anti-inflammatory drugs (aspirin or indomethacin) may be used; corticosteroids are needed only in severe cases.[1-3,6]

NEOPLASTIC PERICARDIAL DISEASE

Metastatic tumors are important because they are responsible for serious pericardial effusion and tamponade. Common malignancies affecting the pericardium are carcinoma of the lung and breast, melanoma, lymphoma, and leukemia. Neoplasms characteristically produce large pericardial effusions and, sometimes, tamponade.

Pericardial metastases can be detected in some cases by echocardiography. Pericardiocentesis is indicated to relieve tamponade, symptomatic pericardial effusion, and for obtaining cytologic specimens. Positive cytologic findings have been reported in 50%-75% of patients with neoplastic pericardial effusion. Open pericardial biopsy taken from suspected loci in the pericardium can be of diagnostic value in up to 90% of the cases with neoplastic involvement. In recurrent pericardial effusion or tamponade, intrapericardial drug administration should be considered such as instillation of a cytotoxic agent or sclerosing agent (e.g., tetracycline). In severe intractable cases, pericardiectomy should be considered. Recently, a new percutaneous balloon dilating catheter was employed to create a nonsurgical pericardial window. This technique was found successful in helping to manage large pericardial effusions, particularly in patients with a malignant condition. It may become the preferred treatment to avoid a more invasive procedure for patients with pericardial effusion and a limited life expectancy.[20,21]

RADIATION PERICARDITIS

Radiation pericarditis may occur early after radiation therapy or many years after exposure. This entity must be diagnosed in patients with neoplastic diseases and differentiated from metastatic involvement of the pericardium because radiation pericarditis has a better prognosis. Sometimes they can be differentiated by cytologic or histologic examination of the fluid and pericardium. Although acute pericarditis and effusion may follow radiation exposure to the heart, effusive constrictive pericarditis is more common.[1,2]

TUBERCULOUS PERICARDITIS

The incidence of tuberculous pericarditis is decreasing in developed countries, excluding AIDS patients. It must be diagnosed in the acute stage, since antituberculous drugs are effective. This condition tends to be associated with large pericardial effusions and, if not treated, progresses to an effusive-constrictive phase and eventually to chronic constrictive pericarditis. Pericardiocentesis can provide positive diagnosis in only 15% of the cases.[1,2,4]

PURULENT PERICARDITIS

Purulent pericarditis is a rare condition which is still a severe disease that is recognized in most patients at necropsy or after severe hemodynamic compromise has developed. The most common microorganisms are streptococci, pneumococci, and staphylococci. Patients with purulent pericarditis are very ill, febrile, and toxic. Empyema remains a common underlying condition and in most of the cases, purulent pericarditis develops in the context of intrathoracic or subphrenic infection or sepsis. The diagnosis of purulent pericarditis is often missed due to 2 main reasons: 1) This disease is associated with features of chest pain and friction rub only in the minority of patients; 2) Clinical feature such as fever, dyspnea or tachycardia may be attributed to the underlying infectious disease. Since this disease is potentially lethal and often missed, a finding of pericardial effusion in a context of infection requires immediate pericardiocentesis to confirm the diagnosis and to obtain cultures. Surgical drainage should be promptly performed to evacuate the purulent fluid and specific antibiotic therapy must be started. Purulent pericarditis tends to progress to constrictive pericarditis despite antibiotic therapy. Constriction develops relatively early in the onset of the disease. In-hospital prognosis depends on the severity of the underlying infectious disease and is relatively good for patients who can be discharged from the hospital.[1,2,4,22]

PERICARDITIS ASSOCIATED WITH AIDS

Pericarditis is common in patients dying of acquired immunodeficiency syndrome. Many of the patients with pericardial disease have concomitant involvement of the myocardium. Recent estimates suggest that in the United States as many as 5,000 patients per year may have cardiac complications resulting from HIV infection.

The clinical spectrum of pericardial involvement ranges from asymptomatic pericarditis with or without effusion to symptomatic pericarditis and tamponade.[23] The pericarditis may be nonspecific by etiology or due to a wide variety of pathogens such as Mycobacterium tuberculosis and Mycobacterium avium, Cryptococcus, Herpes Simplex, Actinomyces, and bacteria such as Staphylococcus aureus. The pericardial involvement may be associated with neoplastic etiology such as Kaposi's sarcoma or lymphoma. AIDS is now a common underlying illness that is associated with large pericardial effusions. The prevalence of pericardial effusion among patients with AIDS is between 16%-40% according to various reports. Among hospitalized patients with HIV associated pericardial effusion, mortality is high: 29%.

In the absence of signs of hemodynamic compromise or inflammation, pericardial effusion still may accompany pleural effusion or ascites in patients with AIDS. Pericardiocentesis should be performed in cases in which the pericardial involvement is a prominent feature of the symptom complex.[1-3,24,25]

UREMIC PERICARDITIS

Uremic pericarditis is associated with advanced chronic renal failure and is a serious complication because it may be associated with tamponade.

Intense hemodialysis is indicated for treatment of uncomplicated uremic pericarditis and results in resolution of pericarditis in 40%-60% of patients. Serial physical examination, chest x-rays, and echocardiograms are useful for follow-up of chronic dialysis therapy in renal patients and for identifying patients with fluid accumulation. Resolution of uremic pericarditis complicated by tamponade is accomplished in most cases by intense hemodialysis in association with pericardiocentesis. Surgical pericardial excision is recommended in patients with recurrent episodes of pericarditis. Although pericardiectomy is a definitive procedure for pericarditis with effusion in the uremic patient, the procedure has a substantial morbidity. Frequently, mild degrees of pericardial effusion are associated with fluid overload, congestive heart failure, and left ventricular dysfunction, which often occurs in chronic renal disease. Cardiac catheterization may be needed to establish whether tamponade is a dominant component in these cases.[1,2,26]

TRAUMATIC HEMOPERICARDIUM

Traumatic hemopericardium can result from penetrating wounds of the heart or as a result of closed chest trauma caused by the steering wheel in automobile accidents. Hemopericardium due to closed chest trauma may be difficult to recognize because it may develop slowly. Pericardial effusions are common following cardiac surgery; uncommonly they are large in size and may cause tamponade, either in the early or late postoperative period. Such effusions causing tamponade may be circumcardiac, but are frequently loculated, in which case 1 or more cardiac chambers is selectively compressed. Cardiac tamponade is rare after cardiac catheterization and pacemaker insertion.

POST-CARDIAC INJURY SYNDROME

Post-cardiac injury syndrome occurs as an inflammatory reaction after either pericardial injury induced in the course of a cardiac operation or trauma to the heart or after the first 14 days of an MI. The incidence of both early postinfarction pericarditis and late post MI pericarditis (Dressler's syndrome) is declining.

Pericardial effusions appear in about 25% of patients after MI, most of them are asymptomatic and do not require specific therapy. There is no absolute contraindication to the use of anticoagulants; however these patients should be followed up carefully by echocardiography. Prominent clinical features include fever, pericarditis, and sometimes pneumonitis and pleuritis. The post-cardiac injury syndrome may occur several days to months after the injury or infarction. Pericarditis may be accompanied by pericardial effusion. The clinical picture mimics acute viral pericarditis, but it is believed to be a hypersensitivity immune reaction after myocardial injury. Patients are generally managed by analgesic anti-inflammatory drugs; in severe disabling or recurring cases, corticosteroids may be effective.[1-3,27,28]

PERICARDIAL EFFUSION ASSOCIATED WITH CONGESTIVE HEART FAILURE

Effusion may accompany heart failure without evidence of pericarditis. In general, pericardial effusion due to heart failure does not lead to tamponade. In 1 study, cardiac disease associated with congestive heart failure was found to be the most common cause of pericardial effusion in patients referred for echocardiography. Parameters of left heart function are markedly abnormal in patients with congestive heart failure and pericardial effusion.[1-4]

REFERENCES

1. Lorell BH, Braunwald E. Pericardial Disease. In: Braunwald E (ed). *Heart Disease: A Textbook of Cardiovascular Medicine*, 4th ed. Philadelphia: WB Saunders; 1992:1465-1527.
2. Shabetai R. Pericardial disease. In: Hurst JW (ed). *The Heart.* New York: McGraw-Hill; 1990:1348-1374.
3. Soler-Soler J, Permanyer-Miralda G, Sagrista-Sauleda J. A systematic diagnostic approach to primary acute pericardial disease. *Cardiol Clin.* 1990;8:609-620.
4. Spodick DH. Pericarditis in systemic disease-Review. *Cardiol Clin.* 1990;8:709-716.
5. Fowler NO. Recurrent pericarditis-Review. *Cardiol Clin.* 1990;8:621-626.
6. Shabetai R. Acute Pericarditis-Review. *Cardiol Clin.* 1990;8:639-644.
7. Feigenbaum H. Pericardial disease. In: Feigenbaum H (ed). *Echocardiography.* Philadelphia: Lea & Febiger; 1976:419 and 4th Ed. 1986:548.
8. Hancock EW. Cardiac tamponade. *Med Clin North Am.* 1979;63:223-237.
9. McGregor M. Pulsus paradoxus. *N Engl J Med.* 1979;301:480-482.
10. Singh S, Wann L, Schuchard G, et al. Right ventricular and right atrial collapse in patients with cardiac tamponade: A combined echocardiographic and hemodynamic study. *Circulation.* 1984;70:966-971.
11. Appleton C, Hatle L, Popp R. Cardiac tamponade and pericardial effusion: Respiratory variation in transvalvular flow velocities studied by Doppler echocardiography. *J Am Coll Cardiol.* 1988;11:1020-1030.
12. Krikorian SG, Hancock EW. Pericardiocentesis. *Am J Med.* 1978;65:808-814.
13. Tavel ME. The jugular pulse tracing: Its clinical application. In: Tavel ME (ed). *Clinical Phonocardiography and External Pulse Recording*, 3rd ed. Chicago: Year Book Medical Publishers; 1978:250-264.
14. Hancock EW. On the elastic and rigid forms of constrictive pericarditis. *Am Heart J.* 1980;100:917-923.
15. Lewis BS. Real time two-dimensional echocardiography in constrictive pericarditis. *Am J Cardiol.* 1982;49:1789-1793.
16. Hatle LK, Appleton CP, Popp RL. Differentiation of constrictive pericarditis and restrictive cardiomyopathy by Doppler echocardiography. *Circulation.* 1989;79:357-370.
17. Klein AL, Cohen GI, Pietrolungo JF, et al. Differentiation of constrictive pericarditis from restrictive cardiomyopathy by Doppler transesophageal echocardiographic measurements of respiratory variations in pulmonary venous flow. *J Am Coll Cardiol.* 1993:22:1935-1943.
18. Tuna IC, Danielson GK. Surgical management of pericardial diseases—Review. *Cardiol Clin.* 1990;8:683-696.
19. Hancock EW. Subacute effusive-constrictive pericarditis. *Circulation.* 1971;43:183-192.
20. Karlstein J, Frishman W. Malignant pericardial diseases: Diagnosis and treatment. *Am Heart J.* 1987;113:785-790.
21. Ziskind AA, Pearce AC, Lommon CC, et al. Percutaneous balloon pericardiotomy for the treatment of cardiac tamponade and large pericardial effusions: description of technique and report of the first 50 cases. *J Am Coll Cardiol.* 1993;21:1-5.
22. Sagrista-Sauleda J, Barrabes JA, Permanyer-Miralda G, et al. Purulent pericarditis: Review of 20 year experience in a general hospital. *J Am Coll Cardiol.* 1993;22:1661-1665.
23. McNulty CM. AIDS and the heart. In: Hurst JW (ed). *New Types of Cardiovascular Diseases.* New York: Igaku-Shoin; 1994:46-62.
24. Kaul S, Fishbein MC, Siegel RJ. Cardiac manifestations of acquired immune deficiency syndrome: a 1991 update. *Am Heart J.* 1991;22:535-544.
25. Eisenberg MJ, Gordon AS, Schiller NB. HIV-associated pericardial effusions. *Chest.* 1992;102:956-958.
26. Rostand SG, Rutsky EA. Pericarditis in end-stage renal disease—Review. *Cardiol Clin.* 1990;8:701-707.
27. Gregoratos G. Pericardial involvement in acute myocardial infarction. *Cardiol Clin.* 1990;8:601-608.
28. Khan AH. The postcardiac injury syndromes—Review. *Clin Cardiol.* 1992;15:67-72.

CHAPTER 27 Infective Endocarditis

Leonard S. Lilly, MD

Infective endocarditis remains a formidable cause of cardiovascular morbidity and mortality despite increased clinical recognition and potent antibiotic therapies. Although this condition may arise in otherwise normal hearts, it is more likely to occur when previous cardiac structural abnormalities exist.[1] Endocarditis may present as an indolent "subacute" form (SBE) or as a more fulminant "acute" syndrome (ABE), depending on the invasiveness of the responsible organism. Clinically, it has become most useful to classify endocarditis into those infections that develop 1) on native heart valves, 2) on prosthetic heart valves, and 3) in IV drug abusers.

ETIOLOGY

Many microorganisms can cause endocarditis;[2] however, streptococcal and staphylococcal species account for the majority of infections on native heart valves (Table 1). The organisms that cause SBE, primarily streptococci found within the body's normal flora, tend to be of low invasiveness, generally establishing infection only when previous cardiac structural abnormalities are present. Streptococcus viridans for example, a normal inhabitant of the oropharynx, is the single most common cause of endocarditis on native valves. Although this organism frequently enters the blood stream during dental work, a documented oral procedure precedes endocarditis less than 20% of the time. More often, transient bacteremia after chewing, tooth brushing, or flossing is likely responsible for endocarditial infection in individuals with predisposing cardiac lesions. Streptococcus bovis endocarditis most often occurs in the elderly, and is often associated with the presence of colonic polyps or intestinal

neoplasms.[3] Enterococcal (S. faecalis) endocarditis develops in association with genitourinary tract infections in young women or prostatic disease in elderly men. In such patients, procedures which result in bacteremia and endocardial infection include urethral catheterization and cystoscopy.

More aggressive organisms, responsible for the fulminant ABE, often infect healthy cardiac valves. Such bacteria are not generally part of the normal flora and include Staphylococcus aureus, gram negative bacilli, and fungal species. These most commonly afflict hospitalized patients and intravenous drug addicts, and gain access to the circulation through diverse sites, including the oral cavity and respiratory tract, the gastrointestinal and genitourinary systems, skin infections and burns, or via indwelling intravenous catheters. Staphylococcus aureus (coagulase-positive staphylococcus) is the main cause of the acute form of endocarditis on native valves and intravenous drug addicts[4] and is a common cause of prosthetic valve endocarditis. S. epidermidis (coagulase-negative staphylococcus) only rarely results in endocarditis of native valves or in drug addicts, but is the most common cause of prosthetic valve infections.[5] Fungal endocarditis is uncommon on native valves in the absence of intravenous drug abuse. However, the incidence is increased in patients with indwelling intravenous catheters who are seriously ill, or for whom glucocorticoids, prolonged antibiotics, or cytotoxic agents are prescribed.[6]

PATHOGENESIS

The subacute form of endocarditis develops in the setting of an underlying cardiovascular

Table 1. Approximate Frequency of Organisms in Infective Endocarditis

ORGANISM	NATIVE VALVE ENDOCARDITIS IN (%)	ENDOCARDITIS IN IV DRUG USERS (%)	EARLY PROSTHETIC VALVE ENDOCARDITIS (%)	LATE PROSTHETIC VALVE ENDOCARDITIS (%)
Streptococci	65	15	10	35
S. viridans	35	5	<5	25
S. bovis	15	<5	<5	<5
enterococcus	10	8	<5	<5
Staphylococci	25	50	50	30
coagulase-positive	23	50	20	10
coagulase-negative	<5	<5	30	20
HACEK group*	5	<5	<1	<5
Gram-negative bacilli	<5	15	15	10
Fungi	<5	5	10	5
Culture-negative	5	<5	<5	<5

Modified from Durak DT. Infective endocarditis. In: Wyngaarden JB, et al (eds). Cecil Textbook of Medicine. (19th ed). Philadelphia: W.B. Saunders; 1992. Orinally from Durak DT. Infective and Noninfective Endocarditis. In: Hurst JW (ed). *The Heart.* 6th Ed. New York: McGraw Hill; 1986:1130-1157.

*HACEK=Haemophilus, Actinobacillus, Cardiobacterium, Eikenella, Kingella.

structural abnormality (Table 2), in which a pressure gradient between 2 cardiac chambers generates turbulent blood flow that traumatizes the surface of the abnormal valve or adjacent endocardium within the lower pressure chamber (e.g., on the left ventricular wall in aortic insufficiency, or the left atrial surface in mitral regurgitation). A sterile platelet-fibrin thrombus (termed nonbacterial thrombotic endocarditis (NBTE)) may then form at the site of endothelial disturbance. Nonbacterial thrombotic endocarditis may also arise in patients with chronic debilitating diseases such as cancer or in areas of intravascular injury by foreign bodies, including intracardiac catheters and prosthetic valves.[7] Subsequent infection develops when a transient bacteremia delivers the offending infectious agent to the sterile platelet-fibrin lesion, where adhesion and multiplication of organisms leads to formation of a vegetation. The factors that determine whether an organism is likely to incite endocarditis relate to: 1) the frequency of bacteremia, 2) the ability of the organism to adhere to the platelet-fibrin thrombus, and 3) the organism's capability to resist host defenses, such as the complement pathway. For example, Streptococcus viridans bacteremia from the oral cavity occurs frequently and the organism easily adheres to platelet-fibrin thrombi such that it is a common cause of endocarditis. Conversely, gram-negative rod bacteremia is also frequent, but these agents do not adhere well and therefore remain a relatively rare cause of endocardial infection.

Once bacterial infection is established, additional deposition of fibrin and platelets forms protective layers which inhibit phagocytic cell host defenses, permitting proliferation of the microorganism and enlargement of the vegetation. Bacteria on the vegetation may then seed back into the circulation acting as a source of continued septicemia.

Although rheumatic valve disease was once the most common condition predisposing to

Table 2. Conditions that Predispose to Endocarditis

Rheumatic valvular disease (even after corrective surgery)

Other acquired valvular lesions:
    Calcific aortic stenosis
    Aortic regurgitation
    Mitral regurgitation
    Mitral valve prolapse (if murmur present, or more than "trace" mitral regurgitation by Doppler)

Obstructive hypertrophic cardiomyopathy ("IHSS")

Congenital heart disease, including:
    Ventricular septal defect
    Patent ductus arteriosus
    Tetralogy of Fallot
    Aortic Coarctation
    Bicuspid aortic valve
    Pulmonic stenosis

Surgically implanted hardware, including:
    Prosthetic heart valves (including bioprosthetic and homograft valves)
    Pulmonary-systemic shunts
    Ventriculo-atrial shunts for hydrocephalus

Previous episodes of endocarditis

---

endocarditis, that cause has declined in industrialized societies. In distinction, endocarditis due to other forms of acquired valvular disease, congenital heart disease, mitral valve prolapse and infections on prosthetic valves have increased in frequency (Table 2). Certain cardiac lesions do not predispose to the subacute form of bacterial endocarditis (Table 3).

The pathogenesis of ABE is less complex in that the organisms involved are highly invasive. Upon gaining access to the circulation, they are required in only small numbers to adhere to endocardium and incite infection, even upon previously healthy cardiac structures.

The appearance of a vegetation relates to the type of invading organism and ranges from small, flat lesions to large, mobile masses such as when fungal species are involved. During effective antimicrobial therapy, healing of the lesion is associated with infiltration of granulocytes which ingest bacteria and cellular debris, and fibroblasts with scar formation. Endothelialization and calcification of the healing lesion may cause structural deformities that result in valvular stenosis or regurgitation, and susceptibility to recurrent infection.

CLINICAL FEATURES

The clinical presentation of infective endocarditis is variable and results from 1) local infection, 2) embolic effects of infected vegetations and 3) the immune response to the infection.

The presentation of SBE is often subtle: low-grade fever accompanied by nonspecific malaise, anorexia and weight loss, generalized weakness, headache, arthralgias and myalgias. A careful history may reveal the portal of bacterial entry, such as recent dental work. The symptoms may mimic an upper respiratory tract infection, and if oral antibiotics are mistakenly prescribed later, blood cultures may be rendered falsely negative. Although these generalized symptoms may last for months, the diagnosis is usually suspected sufficiently early so that "classic" embolic and immune-mediated cutaneous and retinal features of endocarditis (Table 4) only occasionally develop.

The clinical onset of ABE is more explosive: sudden illness is heralded by rigors and high fever, sometimes in association with widely disseminated metastatic infections involving multiple organ systems, especially if Staph. aureus is involved.

Heart murmurs are found in more than 90% of patients with subacute presentations, usually reflecting the predisposing valvular lesions. In ABE, murmurs on presentation are less common but may develop if valvular destruction ensues. Other common physical findings in both forms of endocarditis include pallor due to anemia, splenomegaly, and if congestive heart failure has developed, pulmonary rales and an S_3 on cardiac examination.

Particularly in ABE, fragments of valvular vegetation may dislodge and embolize, most commonly to the brain, kidneys, spleen, mesentery, and coronary arteries with subsequent metastatic infection or infarction of the

Table 3. Cardiac Conditions that do not Predispose to Endocarditis

Isolated ostium secundum atrial septal defect
Previous coronary artery bypass graft surgery
Implanted cardiac pacemaker or defibrillator
More than six months following:
  Ligation and division of patent ductus arteriosus
  Surgical repair of atrial septal defect, without prosthetic patch

involved organ. Large emboli, especially in association with fungal endocarditis, may lodge in major arterial branches and result in the sudden loss of a peripheral pulse. Septic pulmonary emboli may result from right-sided heart valve endocarditis, particularly common in intravenous drug abusers.[8]

One-third of patients manifest neurologic complications during the course of endocarditis,[9] including headache, confusion, and seizures. Focal neurologic abnormalities, such as hemiplegia or hemisensory loss, may result from cerebral emboli and may be the initial presentation of endocarditis. Particularly in ABE, pyogenic organisms may lead to brain abscess formation or purulent meningitis. Intracerebral "mycotic" aneurysms may develop from septic emboli to the arterial wall or by embolic occlusion of the vasa vasorum, and

should be suspected in a patient with endocarditis who describes severe localized headache; intracerebral or subarachnoid hemorrhage may follow. Anticoagulant therapy increases the risk of intracranial hemorrhage in this setting and should be avoided, if possible, in patients with active endocarditis.

Mycotic aneurysms also commonly involve the proximal aorta and arteries to the extremities and viscera. Progressive weakening of the arterial wall and rupture may occur long after successful antibiotic therapy of the initial endocarditis.

Potentially lethal cardiac complications may punctuate the course of both SBE and ABE.[10] Local extension of infection may distort the valve leaflets, chordae tendineae, or supporting structures, resulting in progressive valvular regurgitation and congestive heart failure, the major cause of death in endocarditis. Myocardial abscess formation (more common in ABE than SBE) may extend into the cardiac conduction tissues with resultant AV nodal or intraventricular conduction blocks and arrhythmias. A myocardial abscess may rupture through the interventricular septum or into the pericardiac sac resulting in bacterial pericarditis and cardiac tamponade. In addition, in cases of aortic valve endocarditis, mycotic aneurysms at the sinuses of Valsalva may rupture into the right ventricle or right atrium, creating an acute left-to-right shunt.

Table 4. Cutaneous and Occular Findings in Endocarditis (now uncommon)

Petechiae	Embolic or vasculitic lesions located in conjunctivae, oral cavity, skin
Subungual hemorrhages	Microemboli under the fingernails creating linear splinter-like red streaks which do not extend to the distal nail bed
Osler's nodes	Septic emboli or immune-complex vasculitis which produces erythematous, painful pea-sized nodules in pulp spaces of terminal phalanges, thenar and hypothenar eminences, that persist for hours or days
Janeway lesions	Small, slightly nodular hemorrhages on palms and soles, usually due to septic emboli
Roth's spots	Oval retinal hemorrhages with a pale center

INFECTIVE ENDOCARDITIS IN INTRAVENOUS DRUG ABUSERS

Endocarditis of the ABE variety is an important complication in patients who use illicit intravenous (IV) drugs. Bacteremia in such individuals may arise from microbial contamination of the injected materials or from cellulitis or thrombophlebitis at injection sites.[4] More than 50% of cases of endocarditis in this population are due to Staph. aureus; other commonly involved organisms include Candida and gram-negative bacilli, including Pseudomonas species. Unlike the general population, streptococcal infections account for less than 20% of endocarditis infections in this group. The majority of endocarditis lesions in IV drug abusers develop at previously normal intracardiac sites, and the clinical presentation is that of an acute fulminant infection. Metastatic abscess formation is common, due to the pyogenic organisms involved. Tricuspid valve endocarditis, which afflicts 50%-60% of this group of patients, commonly results in septic pulmonary emboli, reflected by multiple patchy infiltrates on chest x-ray. The aortic valve is affected in 25% of this patient population, the mitral valve in 20%.

The prognosis for an otherwise healthy young drug addict with tricuspid Staph. aureus endocarditis is favorable with intravenous antibiotic therapy. However, the outcome is adversely affected by involvement of the left-sided valves or when gram-negative rods or fungal species are causal.

PROSTHETIC VALVE ENDOCARDITIS

Infections associated with prosthetic heart valves comprise 10%-20% of patients who develop endocarditis. This complication develops in up to 2.2% of patients who have undergone valvular replacement.[5] Infections occur with equal frequency on mechanical and biological prostheses, but endocarditis of artificial aortic valves is much more common than of mitral replacements. In "early" prosthetic valve endocarditis (within the first 60 days following surgery), valvular infection results from intraoperative contamination or bacterial seeding

from pneumonia, urinary tract infection, or mediastinitis. The predominant organism involved is Staph. epidermidis, and there is also a high frequency of Staph. aureus, gram-negative rods, diphtheroids, and fungal species (Table 1). A late form of prosthetic endocarditis, which arises after the first 60 days postoperatively, generally involves the same organisms responsible for endocarditis on native valves, except that Staph. epidermidis is again unusually common, accounting for more than 20% of such infections.

Unlike infections of native heart valves, which usually remain confined to the leaflets, the early variety of prosthetic valve endocarditis frequently extends into perivalvular structures and causes detachment of the sewing ring, perivalvular regurgitation, and congestive heart failure. Local abscess formation at the valve ring occurs in approximately 40% of prosthetic valvular infections; its presence may be suggested by new AV nodal or ventricular conduction blocks due to expansion of the abscess. Less commonly, valvular stenosis may result from encroachment of a vegetation on the prosthetic orifice.

The late form of prosthetic valve endocarditis may be similarly fulminant, however, when organisms of low invasiveness are involved (e.g., streptococci) the course is more often similar to that of native valve subacute endocarditis.

LABORATORY FINDINGS

The diagnosis of endocarditis is confirmed, and appropriate antibiotic therapy selected, by demonstration of the responsible organism by blood cultures. Since bacteremia is continuous in endocarditis, if a single blood culture demonstrates the organism, all are likely to be positive.[11] To minimize confusion by contaminants, at least 3 sets of cultures should be drawn before initiating antibiotics. In SBE, in which immediate therapy is not as crucial as in ABE, blood cultures can be obtained approximately 1 hour apart over a period of several hours. In suspected ABE, however, therapy must not be delayed by even a short time and all blood culture sets should be drawn immediately, from separate venous sites, followed by initiation of empiric antibiotic therapy (see below). Aerobic and anaerobic cultures should be held for 3 weeks to ensure the identification of slow-growing organisms.

Approximately 5% of patients with infective endocarditis have negative blood cultures, and the diagnosis rests on clinical and/or echo-cardiographic findings, as well as the response to empiric therapy. Causes of negative blood cultures include recent antibiotic therapy (within 2 weeks of blood culture),[12] fastidious growth requirements (especially Brucella, Haemophilus parainfluenzae, Chlamydia, Rickettsia and fungal organisms), and technical difficulties, such as inappropriate incubation. Serologic tests can help identify endocarditis caused by Chlamydia, Brucella and Legionella species.

Other laboratory abnormalities are often detected. Normochromic, normocytic anemia is common, particularly in SBE. The white blood cell count may be normal in SBE, but is usually elevated in ABE, with a shift toward less mature forms. In some cases, a gram stain of the peripheral blood buffy coat smear may demonstrate the responsible organism. The erythrocyte sedimentation rate is elevated unless congestive heart failure coexists. Nonspecific immunoglobulin abnormalities are often detected, including the presence of rheumatoid factor (in 25%-50% of patients with SBE but rarely in ABE), and circulating immune complexes in 90%. The latter have been implicated as a cause of arthralgias, skin lesions and acute glomerulonephritis. Microscopic hematuria and proteinuria have been reported in up to 50% of patients due to glomerulonephritis, renal emboli, or metastatic renal abscess.

Transthoracic echocardiography can detect vegetations ≥ 3 mm in size and identifies 60%-80% of valvular vegetations, but a normal study does not exclude the diagnosis. Prosthetic valvular endocarditis may be particularly difficult to image by this technique due to acoustic interference by the implanted material. Transesophageal echocardiography is more sensitive for the detection of native or prosthetic valvular vegetations with a sensitivity greater than 90%, and is particularly useful when endocarditis is strongly suspected clinically but blood cultures and transthoracic imaging are unrevealing.[13] The major role of either echocardiographic technique is in the detection of complications of endocarditis, including flail valve leaflets, ruptured chordae tendineae and perivalvular abscess. In addition, Doppler interrogation identifies and quantifies valvular regurgitation or stenosis due to endocarditis. Some recent studies have suggested that vegetation size determined by echocardiography correlates with the likelihood of embolic events or progressive congestive heart failure.[14]

THERAPY

Before the antibiotic era, infective endocarditis was universally fatal. Antimicrobial and surgical therapies have greatly reduced mortality, but to achieve a cure, appropriate intravenous therapy with bactericidal antibiotics must be administered in high dosage for prolonged periods, in order to eradicate microorganisms deep within the vegetation which are protected from normal host defenses. Since vegetations are avascular, antibiotic penetration can occur only via diffusion from circulating blood as it passes over the lesion. Table 5 lists a compilation of standard recommended antibiotic regimens.

A common problem is that of a patient who presents with suspected endocarditis who has received recent broad spectrum antibiotic therapy. In such patients, blood cultures may not demonstrate the responsible organism until antibiotics are withheld for 24 hours or longer. For individuals with an SBE presentation, treatment can be delayed 2-3 days during which time blood cultures should be drawn daily. However, for individuals with more fulminant symptoms of ABE, antibiotics must be administered as early as possible to avoid life-threatening valve destruction, and empiric therapy is directed against the most aggressive of the likely causal organisms.

In suspected SBE on a native valve, initial therapy, prior to blood culture results, should include coverage against enterococci using intravenous penicillin or ampicillin plus gentamicin (Table 5). In the case of suspected ABE, empiric antibiotics should be directed against Staph. aureus (nafcillin or oxacillin). In an intravenous drug abuser, empiric therapy is

Table 5. Antibiotic Therapy for Common Forms of Endocarditis

ORGANISMS	THERAPY	ALTERNATE THERAPY (PENICILLIN ALLERGY)	DURATION (WEEKS)
Viridans streptococci (penicillin-sensitive) and Streptococcus bovis (MIC* <0.1 µg/ml)	Penicillin G 10-20 million U/day (divided into q4h dosage) (For relapses or complicated courses, add: Gentamicin** 1 mg/kg IV/IM q8h for first 2 weeks)	Vancomycin*** 15 mg/kg IV q12h or Cefazolin 2 g IV q8h	4
	Alternate abbreviated regimen: Penicillin G 10-20 million U/day (divided into q4h dosage) plus Gentamicin** 1 mg/kg IV/IM q8h		2
Streptococci with relative penicillin resistance MIC* >0.1 and <0.5 µg/ml)	Penicillin G 20 million U/day (divided into q4h dosage) plus Gentamicin** 1 mg/kg IV/IM q8h	Vancomycin*** 15 mg/kg IV q12h	4
Enterococci (MIC* ≥ 0.5 µg/ml)	Penicillin G 20-30 million U/day (divided into q4h dosage) [or ampicillin 2 g IV q4h] plus Gentamicin** 1 mg/kg IV/IM q8h	Vancomycin*** 15 mg/kg IV q12h plus Gentamicin** 1 mg/kg IV/IM q8h	4-6
Staph. aureus (methicillin-sensitive)	Oxacilin or nafcillin 2 g IV q4h (some experts also add gentamicin** 1 mg/kg IV/IM q8h for first 3-5 days)	Vancomycin*** 15 mg/kg IV q12h or Cefazolin 2 g IV q6h (some experts also add gentamicin** 1 mg/kg IV/IM q8h for first 3-5 days)	4-6
Staph. aureus (methicillin-resistant)	Vancomycin*** 15 mg/kg IV q12h (some experts also add gentamicin** 1 mg/kg IV/IM q8h for first 3-5 days)		4-6
Staph. epidermidis (methicillin-sensitive) Native valve	Oxacillin or nafcillin 2 g IV q4h	Vancomycin*** 15 mg/kg IV q12 h or Cefazolin 2 g IV q6h	4-6
Prosthetic valve	Oxacillin or nafcillin 2 g IV q4h plus rifampin 300 mg po q8h plus Gentamicin** 1 mg/kg IV/IM q8h for first 2 wk	Vancomycin*** or cefazolin (as above) plus rifampin 300 mg po q8h plus Gentamicin** 1 mg/kg IV/IM q8h for first 2 wk	6

Table 5. Antibiotic Therapy for Common Forms of Endocarditis (continued)			
ORGANISMS	THERAPY	ALTERNATE THERAPY (PENICILLIN ALLERGY)	DURATION (WEEKS)
Staph. epidermidis (methicillin-resistant) Native valve	Vancomycin*** 7.5 mg IV q6h		4-6
Prosthetic valve	Vancomycin*** 7.5 mg IV q6h plus rifampin 300 mg po q8h plus Gentamicin** 1 mg/kg IV/IM q8h for first 2 wk		6

Modified from Bisno AL et al.[16]

* Minimal inhibitory concentration of penicillin G for the organism.
** Each dose of gentamicin should not exceed 80 mg. Desired peak gentamicin level=3 μg/ml. Monitor for ototoxicity and nephrotoxicity, especially if combined with vancomycin. Use IV rather than IM route for patients on anticoagulation therapy.
*** Infuse vancomycin over 1 hr. Desired peak serum level (drawn 1 hr after infusion)=30-45 μg/ml for q12h dosing and 20-35 μg/ml for q6h dosing.

aimed at methicillin-resistant Staph. aureus and gram-negative rods (e.g., vancomycin plus an aminoglycoside). In patients with suspected prosthetic valve endocarditis, therapy is directed against methicillin-resistant Staph. epidermidis, Staph. aureus, and gram-negative rods (vancomycin, gentamicin, and rifampin as shown in Table 5). If endocarditis due to urinary or gastrointestinal sepsis is suspected, initial antibiotics should cover gram-negative bacilli. Once the responsible organism has been definitively identified and sensitivities determined, the antibiotic regimen should be appropriately altered and dosages adjusted such that a 1:8 dilution of the patient's serum, drawn 30 minutes after drug infusion is bactericidal for the infecting organism in culture.[15] If subsequent blood cultures do not demonstrate the responsible organism ("culture-negative" endocarditis), the empiric regimen should be continued if there is a beneficial clinical response.

With the exception of enterococci, most streptococcal species are exquisitely sensitive to penicillin,[16] and high cure rates are expected with 4 weeks of therapy (Table 5). When penicillin is combined with an aminoglycoside, there is a synergistic effect and a more rapid cure rate such that the duration of therapy can be shortened to 2 weeks, and this abbreviated regimen is preferred in young individuals with normal renal function. For patients who have previously suffered penicillin-induced anaphylaxis or hives, vancomycin should be used. For low grade, delayed, or uncertain penicillin allergies, cephalosporins may be used cautiously as shown in the Table.

As Streptococcus bovis bacteremia is associated with malignancies of the gastrointestinal (GI) tract, its presence should prompt GI investigation. Enterococcal endocarditis requires the addition of an aminoglycoside to penicillin for a bactericidal effect. However, in vitro susceptibility testing is necessary, as some enterococcal strains are resistant to aminoglycosides.[17] In such cases, the duration of therapy with penicillin or ampicillin should be prolonged to 6-8 weeks.

Native valve endocarditis due to Staph. aureus or Staph. epidermidis should be treated with a penicillinase-resistant penicillin, such as oxacillin or nafcillin as shown in Table 5.[16]

Some experts add gentamicin for the first 3-5 days to increase the bactericidal effect, although there is no evidence that it improves the clinical outcome nor does it shorten the length of total antibiotic therapy. Methicillin-resistant organisms are immune to all penicillins and cephalosporins and vancomycin therapy is recommended, with or without gentamicin for the first 3-5 days.

Therapy for staphylococcal endocarditis is usually continued for 4 weeks, but should be lengthened to 6 weeks in complicated cases (i.e., when infected emboli have resulted in metastatic infection). Methicillin-resistant Staph. epidermidis infection of prosthetic heart valves should be treated with a combination of vancomycin plus gentamicin plus rifampin for a 6-week course.

The therapeutic approach to other causes of endocarditis (e.g., gram-negative bacilli, anaerobes, Corynebacteria) are directed by in vitro testing of bactericidal drugs. For gram-negative bacilli, therapy usually consists of a third generation cephalosporin plus an aminoglycoside (e.g., cefotaxime 2 grams q6h plus gentamicin 1.7mg/kg q8h) for 4 weeks.

Antimicrobial therapy of fungal endocarditis yields generally disappointing results, especially if the infection affects a prosthetic valve.[6] Amphotericin B is the most potent antifungal agent, but is poorly tolerated due to renal and bone marrow toxicity. Flucytosine, an oral fungistatic drug may be useful in addition to amphotericin B when the organism has demonstrated sensitivity. However, bulky fungal vegetations often form, with local myocardial invasion and peripheral embolization to large arteries, requiring early surgical removal of the infected valve.

Surgical valve replacement in infective endocarditis is necessary when antimicrobial drugs fail to eradicate the infection, or to treat life-threatening structural complications.[18] Absolute indications for surgical interventions include: 1) progressive or refractory congestive heart failure due to valvular dysfunction; 2) persistently positive blood cultures after several days of antibiotics; 3) recurrent major peripheral emboli, with vegetations visualized by echocardiography; 4) myocardial abscess formation, suggested by an otherwise unexplained new electrocardiographic (ECG) conduction abnormality or by echocardiography; 5) ruptured sinus of Valsalva mycotic aneurysm; and 6) fungal endocarditis.

Some experts recommend surgical intervention after a single embolism if a large vegetation ($\geq$ 1cm in diameter) is visualized by echocardiography, but there is little data to support this approach. Other factors that increase the likelihood for surgical therapy include patients with aortic valve involvement, infections due to staphylococci in drug addicts, and prosthetic valve endocarditis. Although it is preferable to treat a patient with antibiotics for several days prior to surgical intervention, when one of the above absolute indications for surgery are present, the operation should not be delayed, as rapid deterioration and a fatal outcome are otherwise likely. Persistence of infection on a newly implanted prosthesis after even just a brief period of antibiotics is uncommon.[19]

The response of prosthetic valve endocarditis (PVE) to antibiotic therapy is often poor, especially if nonstreptococcal species are involved. The ability to eliminate the infection is less compared with native valves[20] and

---

Table 6. Procedures that Warrant Endocarditis Prophylaxis

Dental manipulations that produce gingival bleeding, including professional cleaning

Rigid bronchoscopy or surgery of the upper respiratory tract

Genitourinary procedures, including:
Urethral catheterization (if urinary tract infection present)
Cystoscopy
Prostatectomy
Vaginal delivery (if peripartum infection present)
Vaginal hysterectomy

Gastrointestinal surgery, including cholecystectomy and esophageal dilation

Table 7. Prevention of Endocarditis

PROCEDURE	THERAPY	THERAPY IF PENICILLIN ALLERGIC
Dental or upper respiratory tract	Oral: Amoxicillin 3 g 1 hr prior to procedure; 1.5 g 6 hrs later	Oral: Erythromycin ethylsuccinate 800 mg or erythromycin stearate 1 g po 2 hr prior to procedure; then repeat half the dose 6 hr later or Clindamycin 300 mg po 1 hr before procedure; 150 mg po 6 hr later
	Parenteral: Ampicillin 2 g IV/IM* 30 min prior to procedure; then 1 g IV/IM* 6 hr later (instead of repeat parenteral dose, may substitute amoxicillin 1.5 g po)	Parenteral: Clindamycin 300 mg IV 30 min before procedure; 150 mg IV or po 6 hr later
	Maximum protection (high-risk patient)**: Ampicillin 2 g IV/IM* plus gentamicin 1.5 mg/kg IV/IM* (not to exceed 80 mg) 30 min prior to procedure; repeat once, 8 hr later (instead of repeat parenteral dose, may substitute amoxicillin 1.5 g po, 6 hr after initial dose)	Maximum protection (high-risk patient)**: Vancomycin 1 g IV over 1 hr prior to procedure; repeat dosage not necessary
Gastrointestinal and Genito-urinary Procedures	Ampicillin 2 g IV/IM* plus gentamicin 1.5 mg/kg IV/IM* (not to exceed 80 mg) 30 min prior to procedure; repeat once, 8 hr later (instead of repeat parenteral dose, may substitute amoxicillin 1.5 g po, 6 hr after initial dose)	Vancomycin 1 g IV over 1 hr plus gentamicin 1.5 mg/kg IV/IM* (not to exceed 80 mg) 60 min prior to procedure; may be repeated once, 8 hr later
	Low-risk patients: Amoxicillin 3 g po 1 hr prior to procedure; 1.5 g po 6 hr later	

Modified from Dajani AS et al.[24]

* Use IV rather than IM route for patients on anticoagulation therapy.
** The American Heart Association Committee on endocarditis recommends the use of the oral antibiotic regimen, even in high-risk patients (e.g., prosthetic heart valve); however, some practitioners prefer this parenteral regimen for more intense coverage.

dehiscence of the valve ring, prosthetic dysfunction and myocardial abscess formation are common. Overall mortality is least favorable in the group with "early" prosthetic involvement in which nonstreptococcal species are common. Patients with "late" PVE caused by streptococci can usually be cured by antibiotics alone. Surgical replacement of an infected prosthesis should be performed on an emergent basis if progressive congestive heart failure is demonstrated or if systemic embolization or continued bacteremia occur despite antibiotic therapy. Anticoagulation therapy must be continued in patients with mechanical prostheses; however, there is a risk of intracranial bleeding if cerebral embolization or mycotic aneurysmal rupture should ensue. Therefore, the prothrombin time should be kept in the low therapeutic range, i.e., an international normalized ratio (INR) of approximately 2.5-3.0.

A different surgical approach is sometimes undertaken for intravenous drug abusers with tricuspid valve endocarditis: removal of the infected valve without replacement.[21] The rationale is that an implanted prosthesis is likely to become reinfected with continued IV drug abuse. Although the resultant tricuspid regurgitation can be tolerated for long periods of time, individuals with pulmonary hypertension can develop right heart failure and progressive hepatic congestion.

The importance of daily examination of a patient with endocarditis for new heart murmurs, evidence of heart failure or peripheral emboli, and frequent electrocardiograms to identify new conduction disturbances, cannot be overemphasized.

PREVENTION OF INFECTIVE ENDOCARDITIS

Patients with cardiac lesions that predispose to endocarditis (Table 2) should receive prophylactic antibiotic therapy for invasive procedures likely to result in substantial bacteremia, the most common of which are listed in Table 6. In the case of mitral valve prolapse, antibiotic prophylaxis should be reserved for patients with an audible systolic murmur or more than trivial mitral regurgitation by Doppler.[22]

Given the frequency with which the oropharynx is a source of bacteremia, optimal hygiene should be maintained in patients with a predisposition to endocarditis, particularly in the presence of a prosthetic cardiac valve. Antiseptic mouthwashes (e.g., chlorhexidine) just prior to dental procedures can greatly reduce bacteremia.[23] Home oral irrigation devices should be avoided in patients predisposed to endocarditis because of the frequent bacteremia associated with their use.

The prophylactic antibiotic regimens recommended by the American Heart Association are listed in Table 7.[24] The following procedures generally do not require antibiotic prophylaxis (although some experts prescribe such therapy

if a prosthetic heart valve is present): uncomplicated vaginal delivery (if no evidence of pelvic infection), D&C of the uterus, Cesarean delivery, "in and out" bladder catheterization with sterile urine, barium enema, sigmoidoscopy, flexible bronchoscopy with or without biopsy, fiber optic endoscopy with or without biopsy, endotracheal intubation, percutaneous liver biopsy and diagnostic cardiac catheterization.

In summary, the diagnosis and treatment of bacterial endocarditis remain substantial challenges warranting a high degree of clinical suspicion and vigilant attention to the patient in order to effect a cure and prevent life-threatening complications.

REFERENCES

1. McKinsey DS, Ratts TE, Bisno AL. Underlying cardiac lesions in adults with infective endocarditis. The changing spectrum. *Am J Med.* 1987;82:681-688.
2. Weinberger I, Rotenberg Z, Zacharovitch D, et al. Native valve infective endocarditis in the 1970s versus the 1980s: underlying cardiac lesions and infecting organisms. *Clin Cardiol.* 1990;13:94-98.
3. Leport C, Bure A, Leport J, et al. Incidence of colonic lesions in Streptococcus bovis and enterococcal endocarditis. *Lancet.* 1987;1:748.
4. Scheidegger C, Zimmerli W. Infectious complications in drug addicts: seven-year review of 269 hospitalized narcotics abusers in Switzerland. *Rev Infect Dis.* 1989;11:486-493.
5. Cowgill LD, Addonizio VP, Hopeman AR, et al. Prosthetic valve endocarditis. *Curr Probl Cardiol.* 1986;11:617-664.
6. Rubinstein E, Noriega ER, Simberkoff MS, et al. Fungal endocarditis: analysis of 24 cases and review of the literature. *Medicine.* 1975;54:331-334.
7. Lopez JA, Ross RS, Fishbein MC, et al. Nonbacterial thrombotic endocarditis: a review. *Am Heart J.* 1987;113:773-784.
8. Robbins MJ, Soeiro R, Frishman WH, et al. Right-sided valvular endocarditis: etiology, diagnosis, and an approach to therapy. *Am Heart J.* 1986;111:128-135.
9. Salgado AV, Furlan AJ, Keys TF, et al. Neurologic complications of endocarditis: a 12-year experience. *Neurology.* 1989;39:173-178.
10. Weinstein L. Life-threatening complications of infective endocarditis and their management. *Arch Intern Med.* 1986;146:953-957.
11. Werner AS, Cobbs CG, Kaye D, et al. Studies on the bacteremia of bacterial endocarditis. *JAMA.* 1967;202:199-203.
12. Pazin GJ, Saul S, Thompson ME. Blood culture

positivity: suppression by outpatient antibiotic therapy in patients with bacterial endocarditis. *Arch Intern Med.* 1982;142:263-268.

13. Birmingham GD, Rahko PS, Ballantyne F. Improved detection of infective endocarditis with transesophageal echocardiography. *Am Heart J.* 1992;123:774-781.

14. Mügge A. Echocardiographic detection of cardiac valve vegetations and prognostic implications. *Infect Dis Clin North Am.* 1993;4:877-898.

15. Washington JA. In vitro testing of antimicrobial agents. *Infect Dis Clin North Am.* 1989;3:375-387.

16. Bisno AL, Dismukes WE, Durack DT, et al. Antimicrobial treatment of infective endocarditis due to viridans streptococci, enterococci, and staphylococci. *JAMA.* 1989;261:1471-1477.

17. Eliopoulos GM. Aminoglycoside resistant enterococcal endocarditis. *Infect Dis Clin North Am.* 1993;1:117-133.

18. Karp RB. Role of surgery in infective endocarditis. *Cardiovasc Clin.* 1987;17:141-162.

19. Aslamaci S, Dimitri WR, Williams BT. Operative considerations in active native valve infective endocarditis. *J Cardiovasc Surg.* 1989;30:328-333.

20. Cowgill LD, Addonizio VP, Hopeman AR, et al. A practical approach to prosthetic valve endocarditis. *Ann Thorac Surg.* 1987;43:450-457.

21. Yee ES, Khonsari S. Right-sided infective endocarditis: valvuloplasty, valvectomy or replacement. *J Cardiovasc Surg.* 1989;30:744-748.

22. Lavie CJ, Khandheria BK, Seward JB, et al. Factors associated with the recommendation for endocarditis prophylaxis in mitral value prolapse. *JAMA.* 1989;262:3308-3312.

23. Bender IB, Naidorf IJ, Garvey GJ. Bacterial endocarditis: a consideration for physician and dentist. *J Am Dent Assoc.* 1984;109:415-420.

24. Dajani AS, Bisno AL, Chung KJ, et al. Prevention of bacterial endocarditis. Recommendations by the American Heart Association. *JAMA.* 1990;264:2919-2922.

CHAPTER 28

Cardiac Tumors

Jonathan Leor, MD
Robert A. Kloner, MD, PhD

INTRODUCTION

Tumors of the heart are uncommon.[1,2] The most frequent neoplastic disease of the heart is cardiac involvement by tumor metastases, which is 15 to 60 times more common than primary cardiac tumors.[2,3] However, early diagnosis of primary cardiac tumors, particularly benign cardiac tumors, has paramount importance: immediate surgical removal of the tumor will preclude serious complications unique to primary cardiac tumors and will cure many patients. In recent years, the extensive use of echocardiography, as well as other new noninvasive modalities, has resulted in a significant improvement in the early detection of cardiac tumors. Consequently, there has been an increase in the number of successful therapeutic and palliative procedures in patients with cardiac neoplastic disease.

PRIMARY CARDIAC TUMORS

The incidence of primary cardiac tumors is low: 0.002% to 0.28% of the autopsies in the general population (average, less than 0.1% of the autopsies).[1-4] Approximately 75% of all primary cardiac tumors are benign; the most common (nearly 50%) are myxomas, followed by lipomas, papillary fibroelastomas, rhabdomyomas, and fibromas.[1,2] Twenty-five percent of primary cardiac tumors are malignant, the most common being angiosarcomas and rhabdomyosarcomas.[1,2]

BENIGN PRIMARY TUMORS

LEFT ATRIAL MYXOMA

Myxomas are the most common primary tumor of the heart and account for 30% to 50% of all cardiac tumors.[1,2] Although there has been some debate in the past as to whether these tumors actually represent neoplasms or just well-organized thrombi,[5] studies in which tissue from myxoma was grown in culture showed that the cells had neoplastic properties.[6] These tumors in general are considered benign but occasionally exhibit malignant behavior.[1]

Myxomas tend to arise in the atria from the region of the fossa ovalis: 75% in the left atrium and 18% in the right atrium. Myxomas can also be found in the left (4%) and right (4%) ventricle.[2] Occasionally they are multiple and arise in several cardiac chambers. A small percentage of patients with cardiac myxoma have a complex of features including pituitary adenoma with giganticism or acromegaly, myxoid fibroadenoma of the breast, testicular tumors, and primary pigmented nodular adrenocortical disease with and without Cushing's syndrome.[7-10] It is important to identify this group of patients since they tend to have cardiac myxomas at a young age, a familial occurrence, and an increased incidence of multiple and recurrent cardiac myxomas.[11-13]

Left atrial myxomas typically are pedunculated, mobile, and friable.[1,2] They tend to prolapse through the mitral valve orifice, resulting in obstruction of flow through the valve, or mitral regurgitation.[1,2] The symptoms due to the obstruction and regurgitation, may mimic those of rheumatic mitral valve disease and include dyspnea, orthopnea, paroxysmal nocturnal dyspnea, fatigue, cough, chest pain, and occasionally syncope or sudden death.[1,2] If the tumor becomes lodged in the mitral orifice, acute circulatory failure may occur.[1] Unlike mitral stenosis, the onset of these symptoms is often sudden and may vary with the position of the patient. Due to their friability and intracavitary location, tumor emboli are common, occurring in 20%-50% of patients with atrial myxoma.[1-3] Left atrial myxomas result in systemic emboli, while right atrial myxomas cause pulmonary emboli and pulmonary hypertension.[1,2] If the emboli affect a peripheral vessel, a histologic diagnosis of myxoma can be made by recovering the systemic embolic material.[1]

Systemic symptoms may occur in patients with myxoma. These include fever, weight loss, anemia, general malaise, and arthralgia.[1-3,14-16] It has been postulated that these symptoms result from an immunologic mechanism from products secreted by the tumor, or tumor necrosis.[3] These systemic symptoms plus those of embolization may mimic endocarditis. The presence of splenomegaly favors endocarditis rather than myxoma.

The physical examination of patients with left atrial myxomas reveals a loud S_1 and accentuated pulmonary component of S_2. In addition, an early diastolic sound called a "tumor plop" occurs when the tumor strikes the endocardial wall or when its motion is suddenly halted.[14] This tumor plop usually occurs later and is lower in frequency than an S_3. A low-pitched diastolic rumble due to obstruction of flow through the mitral orifice may mimic the murmur of rheumatic mitral stenosis; a holosystolic murmur at the apex due to mitral regurgitation has also been described. These murmurs typically vary in intensity from time to time or with the patient's position. Friction rubs due to contact of the tumor with the atrial and ventricular endocardium are occasionally present. Examination of the lungs may reveal rales due to pulmonary congestion, and examination of the extremities may show clubbing.

Laboratory studies usually demonstrate anemia, elevated sedimentation rate, hypergammaglobulinemia, leukocytosis, and thrombocytopenia. Chest x-ray findings in patients with left atrial myxoma may include an enlarged left atrium, pulmonary congestion, and calcification within the intracardiac tumor.[17]

The electrocardiogram usually shows a normal sinus rhythm, but may show atrial arrhythmias (atrial fibrillation or flutter), right ventricular hypertrophy, and abnormal P waves.[18]

Two-dimensional transthoracic echocardiography (TTE) and transesophageal echocardiography (TEE) have been extremely useful for assessing the presence of cardiac tumors.[19-21] TEE provides more detail and greater clarity than TTE.[22,23] A left atrial myxoma can be visualized as a mass of echoes in the left atrium during systole. Since myxomas are commonly pedunculated, they prolapse into the left ventricle during diastole, resulting in a mass of echoes behind the anterior leaflet of the mitral valve (Figs. 1, 2).

Radionuclide imaging of the tumors by gated blood pool scanning (resulting in a filling defect),[24] cine-computed tomography (CT),[25] and magnetic resonance imaging (MRI)[26] are helpful if the echocardiogram is inconclusive.

The excellent efficacy and the safety of echocardiography, CT, and MRI usually saves the need for cardiac catheterization. However, cardiac catheterization should be considered if coexisting cardiac disease might affect the surgical procedure or when inadequate information has been obtained by noninvasive methods.[27] Angiography (performed by filming the levo phase of a pulmonary arteriogram in order to avoid dislodging tumor fragments) reveals a mobile left atrial filling defect which may prolapse into the left ventricle during diastole. The promising technique of digital substraction angiography[28] may replace cardiac angiography in the future.

There have been cases of left atrial myxoma associated with arterial aneurysms secondary to myxomatous emboli and peripheral tumor growth. Even after resection of the primary myxoma, benign myxomatous emboli may continue to grow in the periphery (also documented in brain and bone), simulating malignant behavior.[21,29]

RIGHT ATRIAL MYXOMA

Right atrial myxomas constitute about 20% of all myxomas.[1,2] They produce symptoms of right-sided heart failure including peripheral edema, fatigue, ascites, and abdominal discomfort due to obstruction of tricuspid valve flow or tricuspid regurgitation.[30,31] Tricuspid regurgitation is due to actual valve trauma from the tumor or

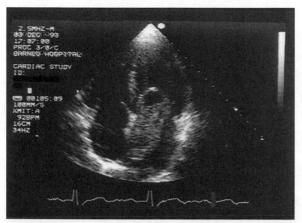 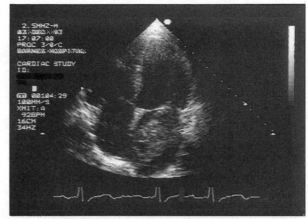

Figure 1. *Transthoracic echocardiogram in the four-chamber view of a large atrial (LA) myxoma. During systole (right panel) the tumor is located in the left atrium, attached to the interatrial septum. During diastole (left panel) the tumor is seen prolapsing across the mitral valve into the left ventricle cavity. (Courtesy of Micha S. Feinberg, MD, Heart Institute, Sheba Medical Center, Tel-Hashomer, Israel)*

interference with normal tricuspid closure. Cyanosis, dizziness, and syncope may be related to body position. Tumor emboli to the pulmonary arteries may result in pulmonary hypertension.[91,92] Physical examination reveals jugular venous distention with a prominent a wave in the jugular venous pulses, hepatosplenomegaly, ascites, peripheral edema, and the murmurs of tricuspid stenosis or tricuspid regurgitation.[33] Friction rubs, clubbing, cyanosis, and signs of superior vena cava obstruction may be present. These findings often mimic those of constrictive pericarditis, rheumatic tricuspid disease, Ebstein's anomaly, and right-sided endocarditis.[11,34] Typical laboratory abnormalities include elevated sedimentation rate, leukocytosis, and hypergammaglobulinemia. If a right-to-left shunt has developed through a patent foramen ovale due to elevated right atrial pressure, polycythemia may occur.[11,34] Electrocardiographic abnormalities may include large P waves, low voltage, and right bundle branch block.[35] Chest x-ray may show right atrial enlargement[34] and intracardiac tumor calcification.[14] The right atrial tumor may be visualized by echocardiography.[36,37] However, TEE may provide more information than transthoracic echocardiography.[36,37] With current noninvasive imaging techniques, cardiac catheterization and angiography are unnecessary and have the risk of tumor dislodgment and pulmonary embolization.

TREATMENT

In view of the threat of tumor embolization, the treatment of both left and right atrial myxomas is immediate surgical excision utilizing cardiopulmonary bypass technique. Cardiac arrest with cardioplegia solution before manipulating the heart can reduce the risk of fragmentation of the friable tumor.[18,38] Complete cure has been documented in long-term follow-up. Recurrence or development of a second cardiac myxoma occurs in about 1% to 5% of cases.[3,12,38a] Many surgeons prefer wide resection of the atrial septum surrounding the attachment of the tumor because recurrence is possible if resection is incomplete. This necessitates the repair of an atrial defect with a Dacron patch.[18,38]

RHABDOMYOMAS

These tumors are the most common cardiac tumors in infants and children.[1,2] They are usually multiple, involve the ventricular walls, and project into the ventricular cavity[39–41] affecting right and left side equally. Rhabdomyomas are not true neoplasms but represent hamartomas, and their histology is characterized by a lack of mitotic figures and glycogenladen immature myocardial cells.[42] Spontaneous regression has been reported.[44,45] Rhabdomyomas commonly occur in association with

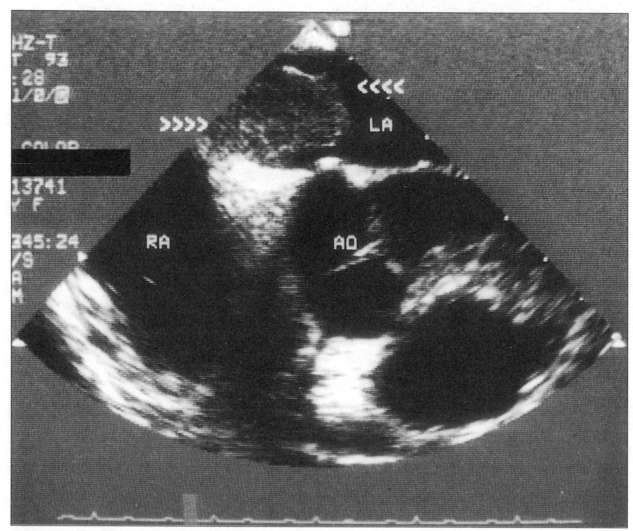

Figure 2. *Transesophageal echocardiogram of a 40-year-old man 4 years after the removal of a left atrial myxoma. A recurrent, large, left atrial (LA) myxoma (arrow) attached to the interatrial septum is seen. AO=Aortic valve; RA=Right atrium. (Courtesy of Zvi Vered, MD, Heart Institute, Sheba Medical Center, Tel-Hashomer, Israel)*

tuberous sclerosis.[18,43] Children with rhabdomyomas may have symptoms and signs related to obstruction of a cardiac chamber or valve orifice, tachyarrhythmias, AV block, and sudden death.[39–41,45] Electrocardiography may show left ventricular hypertrophy, left bundle branch block and tachyarrhythmias. Surgical excision is necessary for treatment of obstruction or arrhythmias.[18,38,45]

FIBROMAS

A fibroma is another benign tumor that most commonly affects infants and children and occurs within the ventricular myocardium.[1,2] Fibromas may be asymptomatic or result in obstruction to intracardiac flow, abnormalities in ventricular contraction, or conduction disturbances leading to sudden death as the presenting symptom.[46–48] Surgical resection is needed for treatment.[46–48]

PAPILLARY FIBROELASTOMA

Papillary fibroelastomas arise from the cardiac valves. They are most frequently seen in patients over 50 years of age. It has been suggested that the origin of these tumors is organized cardiac thrombus.[5,49] Angina or sudden death due to ostial coronary artery occlusion from an aortic valve tumor may be the presenting symptom.[1] The incidence of detection of these tumors is increasing due to the widespread use of echocardiography and TEE.[18] Surgical excision is the recommended therapy.

LIPOMAS

Lipomas may be located within the sub-endocardium, subepicardium, or intramural myocardium. They may be asymptomatic or produce atrioventricular (AV) or intraventricular conduction abnormalities, arrhythmias, and sudden death.[1,2] Impaired ventricular contraction and recurrent pericardial effusion have also been reported.

Diagnosis can be made by echocardiography. When the findings of the echocardiogram are inconclusive, tissue characterization by MRI can provide definite diagnosis.[50] Lipomatous hypertrophy of the atrial septum, an accumulation of nonencapsulated adipose tissues within the interatrial septum, is not considered a true tumor but should be considered in the differential diagnosis. Surgical excision yields excellent long-term results.[18]

MESOTHELIOMAS OF THE AV NODE

Mesotheliomas are rare and unique tumors which tend to be located in the area of the AV node. These slow-growing cystic tumors may cause complete heart block or ventricular fibrillation.[1,2,52] Thus, they should be considered in the differential diagnosis of any case of unexplained sudden death in a young patient.

MALIGNANT PRIMARY TUMORS

Malignant tumors constitute approximately 25% of all primary tumors of the heart and in most cases are sarcomas.[1,2] The most common of these include angiosarcoma, rhabdomyosarcoma, and fibrosarcoma. The development of these tumors is more common in adults and can involve either the atrium or ventricle, but is more common on the right side of the heart. Clinical features include those of progressive right-sided and/or left-sided heart failure, arrhythmias, pericardial effusion, chest pain, and cardiac tamponade.[1-3,18] These tumors may grow rapidly, invading the myocardium, intracardiac chambers and pericardial space, and they often metastasize.[3] They may obstruct either the superior vena cava, resulting in edema of the face and upper extremities, or the inferior vena cava, causing mesenteric, hepatic and lower extremity edema. Most patients have a progressively downhill course and die within weeks to a few years after symptoms are present.[3]

In general, various forms of radiation therapy, chemotherapy, and surgery are palliative and have failed to alter the poor prognosis of cardiac sarcoma.[3] Cardiac transplantation has been utilized in cases of inoperable cardiac neoplasms.[52,53]

METASTATIC TUMORS TO THE HEART

Metastatic tumors to the heart are more common than primary cardiac tumors. Cardiac metastases occur with many types of tumors (carcinoma more commonly than sarcomas) and have been described in 2%-21% of patients dying with malignancy.[54,55] Cardiac metastases, in general, are encountered with widespread systemic tumor dissemination — only rarely are metastases limited to the heart or the pericardium. The most common of these include, in order of frequency, carcinoma of the bronchus, carcinoma of the breast, malignant melanoma, lymphomas, and leukemias.[4] Malignant melanoma has a particular tendency to metastasize to the heart: more than 50% of the cases of this malignancy developed cardiac metastases.[4] Cardiac metastases occur most frequently in patients over the age of 50 years, with an equal gender incidence. The incidence of cardiac metastases is increasing due to the improved therapy and survival of patients with other primary malignancies.[56]

Metastatic tumors are believed to reach the heart by hematogenous, lymphatic spread, or direct invasion. Lymphatic spread is particularly frequent with carcinoma of the bronchus or breast.[4] Intracavitary metastatic tumors are disseminated via the great veins. Thus, metastases from carcinoma of the kidney, testis, liver and uterus invade the right atrium via the vena cava and may mimic myxoma.[18] Metastases from bronchogenic carcinoma may enter the left atrium via the pulmonary veins. Metastases of valvular tissue or the endocardium are unusual, since these structures are avascular. When they occur, it is probably by direct extension. Endocardial and valve metastases may be polypoid and form emboli mimicking myxomas and endocarditis. They can result in valvular stenosis or regurgitation. Pericardial metastases occur more frequently than myocardial metastases and are common in patients with carcinoma of the breast or lung (by lymphatic spread) or mediastinal lymphoma (by direct extension) and in leukemia by hematogenous spread.[18] Pericardial effusions and tamponade or constrictive pericarditis may occur.[4,55] Finally, intramural metastases may be present in either the left or right ventricle. Myocardial infarction has resulted from the metastatic tumor encircling or compressing the epicardial coronary arteries.[57] Myocardial injury may also result from the chemotherapeutic agents and radiation used in the treatment of patients with neoplastic diseases.[4,18,57]

Kaposi's sarcoma, metastatic to the heart, has been described in patients with acquired immune deficiency syndrome (AIDS).[58] This sarcoma has involved the subepithelial adipose tissue adjacent to the coronary arteries, but without evidence of compression of the coronary arteries.[58] Steigman et al[59] recently reported a case of fatal cardiac tamponade due to epicardial Kaposi's sarcoma in a patient with AIDS. In this patient, there was also a nodule of Kaposi's sarcoma involving the endocardial surface of a papillary muscle.

Besides Kaposi's sarcoma, primary non-Hodgkin lymphoma of the heart has been described in patients with AIDS.[60,61] In a report of 2 cases of cardiac lymphoma associated with myocardial and pericardial involvement and arrhythmias in AIDS patients, the pattern and distribution of the tumor suggested de novo origin of the lymphoma of the heart.[62]

Cardiac lymphomas occur in less than 10% of patients with cardiac metastases proven by autopsy.[18] The metastases are not usually a major factor contributing to the death of the patient. Symptoms depend more on the location than the size of the tumor; for example, metastases from hypernephroma may infiltrate the AV node, resulting in complete AV block.[63]

Metastatic tumor to the heart should be suspected when a patient with metastatic disease develops cardiac dysfunction without apparent cause. Common signs and symptoms include those of pericardial involvement including chest pain, persistent pericardial rub, evidence of cardiac tamponade or pericardial constriction, and a rapid increase in heart size. It is important to distinguish malignant pericardial involvement, which can coexist in patients with cancer. Kralstein and Frishman[64] noted that cough, facial swelling, and pericardial tamponade are associated with malignant pericardial disease. Fever, rub, and clinical improvement on non-steroidal anti-inflammatory agents are more suggestive of idiopathic pericarditis. Other common clinical manifestations of cardiac metastases include development of heart block, arrhythmias, changing cardiac murmurs, evidence of obstruction to the great vein orifices, and intractable and unexplained cardiac failure.[4,18] This latter feature may be due to lymphatic obstruction by the tumor, with severe myocardial interstitial edema and secondary pressure on the myofibers resulting in cardiac decompression.

Electrocardiographic abnormalities are common and include ST-T wave changes, which sometimes mimic myocardial infarction (especially when the cardiac metastases produce necrosis); arrhythmias including supraventricular arrhythmias (especially when the metastases involve the atria); AV block and bundle branch block (due to tumor infiltration of the conducting system); abnormal P waves; and reduced QRS amplitude in cases with and without pericardial effusion.[65] The arrhythmias often do not respond to standard therapy. Two-dimensional echocardiography, computer-assisted tomography, and magnetic resonance imaging have been shown to be useful for assessing the presence of cardiac tumors and malignant pericardial involvement. Pericardiocentesis will be needed to treat tamponade but may also be needed to help diagnose malignant infusion. Bloody pericardial fluid with protein concentration of >3 mg/dl and a specific gravity of >1.016 in the absence of myocardial infarction is suggestive of malignant effusion. Positive cytology may be found in 50%-70% of patients. Pericardial biopsy may be needed in cases in which the clinical presentation suggests malignant effusion but in which the pericardial fluid is negative for malignancy.

Rarely, malignant or metastatic tumors may be amenable to surgery. Palliative radiation therapy and systemic chemotherapy may afford symptomatic relief, but radiation to the chest may produce myocardial and pericardial fibrosis and damage to the conduction system, valves and coronary arteries.[4]

Relief of symptoms in cases of malignant pericardial effusion or tamponade can be achieved with percutaneous pericardiocentesis. This procedure can be guided by echocardiography with a low morbidity and mortality.[66] Drainage for several days with an indwelling catheter relieves the effusion without subsequent recurrence. Systemic chemotherapy or radiation therapy is effective in controlling malignant effusions in cases of sensitive tumors such as lymphoma or leukemia. Local sclerotherapy with tetracycline or bleomycine is also effective. Recurrent effusions resulting in tamponade or the presence of pericardial constriction may require surgical pericardiotomy. Recently, percutaneous balloon pericardiotomy has been suggested to provide successful palliation of malignant pericardial effusions and cardiac tamponade.[67]

REFERENCES

1. McAllister HA Jr. Primary tumors and cysts of the heart and the pericardium. *Curr Probl Cardiol.* 1979;4:1-51.
2. McAllister HA Jr, Fenoglio JJ Jr. Tumors of the cardiovascular system. In: *Atlas of Tumor Pathology.* Washington DC: Armed Forces Institute of Pathology, 1978:1-141.
3. Colucci WS, Braunwald E. Primary tumors of the heart. In: Braunwald E (ed). *Heart Disease: A Textbook of Cardiovascular Medicine.* Philadelphia: W.B. Saunders; 1992:1451-1464.
4. Rosenthal DS, Braunwald E. Hematological-oncological disorders and heart disease. In: Braunwald E (ed). *Heart Disease: A Textbook of Cardiovascular Medicine.* Philadelphia: W.B. Saunders; 1992:1752-1760.
5. Sayler WR, Page DL, Hutchins GM. The development of cardiac myxomas and papillary endocardial lesions from mural thrombus. *Am Heart J.* 1975;89:4-17.
6. Seidman JD, Berman JJ, Hitchcock CL, et al. DNA analysis of cardiac myxomas: Flow cytometry and image analysis. *Hum Pathol.* 1991;22:494-500.
7. Vidaillet HJ Jr, Seward JB, Fyke FE III, et al. "Syndrome myxoma": A subset of patients with cardiac myxoma associated with pigmented skin lesions and peripheral and endocrine neoplasm. *Br Heart J.* 1987;57:247-255.
8. Danoff A, Jormak S, Lorber D, et al. Adrenocortical micronodular dysplasia, cardiac myxomas, lentigines, and spindle cell tumors. Report of a kindred. *Arch Intern Med.* 1987;147:443-448.
9. Carney JA, Gordon H, Carpenter PC, et al. The complex of myxomas, spotty pigmentation, and endocrine overactivity. *Medicine.* 1985;64:270-283.
10. Vidaillet HJ Jr, Seward JB, Fyke E III, et al. NAME syndrome (nevi, atrial myxoma, myxoid neurofibroma, ephelides): A new and unrecognized subset of patients with cardiac myxoma. *Minn Med.* 1984;67:695-696.
11. Powers JC, Falkoff M, Heinle RA, et al. Familial cardiac myxoma. Emphasis on unusual clinical manifestations. *J Thorac Cardiovasc Surg.* 1979;77:782-788.
12. McCarthy PM, Piehler JM, Schaff HV, et al. The significance of multiple recurrent and "complex" cardiac myxomas. *Thorac Cardiovasc Surg.* 1986;91:389-396.
13. Carney JA. Differences between nonfamilial and familial cardiac myxoma. *Am J Surg Pathol.* 1985;9:53-55.
14. Peters MN, Hall RJ, Cooley DA, et al. The clinical syndrome of atrial myxoma. *JAMA.* 1974;230:695-701.
15. MacGregor GA, Cullen RA. The syndrome of fever, anemia and high sedimentation rate with an atrial myxoma. *Br Med J.* 1959;2:991-993.
16. Huston KA, Combs JJ Jr, Lie JT, et al. Left atrial myxoma simulating peripheral vasculitis. *Mayo Clin Proc.* 1978;53:752-759.
17. Sharratt GP, Grover ML, Monro JL. Calcified left atrial myxoma with floppy mitral valve. *Br Heart J.* 1979;42:608-610.
18. Hall RJ, Cooley DA, McAllister HA, et al. Neoplastic heart disease. In: Schlant RC, Alexander RW (eds). *The Heart.* New York: McGraw-Hill; 1994:2007-2029.
19. Pechacek LW, Gonzalez-Camid F, Hall RJ, et al. The echocardiographic spectrum of atrial myxoma: A ten year experience. *Texas Heart Inst J.* 1986;13:179-195.
20. Fyke FE III, Seqard JB, Edwards WD, et al. Primary cardiac tumors: Experience with 30 consecutive patients since the introduction of two-dimensional echocardiography. *J Am Coll Cardiol.* 1985;5:1465-1473.
21. Nomeir AM, Watts EE, Seagle R, et al. Intracardiac myxomas: Twenty-year echocardiographic experience with review of the literature. *J Am Soc Echo.* 1989;2:139-150.
22. Reeder GS, Khandheria BK, Seward JB, et al. Transesophageal echocardiography and cardiac masses. *Mayo Clin Proc.* 1991;66:1101-1109.
23. Obeid AI, Marvasti M, Parker F, et al. Comparison of transthoracic and transesophageal echocardiography in diagnosis of left atrial myxoma. *Am J Cardiol.* 1989;63:1006-1008.
24. Bough EW, Boden WE, Gandsman EJ, et al. Radionuclide diagnosis of left atrial myxoma with computed generated functional images. *Am J Cardiol.* 1983;52:1365-1367.

25. Bateman TM, Sethna DH, Whiting JS, et al. Comprehensive noninvasive evaluation of left atrial myxomas using cardiac cine-computed tomography. *J Am Coll Cardiol.* 1987;9:1180-1183.

26. Freedberg RS, Kronzon I, Rumancik WM, et al. The contribution of magnetic resonance imaging to the evaluation of intracardiac tumors diagnosed by echocardiography. *Circulation.* 1988;77:96-103.

27. Fueredi GA, Knechtges TE, Czarnecki DJ. Coronary angiography in atrial myxoma: Finding in nine cases. *Am J Roentgenol.* 1989;152:737-738.

28. Tamari I, Goldberg HL, Moses JW, et al. Left atrial myxoma: Diagnosis by digital substraction angiography. *Cath Cardiovasc Diagn.* 1986;12:26-29.

29. Desousa AL, Muller J, Campbell R, et al. Atrial myxoma: A review of the neurological complications, metastases, and recurrences. *J Neurol Neurosurg Psychiat.* 1978;41:1119-1124.

30. Harvey WP. Clinical aspects of cardiac tumors. *Am J Cardiol.* 1968;21:328-343.

31. Panidis IP, Kotler MN, Mintz GS, et al. Clinical and echocardiographic features of right atrial masses. *Am Heart J.* 1984;107:745-758.

32. Vidne B, Atsmon A, Aygen M, et al. Right atrial myxoma: Case report and review of the literature. *Isr J Med Sci.* 1971;7:1196-1200.

33. Massumi R. Bedside diagnosis of right heart myxomas through detection of palpable tumor shocks and audible plops. *Am Heart J.* 1983;105:303-310.

34. Natarajan P, Vijayanagar RR, Eckstein PF, et al. Right atrial myxoma with atrial septal defect: A case report and review of the literature. *Cathet Cardiovasc Diagn.* 1982;8:267-272.

35. Case Records of the Massachusetts General Hospital, Weekly Clinopathological Exercises. Case 14-1978. *N Engl J Med.* 1978;298:834-842.

36. Mugge A, Daniel WG, Haverich A, et al. Diagnosis of noninfective cardiac mass lesions by two-dimensional echocardiography: Comparison of the transthoracic and transesophageal approaches. *Circulation.* 1991;83:70-78.

37. Vargas-Barron J, Romero-Cardenas A, Villegas M, et al. Transthoracic and transesophageal echocardiographic diagnosis of myxomas in the four cardiac cavities. *Am Heart J.* 1991;121:931-933.

38. Murphy MC, Sweeney MS, Putnam JB Jr, et al. Surgical treatment of cardiac tumors: A 25 year experience. *Ann Thorac Surg.* 1990;49:612-618.

38a. Castells E, Ferran V, Octavio de Toledo MC. Cardiac myxomas: surgical treatment, long term results and recurrence. *J Cardiovasc Surg.* 1993;34:49-53.

39. Mahoney L, Schieken RM, Doty D. Cardiac rhabdomyomas simulating pulmonic stenosis. *Cathet Cardiovasc Diagn.* 1979;5:385-388.

40. Howanitz EP, Teske DW, Qualman SJ, et al. Pedunculated left ventricular rhabdomyoma. *Ann Thorac Surg.* 1986;41:443-445.

41. Spooner EW, Farina MA, Shaher RM, et al. Left ventricular rhabdomyoma causing subaortic stenosis — The two dimensional echocardiographic appearance. *Pediatr Cardiol.* 1982;2:67-71.

42. Fenoglio JJ Jr, McAllister HA, Ferrans VJ. Cardiac rhabdomyoma: A clinopathologic and electron microscopic study. *Am J Cardiol.* 1976;38:241-251.

43. Abushaban L, Denham B, Duff D. 10 year review of cardiac tumors in childhood. *Br Heart J.* 1993;70:166-169.

44. Farooki ZQ, Ross RD, Paridon SM, et al. Spontaneous regression of cardiac rhabdomyoma. *Am J Cardiol.* 1991;67:897-899.

45. Kearney DL, Titus JL, Hawkins EP, et al. Pathologic features of myocardial hamartomas causing childhood tachyarrhythmias. *Circulation.* 1987;75:705-710.

46. Reul GJ, Jr, Howell JF, Rubio PA, et al. Successful partial excision of an intramural fibroma of the left ventricle. *Am J Cardiol.* 1975;36:262-265.

47. Williams DB, Danielson GK, McGoon DC, et al. Cardiac fibroma. Long-term survival after excision. *J Thorac Cardiovasc Surg.* 1982;84:230-236.

48. Reece IJ, Cooley DA, Frazier OH, et al. Cardiac tumors: Clinical spectrum and prognosis of lesions other than classical benign myxoma in 20 patients. *J Thorac Cardiovasc Surg.* 1984;88:439-446.

49. Heath D. Pathology of cardiac tumors. *Am J Cardiol.* 1968;21:315-327.

50. Tuna IC, Julsrud PR, Click RL, et al. Tissue characterization of an unusual right atrial mass by magnetic resonance imaging. *Mayo Clin Proc.* 1991;66:498-501.

51. Manion WC, Nelson WP, Hall RJ, et al. Benign tumor of the heart causing complete heart block. *Am Heart J.* 1972;83:535-542.

52. Dein JR, Frist WH, Stinson EB, et al. Primary cardiac neoplasms. Early and late results of surgical treatment in 42 patients. *J Thorac Cardiovasc Surg.* 1987;93:502-511.

53. Horn M, Phebus C, Blatt J. Cancer chemotherapy after solid organ transplantation. *Cancer.* 1990;66:1468-1471.

54. Deloach JF, Haynes JW. Secondary tumors of the heart and pericardium: Review of the subject and report of one hundred thirty seven cases. *Arch Intern Med.* 1953;91:224-229.

55. Kutalek SP, Panidis IP, Kotler MN, et al. Metastatic tumors of the heart detected by two-dimensional echocardiography. *Am Heart J.* 1985;109:343-349.

56. Lockwood WB, Broghamer WL Jr. The changing prevalence of secondary cardiac neoplasms as related to cancer therapy. *Cancer.* 1980;45:2659-2662.

57. Kopelson G, Herwig KJ. The etiologies of coronary artery disease in cancer patients. *Int J Radiat Oncol Biol Phys.* 1978;4:895-906.

58. Kaul S, Fishbein MC, Siegel RJ. Cardiac manifestations of acquired immune deficiency syndrome: a 1991 update. *Am Heart J.* 1991;122:534-544.

59. Steigman CK, Anderson DW, Macher AM, et al. Fatal cardiac tamponade in acquired immune deficiency syndrome with epicardial Kaposi's sarcoma. *Am Heart J.* 1988;116:1105-1107.

60. Acierno LJ. Cardiac complications in acquired immuno-deficiency syndrome (AIDS): A review. *J Am Coll Cardiol.* 1989;13:1144-1154.

61. Lewis W. AIDS: Cardiac findings from 115 autopsies. *Prog Cardiovasc Dis.* 1989;32:207-215.

62. Balasubramanyam A, Waxman M, Kazal HL, et al. Malignant lymphoma of the heart in acquired immune deficiency syndrome. *Chest.* 1986;90:243-246.

63. Wong DW, Guthaner DF, Gordon EP, et al. Lymphoma of the heart. *Cathet Cardiovasc Diagn.* 1984;10:337-384.

64. Kralstein J, Frishman W. Malignant pericardial disease: Diagnosis and treatment. *Am Heart J.* 1987; 113:785-790.

65. Koiwaya Y, Nakamura M, Yamamoto K. Progressive ECG alterations in metastatic cardiac mural tumor. *Am Heart J.* 1983;105:339-341.

66. Vaiktus PT, Herrmann HC, LeWinter MM. Treatment of malignant pericardial effusion. *JAMA.* 1994;272:59-64.

67. Ziskind AA, Pearce C, Lemmon CC, et al. Percutaneous balloon pericardiotomy for the treatment of cardiac tamponade and large pericardial effusions: Description of technique and report of the first 50 cases. *J Am Coll Cardiol.* 1993;21:1-5.

CHAPTER 29

Evaluation and Management of Hypertension

Allen J. Naftilan, MD, PhD

DEFINITION AND PREVALENCE OF HYPERTENSION

Since systemic arterial pressure fluctuates throughout the day, and the blood pressure in the general population falls in a Gaussian distribution, the limits of normal blood pressure cannot be precisely defined. There is no evidence for a threshold level beyond which cardiovascular risk increases precipitously, but numerous clinical trials have indicated the levels at which treatment of blood pressure decreases risk. The Joint National Committee on the Detection, Evaluation, and Treatment of High Blood Pressure[1] proposes the levels listed in Table 1.

Data from the National Health and Nutrition Examination Survey (NHANES) has demonstrated an increased awareness of hypertension. From 1976-1980 some 73% of hypertensive patients were told they were hypertensive by their physician; from 1988-1991 this has increased to 84%.[1] There was an increase in the estimated total number of people with hypertension from 58 million in 1985 to 80 million in 1990. The prevalence is slightly higher in blacks than whites (38% vs 29%). Also, according to the NHANES survey, a greater percentage of patients are now being treated (56% vs 73%) and more are being controlled (34% vs 55%). This could well account for the solo decrease in mortality from coronary heart disease that has been seen in the past decade.[1] Still, just above half of the patients with documented hypertension are being adequately treated.

PHYSIOLOGY

The major determinants of blood pressure are cardiac output and systemic vascular resistance, both of which are controlled by various neurohumoral mechanisms and the kidney. The autonomic nervous system and the renin angiotensin system are involved in short-term regulation of blood pressure in humans, but the kidney exerts long-term control by regulating sodium balance and extracellular fluid volume. Early in the development of hypertension, elevated blood pressure can result from any circulatory disturbance that increases cardiac output, total peripheral vascular resistance, or both. Initially in essential hypertension, the cardiac output is elevated.[2] Some investigators believe that this increase in cardiac output results in an increase in peripheral resistance, which maintains or even perpetuates the hypertension. Patients with more established, long-standing essential hypertension tend to have normal cardiac output and increased peripheral vascular resistance, findings that support this theory.[3,4] In patients with a long history of hypertension, cardiac output may be decreased. In these cases, the increase in blood pressure is entirely the result of an increase in peripheral vascular resistance.

The development of specific pharmacologic inhibitors of the renin-angiotensin system is an important advance in antihypertensive therapy. Renin is a proteolytic enzyme released by the juxtaglomerular cells in the afferent arterioles of the kidney (Fig. 1).[5] Renin cleaves its substrate in plasma, angiotensinogen, an α_2-globulin synthesized by the liver. Angiotensin I, a decapeptide that is a product of the renin and angiotensinogen reaction, is physiologically inactive and is converted to the octapeptide angiotensin II by angiotensin-converting enzyme (ACE).

Angiotensin II is a potent vasoconstrictor and the primary stimulus for aldosterone secretion by the adrenal cortex. Along with the peripheral

Table 1. Definitions of Hypertension[1]

	SYSTOLIC (MM HG)	DIASTOLIC (MM HG)
Normal	<130	<85
High-Normal	130-139	85-89
Hypertension		
Stage I (mild)	140-159	90-99
Stage II (moderate)	160-179	100-109
Stage III (severe)	180-209	110-119
Stage IV (very severe)	≥ 210	≥ 120

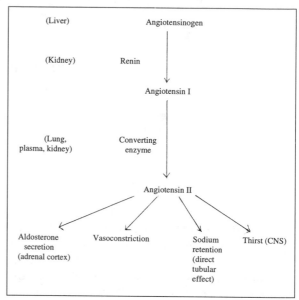

Figure 1. Schematic diagram of renin-angiotensin-aldosterone system

renin-angiotensin system, there are locally active renin-angiotensin systems in the kidney, heart, and blood vessel walls.[6] These local systems may be as, or more, important than the peripheral system in several physiologic functions.

The autonomic nervous system may also be important in the initiation and maintenance of hypertension. Patients with hypertension have exaggerated pressor responses to stress, which may be due to abnormal sympathetic and parasympathetic control mechanisms.[7,8]

EVALUATION OF THE HYPERTENSIVE PATIENT

Evaluation of the hypertensive patient should include a careful history and physical examination as well as screening laboratory tests, with the following goals: 1) proper documentation of hypertension; 2) assessment of cardiovascular risk factors; 3) search for evidence of end-organ damage; and 4) a decision about when to perform a workup for secondary hypertension.

Along with a general physical examination, with particular attention to the cardiovascular and peripheral vascular systems (Table 2), the most critical part of the initial evaluation is accurate determination of blood pressure. During the initial visit, blood pressure should be measured in both the supine and upright positions. At least 3 blood pressure measurements should be taken, at least 5 minutes apart. Proper cuff size is critical. The cuff should be approximately two-thirds the width of the arm,

or 15 cm in an average adult. A cuff that is too short can falsely elevate the readings.[9-11] A rolled sleeve should not constrict the arm, as this can also affect blood pressure. The cuff should be inflated to 20-30 mm Hg above the systolic pressure. The systolic pressure is the point at which the Korotkoff sounds are first heard with every heartbeat. Usually, the diastolic pressure is best recorded at the level at which the heart sounds disappear—Korotkoff phase V.[12] In patients with a high cardiac output and in children, the blood pressure should be measured at the point at which the sounds become muffled—Korotkoff phase IV.[11,12]

With few exceptions, the blood pressure level should be determined from more than 1 office visit before deciding on a treatment plan. Home blood pressure readings are also useful in determining if treatment is necessary. Recently, automatic, portable, 24-hour blood pressure monitors for home use have become available.[13,14] Twenty-four-hour blood pressure monitoring is becoming increasingly utilized. The damage caused by hypertension is generally believed to be a function of the time at which the circulation is exposed to elevated pressures; if this is so, ambulatory 24-hour blood pressure monitoring may be better than office measurements in assessing the need for

---

Table 2. Clinical Evaluation of the Hypertensive Patient

History

    Age, sex, duration of hypertension, response to therapy

    Symptoms of headaches, TIA, CVA, CHF, angina, PVD

    Symptoms of episodic headaches, palpitations, perspiration (pheochromocytoma) muscular weakness, cramps and polyuria (primary aldosteronism), headache and lower extremity claudication (coarctation of aorta)

    Family history of hypertension: history of smoking, diet, exercise, and other risk factors (diabetes, gout)

    Medications: birth control pills, amphetamines (diet and cold capsules, nasal sprays), cocaine abuse, large quantities of licorice, adrenal steroids, thyroid hormones

Physical

    Vital signs including postural BP; arm and leg BP; weight

    Funduscopic examination for retinopathy

    Cardiac and chest examination for heart size, murmurs, and gallops

    Abdominal examination for masses, bruits

    Peripheral vascular examination

    Neurologic examination

    Check for evidence of gout, hyperlipidemia, thyroid disorder, Cushing's syndrome; signs of neurofibromatosis, cafe-au-lait spots

Laboratory (initial)

    Serum potassium and sodium; creatinine or BUN; FBS, cholesterol; ECG; urinalysis

    Additional: CBC, uric acid

TIA=Transient ischemic attack; CVA=Cerebrovascular accident; CHF=Congestive heart failure; PVD=Peripheral vascular disease; FBS=Fasting blood sugar; CBC=Complete blood count; BP=Blood pressure.

---

antihypertensive treatment. Several prospective studies have correlated 24-hour ambulatory pressures versus casual pressures in the clinic with clinical evidence of target organ damage.[15,16] One study of more than 1,000 patients followed for an average of 5 years showed a significant correlation between ambulatory and office blood pressures, but found that ambulatory pressures were an average of 10-15 mm Hg lower than office pressures.[17] Patients who had elevated ambulatory pressures were at greater risk for cardiovascular damage, suggesting that ambulatory measurement may be a good discriminator between high- and low-risk groups within a given level of office blood pressure, especially in mildly hypertensive patients. These and other studies must be further analyzed before the role of ambulatory blood pressure monitoring is clear. Despite this, "casual" blood pressure levels remain important predictors of cardiovascular complications. Indeed, most of the major epidemiologic studies on hypertension and cardiovascular risk use office-casual blood pressure determinations.

The physical examination should include a careful search for evidence of end-organ damage and atherosclerotic vascular disease (i.e., left ventricular [LV] hypertrophy, congestive heart failure, cardiomegaly, evidence of abdominal bruits) and careful examination of the femoral pulses for a pulse delay. Special attention should be given to the opthalmoscopic examination, looking for arteriolar narrowing, hemorrhages, exudates, and possibly, papilledema, especially in the severely hypertensive patient. During neurologic examination, evidence of remote stroke would prompt more rigorous control of blood pressure.

The laboratory examination should evaluate end-organ function, evidence of secondary hypertension, and concomitant risk factors (Table 3). Laboratory procedures should include a hematocrit, urinalysis, electrolytes, BUN, and creatinine to evaluate renal function; and measurement of the patient's blood glucose level, serum uric acid, and total cholesterol and triglyceride levels.[18] If the serum total cholesterol is over 200 mg/dL, a 12-hour fasting serum cholesterol, high-density lipoprotein (HDL) cholesterol, and triglyceride (TG) determination should be performed. Using the formula: low-density lipoprotein (LDL) cholesterol = total cholesterol – HDL cholesterol – TG/5, the atherogenic potential may be predicted.

A chest x-ray is of little value in the routine examination of a hypertensive patient because it has a very low predictive value for cardiac hypertrophy. If a patient has a history of known pulmonary disease or has smoked cigarettes for a long time, a chest x-ray may be useful for evaluating pulmonary pathology. An electrocardiogram (ECG) is recommended as a baseline measure and also to detect LV hypertrophy. The role of echocardiography is unclear, although echocardiography is more sensitive and specific than the ECG for evaluating a patient for LV hypertrophy (Table 4).[19-21] Several studies suggest that LV hypertrophy may be a good predictor of future cardiovascular risk.[21,23,24] However, routine echocardiography in all hypertensive patients is not suggested. Echocardiography may be useful in the patient with long-standing hypertension and evidence of congestive heart failure (HF), to rule out hypertrophic cardiomyopathy rather than poor left ventricular function from prior infarction as a cause of heart failure. Echocardiography is also useful for the patient with borderline hypertension; evidence of mild diastolic dysfunction or LV hypertrophy indicates a need for treatment because these conditions suggest a higher risk of cardiovascular events.

The role of random plasma renin activity (PRA) measurement in the initial assessment of a hypertensive patient should be noted. Essential hypertension may be classified as high, normal, or low renin, and it has been suggested that these classifications may be used to predict cardiovascular complications and guide therapy.[25,26] However, the current consensus is that PRA is not a useful screen, and it is not recommended in the initial assessment of the patient with uncomplicated essential hypertension.[27,28] Although this is true for essential hypertension, a renin profile may be useful to evaluate people for the risk of

Table 3. Baseline Laboratory Tests for Evaluation of Hypertension

TEST	INFORMATION
Complete blood count	Baseline (stress erythrocytosis)
Serum potassium concentration	Pretreatment baseline (diuretic therapy)
	Screening for primary or secondary aldosteronsim (etiology)
Serum creatinine	End-organ function (complication)
	Renal hypertension (etiology)
Fasting blood sugar	Risk factor
Serum cholesterol	Risk factor
Serum uric acid	Baseline (diuretic therapy)
	Indicator of nephrosclerosis (complication)
Electrocardiogram	Risk factor
Urinalysis	Renal hypertension (etiology)
	End-organ function (complications)

Table 4. Left Ventricular Hypertrophy: Electrocardiographic Versus Echocardiographic Assessment

	SENSITIVITY (%)	SPECIFICITY (%)	ACCURACY (%)
ECG criteria			
$SV_1 + RV_5$ or $RV_6 > 35$	33	94	67
RE point score > 4	30	93	65
RE point score > 5	19	96	61
Sokolow-Lyons voltage	21	95	65
$R_aV_L > 11$	7	98	58
$R_1 + S_3 > 25$	8	97	58
Echo criteria			
M-mode; LV mass	93	95	94
Penn-cube method	100	86	90

RE=Romhilt-Estes.

$$\text{Sensitivity (\%)} = \frac{\text{true positives correctly diagnosed}}{\text{total true positives}} \times 100$$

$$\text{Specificity (\%)} = \frac{\text{true negatives correctly diagnosed}}{\text{total true negatives}} \times 100$$

$$\text{Accuracy (\%)} = \frac{\text{positives + negatives correctly diagnosed}}{\text{total tested}} \times 100$$

myocardial infarction. In a recent paper Alderman et al[29] have reported that patients with a high renin profile (obtained by plotting plasma renin activity against urinary excretion of sodium) had a higher risk of myocardial infarction. How this test will be used for total cardiovascular risk profiling remains to be established.

An important and difficult decision in the initial evaluation is whom to evaluate for secondary causes of hypertension. Screening for secondary hypertension should be reserved for selected patients who show 1 of the following features:[18] 1) onset of hypertension at an age younger than 30 years; 2) a rapid onset later in life, sometime after age 50, and no history of essential hypertension; 3) a negative family history of hypertension and a diastolic blood pressure above 110 mm Hg; 4) refractoriness to antihypertensive therapy; 5) features indicative of secondary causes upon initial screening, including hypokalemia (defined as a serum

potassium below 3.5 mEq/L in a patient not taking oral diuretics or below 3 mEq/L in a patient taking diuretics); 6) evidence of an abdominal bruit on physical examination; and 7) history of variable blood pressures with sweating, tachycardia, palpitations, and tremor of the upper extremities, which suggest pheochromocytoma, and 8) use of oral contraceptives by a young woman.

SECONDARY FORMS OF HYPERTENSION

The screening tests for specific forms of hypertension are listed in Table 5.

RENOVASCULAR HYPERTENSION

Renovascular hypertension comprises about 2% of hypertension in adults. Renal artery stenosis usually occurs as a result of atherosclerosis or fibromuscular disease. Atherosclerosis is more

Table 5. Screening Tests for Specific Forms of Hypertension	
DIAGNOSIS	SCREENING TEST
Renovascular hypertension	DSA, captopril renography
	Hypertensive IVP
Primary aldosteronism	Stimulated PRA, 24-hr urine potassium excretion
Cushing's syndrome	Overnight dexamethasone suppression
Pheochromocytoma	24-hr urine metanephrine, VMA, and catecholamines
Renal hypertension	Urinalysis, BUN, creatinine, IVP, ultrasound, urine culture
Coarctation of aorta	Chest x-ray
Hyperparathyroidism	Serum calcium and phosphorus levels
Hyperthyroidism	Serum T4 and thyroglobulin levels

DSA=Digital subtraction angiography; PRA=Plasma renin activity; VMA=Vanillylmandelic acid; IVP=Intravenous pyelogram.

frequently seen in older patients, usually with evidence of diffuse arteriosclerotic disease. Fibromuscular disease is more common in young patients, predominantly women. The hypertension is usually of recent onset. The family history is often negative; an abdominal bruit is present in 50% to 60% of patients with renovascular hypertension. Hypokalemia is seen in 20% of patients and reflects secondary hyperaldosteronism.

Random PRA measurement is of little value in identifying renovascular hypertension. Only 50% to 60% of patients with renovascular hypertension have elevated peripheral plasma renin activity. Basal PRA levels overlap substantially between patients with essential hypertension and those with renal artery stenosis. The stimulated PRA has been used as a screening test by several investigators. This test is performed by sodium restriction (10 mEq sodium for 3 days) plus 2-4 hrs of upright posture, or the simpler intravenous furosemide test (40 mg IV followed by 0.5 hr of upright posture on an unrestricted diet). A PRA level above 10 ng/mL/hr is suggestive of surgically correctable renovascular hypertension. The stimulated PRA test does, however, have a high incidence of false-positive results.

Rapid-sequence "hypertensive" intravenous pyelography (IVP) is used to assess renal morphology and renal blood flow, in evaluating for renovascular hypertension. This technique, first introduced by Maxwell and colleagues[30] in 1964, is performed by injecting an opaque radiocontrast medium; films are then taken at 20 seconds and at 1, 2, 3, 4, 5, 10, 15 and 25 min after the injection. Findings suggestive of obstruction of the main renal artery are: (1) delayed appearance of the opaque medium in the calyces of the involved kidney; (2) increased density of delayed excretion of the contrast medium in the delay films; (3) a decreased pole-to-pole diameter of the kidney (disparity of renal size >1.5 cm); and (4) ureteral notching from enlarged collateral vessels, which is a very important sign of functional stenosis. The IVP has a sensitivity and specificity of 85% to 90%; these are significantly decreased if segmental or bilateral disease is present. In addition, in most centers, rapid-sequence IVPs yield a 15% false-positive rate and a 20% to 25% false-negative rate. The National Heart, Lung, and Blood Institute's cooperative study on renovascular hypertension clearly indicates that rapid-sequence IVP is not helpful in predicting the prognosis from surgery in patients with renal artery stenosis; 40% to 85% of patients with a normal IVP respond favorably to surgery. Thus, rapid-sequence IVP is no longer routinely used in many centers and should only be used when no other test is available.

Digital subtraction angiography (DSA) is a safe and informative procedure. It involves injecting contrast material into the brachiocephalic vein or superior vena cava, or directly into the renal arteries. The image is then digitized by a computer to remove overlying bone, soft tissue, and gas shadows. Digital subtraction angiography does require patient cooperation to minimize motion artifact. It has limited spatial resolution, and renal vessels may be obscured by overlapping mesenteric vessels. Finally images may be nondiagnostic in patients with impaired renal and cardiac function. Overall, DSA has a sensitivity and specificity of 87.6% and 89.5%, respectively, but 7.4% of all renal DSAs are uninterpretable. In experienced centers, DSA may replace rapid-sequence IVP as the initial screening test for renovascular hypertension.

Two pharmacologic tests, the saralasin test and the captopril test, are used to screen for renovascular hypertension. Saralasin is an angiotensin II antagonist with weak agonist properties. At high levels of circulating angiotensin II, saralasin competitively inhibits the binding of angiotensin II to the vascular receptor, diminishing arterial pressure. At low levels of circulating angiotensin II, saralasin can, because of its weak agonist properties, mildly increase arterial pressure. The saralasin infusion test was first described by Hollenberg and Williams.[31] They reported that in 70% of patients with unilateral renal disease, diastolic blood pressure decreased by at least 10 mm Hg in response to this test. Pooling of published data on the test yields an 86% true-positive (determined by improvement or cure 6 months after surgery) and a 14% false-positive rate.[32,33] It is important to note that patients with bilateral renal artery stenosis do not respond to this test.

The test consists of an intravenous infusion of saralasin in 5% dextrose at a constant rate of 0.10-1.0 μg/kg/min for 45 min. A positive response is defined as a sustained decrease in diastolic pressure of at least 10 mm Hg. Plasma renin activity is also measured 30 min after the infusion, and a precipitous rise in PRA may clarify an ambiguous decrease in diastolic blood pressure. The test is most meaningful when it is done after 4 days of sodium restriction (10 mEq diet), with or without the admission of furosemide (40-80 mg). Although early reports suggested a high sensitivity and specificity of the saralasin infusion test, recent evaluations dispute these findings, and the recommendation that the test be used as a routine screening procedure has been challenged.

The captopril test was first reported by Case and Laragh,[34] who examined the responses to both intravenous saralasin and converting enzyme inhibition with teprotide in 47 untreated patients with surgically correctable renovascular hypertension. They found that an exaggerated increase in PRA was a much better indicator of surgically correctable renovascular hypertension than was an exaggerated decrease in blood pressure. The stimulated PRA value was also a much better predictor than the baseline PRA, and vigorous pretest stimulation of the renin-angiotensin system, mainly by salt restriction, diminished the discrimination of patients with renovascular hypertension from those with essential hypertension. However, these initially encouraging results have not been substantiated. In other studies, the sensitivity of the captopril test has ranged from 40% to 100%, and its specificity from 50% to 80%, with a positive predictive value of only 66%.[35–37] This test is complicated by the fact that sodium restriction by the patient, or other drugs that may inhibit renin release, can alter the results.

Captopril renography is based on the finding by Wenting et al[38] that captopril induces a reduction in ^{99m}Tc-diethylenetriamine penta-acetic acid (DTPA) uptake and delays ^{131}I-hippurate excretion. These changes are much more marked in the stenotic than in the contralateral kidney. Geyskes et al[39] reported a high incidence of these captopril-induced changes in ischemic kidneys, and concluded that the following changes could be used as criteria to identify ischemic or functionally stenotic kidneys: a decrease in DTPA uptake relative to the contralateral kidney, a delay in the time to the peak of the hippuran renogram, and a delay in hippuran washout. In this retrospective study, these criteria predicted the antihypertensive response to angioplasty with an 80% sensitivity and 100% specificity. Further studies have confirmed these findings. Sfakianakis et al,[40] and Setari et al[41] have recently reported that the criteria had a sensitivity of 91% with a specificity of 94% in a prospective study. In a recent review Davidson and Wilcox[42] reported scintigraphy with DTPA had sensitivities better than 90% and specificities around 95%. In addition, the presence of scintigraphic abnormalities induced by captopril predicted a cure or improvement in blood pressure in 15 of 18 patients. For these reasons, captopril renography would appear to be the test of choice for screening a selective population for renal artery stenosis. Magnetic resonance imaging (MRI) may soon be a useful test in this disorder. A number of recent studies have reported a sensitivity of 100% and specificity of 94%.[42] This test has only been performed on a small number of patients, however, and further studies will be needed before MRI becomes the test of choice.

Renal arteriography is performed to confirm the diagnosis of renovascular hypertension and to characterize the renal anatomy for consideration of surgery or other therapeutic procedures. Arteriography may reveal: 1) unilateral, bilateral, or multiple stenotic lesions; 2) the location of these lesions (e.g., close to the origin of the renal artery vs just before the bifurcation of the branches vs in segmental branches); 3) the cause of the renovascular hypertension (i.e., atherosclerotic; renal fibromuscular dysplasia; intimal fibroplasia or periarterial fibroplasia); or extrinsic lesions resulting in compression of the renal vasculature; 4) the size of the affected kidney and the contralateral kidney; 5) the presence of collateral vascularity in the affected kidney; and 6) the extent of arteriosclerosis in the abdominal aorta.

Although renal arteriography reveals the anatomy of a lesion, it does not indicate its surgical curability. To determine the physiologic significance of the lesion, differential renal-vein renin measurements are recommended. In a review of the literature, Marks, Maxwell, and colleagues[43,44] reported that of 286 patients with lateralizing ratios of 1:5 and 2:1 and arteriographic evidence of renal artery stenosis, 93% were cured or had significantly less severe hypertension after surgery. In this study, 126 patients with unilateral renal artery stenosis did not have lateralizing renal vein renin values, and 64 of these patients were cured or improved with surgery, leading to a false-negative rate of about 50%. More recent reports confirm these findings and yield a false-positive rate of 14% and a false-negative rate as high as 67%. The causes of nonlateralizing renal vein renin include bilateral renal artery stenosis, volume expansion, nonsimultaneous sampling of renal vein blood, assay error, and a nonsignificant renal artery lesion. To increase the sensitivity of the procedure, drugs that inhibit the secretion of renin (such as ß-adrenergic antagonists, reserpine, clonidine, and methyldopa) should be discontinued from 3 to 5 days before the study. Renin secretion can be further stimulated by a low-salt diet or administration of intravenous furosemide, hydralazine, or a converting enzyme inhibitor, which can accentuate the differences between the two sides.

Stimulation of renin release with a single dose of captopril before the test lowers the false-negative rate,[45] but the number of false-negative responses remains unacceptable. In this test, a single dose of oral captopril (25 mg or 1 mg/kg) is given 1 hr before sampling. A ratio greater than 3.0 predicts a favorable surgical outcome. The test, however, still has a false-negative rate of 40%. The frequency of false-negative results in the renal-vein renin test prompted the recent recommendations in the American Heart Association's Special Report of Office Evaluation of Hypertension.[18] This report recommended that with the advent of angioplasty, differential renal vein renin measurements are probably not necessary, and an attempt at angioplasty to increase revascularization as a diagnostic trial may be more prudent than awaiting the results of differential renal vein renin testing. As discussed earlier, captopril renography may be an even better test of functional significance, and because it is noninvasive, it can be used before arteriography.

MANAGEMENT OF RENOVASCULAR HYPERTENSION

Surgery is usually not recommended for patients with fibromuscular disease. If available, a trial of percutaneous transluminal angioplasty (PTA) is warranted, with close follow-up monitoring of blood pressure, renal function, status of the lesion by DSA, and renal size by ultrasound. We consider PTA the procedure of choice for the very young patient with multiple lesions, because the probability of recurrence elsewhere after surgery is high. In young patients, PTA is technically successful in 87% to 100% of cases. In 80% to 95% of these patients, blood pressure is reduced by PTA as effectively as by surgical revascularization.

Patients with unilateral atherosclerotic stenosis and no associated surgical risks can be treated by drugs, PTA, or surgery. The technical success rate of PTA is lower in patients with atherosclerotic disease than in those with fibromuscular disease. In nonocclusive, nonostial lesions, the success rate is 70% to 90%. Ostial lesions are more difficult to treat, and the success rate of PTA is only 20%. In view of the associated problems of drug therapy (cost, compliance, inconvenience, side effects, and possible progression of disease), we favor surgery or a single trial of PTA before surgery. In patients with diffuse atherosclerosis (particularly involving the abdominal aorta) and associated coronary, cerebrovascular, or pulmonary disease, we prefer a trial of PTA. Revascularization by PTA may be particularly beneficial in high-surgical-risk patients with compromised renal function. Angioplasty can be repeated once or twice, if necessary, in these patients.

High-risk patients with normal renal function may be managed with drugs. However, the patient should be monitored closely for progression of disease and evidence of renal failure or its sequelae. Surgery is usually reserved as a later option in these patients. The benefit rate (cure or improvement) in patients with unilateral focal lesions is about 90%; in those with bilateral, diffuse atherosclerotic lesions, it is 70% to 80%. Figure 2 summarizes a reasonable approach to the evaluation and management of renovascular hypertension. The choice of a screening test depends on the institution but captopril renography may be the test of choice in centers where it is available. With newer studies, however, MRI may replace these tests but further data is needed before it

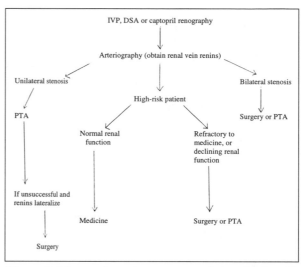

Figure 2. *Diagnosis and management of patients with renovascular hypertension. IVP=Hypertensive intravenous pyelography; DSA=Digital subtraction angiography; PTA=Percutaneous transluminal angioplasty.*

can be recommended for routine use. In patients in whom renal artery stenosis is strongly suspected, renal arteriography may be indicated, even if screening tests are negative.

PRIMARY ALDOSTERONISM

Primary aldosteronism arises from an autonomous hypersecretion of the mineralocorticoid aldosterone by an adrenal adenoma (Conn's syndrome)[46] or from bilateral adrenal hyperplasia. Adrenal adenoma is the more frequent cause. An excessive circulating aldosterone level results in increased renal sodium retention and, usually, potassium excretion. Primary aldosteronism is a rare condition, accounting for less than 1% of cases of hypertension in unselected hypertensive patients.[47] It is usually associated with mild to moderate elevations in blood pressure, but can cause severe, resistant hypertension. It is a difficult and somewhat elusive diagnosis. In its severe form, originally described by Conn, it can cause muscular weakness, polyuria, nocturia, polydipsia, tetany, paresthesia, and headache. The evaluation of primary aldosteronism is outlined in Table 6.

The usual clue to hyperaldosteronism is a low

Table 6. Evaluation of the Patient With Suspected Primary Aldosteronism

TESTS	POSITIVE RESULTS
Hypertension and hypokalemia	$K^+ < 3.5$*
Stop diuretic therapy and give K^+ supplement 1-2 weeks	↓ K^+ persists
24-hr urine K^+ excretion	>30-40 mEq/24 hr
Stimulated PRA	Suppressed
Plasma aldosterone concentration	Elevated
Saline infusion	Plasma aldosterone not suppressed
Abdominal CT scan	Bilateral adrenal hyperplasia or cortical adenoma

* Up to 10% may have a K^+ of 3.5-3.9 mEq/L. CT=Computed tomography; PRA=Plasma renin activity.

serum potassium level, usually defined as a level below 3.5 mEq/L in a patient not taking oral diuretics, or a level below 3 mEq/L in a patient receiving conventional diuretics for treatment of hypertension. In a prospective study of 80 patients with primary aldosteronism, all of whom had spontaneous hypertension, only 73% had spontaneous hypokalemia with a normal salt intake, and only 56% had provoked hypokalemia with a high salt intake for 3 days.[48] Thus, about one-fourth of patients with primary aldosteronism would be missed by using only hypokalemia testing as a screening procedure.

Primary aldosteronism is diagnosed by the finding of inappropriate potassium excretion, an elevated aldosterone level, and suppressed PRA. If a patient suspected of having primary aldosteronism is receiving diuretic therapy, the therapy should be discontinued for at least 2 weeks. Then, if the urinary potassium level is below 20 mEq/24 hr, primary aldosteronism is unlikely even though the serum potassium may be low; a nonrenal loss of potassium is more likely. The urine potassium in cases of primary aldosteronism should exceed 40 mEq/24 hr. Single measurements of PRA and plasma aldosterone are not useful for screening or diagnosis. The diagnosis should be made by assessing 24-hour urinary aldosterone secretion, which should remain at or above 8 μg/24 hr, with a urinary sodium level of 250 mEq/24 hr or more.[18,47,48] To definitively test a patient for primary aldosteronism, 24-hr urinary aldos-

terone secretion should be measured after 3 days of salt loading (approximately 12 g/day).[47,48] Nonsuppressibility of urinary aldosterone levels confirms the diagnosis.

The PRA should also be determined because very high levels of plasma renin can lead to secondary aldosteronsim, which would not be suppressed by sodium loading. An alternative to oral sodium loading is sodium infusion.[49,50] In this procedure plasma aldosterone is measured from venous blood at 8:00 AM, before the infusion of 2 L of normal saline solution over 4 hrs; plasma aldosterone is again measured at noon. Patients must discontinue antihypertensive drug therapy for 2 weeks before this study. It should not be performed in patients with CHF, renal failure, or a history of acute myocardial infarction or stroke in the preceding 6 months. In a study of normal persons, the aldosterone level before infusion of saline solution averaged 30.5 ± 1.1 ng/dL; this level was reduced after saline infusion to 3.4 ± 0.1 ng/dL. In patients with primary aldosteronism the mean aldosterone level at baseline was higher, at 60.9 ± 8.8 ng/dL. Because the baseline aldosterone levels overlapped with values of normal subjects, the test was not useful for identifying patients with primary aldosteronism. After the infusion of saline solution, however, patients with primary aldosteronism had a mean aldosterone value of 36.3 ± 4.2 ng/dL, with no overlap between the 2 groups.

Once primary aldosteronism is diagnosed, it is important to differentiate between a solitary adrenocortical adenoma and bilateral adrenal hyperplasia as the cause. The former is present in 60% to 85% of cases and is surgically curable. Several techniques are available for making this diagnosis. Computed tomographic (CT) scanning can identify adrenal tumors larger than 1.0 cm in diameter and is the most useful test.[51] Patients with bilateral hyperplasia usually have slightly enlarged or normal-appearing glands. Scintigraphic scans with [125]I-19-indocholesterol are no longer used for diagnostic evaluation.

Another approach is direct adrenal-vein sampling via percutaneous catheterization to measure venous aldosterone levels.[52] This method of localizing an adenoma is accurate in more than 90% of cases. Elevated values with less than a twofold difference between the right and left veins suggest bilateral hyperplasia; aldosterone-producing adenomas generally result in a tenfold difference between the sides. In patients with possible primary aldosteronism, abdominal CT scanning should first be performed. If the results are inconclusive, adrenal venous sampling for aldosterone may be indicated.

PHEOCHROMOCYTOMA

Pheochromocytoma should be suspected in a patient, especially a young patient, who has a history of paroxysms of hypertension and other symptoms. The most common symptoms (in addition to labile hypertension) are paroxysms of tachycardia, headaches, palpitations, sweating, and pallor. Other symptoms include medically refractory hypertension that may at times be accelerated, weight loss, abnormal carbohydrate metabolism, and a pressor response to the induction of anesthesia or antihypertensive treatment. The most common screening test for pheochromocytoma is a 24-hour urinalysis for the excretion of vanillylmandelic acid (VMA) or metanephrines, the latter being more reliable.[53,54] In most laboratories, a total metanephrine level above 1.3 mg/24 hr or a VMA level above 7 mg/24 hr is abnormal. Free catechols can also be measured in the urine, although this measurement is somewhat less reliable. Normal values in most

laboratories are 100-150 μg/24 hr. The false-positive rate of the assay increases with the co-administration of many antihypertensive drugs (Table 7) or with any endogenous stimulation of the sympathoadrenal system.[55,56]

An adjunct to measurement of 24-hr urinary VMA, metanephrines, or free catechol excretion, and perhaps a more reliable test, is measurement of plasma catecholamine levels.[56] This test has recently become more widely available and is not hindered by artifacts caused by interference from drugs and angiographic contrast material, or from difficulty in 24-hr urine collections. To draw plasma catechol samples, the patient must be resting and venipuncture avoided for at least 30 min. In patients with pheochromocytoma, plasma catechols are usually elevated to more than 2,000 pg/mL. Urinary catecholamine, VMA, and metanephrine, and plasma catecholamine levels may overlap with normal values. Therefore, other pharmacologic tests have been devised: the clonidine suppression test[57,58] and the

---

Table 7. Substances Interfering With Assays for Catecholamines/Metabolites

Free catecholamines

    Increase: methyldopa, L-dopa, tetracyclines, quinidine, isoproterenol, theophylline

Metanephrines

    Increase: chlorpromazine, monoamine oxidase inhibitors

    Decrease: x-ray contrast media containing methylglucamine (e.g., Renografin, Renovist, Hypaque)

Vanillylmandelic acid (VMA)

    Increase: nalidixic acid, anileridine, nitroglycerin (slight)

    Decrease: monoamine oxidase inhibitors, clofibrate

From Ram CVS, Engelman K. Pheochromocytoma: Recognition and management. In: Harvey WP, et al (eds). *Current Problems in Cardiology*. Chicago: Year Book Medical Publishers; 1979;80:23. With permission.

glucagon stimulation test. In patients whose plasma catechol levels are 500-2,000 pg/mL, the failure of 0.3 mg of clonidine given orally, or of a 25-mg bolus of phentolamine, to suppress catechols by 50% after 3 hrs is a strong indication of the presence of pheochromocytoma.[18,57,58] In the glucagon stimulation test,[18,58] glucagon is administered intravenously in a dose of 1 mg to stimulate secretion of catecholamines by the tumor. An increase in plasma catechol levels to more than 2,000 g/L suggests pheochromocytoma. Care must be taken in administering these pharmacologic tests because they can cause a hypertensive crisis. Phentolamine should be immediately available to counteract this event.

Once a diagnosis of pheochromocytoma is suspected, the tumor should be localized by adrenal CT scanning. The tumor can be localized by this method in 90% of cases.[59] The 10% of pheochromocytomas that are less than 1 cm in diameter (below the resolving power of CT) can be localized using ^{131}I-meta-iodobenzylguanide scanning.[60] False-negative results have been reported for both of these scans, and in a patient who is strongly suspected of having a pheochromocytoma, careful follow-up is indicated. In some cases, selective arteriography with differential venous catheterization and measurements of regional catecholamines may be useful in localizing the tumor when all other tests are negative but the condition is strongly suspected.

Successful treatment for pheochromocytoma requires considerable expertise and should be performed in a center familiar with this disease. Surgical treatment is curative and should be performed in all patients for whom surgery is not contraindicated. Preoperatively, α-adrenergic blockade should be established for at least 1 week prior to surgery. This can be accomplished with either phenoxybenzamine (10-20 mg twice daily) or prazosin (1 to 2 mg 2 to 3 times a day). Once α-blockade is established ß-adrenergic blockade should be started. It is important to remember that it is dangerous to start ß-blockade prior to established α-adrenergic blockade. Labatelol, a mix of α- and ß-blockade, has been used in some patients but has had limited use. Operative mortality is low

(0% to 3%) in centers with a good experience in this procedure. If surgery is not possible ^{131}I-metaiodobenzylguanidine (MIBG) has been used to cause partial regression but most patients relapse in 2 years. Prolonged treatment with α- and ß-blockers can control symptoms for many years and ß-blockade appears to block the catecholamine cardiomyopathy.

CUSHING'S SYNDROME

Cushing's syndrome is produced by an excess of glucocorticoid secretion by adrenal adenoma, carcinoma, or bilateral hyperplasia. Bilateral hyperplasia is often the result of an ACTH-secreting pituitary adenoma or extrapituitary neoplasm (e.g., lung carcinoma). Hypertension is seen in patients with Cushing's syndrome. The pathogenesis of this hypertension is unclear. Glucocorticoid increases hepatic angiotensinogen production, and may increase plasma angiotensin production. Further, there is evidence of increased vascular sensitivity to vasoconstrictor hormones in affected patients. The salt retaining effect of high glucocorticoid levels may also contribute to the development of hypertension. Only patients who have clinical stigmata of Cushing's syndrome, such as truncal obesity, buffalo hump, moon facies, and violaceous striae should be evaluated for this form of hypertension. Treatment is primarily surgical but prior to surgery, pharmacologic treatment with metyrapone, aminoglutethimide, or trilostane for a few weeks is indicated.

A 24-hr urine cortisol excretion assay is a useful screening test for Cushing's syndrome. A more simple alternative is the overnight dexamethasone suppression test, in which 1 mg of dexamethoasone is given at midnight, with the plasma cortisol measured 8 hrs later. Failure of suppression of cortisol (>5 μg/dL) warrants further investigation (Table 8). The next step is the more prolonged dexamethasone suppression test, which involves administration of dexamethasone at 0.5 mg every 6 hrs for 2 days, followed by 2 mg every 6 hrs for 2 more days. Urinary 17-hydroxycorticoid excretion should be measured on the second day of each dose. In patients with Cushing's syndrome, urinary 17-hydroxycorticoid levels are not suppressed

Table 8. Evaluation of the Patient With Suspected Cushing's Syndrome

TEST	RESULTS	CONDITIONS
Overnight dexamethasone suppression: 1 mg at midnight; 8 AM plasma cortisol measurement	>5 μg/dL	Suspected Cushing's syndrome
Standard dexamethasone test		
a) 0.5 mg q6h X 2 days (day 1-2)	≤ 3 mg/24 hr	Normal response
24-hr urine 17-OH corticoid	≥ 3 mg/24 hr	Cushing's syndrome
b) 2 mg q6h X 2 days (day 3-4)	<50% control	Pituitary ACTH excess
24-hr urine 17-OH corticoid day 4	>50% control	Adrenal neoplasia, or nonendocrine ACTH tumor
Metyrapone (750 mg q4h x 14 doses)		
24-hr urine 17-OH corticoid	>2 x increase	Pituitary-hypothalamic dysfunction
Plasma ACTH	<50 pg/mL	Adrenal neoplasia
	>80 pg/mL	Nonendocrine ACTH tumor or pituitary ACTH excess
24-hr urine 17-ketosteroid	>30 mg/24 hr	Adrenal carcinoma
Miscellaneous: skull x-ray, chest x-ray, abdominal or brain CT scan		

below 3 mg/day with a regimen of 0.5 mg dexamethasone every 6 hrs. If Cushing's syndrome is caused by an excess pituitary ACTH drive with bilateral adrenal hyperplasia, the urinary 17-hydroxycorticoid level is suppressed to below 50% of the control value on the second day of a regimen of 2 mg every 6 hrs. In patients whose urinary corticoid excretion is not suppressed, the ACTH level should be measured to differentiate between adrenal neoplasm and adrenal hyperplasia secondary to an ACTH-producing tumor. Patients with adrenal neoplasm have normal to low ACTH levels (<50 pg/mL). Adrenal adenoma can be distinguished from carcinoma on the basis of 24-hr urinary 17-ketosteroid production. Adrenal carcinoma is associated with high urinary 17-ketosteroid excretion (>30 mg/24 hr). Metyrapone testing is also useful in differentiating adrenal tumors from adrenal hyperplasia. Patients with adrenal tumors fail to respond to metyrapone challenge with a rise in urinary 17-hydroxycorticoids. Evaluation of pituitary function by the appropriate roentgenographic and CT scanning procedures, as well as a search for nonendocrine ACTH-producing tumors, may be indicated. In summary, in the presence of clinical stigmata of Cushing's syndrome, the overnight dexamethasone suppression test should reliably detect the disease and confirm the diagnosis. Further workup and management should probably be performed in consultation with an endocrinologist.

COARCTATION OF THE AORTA

Congenital narrowing of the aorta usually occurs beyond the origin of the left subclavian artery or distal to the ligamentum arteriosum. Takayasu's arteritis is an acquired form of coarctation that can also lead to hypertension. Clues from the history and physical examination usually lead to further evaluation for coarctation. Symptoms include headache, epistaxis, and bounding carotid pulsations. Claudication, stroke, and heart failure may occur. Cardiac findings include a thrill in the suprasternal notch, LV hypertrophy, loud A_2, S_4 gallop, and systolic flow murmur that is loudest over the left posterior thorax. A discrepancy between arm and leg blood pressure, with a delayed or absent lower-extremity pulse, is a classic finding. A chest x-ray can confirm the diagnosis by the characteristic rib notching (due to large intercostal collaterals) as well as the "figure 3" sign of the descending aorta.[61] The diagnosis is also confirmed by aortography. Patients with coarctation of the aorta have other, associated cardiac lesions; a bicuspid aortic valve is seen in up to one-third of adolescent and adult patients with coarctation. Treatment is surgical. Depending on the length of the preoperative period, patients only have presistent elevations in blood pressure due to permanent changes in peripheral vascular resistance. There is also an incidence of recurrence depending on surgical technique so these patients require careful follow-up postoperatively.

HYPERTENSION ASSOCIATED WITH ORAL CONTRACEPTIVES

Although blood pressure increases in most women taking oral contraceptives, frank hypertension develops in only 5% within a period of years. The incidence is 3 to 5 times higher than among those who do not use oral contraceptives. The largest increase occurs within the first year, but blood pressure continues to rise over 5 years.[62] The mechanism of oral contraceptive-related hypertension is unknown. Data indicate that plasma volume and cardiac output are increased in healthy women after several months of oral contraceptive use. This may be related to the sodium-retentive effects of estrogen and synthetic progesterone. Hepatic synthesis of angiotensinogen is also stimulated by estrogen. Thus, the rate of angiotensin production increases in the plasma.

Furthermore, sympathetic nervous-system activity may increase, as reflected by high levels of plasma dopamine-ß-hydroxylase. The hypertension is usually mild and reversible. If the blood pressure remains elevated 3 months after discontinuation of oral contraceptives, further workup and therapy should be initiated.

HYPERTENSION RELATED TO RENAL DISEASE

Hypertension can develop with chronic renal failure, renal parenchymal disease without renal insufficiency, acute glomerulonephritis, chronic pyelonephritis, hydronephrosis, or after bilateral nephrectomy. The mechanism of hypertension may be categorized, simplistically, as volume-dependent or renin-dependent. Volume-dependent hypertension is usually responsive to removal of sodium and fluid excess by diuretics or dialysis. Renin-dependent hypertension is usually aggravated by volume depletion and may be responsive to propranolol or α-methyldopa. In some cases, hypertension related to renal disease may be refractory to standard triple therapy. Captopril, minoxidil, and calcium blockers are effective agents for the treatment of refractory hypertension associated with renal insufficiency.

MISCELLANEOUS CONDITIONS

Secondary hypertension may be caused by excessive alcohol intake. A linear, progressive increase in blood pressure has been reported with increasing consumption of alcohol,[63] as has a threshold-type effect.[66] Obesity has been clearly shown to be associated with increases in blood pressure.[65,66] For a patient who is overweight, a weight-reduction program should be recommended and the blood pressure followed closely.

There are also rare endocrine causes of hypertension. Congenital adrenal hyperplasia associated with 11-hydroxylase deficiency or 17-hydroxylase deficiency is associated with hypertension. Systemic hypertension is also seen with hyperthyroidism, hyperparathyroidism, and acromegaly.

CLINICAL PRESENTATION

MALIGNANT HYPERTENSION

Because of the consequences of malignant or accelerated hypertension, it is extremely important for the clinician to recognize the patient who presents with this condition. Usually, the patient presents with a diastolic blood pressure above 120 mm Hg, but the absolute level of blood pressure does not confirm the diagnosis. Headache, often severe and pulsatile, is the most common presenting complaint.[46] The headache may be accompanied by neurologic aberrations known as hypertensive encephalopathy. These include (in addition to headache) nausea, vomiting, blurred vision ranging to transient blindness, seizures, temporary paralysis, altered mental status, and even coma. Focal neurologic deficits may occur, but usually represent other central nervous system disorders that should be rigorously ruled out.[67-69] The cause of hypertensive encephalopathy has been attributed to a breakthrough in cerebral blood flow autoregulation, resulting in forced vaso-dilatation.[68-70]

These pathophysiologic conditions also lead to a change in the retinal arteries. There is both obliteration and rupture of these vessels secondary to the increased blood flow in malignant hypertension. Funduscopic examination, which is essential in these patients, reveals cottonwool exudates, representing ischemic damage to the nerve fibers, as well as flame-shaped hemorrhages due to vessel rupture.[71,72] The increase in intracranial pressure results in papilledema, leading to blurred vision, narrowing of the visual field, transient visual loss, and central scotomas.[72]

A major consequence of malignant hypertension is renal damage, known as malignant nephrosclerosis. Pathologically this condition includes proliferative endarteritis, necrotizing arteriolitis, and a necrotizing glomerulitis.[72,73] The clinical manifestations of these changes consist of proteinuria, microscopic and occasionally gross hematuria, and oliguria progressing even to azotemia.[74] These changes may mimic an acute nephritic or vasculitic process, but are usually less severe. In rare cases a renal biopsy may be needed, especially in the patient without a history of hypertension.

Hematologic and endocrinologic abnormalities are also present. Often, a micro-angiopathic-hemolytic anemia may be present due to changes in the small arterioles. This anemia is often masked initially by hemoconcentration, but becomes apparent once the patient is properly hydrated. Abnormalities of the coagulation system include thrombocytopenia, increased fibrin degradation products, and increases in the concentrations of fibrinogen and factor VIII.[75]

The endocrinologic changes in malignant hypertension are due to activation of the renin-angiotensin-aldosterone system in these patients. This results in hypokalemia and alkalosis, which may persist after the blood pressure has been corrected.[76,77] An abnormal stimulation of antidiuretic hormone, contributing to the volume-depleted state, has also been reported.[78]

Cardiovascular complications are not common, but acute left ventricular decompensation can occur. This is manifested by an enlarged cardiac silhouette on chest x-ray, elevated jugular venous distention, pulmonary congestion on physical examination and on the chest x-ray, and an S_3 gallop. There may also be a murmur of aortic insufficiency due to the elevated blood pressure. If an aortic insufficiency murmur is heard, the possibility of an acute aortic dissection must be considered, because it can be precipitated by extreme elevations of blood pressure.

"BENIGN" HYPERTENSION

Few patients who present with hypertension have accelerated hypertension. Most patients are asymptomatic and their chief complaint is that they were noted to have an elevated blood pressure that was measured for an unrelated reason. The most common complaint of symptomatic patients is headache, often described as an early morning, frontal headache. Although headache is a common complaint in normotensive patients, a number of studies demonstrate that it is more prevalent in patients with hypertension.[79–81] The relationship to migraine headaches is less clear, but in at least 2 studies the incidence of migraine was slightly greater in patients with elevated blood pressures,[82,83] although this has not been confirmed in other series.[81] Two other presenting complaints that are occasionally encountered are dizziness and epistaxis. Whether these complaints are really more common in hypertensive patients is not clear;[84,85] one study suggests that epistaxis is not more frequent in hypertensive patients, although it may be more severe.[85] It is clear that hypertension is usually diagnosed by blood pressure screening of asymptomatic patients, emphasizing the need for accurate and frequent measurement of blood pressure.

CONSEQUENCES OF HYPERTENSION

To fully appreciate the natural history of essential hypertension it is important to examine the statistics before the advent of therapy for this condition, around 1950. In many studies conducted between 1913 and 1946,[86–88] one-third to two-thirds of untreated patients died of heart disease, 15% to 40% died of stroke, 5% to 15% died of uremia, and 10% to 30% died of intercurrent disease. Recently, these natural history studies have been extended to isolated systolic hypertension.[89] In a 20-year study of 2,767 patients, 80% of those with isolated systolic hypertension progressed to definite hypertension as compared with 45% of the normotensive patients. Also, after adjustment for other risk factors, patients with isolated systolic hypertension had an increased risk (odds ratio, 1.39) of development of cardiovascular disease.

Another factor which could affect the natural history of hypertension is the method used to detect the elevation in blood pressure. This has to do with the use of ambulatory blood pressure monitoring to detect hypertension. In a recent report, the National High Blood Pressure Education Program Coordinating Committee[90] has reported on ambulatory blood pressure use and concluded it is useful in a number of instances (Table 9). Most importantly, a number

of small trials have reported that ambulatory monitoring may be more predictive of cardiovascular disease than casual blood pressure. To actually recommend the use of ambulatory blood pressure in all patients is premature but it can be useful in selected patients as indicated in Table 9.

CORONARY ARTERY DISEASE

One of the major consequences of hypertension is an increased incidence of atherosclerosis, usually manifest as coronary artery disease (CAD). The Framingham Study[91,92] showed a striking increase in the incidence of CAD in hypertensive patients, along with smaller increases in claudication, atheroembolic stroke, and congestive failure. The individual risk of cardiovascular disease depends on the associated risk factors present in any given patient. Data from the Framingham Study also reveal the additive risks in hypertensive patients of an elevated cholesterol level, glucose intolerance, cigarette smoking, and LV hypertrophy on the ECG. The cause of this increased risk is not clear, but there appears to be a slight positive correlation between blood pressure and cholesterol level, which may in part explain the findings. Data similar to those

---

Table 9. Clinical Problems in Which Noninvasive Ambulatory Blood Pressure Monitoring is Useful

Borderline hypertension with target organ damage

Evaluation of drug resistance

Episodic hypertension

"Office" or "white-coat" hypertension*

Exclusion of placebo reactors when determining efficacy of antihypertensive drug therapy in controlled clinical trials

*Patients with persistently elevated blood pressures ($\geq$ 140/90 mm Hg) during standardized office visits and normal self-measurements elsewhere.

in the Framingham Study were reported in the Australian Risk Prevalence Study,[93] which revealed a positive correlation between blood pressure and cholesterol levels.

The positive correlation between hypertension and cardiovascular disease brings up one of the more controversial aspects in the treatment of mild to moderate hypertension. As first noted in the Multiple Risk Factor Intervention Trial[94] and, subsequently, in numerous other trials[95,96] patients who were treated for mild to moderate hypertension did not have a drop in cardiovascular events. In the 30% of hypertensive patients who had an abnormal ECG upon entry into the MRFIT trial, cardiovascular and overall mortality were higher in the special-care group than in the usual-care group. Special care included a thiazide diuretic, and this treatment resulted in an increase in plasma LDL levels. This alteration of the lipid profile may explain the results, but this possibility is highly controversial as discussed below.

Although a formal trial has not been conducted, a number of groups have performed meta-analyses of the major trials of mild to moderate hypertension. The first of these[97,98] created regression lines of blood pressure and rates of either stroke or coronary heart disease (CHD). From this they were able to predict that a 5-6 mm Hg drop in diastolic blood pressure should yield a 35 to 40% decrease in stroke and a 20 to 25% decrease in heart disease. When they looked at the actual data from 14 unconfounded clinical trials, stroke was reduced by 42% as predicted, but coronary disease was only reduced by 14%, about half of the expected reduction. This resulted in a number of experts questioning if we were appropriately treating hypertension.

Recently, these conclusions have been questioned. When investigators looked at mortality rates after 10.5 years after the MRFIT trial,[99] they found that mortality rates were lower by 10.6% in the special intervention group and CHD rates were 7.7% lower. This decrease in mortality was primarily due to a 24% reduction in the death rate from acute MI. Also, the TOHMS trial final results[100] found a significant decrease in cardiovascular events and an improved quality of life in patients on drug therapy over an average of 4.4 years of follow-up. In a more recent meta-analyses[101] which included 3 clinical trials completed since the initial analysis in 1990, the authors found a similar reduction of 5-6 mm Hg in usual diastolic blood pressure but the reduction in risk for coronary disease rose from 14% to 16%. The authors conclude that as more data accumulates, the benefit of drug therapy may continue to increase to equal the 20% to 25% predicted risk reduction. Based on these findings JNCV[1] now states that ß-blockers or diuretics are the preferred initial drugs because they have been demonstrated to reduce morbidity and mortality in large clinical trials while other agents have not (see below for details). Obviously, meta-analysis cannot take the place of carefully designed prospective clinical trials and these are currently being conducted.

HYPERTENSIVE HEART DISEASE

Cardiac hypertrophy is another major cardiovascular consequence of hypertension. Classically, cardiac involvement in hypertension is separated into three stages: no clinical evidence of involvement (stage I), left atrial enlargement (stage II), and LV hypertrophy (stage III).[102,103] Only in the final stage, when hypertrophy is present, is cardiac function impaired. These stages were originally determined using ECG criteria, but with the use of echocardiography, they may have to be altered.

Numerous studies, using ECG criteria, show an increased incidence of LV hypertrophy in patients with essential hypertension.[104–106] In the Framingham population, ECG evidence of LV hypertrophy developed in 50% of patients with a systolic blood pressure above 180 mm Hg.[106] Pathologic series demonstrate that the ECG has a sensitivity of 40% to 50% for the detection of LV hypertrophy, as compared with necropsy.[19,20,107] When M-mode echocardiography is compared to true LV weight, however, the sensitivity is 90% to 98%.[21,24]

Risk-factor analysis of the Framingham data shows a great increase in the prevalence of cardiac disease among patients with ECG evidence of LV hypertrophy.[91,92,108] Recent data show that echocardiographic evidence of LV hypertrophy also identifies patients at a higher risk for cardiovascular morbid events.[22] In a small study with an average follow-up of only 5 years, 7 cardiovascular morbid events were observed in 29 hypertensive patients with LV hypertrophy determined by M-mode echocardiography, and 7 events were observed in 111 patients without LV hypertrophy. Although the numbers are small, these data may indicate that echocardiography is needed to more accurately determine an individual patient's cardiovascular risk. In the early stages of LV hypertrophy, increases in LV mass result in a decrease in LV distensibility and a resultant abnormal filling pattern during both passive and active filling.[106,109] Early on, there may also be an increase in cardiac output.[110,111] The abnormal diastolic filling has important clinical implications. Topol et al,[112] in a study of elderly hypertensive patients, reported that among patients with concentric hypertrophy who presented with heart failure, those treated with ß-blockers or calcium-channel blockers did better than those treated with diuretics and vasodilators. It is hypothesized that in patients with LV hypertrophy, a small LV chamber, and normal LV systolic function, volume depletion results in further compromise of the LV cavity and, potentially, a severe hypotensive response. Ultimately, hypertension results in cardiac failure. Hypertension is the leading cause of CHF in the United States.[113] The first studies of antihypertensive treatment, the VA Cooperative Trials,[79,114] demonstrated that treatment can prevent heart failure and thus reduce mortality.

NEUROLOGIC COMPLICATIONS

The Framingham data demonstrate that hypertension is a greater risk factor for cerebral damage than for cardiovascular or renal disease. This typically presents in 3 forms: intraparenchymal hemorrhage, large-vessel atherosclerosis presenting as ischemic strokes and small-vessel disease, and lacunar infarction. The incidence of intraparenchymal hemorrhage has decreased over the past few decades, but this event still accounts for 10% to 14% of strokes.[115,116] This condition has numerous causes, but there is a strong relationship with

hypertension.[116] Most bleeding episodes occur in the cerebral hemispheres, and most patients have associated subarachnoid bleeding.

Ischemic stroke is the most common neurologic complication of hypertension. Control of hypertension has played a major role in the decline in the incidence of stroke in the past 2 decades.[116,117] As discussed above, a number of meta-analyses of large clinical trials have demonstrated a strong decrease in the incidence of stroke of about 40%.[97,98,101] This is what is predicted for the average 5-6 mm Hg decrease in usual diastolic blood pressure and is a major compelling reason to control blood pressure. The prevention of stroke has also been demonstrated in 3 trials of elderly patients.[117–119] This is also true of isolated systolic hypertension where risk of stroke was reduced by 36%.[118]

Not only is the incidence of stroke increased in hypertension, but there is an increased incidence of reversible ischemic attacks. The Italian Multicenter Study[120] revealed a positive correlation between systolic blood pressure and the incidence of transient ischemic attacks (TIAs), but no correlation with diastolic blood pressure. This study also found a positive correlation between systolic blood pressure and the presence of cerebral atherosclerosis. Similar data were reported in the Cooperative Study of Focal Cerebral Ischemia in Young Adults.[121,122] This confirmed the prominent role of hypertension as a risk factor for stroke or TIA along with cardiac disease, oral contraceptives, elevated serum lipids, and smoking.

Small lacunar infarcts are a common autopsy finding in elderly hypertensive patients.[123,124] These infarcts are caused by occlusion of the small penetrating arteries of the circle of Willis. They present as a variety of clinical syndromes; before the advent of antihypertensive therapy, multiple lacunae often resulted in pseudobulbar palsy with emotional instability, a slowed abulic state, and bilateral pyramidal signs.

RENAL DISEASE

Hypertension is one of the most common causes of renal insufficiency and, subsequently, of the need for dialysis.[125] There is also evidence for racial differences in the incidence of end-stage renal disease.[126] In their study, Rostand and colleagues found that the rate of referral for dialysis was 4.2 times greater in blacks than whites. This could reflect a greater predisposition to develop renal disease or a lack of adequate treatment in this group.

The pathology of the renal disease varies. In malignant hypertension the pathology is characterized by fibrinoid necrosis, a process termed arteriolar nephrosclerosis. In essential hypertension, accelerated atherosclerosis of the small- and medium-resistance vessels results in progressive nephrosclerosis. This leads to proteinuria, a loss in renal concentrating ability, and a decrease in creatinine clearance.[127,128] There is also evidence that renal vasoconstriction occurs early in essential hypertension[129] and could increase the progression to end-stage renal disease. The course of the disease is difficult to follow because renal damage by itself can cause hypertension. There is evidence, however, that treatment of blood pressure protects the kidneys.[130]

Special mention should be made of the case of renal function in patients with diabetic nephropathy and proteinuria (urinary protein excretion ≥ 500 mg/day). Two recent studies[131–133] have demonstrated that treatment with angiotensin converting enzyme inhibitors protects against the deterioration in renal function. Clearly, in any diabetic patient with hypertension, strong consideration should be given to treatment with an angiotensin-converting enzyme inhibitor.

OTHER COMPLICATIONS

In the hypertensive patient, accelerated atherosclerosis may result in an increase in peripheral vascular disease.[91] Hypertension is the most important predisposing factor for aortic dissection,[134,135] reported to be present in 70% to 90% of patients with dissections. It apparently occurs more often in distal dissections than in proximal dissections.[136] Aortic aneurysms are also reported to occur more frequently in hypertensive patients than in normotensive persons, probably as a result of the greater frequency of atherosclerosis.[137]

MANAGEMENT OF ESSENTIAL HYPERTENSION

The specific treatment of secondary hypertension has been discussed above and this section will be limited to the treatment of essential hypertension. The Joint National Committee (JNC V)[1] recommends treatment of all patients with a confirmed blood pressure above 140/90 (Table 1) to maintain an arterial blood pressure of 140/90 mm Hg or below. Patients with mild hypertension (diastolic blood pressure 90-99 mm Hg) should have a repeat measurement after 2 months. Patients with high normal blood pressures (diastolic blood pressure 85-89 mm Hg) should be rechecked at yearly intervals. It is important to note that 1 retrospective study showed an increase in cardiac mortality in patients whose mean treated diastolic blood pressure was under 85 mm Hg.[138] More recent data has not supported this finding. In the recent meta-analysis[97,98,101,139] no increase in coronary disease was noted as the blood pressure was lowered below 85 mm Hg. In contrast, Farnett et al[140] studied 13 clinical studies and found a consistent J-shaped relationship between cardiac events and a diastolic blood pressure below 85 mm Hg. More data is obviously needed before a definitive answer can be obtained. At the present time the issue of a J-curve relationship between lowering blood pressure and cardiac events remains controversial.

Again, special mention should be made concerning the treatment of hypertension in the elderly population. A number of recent studies have convincingly shown that this group of patients warrant treatment. In the report on the results of the trial of isolated systolic hypertension in the elderly,[118] which was a trial of over 4,000 patients with systolic blood pressures ranging from 160-219 mm Hg, low-dose diuretic therapy (chlorthalidone), with atenolol added if needed, for blood pressure control, led to a 36% reduction in the incidence of total strokes over a 5-year period. It is clear from this study that isolated systolic hypertension in the elderly patient is easily treatable, with considerable benefit to the patient. Similar results were reported in the

Swedish trial in older patients with hypertension.[119] These investigators found a significant decrease in stroke and mortality up to an age of 84 years with diuretic and ß-blocker therapy. The Medical Research Council trial of treatment of older adults[141] also found a significant reduction in stroke, coronary events and all cardiovascular events in patients treated with a diuretic (hydrochlorothiazide or amiloride). Interestingly, no effect was seen in the ß-blocker group. Based on the above data, JCN V[1] has proposed an algorithm for the treatment of hypertension (Fig. 3).

NONPHARMACOLOGIC THERAPY

A number of lifestyle modifications have been recommended for treatment of mild hypertension. These include:

1. Dietary Modifications. The most consistent approach is dietary changes which include reduced sodium and caloric intake. There is a clear relationship between body weight, blood pressure, and the development of hypertension.[65,142] A reasonable goal is to be within 15% of desirable weight. Although numerous studies show that weight reduction can result in a reliable reduction in blood pressure, the likelihood of a patient achieving this goal and maintaining the reduced body weight is small.[143] A moderate reduction in dietary sodium is also recommended for all hypertensive patients. It is not clear, however, whether this actually results in a substantial reduction in blood pressure.[144–146] Studies have shown that at best, a diet containing 80-157 mmol Na+/24 hr resulted in only a 6 mm Hg mean reduction in systolic blood pressure. Much of the daily sodium intake comes from prepared foods, so proper dietary counseling is important. Sodium restriction is probably best used as an adjunct to medical therapy. Studies reported that a large percentage of patients could reduce or discontinue their medications with moderate sodium restriction.[48,147]

A number of recent studies[148–151] have investigated the effects of combining weight and sodium reduction. They again demonstrated a clear, although modest, reduction in blood

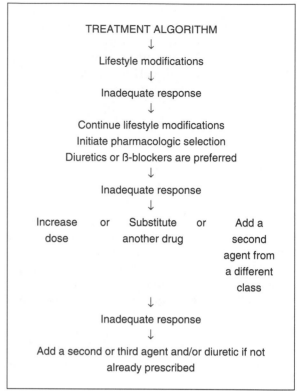

Figure 3. *Algorithm for treatment of hypertension based on JCN V recommendations.*[1]

pressure ranging from 2-7 mm Hg with these therapeutic modalities. Patients should limit sodium intake to less than 100 mMole per day (<2.3 g of sodium or <6 g of sodium chloride). The restriction of sodium is also important since the recent Intersalt trial[152] demonstrated a significant relationship between sodium excretion and blood pressure with populations with low sodium excretion having low mean blood pressures.

2. Restriction of Alcohol. Excessive alcohol intake can increase blood pressure both acutely and chronically.[153,154] A recent large study of 58,218 US female nurses also demonstrated that an alcohol intake greater than 20 g/day had an increased risk of hypertension and the risk increases progressively.[155]

3. Other. The Joint National Committee has also recommended that patients participate in regular exercise, eat a diet high in fiber and low in saturated fat, and avoid tobacco use. Regular exercise has been shown in some studies to lower blood pressure, and a combination of these measures produces an overall reduction in cardiovascular risk.[156,157] The recommendations also urge patients to stop smoking and reduce saturated fat and cholesterol intake to reduce overall cardiovascular risk.

PHARMACOLOGIC THERAPY

The principle of pharmacologic therapy is to inhibit one or several of the factors that can elevate blood pressure, including sodium and volume status, vascular tone, the renin-angiotensin system, and the sympathetic nervous system. In recent years 2 studies have appeared,[148,158] which have investigated the effects of monotherapy in a wide variety of patients. In brief, they found all agents, including diuretics, ß-blockers, α_1-antagonists, calcium blockers, and angiotensin-converting enzyme inhibitors, to be effective. Although some differences were found between patients in quality of life and side effects, no consistent large effects could be found. Based on this type of data and the fact that only diuretics and ß-blockers have been shown to decrease morbidity and mortality from stroke or cardiovascular disease, the JNC V[1] now recommends that first line pharmacologic therapy be either a diuretic or ß-blocker (Fig. 2). If these are not effective then an agent from a different class can be used or added. Table 10 lists commonly used antihypertensive drugs and their effects on serum lipids. Each physician should become familiar with a few agents in each class and use them when appropriate. For individual patients, a particular class may be more effective (Table 11), but this is a general rule and may not be true for each individual patient. Another deciding factor concerning which agent to institute therapy with is the effect on coexisting disease (Table 12).

A particularly controversial topic is the magnitude and importance of the effect of antihypertensive drugs on serum lipids (Table 13). As discussed above, early trials primarily utilizing diuretics and ß-blockers failed to demonstrate the expected benefit on CAD.[97,95,139,159] More recent analyses[101] have

not completely supported this, so avoidance of these agents in an attempt to avoid their effects on lipids cannot be recommended. In a patient who has clearly elevated lipids, lowering serum cholesterol will reduce the frequency of coronary artery events[160–162] and this must be considered in the individual patient taking into full account the increased cost of ACE inhibitors, calcium-channel blockers, or α-blockers, which do not adversely affect the serum lipid profile. Of course, the newer agents avoid problems such as hypokalemia and hyperglycemia seen with diuretics and ß-blockers, but their cost is considerably higher.

In the end, the choice of initial therapy for any individual patient must be tailored for that patient. Considerations such as long-term cost and coexisting diseases must be taken into account. Overall, the goal should be normalization of blood pressure using the agent that is best suited for that patient.

The newest class of antihypertensive drugs are the Angiotensin-II receptor blockers. These agents block the deleterious effects associated with Angiotensin-II (i.e., vasoconstriction, sympathetic activation, aldosterone secretion). Losartan represents the first such agent available in the U.S. It is given once a day, is highly efficient in treating hypertension,[162a] and its adverse effects from treatment are comparable to placebo. Unlike ACE inhibitors, it does not cause cough.

INSULIN RESISTANCE

There is an association between hypertension and obesity with impaired glucose tolerance in humans.[65,163] Recent studies showed that insulin resistance is a feature of untreated, early hypertension. Swislocki et al[164] examined 16 normal and 14 untreated hypertensive patients, and measured their plasma glucose and insulin concentrations during the last 30 minutes of a 180-min infusion of somatostatin, insulin, and glucose. Compared with normal controls, the men with untreated hypertension had higher plasma glucose and insulin concentrations after the oral challenge, thus reconfirming the earlier observation that patients with hypertension are insulin resistant, hyperglycemic, and hyperinsulinemic. Pollare et al[165] demonstrated similar results: they studied

Table 10. Types and Examples of Antihypertensive Drugs

AGENT	DOSE RANGE (MG/DAY)	FREQUENCY OF ADMINISTRATION (TIMES/DAY)	EFFECT ON SERUM LIPIDS	NOTES
Diuretics			↑LDL, ↓HDL, ↑TC	*Thiazide diuretics* may cause hypokalemia,
Chlorothiazide	500-1,000	1-2		hyponatremia, meta-
Chlorthalidone	12.5-50	1-2		bolic alkalosis,
Hydrochlorothiazide (HCTZ)	12.5-100	1-2		glucose intolerance,
Indapamide	1.25-5.0	1		lipid abn., hypercal-
Furosemide	20-600	1-2		cemia, hyperurecemia.
Bumetanide	0.5-2.0	1		*Loop diuretics*—hypo-
Amiloride	5-10	1		kalemia, hyponatremia
Spironolactone	25-100	1-3		blood dyscrasias,
Metolazone (Zaroxolyn)	2.5-5.0	1		otoxicity. *Amiloride and spironolactone* are potassium sparing
Combination Diuretics			↑LDL, ↓HDL, ↑TC	
HCTZ and amiloride	1-2 tabs/day	1		Each tablet contains HCTZ 50 mg, amiloride 5 mg
HCTZ and spironolactone	2-4 tabs/day	1-2		Each tablet contains HCTZ 25 mg, sprionolactone 25 mg
HCTZ and triamterene	1-4 caps/day	1-2		Each capsule contains HCTZ 25 mg, triamterene 50 mg
HCTZ and triamterene	1-2 tabs/day	1-2		Each tablet contains HCTZ 50 or 25 mg, triamterene 75 mg
Adrenergic Inhibitors				
Rauwolfia derivatives				
Reserpine	0.25	1	Neutral	Sedation, dry mouth,
Methyldopa	250-3,000	2-4	Mild ↓HDL	autoimmunity (methyl-dopa), impotence.
Centrally acting agents				
Clonidine	0.1-2.4	2-3	↓TC, ↑HDL	rebound ↑BP
Guanabenz	8-64	1-2	↓LDL, → or ↑HDL, ↓TC	
Guanfacine	1-3	1-2	↓TC, ↑LDL, ← or ↑HDL	
ß-Adrenergic blockers			↔ or ↑TC, ↔ or ↑LDL, ↓HDL (except for those with ISA)	
Acebutolol	200-1,200	1-2	Neutral or slight ↑HDL	Both acebutolol and
Pindolol	10-60	2	Neutral or slight ↑HDL	pindolol have ISA
Atenolol	50-100	1		*ß Blockers* may cause
Metoprolol	100-450	1-2		fatigue, impotence,
Nadolol	40-320	1		bradycardia, worsen
Propranolol	40-640	2-4		AV block, exacerbate
Timolol	20-60	2		CHF, worsen coronary vasospasm, bronchospasm
Mixed α- and ß-blockers				
Labetalol	200-2,400	2	Neutral	

continued

Table 10. Types and Examples of Antihypertensive Drugs (continued)

AGENT	DOSE RANGE (MG/DAY)	FREQUENCY OF ADMINISTRATION (TIMES/DAY)	EFFECT ON SERUM LIPIDS	NOTES
α-blockers			↔ or ↓TC, ↓LDL, ↑HDL	α Blockers may be
Prazosin	2-20	2-3		associated with first
Terazosin	1-20	1-2		dose postural
Doxazosin	1-16	1		hypotension
Vasodilators			Neutral	
Nonspecific				May cause reflex
Hydralazine	20-300	2-4		tachycardia
Minoxidil	5-100	1-2		
Converting enzyme inhibitors			Neutral	Diuretic dose should be decreased when starting ACE inhibitors.
Captopril	50-450	2-3		ACE inhibitors may
Enalapril	5-40	1-2		also be associated
Fosinopril	10-80	1-2		with cough, taste
Lisinopril	10-80	1		disturbance, rarely
Quinapril	10-80	1-2		angioneurotic edema;
Ramipril	2.5-20	1-2		may exacerbate renal
Benazepril	10-80	1-2		insufficiency. Don't use in pregnancy; rarely leukopenia
Angiotensin-II receptor blockers			Neutral	Adverse effects
Losartan	25-100	1		comparable to placebo. Well-tolerated. Use lower dose in volume depletion, liver disease
Calcium blockers			Neutral	Vasodilator side
Diltiazem	80-240	3 4		effects (dizziness,
Diltiazem CD	180-480	1		flushing, headache,
Diltiazem SR	120-360	2		palpitation) less
Nifedipine	30-120	3-4		common with slow
Nifedipine XL (GITS)	30-120	1		release, once-a-day
Nicardipine	30-90	3		calcium blocker
Verapamil	240-480	3-4		preparations.
Verapamil SR	120-480	1-2		Peripheral edema may
Felodipine	5-20	1		occur. Bradycardia,
Isradipine	5-20	2		AV block may occur
Amlodipine	5-10	1		with verapamil, diltiazem. Constipation may occur with verapamil

HDL=High-density lipoprotein; ISA=Intrinsic sympathomimetic activity; LDL=Low-density lipoprotein; TC=Total cholesterol; CHF=Congestive heart failure; SR=Sustained release; GITS=Gastrointestinal therapeutic system; once-a-day preparation.
* Effects of lipids are indicated for classes of drugs, and do not in all cases indicate studies on individual drugs within a class. Short acting nifedipine and diltiazem are not FDA approved for hypertension.

143 newly detected hypertensive patients (of whom 59% were obese), using the euglycemic insulin clamp technique. They assessed insulin sensitivity by measuring both the patients' basal

Table 11. Demographic and Pathophysiologic Determinants of Responses to Antihypertensive Drugs

FACTOR	DIURETICS	β-BLOCKERS	α-BLOCKERS	ACE INHIBITORS	CA++ANAGONISTS
Age (young/old)	More effective in older	More effective in young	Effective in both	More effective in young (?)	More effective in old (?)
Race (white/black)	More effective in black	More effective in white	Effective in both	More effective in white (?)	Effective in both
Sodium-volume	More effective	Less effective	Effective	Less effective	Effective
High renin	Less effective	More effective	Less effective	More effective	Less effective
Increased sympathetic activity	Less effective	More effective	More effective	Effective	Effective

Important: The effectiveness of the various drugs in different groups is *relative*, not absolute. For example, it has been shown recently that ACE inhibitors are effective in black as well as white persons, and that calcium antagonists are effective in young as well as elderly persons.

Modified from Dzau VJ. Evaluation of the clinical management of hypertension. *Am J Med.* 1987;82(suppl IA):36-43.

Table 12. Effects of Antihypertensive Drugs on Coexisting Diseases

DISEASE	DIURETIC	β-BLOCKER	α-BLOCKER	ACE INHIBITOR	CA++ ANTAGONIST
Angina	No effect	Beneficial	No effect	Beneficial (?)	Beneficial
CHF	Beneficial	Worsens	No effect	Beneficial	Beneficial(±) (may worsen)
Arrhythmias	May Worsen	Beneficial	No effect	No effect	Beneficial
COPD	No effect	Worsens	No effect	No effect	Beneficial (?)
Diabetes	May Worsen	May worsen	No effect	Beneficial (?)	No effect

CHF=Congestive heart failure; COPD=Chronic obstructive pulmonary disease.

Modified from Dzau VJ. Evaluation of the clinical management of hypertension. *Am J Med.* 1987;82(suppl IA):36-43.

insulin levels and the rate of glucose disposal after an intravenous glucose tolerance test. Hypertensive patients with normal body weight demonstrated insulin resistance, as indicated by an increased basal insulin level and decreased rate of glucose deposition.

These results may have implications for the treatment of hypertension. Zavaroni et al[166] recently showed that otherwise healthy persons with hyperinsulinemia and normal glucose tolerance test results have an increased risk for CAD as compared with well-matched healthy controls. Because hypertensive patients have an

increased incidence of insulin resistance, this may partly explain the higher incidence of coronary events in this group. It may also alter the treatment of hypertension. The recent report by Pollare et al[167] demonstrated that hydrochlorothiazide, as compared with captopril, had adverse effects on lipid metabolism as well as on glucose metabolism. Using the euglycemic insulin clamp technique, Pollare et al[167] found that hydrochlorothiazide significantly decreased the insulin sensitivity index after 18 weeks of treatment. Captopril had no effect. These results may help explain some of the disparity between

Table 13. Summary of Effects of Antihypertensive Drugs on Serum Lipid Profile

DRUG	TC	LDL	HDL	TRIGLYCERIDE
Thiazide diuretics	↑	↑	↔↓	↑
ß-blockers	↔↑	↔↑	↓	↑
α-blockers	↔↓	↓	↑	↔↓
Sympatholytics	↔	↓	↓	↑
ACE inhibitors	↔	↔	↔	↔
Calcium antagonists	↔	↔	↔	↔

↑=increase; ↓=decrease; ↔=no change; HDL=High-density lipoprotein; LDL=Low-density lipoprotein; TC=Total cholesterol.

Modified from Dzau J. Evaluation of the clinical management of hypertension. *Am J Med*. 1987;82(suppl IA):36-43.

Table 14. Common Drug Interactions in Antihypertensive Therapy

DRUG CLASS	ANTIHYPERTENSIVE AGENT	EFFECT
Tricyclic antidepressants	Clonidine	Attenuate antihypertensive effect
	α-methyldopa	As above
	Reserpine	As above
	Guanethidine	As above
	Bethanidine	As above
Sympathomimetics	Clonidine	Attenuate antihypertensive effect
	α-methyldopa	As above
	Guanethidine	As above
Phenothiazines	α-methyldopa	Paradoxical hypertension
	Guanethidine	Attenuate antihypertensive effect
MAO inhibitors	Guanethidine	Attenuate antihypertensive effect
	α-methyldopa	Paradoxical hypertension
	Reserpine	Paradoxical hypertension
CNS depressants	Clonidine	Increase CNS depression
	α-methyldopa	Increase CNS depression
		Barbiturates reduce α-methyldopa effect
	Reserpine	Increase CNS depression
Miscellaneous		
Digitalis	Diuretics	Hyopkalemia, digitalis toxicity
Warfarin	Thiazides	Increase prothrombin time
Pyridoxine	Hydralazine	Blocks pyridoxine effects
L-dopa	α-methyldopa	Interfere with L-dopa in treatment of Parkinson's disease
	Reserpine	As above
Anesthesia	Central sympatholytics	Hypotension
Digitalis, quinidine	Reserpine	Arrhythmias

CNS=Central nervous system; MAO=Monoamine oxidase.

Table 15. Conditions Associated With Hypertensive Crisis

Hypertensive Emergencies

   Malignant hypertension—eyegrounds reveal hemorrhages, exudates, or papilledema
   Hypertension with acute pulmonary edema
   Hypertensive encephalopathy
   CVA, including hemorrhage and infarction
   Aortic dissection
   Pheochromocytoma with severe hypertension
   Hypertension following tyramine ingestion in patients taking MAO inhibitors
   Severe toxemia or eclampsia

Urgent Conditions Associated With Hypertension

   Accelerated hypertension—eyegrounds reveal hemorrhages and exudates
   Severe hypertension in a patient with myocardial infarction or severe angina
   Occlusive stroke or transient ischemic attack in a hypertensive patient
   Renal failure or significant renal impairment in a hypertensive patient
   Marked hypertensive associated with burns, acute glomerulonephritis, or preeclampsia
   Severe hypertension in patients bleeding postoperatively
   The patient with hypertension, new cardiovascular, or neurologic symptoms
   New patient with DBP >130 mm Hg

CVA=Cerebrovascular accident; DBP=Diastolic blood pressure; MAO=Monoamine oxidase.

---

the effective control of hypertension and the lack of impact of such control on coronary disease prevalence. The mechanisms for the increased cardiovascular risk and increased insulin resistance associated with hypertension are not well understood.

TREATMENT OF REFRACTORY HYPERTENSION

In evaluating patients with treatment-resistant hypertension, one must consider the following factors:

1. Compliance. The most common cause of uncontrolled hypertension is patient non-compliance. This is frequently difficult to document. A careful and thorough history is important, with particular attention to the patient's understanding of the drug regimen and a history of drug side effects. Measurements of plasma or 24-hr urine drug concentrations, and use of pill counts, have been useful in documenting patient non-compliance.

2. Secondary Forms of Hypertension. The possibility of secondary forms of hypertension should be evaluated in all patients who require 3 to 4 agents to control their blood pressure.

3. Drug Interactions. Drug interactions that can result in attenuation of the effect of certain antihypertensives (e.g., tricyclic antidepressants with adrenergic blocking agents) should be excluded. A list of such drug interactions is shown in Table 14.

4. Inappropriate Drug Combinations. In evaluating drug combinations, it is helpful to separate antihypertensive agents into 3 broad classes: diuretics, sympatholytics, and vasodilators. Ordinarily, a second drug from the same class should not be added to a regimen because it may have little or no additional effect. For example, a patient refractory to hydro-

Table 16. Selection of Drugs for Use in Hypertensive Crises*

TYPE OF HYPERTENSIVE CRISIS	DRUG OF CHOICE (PARENTERAL)	DOSAGE (I.V.)	DRUGS TO AVOID (OR USE CAUTIOUSLY)
Hypertensive encephalopathy	Sodium Nitroprusside	0.5-10 μg/kg/min	ß-agonists
	Labetalol	20-80 mg every 5-10 min or 0.5-2 mg/min	Methyldopa
	Diazoxide	50-100 mg every 5-10 min	Clonidine
Cerebral hemorrhage	Sodium Nitroprusside	Same as above	ß-agonists
	Labetalol	Same as above	Methyldopa Clonidine
Acute pulmonary edema	Sodium Nitroprusside	Same as above	Diazoxide
	Nitroglycerin	5-200 μg/min	
	Loop Diuretic		
Aortic dissection	Sodium Nitroprusside + ß-antagonist	Same as above	Hydralazine
	Trimethaphan + ß-antagonist	0.5-5 mg/min	Diazoxide
	Labetalol	Same as above	Minoxidil
Pheochromocytoma or MAO inhibitor with tyramine	Phentolamine	5-10 mg every 5-15 min	
	Labetalol	Same as above	ß-agonists
Malignant hypertension with fundoscopic changes and/or renal compromise	Sodium Nitroprusside	Same as above	
	Labetalol	Same as above	
	Trimethaphan	Same as above	

chlorothiazide, propranolol, and α-methyldopa should be switched to hydrochlorothiazide, propranolol, and hydralazine.

5. Activation of Cardiovascular Compensatory Mechanisms. Certain drugs can activate cardiovascular compensatory mechanisms that may result in the attenuation of the primary action of an antihypertensive drug. For example, hydralazine stimulates the sympathetic nervous system (reflex tachycardia), activates the renin-angiotensin system, and promotes sodium retention. For these reasons, long-term hydralazine monotherapy is ineffective for blood-pressure control. Recent preliminary trials with the calcium blockers amlodipine and felodipine suggested that these agents do not exacerbate CHF, unlike some of the other calcium blockers. It has been postulated that the reason for this may relate to less activation of neurohumoral compensatory mechanisms.[168]

Table 17. Oral Agents Used for Urgent Hypertensive Crises*

DRUG	ROUTE	ONSET	DOSAGE
Nifedipine (not extended release)	Sublingual	5-10 min	10-20 mg every 15-30 min as needed
	Oral	15-20 min	10-20 mg every 30-60 min as needed
Clonidine	Oral	30-60 min	0.1-0.2 mg as needed every hr up to 0.6 mg
Captopril	Oral	15-30 min	25 mg repeated as required
Labetalol	Oral	30 min-2 hrs	200-400 mg every 2-3 hrs as needed

*Reflects common practice and not necessarily approved by FDA, for hypertensive crisis.

HYPERTENSIVE CRISIS

Conditions that are hypertensive emergencies, requiring immediate control of blood pressure, and those that are urgencies, in which hypertension should be controlled over hours to days, must be differentiated. Emergencies are associated with an immediate grave prognosis if blood pressure remains uncontrolled. Rapid-acting parenteral antihypertensive agents are the agents of choice for treatment of patients with a hypertensive emergency, while a rigorous regimen of oral drugs can be used in patients experiencing hypertensive urgency.[169] Table 15 lists the conditions which are associated with hypertensive emergencies and those classified as urgent conditions. The drugs used for hypertensive emergencies are listed in Table 16.

The drugs which can be used in the emergency room for hypertensive urgencies are listed in Table 17. Again, it is important to assure that the patient has no signs of malignant hypertension which would warrant more immediate action and intravenous drugs.

REFERENCES

1. Joint National Committee on Detection, Evaluation, and Treatment of High Blood Pressure (JNC V). The Fifth Report of the Joint National Committee on Detection, Evaluation, and Treatment of High Blood Pressure. *Arch Intern Med.* 1993;153:154-183.
2. Lund-Johansen P. Hemodynamic alterations in hypertension—spontaneous changes and effects of drug therapy. *Acta Med Scand.* 1977;603(suppl):1-14.
3. Julius S, Weder AB, Egan BM. Pathophysiology of early hypertension: Implications for epidemiologic research. In: Gross F, Strassert T (eds). *Mild Hypertension: Recent Advances.* New York: Raven Press; 1979:219.
4. Korner PI. Circulatory regulation in hypertension. *Br J Clin Pharmacol.* 1982;13:95-105.
5. Dzau VJ, Pratt RE. Renin-angiotensin system: Biology, physiology and pharmacology. In: Fozzard HA, Jennings RB, Haber E, et al (eds). *The Heart and Cardiovascular System.* New York: Raven Press; 1986:1031.
6. Dzau VJ. Significance of vascular renin-angiotensin pathway. *Hypertension.* 1986;8:553-559.
7. Jorgensen RS, Houston BK. Family history of hypertension, personality patterns, and cardiovascular reactivity to stress. *Psychosom Med.* 1980;48:102.
8. Bianchetti MG, Beretta-Piccoli C, Weidman P, et al. Blood pressure control in normotensive members of hypertensive families. *Kidney Int.* 1986;29:882-888.
9. Linfors EW, Feussner JR, Blessing CL, et al. Spurious hypertension in the obese patient. Effect of sphygmomanometer cuff size on prevalence of hypertension. *Arch Intern Med.* 1984;144:1482-1485.
10. Manning DM, Kuchirha C, Kaminski J. Miscuffing: Inappropriate blood pressure cuff application. *Circulation.* 1983;68:763-766.
11. Frohlich ED. Recommendations for blood pressure determination by sphygmomanometry. *Ann Intern Med.* 1988;109:612.
12. Finnie KJ, Watts DG, Armstrong PW. Biases in the measurement of arterial pressure. *Crit Care Med.* 1984;12:965-968.
13. Kleinert HD, Harshfield GA, Pickering TG, et al. What is the value of home blood pressure measurement in patients with mild hypertension? *Hypertension.* 1984;6:574-578.
14. Pickering TG, Harshfield GA, Laragh JH. Ambulatory versus casual blood pressure in the diagnosis of hypertensive patients. *Clin Exp Hypertens.* 1985;7A:257-266.
15. Pickering TG, Devereux RB. Ambulatory monitoring of blood pressure as a predictor of cardiovascular risk. *Am Heart J.* 1987;114:925-928.
16. Sokolow M, Wergegar D, Daim HK, et al. Relationship between level of blood pressure measured casually and by portable recorders and severity of complications in essential hypertension. *Circulation.* 1966;34:279-298.
17. Perloff D, Sokolow M, Cowan R. The prognostic value of ambulatory blood pressures. *JAMA.* 1983;249:2792-2798.
18. Gifford RW, Kirkendall W, O'Connor DT, et al. Office evaluation of hypertension. Special report. *Hypertension.* 1989;13:283.
19. Woythaler JN, Singer SL, Kwan OL, et al. Accuracy of echocardiography versus electrocardiography in detecting left ventricular hypertrophy: Comparison with postmortem mass measurements. *J Am Coll Cardiol.* 1983;2:305-311.
20. Casale PN, Devereux RB, Kligfield P, et al. Electrocardiographic detection of left ventricular hypertrophy: Development and prospective validation of improved criteria. *J Am Coll Cardiol.* 1985;6:572-580.
21. Devereux RB, Reichek N. Echocardiographic determination of left ventricular mass in man. Anatomic validation of the method. *Circulation.* 1977;55:613-618.
22. Casale PN, Devereux RB, Milner M, et al. Value of echocardiographic measurement of left ventricular mass in predicting cardiovascular morbid events in hypertensive men. *Ann Intern Med.* 1986;105:173-178.
23. Levy D, Garrison RJ, Savage DD, et al. Left ventricular mass and incidence of coronary heart disease in an elderly cohort. *Ann Intern Med.* 1989;110:101-107.
24. Devereux RB, Alonso DR, Lutas EM, et al. Echocardiography assessment of left ventricular hypertrophy: Comparison to necropsy findings. *Am J Cardiol.* 1986;57:450-458.
25. Helmer OM. Renin activity in blood from patients with hypertension. *J Can Med Assoc.* 1964;90:221.
26. Brunner HR, Laragh JH, Baer L, et al. Essential hypertension: Renin and aldosterone, heart attack and stroke. *N Engl J Med.* 1972;286:441-449.

27. Birkenhager WH, Kho TL, Schalekamp MA, et al. Renin levels and cardiovascular morbidity in essential hypertension. A prospective study. *Acta Clin Belg.* 1977;32:168-172.

28. Kaplan NM. Renin profiles: The unfulfilled promises. *JAMA.* 1977;238:611-613.

29. Alderman MH, Madhavan S, Ooi WL, et al. Association of the renin-sodium profile with the risk of myocardial infarction in patients with hypertension. *N Engl J Med.* 1991;324:1098-1104.

30. Maxwell MH, Gonick HC, Wiita R, et al. Use of the rapid-sequence intravenous pyelogram in the diagnosis of renovascular hypertension. *N Engl J Med.* 1964;270:213.

31. Hollenberg NK, Williams GH. Angiotensin as a renal, adrenal and cardiovascular hormone: Responses to saralasin in normal man and essential and secondary hypertension. *Kidney Int.* 1975;15:529.

32. Dzau VJ, Gibbons GH, Levin DC. Renovascular hypertension: An update on pathophysiology, diagnosis and treatment. *Am J Nephrol.* 1983;3:172-184.

33. Horne ML, Conklin VM, Keenan RE, et al. Angiotensin II profiling with saralasin: Summary of Eaton collaborative study. *Kidney Int.* 1979;15(suppl 9):S115-S122.

34. Case DB, Laragh JH. Reactive hyperreninemia in renovascular hypertension after angiotensin blockade with saralasin or converting enzyme inhibitor. *Ann Intern Med.* 1979;91:153-160.

35. Thibonnier M, Sassano P, Joseph A, et al. Diagnostic value of a single dose of captopril in renin and aldosterone dependent surgically curable hypertension. *Cardiovasc Rev Rep.* 1982;3:1659.

36. Muller FB, Sealey JE, Case DB, et al. The captopril test for identifying renovascular disease in hypertensive patients. *Am J Med.* 1986;80:633-644.

37. Wilcox CS, Williams CM, Smith TB, et al. Diagnostic uses of angiotensin converting enzyme inhibition in renovascular hypertension. *Am J Hypertens.* 1988;1:344S-349S.

38. Wenting GH, Tan-Tjiong HL, Derkx FH, et al. Split renal function after captopril in unilateral and renal artery stenosis. *Br Med J. Clin Res Ed.* 1984;288:886-890.

39. Geyskes GG, Oei HY, Puylaert CB, et al. Renovascular hypertension identified by captopril-induced changes in the renogram. *Hypertension.* 1987;9:451-458.

40. Sfakianakis GN, Bourgoignie JJ, Jaffe D, et al. Single dose captopril scintigraphy in the diagnosis of renovascular hypertension. *J Nuc Med.* 1987;28:1383-1392.

41. Setaro JF, Saddler MC, Chen CC, et al. Simplified captopril renography in diagnosis and treatment of renal artery stenosis. *Hypertension.* 1991;18:289-298.

42. Davidson RA, Wilcox CS. Newer tests for the diagnosis of renovascular disease. *JAMA.* 1992;268:3353-3358.

43. Marks LS, Maxwell MH. Renal vein renin: Value and limitations in the prediction of operative results. *Urol Clin North Am.* 1975;2:311-325.

44. Marks LS, Maxwell MH, Varady PD, et al. Renovascular hypertension: Does the renal vein ratio predict operative results? *J Urol.* 1976;115:365-368.

45. Lyons DF, Streck WF, Kem DC, et al. Captopril stimulation of differential renins in renovascular hypertension. *Hypertension.* 1983;5:615-622.

46. Conn JW, Cohen EL, Lucas CP, et al. Primary reninism, hypertension, hyperreninemia, and secondary aldosteronism due to renin-producing juxtaglomerular cell tumors. *Arch Intern Med.* 1972;130:682-696.

47. Weinberger MH, Grim CE, Hollifield JW, et al. Primary aldosteronsim. Diagnosis, localization, and treatment. *Ann Intern Med.* 1979;90:386-395.

48. Weinberger MH, Cohen SJ, Miller JZ, et al. Dietary sodium restriction as adjunctive treatment of hypertension. *JAMA.* 1988;259:2561-2565.

49. Kem DC, Weinberger MH, Mayes DM, et al. Saline suppression of plasma aldosterone in hypertension. *Arch Intern Med.* 1971;128:380-386.

50. Holland OB, Brown H, Kuhnert LV, et al. Further evaluation of saline infusion for the diagnosis of primary aldosteronism. *Hypertension.* 1984;6:717-723.

51. Abrams HL, Siegelman SS, Adams DF, et al. Computed tomography versus ultrasound of the adrenal gland. A prospective study. *Radiology.* 1982;143:121-128.

52. Vaughan NJ, Jowett TP, Slater JD, et al. The diagnosis of primary hyperaldosteronism. *Lancet.* 1981;1:120-125.

53. Manu P, Runge LA. Biochemical screening for pheochromocytoma: Superiority of urinary metanephrine measurements. *Am J Epidemiol.* 1984;120:788-790.

54. Manger CM, Gifford RW (eds). *Pheochromocytoma.* New York: Springer-Verlag; 1977:398.

55. Bouloux PMG, Perret D. Interference of labetalol metabolites in the determination of plasma catecholamines by HPLC with electrochemical detection. *Clin Chim Acta.* 1985;150:111-117.

56. Bravo EL, Tarazi RC, Gifford RW, et al. Circulating and urinary catecholamines in pheochromocytoma: Diagnostic and pathophysiologic implications. *N Engl J Med.* 1979;301:682-686.

57. Bravo EL, Tarazi RC, Fouad FM, et al. Clonidine-suppression test: A useful aid in the diagnosis of pheochromocytoma. *N Engl J Med.* 1981;305:623-626.

58. Bravo EL. Pheochromocytoma. Current concepts in diagnosis, localization, and management. *Primary Care; Clinics in Office Practice.* 1983;10:75-86.

59. Stewart BH, Bravo EL, Haaga J, et al. Localization of pheochromocytoma by computed tomography. *N Engl J Med.* 1978;299:460-461.

60. Sisson JC, Frager MS, Valk TW, et al. Scintigraphic localization of pheochromocytoma. *N Engl J Med.* 1981;305:12-17.

61. Glancy DL, Morrow AG, Simon AL, et al. Juxtaductal aortic coarctation. Analysis of 84 patients studied hemodynamically, angiographically and morphologically after age 1 year. *Am J Cardiol.* 1983;51:537-551.

62. Stadel BV. Oral contraceptives and cardiovascular disease. *N Engl J Med.* 1981;305:672-677.

63. Klatsky AL, Friedman GD, Armstrong MA. The relationship between alcoholic beverage use and other traits to blood pressure: A new Kaiser-Permanente study. *Circulation.* 1986;73:628-636.

64. Jackson R, Stewart A, Beaglehole R, et al. Alcohol consumption and blood pressure. *Am J Epidemiol.* 1985;122:1037-1044.

65. Chiang BN, Perlman LV, Epstein FH. Overweight and hypertension: A review. *Circulation.* 1969;39:403-421.

66. Haulk R, Hubert H, Fabsitz R, et al. Weight and hypertension. *Ann Int Med.* 1983;98:855.

67. Gifford RW, Westbrook E. Hypertensive encephalopathy: Mechanisms, clinical features, and treatment. *Prog Cardiovasc Dis.* 1974;17:115-124.

68. Bennett C. The syndrome of accelerated or malignant hypertension. *Cardiovasc Med.* 1979;4:1141.

69. Healton EB, Brust JC, Feinfeld DA, et al. Hypertensive encephalopathy and the neurologic manifestations of malignant hypertension. *Neurology.* 1982;32:127-132.

70. Johansson B, Strandgaard S, Lassen NS. On the pathogenesis of hypertensive encephalopathy: The hypertensive breakthrough of autoregulation of cerebral blood flow with forced vasodilation, flow increase and blood-brain barrier damage. *Circ Res.* 1974;34(suppl):167.

71. McLeod D, Marshall J, Kohner EM, et al. The role of axoplasmic flow in the pathogenesis of retinal cotton-wool spots. *Br J Ophthalmol.* 1977;61:177-191.

72. Vaziri ND. Malignant or accelerated hypertension. *West J Med.* 1984;140:575-582.

73. Paronetto F. Immunocytochemical observation on the vascular necrosis and renal glomerular lesions of malignant nephrosclerosis. *Am J Pathol.* 1965;46:901.

74. Schottstaedt MF, Sokolow M. The natural history and course of hypertension with papilledema (malignant hypertension). *Am Heart J.* 1953;45:331.

75. Gavras H, Oliver N, Aitchison J, et al. Abnormalities of coagulation and the development of malignant phase hypertension. *Kidney Int.* 1976;8(suppl):252s.

76. Kahn JR, Skeggs LT, Shumway NP, et al. The assay of hypertension from the arterial blood pressure of normotensive and hypertensive human beings. *J Exp Med.* 1952;95:523.

77. Catt KJ, Cran E, Zimmet PZ, et al. Angiotensin II blood levels in human hypertension. *Lancet.* 1971;1:459-464.

78. Padfield PL, Morton JJ. Proceedings: Application of a sensitive radioimmunoassay for plasma arginine vasopressin pathological conditions in man. *Clin Sci Mol Med.* 1974;47:16p. Abstract.

79. Veterans Administration Cooperative Study Group on Antihypertensive Agents I. Results in patients with diastolic blood pressure averaging 115-129 mm Hg. *JAMA.* 1967;202:1028.

80. Weiss NS. Relationship of high blood pressure to headache, epistaxis, and selected other symptoms. *N Engl J Med.* 1972;287:631-633.

81. Moser M, Wish H, Friedman AP. Headache and hypertension. *JAMA.* 1962;180:115.

82. Walker CH. Migraine and its relationship to hypertension. *Br Med J.* 1959;2:1430.

83. Gardner JW, Moutain CE, Hines EA. The relationship of migraine to hypertension headaches. *Am J Med Sci.* 1940;200:50.

84. Mitchell JRA. Nose-bleeding and high blood pressure. *Br Med J.* 1959;1:25.

85. Shaheen OH. Arterial epistaxis. *J Laryngol Otol.* 1975;89:17-34.

86. Janeway TC. A clinical study of hypertensive cardiovascular disease. *Arch Intern Med.* 1913;12:755.

87. Hunter A, Rogers OH. Mortality study of impaired lives, no. 2. *Trans Acta Soc Am.* 1923;27:738.

88. Bechgard P. Arterial hypertension; a follow-up study of one thousand hypertonics. *Acta Med Scand.* 1946;172(suppl):3.

89. Sagie A, Larson MG, Levy D. The natural history of borderline isolated systolic hypertension. *N Engl J Med.* 1993;329:1912-1917.

90. The National High Blood Pressure Education Program Coordinating Committee. National high blood pressure education program working group report on ambulatory blood pressure monitoring. *Arch Intern Med.* 1990;150:2270-2280.

91. Kannel WB, Schatzbin A. Risk factor analysis. *Prog Cardiovasc Dis.* 1983;26:309.

92. Castelli WP, Anderson K. A population at risk: Prevalence of high cholesterol levels in hypertensive patients in the Framingham study. *Am J Med.* 1986;80(suppl 2A):23-32.

93. MacMahon SW, MacDonald GJ. Antihypertensive treatment and plasma lipoprotein levels. The associations in data from a population study. *Am J Med.* 1986;80(suppl 2A):40-47.

94. Multiple Risk Factor Intervention Trial. Risk factor changes and mortality results. *JAMA.* 1982;248:1465-1477.

95. Houston MC. New insights and new approaches for the treatment of essential hypertension: Selection of therapy based on coronary heart disease risk factor analysis, hemodynamic profiles, quality of life, and subsets of hypertension. *Am Heart J.* 1989;117:911-951.

96. O'Kelly BF, Massie BM, Tubau JF, et al. Coronary morbidity and mortality, pre-existing silent coronary artery disease, and mild hypertension. *Ann Intern Med.* 1989;110:1017-1026.

97. MacMahon S, Peto R, Cutler J, et al. Blood pressure, stroke, and coronary heart disease. *Lancet.* 1990;335:765-744.

98. Collins R, Peto R, MacMahon S, et al. Blood pressure, stroke, and coronary heart disease. Part 2, short-term reductions in blood pressure: overview of randomised drug trials in their epidemiological context. *Lancet.* 1990;335:827-838.

99. Multiple Risk Factor Intervention Trial Research Group. Mortality rates after 10.5 years for participants in the multiple risk factor intervention trial. Findings related to aprior hypotheses of the trial. *JAMA.* 1990; 263(13):1795-1801.

100. Neaton JD, Grimm RH Jr, Prineas RJ, et al, for the Treatment of Mild Hypertension Study Research Group. Treatment of Mild Hypertension Study: Final Results. *JAMA.* 1993;270:713-724.

101. Hebert PR, Moser M, Mayer J, et al. Recent evidence on drug therapy of mild to moderate hypertension and decreased risk of coronary heart disease. *Arch Intern Med.* 1993;153:578-581.

102. Frohlich ED, Tarazi RC, Dustan HP. Clinical-physiological correlations in the development of hypertensive heart disease. *Circulation.* 1971;44:446-455.

103. Dunn FG, Chandraratna P, de Carvalho JG, et al. Pathophysiologic assessment of hypertensive heart disease with echocardiography. *Am J Cardiol*. 1977;39:789-795.

104. Kannel WB, Gordon T, Offurt D. Left ventricular hypertrophy by electrocardiogram. Prevalence, incidence, and mortality in the Framingham study. *Ann Intern Med*. 1989;71:89.

105. Tarazi RC, Levy MN. Cardiac responses to increased afterload. State-of-the-art review. *Hypertension*. 1982;4(suppl II):II-8–II-18.

106. Inouye I, Massie B, Loge D, et al. Abnormal left ventricular filling: An early finding in mild to moderate systemic hypertension. *Am J Cardiol*. 1984;53:120-126.

107. Reichek N, Devereux RB. Left ventricular hypertrophy: Relationship of anatomic, echocardiographic and electrocardiographic findings. *Circulation*. 1981;63:1391-1398.

108. Kannel WB. Prevalence and natural history of electrocardiographic left ventricular hypertrophy. *Am J Med*. 1983;75:4-11.

109. Wikstrand J. Left ventricular function in early primary hypertension. Functional consequences of cardiovascular structural changes. *Hypertension*. 1984; 6(suppl III):III-108-116.

110. Messerli FH, DeCarvalho JGR, Christie B, et al. Systemic and regional hemodynamics in low, normal, and high cardiac output in borderline hypertension. *Circulation*. 1978;58:441-448.

111. Messerli FH, Frohlich ED, Suarez DH, et al. Borderline hypertension: Relationship between age, hemodynamics, and circulating catecholamines. *Circulation*. 1981;64:760-764.

112. Topol EJ, Traill TA, Fortuin NJ. Hypertensive hypertrophic cardiomyopathy of the elderly. *N Engl J Med*. 1985;312:277-283.

113. Kannel WB, Castelli WP, McNamara PM, et al. Role of blood pressure in the development of congestive heart failure. The Framingham Study. *N Engl J Med*. 1972;287;781-787.

114. Veterans Administration Cooperative Study Group on Antihypertensive Agents. Effects of treatment on morbidity in hypertension. II. Results in patients with diastolic pressure averaging 90-114 mm Hg. *JAMA*. 1970;213:1143-1152.

115. Mutlu N, Berry RG, Alpers BJ. Massive cerebral hemorrhage: Clinical and pathological correlations. *Arch Neurol*. 1963;8:644.

116. Wolf PA, Kannel WB, Verter J. Epidemiologic appraisal of hypertension and stroke risk. In: Guthrie GP, Kotchen TA (eds). *Hypertension and the Brain*. New York: Futura; 1984:221.

117. Medical Research Council Working Party. MRC trial of treatment of mild hypertension: Principal results. *Br Med J*. 1985;291:97-104.

118. SHEP Cooperative Research Group. Prevention of stroke by antihypertensive drug treatment in older persons with isolated systolic hypertension. *JAMA*. 1991;265:3255-3264.

119. Dahlöf B, Lindholm LH, Hansson L, et al. Morbidity and mortality in the Swedish trial in old patients with hypertension (STOP-Hypertension). *Lancet*. 1991; 338:1281-1285.

120. Inzitari D, Bianchi F, Pracucci G, et al. The Italian Multicenter Study of Reversible Cerebral Ischemic Attacks. IV. Blood pressure components and atherosclerotic lesions. *Stroke*. 1986;17:185-192.

121. Fieschi C, Prencipe M, Carolie A, et al. Case-control of focal cerebral ischemia in young adults. *Neurology*. 1987;1(suppl):83.

122. Gandolfo C, Loeb C, Moretti C, et al. Patient characteristics in the cooperative study of focal cerebral ischemia in young adults. In: Meyer JS, Lechner H, Reivich M, et al (eds). Proceedings of the World Federation of Neurology, 13th International Salzburg Conference. Amsterdam: Excerpta Medica, International Congress Series 736; *Cerebral Vascular Disease*. 1987;6:77.

123. Fisher CM. Lacunae: Small, deep cerebral infarcts. *Neurology*. 1965;15:774.

124. Fisher CM. The arterial lesions underlying lacunae. *Acta Neuropathol*. 1968;12:1-15.

125. Sugimoto T, Rosansky SJ. The incidence of treated end stage renal disease in the Eastern United States: 1973-1979. *Am J Public Health*. 1984;74:14-17.

126. Rostand SG, Kirk KA, Rutsky EA, et al. Racial differences in the incidence of treatment for end-stage renal disease. *N Engl J Med*. 1982; 306(21):1276-1279.

127. Mujais SK, Emmanouel DS, Kasinath BS, et al. Marked proteinuria in hypertensive nephrosclerosis. *Am J Nephrol*. 1985;5:190-195.

128. Bauer GE, Humphery TJ. The natural history of hypertension with moderate impairment of renal function. *Clin Sci Mol Med*. 1973;45(suppl):191s-193s.

129. van Hooft IMS, Grobbee DE, Derks FHM, et al. Renal hemodynamics and the renin-angiotensin-aldosterone system in normotensive subjects with hypertensive and normotensive parents. *N Engl J Med*. 1991;324:1305-1311.

130. Bergstrom J, Alvestrand A, Bucht H, et al. Progression of chronic renal failure in man is retarded with more frequent clinical follow-ups and better blood pressure control. *Clin Nephrol*. 1986;25:1-6.

131. Björck S, Nyberg G, Mulec H, et al. Beneficial effects of angiotensin-converting enzyme inhibitor on renal function in patients with diabetic nephropathy. *Br Med J. Clin Res Ed*. 1986;293:471-474.

132. Björck S, Mulec H, Johnsen SA, et al. Renal protective effect of enalapril in diabetic nephropathy. *Br Med J*. 1992;304:339-343.

133. Lewis EJ, Hunsicker LG, Bain RP, et al, for the Collaborative Study Group. The effect of angiotensin-converting-enzyme inhibition on diabetic nephropathy. *N Engl J Med*. 1993;329:1456-1462.

134. Lindsay J Jr, Hurst JW. Clinical features and prognosis in dissecting aneurysm of the aorta: A re-appraisal. *Circulation*. 1967;35:880-888.

135. Wilson SK, Hutchins GM. Aortic dissecting aneurysms: Causative factors in 204 subjects. *Arch Pathol Lab Med*. 1982;106:175-180.

136. Slater EE, DeSanctis RW. The clinical recognition of dissecting aortic aneurysm. *Am J Med*. 1976;60:625-633.

137. Cooke JP, Safford RE. Progress in the diagnosis and management of aortic dissection. *Mayo Clin Proc*. 1986;61:147-153.

138. Cruickshank JM, Thorp JM, Zacharias FJ. Benefits and potential harm of lowering high blood pressure. *Lancet*. 1987;1:581-584.

139. Collins R, Peto R, MacMahon S, et al. Blood pressure, stroke, and coronary heart disease. *Lancet*. 1990;335:827-838.

140. Farnett L, Mulrow CD, Linn WD, et al. The J-Curve phenomenon and the treatment of hypertension. Is there a point beyond which pressure reduction is dangerous? *JAMA*. 1991;265:489-495.

141. Medical Research Council Working Party. MRC trial of treatment of hypertension in older adults: principal results. *Br Med J*. 1992;304:405-412.

142. Aristimuno GG, Foster TA, Voors AW, et al. Influence of persistent obesity in children on cardiovascular risk factors: The Bogalusa Heart Study. *Circulation*. 1984;69:895-904.

143. Wing RR, Jeffery RW. Outpatient treatments of obesity. A comparison of methodology and clinical results. *Int J Obesity*. 1979;3:261-279.

144. Parijs J, Joosens JV, Vander Linden L, et al. Moderate sodium restriction and diuretics in the treatment of hypertension. *Am Heart J*. 1973;85:22-34.

145. Richards AM, Nicholls MG, Espiner E, et al. Blood-pressure response to moderate sodium restriction and to potassium supplementation in mild essential hypertension. *Lancet*. 1984;1:757-761.

146. Silman AJ, Locke C, Mitchell P, et al. Evaluation of the effectiveness of a low sodium diet in the treatment of mild to moderate hypertension. *Lancet*. 1983;1:1179-1182.

147. Langford HG, Blaufox MD, Oberman A, et al. Dietary therapy slows the return of hypertension after stopping prolonged medication. *JAMA*. 1985;253:657-664.

148. The Treatment of Mild Hypertension Research Group. The Treatment of Mild Hypertension Study: A randomized, placebo-controlled trial of a nutritional-hygenic regimen along with various drug mono-therapies. *Arch Intern Med*. 1991;151:1413-1423.

149. The Trials of Hypertension Prevention Collaborative Research Group. The effects of nonpharmacologic interventions on blood pressure of persons with high normal levels. Results of the trials of hypertension prevention, phase I. *JAMA*. 1992;267:1213-1220.

150. Hypertension Prevention Trial Research Group. The Hypertension Prevention Trial: Three-year effects of dietary changes on blood pressure. *Arch Intern Med*. 1990;150:153-162.

151. Wassertheil-Smoller S, Blaufox D, Oberman AS, et al. The trial of antihypertensive interventions and management (TAIM) study. Adequate weight loss, alone and combined with drug therapy in the treatment of mild hypertension. *Arch Intern Med*. 1992;152:131-136.

152. Intersalt Cooperative Research Group: Intersalt: an international study of electrolyte excretion and blood pressure. Results for 24 hour urinary sodium and potassium excretion. *Br Med J*. 1988;297:319-328.

153. MacMahon SW, Norton RN. Alcohol and hypertension: Implications for prevention and treatment. *Ann Int Med*. 1986;105:124-126.

154. Kupari M. Acute cardiovascular effects of ethanol: A controlled non-invasive study. *Br Heart J*. 1983;49:174-182.

155. Witteman JCM, Willett WC, Stampfer MJ, et al. Relation of moderate alcohol consumption and risk of systemic hypertension in women. *Am J Cardiol*. 1990;65:633-637.

156. Krotkiewski M, Mandroukas K, Sjostrom L, et al. Effects of long-term physical training on body fat, metabolism and blood pressure in obesity. *Metabolism: Clinical and Experimental*. 1979;28:650-658.

157. Hagberg J, Goldring D, Ehasni A, et al. Effect of exercise training on the blood pressure and hemo-dynamic features of hypertensive adolescents. *Am J Cardiol*. 1983;52:763-768.

158. Materson BJ, Reda DJ, Cushman WC, et al, for the Department of Veterans Affairs Cooperative Study Group on Antihypertensive Agents. Single-drug therapy for hypertension in men: A comparison of six antihypertensive agents with placebo. *N Engl J Med*. 1993;328:914-921.

159. Zusman RM. Alterations to traditional antihypertensive therapy. *Hypertension*. 1986;8:837-842.

160. Lipid Research Clinics (LRC) Program. The Lipid Research Clinics Coronary Primary Prevention Trial results: I. Reduction in incidence of coronary heart disease. *JAMA*. 1984;251:351-364.

161. Lipid Research Clinics (LRC) Program. The Lipid Research Clinics Coronary Primary Prevention Trial results. II. The relationship of reduction in incidence of coronary heart disease to cholesterol lowering. *JAMA*. 1984;251:365-374.

162. Frick MH, Elo O, Haapa K, et al. Helsinki Heart Study: Primary prevention trial with gemfibrozil in middle-aged men with dyslipidemia: Safety of treatment, changes in risk factors, and incidence of coronary heart disease. *N Engl J Med*. 1987;317:1237-1245.

162a. Epstein M. Evolving concepts in the management of hypertension. *Clin Cardiol*. 1995;18(suppl III):III-3–III-11.

163. Jarrett RJ, Keen H, McCartney M, et al. Glucose tolerance and blood pressure in two population samples: Their relation to diabetes mellitus and hypertension. *Int J Epidemiol*. 1978;7:15-24.

164. Swislocki AL, Hoffman BB, Reaven GM. Insulin resistance, glucose intolerance and hyperinsulinemia in patients with hypertension. *Am J Hypertens*. 1989;2:419-423.

165. Pollare T, Lithell H, Berne C. Insulin resistance is a characteristic feature of primary hypertension independent of obesity. *Metabolism*. 1990;39:167-174.

166. Zavaroni I, Bonora E, Pagliara M, et al. Risk factors for coronary artery disease in healthy persons with hyperinsulinemia and normal glucose intolerance. *N Engl J Med*. 1989;320:702-706.

167. Pollare T, Lithell H, Berne C. A comparison of the effects of hydrochlorothiazide and captopril on glucose and lipid metabolism in patients with hypertension. *N Engl J Med*. 1989;321:868-873.

168. Packer M, Nicod P, Khandheria BR, et al. Randomized, multicenter, double-blind, placebo-controlled evalu-ation of amlodipine in patients with mild-to-moderate heart failure. *J Am Coll Cardiol*. 1991;17(2):274A. Abstract.

169. Calhoun EAC, Oparil S. Treatment of hypertensive crisis. *N Engl J Med*. 1990;323:1177-1183.

CHAPTER 30   Pulmonary Hypertension

Demetrios Georgiou, MD
Bruce H. Brundage, MD

Pulmonary hypertension was defined by the World Health organization in 1975 as a mean pulmonary arterial pressure (PAP) of greater than 25 mm Hg at rest and greater than 30 mm Hg during exercise.[1] In the normal adult living at sea level the systolic PAP is 18-25 mm Hg with a diastolic pulmonary pressure of 6-10 mm Hg and a mean PAP of 12-16 mm Hg. When these normal values are exceeded, pulmonary hypertension is diagnosed.

In normal adults, the pulmonary vascular bed is a low-pressure vasculature with low resistance. There are 2 factors which are responsible for this low resistance. First, the pulmonary vasculature is rich in elastic tissue; therefore, an increase in flow will increase the distensibility. Thus, pulmonary vascular resistance (PVR) decreases as flow increases. Second, whenever there is a collapse of vessels in the upper pulmonary lobes, there is an additional recruitment of new vasculature. When there is an increase in flow, these vessels open and therefore PVR is decreased. The ability of the pulmonary vascular bed to distend and expand is probably the explanation for the lack of increase in PAP when cardiac output increases several-fold, for example, during exercise or with a left-to-right shunt of the pre-tricuspid variety such as atrial septal defect (ASD). When medial hypertrophy, intimal fibrosis, and thrombosis of the pulmonary vessels develop, the distensibility of the pulmonary vascular bed is severely reduced; therefore, the number of additional vessels to be recruited is reduced. Under these circumstances even a small increase in flow will markedly increase pulmonary pressures.

The causes of chronic pulmonary hypertension are numerous (Table 1). The most common cause in this country is lung disease, that is, chronic obstructive pulmonary disease (COPD) and interstitial lung disease. Any process that elevates left ventricular (LV) filling pressures such as severe LV systolic dysfunction or valvular disease such as mitral stenosis will induce pulmonary hypertension. Congenital heart disease with left-to-right intracardiac shunt can also produce severe pulmonary hypertension. Another clinical entity that at times may mimic unexplained primary pulmonary hypertension (PPH) is chronic pulmonary embolic disease. Other causes include collagen vascular disease which is a fairly common cause of pulmonary hypertension. Collagen vascular disease may not always represent true vasculitis. Diagnosis of PPH requires exclusion of all other secondary causes. Because the prognosis with PPH is very poor, all potentially treatable causes must be excluded before the diagnosis of primary disease is made.

This chapter will be divided into 2 parts. The first part will review PPH and bring the reader up-to-date in terms of new pharmacologic therapy. Then, the symptomatology and physical findings as well as noninvasive and invasive diagnostic tests will be reviewed. Finally, treatment will be discussed. In the second part the most common causes of secondary pulmonary hypertension such as COPD and other intrinsic lung disease as well as congenital heart disease and chronic pulmonary embolism will be reviewed. Collagen vascular disease, sleep apnea, and obesity-hypoventilation syndrome will be briefly discussed.

PRIMARY (UNEXPLAINED) PULMONARY HYPERTENSION

Primary pulmonary hypertension is a relatively rare disease. The true incidence of this disorder is unknown because many patients remain

Table 1. Etiology of Pulmonary Hypertension

Diseases affecting the airways of the lung and alveoli
   Chronic obstructive pulmonary disease (COPD)
   Chronic bronchitis, bronchiectasis
   Restrictive pulmonary disease
   Cystic fibrosis
Infiltrative or granulomatous disease
   Idiopathic pulmonary fibrosis (Hamman-Rich syndrome)
   Collagen vascular disease
   Sarcoidosis
   Pneumoconiosis
   Hemosiderosis
Upper airway obstruction
Cardiac diseases
   Congenital heart disease causing an increase in pulmonary flow: VSD, PDA, ASD
Increased resistance to pulmonary venous drainage
   Valvular heart disease (mitral valve disease, aortic valve disease)
   Left ventricular failure (cardiomyopathy, coronary artery disease)
   Reduced left ventricular compliance (systemic hypertension, cardiomyopathy)
   Left atrial myxoma
   Cor triatriatum
Pulmonary venous obstruction
   Pulmonary veno-occlusive disease (PVOD)
   Congenital stenosis of the pulmonary veins
Diseases affecting the thoracic cage movement
   Sleep apnea syndrome
   Pleural fibrosis
   Idiopathic hypoventilation
   Kyphoscoliosis
   Neuromuscular disorders
     Poliomyelitis
     Myasthenia gravis
   Obesity-hypoventilation syndrome
     Pickwick syndrome
Pulmonary vascular disease
   Primary pulmonary hypertension (PPH)
   Vasculitides
   Sickle cell disease
   Chronic pulmonary embolism
   Chronic liver disease (cirrhosis)
Infectious etiology
   Human immunodeficiency virus (HIV)
   Autoimmune Deficiency Syndrome (AIDS)

Table 1. Etiology of Pulmonary Hypertension (continued)

Extrinsic compression of the pulmonary vasculature
   Mediastinal tumors
   Aneurysms
   Mediastinal fibrosis
   Granulomata
High-altitude residence disease
Congenital pulmonary defect (pulmonary arteriovenous fistulas)
Toxin-induced pulmonary hypertension
   Aminorex fumarate (appetite suppressant)
   Crotalaria alkaloids
   Intravenous drug use
   L-tryptophan
   Cocaine

VSD=Ventricular septal defect; PDA=Patent ductus arteriosus; ASD=Atrial septal defect.

asymptomatic even when severe pulmonary hypertension is present. In the NIH registry on PPH, 187 patients were enrolled from July 1981 through December 1985.[2] This figure underestimated the true incidence of this disease because only patients who were symptomatic and sought medical attention were enrolled. There is considerable variability in the clinical presentation of this disorder so that patients may remain asymptomatic even when they have severe PPH. Thus, many cases of PPH go undiagnosed or are diagnosed when the disease has progressed to the point of no return. Primary pulmonary hypertension may occur at any age, with the highest incidence in the third and fourth decades. In the NIH registry the mean age of patients enrolled was 36.4 years which is similar to the mean age reported in other studies. Of interest, approximately 20% of the patients were 50 years of age or older at the time of diagnosis in the NIH registry database. This contradicts the previous belief that PPH affects young people exclusively. This contradiction can be explained by the fact that PPH diagnosed in a subject 50-years-old or older probably represents a number of other disease processes that at this time are poorly understood. In terms of sex distribution, in children the incidence of male versus female is equal. After childhood, however, the female to male ratio is 3 to 1. In the NIH registry the female to male ratio was only 1.7 to 1. Familial cases have also been reported.[3] The incidence of familial PPH represented 7% of all cases in the NIH registry.[2] It is thought that the transmission occurs as an autosomal dominant inheritance with incomplete penetrance.

CLINICAL PRESENTATION OF PPH

SYMPTOMS

Often PPH may be diagnosed with hyperventilation, depression, or psychiatric illness. The disorder is characterized by a slow, insidious onset with progressive clinical deterioration. Patients are usually symptomatic for approximately 2 years before they seek medical attention and before the diagnosis is made. Initially, PPH may be well-tolerated. When patients become symptomatic, the disease is already in the advanced stages and the PAP is 2 or 3 times normal.

Symptoms include dyspnea, chest pain or syncope. Dyspnea on exertion is the most common presenting symptom. In fact, 90% of patients enrolled in the NIH registry presented with dyspnea. As the disease progresses, dyspnea becomes evident at rest. Chest pain may present as typical angina. This is a common symptom. The coronary arteries in patients with PPH are usually normal; thus, it is postulated that chest pain occurs as a result of underperfusion of the hypertrophic right ventricle. Syncope was the presenting symptom in 10% of patients according to the NIH registry. The frequency of syncope increases as the disease progresses and its presence usually indicates a poor prognosis. Syncope can occur during exercise and at rest. It is thought that the explanation of syncope during exercise is due to the fact that the patient is unable to increase his or her cardiac output. Arrhythmias are not frequently seen in patients with PPH; the reason being that arrhythmias in patients with low and fixed cardiac output are incompatible with survival. Other less frequently observed symptoms include hemoptysis, cough, and hoarseness which may result from compression of the recurrent laryngeal nerve (Ortner's syndrome) from the enlargement of the pulmonary artery.

PHYSICAL EXAMINATION

On physical examination, the presence of pulmonary hypertension is established when a loud P_2 sound is heard. A right ventricular heave is also frequently palpable. Although the physical examination is helpful for excluding other secondary forms of PPH, the clinical differentiation between PPH and other secondary forms of pulmonary hypertension such as Eisenmenger's syndrome or thromboembolic pulmonary hypertension is often very difficult. When the disease is in the advanced stage, right ventricular failure ensues and on physical examination a murmur of tricuspid regurgitation is heard which increases with deep inspiration, right ventricular S_3 is audible, jugular veins are distended, the liver is pulsatile or enlarged, and ascites and peripheral edema become prominent physical findings. Cyanosis is usually mild but may become a permanent feature of the physical examination when there is presence of right ventricular failure and low cardiac output. Clubbing is not a feature of PPH. When clubbing is present, its presence should alert the physician to the possibility of an undiagnosed congenital cardiac defect or COPD. The lung examination usually demonstrates a clear chest unless pulmonary veno-occlusive disease (PVOD) is present, in which case bilateral rales are usually present due to capillary congestion.

PATHOLOGY

There are 2 different histologic subtypes which cause obstruction at the level of the precapillary arterioles, otherwise known as pulmonary arteriopathy. These are plexogenic pulmonary arteriopathy and thrombotic pulmonary arteriopathy.[4–6] Pulmonary veno-occlusive disease is another pathologic entity causing an obstruction at the level of the pulmonary veins and venules. Plexogenic pulmonary arteriopathy is typical for but not pathognomonic of PPH because it is seen in pulmonary hypertension from other etiologies such as pulmonary hypertension secondary to Eisenmenger's syndrome or to liver cirrhosis. The histologic characteristics of plexogenic pulmonary arteriopathy include concentric laminar intimal fibrosis, often with complete obliteration of the vascular lumen (onion-skin lesions). The sequence of lesions appears to be medial hypertrophy, intimal proliferation and plexiform lesions. Plexiform lesions may represent aneurysmal dilatations of the arterial wall and may look like glomeruli in a small arterial bed or may be a reparative part of lesions in areas of previous fibrinoid necrosis. Plexiform lesions are usually found in advanced stages of PPH. Plexogenic pulmonary arteriopathy has been reported in 28% to 71% of patients with PPH and in 43% of the NIH registry. Plexiform lesions had worse hemodynamics and worse prognosis than patients with thrombotic lesions in the NIH registry.[7] Thrombotic pulmonary arteriopathy was described in 20% to 50% of patients with PPH and in 33% of the NIH registry series. Patients with thrombotic pulmonary arteriopathy often have evidence of recanalized pulmonary thromboembolism which appears as a vascular web. The lesions seen in thrombotic pulmonary arteriopathy include eccentric intimal fibrosis, medial hypertrophy and both fresh and old thrombi. The mechanism of both plexogenic pulmonary arteriopathy and thrombotic pulmonary arteriopathy appears to be due to endothelial cell injury. Recently, Rich and Brundage[8] have proposed that plexogenic pulmonary arteriopathy is associated with abnormalities in endothelial structure and function which may result in impaired release of endothelial relaxing factors. They also suggested that thrombotic pulmonary arteriopathy appears to be the result of injury of endothelial cells that creates a procoagulant environment and widespread eccentric intimal proliferation leading to thrombosis in situ. Pulmonary venous occlusive disease is the least common of all the histopathologic entities. It accounts for less than 10% of the cases of PPH with fewer than 100 cases described so far.[2] The histologic characteristics of this entity are fibrosis and thrombosis of the pulmonary venules with secondary intimal proliferation and medial hypertrophy which may extend back to the arterial bed as well. A clinical observation was made by Rich and colleagues[9] where patients with PVOD were found to have chest x-ray patterns showing interstitial markings similar to mitral stenosis. In the same report these investigators were able to identify 2 predominant types of lung scan patterns: a normal pattern of relatively even distribution of tissue and a diffusely patchy pattern.[9] It was originally thought that the normal pattern represents early disease and the patchy pattern represents late disease. However, when these patients were followed up with serial lung scans over a long period of time, they found that patients whose lung scans were initially normal remained normal until their death, and those patients with patchy scans had unchanging patchy scans.

Wagenvoort and Mulder[10] reported the histologic analysis of 78 patients with plexogenic pulmonary arteriopathy with specific emphasis on the presence and severity of thrombotic lesions. They found that thrombotic lesions are common. However, they proposed that these thrombotic lesions are a complication of the disease rather than a primary pathologic finding. This is in contradiction to the reports suggesting that thrombotic lesions carried in primary plexogenic arteriopathy are an essential part of this disease rather than a complicating feature.[11,12]

PATHOGENESIS OF PPH

The pathogenesis of PPH is not known. Basically, 2 theories have been proposed: abnormal pulmonary vasoconstriction in patients with plexogenic pulmonary arteriopathy and thrombosis in patients with thrombotic pulmonary arteriopathy. The theory in favor of the vasoconstrictive hypothesis was proposed by Wood.[13] It was based upon certain findings that showed medial hypertrophy precedes plexogenic lesions and therefore vasodilator agents may help reduce pulmonary resistance. Furthermore, plexogenic pulmonary arteriopathy has been described in patients with liver cirrhosis[14] and in cases of diet-induced (crotalaria-aminorex) primary pulmonary hypertension. As part of the vasoconstrictive hypothesis, it was suggested that vasoactive substances may reach the pulmonary vessels and cause vasoconstriction. In addition, approximately 10% of patients with PPH have been reported to have Raynaud's phenomenon suggesting a generalized increase in vascular tone.[2] Endothelin-1 (a potent vasoconstrictor) was recently shown to be increased in the endothelial cells of patients with PPH, suggesting that the local production of endothelin-1 may be contributing to the vascular abnormalities associated with this disorder.[15]

On the other hand, thrombi involving the small pulmonary arteries have been found in at least one-third of the patients with PPH, without any evidence of recurrent embolization at autopsy.[7] Therefore, it can be concluded that PPH may be the result of in situ thrombosis caused by endothelial cell abnormalities as well as defective coagulation, fibrinolysis, or platelet abnormalities. This is an attractive hypothesis. However, there is only a small amount of evidence for it. Fuchs and coworkers[16] reported in 13 patients reduced fibrinolytic activity following occlusion of peripheral veins in patients with PPH, which has also been reported in patients with hemophilia chronically receiving Factor 8.[17] Recently, Eisenberg and associates[18] reported elevated levels of fibrinopeptide A in patients with PPH which normalized with institution of heparin in the presence of normal levels of fibrin degradation products and elevated levels of plasminogen activator inhibitor-1, suggestive of acquired fibrolytic defect. Palevsky and colleagues[7] have postulated that the initial insult in PPH patients is at the level of the pulmonary endothelium which may lead to either intimal proliferation with smooth muscle hypertrophy or to intimal proliferation with intravascular thrombosis.

A variety of stimuli, including shear forces, viruses, drugs, and hypoxia can injure the endothelium. Recently, an association between Human Immunodeficiency Virus (HIV) infection and PPH has been reported.[19–21] In a recent paper, Polos and coworkers[21] reported 2 cases with HIV infection and plexogenic pulmonary arteriopathy. One of the 2 cases also demonstrated lymphocytic interstitial pneumonitis (LIP). The authors postulated that the vasculitis (LIP) causes pulmonary constriction thereby inducing pulmonary hypertension. They also suggested that although HIV infection is the most likely mechanism, it is premature to conclude that the HIV infection is the culprit inducing pulmonary hypertension. An increased incidence of PPH has been reported in women taking oral contraceptives,[22] although in the NIH registry, no relationship between pregnancy, oral contraceptive use, and PPH was found.[2]

Rich and associates[23] found positive antinuclear antibodies at titers 1-80 dilutions or greater in 40% of 43 patients with PPH and in only 6% of patients with secondary forms of pulmonary hypertension. In the normal population the incidence of positive antinuclear antibodies is also 6%. In the NIH registry[2] positive antinuclear antibody tests were reported in approximately one-third of the patients. These findings, in addition to the female prevalence of PPH, as well as the presence of Raynaud's phenomenon in about 10% of the patients with PPH and the occurrence of pulmonary hypertension in patients with connective tissue disease, lends support to the possibility that PPH is an autoimmune disease. In conclusion, the exact pathogenetic mechanism that leads to PPH has not yet been identified. With new advances at the cellular and molecular level it appears certain that over the next few decades PPH will be better understood and therefore, we can be cautiously optimistic about the future in terms of deriving new therapeutic strategies.

DIAGNOSTIC TESTS

ROENTGENOGRAM

The initial evaluation of patients with PPH should include noninvasive tests such as chest x-ray, electrocardiogram, echo-Doppler, and a lung scan in order to exclude any secondary causes of pulmonary hypertension. The chest x-ray is the first important screening test in the evaluation of patients with PPH. The findings on the chest x-ray include: enlargement of the main and hilar pulmonary arteries with pruning of the peripheral vasculature.[2,24] An example is shown in Figure 1. The lung fields are generally clear in PPH. Increased brochovascular markings at the bases have been described in PVOD.[25-30] It is important to obtain a good quality, upright posteroanterior and lateral chest x-ray in order to help exclude lung disease as an underlying cause. It is also important to remember that clear lung fields (on a chest x-ray) do not exclude interstitial lung disease as possible etiology.[31]

ELECTROCARDIOGRAPHY

The electrocardiogram frequently will demonstrate right ventricular hypertrophy.[2] The most common findings are right-axis deviation (QRS axis >90), tall R waves in V_1-V_2 with qR patterns suggestive of systemic pulmonary pressures, ST-segment depression, and T-wave inversion in the right precordial leads all indicative of systemic pulmonary pressures including right ventricular strain. Often right bundle branch block may be present. The P waves are tall and peaked, reflecting right atrial enlargement. Atrial arrhythmias are rare. Interestingly, in the NIH registry, none of the 187 patients had arrhythmias. It has been proposed that in PPH, because of low and fixed cardiac output an increased rate and the loss of atrial contraction will produce rapid hemodynamic deterioration incompatible with life.

PULMONARY FUNCTION TESTS

Pulmonary function tests are an essential part of the initial evaluation of patients with PPH in order to rule out obstructive airway disease. Data from the NIH registry demonstrated mild but significant reduction in total lung capacity (89% ±17% predicted) and vital capacity (79% ±19% predicted) confirming the data obtained in previous studies.[32] The diffusion capacity for carbon monoxide is usually reduced because of the increased capillary distance secondary to pulmonary vascular lesions.

Hypoxemia is a routine finding in patients with PPH. The data from the NIH registry demonstrated a mean arterial PO_2 pressure of

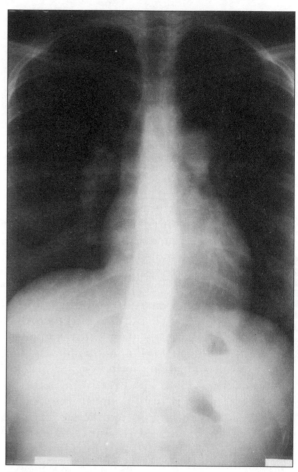

Figure 1. *A posteroanterior projection from a 23-year-old woman with primary pulmonary hypertension clearly demonstrates a prominent main pulmonary artery and hilar pulmonary arteries with oligemia and tapering of the peripheral pulmonary vessels. Mild right atrial enlargement is also present.*

72 ±16 mm Hg because of ventilation perfusion mismatches and in some patients right-to-left shunting across the patent foramen ovale. There is no correlation between pulmonary function tests and PAP.[2] However, an arterial PO_2 of less than 70 mm Hg has been shown to correlate with poor prognosis.[33]

LUNG SCAN

Perfusion tests such as ventilation lung scan are essential in order to exclude chronic pulmonary emboli. The differentiation of PPH from pulmonary hypertension secondary to chronic pulmonary thromboemboli is extremely important since pulmonary thrombectomy has been shown to be safe and effective.[34] The NIH registry series demonstrated that approximately 40% of patients with PPH have a normal lung scan, while 60% have an abnormal scan. The majority have major defects and a minority have a single subsegmental defect. The severity of abnormalities in a lung scan does not correlate with the hemodynamic and physical data.

However, a correlation has been found between perfusion patterns and underlying lesions.[9] Patients with plexogenic pulmonary arteriopathy have a normal perfusion scan, while patients with thrombotic pulmonary arteriopathy and PVOD may have patchy distribution. We believe that the risks associated with lung scans in these patients have been overstated. In the NIH registry there were no morbid clinical events reported with a performance of a lung scan in any of the patients with pulmonary hypertension.[2]

At this time, if pulmonary embolism is strongly suspected, a pulmonary angiogram is important to confirm the diagnosis. Recently, ultrafast computed tomography (CT) has been reported in a retrospective study to have a sensitivity of 95% and a specificity of 80%.[35] These initial results look promising and may obviate the need to perform an invasive test such as pulmonary angiography.

ECHO-DOPPLER

Echocardiography has 2 roles in the assessment of patients with PPH: first, to exclude other valvular and vascular causes of elevated right-sided pressures; second, to quantitatively and qualitatively estimate the hemodynamic abnormalities associated with this disorder. With advances in 2-dimensional echocardiography and echo-Doppler, noninvasive determination of pulmonary pressure has been possible.[36] Estimation of pulmonary pressure requires the detection of tricuspid regurgitation. Echo-Doppler estimation of right ventricular (RV) pressure (RVP) is based upon the formula relating pressure to blood flow velocity: $\Delta P = 4V^2$. By applying this formula to tricuspid regurgitation jets, a pressure gradient between RV and RA during systole can be measured.

Right ventricular systolic pressure (RVSP) can be expressed by the formula: RVSP = ΔP + RAP (right atrial pressure). The reliability of this estimation has been repeatedly documented by several investigators.[36-39] The Doppler estimation of pulmonary pressure, both systolic and diastolic, incorporates the RAP in the calculation. The estimation of RAP adds another source of error and controversy into the measurement. Some investigators have proposed fixed estimates and have suggested adding 10 mm Hg, others 5 mm Hg, and still others 12 mm Hg.[37] In patients without right ventricular failure or severe tricuspid regurgitation, these estimates add only a small error to the measurement. When the RAP is quite elevated, this approach can cause considerable error. Therefore, direct measurement of the height of ventricular venous pulse has been proposed by others.[36] Typically, the echo-Doppler findings in patients with PPH are right ventricular and right atrial dilatation while the LV cavity size is reduced. Using echo-Doppler techniques, Louie et al[40] demonstrated that in patients with PPH the LV is distorted from its usual circular configuration by a flattening of the ventricular septum toward the center of the LV, causing underfilling of the LV during diastole. Right ventricular hypertrophy (RVH) is often present in PPH and the septum usually shows reduced movement as a result of elevated RVP. The use of continuous-wave Doppler studies has been advocated for the noninvasive follow-up of patients with PPH on vasodilator therapy. However, the precision with which Doppler can detect minor changes in PAP is questionable at this time. These measurements have sources of error and are dependent upon the quality of the equipment and the skill of those performing and interpreting the studies. The most important limitation of the technique for the diagnosis of PPH is that the sensitivity falls off with lower levels of pulmonary hypertension.[41]

All of the noninvasive tests mentioned above are useful in the initial evaluation of patients with PPH; however, they have their limitations. In the National Heart, Lung, and Blood Institute (NHLBI) registry,[2] 6% of patients had normal chest roentgenograms, echocardiograms, and electrocardiograms despite the presence of significant pulmonary hypertension on cardiac catheterization. Therefore, if the diagnosis is strongly suspected, right-heart catheterization should be part of a complete evaluation of patients with PPH.

CARDIAC CATHETERIZATION

Cardiac catheterization is an integral part of the initial evaluation of patients with PPH. The goals of catheterization are: first, to directly measure the level of PAP and estimate PVR; second, to exclude any left-to-right shunts or any other significant cardiac disorders affecting the left side of the heart; and third, to test the response of various therapeutic agents. By the time patients with PPH present to the cardiac catheterization laboratory, the mean PAP are frequently between 50-60 mm Hg with increases in RAP.[2,42]

Instrumentation of the PA in patients with PPH may be difficult because of significant tricuspid regurgitation, dilatation of the right-sided chambers, severely elevated PAP, and low cardiac output. The key to a successful right-sided heart catheterization is having the physicians performing the catheterization study be persistent and take their time, sampling multiple areas of the lungs to obtain accurate wedge pressure tracings. Typically patients with PPH have low or normal pulmonary wedge pressure.[2] If the wedge pressure is substantially elevated, left-heart catheterization should be performed to measure the LV end-diastolic pressure directly in order to exclude PVOD causing the impediment of left atrial filling. Other times an elevated wedge pressure may mean an occult mitral valve stenosis. Cardiac catheterization is a relatively safe procedure in patients with PPH. In the NIH registry, 10 out of 187 patients who underwent right heart catheterization experienced severe morbid events, that is, extreme hypotension and hemoptysis during catheterization. However, no deaths occurred as a result of catheterization in the NIH series.[2] Therefore, although right-heart catheterization is an invasive procedure, it carries some risk. In our experience, right-heart catheterization should be part of a complete evaluation, especially when therapeutic interventions are contemplated, such as vasodilator therapy.

LUNG BIOPSY

Patients in the NIH registry with plexiform lesions and PVOD have a worse prognosis than patients with thrombotic lesions, even when differences in baseline hemodynamics are taken into account.[7] Lung biopsy has not been shown to be useful and is still controversial. Open lung biopsy in patients with PPH is associated with an increased risk for complications. There was 1 death reported in the NIH registry. Because of the risks involved and because the knowledge of histologic features has no impact on the management of most patients with PPH, routine lung biopsy is not recommended in the evaluation of these patients.

One of the major difficulties in making an early diagnosis of PPH is that the first symptom, dyspnea — which is the most common symptom — is actually part of normal life. The importance of early diagnosis in these patients cannot be overemphasized, because early diagnosis may offer a substantial benefit to patients with PPH before the disease is fully advanced. Until we better understand the pathogenesis of this lethal disorder, our goal should be to do a thorough work-up, including a history and physical examination, using all the noninvasive tests available in order to diagnose this disorder in the early stages.

PROGNOSIS

Unfortunately, there is very little information except for a few case reports on the duration of the presymptomatic phase. After the onset of symptoms, the survival time is 2–3 years, with shorter times reported in children. The clinical course of PPH is highly variable and cannot be predicted on the basis of clinical presentation and hemodynamic data. Right ventricular failure is a bad prognostic sign and once RV failure takes place, survival beyond 2 years is unlikely. Progression of the disease and clinical deterioration are associated with decreased cardiac output rather than an increased PAP.

Results from the NIH registry demonstrated that variables such as elevated mean RAP (MRAP), elevated mean PAP (MPAP) and decreased cardiac index (CI) were associated with poor survival.[42] Patients with PPH usually die of intractable RV failure or sudden death. Probably the most common mechanism of sudden death is the presence of atrial tachyarrhythmias. Other mechanisms include tachyarrhythmias associated with right ventricular infarction.

THERAPY

Changes in lifestyle such as pregnancy aggravate PPH because of increased volume load, tachycardia, and decreased peripheral resistance not associated with a decrease in PVR. It is well known from the obstetrics literature that both fetal and maternal mortality are extremely high in patients with PPH.[43,44] Therefore patients are strongly advised against pregnancy. Patients with PPH have a variable clinical course and their well-being might change from day-to-day. We advise our patients to follow their symptoms and limit activity on the days when they feel more symptomatic and maximize their activities on days when their symptoms are reduced. Because PPH becomes worse at high altitudes, we advise patients who live at high altitudes to move to sea level and avoid traveling at high altitudes.

OXYGEN SUPPLEMENTATION

Arterial oxygen saturation below 70 mm Hg has been shown to be associated with poor survival and a high incidence of sudden death in patients with PPH.[33] It is thought that hypoxia produces pulmonary vasoconstriction and increases viscosity due to secondary polycythemia. Thus, oxygen supplementation may benefit patients with PPH. However, this benefit has not been documented in controlled studies.[45] Despite the lack of documented beneficial effects, oxygen supplementation is usually prescribed in patients with arterial hypoxemia with the hope to improve exercise tolerance and decrease the risk of myocardial ischemia and arrhythmias.

PHARMACOLOGIC THERAPY

There are 2 categories of pharmacologic agents used in the treatment of PPH: anticoagulants and vasodilators. Digitalis and diuretics are used in patients with right ventricular failure and PVOD to reduce capillary wedge pressure.

The rationale to use anticoagulation therapy is 2-fold: first, thrombi have been found in a majority of patients with PPH at biopsy. The use of anticoagulants has been advocated to hold the progression of the disease even if the thrombus is not the cause of PPH but is the result of endothelial injury. Second, patients who received anticoagulation therapy in a retrospective study[33] had a better survival rate than patients who did not (50% vs 25%, respectively, at 3 years).

Vasodilating agents have been proposed for the treatment of PPH since the early 1950s by Wood,[13] who advanced the hypothesis that PPH was caused by constriction of the pulmonary arteries. Since then, numerous vasodilators have been used in the treatment of PPH: ß-adrenergic agonists, α-adrenergic blockers, direct vasodilators, angiotensin-converting enzyme inhibitors, calcium-channel blockers and prostaglandins (Table 2). Experiences with phentolamine and prazosin have been very limited and disappointing.[46–48] Diazoxide was becoming popular as an effective treatment of severe essential hypertension and a report describing the effect of that agent on patients with PPH suggested that it might be useful.[49] However, when the drug was used more widely, it was shown that several deaths could be attributed to diazoxide.[50] In 1980, Rubin and Peter[51] reported their experience of 4 patients, using oral hydralazine as the treatment for this disorder. However, shortly afterwards Packer and associates[52] reported adverse effects of hydralazine in patients with PPH.

Calcium-channel blockers and prostacyclin appear to hold the most promising results. Rubin and colleagues[53] recently demonstrated that using nifedipine in patients with PPH lowered PVR and improved RV performance. However, the calcium-channel blockers as a group have also been reported to be harmful.[54] In 1985 Rich and coworkers[55] evaluated the response of 23 consecutive patients referred with PPH for the acute administration of either hydralazine or nifedipine. They found a 20% reduction in PVR which was considered a favorable response. Some patients lowered their PVR even less than 20% with a poor clinical course. However, 18 of the 23 patients did respond acutely with lowered pulmonary resistance. Over time it was found that some patients got better, some got worse, and some stayed the same. The other half of the patients were not treated with a vasodilator and again, similar responses were observed: some patients got better, some got worse, and some stayed the same. Survival curves using Kaplan-Meier estimates demonstrated that the patients who had an acute reduction in pulmonary resistance from vasodilators did better than those who did not. But no treatment changed their survival. Recently, Rich and Brundage[56] proposed the use of high-dose calcium-channel blockers based upon their experience in 8 of 13 patients with PPH. Pulmonary vascular resistance and pressure showed only minimal reduction when a standard dose of nifedipine or diltiazem was given, but a larger reduction of 48% in PAP and 60% in PVR was observed when higher doses of calcium blockers were administered. There were no differences in clinical baseline and hemodynamics between respondents and non-respondents. When restudied after 1 year on therapy with calcium-channel blockers, 5 patients maintained a reduction in PAP and a regression of right ventricular hypertrophy was seen by ECG and echocardiography. The chronic oral high-dose calcium-channel blocker administration is determined as follows: nifedipine 10 mg orally is given every hour in a hemodynamically monitored setting until the patient develops gastrointestinal upset, systemic hypotension, or a significant decrease in mean PAP. If this dose is well-tolerated and the patient responds (a reduction in mean PAP of 20% or more than the baseline), then a daily dose of nifedipine is given in divided doses of 6–8 hour intervals. The amount of nifedipine given every 6–8 hours depends upon the dose of nifedipine the patient tolerated. If, for example, the patient tolerated 40 mg of nifedipine and had a good response then the patient would

Table 2. Vasodilators That Have Been or are Currently Used in the Treatment of Primary Pulmonary Hypertension
ß-adrenergic agonists:
Isoproterenol
Terbutaline
α-adrenergic blockers:
Phentolamine
Prazosin
Tolazoline
Direct vasodilators:
Diazoxide
Hydralazine
Angiotensin-converting enzyme inhibitors:
Captopril
Calcium-channel blockers:
Nifedipine
Diltiazem
Prostaglandins (PGI_2) (E_1):
Prostacyclin (Flolan)

receive 40 mg every 6 hours/day for a total of 160 mg. Similarly, diltiazem 60 mg orally can be used acutely to determine the chronic dose. Most recently, calcium-channel blockers have been shown for the first time to improve survival. Rich and colleagues[57] demonstrated that some patients with PPH will respond very well to high doses of calcium-channel blockers associated with a reduction in PAP, PVR and improved quality of life and survival when followed for 5 years. Interestingly, patients who did not respond to the vasodilators and were put on warfarin also had improved survival. The study did not address whether the non-respondents had more advanced vascular disease or a specific histologic type of vascular disease. Therefore, a therapeutic regimen that covers a wide spectrum of abnormalities associated with the pulmonary vascular bed may clearly benefit these patients. A recent multicenter study using prostacyclin (Flolan) randomized 81 patients with PPH. Forty-one patients were randomized to prostacyclin plus conventional therapy and 40 were randomized to conventional therapy alone. Patients were followed for 12 weeks, at the end of which time no deaths were observed in the treatment group, whereas 8 deaths were observed in the conventional therapy group (*P* = 0.0027).[58] In addition, the study demonstrated improvement in exercise tolerance, hemodynamics, and their subjective well-being. This is the first time that prostacyclin has been shown to increase survival. The disadvantage at the present time is that prostacyclin has to be given through a central catheter with continuous infusion. There are adverse effects associated with chronic IV administration such as infection or malfunction of the pump. Prostacyclin is useful as a bridge to lung transplantation.

LUNG TRANSPLANTATION

Lung transplantation is another alternative for patients with severe PPH. Currently, according to the registry of the International Society for Heart Transplant[59] the 1-year survival rate is more than 60%, with a 2-year survival being 55%. Early mortality (<30 days from surgery) remains elevated 20% to 30% due to intra-operative complications such as post-surgical multi-organ failure and infections. Single-lung transplantation appears to have a more favorable result than double-lung transplantation and the number of patients with PPH undergoing single-lung transplant is steadily increasing. In addition, a potential advantage of single-lung transplant over double-lung transplant is the low incidence of chronic obliterative bronchiolitis. Pulmonary transplantation improves survival and function in patients with end-stage PPH.[60] There is a dramatic improvement in PAP and resistance associated with an increase in cardiac output within a few hours following transplant. On the echocardiogram there is regression of RVH as well as on the ECG which usually occurs within a few weeks.

SUMMARY

In summary, several important advances have been made in the field of the management of PPH. With improvements in our understanding of the pathogenetic mechanisms of PPH there is a tendency now to recognize that for in situ thrombosis anticoagulants can be used for patients felt to have underlying pulmonary

thrombosis. Vasodilators in sufficient doses can substantially reduce PAP and PVR which may, in turn, cause a regression of RVH and significant clinical improvement. A major challenge today is the early diagnosis of pulmonary hypertension in these patients when the disease is at a much more controllable stage and to develop new, effective strategies in the treatment of this lethal disorder.

SECONDARY PULMONARY HYPERTENSION

The differential diagnosis of secondary pulmonary hypertension is quite large and includes congenital heart disease such as ventricular septal defect (VSD) causing Eisenmenger's syndrome, valvular heart disease such as mitral stenosis, chronic pulmonary embolism, lung parenchymal disease including connective tissue disorders, COPD, sleep apnea, and other less frequently encountered disorders (Table 1).

CONGENITAL HEART DISEASE

Basically, there are 2 mechanisms of secondary pulmonary hypertension that lead to pulmonary hypertension: pressure overload and volume overload. Pressure overload conditions include PPH and pulmonic valve stenosis. Volume overload includes congenital heart disease with left-to-right shunt causing an increase in pulmonary flow which may eventually lead to Eisenmenger's syndrome. Pre-tricuspid congenital heart disease such as atrial septal defect (ASD) causes an increase in pulmonary flow. However, pulmonary pressures do not increase until late in the course of the disease. On the other hand, post-tricuspid left-to-right shunts such as VSD cause an increase in pulmonary flow as well as an increase in pulmonary pressures early on. The physical examination reflects the underlying congenital heart disease. It is important to note that late in the course of left-to-right shunt such as VSD, the physical examination may not reveal any murmurs and the patient may present with cyanosis due to a right-to-left shunt. When there is evidence of right-to-left shunt with pulmonary pressures at the systemic level, surgery will neither improve symptoms nor decrease pulmonary pressures.

From a pathologic point of view, Heath and Edwards[61] classified pulmonary vascular lesions into 6 grades reflecting a sequential structural change in the pulmonary vascular bed. Grade I shows medial hypertrophy of small muscular pulmonary arteries and arterioles. Grade II is characterized by intimal proliferation. Grade III demonstrates advanced medial thickening with hypertrophy and hyperplasia as well as intimal proliferation and concentric fibrosis that results in the obliteration of many of the small pulmonary vessels. Grade IV is characterized by the so-called "plexiform lesions" seen in the muscular pulmonary arteries and arterioles. Grade V includes complex plexiform as well as angiomatous and cavernous lesions and hyalinization of intimal fibrosis. Finally, Grade VI represents necrotizing arteritis. There is general agreement that Grade I represents the early stage and Grade VI represents the end stage of pulmonary vascular obliterative disease. However, the pathologic lesions in the pulmonary vascular bed may not progress in such an orderly fashion as suggested by the findings of Wagenvoort[62] which indicate that plexiform lesions develop in stages in the areas affected by necrotizing arteritis.

Patients with Eisenmenger's syndrome typically present with dyspnea, fatigue, hemoptysis, or syncope. At times they might complain of atypical chest pain. On physical examination signs of severe pulmonary hypertension include cyanosis and clubbing. In patients with Eisenmenger's syndrome due to patent ductus arteriosus, cyanosis, and clubbing are characteristically found in the lower extremities but not in the upper extremities. The chest x-ray reveals enlargement of the main pulmonary arteries with tapered peripheral vessels and the presence of an enlargement of the RA and the RV. Patients usually die from sudden death. The cause of sudden death is usually either a ventricular arrhythmia, endocarditis, severe heart failure, or severe hemoptysis.[63]

MITRAL STENOSIS

Pulmonary hypertension associated with mitral stenosis initially is the result of an increase in resistance to pulmonary venous drainage and backwards transmission of elevated left atrial pressure (passive). Later, it exhibits marked pulmonary vasoconstriction and anatomic changes in the pulmonary vessels take place (reactive). Pulmonary hypertension in mitral stenosis due to increased PVR may dominate the clinical picture.[64,65] When pulmonary hypertension develops, it may be difficult on physical examination to distinguish a loud pulmonic component of S_2 from an S_2-opening snap interval. The cardiac output decreases and the patients develop dyspnea, becoming worse on exertion.

Noninvasive tests such as echo-Doppler are very useful for the diagnosis of mitral stenosis. At catheterization it is important to distinguish mitral stenosis from PPH and PVOD. In PPH left atrial size and pulmonary capillary wedge pressure are normal and there is no gradient between the wedge and left ventricular pressures. In PVOD, wedge pressure is elevated.

CHRONIC PULMONARY EMBOLISM

It is important to diagnose chronic pulmonary embolism because it may present the same way as PPH. The predominant symptom is unexplained dyspnea on exertion just as it is in PPH. There is an important diagnostic finding on physical examination which is characteristic of chronic thrombotic pulmonary hypertension. On physical examination murmurs are present and are heard over the lung fields. Therefore, because these murmurs are not heard in PPH and rarely in other diseases of pulmonary blood vessels, they are an important diagnostic clue.[66] Other diagnostic tests include pulmonary function tests, lung scans, and echo-Doppler studies.[67] Pulmonary angiography is an essential part of the diagnostic work-up in these patients. In most patients with acute pulmonary embolism the pulmonary embolus usually resolves with time. However, sometimes the thrombus persists causing severe pulmonary hypertension. Today, patients with chronic thromboembolic disease can be treated successfully with thrombectomy.[68,69] Recently, ultrafast CT has been shown to be useful in the detection of pulmonary emboli.[35] Because of its high, special and temporal resolution, ultrafast

CT may be a useful addition in the noninvasive detection of pulmonary emboli. In patients with documented proximal pulmonary artery thrombi, thrombectomy in selected cases provides dramatic improvement. Vasodilators may be effective in some patients with obstruction at the arteriolar level. In patients with both proximal pulmonary emboli and microvascular thrombi, chronic anticoagulation with warfarin, to prevent further progression or extension of thrombi, is recommended.[70]

LUNG PARENCHYMAL DISEASE

The most common condition of parenchymal lung disease leading to hypoxic pulmonary hypertension is COPD. Other conditions include chronic diffuse pulmonary parenchymal disease, inadequate respiratory excursion, and residence at a high altitude. In chronic obstructive lung disease there are 2 clinical entities to consider: patients with predominantly chronic bronchitis and patients with predominant emphysema. Individuals with chronic bronchitis are likely to have manifestations of cor pulmonale,[71] and peripheral edema. Other signs and symptoms may include mental irritability and hypersomnia. A chronic productive cough is characteristic of chronic bronchitis and is almost always present. Long-standing COPD may lead to bronchitis and may cause chronic cor pulmonale. Patients with emphysema may present with a long history of dyspnea upon exertion and markedly decreased lung sounds on physical examination. As the disease progresses, hypoxemia and hypercapnia become manifest in patients with cor pulmonale. Other lung parenchymal disorders that are associated with pulmonary hypertension include a variant of scleroderma, the so-called CREST syndrome, ("calcinosis," Raynaud's phenomenon, esophageal dysmotility, sclerodactyly, and telangiectasia).[72-74] Various other forms of vascular disease have been reported to cause pulmonary hypertension. These entities include Raynaud's phenomenon,[75,76] dermatomyositis,[77] rheumatoid arthritis,[78] as well as systemic lupus erythematosus.[79,80] Another entity, so-called idiopathic pulmonary fibrosis or Hamman-Rich syndrome, has also been reported to cause pulmonary hypertension.[81] In addition, pulmonary hemosiderosis[82] and sarcoidosis[83] have been associated with pulmonary hypertension.

PICKWICK SYNDROME

Obesity-hypoventilation syndrome (Pickwick syndrome) is characterized by obesity, somnolence, edema, and is associated with cor pulmonale. Although the underlying mechanism is not well understood, 2 mechanisms have been postulated: first, inadequate respiratory excursion due to extreme obesity; and second, hypoventilation due to a reduced sensitivity of the central respiratory center.[84-86] Therapy involves weight reduction and progesterone.[87,88]

SLEEP APNEA SYNDROME

This disorder is characterized by very frequent apneic episodes during sleep. These patients rarely reach the deep stages of sleep because of a hypoxic arousal and thus are chronically sleep deprived. There are 3 forms of sleep apnea syndrome: First is a central form of apnea in which there is cessation of all respiratory muscle effort and airflow stops. Second, obstructive apnea, which is characterized by an airway obstruction causing airflow to cease. Characteristically these patients are obese or have other anatomic abnormalities of the upper airway, snore loudly, have morning headaches, daytime hypersomnolence and systemic hypertension. It is believed that the obstruction results from relaxation or discoordination of the buccal and pharyngeal muscles, causing collapse of the walls of the pharynx during inspiration. Third, is a mixed apnea in which airflow and respiratory efforts stop early in the episode.[89-91] The apneic periods occur 40–60 times/hour.[91] This leads to hypoxemia and hypercapnia. Consequently, patients develop cor pulmonale. Chronic hypoxemia results in progressive pulmonary hypertension during sleep and is associated with both brady- and tachyrhythmias.[89] The obstructive form of sleep apnea has been treated with tracheostomy and continuous positive airway pressure (CPAP) applied to the nose during sleep and surgical procedures consisting of removal of enlarged tonsils or adenoids or surgical enlargement of the entrance of the airway.[91] In these patients, any drugs that will suppress the ventilatory stimulus must be avoided.

MISCELLANEOUS CAUSES OF PULMONARY HYPERTENSION

Other less frequently encountered causes of pulmonary hypertension include high-altitude pulmonary edema[92-94] and isolated partial anomalous pulmonary venous drainage.[95] Ingestion of a variety of substances including crotalaria alkaloids and aminorex (an appetite suppressant) have been associated with pulmonary hypertension.[96,97] Finally, hepatic cirrhosis with portal hypertension has been linked with pulmonary hypertension.[98] An association between PPH and portal hypertension has also been reported.[99]

THERAPY OF SECONDARY PULMONARY HYPERTENSION

The underlying cause must always be identified and should be corrected whenever possible. For example, in a patient with congenital heart defect, the shunt must be surgically corrected before there is presence of right-to-left shunt and before significant pulmonary hypertension ensues. In patients with chronic obstructive pulmonary disease, administration of oxygen has been shown to improve survival.[100,101] In an NIH-sponsored study[101] the investigators sought to determine whether survival could improve through continuous oxygen supplementation given day and night compared to nocturnal oxygen therapy alone. On the other hand, a British study[100] sought to demonstrate whether oxygen administration for 15–24 hours a day had a positive impact on survival when it was compared to the group with no oxygen. Both studies clearly demonstrated that survival was better in patients who received oxygen supplementation for the longest part of the day. The criterion most commonly used to initiate chronic oxygen therapy is a PO_2 of 55 mm Hg or less. In patients with mitral stenosis, valve replacement or balloon valvuloplasty should be performed.[102-104] After valve replacement,

symptoms subside and the pulmonary pressure gradually returns to normal.

COR PULMONALE

The term cor pulmonale describes right ventricular dysfunction or hypertrophy secondary to pulmonary hypertension resulting from disorders that affect either the structure or the function of the lungs. An important characteristic of the normal pulmonary circulation is its low resistance and high capacitance in relation to the systemic circulation. Thus, in order for the right ventricle to eject the cardiac output it only needs to employ a small fraction of pressure developed by the left ventricle. Therefore, pulmonary vascular blood flow may increase substantially without a concomitant increase in pulmonary artery pressure. Consequently, pulmonary hypertension sufficient to cause cor pulmonale is almost always indicative of a disease process that has resulted in substantial vasoconstriction or occlusion of the pulmonary arterial tree and it does not result from high cardiac output or increased blood volume.

The causes of cor pulmonale are numerous (Table 1). The most common cause in the United States is chronic obstructive pulmonary disease which includes chronic bronchitis, emphysema, and in some cases, bronchial asthma. It is estimated that 47 million people in the United States alone suffer from chronic lung disease.[105] Together, chronic bronchitis and emphysema account for approximately 30,000 deaths in this country.[106]

DIAGNOSIS

The clinical manifestations of cor pulmonale are often obscured by the signs and symptoms of the underlying pulmonary disease or disorder. Therefore, it is necessary to first recognize the type and severity of the lung disease and then look for the whole syndrome of cor pulmonale. No history is specific for cor pulmonale. Patients with cor pulmonale usually will present with increasing dyspnea, paroxysmal cough, at times syncope, with fluid retention edema, and sometimes ascites. On physical examination the neck veins are distended and prominent a and v waves may be noted with lack of collapse during inspiration suggestive of increased right-sided pressures. Central cyanosis may be present and hypoxia measured by oxygen saturation correlates with the pulmonary artery pressure.[107] On auscultation there is a loud pulmonic closure sound diagnostic of pulmonary hypertension and a right ventricular lift due to right ventricular hypertrophy. In addition, there is usually a right ventricular S_3 gallop heard best at the left sternal edge or in the epigastrium and is accentuated by inspiration. A holosystolic murmur is also present along the lower left parasternal edge and is accentuated by inspiration, indicating tricuspid regurgitation.

THERAPY

The management of cor pulmonale consists primarily of treatment of the underlying disease and oxygen administration in an effort to reduce pulmonary hypertension by improving oxygenation.[108–110] In order to accomplish this goal, reduction in bronchial smooth muscle constriction, rapid drainage of secretions, and treatment of respiratory infections must be carried out through the administration of bronchodilators, ß-agonists, antibiotics, and oxygen supplementation.

Administration of home oxygen has been shown to improve survival in patients with chronic obstructive pulmonary disease. Both the British study[100] and the American NIH study[101] demonstrated that survival was worst in those who did not receive oxygen supplementation and best in those who received oxygen for the longest portion of the day. When chronic oxygen administration is contemplated, caution should be exercised as some patients with COPD may retain CO_2 leading to depression of their ventilatory drive and subsequent hypercapnia. Pulmonary hypertension is the most important variable that contributes significantly to mortality in patients with chronic respiratory disease. The severity of pulmonary hypertension correlates more closely with survival than any other variables studied.[111–113] Patients with severe COPD and FEV_1 (forced expiratory volume in 1 second) < 1 liter but without pulmonary hypertension have a better survival than those without FEV_1 of less than 1 liter but with pulmonary hypertension. In a study by Bishop,[112] less than 10% of patients with a mean pulmonary artery pressure of 45 mm Hg or more survived 5 years. Traver and associates[113] found a 50% mortality rate at 7 years in patients with cor pulmonale and at 13.5 years in those without cor pulmonale in a study of patients with obstructive lung disease.

In an attempt to decrease pulmonary artery pressures, several vasodilatory agents have been used.[46,49,114,115] These agents will inhibit vasoconstriction due to hypoxia and will decrease afterload thereby improving right ventricular function. A calcium-channel blocker, nitrendipine, has been reported to reduce pulmonary vascular resistance and pulmonary artery pressure, and increase cardiac output at 6 weeks.[115]

Although vasodilators will increase right ventricular stroke volume and reduce pulmonary vascular resistance acutely in patients with severe pulmonary hypertension, these hemodynamic benefits last only for a short period of time. None of these agents has been shown to improve survival.[115–118]

Finally, it is important to mention that vasodilator therapy carries significant side effects such as systemic hypotension and worsening of hypoxemia by increasing venous admixture.[52] In addition, calcium-channel blockers may reduce right ventricular contractility.[54] Digitalis therapy in cor pulmonale patients is still controversial. The consensus is that there is no clearcut evidence that digitalis is of substantial benefit unless left ventricular dysfunction coexists.[119]

Diuretics are commonly used for cor pulmonale patients with symptomatic peripheral edema. Clinicians should exercise caution when diuretics are administered as they cause hypokalemia which can induce digitalis toxicity arrhythmias and exacerbate multifocal atrial tachycardia. In addition, since they reduce right ventricular preload, diuretics may cause hypotension.

REFERENCES

1. World Health Organization. *Primary Pulmonary Hypertension.* Hatano S, Strasser T (eds). Geneva: World Health Organization;1975:7-45.
2. Rich S, Dantzker DR, Ayres SM, et al. Primary pulmonary hypertension: A national prospective study. *Ann Intern Med.* 1987;107:216-223.
3. Lloyd JE, Primm PK, Newman JH. Familial primary pulmonary hypertension: Clinical patterns. *Am Rev Respir Dis.* 1984;129:194-197.
4. Wagenvoort CA, Wagenvoort N. Primary pulmonary hypertension: A pathologic study of the lung vessels in 156 clinically diagnosed cases. *Circulation.* 1970;42:1163-1184.
5. Bjornsson J, Edwards WD. Primary pulmonary hypertension: A histopathologic study of 80 cases. *Mayo Clin Proc.* 1985;60:16-25.
6. Pietra GG, Edwards WD, Kay JM, et al. Histopathology of primary pulmonary hypertension. A qualitative and quantitative study of pulmonary blood vessels from 58 patients in the National Heart, Lung and Blood Institute Primary Pulmonary Hypertension Registry. *Circulation.* 1989;80:1198-1206.
7. Palevsky HI, Schloo BL, Pietra GG, et al. Primary pulmonary hypertension. Vascular structure, morphometry and responsiveness to vasodilator agents. *Circulation.* 1989;80:1207-1221.
8. Rich S, Brundage BH. Pulmonary hypertension: A cellular basis for understanding the pathophysiology and treatment. *J Am Coll Cardiol.* 1989;14:545-550.
9. Rich S, Pietra GG, Kieras K. Primary pulmonary hypertension: Radiographic and scintigraphic patterns of histologic subtypes. *Ann Intern Med.*1986;105:499-502.
10. Wagenvoort CA, Mulder PGH. Thrombotic lesions in primary plexogenic arteriopathy. Similar pathogenesis or complication? *Chest.* 1993;103:844-849.
11. Weir EK, Archer SL, Edwards JE. Chronic primary and secondary thromboembolic pulmonary hypertension. *Chest.* 1988;93:149S-154S.
12. Nicod P, Moser KM. Primary pulmonary hypertension: The risk and benefit of lung biopsy. *Circulation.* 1989;80:1486-1488.
13. Wood P. Pulmonary hypertension with special reference to the vasoconstrictive factor. *Br Heart J.* 1958;20:557-570.
14. McDonnell P, Toye P, Hutchins G. Primary pulmonary hypertension and cirrhosis: Are they related? *Am Rev Respir Dis.* 1983;127:437-441.
15. Giaid A, Yanagisawa M, Langleben D, et al. Expression of endothelin-1 in the lungs of patients with pulmonary hypertension. *N Engl J Med.* 1993;328:1732-1739.
16. Fuchs J, Mlczoch J, Niessner H. Abnormal fibrinolysis in PPH. *Eur Heart J.* 1981;2:168. Abstract.
17. Goldsmith GH, Baily RG, Brettler DB, et al. Primary pulmonary hypertension in patients with classic hemophilia. *Ann Intern Med.* 1988;108:797-799.
18. Eisenberg PR, Lucore C, Kaufman M, et al. Fibrino-peptide A levels indicative of pulmonary vascular thrombosis in patients with primary pulmonary hypertension. *Circulation.* 1990;82:841-847.
19. Coplan NL, Shimony RY, Ioachim HL, et al. Primary pulmonary hypertension associated with human immunodeficiency viral infection. *Am J Med.* 1990;89:96-99.
20. Mette SA, Palevsky HI, Pietra GG, et al. Primary pulmonary hypertension in association with human immunodeficiency virus infection. *Am Rev Respir Dis.* 1992;145:1196-1200.
21. Polos PG, Wolfe D, Harley RA, et al. Pulmonary hypertension and human immunodeficiency virus infection. Two reports and a review of the literature. *Chest.* 1992;101:474-478.
22. Kleiger RE, Boxer M, Ingham RE, et al. Pulmonary hypertension in patients using oral contraceptives. A report of six cases. *Chest.* 1976;69:143-157.
23. Rich S, Kieras K, Hart K, et al. Antinuclear antibodies in primary pulmonary hypertension. *J Am Coll Cardiol.* 1986;8:1307-1311.
24. Anderson G, Reid L, Simon G. The radiographic appearances in primary and thromboembolic pulmonary hypertension. *Clin Radiol.* 1973;24:113-120.
25. Dail DH, Liebow AA, Gmelich J, et al. A study of 43 cases of pulmonary veno-occlusive disease. *Lab Invest.* 1978;38:340-350.
26. Thadani U, Burrow C, Whitaker W, et al. Pulmonary veno-occlusive disease. *J Med.* 1975;44:133-159.
27. Kinare SG, Kelkar MD. Pulmonary veno-occlusive disease: A case report. *Angiology.* 1978;29:413-417.
28. Scheiber RL, Dedeker KL, Gleason DF, et al. Radiographic and angiographic characteristics of pulmonary veno-occlusive disease. *Diagn Radiol.* 1972;103:47-58.
29. Rambihar VS, Fallen EL, Cairns JA. Pulmonary veno-occlusive disease: Antemortem diagnosis from roentgenographic and hemodynamic findings. *Can Med Assoc J.* 1979;120:1519-1522.
30. Wagenvoort CA, Wagenvoort N, Takahashi T. Pulmonary veno-occlusive disease: Involvement of the pulmonary arteries and review of the literature. *Hum Pathol.* 1985;16:1033-1041.
31. Epler GR, McLoud TC, Gaensler EA, et al. Normal chest roentgenograms in chronic diffuse infiltrative lung disease. *N Engl J Med.* 1978;298:934-939.
32. Dantzker DR, Bower JS. Mechanisms of gas exchange abnormality in patients with chronic obliterative pulmonary vascular disease. *J Clin Invest.* 1971;64:1050-1055.
33. Fuster V, Steele PM, Edwards WD, et al. Primary pulmonary hypertension: Natural history and the importance of thrombosis. *Circulation.* 1984;70:580-587.
34. Daily PO, Dembitsky WP, Peterson KL, et al. Modifications of techniques and early results of pulmonary thromboendarterectomy for chronic pulmonary embolism. *J Thorac Cardiovasc Surg.* 1987;93:221-233.
35. Teigen CL, Maus TP, Sheedy PF, et al. Pulmonary embolism: Diagnosis with electron beam CT. *Radiology.* 1993;188:839-845.

36. Yock PG, Popp RL. Noninvasive estimation of right ventricular systolic pressure by Doppler ultrasound in patients with tricuspid regurgitation. *Circulation.* 1984;70:657-662.

37. Masuyama T, Kodama K, Kitabatake A, et al. Continuous wave Doppler echocardiographic detection of pulmonary regurgitation and its application to noninvasive estimation of pulmonary artery pressure. *Circulation.* 1986;74:484-492.

38. Berger M, Haimowitz A, VanTosh A, et al. Quantitative assessment of pulmonary hypertension in patients with tricuspid regurgitation using continuous wave Doppler ultrasound. *J Am Coll Cardiol.* 1985;6:359-365.

39. Currie PJ, Seward JB, Chan KL, et al. Continuous wave Doppler determination for right ventricular pressure: A simultaneous Doppler-catheterization study in 127 patients. *J Am Coll Cardiol.* 1985;6:750-756.

40. Louie EK, Rich S, Brundage BH. Doppler echo-cardiographic assessment of impaired left ventricular filling in patients with right ventricular pressure overload due to primary pulmonary hypertension. *J Am Coll Cardiol.* 1986;8:1298-1306.

41. Serwer GA, Cougle AG, Eckerd BM, et al. Factors affecting use of the Doppler-determined time from flow onset to maximal pulmonary artery velocity for measurement of pulmonary artery pressure in children. *Am J Cardiol.* 1986;58:352-356.

42. D'Alonzo GE, Barst RJ, Ayres SM, et al. Survival in patients with primary pulmonary hypertension: Results from a National Prospective Registry. *Ann Intern Med.* 1991;115:343-349.

43. Gleicher N, Midwall J, Hochberger D, et al. Eisenmenger's syndrome and pregnancy. *Obstet Gynecol Surv.* 1979;34:721-741.

44. Jewett JF, Ober WG. Primary pulmonary hypertension as a cause of maternal death. *Am J Obstet Gynecol.* 1956;71:1335-1341.

45. Packer M, Lee WH, Medina N, et al. Systemic vasoconstrictor effects of oxygen administration in obliterative pulmonary vascular disorders. *Am J Cardiol.* 1986;57:853-858.

46. Ruskin JN, Hutter AM Jr. Primary pulmonary hypertension treated with oral phentolamine. *Ann Intern Med.* 1979;90:772-774.

47. Cohen ML, Kronzon I. Adverse hemodynamic effects of phentolamine in primary pulmonary hypertension. *Ann Intern Med.* 1981;95:591-592.

48. Levine TB, Rose T, Kane M, et al. Treatment of primary pulmonary hypertension by alpha adrenergic blockade. *Circulation.* 1980;62:III-26. Abstract.

49. Klinke WP, Gilbert JAL. Diazoxide in primary pulmonary hypertension. *N Engl J Med.* 1980;302:91-92.

50. Rubino JM, Schroeder JS. Diazoxide in the treatment of primary pulmonary hypertension. *Br Heart J.* 1979;42:362-363.

51. Rubin LJ, Peter RH. Oral hydralazine therapy for primary pulmonary hypertension. *N Engl J Med.* 1980;302:69-73.

52. Packer MB, Greenberg B, Massie B, et al. Deleterious effects of hydralazine in patients with primary pulmonary hypertension. *N Engl J Med.* 1982; 306:1326-1331.

53. Rubin LJ, Nicod P, Hillis LD, et al. Treatment of primary pulmonary hypertension with nifedipine: A hemodynamic and scintigraphic evaluation. *Ann Intern Med.* 1983;99:433-438.

54. Packer M, Medina N, Yushak M. Adverse hemodynamic and clinical effects of calcium channel blockade in pulmonary hypertension secondary to obliterative pulmonary vascular disease. *J Am Coll Cardiol.* 1984;4:890-901.

55. Rich S, Brundage BH, Levy PS. The effect of vasodilator therapy on the clinical outcome of patients with primary pulmonary hypertension. *Circulation.* 1985;71:1191-1196.

56. Rich S, Brundage BH. High dose calcium blocking therapy for primary pulmonary hypertension: Evidence for long-term reduction in pulmonary arterial pressure and regression of right ventricular hypertrophy. *Circulation.* 1987;76:135-141.

57. Rich S, Kaufman E, Levy PS. The effect of high doses of calcium channel blockers on survival in primary pulmonary hypertension. *N Engl J Med.* 1992;327:76-81.

58. Long W, Rubin L, Barst R, et al. Randomized trial of conventional therapy alone (CT) vs. conventional therapy + continuous infusions of prostacyclin (CT + PG12) in primary pulmonary hypertension (PPH): A 12-week study. *Am Rev Respir Dis.* 1993;147:4A 538. Abstract.

59. Kriett JM, Kaye MP. The Registry of the International Society for Heart Transplantation: Seventh Official Report, 1990. *J Heart Transplant.* 1990;9:323-330.

60. Williams TJ, Grossman RF, Maurer JR. Long-term functional follow-up of lung transplant recipients. *Clin Chest Med.* 1990;11:347-358.

61. Heath D, Edwards JE. The pathology of hypertensive pulmonary changes in the pulmonary arteries with special references to congenital cardiac septal defects. *Circulation.* 1958;18:533-547.

62. Wagenvoort CA, Wagenvoort N. *Pathology of Pulmonary Hypertension.* New York: John Wiley and Sons; 1977:56-94.

63. Grossman W, Braunwald E. Pulmonary hypertension. In: Braunwald E (ed). *Heart Disease: A Textbook of Cardiovascular Medicine.* Philadelphia: W.B. Saunders; 1992:790-816.

64. Grossman W. Profiles in valvular heart disease. In: Grossman W, Baim DS (eds). *Cardiac catheterization, Angiography and Intervention.* 4th ed. Philadelphia: Lea and Febiger; 1991:557-581.

65. Dexter L. Physiologic changes in mitral stenosis. *N Engl J Med.* 1956;254:829-830.

66. Auger WR, Moser KM. Pulmonary flow murmurs: A distinctive physical sign found in chronic pulmonary thromboembolic disease. *Clin Res.* 1989;37:145A. Abstract.

67. Dittrich HC, Nicod PH, Chow LC, et al. Early changes of right heart geometry after pulmonary thrombo-endarterectomy. *J Am Coll Cardiol.* 1988;11:937-943.

68. Moser KM, Spagg RG, Utley J, et al. Chronic thrombo-

tic obstruction of major pulmonary arteries: Results of thromboendarterectomy in 15 patients. *Ann Intern Med.* 1983;99:299-305.

69. Moser KM, Auger WR, Fedullo PF. Chronic major-vessel thromboembolic pulmonary hypertension. *Circulation.* 1990;81:1735-1743.

70. Rich S, Levitsky S, Brundage BH. Pulmonary hypertension from chronic pulmonary thrombo-embolism. *Ann Intern Med.* 1988;108:425-434.

71. Edelman NH. Cor pulmonale. In: Spittell JA Jr (ed). *Clinical Medicine.* Vol 6. Philadelphia: Harper & Row; 1981:1-13.

72. Salerni R, Rodnan GP, Leon DF, et al. Pulmonary hypertension in the CREST syndrome variant of progressive systemic sclerosis (scleroderma). *Ann Intern Med.* 1977;86:394-399.

73. Follansbee WP, Curtiss EI, Medsger TA, et al. Myocardial function and perfusion in the CREST syndrome variant of progressive systemic sclerosis. *Am J Med.* 1984;77:489-496.

74. Morgan JM, Griffiths M, du Bois RM, et al. Hypoxic pulmonary vasoconstriction in systemic sclerosis and primary pulmonary hypertension. *Chest.* 1991;99:551-556.

75. Seldin DW, Ziff M, DeGraff AV Jr. Raynaud's phenomenon associated with pulmonary hypertension. *Tex State J Med.* 1962;58:654-661.

76. Winters WL Jr, Joseph RR, Lerner N. Primary pulmonary hypertension and Raynaud's phenomenon. *Arch Intern Med.* 1964;114:821-830.

77. Caldwell IW, Aitchison JD. Pulmonary hypertension in dermatomyositis. *Br Heart J.* 1956;18:273-276.

78. Walker WC, Wright V. Pulmonary lesions and rheumatoid arthritis. *Medicine.* 1968;47:501-520.

79. Santini D, Fox D, Kloner RA, et al. Pulmonary hypertension in systemic lupus erythematosus: Hemodynamics and effects of vasodilator therapy. *Clin Cardiol.* 1980;3:406-411.

80. Asherson RA, Mackworth-Young CG, Boey ML, et al. Pulmonary hypertension in systemic lupus erythematosus. *Br Med J.* 1983;287:1024-1025.

81. Muschenheim C. Some observations on the Hamman-Rich disease. *Am J Med Sci.* 1961;241:279-288.

82. Soergel KH, Sommers SC. Idiopathic pulmonary hemosiderosis and related syndromes. *Am J Med.* 1962;32:499-511.

83. Mangla A, Fisher J, Libby DM, et al. Sarcoidosis, pulmonary hypertension and acquired peripheral pulmonary artery stenosis. *Cathet Cardiovasc Diagn.* 1985;11:69-74.

84. Block AJ. Is snoring a risk factor? *Chest.* 1981;80:525-526. Editorial.

85. Rochester DF, Enson Y. Current concepts in the pathogenesis of the obesity-hypoventilation syndrome: Mechanical and circulatory factors. *Am J Med.* 1974;57:402-420.

86. Miller A, Granada M. In-hospital mortality in the Pickwickian syndrome. *Am J Med.* 1974;56:144-150.

87. Lyons HA, Huang CT. Therapeutic use of progesterone in alveolar hypoventilation associated with obesity. *Am J Med.* 1968;44:881-888.

88. Sutton FD, Zwillich CW, Creagh CE, et al. Progesterone for outpatient treatment of Pickwickian syndrome. *Ann Intern Med.* 1975;83:476-479.

89. Cherniack NS. Respiratory dysrhythmias during sleep. *N Engl J Med.* 1981;305:325-330.

90. Millman RP, Fishman AP. Sleep apnea syndrome. In: Fishman AP (ed). *Pulmonary Diseases and Disorders.* 2nd ed. New York: McGraw-Hill; 1991:1347-1362.

91. Strohl KP, Cherniack NS, Gothe B. Physiologic basis of therapy in sleep apnea. *Ann Rev Respir Dis.* 1986;134:791-802.

92. Hultgren HN, Lopez CE, Lundberg E, et al. Physiologic studies of pulmonary edema at high altitude. *Circulation.* 1964;29:393-408.

93. Hackett PH, Creagh CE, Grover RF, et al. High-altitude pulmonary edema in persons without the right pulmonary artery. *N Engl J Med.* 1980;302:1069-1073.

94. Staub NC. Pulmonary edema — Hypoxia and overperfusion. *N Engl J Med.* 1980;302:1085-1086.

95. Saaluke MG, Shapiro SR, Perry LW, et al. Isolated partial anomalous pulmonary venous drainage associated with pulmonary vascular obstructive disease. *Am J Cardiol.* 1977;39:439-444.

96. Kay JM, Smith P, Heath D. Aminorex and the pulmonary circulation. *Thorax.* 1971;26:262-270.

97. Fishman AP. Dietary pulmonary hypertension. *Circ Res.* 1974;35:657-660.

98. Boot H, Visser FC, Thijs JC, et al. Pulmonary hypertension complicating portal hypertension: A case report with suggestions for a different therapeutic approach. *Eur Heart J.* 1987;8:656-660.

99. Robalino BD, Moodie DS. Association between primary pulmonary hypertension and portal hypertension: Analysis of its pathophysiology and clinical, laboratory and hemodynamic manifestation. *J Am Coll Cardiol.* 1991;17:492-498.

100. Stuart-Harris C, Bishop JM, Clark TJH, et al. Long-term domiciliary oxygen therapy in chronic hypoxic cor pulmonale complicating chronic bronchitis and emphysema. *Lancet.* 1981;1:681-685.

101. Nocturnal Oxygen Therapy Trial Group. Continuous or nocturnal oxygen therapy in hypoxemic chronic obstructive lung disease. *Ann Intern Med.* 1980;93:391-398.

102. McKay RG, Lock JE, Keane JF, et al. Percutaneous mitral valvuloplasty in an adult patient with calcific rheumatic mitral stenosis. *J Am Coll Cardiol.* 1986;7:1410-1415.

103. Palacios IF, Lock JE, Keane JF, et al. Percutaneous transvenous balloon valvotomy in a patient with severe calcific mitral stenosis. *J Am Coll Cardiol.* 1986;7:1416-1419.

104. Lock JE, Khalilullah M, Shrivastava S, et al. Percutaneous catheter commissurotomy in rheumatic mitral stenosis. *N Engl J Med.* 1985;313:1515-1518.

105. United States Department of Health and Human Services, National Heart, Lung and Blood Institute, Division of Lung Disease: Progress report; 1980:121.

106. Respiratory Disease. Task force report on prevention,

control and education. Washington, D.C., U.S. Department of Health, Education and Welfare, Public Health Service, National Institutes of Health; 1977:83.

107. Bishop JM, Grass KW. Use of other physiologic variables to predict pulmonary artery pressure in patients with chronic respiratory distress. Multicenter study. *Eur Heart J.* 1981;2:509-517.

108. Ingram R. Chronic bronchitis, emphysema and chronic airways obstruction. In: Wilson JE, Braunwald E, Isselbacher KJ, et al (eds). *Harrison's Principles of Internal Medicine.* 12th ed. New York: McGraw-Hill; 1991:1074-1082.

109. Rubin LJ, Peter RH. Therapy of pulmonary heart disease. In: Rubin LJ (ed). *Pulmonary Heart Disease.* Boston: Martinus Nijhoff; 1984:325-353.

110. Myers KE, Bogden PE. Bronchodilators for patients with ischemic heart disease. *Postgrad Med.* 1989;86:324-326.

111. Burrows B, Kettel LJ, Niden AH, et al. Patterns of cardiovascular dysfunction in chronic obstructive lung disease. *N Engl J Med.* 1972;286:912-918.

112. Bishop JM. Hypoxia and pulmonary hypertension in chronic bronchitis. *Progr Resp Dis.* 1975;9:10-14.

113. Traver GA, Cline MG, Burrows B. Predictors of mortality in chronic obstructive pulmonary disease: A 15-year follow-up study. *Am Rev Respir Dis.* 1979;119:895-902.

114. Rubin LJ. Vasodilator therapy (general aspects). In: Fishman AP (ed). *The Pulmonary Circulation: Normal and Abnormal.* Philadelphia: University of Pennsylvania Press; 1990:479-483.

115. Rubin LJ, Moser K. Long-term effects of nitrendipine on hemodynamics and oxygen transport in patients with cor pulmonale. *Chest.* 1986;89:141-145.

116. Biernacki W, Prince K, Whyte K, et al. The effects of six months of daily treatment with the ß-2 agonist oral pributerol on pulmonary hemodynamics in patients with chronic hypoxic cor pulmonale receiving long-term oxygen therapy. *Am Rev Respir Dis.* 1989; 139:492-497.

117. Morley TF, Zappasodi SJ, Belli A, et al. Pulmonary vasodilator therapy for chronic obstructive pulmonary disease and cor pulmonale. *Chest.* 1987;92:71-76.

118. Vestri R, Philip-Joet F, Surpas P, et al. One-year clinical study on nifedipine in the treatment of pulmonary hypertension in chronic obstructive lung disease. *Respiration.* 1988;54:139-144.

119. Mathur PN, Powles ACP, Pugsley SO, et al. Effect of digoxin on right ventricular function in severe chronic airway obstruction. *Ann Intern Med.* 1981;95:283-288.

CHAPTER 31

Pulmonary Embolism

Samuel Z. Goldhaber, MD

EPIDEMIOLOGY

Pulmonary embolism (PE) and deep venous thrombosis (DVT) account for more than 250,000 hospitalizations per year in the United States and, therefore, constitute a very common cardiovascular and cardiopulmonary illness. Since most cases of venous thrombosis are not recognized clinically, the frequency of hospitalization represents the "tip of the iceberg." Pulmonary embolism causes or contributes to as many as 50,000 deaths per year in the United States, a rate that has probably remained constant for the past 3 decades. Estimated annual charges for diagnosis and treatment of venous thrombosis in the United States are $2.9 billion.[1] These charges do not include the cost of time lost from work, discomfort from chronic pulmonary hypertension due to pulmonary embolism, and the value placed on the loss of life.

Patients suspected of pulmonary embolism should be assessed for the presence of common risk factors for venous thrombosis (Table 1). Many patients with an underlying hypercoagulable state[2-5] will not manifest venous thrombosis unless stressed by immobilization, surgery, or other commonly acquired risk factors. Young patients, especially those with recurrences, should be worked up with blood tests to detect the presence of a hypercoagulable state (Table 2). Such testing is best deferred to the outpatient setting rather than undertaking such an evaluation during the initial in-hospital presentation.

PREVENTION

Pulmonary embolism is easier and less expensive to prevent than it is to diagnose or treat.[6] Virtually all hospitalized patients should receive prophylactic measures against venous thromboembolism.[7-10] For every 1,000,000 patients undergoing general, orthopedic, or urological surgery, preventive measures will both improve patient outcomes and reduce total health care costs by about $60 million.[1]

As many as 30% of pulmonary embolisms among postoperative patients may occur as late as 1 month after discharge from the hospital.[11] In the United States, there are about 400,000 elective total hip or knee replacements annually as well as about 400,000 coronary artery bypass operations. These types of surgery, in particular, continue to be associated with high rates of venous thrombosis. Each patient's level of risk for PE should be assessed to determine whether to use mechanical, pharmacologic, or combined prevention modalities (Table 3). Because the risk of PE continues after discharge from the hospital, prophylaxis should be continued at home among those patients at moderate or high risk for venous thromboembolism.

Despite the availability of effective measures to curb venous thromboembolism, prophylaxis continues to be underutilized, even among high-risk hospitalized patients. In a survey of 16

Table 1. Common Risk Factors for Venous Thrombosis

Surgery/Trauma/Immobilization
Obesity
Increasing age
Pregnancy/Postpartum/Oral contraceptives
Cancer, especially adenocarcinoma
Spinal cord injury/stroke
Inflammatory bowel disease
Indwelling central venous catheter
Prior venous thrombosis

Table 2. Hypercoagulable States Associated With Venous Thrombosis

HYPERCOAGULABLE STATE	COMMENTS
Genetic Predisposition or Family History	Obtaining a careful family history is more cost effective than obtaining blood tests to screen for an inherited hypercoagulable state.
Protein C Deficiency	By age 45, 50% of heterozygotes and 10% of normal relatives can be expected to have an episode of venous thrombosis. About half of thrombotic events are associated with immobilization or surgery.[2]
Poor anticoagulant response to activated protein C	The most exciting and far-reaching discovery in this field. Normally, add a known amount of activated protein C to plasma and observe prolongation of the activated partial thromboplastin time (PTT). However, if the PTT prolongation is less than twice control, patients have a poor anticoagulant response. This abnormality was detected in 21% of unselected consecutive patients (<70 years old) with venous thrombosis and only among 5% of controls.[3] The finding is due to a mutation in the Factor V gene.
Protein S deficiency	Protein S is a cofactor for protein C. In a cohort of 141 venous thrombosis patients <45 years old, 5% had this defect.[4]
Antithrombin III deficiency	In a cohort of 141 venous thrombosis patients <45 years old, 3% had this defect.[4] In another cohort of 280 patients with acute deep venous thrombosis, 1% had this defect.[5]
Presence of lupus anticoagulant	Acquired; usually not associated with lupus; often found in patients whose baseline PTT is elevated.
Presence of anticardiolipin antibodies	May be elevated in patients who also have lupus anticoagulant; associated with venous thrombosis and with patients who have recurrent first trimester miscarriages.
↑ Prothrombin fragment $F_{1.2}$	Levels will decrease toward normal with warfarin.

short-stay hospitals in central Massachusetts,[12] only 32% of patients at high risk for venous thrombosis received prophylaxis. The rates of prophylaxis varied widely, from 9%-56% at the different hospitals. Patients received prophylaxis at teaching hospitals more often than at nonteaching hospitals. Fixed low-dose subcutaneous heparin was utilized in about four-fifths of the patients who did receive preventive measures. Prevention programs should be established at all hospitals, with nurses and physicians collaborating to establish protocols that are streamlined and standardized.[13]

Prevention options are broad and include mechanical, pharmacologic, or combined modalities (Table 3). Graduated compression stockings (GCS) and intermittent pneumatic compression (IPC) have complementary mechanisms. Graduated compression stockings provide continuous stimulation of blood flow and prevent perioperative venodilation of the legs. They are inexpensive, uncomplicated, and free of serious complications such as hemorrhage. In randomized trials evaluating GCS for prevention of venous thrombosis after non-orthopedic surgery (general surgery, gynecologic surgery, or neurosurgery), there is an overall reduction of 72% in the likelihood of

Table 3. Prevention Options

Mechanical	Graduated compression stockings (GCS)
	Intermittent pneumatic compression (IPC)
	Combined GCS and IPC
	Inferior vena caval filter
	Closure of patent foramen ovale
Pharmacologic	Unfractionated heparin
	Low molecular weight heparin
	Warfarin
Combined Mechanical + Pharmacologic	GCS plus heparin
	IPC plus heparin
	IPC plus warfarin

having a DVT.[14] Intermittent pneumatic compression devices compress the veins more forcefully than GCS, but for a relatively brief period, and also stimulate the endogenous fibrinolytic system. Low-molecular weight heparin, approved by the Food and Drug Administration (FDA) in 1993, is the most recent innovation in pharmacologic prophylaxis of venous thrombosis.

Subcutaneous administration of unfractionated heparin has become the standard prophylaxis measure during the past 2 decades. Collins and colleagues pooled the data from 78 randomized controlled unfractionated heparin trials with 15,598 patients undergoing surgery.[15] There was a 40% reduction in nonfatal PE and 64% reduction in fatal PE among patients prophylaxed with heparin. Patients assigned to heparin had about one-third as many DVTs as control patients, regardless of whether they had undergone general, urological, elective orthopedic, or trauma surgery. Although there was no significant difference in fatal hemorrhage between the heparin and control groups, an absolute excess in important bleeding of about 2% occurred among patients assigned to heparin — especially in those who underwent urological procedures.

Low-molecular weight heparins exhibit less binding to plasma proteins and to endothelial cells than unfractionated heparin. Conse-

quently, they tend to have a more predictable dose-response, more dose-independent mechanism of clearance, and longer plasma half-life than unfractionated heparin. In most prevention trials, low-molecular weight heparins are administered as once- or twice-daily subcutaneous injections in fixed or weight-adjusted doses, without laboratory monitoring or dose adjustment. For prophylaxis in elective hip surgery, low-molecular weight heparins have consistently performed well compared with other prevention modalities.[16] In 1993, the FDA approved the low-molecular weight heparin, enoxaparin, for prophylaxis against venous thrombosis among patients undergoing elective total hip replacement.[17] The approved dose is 30 mg subcutaneously twice daily for 10-14 days.

Most North American orthopedic centers currently use adjusted dose warfarin, target International Normalized Ratio (INR) of 2.0-3.0, to help prevent venous thrombosis in elective total hip replacement. At Brigham and Women's Hospital, we begin warfarin and an IPC device simultaneously because it takes 3-5 days for the warfarin to become effective. We continue adjusted dose warfarin for approximately 6 weeks. Warfarin and low-molecular weight heparin were compared to prevent venous thrombosis in a randomized trial[18] of 1,207 patients undergoing elective total hip or total knee replacement. Disappointingly, both strategies resulted in surprisingly high rates of venographically proven DVT. Although the rate of isolated calf-vein thrombosis was slightly higher in the warfarin-treated patients, the major bleeding complication rate was 3 times higher among those who received low-molecular weight heparin.

Pulmonary embolism is no longer considered a very rare complication of coronary artery bypass grafting (CABG). In a review of 819 consecutive patients undergoing CABG (without other concomitant cardiac surgery),[19] 4% were found to have suffered postoperative pulmonary embolism according to autopsy, angiography, or high probability lung scanning. The majority were identified during the second postoperative week. Of those with PE, 19% died, compared with an operative mortality of 3% among those without PE. In a case series of 29 patients who had undergone uncomplicated CABG at Brigham and Women's Hospital, leg ultrasonography was obtained prior to hospital discharge.[20] Although none had postoperative signs or symptoms suggestive of DVT, ultrasonography detected DVT in 48% of the patients. In all but 1, the DVT was limited to the calf veins. Unexpectedly, half of the venous thrombi occurred in the leg contralateral to the saphenous vein harvest site.

Venous thrombosis is almost certainly a problem among hospitalized medical patients as well as those who undergo surgery. To determine the prophylaxis rate in the Medical Intensive Care Unit (MICU), we undertook a prospective survey at Brigham and Women's Hospital of 152 consecutive MICU patients.[21] Of the 152 patients, 88% had at least one risk factor and 53% had multiple risk factors for venous thrombosis. Overall, 67% received no prophylaxis. Of those who did receive some form of prophylaxis, there was an average delay of 2 days in the MICU before instituting preventive measures.

DIAGNOSIS

Pulmonary embolism may be quite difficult to diagnose despite the availability of lung scanning and pulmonary angiography. Thus, appreciation of the clinical setting for possible PE and maintenance of a high degree of clinical suspicion are of paramount importance. The most common symptoms and signs of PE are nonspecific: dyspnea, tachypnea, chest pain, and tachycardia. Usually, patients who present with severe chest pain or with hemoptysis have anatomically small PE near the periphery of the lung, where nerve innervation is greatest and where pulmonary infarction is most likely to occur due to poor collateral circulation. Ironically, patients with life-threatening PE often have a painless presentation characterized by dyspnea, syncope, or cyanosis.

Pulmonary embolism should be suspected in hypotensive patients when: 1) there is evidence of, or there are predisposing factors for, venous thrombosis and, 2) there is clinical evidence of acute cor pulmonale (acute right ventricular failure) such as distended neck veins, an S_3 gallop, a right ventricular heave, tachycardia, or tachypnea, especially if 3) there is electrocardiographic evidence of acute cor pulmonale manifested by a new $S_1 Q_3 T_3$ pattern, new incomplete right bundle branch block, or right ventricular ischemia.[8]

LABORATORY AND IMAGING TESTS

The chest x-ray and electrocardiogram help exclude diseases such as lobar pneumonia, pneumothorax, or acute myocardial infarction that can have similar clinical presentations. However, such patients can have concomitant

Lung Scan Category	CLINICAL PROBABILITY (%)							
	80–100% #PE/#PTS (%)		20–79% #PE/#PTS (%)		0–19% #PE/#PTS (%)		**0–100%** #PE/#PTS (%)	
High	28/29	(96)	70/80	(88)	5/9	(56)	**103/118**	**(87)**
Intermediate	27/41	(66)	66/236	(28)	11/68	(16)	**104/345**	**(30)**
Low	6/16	(40)	30/191	(16)	4/90	(4)	**40/296**	**(14)**
Very Low	0/5	(0)	4/62	(6)	1/61	(2)	**5/128**	**(4)**
Total	61/90	(68)	170/569	(30)	21/228	(9)	**252/887**	**(28)**

Table 4. PIOPED: Pulmonary Embolism Status

Adapted with permission from the PIOPED Investigators: Value of the ventilation/perfusion scan in acute pulmonary embolism. *JAMA.* 1990;263:2757.

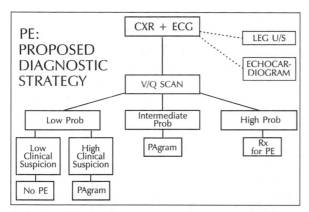

PE: PROPOSED DIAGNOSTIC STRATEGY

CXR + ECG → LEG U/S, ECHOCARDIOGRAM
→ V/Q SCAN → Low Prob, Intermediate Prob, High Prob
Low Prob → Low Clinical Suspicion (No PE), High Clinical Suspicion (PAgram)
Intermediate Prob → PAgram
High Prob → Rx for PE

Figure 1. Suggested diagnostic strategy for investigation of suspected pulmonary embolism. Please refer to text. U/S=Ultrasound. Reprinted with permission from Goldhaber SZ. Recognition and management of pulmonary embolism. Heart Disease and Stroke. *1993;2:142-146.*

PE. Unfortunately, neither room air arterial blood gases nor calculation of the alveolar-arterial oxygen gradient helps to differentiate patients with a confirmed PE at angiography from those with a normal pulmonary angiogram.[22] Therefore, arterial blood gases should not be obtained as a screening test in patients suspected of PE. The most promising blood test for screening is an abnormally elevated level of plasma D-dimer (>500 ng/ml) performed with an ELISA assay, which has a more than 90% sensitivity for angiographically proven PE.[23]

Ventilation-perfusion (V-Q) lung scanning should be the principal diagnostic test when PE is being seriously considered (Fig. 1).[24] The V-Q scan is most useful if it is clearly normal or if it demonstrates a pattern suggestive of a high probability for PE. Intermediate probability scans or low probability scans with high clinical suspicion do not exclude PE (Table 4).[24] Patients in these latter categories may require pulmonary angiography.

A constant intraluminal filling defect seen in more than one projection is the most reliable feature to diagnose PE among patients undergoing pulmonary angiography. This procedure can almost always be accomplished safely if: 1) Selective angiography is performed, with the perfusion lung scan serving as a road map to the angiographer; 2) Soft flexible catheters with side holes are employed, rather than stiff catheters

with end holes; and 3) A low osmolar contrast agent is utilized to minimize the transient hypotension and the transient heat and coughing sensation that often occurs with conventional radiocontrast agents.[8]

Ultrasonography of the leg veins is usually accurate in diagnosing proximal leg DVT in symptomatic outpatients and may sometimes serve as a useful surrogate for PE. However, even high resolution compression ultrasonography of the legs with color Doppler imaging may be insensitive for DVT diagnosis among asymptomatic inpatients, especially those who have undergone recent total hip or total knee replacement.[25] Overall, one-third to one-half of patients with PE have no ultrasound or venogram evidence of leg DVT. Therefore, if clinical suspicion of PE is high, patients without clinical or imaging evidence of DVT should still be examined for PE.

Among hemodynamically unstable patients, bedside echocardiography may suggest PE if the following constellation of findings is present: right ventricular dilatation and hypokinesis; bowing of the interventricular septum into the left ventricle; tricuspid regurgitation; and preserved left ventricular function. Echocardiography in this setting can also help to exclude other life-threatening conditions, such as ventricular septal rupture, aortic dissection, and pericardial tamponade. Nevertheless, patients can have a normal echocardiogram despite an anatomically extensive PE. Therefore, echocardiography must be considered an ancillary rather than a principal diagnostic test.

THERAPY

When PE is strongly suspected on clinical grounds, heparin should be initiated with a bolus of 5,000-10,000 units followed by a continuous intravenous infusion of approximately 1,250 units/hour while the diagnostic work-up is pursued. The partial thromboplastin time (PTT) should be targeted to 1.5 to 2.5 times control. Failure to use heparin in adequate doses can prolong the hospital stay, predispose to recurrent PE, and increase the costs of medical care. Bleeding and thrombocytopenia are the major side effects of short-term heparin administration.

Oral anticoagulation with warfarin (Coumadin®) can be started as soon as the PTT is within the therapeutic range. Patients should receive at least 5 days of heparin while an adequate level of oral anticoagulation is established. The prothrombin time, utilized to adjust the dose of oral anticoagulation, should be reported according to the International Normalized Ratio (INR), not the prothrombin time ratio or the prothrombin time expressed in seconds.

The INR is essentially a "corrected" prothrombin time that adjusts for the several dozen assays used in North America and Europe. For example, within North America, a prothrombin time of 18 seconds and prothrombin time ratio of 1.5 at 1 laboratory could be equivalent to a prothrombin time of 22 seconds and prothrombin time ratio of 1.8 at another laboratory. The same blood specimen in some European laboratories might yield a prothrombin time of 30 seconds and prothrombin time ratio of 2.5. Nevertheless, the INR for this same blood sample would be 3.0 at all laboratories, despite the three markedly different prothrombin time ratios and prothrombin times given in this example.[8]

For pulmonary embolism patients, I use a target INR of 3.0 to 4.0. and usually prescribe warfarin for 12 months. Lifelong anticoagulation may be required in patients with persistent risk factors, such as massive obesity or cancer. The most frequent outpatient complication of warfarin therapy that I observe is alopecia, which resolves after warfarin is discontinued.

THROMBOLYTIC THERAPY

Thrombolytic therapy may be a very useful adjunct to heparin in patients who have either hemodynamic instability or a normal systemic arterial pressure with echocardiographic evidence of right ventricular dysfunction (Fig. 2). However, contraindications to thrombolysis (such as intracranial disease, recent surgery, or trauma) will preclude its use, in some patients who can safely receive heparin alone.

To test whether thrombolysis followed by heparin more rapidly reverses right ventricular dysfunction and restores pulmonary tissue perfusion than heparin alone, our multicentered Pulmonary Embolism Research Group randomized 101 hemodynamically stable patients to rt-PA 100 mg/2h followed by intravenous heparin vs heparin alone.[26] The initial systolic arterial pressure was at least 90 mm Hg in every patient whom we studied. Only 20% of the patients underwent diagnostic pulmonary angiograms. The others were enrolled on the basis of high probability lung scans. Serial echocardiograms were obtained at baseline, 3 hours, and 24 hours. Pulmonary perfusion scans were obtained at baseline and 24 hours.

At baseline, about one-half of the patients with PE had entirely normal right ventricular function. Qualitative assessment of right ventricular wall motion at baseline versus 24 hours demonstrated that 39% of the rt-PA patients improved and 2.4% worsened, compared with 17% improvement and 17% worsening among those who received heparin alone ($P = 0.005$). Quantitative assessment showed that rt-PA patients had a significant decrease in right ventricular end-diastolic area during the 24 hours after randomization compared with none among those allocated to heparin alone ($P = 0.01$). Patients receiving rt-PA also had an absolute

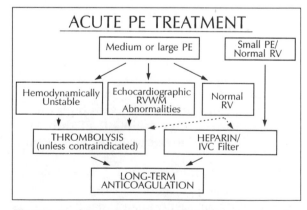

Figure 2. Suggested management strategy for pulmonary embolism. Refer to text. RVWM=Right ventricular wall motion. Reprinted with permission from Wolfe MW, Skibo LK, Goldhaber SZ. Pulmonary embolic disease: Diagnosis, pathophysiologic aspects, and treatment with thrombolytic therapy. Curr Probl In Cardiol. 1993;18:585-636.

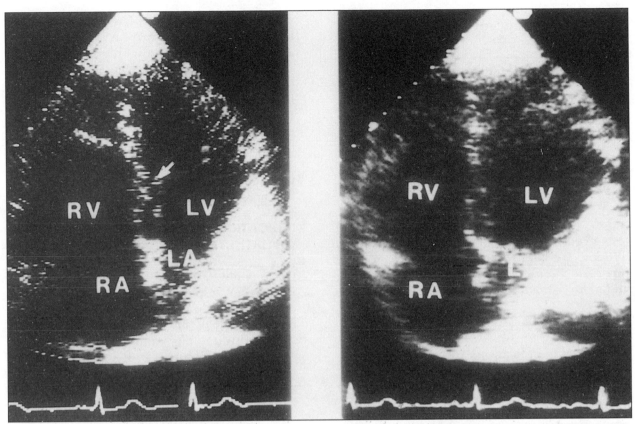

Figure 3. Echocardiograms (4 chamber view) in a 53-year-old previously healthy ophthalmologist with a high probability lung scan for pulmonary embolism. (Left Panel) Right ventricular enlargement before treatment. The right ventricular end diastolic area was 42.9 cm², and the interventricular septum (arrow) was displaced toward the left ventricle. The Echocardiogram Panel, which was not aware of the timing of the echocardiogram or of the patient's assignment to rt-PA therapy, graded this examination as showing moderately severe right ventricular hypokinesis. (Right Panel) Three hours after initiating rt-PA therapy, the right ventricle normalized in size (with a planimetered area of 25.7 cm²), and the interventricular septum resumed its normal configuration. The Echocardiogram Panel, which was not aware of the timing of the echocardiogram or of the patient's assignment to rt-PA therapy, graded this examination as showing normal right ventricular wall motion.

improvement in pulmonary perfusion of 14.6% at 24 hours, compared with 1.5% improvement among heparin alone patients (*P* < 0.0001).

Most importantly, no clinical episodes of recurrent PE occurred among rt-PA patients, but there were 5 (2 fatal and 3 nonfatal) clinically suspected recurrent PEs within 14 days in patients randomized to heparin alone (*P* = 0.06). All 5 presented initially with right ventricular hypokinesis on echocardiogram. This latter observation suggests that echocardiography may help identify a subgroup of patients with PE at high risk of adverse clinical outcomes if treated with heparin alone. Such patients, in particular, would appear to be

excellent candidates for thrombolytic therapy in the absence of contraindications (Fig. 3). Our findings suggest that rapid improvement of right ventricular function and pulmonary perfusion, accomplished with thrombolytic therapy followed by heparin, may lead to a lower rate of death and recurrent PE, especially among patients who present with right ventricular hypokinesis.

There are currently 3 FDA-approved thrombolytic regimens from which to choose (Table 5). Heparin is not administered concomitantly and is simply restarted without a bolus at the conclusion of thrombolysis administration. Because thrombolysis dosing regimens are fixed, no coagulation

---

Table 5. FDA Approved Thrombolytic Regimens for PE

Streptokinase: 250,000 IU as a loading dose over 30 minutes, followed by 100,000 U/hr for 24 hours — approved in 1977.

Urokinase: 2,000 IU/lb as a loading dose over 10 minutes, followed by 2,000 IU/lb/hr for 12-24 hours — approved in 1978.

rt-PA: 100 mg as a continuous peripheral intravenous infusion administered over 2 hours — approved in 1990.

---

tests need be obtained during the thrombolytic infusion. We have recently learned how to make thrombolytic therapy safer, more streamlined, and more economical (Table 6).

INFERIOR VENA CAVAL FILTER

The 2 major indications for placement of an inferior vena caval (IVC) filter are: 1) active, clinically important bleeding that prohibits the use of heparin, and 2) recurrent PE despite adequate heparin therapy. An IVC filter is also useful in hemodynamically compromised patients who cannot be treated with thrombolytic therapy. It should be kept in mind, however, that an IVC filter prevents PE, not DVT. Therefore, anticoagulation should also be utilized, if possible, to prevent propagation of the venous thrombus. Despite placement of an IVC filter, there is a small possibility of recurrent PE through collateral venous channels that may develop.

INDICATIONS FOR SURGERY OR CATHETER-BASED INTERVENTION

Occasionally, a patient with an acute, massive PE may not respond to thrombolytic therapy or may have absolute contraindications to its use. Such individuals should be evaluated for acute surgical pulmonary embolectomy,[27] suction catheter embolectomy,[28] or mechanical fragmentation of thrombus with a pulmonary artery catheter.[29] Patients with chronic pulmonary

---

Table 6. New Concepts in Pulmonary Embolism Thrombolysis

VARIABLE	OLD	NEW
	PE THROMBOLYSIS	
Diagnosis	Mandatory pulmonary angiogram	High probability lung scan or suggestive echocardiogram (if hypotensive) or angiogram
Indications	Hypotension; hemodynamic instability	Hypotension or normotension with accompanying right ventricular hypokinesis
Time window	5 days or less	14 days or less
Agents	Streptokinase (SK) or urokinase (UK)	rt-PA or SK or UK
Dosing regimens	24h SK or 12-24h UK	100 mg/2h rt-PA (FDA approved) or 3,000,000 U/2h UK (not FDA approved) or 1,500,000 U/1h SK (not FDA approved)
Route	Via pulmonary artery catheter	Via peripheral vein
Coagulation tests	"DIC screens" every 4-6h during infusion	PTT at conclusion of thrombolysis
Location	Intensive Care Unit	Intermediate Care Unit

hypertension due to prior PE may be virtually bedridden with breathlessness due to high pulmonary arterial pressures. They should be considered for pulmonary thromboendarterectomy which, if successful, can reduce, and at times even cure, pulmonary hypertension.[30]

EMOTIONAL SUPPORT

Although PE can be as devastating emotionally as myocardial infarction, the burden on PE patients may be greater because the general public does not understand PE as well, particularly regarding the possibility of long-term disability and incomplete recovery. Young patients with PE repeatedly voice a common theme. Although they appear healthy, they often have difficulty expressing their fears and feelings about their potentially life-threatening illness to close family and friends.

Virtually all patients with PE will wonder why they were stricken with the illness and whether they have an underlying coagulopathy or "bad genes" that predisposed them to it, even if a specific hypercoagulable state can not be identified. When anticoagulation is discontinued after an "adequate" course of therapy, patients will be fearful of recurrent PE and may resist attempts to be weaned from warfarin. We may be able to ease the emotional burden of PE by taking the time to discuss the implications of the illness with the patient and family. In our clinical practice, we began a Pulmonary Embolism Support Group which is co-led by a nurse-physician team and which meets on 1 weeknight every 3 weeks. Although these sessions have an educational component, the major emphasis is discussing the anxieties and living difficulties that occur in the aftermath of pulmonary embolism.

REFERENCES

1. Landefeld CS, Hanus P. Economic burden of venous thromboembolism. In: Goldhaber SZ (ed). *Prevention of Venous Thromboembolism.* New York: Marcel Dekker; 1993:69-85.
2. Allaart CF, Poort SR, Rosendaal FR, et al. Increased risk of venous thrombosis in carriers of hereditary protein C deficiency defect. *Lancet.* 1993;341:134-138.
3. Koster T, Rosendaal FR, de Ronde H, et al. Venous thrombosis due to poor anticoagulant response to activated protein C: Leiden Thrombophilia Study. *Lancet.* 1993;342:1503-1506.
4. Gladson CL, Scharrer I, Hach V, et al. The frequency of type I heterozygous protein S and protein C deficiency in 141 unrelated young patients with venous thrombosis. *Thromb Haemost.* 1988;59:18-22.
5. Heijboer H, Brandjes DPM, Büller HR, et al. Deficiencies of coagulation-inhibiting and fibrinolytic proteins in outpatients with deep-vein thrombosis: *N Engl J Med.* 1990;323:1512-1516.
6. Goldhaber SZ. Practical aspects of venous thromboembolism prevention: An overview. In: Goldhaber SZ (ed). *Prevention of Venous Thromboembolism.* New York: Marcel Dekker; 1993:129-144.
7. National Institutes of Health Consensus Conference. Prevention of venous thrombosis and pulmonary embolism. *JAMA.* 1986;256:744-749.
8. Goldhaber SZ, Morpurgo M, for the WHO/ISFC Task Force on Pulmonary Embolism. Diagnosis, treatment, and prevention of pulmonary embolism. Report of the WHO/International Society and Federation of Cardiology Task Force. *JAMA.* 1992;268:1727-1733.
9. European Consensus Statement. Prevention of Venous Thromboembolism. *International Angiology.* 1992;11:151-159.
10. Thromboembolic Risk Factors (THRIFT) Consensus Group. Risk of and prophylaxis for venous thromboembolism in hospital patients. *Br Med J.* 1992;305:567-574.
11. Huber O, Bounameaux H, Borst F, et al. Postoperative pulmonary embolism after hospital discharge. An underestimated risk. *Arch Surg.* 1992;127:310-313.
12. Anderson FA Jr, Wheeler HB, Goldberg RJ, et al. Physician practices in the prevention of venous thromboembolism. *Ann Intern Med.* 1991;115:591-595.
13. Morrison RB. Nurse and physician collaborative responsibility. In: Goldhaber SZ (ed). *Prevention of Venous Thromboembolism.* New York: Marcel Dekker; 1993:577-582.
14. Wells PS, Lensing AWA, Hirsh J. Graduated compression stockings in the prevention of postoperative venous thromboembolism. A meta-analysis. *Arch Intern Med.* 1994;154:67-72.
15. Collins R, Scrimgeour A, Yusuf S, et al. Reduction in fatal pulmonary embolism and venous thrombosis by perioperative administration of subcutaneous heparin. Overview of results of randomized trials in general, orthopedic, and urologic surgery. *N Engl J Med.* 1988;318:1162-1173.
16. Mohr DN, Silverstein MD, Murtaugh PA, et al. Prophylactic agents for venous thrombosis in elective hip surgery. Meta-analysis of studies using venographic assessment. *Arch Intern Med.* 1993;153:2221-2228.
17. Enoxaparin — A low-molecular-weight heparin. *Medical Letter.* 1993;35:75-78.
18. Hull R, Raskob G, Pineo G, et al. A comparison of subcutaneous low-molecular-weight heparin with warfarin sodium for prophylaxis against deep-vein thrombosis after hip or knee implantation. *N Engl J Med.* 1993;329:1370-1376.

19. Josa M, Siouffi SY, Silverman AB, et al. Pulmonary embolism after cardiac surgery. *J Am Coll Cardiol.* 1993;21:990-996.

20. Reis SE, Polak JF, Hirsch DR, et al. Frequency of deep venous thrombosis in asymptomatic patients with coronary artery bypass grafts. *Am Heart J.* 1991;122:478-482.

21. Keane MG, Ingenito EP, Goldhaber SZ. Utilization of venous thromboembolism prophylaxis in the Medical Intensive Care Unit. *Chest.* 1994. In press.

22. Stein PD, Terrin ML, Hales CA, et al. Clinical, laboratory, roentgenographic, and electrocardiographic findings in 21 patients with acute pulmonary embolism and no pre-existing cardiac or pulmonary disease. *Chest.* 1991;100:598.

23. Goldhaber SZ, Simons GR, Elliott CG, et al. Quantitative plasma D-dimer levels among patients undergoing pulmonary angiography for suspected pulmonary embolism. *JAMA.* 1993; 270:2819-2822.

24. PIOPED Investigators. Value of the ventilation/perfusion scan in acute pulmonary embolism. Results of the Prospective Investigation of Pulmonary Embolism Diagnosis (PIOPED). *JAMA.* 1990;263:2753-2759.

25. Davidson BL, Elliott CG, Lensing AWA for the RD Heparin Arthroplasty Group. Low accuracy of color Doppler ultrasound in the detection of proximal leg vein thrombosis in asymptomatic high-risk patients. *Ann Intern Med.* 1992;117:735-738.

26. Goldhaber SZ, Haire WD, Feldstein ML, et al. Alteplase versus heparin in acute pulmonary embolism: randomised trial assessing right ventricular function and pulmonary perfusion. *Lancet.* 1993;341:507-511.

27. Meyer G, Tamisier D, Sors H, et al. Pulmonary embolectomy: A 20-year experience at one center. *Ann Thorac Surg.* 1991;51:232-236.

28. Timsit J-F, Reynaud P, Meyer G, et al. Pulmonary embolectomy by catheter device in massive pulmonary embolism. *Chest.* 1991;100:655-658.

29. Brady AJB, Crake T, Oakley CM. Percutaneous catheter fragmentation and distal dispersion of proximal pulmonary embolus. *Lancet.* 1991; 338:1186-1189.

30. Moser KM, Auger WR, Fedullo PF. Chronic major-vessel thrombembolic pulmonary hypertension. *Circulation.* 1990;81:1735-1743.

CHAPTER 32

Pregnancy and Heart Disease

John H. McAnulty, MD

A cardiac care unit nurse for 10 years, always logical and calm, and 7 months into her second pregnancy—could she be this frightened? She is (the very day this paragraph is written), and it's about what the pregnancy will do to her heart and what her heart will do to her pregnancy. She, of course, knows too much. She has heard of a peripartum cardiomyopathy and is for some reason convinced that her labor will cause it. She is wrong about that (we believe), but she still is an appropriate representative of a prospective parent—easily worried about the effects of pregnancy on her health and worried about the baby. She knows about her ventricular ectopy. It has to be bad for the baby! She's probably wrong again, but again, this is an example of how pregnancy raises issues that we ordinarily do not consider when taking care of a patient: an example of the apprehension that surrounds heart disease and pregnancy.

Others are affected whenever we care for a patient. Management of the pregnant woman emphasizes this in an even more tangible, more direct, way. The developing fetus depends entirely on the mother for an adequate supply of nutrients and oxygen. With remarkable cardiovascular and volume changes during pregnancy, a mother can provide this support. Her commitment to the fetus is exceptional. As much as she gives, however, there are limits. When the mother requires a redistribution of blood volume, it is diverted away from the uterus and the fetus first. For the most part, in the woman with a normal cardiovascular system, blood flow to the fetus is adequate, even when she goes through periods of physical and emotional stress. In the woman with heart disease, when uterine flow may already be

marginal, the chance of inadequate uterine perfusion increases. The fetus is vulnerable. Still, pregnancy can be successful, even in the woman with heart disease.

This chapter will address—often too briefly and with biases—the approach to heart disease and pregnancy. Relatively lightly referenced, those listed are in turn referenced and will take an interested reader still further into this fascinating subject.

IMPORTANT PRINCIPLES

Caring for a patient should not be made trivial by relating it to a game, but a game can serve as an analogy in 1 sense—it is important to know the rules before playing.

HEALTH PRIORITIES

The mother's health and safety is the highest priority. The fetus should be considered with all interventions, but maternal needs should always take precedence.

PATIENT FRAGILITY

Pregnant women with heart disease are at risk of hemodynamic embarrassment. Management is specialized enough that availability to individuals with the greatest experience in working with these patients is appropriate. A team comprising the obstetrician, pediatrician, delivery anesthesiologist, and cardiologist should be informed and available. In essence, this is a recommendation to call for help when caring for these patients.

637

IDENTIFICATION OF WOMEN WITH HEART DISEASE AT PARTICULARLY HIGH RISK

Most women with heart disease are at increased risk during pregnancy. The danger for some is so great that avoidance or interruption of pregnancy is recommended (Table 1). As each abnormality is discussed in this chapter, hopefully this seemingly harsh approach will be understood and supported. Cardiovascular abnormalities having a 5% to 50% maternal mortality rate are often associated with or defined by cyanosis, an increased hemoglobin level, increased pulmonary artery pressures, the presence of a prosthetic valve, or significant ventricular dysfunction.

CARDIOVASCULAR CHANGES OF A NORMAL PREGNANCY

After the just-completed sobering paragraph, it is worth switching to a review of the remarkable cardiovascular changes of a normal pregnancy. In order to enjoy the opportunity of caring for the woman with heart disease and, more importantly, to manage her appropriately, some understanding of the normal physiologic changes of pregnancy is helpful.

CARDIAC OUTPUT AND ITS DISTRIBUTION

The resting cardiac output increases by almost 50% above the nonpregnancy level by the 20th week of pregnancy.[1-4] From that point in pregnancy, it is greatly affected by position. Late in pregnancy, with the woman on her back, the uterus interferes sufficiently with return of inferior vena caval blood flow to the heart that the cardiac output falls to a level approximately 25% above baseline. On occasion, this fall in venous return, in combination with the failure of maternal heart rate and arterial vascular resistance to respond appropriately, results in syncope— the "supine hypotension syndrome" of pregnancy. When the cardiac output is measured with the woman on her left side it remains about 40% to 50% above normal until the time of labor when it increases another 40% to 50% with each contraction (approximately 9 L/min).[5] It falls by 30% to 40% with epidural

Table 1. Cardiovascular Abnormalities Placing a Mother and Infant at High Risk
ADVISE AVOIDANCE OR INTERRUPTION OF PREGNANCY:
Pulmonary hypertension Dilated cardiomyopathy with congestive failure Marfan's syndrome with dilated aortic root Cyanotic congenital heart disease Symptomatic obstructive lesions
CONSIDER AVOIDANCE OF INTERRUPTION OR PREGNANCY:
Prosthetic valve Coarctation of the aorta Marfan's syndrome Dilated cardiomyopathy in asymptomatic women

anesthesia and slightly more with general anesthesia.[6] Immediately after delivery, another rise in cardiac output is followed by a fall over hours to days, and within a few weeks it is normal.

As the product of stroke volume and heart rate, the cardiac output increase is a result of both. The heart rate increases by approximately 20 beats/min in a steady fashion throughout pregnancy (although rarely reaches resting levels greater than 100 beats/min). Stroke volume also gradually increases, but is strongly affected by position. The increase in both might be expected to be poorly tolerated in specific cardiovascular abnormalities; for example, mitral stenosis where the shortened diastole of a tachycardia as well as the increased stroke volume could and occasionally do, result in pulmonary edema.

The maternal systemic vascular resistance falls during the first trimester, with an associated 10 mm Hg fall in mean arterial pressure. Both rise to nonpregnant levels by term. The pulmonary vascular resistance and pressures seem to fall to about the same degree. This is important when considering the effects that pregnancy might have on women with intracardiac left to right shunts. In general, the degree of shunting is not significantly altered by pregnancy.

The increase in cardiac output does not simply go to the enlarging uterus, but some does. At rest, uterine blood flow in nonpregnant women is approximately 100 mL/min (2% of the cardiac output). In the normal pregnancy, this increases to approximately 1200 mL/min at term (17% of the cardiac output).[7,8] The remainder of the increase in cardiac output is distributed mainly to the kidneys, the skin, and to the breasts.

Heart disease, and treatment for it, can greatly affect uterine blood flow. For the most part, the uterine blood vessels are maximally dilated during pregnancy, and there is little favorable local autoregulation that can improve blood flow. If uterine blood flow is to improve, it has to be the result of increased maternal arterial perfusion pressure and flow. Conversely, uterine blood flow can fall for many reasons. The most important is a fall in maternal perfusion pressure. In a woman with heart disease where total flow may already be compromised, uterine flow is the most vulnerable. Catecholamine excess (or increased sensitivity to catecholamines) uterine contractions, maternal medications that alter blood pressure and cardiac output and pulmonary ventilation can all significantly decrease blood flow to the uterus.

VOLUME CHANGES DURING PREGNANCY

Total body water volume increases steadily throughout a normal pregnancy, adding 6 to 8 liters at term. This is accompanied by retention of 500 to 900 mEq of sodium. Most of the fluid is extracellular and extravascular, but the blood volume also increases steadily throughout pregnancy, reaching levels approximately 40% above normal by the time of delivery.[9] Since the plasma volume increases by 50% and the red blood cell volume rises by 20%, in a normal pregnancy, there is a fall in hematocrit to values in the range of 32% to 36%. (Iron supplementation during pregnancy is encouraged.)

VASCULAR CHANGES DURING PREGNANCY

It might be assumed that the increase in volumes just mentioned would result in increased intravascular pressures. It does not. This is the result of a generalized increase in vascular capacitance in both the venous and

arterial beds. An advantage of this increased vascular compliance is the protection against rising pressures as the volumes increase. A disadvantage is that there appears to be increased vascular fragility; vascular accidents, when they do occur, commonly do so during pregnancy.

CHANGES IN THE HEART

Whereas many of the hemodynamic changes are the results of volume and vascular alterations, the heart does change. The stroke volume increases by 25%, but the ejection fraction does not. This means the heart must enlarge (since the ejection fraction is the stroke volume divided by the end-diastolic volume). Echocardiographic studies have shown that this does occur although the enlargement is only mild, a clue that in addition to enlargement, there is some reconfiguration of the heart.[10,11] This contributes in part to the change in cardiac appearance on the chest x-ray.

EXERCISE AND PREGNANCY

The cardiovascular response to exercise is also different in the pregnant woman. The overall oxygen consumption is increased for any given level of exercise.[12,13] The cardiac output is also increased at any given level and the maximum cardiac output is reached at lower levels of exercise during pregnancy when compared with nonpregnant women. The increase in cardiac output exceeds that of the oxygen consumption, indicating that the arterial–venous oxygen difference at each work level is wider during pregnancy. This suggests that oxygen is supplied to the periphery somewhat less efficiently in the pregnant woman as compared with the nonpregnant woman. It also suggests that maternal cardiac reserve is lowered during pregnancy and, in turn that there is shunting of blood away from the uterus at the time of exercise. Animal models suggest that this does occur.

These observations have raised questions about the value and risk of exercise during pregnancy. It has been observed that mothers who work in a standing position during pregnancy may have infants that are smaller than expected, a possible long-term disadvantage to the child.[14] It may not be appropriate to expect the same for recreational exercise. For the mother, exercise carries the usual advantages of physical and emotional well being. The overall effects on the fetus are less clear although there have been some studies examining this issue. Maternal hemodynamics and perfusion of the uterus are affected by the type of exercise. For example, swimming causes less fetal bradycardia (a marker for fetal hypoperfusion) than the same level of cycling.[15] There is no known adverse effect from either. Routine and regular endurance aerobic exercise has been associated with a reduction in birthweight.[16] This reduction is the result of a decrease in neonatal fat, and again it is not clear if this is a disadvantage. In any event, in women with heart disease, where cardiac output may already be compromised, the further demands of exercise may result in a decrease in uterine perfusion. It seems best to at least advise limitation of exercise to a level below that which causes symptoms.

CAUSES OF CARDIOVASCULAR CHANGES IN PREGNANCY

This heading implies we know the causes, which may in part be true. Since many of the changes occur before the metabolic needs of the mother and fetus increase, it seems that metabolic needs cannot be the driving force alone. Currently, it seems that increases in circulating hormones are most responsible for the cardiovascular changes.[17] The known increase in circulating steroid hormones not only increase venous and arterial distensibility but also cause relaxation of the connective tissue in the heart. They, along with increases in prostaglandins, atrial naturetic peptide and changes in the renin–angiotensin system are probably responsible for most of the volume changes as well.[18]

CLINICAL ASSESSMENT OF THE PREGNANT WOMAN

Recognition of heart disease during pregnancy is difficult. During a normal pregnancy, women often note fatigue, dyspnea, orthopnea, chest discomfort, palpitations, and pedal edema. It is often unclear when these symptoms cross the line of being acceptable. However, dyspnea that is severe enough to limit day-to-day activities, orthopnea and paroxysmal nocturnal dyspnea (PND), which interfere regularly with sleep, syncope with exertion, or hemoptysis, cannot be considered normal and require evaluation. Chest pain associated with activity and relief by rest should at least keep the consideration of myocardial ischemia open as, on occasion, this does occur in pregnant women.

The physical exam may also be difficult. In a normal pregnancy, pedal edema is common, a third heart sound is the rule, and a systolic murmur is not unusual. However, findings that should increase the index of suspicion for heart disease are a systolic murmur that is more than grade 3/6 in intensity or any diastolic murmur. When listening for murmurs, it is important to exclude bruits originating in the internal mammary arteries (the mammary souffle) and venous hums. Both have systolic and diastolic components and are common in normal pregnancies. Cyanosis and clubbing, no matter what the cause, are abnormal.

MANAGEMENT OF HEART DISEASE

Once heart disease is recognized, management should be influenced by pregnancy and should be individualized. Some aspects of the use of diagnostic and treatment modalities apply in all cases.

DIAGNOSTIC STUDIES

It is always preferable to assess a woman's cardiac status using the history and physical examination alone, but on occasion, testing is necessary. Some tests put the mother as well as the fetus and subsequent live-born children at risk. All are expensive. Maternal apprehension is the rule. Misinterpretation is common. Still, when essential, the studies should be performed (and interpreted by individuals familiar with the changes of a normal pregnancy).

Radiographic Procedures

Radiographic exposure can alter the development of the fetus and may increase the chance of subsequent malignancy in the child. Before an x-ray procedure, a woman of childbearing age should be questioned about the possibility of pregnancy. If an x-ray is required during pregnancy, the fetus should be shielded with a lead screen. A standard chest x-ray has not been associated with any recognizable increase of congenital deformities or malignancies (fetal exposure has been estimated to be less than 40 mrad). Interpretation of a chest x-ray should take into consideration the changes expected in a normal pregnancy—an increase in systolic and diastolic volumes and some increase in pulmonary vascular markings.

Electrocardiography

There are no recognized risks to the mother or the fetus with this procedure. The occasional difficulty of recognizing normal variations in young women can be made more difficult by the pregnancy. Mild, inferior-wall ST-T abnormalities are of no recognized clinical significance; anterior changes should not exceed those expected in a normal young woman. A horizontal QRS axis is common, but true left-axis deviation is not—it is a clue for heart disease.

Echocardiography

In association with evaluation of flow by Doppler ultrasound, echocardiography is excellent for the assessment of ventricular function, valve abnormalities, and intracardiac shunts. This, in combination with its proved safety, make it particularly helpful—and particularly seductive. It is expensive (usually over $500), and again misinterpretation is not uncommon. There is little information about the role or safety of transesophageal echo but when indicated, it would seem that the major risk would be from the anesthetic agent.

Radionuclide Studies

Some radionuclides are known to cross the placenta, and others that bind to albumin can unbind and cross as well. It has been estimated that radiation exposure by the fetus would be small (<0.8 rad; a dose <5 rad is unlikely to result in any fetal malformation, even at critical development periods). Still, radionuclide imaging should be limited to the situations where it is absolutely essential.

Magnetic Resonance Imaging

Evaluation of noncardiovascular diseases with this technique in pregnancy has shown no adverse effects. It would appear that cardiovascular imaging could be used if necessary (remembering, as always, that the procedure should not be performed in women with implanted pacemakers or defibrillators until its implications are better understood).

CARDIOVASCULAR DRUGS AND PREGNANCY

There is so little information about drugs and pregnancy that rigid recommendations are inappropriate. We do know that almost all cross the placenta and are excreted in breast milk. Many have pharmacologic effects on the fetus (this on occasion is used for fetal therapy), and some may be dangerous to the fetus.[19]

Diuretics

For treatment of hypertension or clinical congestive heart failure, the use and choice of diuretics should be the same during pregnancy as at other times. Diuretics should not be used to treat simple pedal edema; they may cause preeclampsia.

Inotropic Agents

Indications for the use of digoxin are not changed by pregnancy. Efficacy and toxicity are best judged by clinical and electrocardiographic criteria. A given dose can be expected to result in a lower circulating level during pregnancy, mainly the result of the increased volume of distribution. Recent recognition of the existence of digoxin-like substances in pregnant women make interpretation of some assay results difficult. The drug crosses the placenta and is excreted in breast milk with the concentration being somewhat lower than that in the blood.

In extreme cases, the intravenous inotropic agents—epinephrine, dopamine, or dobutamine—may be required. All cause uterine blood vessel constriction, but if successful, they increase cardiac output. In balance, the overall effect on the fetus is unclear. If required for maternal safety, the drugs should be used. There is no information about the effect of drugs that act partially or completely by inhibiting phosphodiesterase activity.

Ritodrine and terbutaline are ß-agonists (and thus inotropic agents). It has been of interest that when they are used to treat premature labor, they have been shown to cause pulmonary edema. Whereas their value in quieting the uterus has recently been questioned, if the drugs are used and if pulmonary edema develops, stopping administration can reverse the complication.

Vasopressor Agents

Dopamine, dobutamine, and epinephrine may be used as vasoconstricting agents. When a pure vasoconstrictive effect is desired, ephedrine sulfate is preferable: It has little cardiac effect and increases maternal blood pressure without decreasing uterine blood flow.

Vasodilator Drugs

A controversial first recommendation—when maternal safety is threatened by a hypertensive crisis, acute valvular regurgitation, or severe ventricular dysfunction—nitroprusside is the vasodilator drug of choice. This recommendation is made despite a paucity of information about its use during pregnancy. The reasons are that it is highly effective, works instantaneously, is easily titrated, and its effects dissipate immediately when the drug is stopped. The metabolite, cyanide, has been detected in the fetus, but it has not been demonstrated to be a significant problem; it is a reason to limit the duration of use of this drug whenever possible. Intravenous nitroglycerin and hydralazine or sublingual nitroglycerin or nifedipine have also been used in emergency situations without adverse effects.

Chronic vasodilation for treatment of hypertension, valve regurgitation, or ventricular dysfunction can be achieved with hydralazine, nitrates, or nifedipine. Angiotensin-converting-enzyme inhibitors should not be used during pregnancy, because they increase the risk of fetal renal development abnormalities and there is some concern about teratogenicity.[20] They can, however, be used at the time of labor and delivery.

ß-Blocker Agents

ß-Receptor stimulation promotes uterine relaxation. Thus, one concern about the use of ß-blockers during pregnancy is that they will cause premature labor. Other concerns are that the drug will cause intrauterine growth retardation or will cause metabolic abnormalities. However, use of the ß-blocking agents in thousands of patients during pregnancy has not led to the observation of an increase in these problems compared with women not taking the drugs. There are anecdotal observations and theoretic reasons that the ß1-selective agents may even further minimize any potential risks to the fetus. With these thoughts in mind, the ß-blocker preparations can be used effectively for treatment of hypertension and supraventricular tachyarrhythmias. A child born to a mother who is taking ß-blocker therapy should be observed closely in the newborn period for hypoglycemia, delayed respirations, or bradycardia.[19,21]

Calcium-Channel Blocking Agents

Calcium antagonists can also be used as vasodilators. Detrimental fetal effects have not been described with nifedipine or verapamil (and actually both have been used to treat maternal hypertension and supraventricular arrhythmias). There is no reported experience with diltiazem or more recently introduced agents during pregnancy.

Antiarrhythmia Agents

Because it has been available longer than any other antiarrhythmia drug, quinidine has been used most often in pregnancy. Equally as effective (or ineffective) as it is in nonpregnant women, it has not clearly been associated with adverse fetal effects. Neither it nor the other antiarrhythmic drugs have been well evaluated. As always, the drugs should be avoided unless required for unacceptable maternal symptoms or danger.

Antithrombotic Agents

Warfarin is contraindicated during pregnancy.[22] It crosses the placenta and has a 5% to 25% chance of causing fetal abnormalities. Its teratogenic effect is greatest in the first trimester.[23] Some recommend warfarin (when anticoagulation is required) in the second and third trimester, but heparin therapy throughout pregnancy seems optimal. Heparin has the inherent advantage of not crossing the placenta, and long-term subcutaneous use is feasible, well tolerated and effective. Of the antiplatelet agents, only aspirin has been evaluated. There has been controversy about its use, but in general, it is well tolerated. If possible, it is preferable to stop antithrombotic drugs before delivery.

CARDIOVASCULAR COMPLICATIONS

Individualized therapy is always required but general recommendations for treatment of the cardiovascular complications apply no matter what the underlying cause.

LOW CARDIAC OUTPUT SYNDROME

Why begin with this complication when it is generally fluid overload (congestive heart failure) that has been most emphasized as a problem in patients with organic heart disease? Although volume overload may indeed be a problem requiring treatment, it is the low cardiac output syndromes that are more dangerous. This is particularly true in pregnancy. Always ominous, this is particularly

so in women with obstructive lesions—pulmonary hypertension, mitral stenosis, aortic stenosis, and hypertrophic obstructive cardiomyopathy. Recognized by signs of poor perfusion (obtundation, hypotension, tachycardia, peripheral vascular constriction, decreased urine output), it is most often the result of a relative depletion of central vascular volume. Measures to protect the woman against this syndrome are listed in Table II. Abnormalities other than hypovolemia should be considered (cardiac tamponade, severe myocardial dysfunction), but when in doubt, administration of fluid is essential. This syndrome is particularly dangerous just after delivery: Women at high risk should be monitored for 48 to 72 hours with specific attention to this issue. In some, if volume status is uncertain, intravascular pressure monitoring lines are appropriate.

CONGESTIVE HEART FAILURE

Though relegated to second in the list of cardiovascular complications in this chapter, congestive heart failure is not uncommon. Treatment should be as in the nonpregnant woman. If a woman develops pulmonary edema, particularly when it is caused by myocardial dysfunction or severe valvular regurgitation, treatment should be given with oxygen, morphine, parenteral diuretics, and nitroprusside. Note again that nitroprusside is mentioned: This is for the reasons listed earlier and despite potential concerns about its effect on a fetus. Chronic congestive heart failure can be treated in a standard fashion, but one must remember to avoid the angiotensin-converting-enzyme inhibitors.

PULMONARY HYPERTENSION

Pregnancy is contraindicated in women with pulmonary hypertension. Still, pregnancy does occur in women with the disorder. In some, the pulmonary hypertension is not recognized. Others elect to proceed despite the risk.[24] This is one of those lesions with up to a 50% maternal mortality and an even higher fetal loss. When pulmonary hypertension is recognized, interruption of pregnancy is recommended. Again, if this is not possible or not accepted, management should focus on a number of issues. The first is to assiduously avoid hypovolemia (Table II). Predelivery volume loading with maintenance of a high central venous pressure (CVP) for 48 to 72 hours postdelivery is essential. At the time of labor and delivery (or general surgery), central venous and arterial pressure lines should be used for pressure monitoring, for administration of fluids and medications, and for blood gas analysis. Intensive care unit monitoring should last for 72 to 96 hours after delivery. Oxygen will maintain optimal arterial saturation and minimize pulmonary artery constriction.

ARRHYTHMIAS

In the woman with heart disease, an arrhythmia has the usual potential of creating symptoms or danger for the mother and is likely to decrease uterine perfusion. These are reasons that treatment (versus no treatment) might best be applied a little earlier in the pregnant woman as compared with when it might otherwise be done. Otherwise, the same rules of treatment apply. No rhythm should be treated until documented. The benefit of treatment should always be weighed against the potential risk of treatment.

Tachyarrhythmias

Whether or not tachyarrhythmias are more frequent during pregnancy remains uncertain, but they, nevertheless, are common. Treatment should be as in the nonpregnant woman, but also consider that ventricular and atrial premature beats are a reason to consider an underlying cause and may be a reason to recommend a decrease of stimulant beverages or medicines; no other treatment is needed.

Sinus Tachycardia

A sinus rhythm exceeding 100 beats/min at rest is unusual and is a reason to consider and look for an underlying cause.

Table 2. Protection Against Hypovolemia

DAY TO DAY MEASURES:

Avoid dehydration
Leg elevation when sitting or supine
Left lateral position when supine
Full leg stockings
Avoid volume depleting drugs—diuretics, vasodilators

LABOR AND DELIVERY OR SURGERY MEASURES:

Left lateral position when feasible
Volume preloading—1,500 mL of glucose free normal saline
Avoid volume depleting drugs
Anesthesia:
 favor regional: serial small boluses if general required; emphasis on benzodiazepines and narcotics
Intravascular pressure monitoring during procedure and for next 72 hours in high-risk patients

Atrial Tachycardia

The types occurring in paroxysms—paroxysmal atrial tachycardia (PAT) or paroxysmal supraventricular tachycardia (PSVT)—may occur more frequently during pregnancy.[25] This appears to be true whether the mechanism is the result of an accessory atrial ventricular pathway (Wolff–Parkinson–White syndrome if there is evidence of antegrade conduction on the sinus rhythm electrocardiogram) or to dual atrioventricular nodal pathways. It is as important during pregnancy, as at other times, to explain to the woman that this is not acquired or degenerative heart disease, but rather a congenital problem and management should be as in the nonpregnant woman. If radiofrequency catheter ablation is to be considered, it is optimal to wait until the completion of pregnancy because of the radiation exposure accompanying the procedure.

Atrial flutter and fibrillation are more likely to be attributable to and associated with organic heart disease. Their management should not be changed by pregnancy. Thromboemboli are always the greatest concern with these rhythms but are uncommon in women of childbearing age. However, if the rhythms are associated with significant left ventricular dysfunction, the problem should be addressed: Warfarin should be avoided during pregnancy, and the decision should be made regarding home administration of heparin or an aspirin tablet.

Ventricular rhythms can occur during pregnancy. It is of interest that much of the reported ventricular tachycardia fits the criteria of being the type that comes from the right ventricular outflow tract. Not only is this rhythm potentially amenable to ablation therapy (again this should be considered only after pregnancy because of the radiation involved), but it is reasonably responsive to ß-blocker therapy — the initial treatment of choice. If a ß-blocker does not work, quinidine or flecainide can be used, with the usual uncertainty about their effects on pregnancy. Whether required for supraventricular tachycardias or ventricular tachycardias, cardioversion can be performed in the standard fashion, with the major risk to the mother or the baby being from the anesthetic.

An episode of ventricular fibrillation during pregnancy requires all available therapy—any maneuvers that can be performed with the woman rolled somewhat toward her left are preferable and immediate cesarian section should be considered if the pregnancy is greater than 30 weeks in duration.

Bradyarrhythmias

These also have been noted during pregnancy. If required, pacemakers can and should be inserted.

HYPERTENSION

Approximately 1% to 2% of women are hypertensive before pregnancy, and another 5% to 7% develop hypertension during their pregnancy. The latter has been called pregnancy-induced hypertension (a term not liked by all in this field). If accompanied by proteinuria, the woman has the syndrome of preeclampsia, and if this in turn is associated with seizures, the woman has eclampsia. The rules for appropriate

blood pressure control are not fully established. A systolic pressure of less than 140 mm Hg and a diastolic pressure of less than 90 mm Hg are feasible and reasonable. Angiotensin-converting-enzyme inhibitors should not be used, but other antihypertension drugs can be used in a standard fashion. In a woman presenting with a hypertensive crisis, standard emergent care is appropriate; again, nitroprusside makes the most sense.

BACTERIAL ENDOCARDITIS

The best therapy for bacterial endocarditis is prevention. Although it is not clear that antibiotic prophylaxis at the time of dental or surgical work is preventative in any patient, its use is as appropriate during pregnancy as at other times.[26] A committee of the American Heart Association has leaned away from recommending antibiotics for routine labor and delivery, but many working with women with heart disease disagree. It is recommended that antibiotics be started with labor and continued for 24 hours after delivery (recognizing that false labor will result in intermittent stuttering of antibiotic therapy). This applies in women with valve disease and most congenital heart disease. Antibiotics are not indicated in women with an atrial septal defect (ASD) or in those with surgically closed atrial or ventricular septal defects (VSDs).

THROMBOEMBOLIC COMPLICATIONS

In the woman at high risk for thromboembolic complications (i.e., those who have had an embolus, those with severe ventricular dysfunction, and those with atrial fibrillation in combination with ventricular dysfunction) preventive therapy is appropriate. During pregnancy, the woman should be instructed in the use of subcutaneous heparin because of the previously mentioned concerns of warfarin use.

PERICARDIAL DISEASE

If pericarditis is recognized, a search for the usual underlying causes is appropriate, and management with anti-inflammatory therapy is as appropriate as in nonpregnant women. Rarely, tamponade develops during pregnancy, but treatment should not be changed by the pregnancy.

SURGERY, LABOR, AND DELIVERY

Not exactly cardiovascular complications, these are of significance in women with heart disease. If nonobstetric surgery is required, (as it is in up to 2% of all pregnancies), and with labor and delivery, consideration of the need for antibiotic prophylaxis is appropriate in women with structural heart disease. Local or epidural anesthesia is almost always preferable to general anesthesia. If general anesthesia is required, one should consider the potential disadvantages of select anesthetic agents (e.g., those drugs with myocardial depressant effects should be avoided in women with ventricular dysfunction). If cardiac surgery is required, expertise in management of cardiopulmonary bypass during pregnancy is required.[27]

CARDIOVASCULAR DISEASE

RHEUMATIC FEVER

Worldwide, rheumatic fever and its consequences, in particular mitral stenosis, is still the most common cause of heart disease in pregnancy.[28] Rheumatic fever itself may occur during pregnancy—most commonly in the first trimester. The diagnosis is as difficult as in any other patient. Use of the revised Jones criteria in combination with evidence of a recent streptococcal infection (an elevated antistreptolysin–O titer) can help with the diagnosis. Individuals with previous rheumatic fever, particularly those with heart involvement, are most likely to get the disease. It is these patients in whom the diagnosis should be most strongly considered. If rheumatic fever does occur, a course of antibiotic therapy may decrease the severity and is recommended. Anti-inflammatory therapy (aspirin and, if necessary, steroids) is recommended for extreme arthritis. Prevention is better than treatment; antibiotic prophylaxis is effective.[29]

VALVE DISEASE

Mitral Stenosis

Mitral stenosis remains the leading cause of cardiac death during pregnancy and it is even more commonly the cause of cardiac symptoms. Given the pathophysiology of the stenosis, it is not surprising that the hemodynamic changes of pregnancy are not well tolerated. The increased cardiac output trying to pass through a stenotic valve can increase left atrial pressure. This can be sufficient to cause pulmonary edema or hemoptysis. An already precarious situation can be exacerbated by the sudden onset of atrial fibrillation with its rapid ventricular response, further compromising diastole and the time to empty the left atrium. Although hypervolemia and atrial fibrillation can put a woman at risk of pulmonary edema, the other extreme, hypovolemia, may also be dangerous in mitral stenosis. A reduction in left atrial filling pressure can result in a significant fall in cardiac output. Fatigue, dyspnea, orthopnea, or hemoptysis suggest heart disease, and the typical loud first heart sound, opening snap, and diastolic rumble should lead to the diagnosis. Echocardiography with Doppler flow measurements can confirm the diagnosis and quantify the degree of stenosis.

If symptoms develop during pregnancy, hypervolemia, or hypovolemic states should be treated. If these measures, in combination with rest, are not effective, balloon valvuloplasty or surgical commissurotomy can be performed.

Mitral Regurgitation

Most interesting of all the valve lesions because it can result from alteration of any part of the mitral apparatus, mitral regurgitation, no matter what its cause, is generally well tolerated during pregnancy. If congestive heart failure should occur, treatment should be as previously described. One cause of mitral regurgitation, mitral valve prolapse, requires further discussion, not because the regurgitation itself is different but because it is so common. Whereas pregnancy can alter the physical examination findings, making them more or less prominent, the rare complications of arrhythmias, emboli, endocarditis, or severe regurgitation are not clearly influenced by pregnancy nor does the valve lesion itself influence pregnancy.

Aortic Regurgitation

The management of aortic insufficiency is as difficult during pregnancy as at other times. Fortunately, pregnancy is generally well tolerated. If the mother is symptomatic or if there are signs of hemodynamic decompensation (clinical congestive heart failure or cardiac chamber enlargement by echocardiography) the treatment described earlier is appropriate, with emphasis on the use of afterload reduction. Because the angiotensin-converting-enzyme inhibitors are contraindicated, hydralazine and/or nifedipine are the initial agents of choice. If aortic insufficiency is caused by endocarditis, and infection cannot be readily controlled, emergency surgery should be used as in nonpregnant patients.

Aortic Stenosis

Since aortic stenosis is more common in men, pregnant women are infrequently affected. When they are, there has been a concern about high maternal as well as fetal mortality. A recent series has suggested, however, that the lesion is reasonably well tolerated, with little or no maternal mortality or fetal loss.[30] There is a 5% chance that a live-born infant will have congenital heart disease. Maternal mortality has been associated with situations in which low cardiac output syndrome and hypovolemia are common—with abortions and at the time of delivery. Whereas hypovolemia should be prevented, it is also necessary on occasion to treat congestive heart failure; This should be done in the standard fashion. If severe symptoms persist despite standard treatment, a balloon valvuloplasty or surgery can be performed, even during pregnancy.

Tricuspid Valve Disease

Echocardiography frequently reveals tricuspid regurgitation during pregnancy, but clinically significant disease is unusual. When present, it is most often caused by endocarditis related to intravenous drug use. Pregnancy is well tolerated in patients with tricuspid regurgitation, and specific treatment is not required. Isolated tricuspid valve stenosis is so rare that a discussion cannot be based on experience. Stenosis is occasionally observed in women with Ebstein's syndrome or in women with prosthetic heart valves (see below for both of these). The treatment should be similar to that described for mitral stenosis, again emphasizing the need to avoid hypovolemia.

Pulmonary Valve Disease

Pulmonary valve stenosis is almost exclusively congenital in origin. It has generally been recognized and corrected during childhood with surgery or increasingly with balloon valvuloplasty. On occasion, pulmonary valve stenosis is first noted during pregnancy. Specific treatment is not required if the woman is asymptomatic. Still, it is another abnormality where attention to maintenance of a normal or high venous pressure is appropriate.

Pulmonary valve insufficiency is almost always secondary to previous surgery—particularly after surgery for previous pulmonary valve stenosis or for tetralogy of Fallot. It is well tolerated during pregnancy.

Prosthetic Heart Valve

Thousands, if not millions, of lives have been improved or saved since the first insertion of the prosthetic heart valve in 1960. Still, introduction of this approach immediately introduced a new disease—prosthetic heart valve disease. Even today, this disease, consisting of thromboembolic complications, anticoagulation complications, endocarditis, valve dysfunction, reoperation, or death occurs at a rate of 5% per year. There is some concern that pregnancy can accelerate or exacerbate some of these problems. Whereas it is appropriate to operate on a woman with significant valve regurgitation or stenosis before pregnancy, if a prosthesis is needed, it is still difficult to know whether to choose a mechanical prosthesis or a tissue prosthesis. Selection of the former dictates the need for continuous full anticoagulation. Since warfarin is contraindicated during pregnancy, a woman with a mechanical prosthesis requires subcutaneous heparin. A tissue prosthesis has the advantage of avoiding the issue of anticoagulation, but tissue valves in young people rapidly become dysfunctional, resulting in the high likelihood of reoperation within 10 years. The problems are sufficient in each case to be certain that prospective parents are informed and to raise the consideration of avoidance of pregnancy or even interruption of pregnancy should it occur. In the woman electing to continue with pregnancy, cardiac complications, if they occur, could be treated as previously described.

CONGENITAL HEART DISEASE

In the United States, congenital heart disease has become the most common type of heart disease associated with pregnancy. This is attributable, in part, to a decline in rheumatic fever but, also, because the population of women with congenital heart disease is increasing. In the past, women with congenital heart disease did not make it to child-bearing age, and many of those who did were not capable of conception. If either parent has a congenital abnormality, offspring have a 2% to 15% chance of having a congenital abnormality, depending on the parental lesion (compared with a 0.8% increase of all live births in this country.)[31,32] Observations that the chance of congenital heart disease in the offspring is greater if it is the mother who is affected rather than the father (not agreed upon by all)[33] suggest something other than gene expression alone is involved. However, genetics predominate, particularly when a trait is autosomal dominant, giving a child a 50% chance of being affected (e.g., hypertrophic obstructive cardiomyopathy or Marfan's syndrome). In summary, congenital heart disease is already common and will become even more so in future generations.

Which congenital heart disease is most commonly associated with pregnancy? In this country, it is probably an abnormality that has been altered ("corrected") with surgery or catheters. Generally, the intervention has improved the mother's condition, making

pregnancy safer for the mother and the fetus. Often, some residual stenosis, regurgitation, shunting, or exposed prosthetic material persists and late myocardial dysfunction or arrhythmias may occur.

INTRACARDIAC SHUNTS

Women with a left-to-right shunt tolerate pregnancy, labor and delivery. A right-to-left shunt, however, is associated with high maternal and fetal mortality.

Left-to-Right Shunts

The volume of blood shunted from left to right in a woman with an intracardiac defect is influenced most by the balance of resistances in the systemic and pulmonary vascular beds. As mentioned earlier, the resistance declines early during pregnancy and gradually rises proportionally in both vascular beds. Thus, the degree of shunting does not change significantly. The potential complications of left-to-right shunting include right ventricular failure, pulmonary hypertension, and arrhythmias. In addition, the shunt sight can act as a source of systemic emboli—a paradoxical embolus. It is not clear that any of these are exacerbated by pregnancy. The chance of the offspring having congenital heart disease is approximately 4%, an incidence not changed by surgical closure of the shunt site.

Atrial Septal Defects (ASD)

Because women with an ASD may have few or no symptoms and because the classical physical exam findings of a fixed split second heart sound and systolic murmur at the base may be subtle or missed, an ASD may first be recognized at the time a woman is pregnant. The more common ostium secundum defect is well tolerated during pregnancy. An ASD caused by an endocardial cushion defect (ostium primum defect) is more likely to be associated with other cardiac abnormalities (e.g., an associated VSD or a cleft mitral valve) and the risk of a cardiac complication is somewhat higher. In either case, the occasional complications of heart failure or arrhythmias can be treated in the standard fashion. Antibiotic prophylaxis against endocarditis is not required for simple ASD—it should be considered in those with associated valvular abnormalities.

Ventricular Septal Defects (VSD)

Because of the prominent murmur, this abnormality is more likely (than an ASD) to be recognized in a child. Up to 50% of the VSDs close spontaneously before age 5, and it is likely that the remainder will have been closed with surgery before a women reaches child-bearing age. On occasion, a woman with a VSD that has not been corrected does become pregnant, and in general, pregnancy is well tolerated. If complications occur, they should be treated as previously described—antibiotic prophylaxis at the time of labor and delivery is recommended.

Patent Ductus Arteriosus (PDA)

Like in ASD, patent ductus arteriosus can also go undetected and perhaps first noticed at a time a woman is of child-bearing age. Like the other common left-to-right shunts, it too is well tolerated during pregnancy. Antibiotic prophylaxis against endocarditis should be provided at the time of labor and delivery.

Right-to-Left Shunt–Associated Cyanosis

No matter where the sight, these shunts are associated with high maternal and fetal mortality. The hallmark of these shunts is cyanosis, often with a secondary increase in hemoglobin. The shunts are invariably associated with other cardiac (and often noncardiac) abnormalities.[31,34]

Elevated Pulmonary Vascular Resistance. Right-to-left shunting may be the result of an elevated pulmonary vascular resistance, i.e., Eisenmenger's syndrome. Because pregnancy in affected women is associated with a 50% maternal mortality and a still greater fetal loss, pregnancy is inadvisable, and interruption is recommended if it does occur. If the parents continue with the pregnancy, meticulous

attention to the avoidance of hypovolemia (Table 2) is essential. Maternal deaths frequently occur with attempts to interrupt the pregnancy, with surgical procedures and at the time of delivery as well as in the 48 to 72 hours postdelivery. At these times, intravascular right atrial and arterial pressure monitoring lines can be helpful (again, requiring meticulous efforts to avoid air through or thrombus formation, on the catheters). The use of low-dose continuous oxygen throughout the pregnancy can improve maternal comfort and favorably affects pulmonary vascular resistance.

Normal Pulmonary Vascular Resistance. If left-to-right shunting occurs as a result of obstruction to pulmonary outflow with a normal pulmonary vascular resistance, the long-term consequences to the woman are better, because it is a potentially correctable abnormality. The most common syndrome with this physiology is tetralogy of Fallot. If a woman with this syndrome becomes pregnant before surgical correction, interruption is advisable. With this lesion, it is not pulmonary vascular resistance but rather alterations in systemic vascular resistance that determine the amount of shunting. A fall in systemic vascular resistance can result in increased right-to-left shunting, with significant hypoxia. Hypotension, if it should occur, can be treated with volume and with a vasoconstrictive agent (e.g., ephedrine).

It is preferable that tetralogy of Fallot be surgically corrected before pregnancy. When this is done, pregnancy is tolerated without clear increased risk to the mother, and fetal loss does not exceed what might otherwise be expected. The child does continue to have an increased chance of having congenital heart disease.

VENTRICULAR OUTFLOW TRACT OBSTRUCTION

Right Ventricular Outflow Tract Obstruction

The 2 most common forms, pulmonary valve stenosis and pulmonary vascular hypertension have already been discussed. Other causes include peripheral pulmonary artery stenosis (one of the features of the rubella syndrome) and subpulmonic valve muscular thickening. In general, unless severe and associated with right ventricular hypertrophy, the lesions are well tolerated during pregnancy. Hypovolemic states should be avoided.

Left Ventricular Outflow Tract Obstruction

Aortic valve stenosis has already been discussed. Supra-aortic valve stenosis and subaortic webs may be difficult to distinguish from aortic valve stenosis—an echocardiogram can define the site of the obstruction. Experience in pregnant patients with these lesions is small, but it would seem that the recommendations given for aortic valve stenosis would apply. (Hypertrophic obstructive cardiomyopathy, previously called idiopathic hypertrophic subaortic stenosis, a common and important form of left ventricular outflow tract obstruction, is discussed under cardiomyopathies.)

Coarctation of the aorta is a form of left ventricular outflow obstruction that has some unique features related to pregnancy. It is associated with a 3% to 8% chance of maternal mortality, usually the result of intrathoracic or intracranial vascular rupture generally late in pregnancy at the time of labor and delivery. The risk is sufficient to recommend avoidance (until surgical correction) or interruption of pregnancy. If the recommendations are not accepted, control of blood pressure in an attempt to minimize the chance of vascular rupture is recommended. It is difficult to know how aggressive treatment should be. The lowest asymptomatic pressure obtainable would seem optimal for the mother, but this may critically reduce an already compromised uterine blood flow. With some arbitrariness, we recommend keeping the systolic pressure in the right arm less than 140 mm Hg. Correction of the lesion before pregnancy seems to decrease the chance of maternal and fetal mortality and morbidity.[35]

COMPLEX LESIONS

Ebstein's Anomaly

With its hallmark being a tricuspid valve that is displaced into the right ventricular cavity,

Ebstein's anomaly is actually a spectrum of problems. Some women have only mild valve displacement and are never affected by their heart abnormality. Associated abnormalities are common, and it is these that seem to influence pregnancy (i.e., right ventricular hypoplasia, obstruction of the right ventricular outflow tract, and an ASD [which, in combination with right ventricular disease, can lead to right-to-left shunting]). Accessory atrioventricular rhythm pathways (Wolff–Parkinson–White syndrome) occur in 10%. Unless these women have cyanosis, their ability to tolerate pregnancy is excellent, and the occasional complications of heart failure or arrhythmias can be managed as previously described.[36]

Transposition of the Great Arteries

As strange as it seems, this seemingly most complex (and most cyanotic) of heart diseases does not necessarily prevent a successful pregnancy. Incompatible with life if there are no associated shunts, women who reach childbearing age certainly have declared themselves as "survivors," and they are able to conceive. With cyanosis, the maternal mortality is high, and the fetal viability is compromised, but successful pregnancies have occurred. However, the risk to mother and fetus is so great that pregnancy should be avoided or interruption recommended until after surgical correction.[37]

Marfan's Syndrome

Women with this autosomal dominant disease are at risk of cardiovascular complications, and this is especially likely during pregnancy. Maternal mortality rates between 4% and 50% have been reported, and the deaths are due almost exclusively to vascular dissection or rupture. This, the expected shorter than usual maternal lifespan even if pregnancy is tolerated, and the 50% likelihood that the child will have the same disease, are reasons to recommend the avoidance of pregnancy in women with this syndrome. If the aortic root is not dilated (i.e., <4 cm wide on echocardiography), some suggest the maternal risk is low enough that pregnancy need not be discouraged.[38] If pregnancy does occur, attention to prevention of hypertension is particularly important, keeping the systolic blood pressure at 120 mm Hg or less. This is one lesion where cesarian section is strongly preferred over vaginal delivery to avoid the hypertension associated with prolonged contractions during labor.

MYOCARDIAL DISEASE— CARDIOMYOPATHIES

During pregnancy as in other clinical situations, it is helpful to divide cardiomyopathies into those that are dilated and those that are hypertrophic.

Dilated Congested Cardiomyopathies

Women with a dilated cardiomyopathy should be advised to avoid pregnancy, and depending on the severity of the disease, interruption of the pregnancy should be recommended. This recommendation is not based on the results of a definitive prospective clinical trial but rather from the observation that no matter what the type of associated heart disease, it is ventricular dysfunction that is often associated with maternal morbidity and mortality.[39] Maternal mortality can approach 10%. It is not clear that the known complications of heart failure, systemic emboli, or arrhythmias are made more severe by pregnancy, but each can occur; if so, treatment for each should be as previously described. Whereas recent studies have shown that prophylactic use of angiotensin-converting-enzyme inhibitors may decrease the chances of heart failure and may improve survival, these drugs are contraindicated in pregnancy and should be avoided. Substitution with hydralazine may be effective (although not of proved value). Warfarin is generally recommended for individuals with dilated cardiomyopathies; it is contraindicated during pregnancy, and the women should be switched to subcutaneous heparin.

Pregnancy may cause myocardial disease; this is thought to be the case if it is first recognized in the third trimester of pregnancy or in the postpartum period. This "peripartum cardiomyopathy" may occur more often in black women, in women with hypertension, and with multiparity. Management should be the same as in other dilated cardiomyopathies. If a woman does develop peripartum cardiomyopathy, advice about subsequent pregnancies is difficult; if any residual remains, most cardiologists would advise against further pregnancies.

Hypertrophic Cardiomyopathies

When the hypertrophy is concentric, the effects on pregnancy are unknown. When caused by hypertension or left ventricular outflow tract obstruction, treatment of those causes should be as previously described. If an unexplained finding, no specific treatment is recommended. In either case, hypovolemia should be avoided.

"Asymmetric" hypertrophic cardiomyopathies (including idiopathic hypertrophic subaortic stenosis [IHSS] or hypertrophic obstructive cardiomyopathy) are becoming more common—they may become the most common form of congenital heart disease given the autosomal dominant transmission of the disease. It is not clear that the 0.5% to 5.5% yearly risk of sudden death with hypertrophic obstructive cardiomyopathy is affected by pregnancy, but 1 death has been reported.[39] It is interesting to consider the physiology of this abnormality as it relates to pregnancy. The ventricular dilation and hypervolemic states might be considered an advantage. Conversely, the sudden shifts of volume with the potential of hypovolemia could lead to worsening of outflow tract obstruction and potentially exacerbate symptoms and complications. Despite there concerns, pregnancy is generally well tolerated. The suggestion that ß-blockers be used at the time of labor and delivery has not been universally accepted and these drugs should be reserved for those with unacceptable symptoms.

CORONARY ARTERY DISEASE

In young women, it seems inappropriate to consider coronary artery disease, but it can occur. In women with severe familial hyperlipidemia, diabetes, or hypertension and smoking history, it may be caused by atherosclerosis, but other etiologies include spasm, vasculitis, dissection or thromboemboli. The increasing prevalence of Kawasaki's disease suggests it may be a cause as well. Coronary artery disease can usually be managed with medical therapy. On rare occasions angioplasty or surgery is required.

CARDIAC TRANSPLANTATION

Transplant recipients are often women of child-bearing age. Normal and successful pregnancies have been reported. The mother and the fetus, however, are at potential risk from immuno-suppressive therapy, infection, and maternal heart failure. All of these and a possible shortened lifespan for the mother are reasons to consider whether pregnancy is advisable.

CONCLUSIONS

Probably, at best, it can be hoped that this chapter is a reasonable starting point for an understanding of the heart and heart disease during pregnancy. There is, relatively, so little known that it will be important (and exciting) for all of us to grow with the subject.

REFERENCES

1. Ueland K, Novy MJ, Peterson EN, et al. Maternal cardiovascular dynamics: IV. The influence of gestational age on the maternal cardiovascular response to posture and exercise. *Am J Obstet Gynecol.* 1969;104:856-864.
2. Capless EL, Clapp JF. Cardiovascular changes in early phase of pregnancy. *Am J Obstet Gynecol.* 1989;161:1449-1453.
3. Easterling TR, Bendetti TJ, Schmucker BC, et al. Maternal hemodynamics in normal and preeclamptic pregnancies: A longitudinal study. *Obstet Gynecol.* 1990;76:H1060-H1065.
4. Clark SL, Cotton DB, Pivarnik JM, et al. Position change and central hemodynamic profile during normal third-trimester pregnancy and post partum. *Am J Obstet Gynecol.* 1991;164:883-887.
5. Robson S, Dunop W, Boys R, et al. Cardiac output during labor. *Br Med J.* 1987;295:1169-1172.
6. James C, Banner T, Caton D. Cardiac output in women undergoing cesarean section with epidural or general anesthesia. *Am J Obstet Gynecol.* 1989;160:1178-1184.
7. Toresen M, Wesche J. Doppler measurements of changes in human mammary and uterine blood flow during pregnancy and lactation. *Acta Obstet Gynecol.* 1988;67:741-745.
8. Thaler I, Manor D, Itskovitz J, et al. Changes in uterine blood flow during human pregnancy. *Am J Obstet Gynecol.* 1990;162:121-125.
9. Hytten FE, Paintin DB. Increase in plasma volume during normal pregnancy. *J Obstet Gynecol Br Commonw.* 1963;70:402-407.
10. Katz R, Karliner JS, Resnik R. Effects of a natural volume overload state (pregnancy) on left ventricular performance in normal human subjects. *Circulation.* 1978;58:434-441.
11. Morton MJ, Tsang H, Hohimer AR, et al. Left ventricular size, output and structure during guinea pig pregnancy. *Am J Physiol.* 1984;246:R40-R48.
12. Morton MJ, Paul MS, Campos FR, Hart MV, Metcalfe J. Exercise dynamics in late gestation: Effects of physical training. *Am J Obstet Gynecol.* 1985;152:91-97.
13. Guzmen CA, Caplin R. Cardiorespiratory response to exercise during pregnancy. *Am J Obstet Gynecol.* 1970;108:600-605.
14. Naeye RL, Peters EC. Working during pregnancy: Effects of the fetus. *Pediatrics.* 1982;69:724-727.
15. Watson WJ, Katz VL, Hackney AC, Gall MM, McMurray RG. Fetal responses to maximal swimming and cycling exercises during pregnancy. *Obstet Gynecol.* 1991;77:382-386.
16. Clapp JF III, Capeless EL. Aortic function during normal human pregnancy. *Am J Obstet Gynecol.* 1986;154:887-891.
17. Magness RR, Parker CR, Jr, Rosenfeld CR. Does chronic administration of estradiol-17b (E2) reproduce the cardiovascular effects of pregnancy in non-pregnant ovariectomized sheep? Program and Abstracts, Endocrine Society 67th Annual Meeting, 1985, p 160.
18. Schrier RW. Pathogenesis of sodium and water retention in high-output and low-output cardiac failure, nephrotic syndrome, cirrhosis and pregnancy. *N Engl J Med.* 1988;319:1065-1072.
19. Ueland K, McAnulty JH, Ueland FR, et al. Special consideration in the use of cardiovascular drugs. *Clin Obstet Gynecol.* 1981;24:809-823.
20. Hanssens M, Keirse MJ, Vankelecom F, Van Assche FA. Fetal and neonatal effects of treatment with angiotensin converting enzyme inhibitors in pregnancy. *Obstet Gynecol.* 1991;78:128-135.
21. Frishman WH, Chesner M. Beta-adrenergic blockers in pregnancy. *Am Heart J.* 1988;115:147-152.
22. Hall JT, Pauli Rm, Wilson KM. Maternal and fetal sequelae of anticoagulation during pregnancy. *Am J Med.* 1980;68:122-140.
23. Iturbe-Alessio I, Fonseca MC, Mutchinik O, et al. Risks of anticoagulant therapy in pregnant women with artificial heart valves. *N Engl J Med.* 1986;315:1390-1393.
24. Gleicher N, Midwall JJ, Hochberger D, et al. Eisenmenger's syndrome and pregnancy. *Obstet Gynecol Surv.* 1979;34:721-741.
25. Tawam M, Levine J, Mendelson M, et al. Effect of pregnancy on paroxysmal supraventricular tachycardia. *Am J Cardiol.* 1993;72:838-840.

26. Prevention of Bacterial Endocarditis: Recommendations by the American Heart Association by the Committee on Rheumatic Fever, Endocarditis and Kawasaki Disease. *JAMA*. 1990;264:2919-2922.

27. Metcalf JM, McAnulty JH, Ueland K. *Heart Disease and Pregnancy*. 2nd Ed. Boston: Little, Brown; 1986.

28. McAnulty JH. Rheumatic heart disease. In: Geicher N, Gall SA, Sibai BM, et al (eds). *Principles and Practice of Medical Therapy in Pregnancy*, 2d Ed. Norwalk, CT: Appleton and Lange; 1992:783-788.

29. Dajani AS, Bisno AL, Chung KJ, et al. Prevention of rheumatic fever. *Circulation*. 1988;78:1082-1086.

30. Lao TT, Sermer M, MaGee L, et al. Congenital aortic stenosis and pregnancy—a reappraisal. *Am J Obstet Gynecol*. 1993;169:540-545.

31. Whittemore R, Hobbins JC, Engle MA. Pregnancy and its outcome in women with and without surgical treatment of congenital heart disease. *Am J Cardiol*. 1982;50:641-651.

32. Nora JJ, Nora AH. The evolution of specific genetic and environmental counseling in congenital heart diseases. *Circulation*. 1971;57:205-213.

33. Whittemore R, Wells JA, Castellsague X. A second-generation study of 427 probands with congenital heart defects and their 837 children. *J Am Coll Cardiol*. 1994;23:1459-1471.

34. Presbitero P, Somerville J, Stone S, et al. Pregnancy in cyanotic congenital heart disease outcome of mother and fetus. *Circulation*. 1994;89:2673-2676.

35. Pitkin RM, Perloff JK, Koos BJ, et al. Pregnancy and congenital heart disease. *Ann Intern Med*. 1990;112:445-454.

36. Connolly H, Warnes CA. Ebstein's Anomaly: Outcome of pregnancy. *JACC* 1994;23:1194-1198.

37. Lao TT, Sermer M, Colman JM. Pregnancy following surgical correction for transposition of the greater arteries. *Obstet Gynecol*. 1994;83(5Pt1):665-668.

38. Pyeritz RE. Maternal fetal complications of pregnancy in the Marfan syndrome. *Am J Med*. 1981;71:784-790.

39. McAnulty JH, Morton MJ, Ueland K. The heart and pregnancy. *Curr Probl Cardiol*. 1988;95:586-587.

CHAPTER 33

Aortic and Peripheral Arterial Disease

Marc A. Pfeffer, MD, PhD

AORTIC DISEASE

As with any other viable tissue, the aorta is subject to systemic diseases, trauma, and degenerative changes, as well as congenital anomalies. Since even a grossly diseased aorta may perform the function of transmitting blood from the left ventricle to branch arteries, it is not uncommon for severe aortic diseases to be asymptomatic. On the other end of the spectrum, the first clinical manifestation of aortic disease may be a catastrophic interruption in the integrity of this major arterial conduit. This discussion is concerned with diseases of the aorta that produce aneurysms and thereby threaten rupture, or produce vascular occlusion as another serious manifestation of aortic disease.

The media of the large arteries have a high content of elastic fibers and smooth-muscle cells. During the aging process, these cells and fibers degenerate and are replaced by fibrous tissue.[1] This histologic change produces the well-known reduced aortic distensibility of aging and results in systolic hypertension and a greater workload on the left ventricle in elderly persons. Medionecrosis, defined as a focal loss of nuclei in the media, also has been described as an aging process of the aorta. These changes of the aorta are believed to represent injury and repair processes resulting from the continuous hemodynamic impact to which the aorta is subjected.

Another important histologic alteration of the media of the aorta is seen in idiopathic cystic medial necrosis. The histologic appearance of cystic medial necrosis is a focal loss of the normal elastic and fibromuscular elements of the media with replacement by amorphous ground substance. Although the etiology of cystic medial necrosis is truly idiopathic, the association with Marfan's syndrome and other genetically transmitted disorders of connective tissue matrix underscore the hereditary defect in elastin-collagen formation. The histologic changes in the aorta are, of course, a combination of degenerative and hereditary influences, since the importance of these changes that result in the loss of the normal laminar pattern of fibrous-elastin elements and smooth muscle is the resultant weakening of the arterial wall. Such changes may result in localized dilatation of the vessel or aneurysm. Once initiated, an aneurysm promotes its own expansion by the LaPlace relationship, in which wall stress is directly proportional to the product of the vessel radius and distending pressure divided by wall thickness. Thus, dilatation (increase in radius) at a site of medial weakness can increase wall tension without altering blood pressure, thereby promoting further expansion and thinning, which may lead to fatal rupture of a major vessel. The deleterious combination of both increased radius and pressure underscore the critical importance of blood pressure control.

Aneurysms may occur at any location along the aorta, from the Sinuses of Valsalva to the terminal bifurcation into the iliac arteries. The three important causes of aortic aneurysms are atherosclerosis, cystic medial necrosis, and syphilis. With the dramatic decrease in the incidence of tertiary syphilis, atherosclerotic aneurysms are now by far the most prevalent aortic aneurysms.[2] Although atherosclerosis is generally considered as an intimal process, secondary medial weakening is produced by the destruction of elastic and fibromuscular support structures.

655

ATHEROSCLEROTIC ANEURYSMS

ABDOMINAL AORTIC ANEURYSMS

Most atherosclerotic aneurysms occur in the abdominal aorta, where more than 90% of aneurysms are caused by atherosclerosis.[2] Typically, these aneurysms are fusiform, located beneath the renal arteries, and may extend beyond the aortic bifurcation into the iliac arteries. Aside from the ever-present risk of rupture, these aneurysms usually contain mural thrombi and are potential sites for the formation of emboli to the lower extremities.

Although patients with unruptured abdominal aortic aneurysms are usually asymptomatic, the presence of dull abdominal or back pain, or awareness of an abdominal pulsation in an elderly person with other evidence of cardiovascular disease, should alert the examiner to the possibility of an aortic aneurysm. Physical examination may disclose a pulsatile abdominal mass, bruit, or evidence of peripheral arterial occlusive disease. In many instances, aortic aneurysms are first detected by abdominal roentgenograms or ultrasound examinations performed for unrelated reasons. Not infrequently, the aneurysm is outlined by calcification of the atherosclerotic plaque. Abdominal ultrasound examination is a reliable method of not only detecting and quantitating the extent of the aneurysm, but also providing a convenient noninvasive means of sequentially following abdominal aortic aneurysms.

The major clinical problem with asymptomatic abdominal aortic aneurysm, or with any asymptomatic aneurysm, is assessing the risk of surgical repair versus that of a life-limiting rupture. In practical terms, the question is, "is the affected individual likely to die with or from the aneurysm?" To make this assessment, the health status of the patient must be related to characteristics of the aneurysm. Although the actual frequency of death due to rupture in patients with abdominal aortic aneurysms is controversial, compilations of both autopsy and clinical studies indicate that in about one-third of these patients, death was attributed to a ruptured aneurysm.[3] One consistent conclusion is that the likelihood of rupture increases with the size of the aneurysm. The incidence of rupture of aneurysms larger than 6 cm in diameter approaches 50%, whereas rupture of aneurysms less than 5 cm was considered uncommon. An autopsy series by Darling and coworkers confirmed this high rate of rupture of large aneurysms; however, the series also yielded a 23% rate of rupture of aneurysms of only 4-5 cm in diameter.[4] Since surgical mortality for patients who present with a ruptured abdominal aneurysm remains high, the medical task is to select patients at risk for rupture for elective surgery.[5]

With the progressive reduction in operative mortality, surgical treatment of the asymptomatic patient with an abdominal aortic aneurysm has become even more attractive.[5,6] The operative mortality in experienced centers is 1%-4% for elective resection of an abdominal aneurysm. This figure is impressive when one considers that the surgery is usually performed on elderly patients with diffuse atherosclerosis. Intravascular stents are being actively evaluated and, if effective, may provide an alternative for a highly selected group at high operative risk.

The clinical decision regarding resection of an aneurysm must be tailored to each patient. However, a reasonable framework is to recommend surgery for patients with aneurysms ≥ 5 cm in diameter, or for symptomatic patients with even smaller aneurysms. Aneurysms 4-5 cm in diameter should not be considered benign, because there is still a definite risk of rupture.[6] One may recommend elective resection or a more conservative course of frequent evaluation of the size of the aneurysm by ultrasound.[7,8] An increase in cross-sectional diameter of 0.5 cm over 3-6 months is an indication for surgery even in relatively small aneurysms. In all cases, this decision should be individualized with consideration for not only the patient and characteristics of the aneurysm, but also the local surgical expertise.

In any event, the abdominal aortic aneurysm should be considered a manifestation of diffuse atherosclerosis. Patients with abdominal aortic aneurysms are at high-risk of other serious cardiovascular events. All efforts should therefore be directed at reducing modifiable risk factors.

THORACIC AORTIC ANEURYSMS

In the past half century, the etiology of the majority of aneurysms of the thoracic aorta has shifted dramatically from syphilitic to atherosclerotic. In a large autopsy series compiled from the mid-1920s to the mid-1950s, more than 80% of the aortic aneurysms were attributed to syphilis. More than 90% of these syphilitic aneurysms were located in the thoracic aorta and usually involved the ascending aorta. However, in a review of 100 consecutive cases of ascending aortic aneurysms operated on by DeBakey's group,[9] only 9% were attributed to syphilis. Secondary degenerative changes in the media produced by atherosclerosis accounted for 69% of the ascending aortic aneurysms. In 22 of the 100 patients, the ascending-aortic aneurysms were believed to be due to cystic medial necrosis, and 6 patients demonstrated skeletal stigmata of Marfan's syndrome.

Marfan's syndrome represents an autosomal dominant transmitted disorder of connective tissue, with a constellation of musculoskeletal, ocular, and cardiovascular abnormalities.[10,11] These patients are usually tall, with long extremities (span exceeds height), and elongated fingers and toes (arachnodactyly). A high-arched palate, pectus excavatum, and kyphoscoliosis are other musculoskeletal abnormalities associated with the syndrome. Lax ligaments, including the suspensory ligament of the lens, may result in subluxation of the lens (ectopia lentis). Indeed in recent years this biochemical defect in fibrillin in patients with the Marfan's syndrome[12] has been linked to a specific gene defect[13,14] which was previously localized to the long arm of chromosome 15.[15] Fibrillin, a large glycoprotein, is a major component of microfibrils that provide the scaffold for elastin. Dermal fibroblasts cultured from patients with Marfan's syndrome demonstrated abnormalities in fibrillin fibers which resulted in a failure of tissue culture to produce the normal network of fibrous materials.[16]

The cardiovascular abnormalities, which may include "floppy" redundant mitral valves and degenerative changes in the media of the major vessels, account for most of the premature deaths in affected persons. The medial degeneration characteristically involves the aortic ring and sinuses. Aortic regurgitation or rupture, and/or medial dissection of the aorta are grave consequences of the focal loss of elastic and fibromuscular elements in the aortic wall. The terms anuloaortic ectasia and idiopathic cystic medial necrosis are often used to describe similar aortic conditions without other musculoskeletal stigmata of Marfan's syndrome. Other families have been characterized with the proximal aortic weakness and complications as the only manifestation of an inheritable connective tissue disorder. The effectiveness of chronic ß-adrenergic blockade as prophylactic therapy in patients with Marfan's syndrome to attenuate aortic dilatation and clinical complications was recently demonstrated.[17] The clinical approach to aneurysms of the thoracic aorta, whether atherosclerotic, luetic, or inherited collagen weakness, should be directed to the basic clinical question of whether the aneurysm poses such a threat to survival that surgical resection must be undertaken.

As with abdominal aortic aneurysms, several associated factors appear to greatly reduce the 5-year survival rate of persons with thoracic aortic aneurysms. A vessel diameter of 6 cm or larger, associated atherosclerotic disease manifested in other regions, hypertension, and the presence of symptoms all appear to adversely alter the natural history of thoracic aortic aneurysms.

Thoracic aneurysms are more likely to produce symptoms than abdominal aneurysms. Pain described as a deep throbbing or aching sensation was the presenting symptom of 18 of the 107 patients with aneurysms of the thoracic aorta reported by Joyce et al.[18] Other presenting symptoms included cough and dyspnea from compression of the tracheo-bronchial tree, dysphagia from extrinsic compression of the esophagus, and hoarseness from involvement of the recurrent laryngeal nerve. Symptoms in patients with ascending aortic aneurysms may also reflect the commonly associated aortic regurgitation due to dilatation of the aortic ring.

In patients with ankylosing spondylitis, even limited aortic involvement may lead to severe aortic insufficiency. In this relatively benign rheumatologic condition, a very limited area of the aorta behind the sinuses and into the leaflets may be involved by an adventitial infiltrate clustering around the vasa vasora, as in syphilitic aortitis. Because of the critical location of this limited aortic involvement, severe aortic regurgitation may be produced which, when present, is the leading cause of cardiovascular morbidity in this otherwise benign disease.[19]

Advances in prosthetic valves and synthetic grafts and in cardiopulmonary bypass procedures have reduced the mortality and morbidity rates of even complex aortic reconstruction by experienced thoracic surgeons. Surgical intervention is urgent in patients with large symptomatic aneurysms. In patients who have smaller asymptomatic aneurysms but who do not have aortic insufficiency, the risk of surgery must be weighed against the risk of the continued presence of the aneurysm. In patients with Marfan's syndrome, prophylactic repair of asymptomatic ascending aortic aneurysms even less than 6 cm is recommended.[17] Care of these young individuals at high-risk of urgent cardiovascular complications should involve experienced tertiary care centers.

AORTIC DISSECTION

Perhaps the most catastrophic of all diseases of the aorta is acute dissection. A compilation of almost 1,000 untreated patients experiencing such dissection revealed a 50% mortality rate within 48 hours after the onset of pain. Before effective treatment was available, 90% of the patients died within 3 months of acute aortic dissection. During the past quarter-century, advances in diagnostic, medical, and surgical practices have so altered this grim prognosis that one can now expect to save 70% to 80% of patients presenting with acute aortic dissections.[20]

The fundamental pathologic lesion in aortic dissection is a cleavage of the aortic media by a dissecting hematoma. Degenerative changes in the media of the aorta, whether from congenital defects or changes produced by aging and hypertension, are the predisposing factors for aortic dissection. With each cardiac contraction, the ascending aorta and the aorta just distal to

the left subclavian artery are flexed by the sudden installation of blood from the left ventricle into the arterial tree. In some patients, these forces produce an intimal tear, permitting blood to enter the weakened media. Once initiated, the dissecting hematoma may propagate rapidly, involving a variable length of the aorta. The aortic media is cleaved into a thin outer wall surrounding a false channel. This thin outer wall is all that protects the aorta against fatal rupture and extravasation of blood. The propagation of the dissecting hematoma has been shown in experimental animals to depend on the rate of change in arterial pressure (dP/dt) and the level of blood pressure.[21] Untreated, a dissecting hematoma almost invariably progresses to rupture and death. Hemopericardium with cardiac tamponade and hemothorax are the most frequent fatal complications.[22] Aside from outright rupture, the medial hemorrhage may distort the aortic annulus and produce aortic regurgitation. Occlusion of a major branch artery is yet another major complication of aortic dissection. The false channel may so compress the lumen of the true channel as to produce arterial insufficiency of the region supplied by the branch vessel. In aortic dissection, renal, splanchnic, cerebral, and even coronary ischemia may be encountered as a consequence of compression of the vital arteries.

As with other catastrophic disease processes, a rapid and accurate diagnosis is essential so that life-sustaining therapy can be immediately instituted. Severe pain is the outstanding clinical feature that should alert the physician to the possibility of aortic dissection. The pain is usually characterized as sharp and tearing; however, it may mimic the pain of a myocardial infarction. It may be localized in the anterior chest or interscapular region and, particularly in distal dissections, may occur simultaneously in several regions both above and below the diaphragm. In some instances, because of an altered state of consciousness, pain is not perceived, and therefore, is not a presenting symptom. Neurologic symptoms indicative of cerebral ischemia represent an ominous presentation of aortic dissection.

Patients with acute aortic dissection characteristically appear in overt distress. Arterial pressure is usually elevated at the time of presentation. Hypotension is suggestive of proximal dissection or aortic rupture. Occlusion of an arterial branch of the aorta by compression of the true lumen produces the reduced or absent arterial pulse found in about one-third of patients with aortic dissections. Therefore, careful examination of the carotid, brachial, radial, and femoral arteries is important. A murmur of aortic regurgitation is detected in about one-third of patients with aortic dissections. It usually indicates proximal dissection with loss of annular support.

The electrocardiogram in aortic dissection may be abnormal but is usually nonspecific. Because of the patient population, left ventricular hypertrophy with or without evidence of strain or ischemia is more common. However, severe chest discomfort in the absence of electrocardiographic evidence of acute myocardial necrosis should raise the suspicion of aortic dissection.

Plain films of the chest may provide findings suggestive of aortic dissection. The most common abnormalities are in the region of the aortic knob. In one study of patients with aortic dissection, findings of an increased aortic diameter, double density as a result of posterior aortic enlargement, or deviation of the trachea to the right were reported in more than one-half of the cases. Mediastinal widening or displacement of calcified intima by more than 1 cm was noted in only 11% and 7%, respectively, of the plain films of patients with confirmed dissections. In this study, the plain chest films were not suggestive of aortic disease in 20% of the patients with confirmed aortic dissection.[23] Therefore, the lack of chest x-ray evidence of a mediastinal process should not derail a rapid diagnostic evaluation.

Although aortography has been the standard procedure for confirming the diagnosis of aortic dissection, the prompt use of newer, noninvasive methods has shown considerable effectiveness. The objective of these diagnostic procedures is to determine first and foremost the presence of a dissection. Second, the objectives are to determine the origin of the dissection as well as to define the extent of the dissecting hematoma

and specifically determine whether the ascending aorta is involved. The most common angiographic finding is opacification of the false channel, creating a double lumen. Magnetic resonance imaging (MRI) and computer axial tomography (CAT) scanning have emerged as sensitive and specific means of obtaining the anatomic information needed to guide management decisions in aortic dissection.[24,25] However, the speed at which these modalities can be implemented in critical situations has been a major limitation. Although routine transthoracic echocardiography did not have the diagnostic accuracy on which to base major medical-surgical decisions regarding possible aortic dissection, adding transesophageal echocardiography has dramatically increased the sensitivity and specificity of echocardiography in the imaging of aortic dissection.[25] The specific diagnostic modality employed will depend on the expertise at a particular center and the ability to effect a prompt study of and provide definitive information about the condition of these critically ill persons.

Treatment of aortic dissection has progressed dramatically in the past 25 years. In 1955, DeBakey and coworkers described a surgical approach to dissecting aneurysms. By the mid-1960s, they reported a 74% survival rate in an extensive series of patients with dissections. Based on this experience, DeBakey defined specific surgical approaches to aortic dissection according to the origin and extent of the dissection.[26] Type I dissections begin at the ascending aorta and extend to the abdominal aorta; type II dissections are localized to the ascending aorta and aortic arch; and type III dissections begin just distal to the left subclavian artery and extend to below the diaphragm (Fig. 1). The early results of other surgical series are not as impressive as those of DeBakey's group.

Wheat and coworkers reported encouraging results with intensive medical therapy in patients with acute aortic dissection.[27] They reasoned that the complications of aortic dissection were produced by the progression of the medial hematoma and not the initial intimal tear itself. Hydrodynamic modeling of the forces in the arterial system underscored the importance of the rate of rise of arterial

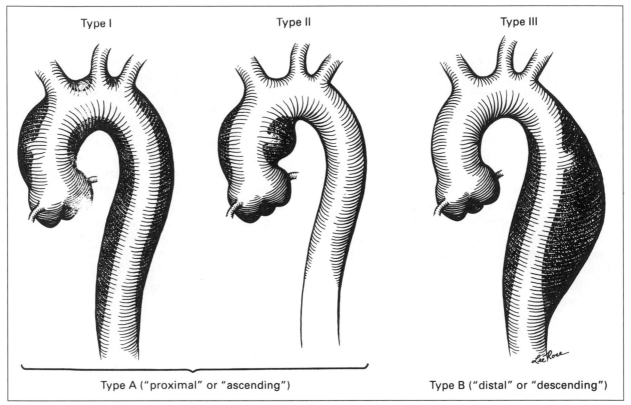

Type I   Type II   Type III

Type A ("proximal" or "ascending")   Type B ("distal" or "descending")

Figure 1. *Classification of Aortic Dissections. Type I in previous DeBakey classification. Type I and II involve the ascending aorta are now pragmatically lumped together as Type A (proximal or ascending aorta) involvement. Type III does not involve the ascending aorta and propogates from beyond the left subclavian artery. These dissections are termed "Type B" or distal or descending dissections. From Massumi A. Clinical recognition of aortic dissection.* Tex Heart Inst J. *1990;17:254-256. With permission.*

pressure, not just the level of blood pressure, as the major factors determining the propagation of the hematoma to rupture and death. Pharmacologic attempts to halt progression of the medial hematoma are therefore directed at reducing the steepness of the pulse wave (dP/dt) and reducing arterial pressure. By the late 1960s, Wheat had used medical therapy in more than 50 patients with survival rates as impressive as in DeBakey's original surgical series.

By the early 1970s, as more experience was gained with both surgical and medical therapies, it was apparent that neither blanket surgical nor medical strategies provided optimal management for patients with aortic dissection. A new classification was developed that remains of both therapeutic and prognostic importance: type A dissections originate in the ascending aorta (DeBakey I and II) and type B dissections begin

after the left subclavian artery (DeBakey III).[28] Roughly two-thirds of aortic dissections are type A and one-third are type B.

Recent results indicate that surgery is the treatment of choice for proximal (type A) aortic dissections. In general, in patients with acute dissection originating or involving the ascending aorta, medical therapy alone has been extremely disappointing. In contrast, patients with type A dissections who were treated surgically had a 70%-80% survival rate. With ascending aortic involvement, the potential for retrograde dissection and fatal pericardial tamponade is great, and prompt surgical intervention is indicated.[28,29]

In contrast, patients with type B, or dissecting hematoma distal to the left subclavian artery not involving the ascending aorta, immediate surgical intervention did not improve survival.[28,30] In patients with distal dissections the surgical survival was either not as good or equivalent to that of the medically treated group.[29] An important caveat is that many medically treated patients with distal dissections did undergo surgical intervention as a result of complications. Therefore, in the uncomplicated distal dissection, medical therapy remains an option with the understanding that surgical consultation and possible intervention be available.

Using recent, carefully documented experiences, a unified plan can be suggested that will provide for the optimal management of patients with acute aortic dissection. Patients suspected of having an aortic dissection should be treated immediately to halt progression of the dissecting hematoma. This therapy should reduce arterial pressure to the lowest level commensurate with organ perfusion and reduce the rate of rise of arterial pressure. The ganglionic blocking agent, trimethaphan, has been used effectively for this purpose. Alternatively, use of the vascular smooth-muscle dilator, nitroprusside, in combination with a ß-adrenergic blocking agent such as propranolol, provides therapy designed to arrest the progression of the dissecting hematoma. Esmolol as a titratable intravenous ß blocker is being increasingly utilized.

While attempting to control pain and blood pressure, a prompt diagnostic procedure must be obtained. Although the aortogram was the gold standard to confirm the diagnosis and determine whether the dissecting hematoma involves the ascending aorta, the improvements in noninvasive imaging have increased the options. At this level of suspicion the front line clinician should be aided by specialists with imaging and surgical expertise in aortic dissection. The urgency of establishing a prompt diagnosis requires a working knowledge of each specific institution's capabilities rather than literature-cited experience. The presence of cardiac surgeons during the diagnostic evaluation can limit precious time often wasted on supplemental, not critical, imaging data. Identification of a proximal dissection constitutes an urgent indication for surgical therapy.

Patients with distal dissections not involving the ascending aorta (type B) may do somewhat better initially with medical therapy. If no complications are encountered in patients with type B dissections, intravenous antihypertensive agents can be replaced by an oral regimen, which should include a ß-adrenergic blocking agent. If a patient with a distal dissection undergoing intensive medical therapy has complications, surgical intervention is required. Indications for surgical intervention in patients with distal dissection are: evidence of continued propagation of the hematoma, continued pain, new aortic insufficiency murmur, and signs of occlusion of a major branch of the aorta, such as new neurologic findings, loss of an arterial pulse, or inability to control pressure. Indications of impending rupture of the dissecting hematoma, such as increasing size of the aneurysm and blood in the pleural space or pericardium, are other indications for prompt surgical intervention, even in patients initially stabilized with type B acute dissections.

If a medically or surgically treated patient has survived the acute phase of dissection, careful follow-up evaluations should be performed. Impressive 5-year survival rates have been reported for both medically and surgically treated patients who have survived the acute phase of aortic dissection.

In summary, in the past 25 years, much progress has been made in the management of acute aortic dissection. One can now expect a 70%-80% survival rate in a condition that was once almost always fatal.

OCCLUSIVE DISEASES OF THE AORTA AND PERIPHERAL VESSELS

Atherosclerosis is the cause of chronic occlusive arterial disease in 95% of cases. The infrarenal abdominal aorta and its iliac branches are the common sites of extensive atherosclerosis that produce chronic ischemia of the lower limbs. A dynamic state exists between progressive occlusive disease and development of collateral channels. As with coronary artery disease (CAD), ischemia is a result of an imbalance between oxygen delivery and utilization.

Intermittent claudication, the discomfort in

the limbs that occurs with exercise and is relieved by rest, is usually the first symptom of chronic occlusive arterial disease. This ischemic pain is usually indicative of severe multi-segmental occlusive disease. With severe occlusive disease, nonobstructing factors that reduce oxygen delivery, such as reduced cardiac output, relative hypotension, and anemia, may enhance peripheral ischemia. In the patient awakened by an aching numbness from a distal limb, the slight increase in arterial inflow produced by the gravitational effect of hanging the extremity over the edge of the bed may be sufficient to relieve the ischemic pain. In its most severe form, chronic occlusive arterial disease may present as ischemic ulceration with gangrene as an end stage. The hallmark of the physical examination of patients with chronic occlusive arterial disease is a diminished peripheral pulse. Bruits may or may not be heard. Postural color changes such as pallor on elevation and rubor on dependency of the extremity are indicative of moderate to severe arterial insufficiency. Nutritional atrophy of skin and nails should be noted.

Noninvasive assessment of the arterial inflow to the extremity provides a more standardized diagnostic assessment. An index of Doppler-determined systolic pressures in the tibial and brachial arteries provides a quantitative assessment of the degree of chronic occlusive arterial disease. A resting tibial over brachial systolic arterial pressure ratio or ankle/arm index provides an objective assessment of the severity of the arterial occlusive disease to the lower extremity.

In considering treatment options, both the patient and physician must be aware that intermittent claudication in and of itself does not alter life expectancy. However, the finding of peripheral vascular disease should alert the physician to coexisting atherosclerotic disease which is associated with reduced survival.[31,32] The limitation of activity imposed by the exercise-induced pain may be acceptable to the patient. However, the intermittent claudication may so disable the patient that elective revascularization to improve the quality of life may be desired. Also, revascularization may be urgently recommended to avoid the possible

loss of a limb. Recent transcatheter approaches (transluminal angioplasty, laser-assisted angioplasty, and atherectomy) to peripheral vascular disease continue to evolve and offer a nonsurgical option especially for predominant aortoiliac involvement.

A detailed medical evaluation is most important in all patients considered for arterial reconstructive surgery. Patients with symptoms of atherosclerosis in the extremities usually have coexisting cardiac and respiratory disease. In obtaining a cardiac history from these patients, the physician must be aware that the functional limitations produced by the peripheral vascular disease may mask significant CAD. Indeed, many physicians perform exercise tests for ischemic cardiac changes before vascular reconstructive surgery, even though the test is usually limited by claudication. In a recent study, dipyridamole-thallium screening did not add predictive information of postoperative adverse-cardiovascular events.[33] Preoperative ambulatory ST-segment monitoring for ischemic episodes has been useful in identifying high-risk individuals without exercise testing.[34] If there is clinical evidence of impressive myocardial ischemia at low exercise levels or on ambulatory monitoring, coronary angiography may be recommended prior to elective vascular surgery. Despite newer modalities to detect myocardial ischemia, the basic approach for the need for preoperative myocardial revascularization remains based on sound clinical judgment.

Patients with chronic occlusive arterial disease should be instructed to provide meticulous care and avoid trauma to their ischemic extremities. It is not uncommon for urgent bypass surgery, or even amputation, to be required because of avoidable injury to an ischemic extremity in a person considered to have relatively poor operative risk. Cigarette smoking is strongly contraindicated, as evidenced by the 10-fold greater amputation rate among patients with chronic occlusive arterial disease who continue to smoke compared with those who stop. Vasodilator therapy is generally ineffective. Pentoxifylline, by making red blood cells more deformable and thereby increasing post-stenotic blood flow, purportedly prolongs the time to onset of leg pain during exercise testing in patients with intermittent claudication. However, the subjective clinical responses to this therapy have not been impressive.

Arterial reconstructive surgery should be considered in suitable candidates to improve a disabling lifestyle, relieve pain at rest, or — the most urgent indication — prevent tissue necrosis and amputation.

In appropriate patients, percutaneous transluminal angioplasty provides an excellent alternative to reconstructive surgery. Long-term patency appears better for iliac than for femoral angioplasty, with approximately 80% and 60% 3-5 year patency rates, respectively.[35] Experience with the newer atherectomy catheters and laser probe therapy is too recent to determine long-term outcome. However, intravascular stents appear promising for longer durations of patency, especially in larger arteries.

TAKAYASU'S ARTERITIS

Takayasu's arteritis, or pulseless disease, is a rare, nonspecific inflammatory process of unknown etiology affecting segmental areas of the aorta and its main branches. The disease process results in a marked thickening of the arterial wall, which eventually produces occlusions of major branches of the aorta. Takayasu's arteritis has been linked to rheumatic fever, syphilis, and tuberculosis; however, the evidence for each of these associations is sketchy. Unlike giant cell (temporal) arteritis, which usually afflicts elderly men, Takayasu's arteritis is a disease of young persons. It is far more prevalent among women; the female-to-male ratio is 9:1. Although typically described as a disease of young Oriental women, Takayasu's arteritis has a worldwide distribution.

Several classifications of regional involvement of the aorta and major branches have been described. The most common areas of the arterial tree to be involved with the proliferative process are the aortic arch, including the origins of the brachiocephalic arteries, and the thoracoabdominal aorta, including the renal arteries.[36]

The symptoms and signs of arterial occlusive disease are usually preceded by an initial systemic illness presenting with fever, weight loss, arthralgias, and fatigue. In the chronic phase, the young patient presents with cardiovascular and neurologic symptoms related to arterial obstruction. Absent pulses and vascular bruits are almost always found. Hypertension was reported in 72% of a recent series of 107 patients with Takayasu's arteritis.[37] Renal artery involvement caused hypertension in the majority of cases. The clinical course of this devastating arteritis is unpredictable. During the acute phase, intravenous gamma globulin therapy appears to reduce the extent of coronary artery involvement. At present, therapy is directed only at the manifestations of the disease process: steroids for constitutional symptoms; antihypertensive therapy; and possible anticoagulation therapy. The frequent need for both surgical and transcatheter vascular bypass procedures to restore blood flow to vital organs requires detailed serial evaluations.[38]

REFERENCES

1. Schlatmann TJ, Becker AE. Pathogenesis of dissecting aneurysm of aorta. Comparative histopathologic study of significance of medial changes. *Am J Cardiol.* 1977;39:21-26.
2. Reed D, Reed C, Stemmermann G, et al. Are aortic aneurysms caused by atherosclerosis? *Circulation.* 1992;85:205-211.
3. Szilagyi DE, Smith RF, DeRusso FJ, et al. Contribution of abdominal aortic aneurysmectomy to prolongation of life. *Ann Surg.* 1966;164:678-699.
4. Darling RC, Messina CR, Brewster DC. Autopsy study of unoperated abdominal aortic aneurysms. The case for early resection. *Circulation.* 1977;56(S2):161-164.
5. Ernst CB. Abdominal aortic aneurysm. *N Engl J Med.* 1993;328:1167-1172.
6. Katz DA, Littenberg B, Cronenwett JL. Management of small abdominal aortic aneurysms: early surgery vs watchful waiting. *JAMA.* 1992;268:2678-2686.
7. Nevitt MP, Ballard DJ, Hallett JW. Prognosis of abdominal aortic aneurysms. *N Engl J Med.* 1989;321:1009-1014.
8. Masuda Y, Takanashi K, Takasu J, et al. Expansion rate of thoracic aortic aneurysms and influencing factors. *Chest.* 1992;102:461-466.
9. DeBakey ME, Noon GP. Aneurysms of the thoracic aorta. *Mod Concepts Cardiovasc Dis.* 1975;44:53-58.
10. Pyeritz RD, McKusick VA. The Marfan syndrome: diagnosis and management. *N Engl J Med.* 1979;300:772-777.

11. Pyeritz RE. Marfan syndrome. *N Engl J Med.* 1990;323:987-989.
12. Hollister DW, Godfrey M, Sakai LY, et al. Immuno-histologic abnormalities of the microfibrillar-fiber system in the Marfan syndrome. *N Engl J Med.* 1990;323:152-159.
13. Pereira L, D'Alessio M, Ramirez F, et al. Genomic organization of the sequence coding for fibrillin, the defective gene product in Marfan syndrome. *Hum Mol Genet.* 1993;2:961-968.
14. Dietz HC, Cutting GR, Pyeritz RE, et al. Marfan syndrome caused by a recurrent de novo missense mutation in the fibrillin gene. *Nature.* 1991;352:337-339.
15. Kainulainen K, Pulkkinen L, Savolainen A, et al. Location on chromosome 15 of the gene defect causing Marfan syndrome. *N Engl J Med.* 1990;323:935-939.
16. Milewicz DM, Pyeritz RE, Crawford ES, et al. Marfan syndrome: defective synthesis, secretion, and extracellular matrix formation of fibrillin by cultured dermal fibroblasts. *J Clin Invest.* 1992;89:79-86.
17. Shores J, Berger KR, Murphy EA, et al. Progression of aortic dilatation and the benefit of long-term beta-adrenergic blockade in Marfan's syndrome. *N Engl J Med.* 1994;330:1335-1341.
18. Joyce JW, Fairbairn JFI, Kincaid OW, et al. Aneurysms of the thoracic aorta. *Circulation.* 1964;29:176-181.
19. Bulkley BH, Roberts WC. Ankylosing spondylitis and aortic regurgitation. Description of the characteristic cardiovascular lesion from study of eight necropsy patients. *Circulation.* 1973; 48:1014-1027.
20. Cooley DA. Surgical management of aortic dissection. *Tex Heart Inst J.* 1990;17:289-301.
21. Wheat MW, Jr. Acute dissecting aneurysms of the aorta: diagnosis and treatment-1979. *Am Heart J.* 1980;99:373-387.
22. Roberts WC. Aortic dissection: anatomy, consequences, and causes. *Am Heart J.* 1981;101:195-214.
23. Earnest F, Muhm JR, Sheedy PF. Roentgenographic findings in thoracic aortic dissection. *Mayo Clin Proc.* 1979;54:43-50.
24. Nienaber CA, von Kodolitsch Y, Nicolas V, et al. The diagnosis of thoracic aortic dissection by noninvasive imaging procedures. *N Engl J Med.* 1993;328:1-9.
25. Cigarroa JE, Isselbacher EM, DeSanctis RW, et al. Diagnostic imaging in the evaluation of suspected aortic dissection. Old standards and new directions. *N Engl J Med.* 1993;328:35-43.
26. DeBakey ME, Henly WS, Cooley DA, et al. Surgical management of dissecting aneurysms of the aorta. *J Thorac Cardiovasc Surg.* 1965;49:130-149.
27. Wheat MW Jr, Palmer RF, Bartley TD, et al. Treatment of dissecting aneurysms of the aorta without surgery. *J Thorac Cardiovasc Surg.* 1965;50:364-373.
28. Miller DC, Stinson EB, Oyer PE, et al. Operative treatment of aortic dissections. Experience with 125 patients over a sixteen-year period. *J Thorac Cardiovasc Surg.* 1979;78:365-382.
29. Crawford ES, Kirklin JW, Naftel DC, et al. Surgery for acute dissection of ascending aorta. Should the arch be included? *J Thorac Cardiovasc Surg.* 1992;104:46-59.
30. Glower DD, Fann JI, Speier RH, et al. Comparison of medical and surgical therapy for uncomplicated descending aortic dissection. *Circulation.* 1990;82(suppl IV):IV39-IV46.
31. Criqui MH, Langer RD, Fronek A, et al. Mortality over a period of 10 years in patients with peripheral arterial disease. *N Engl J Med.* 1992;326:381-386.
32. Vogt MT, Cauley JA, Newman AB, et al. Decreased ankle/arm blood pressure index and mortality in elderly women. *JAMA.* 1993;270:465-469.
33. Baron JF, Mundler O, Bertrand M, et al. Dipyridamole-thallium scintigraphy and gated radionuclide angiography to assess cardiac risk before abdominal aortic surgery. *N Engl J Med.* 1994;330:663-669.
34. Raby KE, Barry J, Creager MA, et al. Detection and significance of intraoperative and postoperative myocardial ischemia in peripheral vascular surgery. *JAMA.* 1992;268(2):222-227.
35. Tegtmeyer CJ, Hartwell GD, Selby JB, et al. Results and complications of angioplasty in aortoiliac disease. *Circulation.* 1991;83(suppl I):I53-I60.
36. Gersony WM. Diagnosis and management of Kawasaki disease. *JAMA.* 1991;265:2699-2703.
37. Lupi-Herrera E, Sanchez-Torres G, Marcushamer J, et al. Takayasu's arteritis. Clinical study of 107 cases. *Am Heart J.* 1977;93:94-103.
38. Dajani AS, Taubert KA, Takahashi M, et al. Guidelines for long-term management of patients with Kawasaki disease. Report from the Committee on rheumatic fever, endocarditis, and Kawasaki disease, Council on cardiovascular disease in the young, American Heart Association. *Circulation.* 1994;89:916-922.

CHAPTER 34

Cardiovascular Problems in Patients With Primarily Noncardiac Diseases

Marlo F. Leonen, MD
James D. Marsh, MD

The internist or cardiologist is frequently asked to see patients who have primarily noncardiac disorders but are suspected of having some cardiovascular complication arising from their primary disease or its therapy. Many disorders have secondary manifestations that involve the pericardium, myocardium, epicardium, valves, great vessels, coronary arteries, or the neurohumoral regulation of the heart and circulation. This chapter discusses the recognition and management of cardiovascular manifestations of primarily noncardiac diseases.

RHEUMATOID, BONE AND CONNECTIVE TISSUE DISORDERS

PAGET'S DISEASE

Paget's disease (osteitis deformans) is a skeletal abnormality that afflicts between 1% and 3% of the U.S. population over the age of 40 years. Cardiac manifestations of Paget's disease can include high-output congestive heart failure (CHF) and metastatic calcification of the cardiac skeleton, producing varying degrees of conduction abnormalities. For many years arteriovenous fistulas were believed to be present in the bone marrow of patients with this disorder. However, radiolabeled macro-aggregated-albumin studies show that no true arteriovenous fistulas are present.[1] Instead, cutaneous and soft-tissue vasodilatation frequently accounts for increased flow to an extremity. In some patients, the blood flow through the involved extremity is 9 times the normal level.[2,3]

Paget's disease most frequently presents in elderly patients. However, the most common causes of congestive heart failure in patients with Paget's disease are also the usual causes in an elderly population, such as ischemic or hypertensive heart disease, and not high-output heart failure. High-output symptoms respond well to a pulse of steroids, such as prednisone at 60 mg/day. Hemodynamic improvement is usually evident within 3 or 4 days.

RHEUMATOID ARTHRITIS

Involvement of cardiac structures in rheumatoid arthritis is very common but usually subclinical (Table 1). Nodular granulomas are the characteristic pathologic lesions involving the myocardium, endocardium, and valves. Granulomas sometimes involve the conduction system and produce varying degrees of heart block. The most frequent electrocardiographic abnormality in patients with rheumatoid arthritis is first-degree atrioventricular (AV) block. Rheumatoid granulomas may involve the cardiac valves, but very rarely produce enough distortion of the valve structure to cause regurgitation or stenosis of any hemodynamic significance. Myocarditis and coronary arteritis may be present at necropsy, but they rarely cause clinical symptoms.

In approximately 30% of patients with rheumatoid arthritis, the pericardium is involved at necropsy or on echocardiographic study. However, pericarditis is clinically evident in only about 2%-5% of patients with rheumatoid arthritis, and usually follows a benign course, responding to moderate doses of steroids. Rarely, pericarditis is severe, producing either constriction or tamponade. Needle pericardiocentesis is often technically difficult to perform because of the markedly thickened pericardium and the tendency for loculation of pericardial effusions. When pericardial fluid is obtained, complement levels and glucose are frequently depressed, as they are in fluid from other serous spaces in

Table 1. Cardiovascular Manifestations of Rheumatoid Diseases

DISEASE	PERICARDITIS	FIBROSIS	MYOCARDITIS/ ENDOCARDITIS	↑ BP	VALVES INVOLVED	CONDUCTION ABNORMALITIES	GRANULOMAS
Rheumatoid arthritis	+ +	+	+		AoV MV	+	Nodular granulomas
SLE	+ + + +	+ +	+ + +	+ +	AoV MV	+	Microvasculitis
Periarteritis nodosa		+ +		+ + + +			Necrotizing vasculitis
Scleroderma	+ +	+ + + +	+	+ + + +		+ + +	Vascular fibrosis

AoV=Aortic valve; BP=blood pressure; MV=Mitral valve; SLE=Systemic lupus erythrmatosus.

rheumatoid arthritis. Intrapericardial injection of corticosteroids may provide temporary improvement but will not prevent recurrence.[4] Surgical pericardiectomy is rarely required but should be undertaken if clear-cut tamponade is present. Unfortunately, patients requiring pericardiectomy for rheumatoid pericarditis have high perioperative morbidity and mortality, largely due to their poor wound-healing and underlying state of debility.

SYSTEMIC LUPUS ERYTHEMATOSUS

Cardiac manifestations of systemic lupus erythematosus (SLE) are numerous (Table 1). The underlying pathologic abnormality is diffuse microvasculitis. Cardiac involvement is very common at necropsy, although clinical cardiac involvement is present in only about half of cases.[5] Systemic lupus erythematosus produces pancarditis, with involvement of the pericardium most evident clinically. Approximately 30% of all patients with SLE have clinical symptoms of pericarditis, and another substantial proportion may have findings of pericarditis on auscultation or on electro-cardiograph (ECG). Inflammation of the pericardium may be pronounced, involving the pericardium, epicardium, and occasionally even the sinoatrial (SA) and AV nodes, with destruction of conducting fibers and resulting arrhythmias and conduction blocks. Pericardial

constriction or tamponade occurs in a small but important number of patients. Corticosteroids usually control the symptoms of pericarditis. No compelling evidence shows that administration of steroids prevents progression to constriction. Patients with refractory pericardial symptoms may rarely require pericardiectomy.

The myocarditis of SLE is due to segmental arteritis of the small arteries in the myocardium. Subclinical myocarditis is common. It produces fibrinoid necrosis in small vessels, although actual necrosis of myocardial cells is rare. In SLE, arteritis of the major coronary arteries leading to a clinical myocardial infarction is a very rare event. However, the incidence of atherosclerotic coronary artery disease may be somewhat higher in patients with SLE. In these patients, clinical myocardial ischemia or necrosis is far more likely to be due to typical large-vessel coronary artery disease than to arteritis. Thus, patients with signs of myocardial ischemia are best treated with conventional measures rather than with a pulse of steroids as a first approach.

Libman-Sacks endocarditis is observed at necropsy in 50% of SLE cases. These verrucous excrescences on valve leaflets are comprised of degenerating valve tissue. A prospective echocardiographic study found that 18% of patients with SLE had heart valve abnormalities. Those with Libman-Sacks vegetations had a relatively benign course, whereas 80% of those with rigid, thickened valves required surgery over a 5-year period.[6] In view of the frequent valve abnormalities in SLE patients, and the frequency of immunosuppressive therapy with steroids, antibiotic prophylaxis for endocarditis is recommended. In patients with SLE, the presence of a high titer of anticardiolipin antibodies is highly predictive of structural heart disease, including valvular, pericardial, or myocardial abnormalities.[5] Moreover, even in the absence of anticardiolipin antibodies, patients with SLE very commonly have subclinical diastolic dysfunction[7] that may be related to concomitant hypertension.

Children born to mothers with SLE are at risk for congenital heart block, due to transplacental transfer of maternal antibodies.

PERIARTERITIS NODOSA

Necrotizing vasculitis of muscular arteries is the pathologic hallmark of periarteritis nodosa (Table 1). Gross nodularity of the involved vessels is apparent at necropsy. The vasculitis may produce infarction of an involved organ and, when coronary arteries are involved, as they frequently are, myocardial necrosis may occur. Clinically recognized acute myocardial infarction caused by periarteritis nodosa is uncommon, although clinically unrecognized events are frequent, as patchy fibrosis of the myocardium is common and contributes to the dilation of the left ventricle that frequently occurs. Small aneurysms of coronary arteries are present, particularly at bifurcations; on occasion, they may rupture and produce hemopericardium. Pericarditis is uncommon in periarteritis nodosa, as is endocarditis.[8]

The clinical picture of cardiac involvement in periarteritis nodosa is most frequently dominated by the effects of hypertension resulting from renal involvement. Indeed, CHF secondary to hypertension and renal involvement is a very common cause of death.

SCLERODERMA (PROGRESSIVE SYSTEMIC SCLEROSIS)

In this systemic fibrosing disease, visceral rather than skin involvement is the main determinant of the clinical course. There is gradual obliteration of small vessels with extensive fibrosis and scarring. Progressive systemic sclerosis often involves the heart pathologically, although clinical involvement is less often appreciated (Table 1). A pancarditis is produced, with pericarditis and asymptomatic myocarditis common, whereas endocardial thickening is unusual. Intimal sclerosis of small intramural coronary arteries produces ischemia and focal areas of myocardial necrosis and fibrosis. Focal fibrosis frequently causes conduction abnormalities; if fibrosis is extensive, cardiomyopathy may result.

Relative myocardial ischemia is common in scleroderma. Single photon emission computed tomography (SPECT) and thallium myocardial perfusion studies demonstrate areas of poor perfusion that improve with vasodilator therapy, including therapy with calcium channel blockers and angiotensin-converting enzyme (ACE) inhibitors. It is not certain whether the improvement in perfusion is due to the action of these drugs on intramyocardial arterioles or due to their peripheral vasodilating effects.[9,10]

Direct cardiac involvement is often overshadowed by cardiac effects of both pulmonary and systemic hypertension. Both right-and left-ventricular failure are common. If CHF develops, either from hypertension or direct myocardial involvement, the prognosis is poor. Conduction abnormalities usually indicate primary myocardial involvement.

Specific treatment is not entirely satisfactory. Corticosteroids have a beneficial effect on pericarditis in scleroderma, and there have been reports of calcium-channel blockers improving myocardial and pulmonary blood flow. Conduction disturbances occasionally require management with a permanent pacemaker. Aggressive management of hypertension in scleroderma is essential.

ANKYLOSING SPONDYLITIS

Dilatation of the aortic root and fibrosis of the aortic valve cusps produce incompetence of the aortic valve in approximately 10% of patients with ankylosing spondylitis. Fibrosis usually occurs at the base of the valves but can extend into the conduction system, causing conduction defects. Aortic regurgitation may become severe and valve replacement may be necessary. Even in the absence of significant aortic regurgitation, Doppler echocardiographic studies frequently demonstrate diastolic dysfunction in these patients.[11]

DERMATOMYOSITIS

Dermatomyositis involves primarily the skin and skeletal muscles. Clinical cardiovascular manifestations are unusual, although pathologic abnormalities are frequently present. Degeneration and fibrosis occur primarily in the conduction system and occasionally in scattered areas of myocardium. While these effects are usually asymptomatic, arrhythmias and heart block have been observed, and repolarization abnormalities are frequently present on the electrocardiogram.

KAWASAKI SYNDROME (MUCOCUTANEOUS LYMPH NODE SYNDROME)

Kawasaki syndrome is an idiopathic, acute febrile illness of children associated with fever, rash, peripheral edema, dry fissured lips, strawberry tongue, conjunctival congestion, cervical lymphadenopathy, and cardiac involvement. Coronary artery aneurysms develop in approximately 30% of children with the syndrome and thrombosis of the coronary arteries is the major cause of death. Two-year follow-up coronary arteriography in children with aneurysms shows resolution in half of the cases. Randomized studies show that therapy with intravenous gamma globulin plus aspirin significantly reduces the incidence of coronary artery abnormalities when administered early.

In the United States, Kawasaki's disease has been prevalent for a sufficient number of years so that patients affected as children are coming to the attention of adult cardiologists and internists. The major concern with these patients is that the aneurysmal dilatation of the coronary arteries have often transformed to obstructive lesions. For unclear reasons, right coronary aneurysms are more likely to undergo transformation than lesions in other vessels. In this young age group, development of collateral vessels is often exuberant.[12] Although it is tempting to perform "prophylactic" angioplasty on focal lesions that have undergone transformation from aneurysm to stenosis, such lesions are at higher than usual risk for restenosis and at present there is no compelling evidence that such interventions are warranted.

MARFAN'S SYNDROME

Cardiovascular manifestations of Marfan's syndrome are prominent and frequently determine the fate of patients with the syndrome (Table 2). It is caused by missense mutations in the fibrillin gene (FBN1). Cystic medial necrosis is present in the aorta, with degeneration of the elastic elements. The ascending aorta is frequently dilated, as is the aortic annulus. Sinuses of Valsalva may become grossly enlarged; the proximal pulmonary artery is often dilated. Chronic aortic dissection and tearing with dissection are frequently found. Dilatation of the aortic valve annulus leads to chronic aortic regurgitation, with left ventricular dilatation and hypertrophy as a consequence. The mitral valve may have intrinsic abnormalities as well, with redundancy of the mitral valve leaflets often seen by echocardiography. The chordae tendineae are often elongated, and occasionally there is frank fenestration of the mitral valve leaflets. In patients with Marfan's syndrome, death from a cardiac cause is very common, coming from aortic dilatation, dissection, or rupture in most patients. Mitral regurgitation may be the dominant clinical feature, although somewhat less frequently than aortic regurgitation. Because of markedly altered hemodynamics and turbulent blood flow, endocarditis may be a complication. Ventricular conduction abnormalities have also been reported.

The cardiovascular management of a patient with Marfan's syndrome is directed toward minimizing the hemodynamic stress in the arterial tree. To this end, ß-adrenergic blockers are often used. Replacement of the ascending aorta with a Dacron graft-valve conduit before severe dilatation and aortic regurgitation evolve appears to improve the prognosis in patients with progressive aortic root dilatation (>6 cm in diameter).[13] In experienced hands, these major surgical repairs, usually involving aortic valve and at least partial aorta replacement, have acceptable short-term mortality of 6% at 30 days.[14] About one-quarter of patients with ascending aortic operations require reoperation. The prognosis remains guarded for patients with Marfan's syndrome. Following operation the 10-year survival is approximately 50%.

MISCELLANEOUS CONNECTIVE TISSUE DISORDERS

Not surprisingly, all of the connective tissue disorders affect the heart and vascular system (Table 2). Due to valvular involvement, endocarditis prophylaxis is generally recommended.

Osteogenesis imperfecta affects type 1 collagen, which is responsible for structural support. The spectrum of cardiac manifestations of this condition is similar to that of Marfan's syndrome except that clinical cardiac involvement is much less frequent and severe.

Ehlers-Danlos syndrome is characterized by defective collagen synthesis, leading to weakness in arterial walls, cardiomegaly, and valvular heart disease. Affected patients have a high incidence of aortic and peripheral vascular dissection and rupture, both spontaneously and secondary to minimal trauma. Therefore, arterial catheterization, including placement of radial arterial lines, should be avoided.

Pseudoxanthoma elasticum is characterized by dysplasia of the elastic tissue with an increase in elastic fibers that are structurally abnormal and have a propensity to calcify. This results in abnormally calcified and thickened vessels, causing coronary artery disease, peripheral vascular disease, and hypertension (renal artery involvement). Pseudoxanthoma elasticum may produce focal stenoses of the epicardial coronary arteries and other medium-sized arteries, including the internal mammary artery. Accordingly, if coronary artery bypass grafting (CABG) is required in these patients, vein grafts should be used exclusively as conduits.

Endocardial involvement results in restriction to filling, with ensuing CHF and valvular abnormalities. Indeed, echocardiography can demonstrate endocardial calcification, which can be a source for thromboembolism.[15] Because these patients have a high incidence of gastrointestinal bleeding, anticoagulation is contraindicated.

Hurler's syndrome is due to abnormal mucopolysaccharide metabolism producing abnormal collagen fibers. Cardiac chambers may be dilated, valves and chordae thickened, and coronary arteries narrowed.

MUSCULAR DYSTROPHIES

Cardiac involvement may be seen with the hereditary familial muscular dystrophies. Duchenne's and Becker's muscular dystrophies, the 2 most common forms, are caused by abnormalities on the dystrophin gene located at chromosome Xp21. In Duchenne's X-linked muscular dystrophy there is selective necrosis and fibrosis of the posterobasal and lateral left ventricle, accounting for the characteristic

---

Table 2. Cardiovascular Manifestations of Connective Tissue Disorders

SYNDROME	AOV	MV	SITES OF INVOLVEMENT		
			ASCENDING AORTA	PERIPHERAL ARTERIES	CARDIAC CHAMBERS
Marfan's	++++	+++	++++		
Osteogenesis imperfecta	+++	++	+++		
Ehlers-Danlos		+	++	+++	
Pseudoxanthoma elasticum	++	+++		++++	Restriction
Hurler's	++	++			Dilation

AOV=Aortic valve involvement; MV=Mitral valve involvement.

electrocardiographic pattern of tall R waves in the right precordial leads, with an increased R/S ratio and deep Q waves in the lateral leads. Affected patients may develop arrhythmias (usually atrial) and CHF, which is rapidly progressive. The incidence of cardiac involvement with Duchenne's muscular dystrophy is high[16] and contributes to death in about 10% of affected boys. There is also a lower incidence of cardiomyopathy in woman carriers. Becker's muscular dystrophy less commonly has an overt cardiomyopathy as part of its presentation. However, an echocardiographic study has reported a high incidence of subclinical left ventricular dysfunction and dilatation. The LV dysfunction is severe at times, and not age-related.[17]

Myotonic muscular dystrophy is an autosomal dominant disease whose cardiac manifestations are due primarily to involvement of the His-Purkinje system. Conduction block, which may be life-threatening, may develop. The electrocardiogram shows prominent Q waves in the anterior precordial leads. Syncope and sudden death due to ventricular trachycardia has been reported.

Friedreich's ataxia is an autosomal recessive disorder that may be associated with a wide spectrum of cardiac abnormalities. On the basis of electrocardiographic and echocardiographic studies, 95% of patients have cardiac involvement. Electrocardiographic abnormalities include right-axis deviation (40%), a tall R wave in lead V1 (20%), abnormal inferior Q waves (14%), and left ventricular hypertrophy (16%). Twenty percent of patients have echocardiographic evidence of left ventricular hypertrophy, and 7% have globally decreased left ventricular function.[18]

HEMATOLOGIC/ONCOLOGIC DISEASES

SICKLE-CELL DISEASE

Cardiac manifestations of sickle cell disease are principally the sequelae of chronic anemia and chronic hypoxemia. Pulmonary arterial thrombosis in situ occurs frequently in patients with sickle-cell anemia, with resulting arteriovenous shunting and systemic oxygen desaturation. Cardiovascular findings are principally those of a hyperdynamic circulation. However, the additional burden of arterial desaturation for any given hemoglobin concentration produces auscultatory and hemodynamic findings which are more prominent than in other forms of anemia.

At necropsy, most hearts of patients with sickle-cell disease are found to have cardiac hypertrophy and ventricular dilatation. The right and left ventricle generally remain compensated in a high cardiac output state until the appearance of an intercurrent problem, at which time symptoms of CHF may develop.[19]

Although pulmonary infarction is common and often causes a painful crisis, pulmonary hypertension is infrequent, and the incidence of cor pulmonale is not increased in patients with sickle-cell disease. Chest pain in painful crises may mimic the pain of myocardial ischemia, and repolarization abnormalities are very common on the electrocardiogram. Myocardial infarction due to sickling and thrombosis in situ is exceedingly rare, although it has been reported to occur. Interestingly, autopsy studies seem to show that coronary atherosclerosis may be less common in patients with sickle-cell disease as compared to the general adult population.[20]

NEOPLASTIC DISEASE

Pericardial metastases are seen most often in patients with lymphoma, leukemia, carcinoma of the lung, and carcinoma of the breast. Distinguishing metastatic disease from radiation-induced pericarditis may be difficult. Although it is a less common malignancy, malignant melanoma often metastasizes to the pericardium. Occasionally this can lead to tamponade, which must be relieved by a drainage procedure (transcutaneously or surgically). The dramatic black appearance of the effusion can help one make a rapid diagnosis of the etiology of the effusion.

Radiation therapy can affect the entire heart, although the most common complication is pericarditis. The risk of pericarditis is related to the dose of radiation and quantity of heart within the radiation field. The incidence of pericarditis peaks at approximately 6 months, although symptoms may occur up to 10 years later.[21] Less common complications of radiation therapy include constrictive pericarditis, endocardial fibrosis, and accelerated coronary artery disease.

Multiple myeloma is associated with amyloid deposits in the myocardium, leading to a restrictive cardiomyopathy that is refractory to therapy. A high cardiac output syndrome in multiple myeloma has been described as well.[22] The etiology of the high-output state remains obscure. The cardiac output can be elevated to 2 to 3 times normal in patients at rest, a degree of elevation of cardiac output that is greater than that which can be ascribed to the concomitant anemia.

CHEMOTHERAPEUTIC AGENTS

Important chemotherapeutic agents known to have cardiovascular effects include the anthracycline drugs, 5-fluorouricil (5-FU), cyclophosphamide, interferon, interleukin-2, and paclitaxel. The anthracycline drugs doxorubicin (Adriamycin) and daunorubicin (Cerubidine) produce both early and late cardiac effects. Early manifestations of cardiotoxicity include arrhythmias, nonspecific electrocardiographic changes, and rare idiosyncratic episodes of myocarditis and acute LV dysfunction. Late cardiotoxicity is characterized by a dose-dependent cardiomyopathy that occurs with increasing frequency after cumulative doses greater than 500 mg/m². This cardiomyopathy occasionally (about 5% of patients) occurs at lower doses. The cardiomyopathy has a highly variable course, with some patients spontaneously improving, some stabilizing with poor ventricular function, and other patients dying with progressive, refractory heart failure.

The spectrum of 5-FU cardiomyopathy ranges from angina (with or without ischemic electrocardiographic changes) to myocardial infarction, induction and worsening of supraventricular and ventricular arrhythmias, and potentially reversible myocardial depression. Although in documented cases angina and ECG changes are often reproducible, simulating an ischemic event,

significant CAD or vasospasm is not often substantiated and the exact mechanism remains elusive.[23]

Administration of high doses of cyclophosphamide is associated with a toxic, often fatal pericardiomyopathy. Histopathologically, endothelial injury and hemorrhagic myocarditis are found at necropsy.[24]

Interferon has been shown to produce non-dose-related cardiovascular effects, more commonly in patients with history of coronary artery disease (CAD) or previous chemotherapy with drugs known to be cardiotoxic. It has been reported to induce atrial arrhythmias, dilated cardiomyopathy, myopericarditis, and symptoms of ischemic heart disease.[25]

Therapy with high doses of interleukin-2 induces hemodynamic changes consistent with a high-output and low-resistance state similar to changes noted during the early phase of septic shock.[26] These effects may be responsive to the infusion of pressor agents such as dopamine or phenylephrine.

Finally, paclitaxel (Taxol) produces asymptomatic bradycardia in 29% of patients. Uncommonly, it produces conduction abnormalities including AV conduction and bundle-branch blocks.[27] Fortunately, these abnormalities are usually of no clinical importance in this setting.

CEREBROVASCULAR DISEASE

Not only does the heart play a role in the pathogenesis of cerebrovascular disease, but it also often reflects active intracerebral processes. The manifestations are principally disturbances of cardiac conduction and rhythm. Ninety percent of patients with strokes who are carefully monitored for the first 3 days demonstrate electrocardiographic abnormalities. Sinus bradycardia may be present; at times it may be symptomatic and require pharmacologic or pacemaker intervention. Sinus tachycardia, atrial fibrillation, arterial flutter, supraventricular tachycardia, ventricular tachycardia, and conduction abnormalities are also frequently reported. Perhaps the most characteristic electrocardiographic changes of cerebrovascular disease are caused by subarachnoid hemorrhage or spontaneous intra-cranial hemorrhage. These changes may closely simulate acute myocardial ischemia, with ST elevation and symmetric T-wave inversion. The classic "cerebral T waves" occur in these disorders and are manifested by deep and markedly symmetric T-wave inversion. Frequently, prominent U waves are present and there is QT prolongation. The etiology of the repolarization abnormalities is not clear, but it is not simply related to increased cerebrospinal fluid pressure. One common cardiac sign of increased intracerebral pressure is the Cushing reflex, with elevation of blood pressure and bradycardia, at times marked.[28]

Intrinsic cardiac disease is often involved in the pathogenesis of cerebral events. Cerebral emboli often occur in patients with abnormal valves (prosthetic valves, rheumatic heart disease, and bacterial and marantic endo-carditis), atrial fibrillation, left atrial myxomas, left ventricular aneurysms, recent myocardial infarction, and from paradoxical emboli from the venous system and right heart. In a young person with an unexplained embolic stroke, it is not rare that an intra-atrial shunt, due either to a previously unsuspected atrial-septal defect or patent foramen ovale, is present.[29] Young patients with stroke warrant very careful examination by Doppler and contrast echocardiography. Surgical or transcatheter closure of the shunt may be indicated if the shunt is implicated in an embolic event. In patients for whom the cause of stroke is uncertain (cryptogenic stroke), detailed cardiac imaging may be of particularly high yield. A patent foramen ovale is present in 20% to 30% of patients with cryptogenic stroke, suggesting, but not proving, that a paradoxical embolus may have occurred. Transthoracic echocardiography is often inadequately sensitive for detecting intra-atrial shunts. Transesophageal echocardiography with venous contrast injection is highly sensitive and specific for ASDs and patent foramen ovale. At some centers it is routine practice to perform a transesophageal echocardiography with contrast injection on every young cryptogenic stroke patient.[30]

In evaluating a patient with a recent cerebrovascular accident, one must be aware

that 12%-30% of these patients have had a recent myocardial infarction. Coincidence of myocardial infarction and stroke is particularly common in patients over age 65. The diagnosis of recent myocardial infarction in this setting is sometimes subtle, since an accurate history is not often available, and the clinician may be inclined to attribute electrocardiographic abnormalities to the cerebral event. However, elevation of the muscle/brain (MB) fraction of the serum creatine kinase (CK) level may be helpful in making the diagnosis.

Thrombolytic therapy for early reperfusion in stroke is gaining wider acceptance. Cardiologists and internists are now being called upon to assist neurologists in managing such patients because of their greater familiarity with lytic therapy. It is mandatory to obtain a cerebral computed tomography (CT) scan without contrast to exlude intracranial hemorrhage prior to administration of lytic therapy. Initial studies suggest that lytic therapy within three hours of a thrombotic stroke is relatively safe, but later lytic therapy may carry a higher risk of intracerebral hemorrhage. The sequelae following thrombolysis of intracerebral thrombus is generally similar to that following coronary thrombolysis. Bleeding at sites of instrumentation is the most common problem. Although many of these patients have concomitant CAD, destabilization of the coronary situation does not appear to be a major problem in this setting.

PSYCHOTROPIC DRUGS

TRICYCLIC ANTIDEPRESSANTS

Tricyclic antidepressants (TCAs) act by blocking reuptake in the synaptic clefts of both central and peripheral neurons, thereby augmenting neurotransmitter availability at postsynaptic receptors. Vascular and cardiac side effects are a result of their sympathomimetic action (tachy-cardia), α-adrenergic blockade (hypotension), and quinidine-like effects (arrhythmia and conduction abnormalities).

Resting heart rate increases to some extent in nearly all patients receiving TCAs. A degree of postural hypotension is almost universal, and in

24% of cardiac patients receiving TCAs the hypotension causes marked symptoms. This is particularly common in patients with CHF. Postural hypotension is often attenuated after the first several days of therapy. TCAs have, in varying degrees, properties of type IA antiarrhythmic agents. This may be manifest by suppression of ventricular premature beats and, in higher doses, conduction abnormalities and depression of myocardial contractility. Electrocardiographic changes include prolongation of the PR, QRS and QT segments, T-wave abnormalities, and development of AV block. Patients with pre-existing AV block are at increased risk for conduction abnormalities. TCAs may also exacerbate atrial and ventricular arrhythmias, analogous to the potential proarrhythmic effect of type IA antiarrhythmic agents.

When starting patients on a TCA, the clinician should obtain a baseline ECG and then a follow-up ECG to monitor for conduction abnormalities (particularly in patients with pre-existing AV block), and for QTc prolongation to >0.50 seconds, which, if present, should prompt a reduction in dosage.

Widening of the QRS interval is the most reliable marker for complications of TCA overdose, with seizures occurring only in patients with QRS duration of 0.16 seconds or more.[31] Acidosis potentiates the toxicity of TCAs and administration of sodium bicarbonate to correct the acidosis is first-line treatment for cardiovascular complications. The management of TCA toxicity includes use of the anticholinesterase agent, physostigmine, for atrial tachyarrhythmias; lidocaine, for ventricular arrhythmias; and fluid boluses and α-adrenergic agonists such as norepinephrine for profound hypotension.

MONOAMINE OXIDASE (MAO) INHIBITORS

This class of antidepressants commonly produces some degree of postural hypotension. Conversely, a hypertensive crisis is a major hazard. This can be induced by ingesting food containing tyramine or from the administration of sympathomimetic amines. The management of a hypertensive crisis for patients taking MAO inhibitors involves the administration of an α-adrenergic blocker such as prazosin. Intravenous sympathomimetic amines (such as dopamine) should be assiduously avoided in patients taking MAO inhibitors. MAO-inhibitor therapy must be discontinued well in advance of any surgical procedure in which the use of pressors might be required.

SEROTONIN-UPTAKE INHIBITORS

In contrast to the TCAs, newer generation antidepressants like fluoxetine (Prozac) and sertraline (Zoloft) have little or no affinity for cholinergic receptors, acting mostly by inhibition of reuptake of serotonin at CNS sites. Studies on fluoxetine show that it has no significant effect on the baseline ECG, except for a small decrease in resting heart rate. However, rare case reports of dysrhythmias, including supraventricular tachycardia, atrial fibrillation and flutter have been reported.[32] The exact mechanism of this phenomenon remains to be elucidated. Because serotonin produces direct unopposed vasoconstriction in endothelium damaged by CAD, concern about precipitation of unstable angina and myocardial infarction has been raised, although thus far, no direct drug-related clinical events have been demonstrated, despite wide experience with this class of drugs.

ANTIPSYCHOTICS

The cardiovascular effects of antipsychotic medications are similar to those of TCAs. Prominent among the effects are α-adrenergic blockade producing orthostatic hypotension, anticholinergic effects causing tachycardia, and a quinidine-like effect on the heart. Haloperidol should be considered for agitated patients with cardiac disease who require an antipsychotic agent. Haloperidol has fewer anticholinergic and α-blocking effects than thioridazine (Mellaril), which should be avoided. In addition, a specific toxic cardiomyopathy has been reported for phenothiazines. Management of the toxic effects of phenothiazines is similar to that for TCAs. In patients with TCA and phenothiazine toxicity, the use of type IA antiarrhythmic drugs should be avoided, as they may worsen conduction abnormalities.

LITHIUM

Lithium carbonate is frequently very effective for the management of manic-depressive illnesses. It has minimal important cardiotoxicity and blood pressure effects. Lithium can cause electrocardiographic abnormalities that resemble those of hypokalemia, since it partially displaces intracellular potassium. Flattening and inversion of the T wave may be seen. However, this is not an indication to discontinue the drug. Patients with CHF are at increased risk of lithium toxicity due to decreased renal clearance and increased plasma levels of lithium caused by thiazide diuretics. In these patients, serum lithium concentrations must be closely monitored.

SEDATIVE-HYPNOTIC DRUGS

In therapeutic doses, sedative-hypnotic drugs have minimal cardiovascular effects. Intentional overdosing with these drugs can, however, result in hypotension and pulmonary edema due to increased capillary permeability.

NARCOTICS

Narcotic overdose produces centrally- and peripherally-mediated increases in vagal tone and decreases in sympathetic tone, causing bradycardia and hypotension, in addition to the triad of decreased mental status, miosis, and respiratory depression. The specific narcotic antagonist naloxone is an important first-line of therapy. As with the sedative-hypnotic class of drugs, noncardiogenic pulmonary edema can occur with narcotics.

COCAINE

Cocaine produces clinical effects by inhibiting catecholamine reuptake at nerve presynaptic sites, producing membrane anesthetic actions through blockage of sodium channels, and by direct vasotonic effects by enhancing calcium influx across cell membranes. Studies have demonstrated alterations in platelet-endothelial cell function and changes in immune function of natural killer cells.[33] The spectrum of cardiovascular complications of cocaine abuse include acute ischemic syndromes and nonischemic myocardial dysfunction such as myocarditis and cardiomyopathy. Cocaine can induce ventricular arrhythmias including ventricular tachycardia (VT) and ventricular fibrillation (VF), and can lead to sudden arrhythmic death.

Numerous reports of myocardial infarction temporally related to cocaine use have been documented in the literature, 12% of which are ultimately fatal.[34] The typical patient is a young male (average age, 34), a cigarette smoker with no other risk factors for atherosclerosis. There has been no demonstrable relation to the dose, pattern, and frequency of cocaine use. It is becoming clear from clinical and autopsy studies that the relation between cocaine and myocardial infarction (MI) is multifactorial and cannot be explained by 1 single action of cocaine. One-third of patients who undergo coronary angiographic studies have normal epicardial arteries. Experimental studies have implicated coronary spasm both from adrenergic and nonadrenergic mechanisms to be responsible for inciting acute ischemia. About one-third of patients withdrawing from cocaine have demonstrated ST-segment elevations with ambulatory ECG monitoring, strongly supporting the role of coronary vasomotion induced by cocaine and its metabolites. Histopathologic studies have also underscored the role of thrombus formation and accelerated atherosclerosis. Cocaine has been shown in vitro to enhance platelet thromboxane production and platelet aggregation. Furthermore, the possibility of procoagulant effects have been demonstrated in a patient with depleted protein C and antithrombin-III levels in association with cocaine use.

Careful monitoring is recommended in a patient presenting with chest pain associated with cocaine use. Occasionally early angiography may be necessary in difficult cases not responsive to usual measures. The use of calcium-channel blockers is theoretically useful to alleviate the possibility of spasm, although the use of ß-blockers is not necessarily contraindicated because of their generally beneficial effects in a hyperadrenergic state. The patient with an evolving myocardial infarction is treated similarly — aspirin should be given and thrombolytic drugs administered — provided the usual contraindications such as a suspected neurologic event or uncorrected hypertension are carefully excluded.

Cocaine produces direct myocardial depressant effects and clinical case reports show an acute nonischemic cardiomyopathy responsive to cocaine withdrawal. Chronically, there exists a "cocaine-related cardiomyopathy," the pathophysiology of which seems to be multifactorial. Pathologic studies have provided evidence of myocarditis with striking eosinophilic involvement in some cases whereas, findings of contraction band necrosis similar to those reported in cases of pheochromocytoma have also been reported. Acute management with pressor agents or IABP, if necessary, should be used to support the patient during transient myocardial dysfunction. For patients with dilated cardiomyopathy secondary to cocaine use, usual regimens for treatment of systolic dysfunction should be used.

Cocaine-induced ventricular arrhythmias have been postulated to result from cocaine's local anesthetic effects on cardiac membranes. Cocaine blocks sodium channels, producing slowed conduction and unidirectional block, substrate for reentrant arrhythmias. Although animal studies have not, as of yet, convincingly shown that cocaine definitely produces malignant ventricular arrhythmias, clinical experience supports the presence of cocaine at least contributing to arrhythmias in some patients. The management of ventricular tachycardia in the setting of cocaine abuse is directed toward correction of metabolic factors such as electrolyte imbalances, hypoventilation, and seizures. Beta-blockers are potentially helpful. However, other antiarrhythmic drugs should be employed with caution because many of these patients will already have prolongation of their QT interval.

Finally, there are rare cardiac complications of cocaine use: aortic rupture presumably from cocaine-induced increase in blood pressure, infective endocarditis as a result of intravenous drug use, and pneumopericardium secondary to free-base inhalation and positive ventilatory pressure. The concomitant use of alcohol and cocaine has been thought by some to be primarily responsible for the deaths that occur among cocaine abusers, principally by producing cocaethylene, a metabolite with proarrhythmic properties.

STIMULANTS

Although differing in basic pharmacologic properties, amphetamines, phencyclidine, and marijuana have similar cardiovascular effects. Each of these agents may produce a relative hyperadrenergic state with hypertension and tachyarrhythmias.

RENAL AND ELECTROLYTE ABNORMALITIES

Renal disease and cardiac function are inextricably linked, as the kidneys ultimately determine extracellular fluid volume and intravascular volume. The heart must circulate the volume of fluid that the kidneys have regulated.

ACUTE RENAL FAILURE

Three principal aspects of acute renal failure have cardiovascular sequelae: altered fluid volume, hypertension, and metabolic abnormalities. Fluid overload in acute renal failure can usually be managed by zealous attention to fluid intake and the use of potent loop diuretics. Occasionally, ultrafiltration may be required.

Hypertension is often "volume-dependent," with blood pressure exquisitely responsive to a reduction in intravascular volume. Methyldopa, ß-blockers, hydralazine, and calcium-channel blockers may be used in usual doses because they do not critically depend on renal function for their clearance.

Recognition and management of electrolyte abnormalities in acute renal failure is critically important because such abnormalities in this setting may produce life-threatening arrhythmias and conduction abnormalities (see following discussion of electrolytes).

CHRONIC RENAL FAILURE

End-stage renal disease presents a panoply of cardiovascular complications, and indeed, success or failure in management of the cardiovascular complications of renal diseases often determines the patient's survival. Hypertension is a significant problem in most patients with end-stage renal failure. As in acute renal failure, the hypertension is frequently "volume dependent." A subset of patients with end-stage renal failure have exceedingly high plasma-renin activity, and alterations of intravascular volume make little difference in blood pressure control. In some patients with chronic renal failure, baroreceptor function is altered significantly. Nonetheless, with the addition of ACE inhibitors, hypertension can be controlled subsequent to control of intravascular volume and judicious use of other anti-hypertensive medications.

Accelerated atherogenesis is common in patients with end-stage renal disease. This process is multifactorial, with probable contributions by the elevated triglyceride levels and decreased high-density lipoprotein (HDL) levels found in these patients, by hypertension, and by diabetes mellitus.

Pericarditis is a common complication of both acute and chronic renal failure. Echocardiography frequently reveals a small, asymptomatic effusion in patients with chronic renal failure. Clinically, pericarditis may be diagnosed by characteristic symptoms of positional pleuritic precordial pain and by the presence of a precordial friction rub. Characteristic electro-cardiographic abnormalities include ST elevation without reciprocal ST depression. In patients undergoing dialysis, one suggestive sign of some degree of constriction or pericardial tamponade is marked hypotension as intra-vascular volume is reduced. The pericardial effusion tends to be fibrinous and hemorrhagic, and systemic heparinization for dialysis may augment hemorrhage into the pericardium and lead to tamponade. Therefore, in patients with active pericarditis, regional heparin administration may help to prevent this problem. When an effusion produces tamponade, pericardio-centesis can rapidly relieve the symptoms; often, catheter drainage of the pericardium is needed. With vigorous dialysis, the size of the effusion can usually be reduced, and pericardiectomy is not usually required.

Dialysis introduces additional demands on the cardiovascular system. At initiation of dialysis, the extracellular potassium concentration often rapidly decreases, the extracellular ionized calcium concentration rapidly increases, and transient hypoxemia develops, with a decrease in PO_2 of 10-15 mm Hg. Dialysis patients are frequently receiving digoxin, and this combination of electrolyte and metabolic alterations sets the stage very effectively for signs and symptoms of digitalis toxicity despite "normal" serum digoxin levels. This can best be managed by the very cautious use of digoxin in these patients, maintenance of a relatively high potassium level in the dialysis bath at the initiation of dialysis, and supplemental oxygen if indicated. Most patients undergoing chronic hemodialysis have 1 or more arteriovenous fistulas or shunts for circulatory access. In patients with symptoms of CHF who no longer require their arteriovenous shunt, closure of the shunt is often beneficial. The presence of vascular access for dialysis also increases the incidence of infectious endocarditis due to shunt or fistula infections.

Patients with chronic renal failure may occasionally benefit from cardiac valve replacement or CABG, partly because of the hemodynamic ravages of chronic renal failure as well as the rapid progression of atherosclerosis. When scrupulous attention is paid to electrolyte balance, fluid replacement, and arrhythmias, these procedures can be undertaken with only a modestly higher risk of morbidity and mortality over that expected for the general population.[35] Surgical correction of these important cardiac lesions may make subsequent clinical management substantially smoother.

ELECTROLYTE ABNORMALITIES

Abnormalities of potassium balance may have critical cardiac manifestations. The presence of CHF itself alters potassium balance, as there is enhanced exchange of sodium for hydrogen and potassium ions in the renal distal tubule under the influence of the excess aldosterone associated with heart failure. In addition, many diuretics increase sodium delivery to the distal tubule, thereby enhancing potassium wasting.

Potassium replacement in CHF should be in the form of potassium chloride, because potassium excretion is augmented and accompanied by alkalosis.

Hyperkalemia may have catastrophic cardiac effects. The earliest electrocardiographic effects of hyperkalemia (Table 3) are peaked symmetric T waves, followed by broadening of the QRS complex and prolongation of the PR interval. This can occur with a serum potassium level <6.5 mEq, and is usually present at potassium levels >8 mEq. As the serum potassium level increases, atrial excitability is suppressed, followed by complete AV dissociation, ventricular fibrillation, or asystole. These electrocardiographic and electrophysiologic changes are potentiated by hyponatremia or hypocalcemia. Mild elevations in the potassium level decrease the rate of spontaneous diastolic depolarization of all pacemaker fibers; ectopic pacemakers are more sensitive than the SA node, with the resulting antiarrhythmic effect of mild hyperkalemia. When hyperkalemia has abolished atrial activity, broadened the QRS, and altered repolarization so that the electrocardiogram has developed a sine-wave pattern, a true medical emergency exists. Ten to 20 ml of 10% $CaCl_2$ should be administered intravenously while the electrocardiogram is continuously monitored. This helps to correct some of the electrophysiologic abnormalities produced by hyperkalemia, but does not lower the serum potassium level. Administration of $NaHCO_3$ (1-2 ampules, 44-88 mEq), followed by 50 ml of D50W and 10 units of regular insulin, lowers extracellular potassium concentrations within 15 minutes; the effect lasts for a few hours. However, the total body potassium level is not altered by this regimen. Sodium polystyrene sulfonate (Kayexalate), a cation exchange resin, should be administered orally or rectally in a dose of 50 g. When it is administered orally, it should be combined with sorbitol to avoid gastrointestinal inspissation. This resin will bind potassium (1 mEq/g resin), effectively lowering total body potassium stores.

Hypokalemia has important cardiac effects as well, although by itself it is less life-threatening than hyperkalemia. A low potassium level has a mildly negative inotropic effect. On the electrocardiogram, T waves are flattened or inverted and U waves may become more prominent. TU fusion produces pseudo-QT prolongation. The correlation between serum potassium level and electrocardiographic findings for both hypo- and hyperkalemia is rough, and may vary with the acuity of the change in serum levels. Hypokalemia increases arrhythmogenicity, in particular, the digitalis-toxic arrhythmias, and should be avoided in patients receiving cardiac glycosides.

Chronic elevations of the serum calcium level may produce ectopic calcification of the cardiac skeleton and varying degrees of heart block. The electrophysiologic effects of hypercalcemia include augmented contractility, shortened systole, and decreased automaticity. The electrocardiographic manifestations are a slight increase in the PR and QRS intervals and shortening of the QT interval. Hypercalcemia can be managed in the short term by sodium chloride infusion and furosemide administration. Hypocalcemia may prolong the QT interval and shorten the PR and QRS intervals.

Elevated serum magnesium levels in

Table 3. Electrocardiographic Manifestations of Electrolyte Abnormalities

	INTERVAL			T WAVE	U WAVE	ATRIAL ACTIVITY	VPB FREQUENCY
	PR	QRS	QT				
↑K+	↑	↑		↑		↑ or ↓	↓
↓K+		↑	↑*	↓	↑		↑
↑Ca++	↑	↑	↓				
↓Ca++	↓	↓	↑				

*QU prolongation; VPB=Ventricular premature beat.

experimental preparations decrease cardiac conduction and ventricular irritability. There are no diagnostic electrocardiographic findings of hypermagnesemia. Hypomagnesemia may be associated with atrial and ventricular arrhythmias, and the correction of hypomagnesemia may be an effective strategy for control of arrhythmias.

Alterations in serum pH have no direct electrocardiographic effects but are associated with alterations in potassium and calcium concentrations. Marked acidosis has an important negative inotropic effect, decreases the ventricular response to epinephrine, and lowers the ventricular fibrillation threshold. Correction of acidosis is frequently critical in cardiac defibrillation.

Hypophosphatemia may be related to depressed intracellular concentrations of high-energy phosphate compounds.

In any patient with new arrhythmias, electrolyte levels should be checked in a search for a readily reversible precipitating cause. In particular, patients with torsades de pointes tachycardia should have their serum potassium, calcium, and magnesium levels checked, because low concentrations are associated with prolongation of the QT interval.

ENDOCRINOLOGIC ABNORMALITIES

HYPERTHYROIDISM

Palpitations, dyspnea, tachycardia, and hypertension occur in about 30% of patients with hyperthyroidism, and can be the only symptoms in those with the so-called "apathetic hyperthyroidism." Supraventricular arrhythmias, particularly atrial fibrillation, occur in approximately 20%. Echocardiographic or radionuclide assessment of ventricular function reveals hyperdynamic ventricles. Symptoms of CHF may be due to a high output state and relative myocardial ischemia. In general, however, cardiovascular symptoms are due to underlying cardiac disease and rarely due to hyperthyroidism alone.

One physical finding helpful in making the diagnosis of hyperthyroidism is the minimal diminution in heart rate while the patient sleeps. Patients may also have a midsystolic scratch present at the left upper sternal border, believed to be secondary to hyperdynamic rubbing of the pericardial and pleural surfaces.

Pharmacologic management of cardiovascular signs and symptoms of hyperthyroidism may be difficult until the underlying hyperthyroid state is treated. Patients are relatively refractory to the effects of digoxin. Thirty percent of hyperthyroid patients in atrial fibrillation rendered euthyroid will convert to sinus rhythm. Indeed, treatment of the hyperthyroidism may be dramatically effective for most cardiovascular symptoms. In the short term, ß-adrenergic blockade may ameliorate many of the signs of a hyperdynamic circulation. The combination of ß-blockers and digoxin is often effective in regulating the ventricular response in atrial fibrillation, while avoiding dose-dependent adverse effects of either medication.

HYPOTHYROIDISM

In studies of hypothyroid animals, myocardial contractility is decreased. In severe, long-standing hypothyroidism there is myofibrillar swelling with interstitial fibrosis, and the heart may become grossly dilated. It is uncommon for hypothyroidism to be prolonged and severe enough to produce symptoms of CHF in humans. It is believed that the mild reduction in myocardial contractility in hypothyroid patients is compensated for by the decreased demands placed on the heart. The presence of effusions more likely represents altered capillary permeability rather than myocardial failure. One-third of patients with myxedema have pericardial effusions, only rarely leading to tamponade.

Electrocardiographic findings include bradycardia, prolongation of the QT interval, decreased electrical voltage, and a three-fold greater incidence of conduction disturbances.

Serum cholesterol and triglyceride levels are often elevated in hypothyroid patients. This may contribute to the increased incidence of atherosclerosis in these patients. Evaluation of chest pain in a hypothyroid patient can be perplexing, as hypothyroidism itself can cause modest elevations in the serum creatine kinase level.

Hypothyroidism frequently occurs in elderly

patients who may have underlying ischemic heart disease or other important cardiac disorders. Therefore, thyroid replacement therapy must proceed cautiously so as not to induce severe angina or myocardial necrosis. Should severe, medically-refractory angina develop during thyroid replacement, coronary revascularization may then be required.

ORAL CONTRACEPTIVES

The use of oral contraceptives is associated with a three-fold increased risk of myocardial infarction. Platelet adhesiveness is increased, concentrations of clotting factors increase, and levels of antithrombin III decrease, all of which increase the risk for thromboembolic disease. Once oral contraceptive therapy is discontinued, the risk reverts to baseline.[36]

DIABETES

Although diabetes is one of the major risk factors for coronary atherosclerosis, the Framingham study revealed that diabetics have an increased incidence of CHF not attributable to CAD. Diabetic cardiomyopathy is a poorly understood and not uncommon syndrome. The cellular and molecular basis is still unclear. In asymptomatic patients, 2D echocardiography demonstrates abnormalities in diastolic function, with a decrease in left ventricular ejection time and a prolonged pre-ejection period, indicating reduced LV compliance.[37] This may lead to symptomatic cardiomyopathy not attributable to microvascular cardiac disease. Abnormalities in systolic function may also be present, initially manifesting as a diminished contractile response to exercise, then as frank CHF.

Apart from attention to blood sugar control, management consists of the usual approaches to systolic and diastolic heart failure; ACE-inhibition is a particularly attractive strategy because of its additional benefits in preserving renal function.

PHEOCHROMOCYTOMA

Cardiac pheochromocytomas are rare. 125I-MIBG scintigraphy or angiography most commonly demonstrates involvement of the roof of the left atrium.[38] A catecholamine-induced dilated cardiomyopathy, although rare, is sometimes associated with pheochromocytomas. Patients uncommonly present with clinical heart failure. The characteristic histologic finding is contraction band necrosis of cardiocytes, similar to those found in patients dying of intracerebral catastrophes, tetanus, drowning, or cocaine abuse. The reduction of myocardial function is thought to be a consequence of ß-receptor downregulation and patchy myocardial necrosis. Improvement in LV function has been shown following surgical removal of the tumor. Preoperatively, adequate α-blockade with phenoxybenzamine or prazosin controls blood pressure and allows correction of existing hypovolemia.

Beta-blockers may be used to control supraventricular arrhythmias or tumor-related tachycardia but should not be used without prior establishment of adequate α-blockade. Limited clinical studies suggest that captopril may also be effective in this setting.[39]

ACQUIRED IMMUNODEFICIENCY SYNDROME

The cardiologist will become increasingly involved in the team approach to the management of patients with Acquired Immunodeficiency Syndrome (AIDS). Although a cardiac mode of death continues to be uncommon for patients with AIDS, cardiac complications are being recognized more frequently. A large autopsy series described cardiac findings in more than half of the cases of patients dying of AIDS and AIDS-related complex.[40] Moreover, the largest echocardiographic series in the United States reports a 64% prevalence of cardiac abnormalities in hospitalized patients with AIDS.[41]

AIDS-related cardiac disease may involve the pericardium, myocardium, or the endocardium. Symptomatic involvement occurs most often in the end stage of the disease, presumably due to opportunistic infection and/or secondary malignancies. Recent studies support several mechanisms of myocardial disease in AIDS. However, whether it is as a result of direct HIV myocardial involvement, the resultant immunosuppression, or an undefined pathogen remains unsettled.

Table 4. Cardiac Manifestations in AIDS

Pericardial Effusion
     Small, asymptomatic
     Medium to large
     Hemodynamically compromising
Myocarditis
     AIDS-associated
     Secondary (Toxoplasma, Cryptococcus,
     Mycobacteria)
     Idiopathic
Dilated Cardiomyopathy
     Myocarditis
     Drug-related (Interferon-α, Doxorubicin)
Right Ventricular Hypertrophy of the Myocardium
Neoplastic Involvement of the Heart
     Kaposi's Sarcoma
     Malignant Lymphoma
Nonbacterial Thrombotic Endocarditis

PERICARDIAL EFFUSION

A pericardial effusion is an incidental echocardiographic finding in most cases and is usually small and without clinical consequence. Uncommonly, patients present with moderate to large volume effusions and echocardiographic evidence of hemodynamic compromise. Clinical tamponade is treated in the usual manner with transcatheter drainage or pericardiectomy followed by specific drug therapy if an etiologic agent is identified (i.e., tuberculous pericarditis). However, some patients who have moderate to large effusions associated with mild right atrial collapse on 2D echocardiography have been reported to respond to nonsteroidal anti-inflammatory drugs. In the majority of asymptomatic effusions, culture of pericardial fluid is unrevealing.[42]

MYOCARDITIS

Histological evidence of myocarditis is found in about half of necropsy patients dying of AIDS.[43] In AIDS-associated myocarditis, the histologic findings most frequently described are nonspecific (lymphocytic) inflammatory infiltrates without myocyte damage. Secondary myocarditis due to identifiable pathogens is found in the minority of cases, most commonly as a result of toxoplasma, cryptococcal, or mycobacterial infections. In patients with a histologic pattern of myocardial necrosis without inflammation, postulated mechanisms include direct infection with viral agents such as cytomegalovirus (CMV) as well as HIV itself.

DILATED CARDIOMYOPATHY

In an AIDS patient presenting with dyspnea out of proportion to known pulmonary disease, dilated cardiomyopathy should be considered as the cause of the symptoms. The prevalence of myocardial dysfunction in AIDS is estimated to be about 20%-30% and AIDS is increasingly recognized as an important etiologic factor in dilated cardiomyopathy. Although it is postulated that myocarditis contributes to a large proportion of these cases, myocardial dysfunction as a result of drug therapy, particularly that of interferon-α and doxorubicin used in the treatment of Kaposi's sarcoma should always be borne in mind. The role of endomyocardial biopsy in the management of patients with AIDS who have a dilated cardiomyopathy remains undefined.

RIGHT VENTRICULAR HYPERTROPHY

Cardiomegaly predominantly due to right ventricular hypertrophy (RVH) is found in about one-third of patients with cardiac involvement at autopsy. This finding correlates with the presence of pulmonary interstitial diseases prevalent with AIDS including diffuse alveolar damage and opportunistic infections.

NEOPLASTIC INVOLVEMENT OF THE HEART

The 2 most common neoplasms associated with AIDS that affect the heart are Kaposi's sarcoma and malignant lymphoma. Cardiac Kaposi's sarcoma has a predilection for the epicardium and the subepicardial fat, although pericardial involvement causing effusion and also myocardial invasion have been reported. Lymphomatous infiltration of the myocardium may be diffuse or result in discrete isolated lesions. In the majority of cases, neoplastic involvement of the heart occurs as part of a widely disseminated, systemic process.

NONBACTERIAL THROMBOTIC ENDOCARDITIS

Although most often diagnosed postmortem, the most common endocardial lesion in AIDS is nonbacterial thrombotic (marantic) endocarditis. Friable vegetations, consisting of platelets within a fibrin mesh and a few inflammatory cells can result in systemic or pulmonary embolization with resultant end-organ damage. Interestingly, infective endocarditis and healed bacterial endocarditis do not seem to be more frequent in patients with AIDS.

REFERENCES

1. Rhodes BA, Greyson ND, Hamilton CR, et al. Absence of anatomic arteriovenous shunts in Paget's disease of the bone. *N Engl J Med.* 1972;287:686-689.
2. Criscitiello MG, Ronan JA, Besterman EMM, et al. Cardiovascular abnormalities in osteogenesis imperfecta. *Circulation.* 1965;31:255-262.
3. deDeuxchaisnes CN, Krane SM. Paget's disease of bone: Clinical and metabolic observations. *Medicine.* 1964;43:233-266.
4. Escalante A, Kaufman RL, Quismorio FP, et al. Cardiac compression in rheumatoid pericarditis. *Sem Arthritis Rheum.* 1990;20:148-163.
5. Nihoyannopoulos P, Gomez PM, Joshi J, et al. Cardiac abnormalities in systemic lupus erythematosus. Association with raised anticardiolipin antibodies. *Circulation.* 1990;82:369-385.
6. Galve E, Candell-Riera J, Pigrau C, et al. Prevalence, morphologic types, and evolution of cardiac valvular disease in systemic lupus erythematosus. *N Engl J Med.* 1988;319:817-823.
7. Leung WH, Wong KL, Lau CP, et al. Doppler echocardiographic evaluation of left ventricular diastolic function in patients with systemic lupus erythematosus. *Am Heart J.* 1990;120:82-87.
8. Holsinger DR, Osmundson PJ, Edwards JE. The heart in periarteritis nodosa. *Circulation.* 1962;25:610-618.
9. Duboc D, Kahan A, Maziere B, et al. The effect of nifedipine on myocardial perfusion and metabolism in systemic sclerosis. A positron emission tomographic study. *Arthritis Rheum.* 1991;34:198-203.
10. Kahan A, Devaux JY, Amor B, et al. The effect of captopril on thallium 201 myocardial perfusion in systemic sclerosis. *Clin Pharmacol Ther.* 1990;47:483-489.
11. Gould BA, Turner J, Keeling DH, et al. Myocardial dysfunction in ankylosing spondylitis. *Ann Rheum Diseases.* 1992;51:227-232.
12. Onouchi Z, Hamaoka K, Kamiya Y, et al. Transformation of coronary artery aneurysm to obstructive lesion and the role of collateral vessels in myocardial perfusion in patients with Kawasaki disease. *J Am Coll Cardiol.* 1993;21:158-162
13. Gott VL, Pyeritz RE, Magovern GJ, et al. Surgical treatment of aneurysms of the ascending aorta in the Marfan syndrom. *N Engl J Med.* 1986;314:1070-1074.
14. Svensson LG, Crawford ES, Coselli JS, et al. Impact of cardiovascular operation on survival in the Marfan patient. *Circulation.* 1989;80:1233-1242.
15. Rosenzweig BP, Guarneri E, Kronzon I. Echoαcardiographic manifestations in a patient with pseudoxanthoma elasticum. *Ann Intern Med.* 1993;119:487-490.
16. Muntoni F, Cau M, Ganau A, et al. Deletion of the dystrophin muscle-promoter region associated with x-linked dilated cardiomyopathy. *N Engl J Med.* 1993;329:921-925.
17. Steare SE, Dubowitz V, Benatar A. Subclinical cardiomyopathy in Becker muscular dystrophy. *Br Heart J.* 1992;68:304-308.
18. Child JS, Perloff JK, Bach PM, et al. Cardiac involvement in Friedreich's ataxia: A clinical study of 75 patients. *J Am Coll Cardiol.* 1986;7:1370-1378.
19. Gerry JL, Bulkley BH, Hutchins GM. Clinicopathologic analysis of cardiac dysfunction in 52 patients with sickle cell anemia. *Am J Cardiol.* 1978;42:211-216.
20. Barrett O, Saunders DE, McFarland DE, et al. Myocardial infarction in sickle cell anemia. *Am J Hematology.* 1984;16:139-147.
21. Ikaheimo MJ, Niemela KO, Linnaluoto MM, et al. Early cardiac changes related to radiation therapy. *Am J Cardiol.* 1985;56:943-946.
22. McBride W, Jackman JD, Gamon RS, et al. High-output cardiac failure in patients with multiple myeloma. *N Engl J Med.* 1988;319:1651-1653.
23. Robben NC, Pippas AW, Moore JO. The syndrome of 5-fluorouracil cardiotoxicity. *Cancer.* 1993;71:493-509.
24. Gottdiener JS, Appelbaum FR, Ferrans VJ, et al. Cardiotoxicity associated with high-dose cyclophosphamide therapy. *Arch Intern Med.* 1981;141:758-763.
25. Sonnenblick M, Rosin MB. Cardiotoxicity of interferon. *Chest.* 1991;99:557-561.
26. Gaynor ER, Vitek L, Sticklin L, et al. The hemodynamic effects of treatment with interleukin-2 and lymphokine-activated killer cells. *Ann Intern Med.* 1988;109:953-958.
27. Rowinsky EK, Eisenhauer EA, Chaudhry V, et al. Clinical toxicities encountered with paclitaxel (taxol®). *Semin Oncol.* 1993;20:1-15.
28. Dimant J, Grob D. Electrocardiographic changes and myocardial damage in patients with acute cerebrovascular accidents. *Stroke.* 1977;8:448-455.
29. Lechat P, Mas JL, Lascault G, et al. Prevalence of patent foramen ovale in patients with stroke. *N Engl J Med.* 1988;318:1148-1152.
30. Di Tullio M, Sacco RL, Venketasubramanian N, et al. Comparison of diagnostic techniques for the detection of a patent foramen ovale in stroke patients. *Stroke.* 1993;24:1020-1024.
31. Boehnert MT, Lovejoy FH. Value of the QRS duration versus the serum drug level in predicting seizures and ventricular arrhythmias after an acute overdose of tricyclic

antidepressants. *N Engl J Med.* 1985;313:474-479.

32. Buff DD, Brenner R, Kirtane SS, et al. Dysrhythmia associated with fluoxetine treatment in an elderly patient with cardiac disease. *J Clin Psychiatry.* 1991;52:174-176.

33. Laposata EA. Cocaine-induced heart disease: mechanisms and pathology. *J Thorac Imaging.* 1991;6:68-75.

34. Isner JM. Cardiovascular complications of cocaine. *Curr Probl Cardiol.* 1991;2:95-123.

35. Lamberti JJ, Cohn LH, Collins JJ. Cardiac surgery in patients undergoing renal dialysis or transplantation. *Ann Thorac Surg.* 1975;12:135-141.

36. Stampfer MJ, Willett WC, Colditz GA, et al. A prospective study of past use of oral contraceptive agents and risk of cardiovascular diseases. *N Engl J Med.* 1988;319:1313-1317.

37. Shapiro LM. Echocardiographic features of impaired ventricular function in diabetes mellitus. *Br Heart J.*

1982;47:439-444.

38. Jebara VA, Sousa M, Farge A, et al. Cardiac pheochromocytomas. *Ann Thorac Surg.* 1992;53:356-361.

39. Salathe M, Weiss P, Ritz R. Rapid reversal of heart failure in a patient with phaeochromocytoma and catecholamine-induced cardiomyopathy who was treated with captopril. *Br Heart J.* 1992;68:527-528.

40. Lewis W. AIDS: cardiac findings from 115 autopsies. *Prog Cardiovasc Dis.* 1989;23:207-215.

41. Himelman RB, Chung WS, Chernoff DN. Cardiac manifestations of human immunodeficiency virus infection: a two-dimensional echocardiographic study. *J Am Coll Cardiol.* 1989;13:1030-1036.

42. Kaul S, Fishbein MC, Siegel RJ. Cardiac manifestations of acquired immune deficiency syndrome: a 1991 update. *Am Heart J.* 1991;122:535-544.

43. Anderson DW, Virmani R, Reilly JM, et al. Prevalent myocarditis at necropsy in the acquired immuno-deficiency syndrome. *J Am Coll Cardiol.* 1988;11:792-799.

35 Noncardiac Surgery in the Cardiac Patient

Thomas H. Lee, MD
Lee Goldman, MD

Although cardiology consultants are frequently asked to "clear" a patient for surgery, their role is considerably more complex. The consultant should be prepared to assess the individual patient's risk of cardiac complications; determine whether specialized testing may be appropriate to refine this risk assessment; recommend risk reduction strategies; and participate in postoperative medical management. This chapter addresses these specific tasks and reviews approaches to common perioperative problems.

ASSESSMENT OF RISK

The aging of the population has led to an increase in the prevalence of chronic diseases (e.g., diabetes, ischemic heart disease) in surgical patients. Despite this trend toward higher-risk patients, the overall risk of cardiac complications with noncardiac surgery remains low and has probably decreased over the last 20 years. The risk of perioperative myocardial infarction (MI) is now only about 0.1% and cardiac deaths occur in only about 0.04% of general surgical patients.

These risks are not homogeneous, however, and identification of higher-risk candidates who may warrant special management strategies should be based upon a preoperative cardiac evaluation that includes a history, physical examination, and electrocardiogram, and, in selected patients, a chest x-ray, and a serum chemistry evaluation of renal function. Because noncardiac conditions such as chronic renal failure, diabetes, and cerebrovascular disease may also indicate an increased risk for cardiovascular complications, the cardiology consultant must perform this evaluation from the perspective of an internist as well as a subspecialist. This general database is intended to identify conditions associated with an increased risk of anesthesia and surgery.

CORONARY ARTERY DISEASE

The most important predictor of cardiac complications remains ischemic heart disease, with recent acute MI carrying an especially high risk. Analysis of pooled data from the 1960s and 1970s showed that recurrent MI or cardiac death occurred in about 30% of patients who underwent noncardiac surgery within 3 months after acute MI and about 15% of patients who underwent surgery within 3 to 6 months (Table 1). Complication rates were stable, about 5%, if more than 6 months had elapsed after acute MI. However, more recent data indicate that this risk has fallen, and with careful patient selection and perioperative invasive hemodynamic monitoring, reinfarction rates have been reported to be as low as about 6% within the first 3 months after an MI and 2% at 3 to 6 months after the MI.[1,2] Patients with a non-Q-wave infarction have complication rates similar to those of patients with Q-wave infarctions.

Because elective noncardiac surgery is usually deferred in postinfarction patients or in patients with unstable angina, a much more common and difficult challenge for the cardiology consultant is assessing perioperative risk for patients with stable angina. This risk is low if the patient's ischemic symptoms are truly stable, but physicians may be misled by self-reported histories of the frequency of angina, because patients may voluntarily reduce their activity levels to avoid cardiac or noncardiac symptoms. Some clinicians have advocated aggressive evaluation of the extent of coronary disease, including angiography and possible bypass graft surgery for every operative patient with angina or a history of MI. They cite nonrandomized data demonstrating that patients with New York Heart Association class I or II anginal symptoms have higher mortality rates with noncardiac surgery if they have not undergone previous coronary artery bypass graft (CABG) surgery. However, the operative mortality risk of elective CABG surgery would erase any potential benefit of this strategy in patients with mild stable angina. Thus, instead of routine angiography, evaluation of patients with stable angina should focus on assessment of the threshold at which ischemia is induced. This assessment sometimes requires the use of specialized cardiac tests (see later).

Data on patients with unstable angina who undergo noncardiac surgery are scanty, but unstable angina is known to be a poor prognostic factor for patients undergoing CABG surgery, and its impact on noncardiac surgical mortality is also deleterious. Therefore, elective surgery should be postponed until ischemic symptoms are stabilized, and noninvasive and invasive testing should be considered in the interim. If the operation cannot be delayed, the patient should undergo the procedure with appropriate hemodynamic and electro-cardiographic monitoring.

CONGESTIVE HEART FAILURE

Because anesthesia and surgery are associated with rapid changes in the volume status, patients with preoperative congestive heart failure (CHF) are clearly at increased risk for a postoperative exacerbation or other cardiac events. The new onset of pulmonary edema occurs in about 16% of patients whose signs or symptoms of CHF persist up to the time of operation, with even higher risk (23%-35%) among patients who have jugular venous distention or an S_3 gallop at the time of the preoperative evaluation, or have a history of pulmonary edema.[3] Patients who have a history of heart failure but are not in failure at the time of surgery have about a 6% risk of pulmonary edema, which suggests that treatment of manifestations of heart failure before surgery may reduce complication rates. However, because many anesthetic agents cause arterial and venous vasodilation, over-diuresis may lead to hypotension; thus, diuretic therapy should probably be withheld if patients demonstrate orthostatic changes in blood pressure and heart rate. New onset of pulmonary edema or heart failure is rare in patients with no history of heart failure, and, when it occurs, is related to a postoperative MI in about 30% of cases.

VALVULAR HEART DISEASE

Patients with preoperative valvular heart disease have about a 20% risk of new or worsened heart failure developing in the perioperative period; these patients are often candidates for preoperative noninvasive cardiac testing. The most important lesion to diagnose is severe aortic stenosis, a lesion which is increasing in prevalence as the population ages and which has historically been associated with risks of perioperative mortality as high as 13%. Evaluation and management of patients with

Table 1. Risk of Reinfarction from Surgery in Post-MI Patients

MONTHS AFTER PRIOR MI	POOLED DATA PRE-1976	RAO ET AL 1983*	SHAH ET AL 1990**
0–3	31%	6% (3/52)	4% (1/23)
4–6	15%	2% (2/86)	0% (0/18)
>6	5%	1.5% (9/595)	6% (10/174)

* Rao TLK.[1]
**Shah KB et al.[2]

suspected aortic stenosis is evolving, however, because echocardiography with Doppler analysis allows reliable noninvasive diagnosis of this lesion. Noncardiac surgery has been performed with careful hemodynamic monitoring in small series of selected patients with critical aortic stenosis, with acceptable rates of major complication;[4] thus, it is preferable to embark on surgery without aortic valve replacement or balloon valvuloplasty if the patient does not have symptoms from the aortic valve disease, and even in some patients with symptoms. In patients with advanced symptoms, however, an aortic valve procedure should be strongly considered before noncardiac surgery. If the noncardiac surgery is urgent, balloon aortic valvuloplasty can serve as a way to reduce the severity of the aortic stenosis for several months and permit the noncardiac surgery to be performed. Aortic valve replacement could subsequently be considered on an elective basis.

In patients with mitral stenosis, supraventricular tachyarrhythmias may develop and precipitate CHF and ischemia. Digitalis administration, which may not prevent atrial tachyarrhythmias but may decrease the rate of ventricular response should one occur, can be started preoperatively in patients who have mitral stenosis and are in sinus rhythm. Increasingly, however, many physicians opt to treat atrial arrhythmias, when they arise, with intravenous administration of drugs that slow conduction through the atrioventricular node, such as verapamil or adenosine. In patients with chronic aortic and mitral regurgitation, the left ventricle is subjected to high volume loads that may impair contractility. These patients are not as sensitive to small shifts in hemodynamic status as are those with critical aortic stenosis, and they can often be managed without hemodynamic monitoring during the perioperative period if they are not in CHF at the time of the preoperative evaluation.

Patients with any of these valvular abnormalities or with prosthetic valves should receive appropriate antibiotic prophylaxis before procedures that are associated with bacteremia. In addition, patients with prosthetic valves who receive chronic anticoagulation therapy may require special management strategies (see later).

ARRHYTHMIAS

Patients with preexisting rhythm disorders are at increased risk for cardiac complications, but much of this increased risk is due to underlying ischemic or valvular heart disease, or CHF. Thus, patients with ventricular arrhythmias and myocardial dysfunction are at higher risk for perioperative CHF and cardiac death, and there are no data that suggest that prophylactic antiarrhythmic therapy lowers these risks. Arrhythmias and conduction abnormalities that occur in these patients during the perioperative period can usually be managed as they arise, and pharmacologic interventions or pacemakers should be reserved for cases in which patients meet indications for these therapies. In general, in patients without evidence of structural heart disease, ventricular premature contractions are not associated with increased risk of cardiac death or morbidity, and their prognostic importance for predicting perioperative complications is also probably small.

OTHER RISK FACTORS

The risk of cardiac complications increases in an almost linear fashion with age, so that the risk of perioperative cardiac death is about 10 times higher for patients over age 70 than for patients below 70.[3,5] The increase in perioperative risk among the elderly persists even after adjustment for their higher prevalence of cardiac disease and other conditions. Risk assessment may be hindered by the inability of many elderly patients to undergo treadmill exercise testing. Because the risk of cardiac complications is highest in patients who cannot exercise, alternative tests for evaluating the inducibility of ischemia may be especially appropriate.

The type and timing of the surgery are also major correlates of perioperative cardiovascular risk. Major intra-abdominal, intrathoracic or aortic procedures are associated with higher risks than other types of operations, probably because of several factors, including the prevalence of underlying coronary artery disease (CAD); the seriousness of the surgery; the degree of respiratory compromise and postoperative pain; and the fluid and electrolyte

Table 2. Multifactorial Index of Cardiac Risk in Noncardiac Surgery

PARAMETER	POINTS
History	
Myocardial infarction within 6 months	10
Age over 70 years	5
Physical examination	
S_3 or jugular venous distention	11
Important aortic stenosis	3
Electrocardiogram	
Rhythm other than sinus or sinus plus APBs on last preoperative electrocardiogram	7
More than 5 premature ventricular beats/min at any time preoperatively	7
Other factors	
Poor general medical status*	3
Intraperitoneal, intrathroacic, or aortic surgery	3
Emergency operation	4
TOTAL	53

APB=Atrial premature beat.

*Electrolyte abnormalities (potassium <3.0 mEq/l or HCO_3 <20 mEq/l); renal insufficiency (blood urea nitrogen >50 mg/dl or creatinine >3.0 mg/dl); abnormal blood gases (pO_2 <60 mm Hg or pCO_2 >50 mm Hg); abnormal liver status (elevated serum asparate transaminase or signs on physical examination of chronic liver disease); or any condition that has caused the patient to be chronically bedridden.

Adapted from Goldman L, et al.[5]

shifts associated with these procedures. The risk of any operation increases about 4-fold if it is performed emergently instead of electively, probably because of general medical problems that cannot be corrected before emergency operations. Abnormalities such as hypoxia, carbon dioxide retention, acidosis, hypokalemia, elevated liver function enzyme levels, and evidence of renal failure are all associated with increased risk.

Finally, the aging of the population has led to the performance of procedures upon an increasing number of patients with one or more comorbid noncardiac medical conditions, such as diabetes and chronic renal insufficiency. Preliminary data indicate that these factors may be independently associated with increased risk for cardiac complications, although the importance of these conditions compared with other known risk factors remains to be determined.

MULTIVARIATE ASSESSMENT OF RISK

Integrating the impact of the presence of more than 1 of these factors into a single overall risk estimate can be performed using a multivariate index of cardiac risk in noncardiac surgery that was derived from data on 1,001 patients at a single hospital in the mid 1970s.[5] Nine independently important factors were identified (Table 2). Points were assigned to each factor that can be used to place patients into approximate risk classes (Table 3). In the original series of patients, more than one-half of all patients were placed into risk class 1, and the risk of life-threatening or fatal cardiac complications in such patients was less than 1%. In risk classes II and III, the rate of complications increased, but only 2% of patients died perioperatively. Only 18 patients were in risk Class IV, but more than 50% died of cardiac causes. A revised index has suggested the

Table 3. Prospective Performance of the Cardiac Risk Index

CLASS		NO. OF PATIENTS		LIFE-THREATENING COMPLICATIONS*		CARDIAC DEATH	
(Points)		MGH	Toronto	MGH	Toronto	MGH	Toronto
I	(0–5)	537	590	<1%	<1%	<1%	<1%
II	(6–12)	316	453	5%	2%	2%	1%
III	(13–25)	130	74	12%	11%	2%	4%
IV	(>25)	18	23	22%	4%	56%	26%

MGH=Original series at Massachusetts General Hospital (Goldman et al. 1977).
Toronto=Prospective evaluation by Zeldin in Toronto (*Can J Surg.* 27:402, 1984).
*Documented intraoperative or postoperative myocardial infarction, pulmonary edema, or ventricular tachycardia without progression to cardiac death.

addition of factors to account for prior histories of Class III or IV angina, remote MI, and pulmonary edema (Table 4).[6,7]

In prospective testing at other institutions in varying patient populations,[6–9] the original index has been shown to separate patients reliably into risk groups, although recent data indicate that mortality rates as low as 8% can be achieved in risk Class IV patients through patient selection and hemodynamic monitoring.[10]

Because the risk index may underestimate the rate of cardiac complications in certain higher-risk populations such as patients undergoing abdominal aortic aneurysm surgery,[11] the index may be more appropriately used in a Bayesian manner that takes into consideration the patient's prior probability of complications (Table 5).[2,6,7]

SPECIALIZED TESTS FOR PREOPERATIVE RISK ASSESSMENT

Patients with evidence of ischemia during exercise tolerance testing have higher rates of

Table 4. Modified Multifactorial Index

PARAMETERS		POINTS
MI:	<6 months ago	10
	>6 months ago	5
Angina:	Class III	10
	Class IV	20
Unstable angina within 6 months		10
Pulmonary edema: ever		5
	<1 week ago	10
Suspected critical aortic stenosis		20
Rhythm other than sinus or sinus plus APBs on last preop ECG		5
More than five PVC/min at any time		5
Poor general medical status		5
Age over 70		5
Emergency operation		10

From Detsky AS, et al.[6]

cardiac complications with noncardiac surgery, but whether exercise test results add information to data from a careful history is unclear. Patients with stable angina usually do well if angina is their only risk factor, and patients with severe symptoms of ischemic heart disease at a low level of exertion are candidates for catheterization and consideration of revascularization with angioplasty or CABG. However, the clinician must determine whether patients with apparently stable angina are active enough to increase cardiovascular work to a level similar to that of surgery. If the patient's threshold for inducibility of ischemia is uncertain, an exercise test, with or without thallium scintigraphy, may provide important information. Patients who can appropriately raise their heart rates with exercise or perform a reasonable amount of exercise are clearly at lower risk for complications, even if they have electrocardiographic changes at peak exercise.[13,14]

Many patients cannot undergo adequate treadmill exercise testing due to poor conditioning or noncardiac disorders, but several new techniques have been evaluated for their ability to predict perioperative cardiac complications in these patients. The most extensive experience to date is with vascular surgery patients who have undergone thallium scintigraphy using dipyridamole to induce ischemia. Dipyridamole increases flow in areas perfused by nonstenotic coronary arteries, so that flow to myocardium supplied by stenotic arteries may diminish because of a coronary "steal" syndrome or peripheral vasodilatation. These differences in flow can be detected with radionuclides such as thallium, which will be present in lower concentrations in areas of the heart in which flow does not increase.

Several studies of patients who have been referred for dipyridamole-thallium testing have demonstrated that patients who do not have evidence of ischemia on testing have a low risk for cardiac complications during subsequent vascular surgery.[15–17] But this test, and other tests for inducible ischemia, tend to be abnormal in many patients who will not have complications — hence, the positive predictive value of the test (that is, the percent of patients with an abnormal result who go on to have complications) has been about 30% or less in most studies, including selected patients undergoing elective hip surgery.[18]

When used in consecutive, unselected

Table 5. Use of the Multifactorial Cardiac Risk Index in Patient Subgroups With Different Baseline Risks of Cardiac Complications

PATIENT TYPE	APPROXIMATE BASELINE RISK: MAJOR CARDIAC COMPLICATIONS	ADJUSTED CARDIAC COMPLICATION RISK USING MULTIFACTORIAL INDEX			
		I	II	III	IV
Minor surgery	1%	0.3%	1%	3%	19%
Unselected consecutive patients >40 years old who have major noncardiac surgery	4%	1.2%	4%	12%	48%
Patients undergoing abdominal aortic aneurysm surgery or who are >40 years old and have high-risk characteristics that generally generate medical consultations before major noncardiac surgery	10%	3%	10%	30%	75%

Adapted from Goldman L.[12]

patients, however, dipyridamole-thallium scanning appears to be much less useful.[19] Therefore, if the test is to be used, it should be preceded by a clinical evaluation to stratify patients into groups with high, medium, and low risks for complications. Dipyridamole-thallium testing appears to be most useful for patients who have an intermediate risk for postoperative cardiac ischemic events,[15] as evidenced by factors such as age, diabetes, prior MI, and ventricular arrhythmias. Dipyridamole-thallium is unlikely to be beneficial for patients with a low risk for complications, and a definitive evaluation of coronary disease with cardiac catheterization is likely to be appropriate for patients with a very high clinical risk for complications regardless of the result of the dipyridamole-thallium scan. In the intermediate risk group, however, dipyridamole-thallium test results can influence management.

These same principles are probably applicable to other noninvasive testing technologies that use pharmacological stresses to provoke ischemia. Alternative pharmacological agents include dobutamine and adenosine, and echocardiography can be used instead of radionuclide scintigraphy to detect ischemia.[20,21] These testing technologies have not been directly compared in large prospective trials, so there are not sufficient data to identify which if any is the "best" test for prediction of perioperative cardiac risk. Their diagnostic accuracy is heavily dependent on operator experience, however, so that whichever test is most routinely available to clinicians may be the best choice.

An alternative is ambulatory ischemia monitoring, which uses electrocardiographic monitoring equipment similar to that frequently used for arrhythmia detection. Preoperative electrocardiographic ischemia identifies patients with an increased risk for cardiac complications after vascular surgery with sensitivity, specificity, and positive predictive value similar to those for dipyridamole-thallium testing.[22-25]

Patients undergoing vascular surgery who have a low ejection fraction detected by radionuclide angiography have higher complication rates.[26,27] However, several reports have suggested that this test does not add substantial

information beyond that available through a clinical assessment.[13,28]

RISK REDUCTION STRATEGIES

Several of the factors associated with increased cardiac risk in noncardiac surgery may be "controlled." For example, delaying an operation until 3 to 6 months after MI may decrease the risk of perioperative cardiac complications. However, emergent and urgent operations (e.g., resection of a possibly malignant lesion) often cannot be delayed. Therefore, clinicians are often required to weigh the risks of surgery against nonsurgical management.

Although no controlled trials have studied this issue, some data suggest that preoperative control of CHF reduces the risk of postoperative pulmonary edema or worsened CHF. Because both general and spinal anesthetic agents may induce intraoperative hypotension if the patient is volume-depleted, preoperative diuresis must not result in dehydration. Such over-diuresis can be avoided by monitoring the patient's blood urea nitrogen and creatinine levels and by carefully assessing postural blood pressure and pulse changes.

Because of the potential hemodynamic consequences of small volume shifts in patients with critical aortic stenosis, suspicious murmurs must be evaluated preoperatively with a careful history and physical examination, and if the data are consistent with aortic stenosis, echocardiography should be performed. Echocardiography supplemented by Doppler analysis can usually identify critical aortic stenosis; only rarely is cardiac catheterization required. Determining whether patients with aortic stenosis have symptoms as a result of the lesion may be more difficult, because noncardiac conditions may limit exertional capacity. Therefore, detailed questioning about the patient's ability to perform specific tasks should be conducted.

The optimal management of patients with known coronary disease remains complex. Patients who survive successful coronary revascularization with percutaneous transluminal coronary angioplasty (PTCA)[29] or CABG surgery[30] usually do well with subsequent noncardiac surgery. However, the intrinsic risks of each of these procedures are in the 1% to 2% range; a range that makes the risk of coronary revascularization followed by noncardiac surgery in patients with stable class I-II angina similar to the expected risks of cardiac death with the noncardiac surgery itself.[30,31] Nevertheless, there is general agreement that patients with unstable or crescendo angina should not undergo noncardiac surgery until the angina is controlled, unless immediate surgery is imperative. Because long-term follow-up studies show that patients with abnormal noninvasive tests for ischemia have poorer cardiac prognoses, many clinicians currently advocate consideration of coronary angiography for patients with markedly abnormal test results not so much to reduce perioperative risk as to improve long-term survival. The impact of this approach has not been demonstrated in interventional studies.

Effective treatment of a patient's general medical problems is also likely to decrease operative risk by reducing cardiac stress. The consulting cardiologist may recommend that surgery be delayed until such problems can be corrected.

Although hypertension is not an independent risk factor for perioperative cardiac complications, hypertensive patients are more likely to have labile blood pressures during anesthesia and surgery.[32] At one time, it was felt that this lability might be reduced by discontinuing antihypertensive medications several days before surgery or by aggressively controlling blood pressure before surgery. More recent data suggest, however, that neither of these 2 extremes is correct. Thus, antihypertensive medications may be continued until surgery, and surgery need not be delayed in patients with moderate persistent hypertension until better control is achieved. The cardiology consultant should follow the patient postoperatively, however, to ensure that he or she is receiving an effective antihypertensive regimen.

Anesthesiologists are usually more familiar with the risks and benefits of various agents and techniques than internal medicine physicians, so the cardiology consultant rarely plays a major role in these choices. Spinal anesthesia causes as much peripheral vasodilation and subsequent hypotension as does general anesthesia. Furthermore, any anesthetic technique that does not effectively eliminate pain will be associated with markedly increased cardiac demands. Spinal anesthesia may also be preferable for patients with important pulmonary disease in whom postoperative hypoxia or other pulmonary problems might increase cardiac demands.

The selection of general anesthetic agents is not nearly as critical as formerly believed. Halothane, which causes both myocardial depression and peripheral vasodilation, is the agent most frequently associated with hypotension, and it should be used cautiously in patients who have other risk factors for intraoperative hypotension. In patients with hypertrophic cardiomyopathy (idiopathic hypertrophic subaortic stenosis) or with right-to-left shunts, peripheral vasodilation during anesthesia may be especially hazardous. Ketamine, which has a sympathomimetic effect, is often recommended for such patients; alternatively, an α-adrenergic agent may be used to increase systemic vascular resistance.

An important development in recent years has been the use of electrocardiographic ischemia monitoring in the perioperative period to detect patients at high risk for subsequent severe cardiovascular complications. Postoperative myocardial ischemia is associated with at least a 2.8-fold increase in the odds of adverse cardiac outcomes,[25] and electrocardiographic ischemia usually precedes cardiac events.[22,23] Prolonged untreated ischemia is especially noteworthy.[33] These data suggest that "real time" ischemia monitoring may become a strategy for reducing complications.

An aggressive intervention that may be useful for reducing overall risk for some subsets of patients is the deliberate increase of oxygen delivery using volume-loading and inotropic agents. This strategy evolved from the observation that patients who died after traumatic or surgical shock tended to have low oxygen delivery despite their increased metabolic needs. A recent randomized clinical trial showed that high-risk surgical patients who had their oxygen delivery index increased to more than 600 ml/min per square meter by use of an inotropic infusion had a reduction in mortality compared to patients who received usual care (6% vs 22%).[34] The routine use of such techniques for elective abdominal aortic aneurysm surgery remain controversial.[35,36] The presumed mechanism for this intervention is the prevention of multi-organ failure due to regional hypoperfusion.

COMMON PERIOPERATIVE QUESTIONS AND COMPLICATIONS

One of the major roles of the cardiology consultant is to anticipate common problems that may develop in the perioperative period. The delineation of such problems and the description of contingency plans are often more helpful to surgical and anesthesia colleagues than calculations of overall perioperative risk.

ISCHEMIC HEART DISEASE

Numerous strategies have been suggested for integrating available data into a sensible approach to the preoperative evaluation of patients with known or suspected coronary heart disease (CHD).[31,37–40] In our opinion, for both the postinfarction patient and the patient with angina, a key determinant of surgical risk is functional status. In general, patients who are in functional Class I or early Class II (which implies that they can do exercise equivalent to carrying 2 grocery bags up a flight of stairs) can achieve a heart rate and blood pressure equivalent to what would be expected with general anesthesia and surgery. If such an activity level can be achieved, the risk of perioperative infarction is probably no higher than 1%-4%. In such patients, the two principal approaches — continued medical management and "prophylactic" coronary revascularization — have apparently equivalent morbidity and mortality risks. Thus, routine revascularization does not currently appear to be warranted for patients with stable coronary symptoms and a good exercise capacity.

If the patient's functional status can be determined accurately by a good medical history, exercise testing is not routinely necessary. If the history is not definitive, exercise testing is helpful in determining functional status. In such cases, decisions about the safety of surgery should depend more on the patient's ability to exercise than on the magnitude of ST-segment depression, since perioperative risk is probably more related to physiologic status than to the underlying coronary anatomy per se (although the latter may be an important long-term prognostic factor). In patients who cannot exercise, dipyridamole-thallium scintigraphy, stress echocardiography, or ambulatory electro-cardiographic monitoring are alternative strategies for determining the patient's level of ischemia and for determining risk. However, current data are not sufficient to mandate that patients who have positive results on either of these 2 tests must have preoperative coronary arteriography and revascularization.[41] Nevertheless, the adverse long-term prognostic significance of markedly abnormal test results makes consideration of an invasive evaluation reasonable even if it is unlikely to change the risk associated with the planned surgery.

Patients who have more severe angina should be routinely considered for coronary arteriography before undergoing elective noncardiac surgery. The physician should, as noted earlier, concentrate more on the patient's functional status than on the frequency of angina, since very active patients may have relatively more-frequent angina whereas patients with angina on very minimal activity may so curtail their exertion that their angina decreases in frequency.

PREMATURE VENTRICULAR CONTRACTIONS

Patients with ventricular arrhythmias have an increased risk of cardiac complications with surgery, but most of these complications are related to ischemia and CHF rather than to uncontrolled ventricular arrhythmias. Therefore, therapeutic interventions in patients with arrhythmias should usually be directed toward the underlying coronary artery disease or cardiomyopathy, and antiarrhythmic therapy should be reserved for patients who meet criteria for chronic antiarrhythmic therapy.

Accordingly, prophylactic lidocaine is usually recommended for patients with a history of symptomatic ventricular arrhythmias, a history of cardiac arrest, or very high-grade degrees of asymptomatic ventricular arrhythmia. Patients with less severe ventricular arrhythmias may be given lidocaine intraoperatively if arrhythmias compromise cardiac function. Because many ventricular arrhythmias during surgery result from inadequate anesthesia, hypoxia, myocardial ischemia, or fluid and electrolyte imbalance, the identification and correction of such problems is more appropriate than is reliance on the antiarrhythmic effects of drugs such as lidocaine. It should be remembered that anesthesia may obscure the usual neurologic warnings of lidocaine overdose.

PATIENTS TAKING ß-ADRENERGIC BLOCKING AGENTS

Concerns that ß-adrenergic blocking agents blunt sympathetic responses during the perioperative period have been allayed by data indicating that patients taking propranolol usually respond appropriately to surgical stresses and that supplemental isoproterenol can be used to overcome the negative inotropic and chronotropic effects of these drugs. Thus, patients being treated with ß-adrenergic blockers for hypertension or angina can usually be maintained on their medications until, and often including, the morning of surgery. Perioperative hypotension or bradycardia in these patients should not be treated with α-adrenergic agents or catecholamines with mixed α- and ß-adrenergic effects (e.g., epinephrine), since unopposed α-adrenergic effects may lead to a hypertensive crisis.

In patients who must discontinue use of ß-adrenergic blocking agents, the risk of a symptomatic rebound in sympathetic activity after abrupt cessation is small, but patients may be hypersensitive to sympathetic stimuli after the drug is discontinued. The timing of this hypersensitivity varies with different ß-adrenergic blocking agents, with longer half-lives leading to delays in the withdrawal phenomenon. Thus, in many patients, oral therapy can be resumed before the drug is cleared completely. Rarely does a patient require intravenous propranolol or metoprolol. An alternative is esmolol, a short-acting ß-adrenergic blocking agent, which can be given with a loading infusion of 500 mcg/kg/min for 1 min followed by a 4-min maintenance infusion of 50 mcg/kg/min. If the desired therapeutic effects have not been achieved, this maintenance infusion can be increased to 100-200 mcg/kg/min.

PROPHYLACTIC DIGITALIS

Patients who develop new perioperative supraventricular tachyarrhythmias during digitalis administration do so at a lower rate than that seen in patients who have not taken digitalis. Therefore, preoperative initiation of digitalis is often considered in patients who are at risk of these arrhythmias, including elderly patients undergoing pulmonary surgery, patients with valvular heart disease, and patients who have CHF. However, intravenous calcium-channel blocking agents that slow conduction through the atrioventricular node (e.g., verapamil, 5-10 mg given as an intravenous bolus over 2 min) provide an acute alterative that can be reserved for the occurence of tachyarrhythmias.

Digitalis is the only routinely available oral inotropic agent, and it has been shown to prevent the myocardial depression caused by general anesthetic agents. However, prophylactic digitalis is not recommended for prevention of perioperative heart failure in patients at risk for this complication.

ANTICOAGULANT THERAPY

Management of patients receiving chronic anticoagulant therapy is determined by the indication for anticoagulation. Patients taking prophylactic anticoagulants for prevention of systemic emboli in the setting of atrial fibrillation or rheumatic heart disease or for the prevention of deep-venous thrombosis can usually discontinue warfarin therapy several days preoperatively, allowing the prothrombin time a period to decline to normal or near-normal, and then have anticoagulation restarted several days postoperatively. Patients who undergo anticoagulation because of prosthetic heart valves can follow a similar regimen, except that heparin is often started within 48 hours postoperatively and continued until warfarin has resulted in an appropriate prothrombin time.

Patients who have caged-disk valves (e.g., Harken prostheses) have another reason to be at especially high risk of thromboembolism, even with brief discontinuation of anticoagulant use. They may be admitted 2 to 3 days before surgery and receive intravenous heparin while the prothrombin time decreases. If a long preoperative hospitalization is not possible, the effect of warfarin may be reversed pharmacologically about 24 hours preoperatively, and low dose heparin may be initiated at the same time; then, full-dose heparin can be started 12-24 hours postoperatively and continued until the patient can resume oral warfarin. It is always easier to reverse heparin rapidly (with protamine) than to reverse the effects of oral vitamin K antagonists.

PACEMAKERS

Prophylactic temporary pacemakers are usually indicated only in patients who meet criteria for placement of a permanent pacemaker. Patients with asymptomatic bifascicular or trifascicular block are at risk for development of complete heart block, but such events rarely occur during the perioperative period unless the patient has a new MI. When autonomic instability associated with intubation and surgery leads to second- or third-degree heart block or hemodynamically significant sinus bradycardia, intravenous atropine usually restores normal conduction and rate.

If implantation of a permanent pacemaker is indicated, it can be implanted before the operation if the planned surgery is elective. If the operation is urgent or emergent, a temporary pacemaker can be used. If the planned procedure may lead to a bacteremia, a temporary pacemaker may be used perioperatively to avoid contamination of a permanent device.

An exception to this conservative approach to the use of temporary pacemakers may be made for patients with preoperative left bundle branch block who are undergoing placement of

a pulmonary artery catheter. This procedure is associated in about 5% of cases with the transient development of right bundle branch block, which, superimposed on a left bundle branch block, could lead to complete heart block. Thus, a method of ventricular pacing should be readily available before right-heart catheterization in this patient population.

A potentially fatal intraoperative problem for patients with permanent pacemakers is inhibition of demand pacemakers by electrocautery. If electrocautery is used, frequency and duration should be limited to 1-second bursts 10 seconds apart, and the ground plate should be placed as far from the pacemaker pulse generator as possible. Placing a magnet over many types of pacemakers switches them into a mode in which the heart is paced at a fixed rate, but because programming of more sophisticated devices may vary, it is important to determine before surgery the pacemaker type and model number, its response to electrical interferences, and reprogramming methods. During periods of electrocautery, the electrocardiogram may be useless for monitoring heart rhythm, and an alternative such as direct palpation of the radial pulse should be used.

PROPHYLACTIC ANTIBIOTICS

Patients with valvular heart disease, prosthetic valves, many forms of congenital heart disease, and arterial abnormalities such as arteriovenous shunts should receive appropriate antibiotic prophylaxis for the type of bacteremia that might be expected based on the site of surgery.[42] In general, antibiotic prophylaxis should begin 6-24 hours preoperatively and be continued for no more than about 48 hours postoperatively.

SPEED AND EXTENT OF SURGERY

After adjusting for the type of operation, there is no correlation between the length of surgery and the development of cardiac complications. Thus, there is no evidence that planned operations should be shorter in patients with cardiac disorders, although it is sometimes appropriate to choose a less ambitious procedure (e.g., a cholecystotomy instead of a cholecystectomy) in the patient with acute cardiac decompensation. Laparoscopic procedures are still too new to permit reliable estimates of their cardiac risk, but early experience has demonstrated that the cardiac risk associated with these procedures is not trivial. Hence, consultants should not be lulled into complacency by the prospects of a laparoscopic procedure.

Many cardiac complications occur when patients are experiencing postoperative pain, fluid shifts, hypoxia, and other stresses. Thus, intraoperative management should be planned to minimize these postoperative risks.

INTRAOPERATIVE MONITORING

Because marked changes in blood pressure or volume status contribute to the development of myocardial ischemia and other cardiac complications, careful intraoperative monitoring is important in the management of patients with cardiovascular disease. A pulmonary artery catheter or a radial artery catheter may be helpful in patients with substantial left ventricular dysfunction, recent preoperative MI or other unstable CAD syndromes, aortic stenosis, or other high-risk factors. Patients who are candidates for interventions aimed at increasing oxygen delivery through the use of volume infusions and/or inotropic agents should undergo hemodynamic monitoring while these treatments are being administered.

INTRAOPERATIVE BRADYCARDIA

Intraoperative bradycardias are usually the result of vagal stimulation, and if arrhythmias such as sinus bradycardia or nodal rhythms do not cause hypotension, ischemia or inadequate perfusion, no therapy is necessary. Otherwise, these arrhythmias can be treated with changes in anesthetic technique, small doses of intravenous atropine, or, occasionally, small doses of ß-adrenergic agents. Such arrhythmias are almost always benign and short-lived and do not correlate with more serious perioperative cardiac complications.

PERIOPERATIVE HYPERTENSION

Perioperative hypertension, defined as a systolic blood pressure of >200 mm Hg or an increase in systolic pressure of >50 mm Hg, occurs in about 5% of patients without a preoperative history of hypertension and in about 25% of patients with a preoperative history of hypertension. These hypertensive episodes are common during intubation, during periods of inadequate anesthesia and in the recovery room as the patient begins to wake up.

Although cardiology consultants may recommend adjustments in the antihypertensive regimen if preoperative blood pressure control is not satisfactory, the risk of perioperative hypertension is not definitely reduced by such measures. Episodes can usually be reversed when they occur by changes in anesthetic technique in the operating room or by correcting the hypoxia, fluid overload, or inadequate postoperative analgesia that has precipitated the hypertension.

If these measures fail, antihypertensive agents may be administered. Intravenous nitroprusside is the best means of controlling hypertension gradually and effectively, and it can be administered in the recovery room or intensive care unit setting. Labetalol has α-and ß-adrenergic blocking effects, may be given as a 20-80 mg intravenous bolus every 10 minutes or as a 2 mg/min infusion, and can be expected to take effect within 5-10 minutes. Nifedipine can be administered sublingually to titrate blood pressure acutely. Intravenous methyldopa, an older but effective alternative, is usually given as 500 mg every 6 hours; it will not manifest its pharmacologic effects for about 6 hours, but is often enough to control moderate blood pressure elevations. Hydralazine, a vasodilator that can be given intramuscularly or intravenously, is an effective antihypertensive drug, but it often precipitates supraventricular tachycardia; hence, it should not be used unless other measures have failed, and it should usually be combined with an intravenous ß-blocker to control tachycardia.

VALVULAR HEART DISEASE

Careful perioperative fluid control is especially important in patients with valvular heart disease because of their increased risk of CHF. In addition, in patients with mild-to-moderate mitral stenosis who are asymptomatic, pulmonary edema may develop if marked tachycardia develops during the perioperative period, making adequate anesthesia essential in these patients.

HYPERTROPHIC OBSTRUCTIVE CARDIOMYOPATHY

Patients with hypertrophic obstructive cardiomyopathy (formerly idiopathic hypertrophic subaortic stenosis, or IHSS) may develop hypotension if they become volume depleted, receive ß-adrenergic agents or vasodilators, or develop tachyarrhythmias. Intravenous propranolol or verapamil can be used to reduce left ventricular outflow obstruction and to improve diastolic filling of the left ventricle. Diuretics may worsen outflow obstruction and hence, worsen CHF.

MITRAL VALVE PROLAPSE

There is no evidence that patients with mitral valve prolapse are at increased risk for cardiac complications with surgery. Patients whose prolapse is accompanied by an audible murmur of mitral regurgitation should receive prophylactic antibiotic therapy, but antiarrhythmic or other therapy should be administered only if the patient meets routine indications for them.

POSTOPERATIVE MEDICAL MANAGEMENT

Recent studies show that most perioperative MIs occur within 48 hours of surgery, but postoperative complications such as CHF and hypertension frequently occur three to five days after surgery, when extravascular fluid returns to the intravascular space, thus increasing cardiac preload and work. Consequently, cardiology consultants should follow patients for at least 5 days after major surgery. During this postoperative period, the consultant can assist with the management of any acute postoperative complications and help to plan chronic therapy for conditions such as hypertension, CHF, or arrhythmias.

POSTOPERATIVE MYOCARDIAL ISCHEMIA AND INFARCTION

Because of anesthesia and noncardiac postoperative pain, only about one-half of postoperative infarctions are accompanied by a complaint of chest pain. Nevertheless, most postoperative MIs are associated with some symptoms or signs: decreased blood pressure, CHF, arrhythmias, or a change in mental status. Electrocardiograms may reveal asymptomatic ischemia, but their interpretation may be complicated by the high prevalence of ST-segment or T-wave changes of doubtful significance in postoperative patients. ST-T wave changes are probably more likely to reflect ischemia if they are prolonged in duration.

Similarly, cardiac enzyme levels may be difficult to interpret because the trauma of surgery can be expected to lead to abnormalities of creatine kinase (CK), lactate dehydrogenase (LDH), and LDH isoenzyme levels. Creatine-kinase MB (CK-MB) is usually unaffected by noncardiac surgery if measured in its usual serial manner, but the definitive diagnosis of MI may still be difficult in many cases.[43] Some investigators recommend that a combination of enzymatic and electrocardiographic criteria be used. Newer enzyme assays such as the cardiac troponins I and T[44] appear to improve diagnostic accuracy in the setting of noncardiac surgery.

POSTOPERATIVE HEART FAILURE

Congestive heart failure is often precipitated by postoperative surgical problems that increase myocardial demands, but some uncomplicated patients develop mild heart failure about 12-36 hours postoperatively, when mobilization of intraoperative fluid begins. Diuretic therapy is usually sufficient to manage these volume shifts, but all patients with postoperative heart failure should be evaluated carefully to determine whether a perioperative MI may have contributed to their failure.

POSTOPERATIVE ARRHYTHMIAS

The new onset of supraventricular tachy-arrhythmias or the development or worsening of ventricular arrhythmias in the postoperative period may be due to increased sympathetic tone in response to surgery, but may also reflect coexisting medical problems. New supraventricular tachyarrhythmias are associated with other cardiac disorders in about 50% of cases, but with abnormalities, such as infection, hypoxia, and new intravenous medications in many patients.

In general, new postoperative supraventricular tachyarrhythmias do not require cardioversion, because most resolve either with the continuation of the patient's chronic cardiac medications or with treatment with intravenous verapamil or digitalis. Electrical cardioversion should be used only if cardiac output is compromised or evidence of ischemia develops.

REFERENCES

1. Rao TLK, Jacobs KH, El-Etr AA. Reinfarction following anesthesia in patients with myocardial infarction. *Anesthesiology.* 1983;59:499-505.
2. Shah KB, Kleinman BS, Sami H, et al. Reevaluation of perioperative myocardial infarction in patients with prior myocardial infarction undergoing noncardiac operations. *Anesth Analg.* 1990;71:231-235.
3. Goldman L, Caldera DL, Southwick FS, et al. Cardiac risk factors and complications in noncardiac surgery. *Medicine.* 1978;47:357-370.
4. O'Keefe JH, Shub C, Rettke SR. Risk of noncardiac surgical procedures in patients with aortic stenosis. *Mayo Clin Proc.* 1989;64:400-405.
5. Goldman L, Caldera DL, Nussbaum SR, et al. Multifactorial index of cardiac risk in noncardiac surgical procedures. *N Engl J Med.* 1977;297:845-850.
6. Detsky AS, Abrams HB, McLaughlin JR, et al. Predicting cardiac complications in patients undergoing noncardiac surgery. *J Gen Intern Med.* 1986;1:211-219.
7. Detsky AS, Abrams HB, Forbath N, et al. Cardiac assessment for patients noncardiac surgery. A multifactorial clinical risk index. *Arch Intern Med.* 1986;146:2131-2134.
8. Zeldin RA. Assessing cardiac risk in patients who undergo noncardiac surgical procedures. *Can J Surg.* 1984;27:402-404.
9. Michel LA, Jamart J, Bradpiece HA, et al. Prediction of risk in noncardiac operations after cardiac operations. *J Thorac Cardiovasc Surg.* 1990;100:595-605.
10. Shah K, Kleinman B, Rao T, et al. Reduction in mortality from cardiac causes in Goldman Class IV patients. *J Cardiothorac Anesth.* 1988;2:789-791.
11. Jeffrey CC, Kunsman J, Cullen DJ, et al. A prospective evaluation of cardiac risk index. *Anesthesiology.* 1983;58:462-464.
12. Goldman L. Multifactorial index of cardiac risk in noncardiac surgery: Ten-year status report. *J Cardiothorac Anesth.* 1987;1:237-244.
13. Gerson MC, Hurst JM, Hertzberg VS, et al. Cardiac prognosis in noncardiac geriatric surgery. *Ann Intern Med.* 1985;103:832-837.
14. McPhail N, Calvin JE, Shariatmadar A, et al. The use of preoperative exercise testing to predict cardiac complications after arterial reconstruction. *J Vasc Surg.* 1988;7:60-68.
15. Eagle KA, Coley CM, Newell JB, et al. Combining clinical and thallium data optimizes preoperative assessment of cardiac risk before major vascular surgery. *Ann Intern Med.* 1989;110:859-866.
16. Brown KA, Rowen M. Extent of jeopardized viable myocardium determined by myocardial perfusion imaging best predicts perioperative cardiac events in patients undergoing noncardiac surgery. *J Am Coll Cardiol.* 1993;21:325-330.
17. Lette J, Waters D, Champagne P, et al. Prognostic implications of a negative dipyridamole-thallium scan: results in 360 patients. *Am J Med.* 1992;92:615-620.
18. Coley CM, Field TS, Abraham SA, et al. Usefulness of dipyridamole-thallium scanning for preoperative evaluation of cardiac risk for nonvascular surgery. *Am J Cardiol.* 1992;69:1280-1285.
19. Baron JF, Mundler O, Bertrand M, et al. Assessment of cardiac risk before abdominal aortic surgery with dipyridamole-thallium scintigraphy and gated radionuclide angiography. *N Engl J Med.* 1994;330:663-669.
20. Tischler MC, Lee TH, Hirsch AT, et al. Prediction of major cardiac events after peripheral vascular surgery using dipyridamole echocardiography. *Am J Cardiol.* 1991;68:593-597.
21. Poldermans D, Fioretti PM, Forger T, et al. Dobutamine stress echocardiography for assessment of perioperative cardiac risk in patients undergoing major vascular surgery. *Circulation.* 1993;87:1506-1512.
22. Raby KE, Goldman L, Creager MA, et al. Correlation between preoperative ischemia and major cardiac events after peripheral vascular surgery. *N Engl J Med.* 1989;321:1296-1300.
23. Raby KE, Barry J, Creager MA, et al. Detection and significance of intraoperative and postoperative myocardial ischemia in peripheral vascular surgery. *JAMA.* 1992;268:222-227.
24. Fleisher LA, Rosenbaum SH, Nelson AH, et al. The predictive value of preoperative silent ischemia for postoperative ischemic cardiac events in vascular and nonvascular surgical patients. *Am Heart J.* 1991;122:980-986.
25. Mangano DT, Browner WS, Hollenberg M, et al. Association of perioperative myocardial ischemia with cardiac morbidity and mortality in men undergoing noncardiac surgery. *N Engl J Med.* 1990;323:1781-1788.

26. Pasternack PF, Imparato AM, Riles TS, et al. The value of the radionuclide angiogram in the prediction of perioperative myocardial infarction in patients undergoing lower extremity revascularization procedures. *Circulation.* 1985;72(suppl 2):13-17.

27. Rose EL, Liu XJ, Henley M, et al. Prognostic value of noninvasive cardiac tests in the assessment of patients with peripheral vascular disease. *Am J Cardiol.* 1993;71:40-44.

28. Franco CD, Goldsmith J, Veith FJ, et al. Resting gated pool ejection fraction: A poor predictor of perioperative myocardial infarction in patients undergoing vascular surgery for infrainguinal bypass grafting. *J Vasc Surg.* 1989;10:656-661.

29. Huber KC, Evans MA, Bresnahan JF, et al. Outcome of noncardiac operations in patients with severe coronary artery disease successfully treated preoperatively with coronary angioplasty. *Mayo Clin Proc.* 1992;67:15-21.

30. Foster ED, Davis KB, Carpenter JA, et al. Risk of noncardiac operation in patients with defined coronary disease: The Coronary Artery Surgery Study (CASS) registry experience. *Ann Thorac Surg.* 1986;41:42-50.

31. Ashton CM, Petersen NJ, Wray NP, et al. The incidence of perioperative myocardial infarction in men undergoing noncardiac surgery. *Ann Intern Med.* 1993;118:504-510.

32. Goldman L, Caldera DL. Risks of general anesthesia and elective operation in the hypertensive patient. *Anesthesiology.* 1979;50:285-292.

33. Landesberg G, Luria MH, Cotev S, et al. Importance of long-duration postoperative ST-segment depression in cardiac morbidity after vascular surgery. *Lancet.* 1993;341:715-719.

34. Boyd O, Ground RM, Bennett ED. A randomized clinical trial of the effect of deliberate perioperative increase of oxygen delivery on mortality in high-risk surgical patients. *JAMA.* 1993;270:2699-2707.

35. Berlauk JF, Abrams JH, Gilmour IJ, et al. Preoperative optimization of cardiovascular hemodynamics improves outcome in peripheral vascular surgery. A prospective, randomized clinical trial. *Ann Surg.* 1991;214:289-299.

36. Ellis JE. Con: Pulmonary artery catheters are not routinely indicated in patients undergoing elective abdominal aortic reconstruction. *J Cardiothorac Vasc Anesth.* 1993;7:753-757.

37. Goldman L, Braunwald E. General anesthesia and noncardiac surgery in patients with heart disease. In: Braunwald EB (ed). *Heart Disease.* Fourth Edition. Philadelphia: WB Saunders; 1992:1708-1720.

38. Fleisher LA, Barash PG. Preoperative cardiac evaluation for noncardiac surgery: a functional approach. *Anesth Analg.* 1992;74:586-598.

39. Wong T, Detsky AS. Preoperative cardiac risk assessment for patients having peripheral vascular surgery. *Ann Intern Med.* 1992;116:743-753.

40. Massie BM, Mangano DT. Assessment of perioperative risk: Have we put the cart before the horse? *J Am Coll Cardiol.* 1993;21:1353-1356.

41. Goldman L. Research in cardiac nuclear medicine: The difficult but critical next step. *J Nuclear Cardiol.* 1994;1:210-212. Editorial.

42. Dajani AS, Bisno AL, Chung KJ, et al. Prevention of bacterial endocarditis. Recommendations by the American Heart Association. *JAMA.* 1990;264:2919-2922.

43. Charlson ME, MacKenzie CR, Ales KL, et al. The postoperative electrocardiogram and creatine kinase: implications for diagnosis of myocardial infarction after noncardiac surgery. *J Clin Epidemiol.* 1989;42:25-34.

44. Adams JE, Sicard GA, Allen BT, et al. Diagnosis of perioperative myocardial infarction with measurement of cardiac troponin I. *N Engl J Med.* 1994;330:670-674.

36 Perioperative Evaluation of the Cardiac Surgical Patient and Cardiac Transplantation

Gilbert H. Mudge, Jr, MD

Cardiology is the most surgically oriented of all medical sub-specialties. The properly trained cardiologist is always assessing the timing of surgical intervention in patients with valvular heart disease, is reappraising medical therapy and symptomatic status in patients with angina pectoris, and must be critical of potential benefits and pitfalls for emergency operative intervention. A working relationship among the cardiologist, cardiothoracic surgeon, and anesthesiologist is mandatory so that patients receive expeditious surgical intervention when so indicated, and so that common cardiologic problems can be easily addressed post-operatively. This chapter reviews certain aspects of the perioperative care of patients undergoing both valvular replacement and coronary artery bypass grafting. Subtleties of perioperative care that enhance the cardiologist's contribution to postoperative management are emphasized. Cardiac transplantation is also reviewed, with emphasis placed upon criteria for trans-plantation.

PERIOPERATIVE EVALUATION

It is assumed that the cardiologist is satisfied with the preoperative cardiac evaluation that has led to the decision for surgical intervention. Although the physiology or anatomy may justify surgical approach, there are secondary factors that also contribute to defining morbidity and mortality which must be addressed with the patient and family and be considered in the ultimate recommendation for surgical intervention.[1] Emergency intervention carries a higher morbidity/mortality than elective procedures. The older patient is prone to more postoperative complications, although more recent data suggest that improved results can be achieved in the elderly patient population.[2] Patients with advanced left ventricular dysfunction or symptomatic congestive heart failure, and critical left main stenosis, are also predisposed to a slightly higher morbidity. It might also be argued that morbidity and mortality are enhanced in the female gender. Although such analysis remains controversial, it can also be acknowledged that females undergoing surgical revascularization are generally older and may have more advanced pathology to account for the higher complication rate. Other factors including especially obesity and diabetes will predict perioperative complications such as prolonged intubation, mediastinal infection, and delayed ambulation.

Special considerations also have to be entertained for the patient undergoing repeat sternotomy. What were complications encountered in the previous operative experience? Are there any reasons to avoid sternotomy, favoring a right lateral thoracotomy for mitral valve repair or left lateral thoracotomy for surgical revascularization in the distribution of the left circumflex artery? Will the healing of the sternotomy be compromised by surgical modification of the anterior thoracic arteries?

Cardiac examination of patients with surgical valvular heart disease or coronary artery disease, with or without left ventricular dysfunction, is not emphasized here. However, several aspects of the general physical examination must not be overlooked during final preoperative evaluation.

In a patient being considered for valve replacement, a careful oral examination is required, and carious teeth must be removed. Since 1 of the most serious complications of prosthetic valve replacement is superimposed bacterial endocarditis, all necessary dental procedures should be completed before surgical intervention; a full mouth extraction and complete healing of the gum may be required in extreme cases before elective valve replacement.

Patients undergoing coronary artery bypass surgery or mitral valve replacement should be carefully examined for evidence of non-surgical aortic insufficiency. This is best assessed with Doppler flow analysis. Patients with hemo-dynamically insignificant aortic insufficiency may develop ventricular distension when they are placed on bypass, for central aortic perfusion will distend the left ventricle and extensive subendocardial damage may ensue. Postoperative intra-aortic balloon support is also contraindicated in this situation. Accordingly, the surgeons should be advised when such insufficiency is suspected.

The peripheral circulation should be scrutinized preoperatively. Blood pressure should be assessed in both arms and peripheral pulses assessed in all extremities. The role of carotid surgery in the asymptomatic patient who is to undergo cardiac surgery is debatable, but a complete history for transient cerebral ischemia should be recorded. Patients with asymptomatic carotid bruits should undergo non-invasive evaluation of their carotid, with digital subtraction angiography or carotid angiography if so indicated. Because patients are often perfused at a non-pulsatile pressure of 50 mm Hg while on cardiopulmonary bypass, uncertainties about the carotid circulation must be clarified. Carotid endarterectomy followed by cardiopulmonary bypass can be effectively and safely performed in patients with high-grade symptomatic carotid disease who require cardiac surgical intervention.[3] If not performed, major neurologic insult may occur following the hypotension required for cardiopulmonary bypass.

The abdominal aorta should be examined for bruits, and the competency of the iliofemoral system checked. This is particularly important in patients who might require transient intra-aortic balloon counterpulsation after surgery. Significant peripheral vascular disease may preclude femoral artery cannulation for initiation of cardiopulmonary bypass. Women who have undergone left radical mastectomy may not be candidates for utilization of the

internal thoracic arteries as conduits; compromised thoracic arterial blood supply may prevent adequate sternal and wound healing.

A careful gastrointestinal, renal, and neurologic history and examination is likewise required; the latter is particularly important should any question regarding alteration in neurologic status arise after surgery. History of gastrointestinal bleeding must be specifically excluded in any patient who might receive a prosthetic valve. The nutritional status should be carefully assessed, and surgery postponed if possible when the patient has severe cachexia. In such instances, preoperative nutritional supplementation may reduce postoperative complications of respiratory failure and delayed ambulation. Venous status should be examined carefully in patients who are to undergo aortocoronary artery bypass surgery. A history of venous ligation or remote history of thrombophlebitis should be underscored in the admitting note. If arm veins are to be used as conduits, they should not be used preoperatively for intravenous therapy. Patients with tinea pedis may have recurrent lower-extremity cellulitis after revascularization surgery that uses saphenous vein conduits.

Conventional laboratory studies are mandatory in preoperative evaluation. The patient should be carefully screened for any perioperative bleeding tendency. Patients with chronic obstructive lung disease or a long-term history of cigarette smoking should have a pulmonary function test; this will help in planning postoperative extubation and pul-monary care. The conventional indices of hepatic function should be carefully scrutinized in patients with advanced right heart failure. Thyroid studies should be performed for patients with underlying atrial fibrillation. Stool guaiacs for occult blood are mandatory because they may help direct the choice of prosthetic valve. Chronic renal failure with hemodialysis is not a contraindication to cardiopulmonary bypass, but compromised renal function that has not yet required hemodialysis may be reason for reconsideration of surgery; hypotension and nonpulsatile blood flow that occur during cardiopulmonary bypass may exacerbate renal dysfunction. There is preliminary evidence that a cardiopulmonary bypass machine capable of pulsatile blood flow will help in preserving borderline renal function.

Patients who are to undergo elective surgery may be candidates for autologous blood donations. While policies vary from blood bank to blood bank, patients with chronic stable angina can make such donations under careful supervision; saline replacement may be necessary. Patients with unstable ischemia, recurrent congestive heart failure, tight aortic stenosis or critical left main coronary artery disease are usually not considered acceptable candidates for autologous donations.

The results of cardiac catheterization must be carefully reviewed before the final decision regarding surgery. In patients with severely compromised left ventricular function with high left ventricular end-diastolic pressure and pulmonary capillary wedge pressure, elevation of pressure can be expected to persist or become more marked during the early postoperative stages.

Two other aspects of the results of cardiac catheterization should be emphasized. First, right atrial pressure should be noted as a rough approximation of right ventricular function and estimation of the degree of tricuspid regurgitation. Many patients with right coronary artery disease have sustained subclinical right ventricular infarctions. Right ventricular dysfunction may be exacerbated in the early postoperative stages, especially if pulmonary function is abnormal.[4] A right atrial pressure greater than 10 mm Hg should alert the cardiologist that right ventricular dysfunction and tricuspid regurgitation is present and that enhanced volume may be required during the first 48 hours after surgery. This need can obviously be further assessed with Doppler echocardiography.

Second, pulmonary artery pressure should be noted. In many patients with mitral valve disease and associated pulmonary hypertension, pulmonary artery pressure will be persistently elevated during the initial postoperative days. This is identified by a pulmonary artery diastolic pressure that exceeds the mean pulmonary capillary wedge pressure by 10 mm Hg. This condition not only necessitates extremely high right atrial filling pressures, but may also be exacerbated by hypoxia. These patients must be well oxygenated, and a pulmonary vasodilator, such as isoproterenol, should be considered in their early pharmacologic regimen. Intravenous nitrate preparations have also been reported to be helpful in such situations.[5] Patients with severe pulmonary hypertension whose pulmonary artery diastolic pressure equals pulmonary capillary wedge pressure usually have rapid resolution of pulmonary hypertension when the pulmonary capillary wedge pressure is reduced after mitral valve replacement.

Most medications can be safely continued right up until the time of surgery. Some surgical centers administer digoxin during the last preoperative day, not only for inotropic support but also to control atrial fibrillation should it occur postoperatively.[6,7] But it might be argued that postoperative electrolyte imbalance and enhanced catecholamine state will result in digitalis toxicity. Diuretic therapy can also be continued, bearing in mind that many patients receiving long-term diuretic therapy have relative total body potassium depletion although serum potassium levels are normal. Since hypokalemia may account for many early postoperative ventricular arrhythmias, additional potassium supplementation should be considered in the final preoperative days for patients receiving large doses of diuretics.

Beta-adrenergic blocking agents are usually administered to patients until the day of coronary artery revascularization. In most patients with a left ventricular ejection fraction >0.40, ß-adrenergic blocking therapy can be continued until the time of surgery.[8,9] By so doing, "rebound" is avoided against postoperative arrhythmias.[10] In patients with compromised left ventricular function, ß-adrenergic blocking agents are best discontinued for at least 24 hours before surgery, as long as the patient's activity is curtailed and adequate nitrate administration is maintained to protect against recurrent myocardial ischemia.

There is no current contraindication to continued use of calcium-channel blocking agents up to the time of surgery. This is mandatory if part of a patient's clinical presentation is coronary artery vasospasm superimposed upon a high-grade fixed obstructive lesion. Sudden withdrawal of a calcium-channel blocking agent can exacerbate coronary artery vasospasm, provoking a preoperative myocardial infarction.[11] Since 1 of their potential pharmacologic effects is to uncouple myocardial excitation from subsequent contraction, calcium-channel blocking agents may have profound negative inotropic effects during the early hours after cardiopulmonary bypass in patients with severe left ventricular function. Indications for use of diltiazem, verapamil and high-dose ß-blocking therapy should be questioned preoperatively. The negative chronotropic effects of both agents may be compounded by hypothermia as the patient is weaned from cardiopulmonary bypass; junctional heart rates of 25-30 beats/min are frequently seen in this setting and are often unresponsive to isoproterenol infusion or atropine; pacing may be required for 24-36 hours postoperatively.

Conventional anticoagulation with warfarin obviously must be discontinued so that the prothrombin time and partial thromboplastin time return to normal before surgery. Patients with absolute indications for anticoagulation must be switched to heparin. Aspirin may be associated with postoperative bleeding and should be avoided if possible 72 hours before surgery, but will be rapidly reinstituted postoperatively to improve graft patency in patients undergoing revascularization.[12] The safety of other antiplatelet agents in the final preoperative hours is unclear. Dipyridamole was administered preoperatively to patients undergoing myocardial revascularization without resulting in excessive postoperative bleeding,[13] but the incremental benefit of this to aspirin therapy is uncertain.

Most conventional oral antiarrhythmics can be continued up to the time of surgery, and replaced with intravenous preparations if needed, as determined by the anesthesiologist. There is little evidence that antiarrhythmics should be initiated as prophylaxis against postoperative arrhythmias. Amiodarone has substantial clinical and subclinical pulmonary toxicity, and its administration has been associated with persistent and prolonged hypoxia after cardiopulmonary bypass. The indications for its use should be carefully reviewed with the surgeons before surgical interventions. The indications for other antiarrhythmics agents with potent negative inotropic effects should also be reassessed perioperatively.

INTRAOPERATIVE CONSIDERATIONS

The choice of anesthetic agents is best deferred to the anesthesiologist. Because many anesthetics reduce both preload and afterload, patients may often require enhanced volume administration early postoperatively. Such anesthesia may be dangerous in patients whose cardiac output is dependent on their preload status, such as patients with critical aortic stenosis, when left ventricular stroke volume depends on left ventricular filling volume; patients with right-to-left shunts will have shunting increase. Reductions in peripheral vascular resistance should be treated with both volume expansion and administration of pressor agents during induction of anesthesia.

The cardiologist must be thoroughly familiar with the techniques of thoracotomy, of placing the patient on the pump oxygenator, of the surgical procedure itself, and of weaning the patient from cardiopulmonary bypass. The sternotomy and cardiac dissection must be done with extreme care in any patient undergoing reoperation and who has a patent vein graft or internal thoracic artery to the left anterior descending artery; interruption of this conduit during surgical dissection can be disastrous. The aortic arch is usually cannulated to receive the arterial input from the pump oxygenator. Femoral artery cannulation is often indicated in patients with severely compromised left ventricular function or prior sternotomy so that partial cardiopulmonary bypass support may be given during sternotomy. Femoral artery cannulation might also be required if the surgery involves the aortic arch itself. Cannulation of the aortic arch saves time by avoiding groin dissection, but it must be done with extreme care, particularly in elderly patients with fragile calcified aortas. Dissection from an aortic cannulation usually has dire consequences.

The venous return to the oxygenator is usually obtained from the vena cava via the right atrium. Once venous and arterial cannulas are in place, the patient may be cooled to approximately 28°C, with supplemental topical cardiac hypothermia applied during the time that the aorta is cross-clamped. Left ventricular distention must be prevented during the time of aortic cross-clamp; a left ventricular vent may be required. The cardiologist should also be familiar with the technique that the surgeon uses to remove air from the left heart and aorta before left ventricular ejection is permitted. The pump oxygenator usually maintains a blood flow of 2.0-2.5 l/min/m², which generates a mean non-phasic blood pressure of 50-60 mm Hg. Lower blood flows are permitted with more intense cooling, and total circulatory arrest may be feasible at 20°C for brief periods.

When the surgical procedure is complete, monitoring lines are inserted before the patient is weaned from cardiopulmonary bypass. The exact line used will often depend on the preference of the anesthesiologist or surgeon. Percutaneous pulmonary artery catheters are always feasible; direct left atrial lines inserted into the posterior aspect of the left atrium via the pulmonary veins provide a precise definition of hemodynamics for the first 48 postoperative hours. These can be brought out easily through a small skin incision and pulled before the chest tubes are removed. Right atrial lines may be similarly inserted by the surgeons, with minimal complications during their removal. Once both right and left heart pressures are measured, the surgeon weans the patient from cardiopulmonary bypass. Anterior and posterior mediastinal chest tubes are then inserted; additional chest tubes may be required if the pleural cavities have been entered. The pericardium is usually left open. Atrial and ventricular pacing wires are attached and brought out through the skin. The former wires are particularly helpful in the postoperative management of patients with hypertrophied, noncompliant ventricles that respond to A-V sequential pacing, and in diagnosis and treatment of postoperative supraventricular tachycardias. The sternum is then reapproximated, the skin is closed, and the patient is returned to the recovery room intubated, with need for continued ventilatory support.

POSTOPERATIVE CARE

HEMODYNAMIC MONITORING AND SUPPORT

The presence of an arterial monitor, potential right and left atrial lines, and perhaps a pulmonary artery catheter simplifies the close hemodynamic monitoring required for patients after cardiopulmonary bypass. The right atrial line may be a venous access; the left atrial line must never be so used in order to avoid systemic arterial embolization.

The postoperative care of the patient with advanced left ventricular dysfunction requires the close cooperation between cardiac surgeon, anesthesiologist, and cardiologist. In many instances when preoperative assessment suggests a high risk for postoperative left ventricular dysfunction, intra-operative placement of intra aortic balloon device is entirely justified. This often expedites weaning from cardiopulmonary bypass, and makes the hemodynamic management of the patient in the first 48 hours postoperatively somewhat easier. More aggressive strategies for the patient with severe left ventricular dysfunction in the operating room include maintenance of extra-corporeal oxygenation systems, and employment of right and left ventricular assist devices. Recent technological advances of the left ventricular assist device suggest that this may be a suitable option in patients who are high risk for conventional surgery, and may be a satisfactory means of stabilizing the patient's overall medical status, serving as an effective bridge to heart transplantation.

Persistent hypoxia may not be secondary to left ventricular dysfunction, but adult respiratory distress syndrome. This patient population is predisposed to it, for there is a direct correlation between the duration of cardiopulmonary bypass, and the ultimate abnormalities within the pulmonary vasculature that lead to enhanced capillary permeability and increased interstitial pulmonary edema. The ultimate management of such a problem includes prolonged mechanical ventilation with positive end expiratory pressures, maximizing cardiac function by reducing pulmonary venous pressures, and ample nutritional support.

Postoperative pulmonary dysfunction also emerges as a primary problem that requires identification in the early postoperative state. This patient population is predisposed to such pulmonary failure due to associated chronic obstructive pulmonary disease, sternal incision and the potential for development of pleural effusions. In addition, there may be diaphragmatic dysfunction when the phrenic nerve is interrupted, an occurrence most often seen when there is mobilization of both internal thoracic arteries for revascularization.

Postoperative hypotension is the most common hemodynamic problem in the first hours after surgery. During the first hours after coronary artery bypass surgery, patients may have enormous volume requirements. Such enhanced fluid requirements are most often due to systemic venous vasodilation; a less likely reason is transient right ventricular dysfunction. During the final phases of cardiopulmonary bypass, with a body temperature of 28°C, there is a significant vasoconstriction with increased systemic vascular resistance. As the patient's temperature returns to normal, vasodilation increases volume requirements. Patients with normal left ventricular function and an uncomplicated postoperative course often require 6-7 liters of fluid before their condition stabilizes. The choice of type of volume is made in conjunction with the surgeons; the patient should receive available blood from the pump oxygenator. Pharmacologic inotropic support usually does not need to be added to the patient's intravenous regimen until adequate right and left atrial filling pressures are achieved. Daily weights during the first postoperative week and comparison to preoperative weight constitute an important means of assessing fluid balance.

Hypotension associated with high left-atrial filling pressures should be treated with inotropic support. Many patients may have inappropriately high systemic vascular resistance with depressed left ventricular function and borderline hypotension; combined inotropic support with afterload reduction in such

patients is justified. During the first 24 hours after surgery, intravenous nitroprusside and dopamine are often adequate. Patients should be closely monitored for arrhythmias, which can be precipitated by inotropic agents such as dopamine and epinephrine. There is some evidence that dopamine has equal positive inotropic effect to dobutamine with greater afterload reduction capability; these characteristics may justify single drug therapy in patients with severely depressed left ventricular function.[14]

Perioperative pericardial tamponade is not an infrequent cause of postoperative hypotension, and should be at the top of any differential diagnosis that does not respond to conventional therapy. While all patients may have some degree of pericardial effusion postoperatively, this can be rapidly assessed with echocardiographic techniques. The presence of diminished heart sounds, pulsus paradoxus, and kinking of the anterior mediastinal chest tube with variable drainage, should all raise suspicion. Echocardiographic evaluation is mandatory in such instances, and early postoperative tamponade is probably best addressed surgically with either a subxyphoid incision or reopening the sternal incision.

Systemic hypertension after coronary artery bypass surgery or aortic valve replacement is reported to occur in 30%-50% of patients undergoing myocardial revascularization.[15,16] Hemodynamic studies indicate that this is related to an increase in total peripheral vascular resistance without change in cardiac output; an increase in resting α-adrenergic vasoconstrictor tone is postulated as the mechanism. Plasma epinephrine and norepinephrine levels are documented to increase substantially in the early postoperative course;[17] the renin-angiotensin system has also been incriminated, and converting enzyme inhibitors have been used successfully to control blood pressure.[18] There is no correlation with a history of hypertension or previous propranolol dosage. Most patients become hypertensive within 2 hours after surgery, the hypertension abating 48-72 hours later. Aggressive therapy of this acute hypertension is indicated for several reasons. Not only does myocardial oxygen consumption increase as a result of the enhanced blood pressure, but the degree of postoperative bleeding, both from the aortic cannulation site and from saphenous vein graft anastomosis, can be related to the blood pressure. Chest tube drainage often resolves when postoperative hypertension is controlled. Because postoperative hypertension is a transient hemodynamic phenomenon during the first 48 postoperative hours, intravenous therapy with sodium nitroprusside is often indicated to lower the systolic pressure to 120 mm Hg. This therapy can be easily tapered as the hypertension resolves. Should blood pressure elevation persist for more than 48 hours postoperatively, calcium-channel blocking agents, converting-enzyme inhibitors or ß-blocking agent may be administered. Almost all patients who are normotensive during preoperative evaluation can be tapered off antihypertensive medication before hospital discharge.

Postoperative bleeding should be carefully monitored by the anterior and posterior mediastinal chest tube drainage. Adequate protamine sulfate should be administered to reverse the heparin given when the patient was on the pump oxygenator. Protamine sulfate may produce peripheral vasodilation and hypotension, thus enhancing initial postoperative volume requirements. Platelet count should also be carefully monitored. In most patients with a normal preoperative platelet count, that count will drop to 60,000-70,000 secondary to destruction from the pump oxygenator and most coagulation factors are reduced by hemodilution. Platelet transfusions are rarely required. Some surgeons will control mediastinal bleeding with positive end-expiratory pressure from the respiratory ventilator, but this should be avoided in patients with chronic obstructive pulmonary disease or with complex congenital heart diseases. Elevation of alveolar pressure in the former population may enhance the risk of pneumothorax; elevation of right atrial pressure in the latter should be avoided. If bleeding continues at 200-300 ml/hr for 4 hours after initial chest closure, surgical re-exploration is usually required.

More recent improvements in surgical technique may reduce postop bleeding problems. These include increasing use of anti-fibrinolytic agents, aminocaproic acid and tranexamic acid, and the serene protease inhibitor, trasylol. In addition, there are surface coated devices in which heparin is covalently bonded to bioactive surfaces. This reduces heparin requirements, and blunts both platelet destruction and complement activation of neutrophils.

CARDIAC ARRHYTHMIAS

Significant ventricular arrhythmias often occur after valvular or revascularization surgery.[19] Such dysrhythmias have many causes: direct trauma to the ventricle, hypoxia, depressed left ventricular function, anesthetic agents, endogenous or exogenous catecholamine stimulation, electrolyte or acid-base abnormality, and, more often, the underlying disease process itself. Since maximal depression of left ventricular function does not occur for 18-24 hours after cardiopulmonary bypass, all ventricular premature contractions occurring more frequently than 10 per minute in the first 48 postoperative hours should be treated with intravenous therapy, after correcting transient causes such as hypoxia, hypokalemia, acidosis, or alkalosis. The possibility of digitalis toxicity must not be overlooked. Lidocaine is often preferred as the initial intravenous anti-arrhythmic agent, because depression of myocardial contractility and peripheral vasodilation are far less marked than with equivalent doses of procainamide or the newer parenteral antiarrhythmic agents. If a patient is refractory to lidocaine administration, intravenous procainamide can be administered, and the patient can then be switched to an oral preparation if needed. Diphenylhydantoin, bretylium tosylate, or amiodarone may also be considered as intravenous agents should patients have refractory high-grade and life-threatening ventricular ectopic activity. A patient with persistent life-threatening ventricular ectopic activity for more than 72 hours postoperatively must be aggressively treated. Full electrophysiologic testing may be required in the last postoperative course, but is probably not justified if the arrhythmias are controlled in the 24-48 hours postoperatively; many of the early postoperative arrhythmias are secondary to the transient and correctable causes mentioned above.[20]

All patients who require intravenous antiarrhythmic therapy for ventricular ectopic activity should receive 24 hours of continuous monitoring in the final postoperative days before discharge. Significant ventricular ectopic activity, including couplets, multiform ventricular premature beats, or brief ventricular tachycardia, is usually suppressed by oral therapy for at least 6 weeks after surgery, although the value of this practice is unproved except perhaps in patients suspected of having a perioperative myocardial infarction.

Supraventricular tachycardias are also common after valvular or coronary bypass surgery. Atrial premature beats are typical, and transient atrial flutter or fibrillation is reported to occur in as many as 30% of patients who were in normal sinus rhythm preoperatively.[21,22] Most of these atrial dysrhythmias can be easily converted to sinus rhythm and controlled with conventional antiarrhythmic therapy. Cardioversion is rarely needed. The atrial electrode should be used if the diagnosis of any supraventricular tachycardia is equivocal; the atrial wire can be connected to the precordial lead of an electrocardiogram and atrial activity recorded. Causes of recurrent supraventricular tachycardia in the early postoperative course must be carefully considered. Hypoxia, persistent pulmonary infiltrates, pericarditis, gastric dilatation, anemia, fever, or right or left atrial cannulas are often the cause.

Rapid supraventricular tachycardias that cause hemodynamic embarrassment should be immediately treated by cardioversion. Little additional anesthesia is usually required in the first 12 postoperative hours; 5-10 mg of intravenous diazepam is usually adequate. Supraventricular tachycardias in patients who have undergone valve replacement should be treated with either quinidine or procainamide. Among patients who have such dysrhythmia after coronary artery bypass surgery, low-dose ß-adrenergic blockade or verapamil are extremely

effective and safe[23] and form the justification for prophylactic use of ß-adrenergic blocking agents postoperatively. Esmolol, the ultra-short-acting cardioselective ß-blocker is especially useful in this instance.

Atrial flutter with rapid ventricular response may severely compromise the patient's condition. Rapid atrial pacing is safe and atraumatic in this condition and can be considered if an atrial wire is in place.[24] The atrial rate should be increased to 125% of the underlying atrial arrhythmia. When pacing is abruptly terminated, normal sinus rhythm or atrial fibrillation often follows, the latter more easily controlled than atrial flutter with intravenous digoxin or verapamil. In patients with postoperative atrial fibrillation who were in normal sinus rhythm preoperatively and maintain normal sinus rhythm for 5 to 6 weeks after surgery, antiarrhythmic therapy can be discontinued.

Many patients with mitral valve disease and chronic atrial fibrillation preoperatively may have normal sinus rhythm postoperatively. In such patients, the left atrium has often been inspected for thrombi. While most of these patients may revert to their atrial arrhythmia during the first postoperative week, antiarrhythmic therapy should be administered to try to maintain a sinus mechanism. In patients with an aortic porcine heterograft, maintenance of normal sinus rhythm might obviate the need for long-term anticoagulation.

The possibility of digitalis toxicity should always be considered as a cause of arrhythmias, and digoxin levels should be checked when clinically indicated. This is particularly important after quinidine therapy is instituted.

Third-degree heart block is a rare complication of open heart surgery, more common after repair of ventricular septal defect and endocardial cushion defect. In adults, debridement of a heavily calcified aortic valve may produce complete heart block by disrupting the conduction system below the noncoronary cusp. This is often recognized in the operating room and treated with ventricular wires. In patients with evidence of bifascicular conduction abnormalities preoperatively or a complete heart block on the operating table, a permanent epicardial wire can be brought down to a subcutaneous subxyphoid pouch. These can easily be retrieved and attached to a pacemaker if normal conduction is not spontaneously restored after surgery. Nodal rhythms are a common conduction abnormality, particularly after mitral valve and aortic valve replacement. Nodal rhythms are usually well tolerated if the rate is adequate, but can always be treated with overdrive pacing or isoproterenol infusion. Such nodal rhythm disturbances usually last 48-72 hours and resolve spontaneously.

MYOCARDIAL INFARCTION

Intraoperative myocardial infarction is a complication that must be addressed within the first 48 hours after surgery. Perioperative infarction is documented in about 10% of patients,[25] reflecting a compilation of potential problems that include extent of disease, anastomotic considerations, thrombosis, embolism, myocardial protection, left ventricular hypertrophy, enhanced myocardial oxygen demand and postoperative hypotension or hypoxia. The appearance of new Q waves should be interpreted as evidence of infarction, and little clinical emphasis should be placed on the changes in ST-segment or T-wave contour or modest elevation of postoperative creatine kinase (CK) levels. Such ST-segment elevation may resolve when the anterior and posterior mediastinal chest tubes are removed. Post-pericardiectomy ST-T wave abnormalities may persist for 6 months after surgery. Conventional myocardial enzyme levels are often elevated following cardiac surgery; a CK of 600-800 IU/l is not unusual and may be associated with trace elevation of the CK-MB fraction. The CK-MB isoenzyme is frequently found in patients who have required direct conversion of ventricular fibrillation to sinus rhythm in the operating room with paddles placed upon the heart. An SGOT greater than 100 IU/l coupled with a CK above 1,000 IU/l with CK-MB more than 30 IU/l should be considered evidence of subendocardial myocardial infarction. The development of new regional wall motion abnormalities on echocardiogram is presumptive evidence for perioperative infarction.

Most such infarctions are subendocardial and do not cause major hemodynamic compromise, and the patients can usually be ambulated and managed postoperatively without undue complication. Those patients at risk with perioperative myocardial infarctions include the elderly, those with preoperative myocardial infarctions, advanced left ventricular dysfunction, or persistent postoperative ventricular dysrhythmias. A perioperative myocardial infarction is also an adverse prognostic indicator in those patients with incomplete surgical revascularization and advanced left ventricular dysfunction. Perioperative infarction with major hemodynamic compromise should be treated with conventional therapy, including proper inotropic support, and intra-aortic balloon counterpulsation if necessary. Patients with perioperative infarctions are usually not considered candidates for emergency revascularization and can certainly not receive thrombolytic therapy.

PRE- AND POST-DISCHARGE CARE

Patients are usually slowly ambulated 48 to 72 hours after surgery. A low grade, unexplained fever is common, and can be safely monitored if routine causes such as drug reaction, atelectasis, phlebitis at intravenous access site and occult infection are considered and excluded. Early rehabilitation 48 to 72 hours following surgery includes walking and range of motion exercises. If the postoperative course is uncomplicated, discharge can be anticipated on the seventh to tenth postoperative day or even earlier in uncomplicated instances. In patients who have undergone coronary artery bypass surgery, the leg incisions are often the primary source of discomfort. The physical examination should be directed toward evidence of congestive heart failure, pulmonary consolidation, atelectasis, pericardial rub, pericardial tamponade (evidence of pulsus paradoxus should be sought), and thrombophlebitis. The incidence of post-pericardiectomy syndrome is low, about 5% in most series. Unexplained fever, chest pain, and pericardial rub are indications for treatment with nonsteroidal anti-inflammatory agents, but renal function should be carefully monitored if these agents are used. Other postoperative complications include wound infection, pulmonary embolism, cerebrovascular accident, urinary tract outlet obstruction, complications from use of intra-aortic balloon pump, and hepatitis resulting from transfusion.

Indefinite anticoagulation is required for all mechanical prosthetic valves.[26] A porcine xenograft valve placed in the aortic position does not require anticoagulation therapy, but a patient with a porcine xenograft in the mitral position and normal sinus rhythm usually receives anticoagulation for 6 weeks after surgery. If normal sinus rhythm is maintained, then anticoagulation therapy can be discontinued without undue risk of thromboembolic complications.[27] Patients with chronic atrial fibrillation should receive anticoagulation indefinitely, irrespective of the type of valve used. Anticoagulation can be started 48 hours after surgery, once the chest tubes and atrial cannulae have been removed.

Early evidence suggests that aggressive antiplatelet therapy should be initiated in patients with coronary artery disease. Studies of sulfinpyrazone therapy[28] and of combined aspirin/dipyridamole therapy[13] showed that graft closure rate can be reduced 3%-4% after coronary artery revascularization; patients who received placebo therapy had a graft closure rate of 9%-10%. In the study with aspirin/dipyridamole, dipyridamole was initiated before surgery and aspirin instituted as soon as mediastinal bleeding ceased. The Veterans Administration Cooperative Study showed little additional benefit with dipyridamole over aspirin alone. When one takes this study into account with the recent studies on unstable angina[29] and the natural history of coronary artery disease,[30] it seems reasonable to suggest that after surgical revascularization all patients should receive enteric aspirin therapy unless it is specifically contraindicated.

Before discharge, the patient's physical examination should be carefully noted in the record; a postoperative echocardiogram evaluating prosthetic valve function has been advocated as a baseline control observation. The physician should check the stability of the sternum, placing fingers on either side of the incision and asking the patient to cough.

Patients must be instructed regarding the complications of anticoagulation and prophylaxis for subacute bacterial endocarditis as so indicated. In patients with significant left ventricular dysfunction, the diuretic regimen and sodium intake must be carefully adjusted.

Patients are encouraged to slowly increase their daily activity as comfort and energy permit. Most patients continue to experience variable degrees of fatigue for 4-6 weeks after surgery, with residual leg and sternal discomfort; resumption of normal activity usually is not recommended until 8 weeks postoperatively. An active rehabilitation program may not be practical until discomfort is fully resolved, and evaluation of operative success by exercise tolerance study is of little benefit until the ST-segment and T-wave abnormalities have resolved and the patient is completely comfortable. Stress thallium studies may be indicated if chronic ST-segment abnormalities prevent adequate electrocardiographic interpretation.

Most patients should be seen at least once a year by a cardiologist after open heart surgery. Risk factors that contribute to the development of coronary artery disease cannot be ignored. Cigarette smoking must cease, blood pressure must be controlled, and plasma lipid level elevations must be aggressively pursued. Recognizing that coronary artery bypass surgery is a palliative procedure, such patients should be carefully followed for evidence of recurrent myocardial ischemia. Those with valve replacement must be carefully followed for evidence of paravalvular leaks or primary valve dysfunction and carefully instructed in antibiotic prophylaxis for subacute bacterial endocarditis.

CARDIAC TRANSPLANTATION

Despite the recent advances with converting enzyme inhibitor therapy and more aggressive afterload reduction, the mortality for Class IV congestive heart failure continues to be approximately 30% in the first year of follow-up.[31] Since 1-year survival after cardiac transplantation can now exceed 90%, cardiac transplantation has become a reasonable option for the patient with end-stage congestive heart failure.[32] The operation is available in more than 150 heart transplant centers within the United States; access on the basis of geographic location is no longer a consideration. However, at the same time that the medical capabilities with immunosuppressive therapy achieve impressive long-term results, new ethical issues have been addressed regarding cardiac transplantation that need to be resolved. There are approximately 40,000-50,000 individuals per year who meet current criteria for cardiac transplantation,[33] but yet the donor supply has been stable at 2,200 hearts for the last several years. Hence, 1 in 20 potential recipients will receive an organ. For those that do receive hearts, the median waiting time within the United States exceeds 9 months. Given these disparities, it is important that the selection criteria for cardiac transplantation be critically examined.

The standard selection criteria include progressive, symptomatic congestive heart failure, an escalating medical regimen with recurrent hospitalizations for congestive heart failure, no secondary exclusion criteria that might include diabetes, hepatic disease, or renal impairment, or clinically significant peripheral vascular disease, an adequate psychosocial profile and suitable chronologic to physiologic age. While most centers use 60 as an arbitrary age cut off, patients up to the age of 65 who are otherwise in excellent health have been considered.[34] Refractory angina with inoperable coronary artery disease, but preserved left ventricular function, or life-threatening ventricular ectopic activity are generally not considered acceptable indications for transplantation.

Whatever the cause of the patient's terminal illness, symptoms of congestive heart failure should be refractory to conventional medical therapy, limiting the patient with ordinary daily activity or occurring at rest, in order to consider the patient for transplantation. Simple documentation of advanced left ventricular dysfunction is not an indication, for some patients may be very well compensated for years before presenting with a terminal condition. Circulating catecholamines[35] and serum sodium[36] are poor prognostic indicators, as is poor exercise capacity.[37]

Secondary medical conditions may serve as general exclusion criteria. Patients with an active infectious process cannot receive the intense immunosuppressive therapy required after transplantation. Those with clinically significant cerebral and peripheral vascular disease may have limited rehabilitation potential. Insulin-dependent diabetes with secondary retinopathy or nephropathy is a relative contraindication to cardiac transplantation. Most cardiac transplant centers recognize that simple glucose intolerance, without other organ involvement, can be easily managed; it often becomes initially manifest when the patient is placed on high-dose steroid therapy.

The presence of pulmonary embolism with residual scar formation predisposes patients to cavitation at the site of infarction, and serves as a relative contraindication to cardiac transplantation. Clinically active chronic obstructive pulmonary disease, including chronic bronchitis and bronchiectasis, will only be exacerbated with aggressive immunosuppressive therapy. The differentiation between advanced obstructive or restrictive pulmonary disease and severe congestive heart failure is not often easily established by pulmonary function studies; severe congestive heart failure may simulate restrictive physiology. Patients with an FEV1/FVC ratio <45% of predicted value are at relatively high risk for post-transplant pulmonary problems. When such patients are being considered for transplantation, pulmonary function studies while a patient is in congestive heart failure must be compared with those that might have been obtained before the clinical presentation of congestive heart failure.[38]

Clinically active peptic ulcer disease will certainly be exacerbated with high-dose steroid administration, and serves as a relative exclusion criterion, as does the presence of any other coexisting systemic illness that might limit life expectancy. Preexisting malignancy should not be an absolute contraindication to cardiac transplantation if such malignancy is judged to be cured by the usual clinical criteria. This consideration becomes particularly germane to patients who present with adriamycin cardiotoxicity, having been cured of the primary neoplastic disease by conventional clinical guidelines.

Psychosocial support is an important consideration, as is the patient's ability to follow a complicated medical regimen. In persons with active and continued drug or alcohol abuse, poor compliance makes the complicated postoperative follow-up impossible. Intensive counseling is mandatory in any patient with a history of such abuse.

All potential recipients are screened for preformed antibodies to potential donors' lymphocytes. The presence of such antibodies predicts a high likelihood of acute rejection at the time of cardiac transplantation. A candidate who has high titer of such preformed antibodies may be very difficult to match with potential donors.

Potential recipients require careful right heart catheterization at least 6 months before heart transplantation. Pulmonary hypertension, with a pulmonary vascular resistance of 480-600 dynes-sec-cm^{-5} is an absolute contraindication to conventional orthotopic cardiac transplantation.[39] With high pulmonary vascular resistance, the new heart can be expected to develop acute right ventricular failure; this complication accounts for approximately 5% of all intra-operative deaths. In patients who have an elevated pulmonary vascular resistance, this condition must be further assessed with acute afterload reduction with nitroprusside, or prostaglandin E-1 at the time of cardiac catheterization. Patients whose pulmonary vascular resistance can decrease are usually suitable for orthotopic transplantation.

LIMITATIONS OF CURRENT SELECTION CRITERIA

These criteria for cardiac transplantation have many limitations. They form exclusion criteria rather than inclusion criteria; none of these criteria really provide an objective assessment of prognosis, nor differentiate the prognosis in patients presenting with advanced left ventricular dysfunction. Moreover, clinical improvement may occur in patients who are placed on waiting lists, but yet there is no systematic way to "de-select" or "de-list" these

patients, in an equitable fashion when their clinical condition has stabilized. In addition, it is now acknowledged that insufficient emphasis has been placed on the patient who is felt to be too well to need transplantation during initial evaluation. Such a population continues to have a very high mortality. Other dilemmas include the misperception that cardiac transplantation is a low risk surgical procedure. With an intra-operative mortality of less than 5%, it is at times favored over other higher risk surgical interventions, such as repeat revascularization surgery or high risk valve replacement. The selection criteria do not address the issue of retransplantation. Given the limitation of the donor supply, how may hearts is a patient entitled to? Should a patient who develops allograft coronary artery disease following heart transplantation take precedent over an individual waiting with end stage heart failure? Current clinical criteria do not address these important issues.

The criteria should also focus upon survival, and not on functional capacity. Moreover, at the present time, prioritization for hearts is often based upon waiting times for recipients, which selects cardiac transplantation for those patients who have a demonstrated survival without the operation. If 2 patients are of the same blood group and same body size, 1 patient waiting 1 year for a heart transplant, the other waiting 1 week for a heart transplant, the organ will be allocated to the individual waiting 1 year. This current procedure seems counter-intuitive to the natural history of the disease, for it thus allocates organs to an individual who may not need it for long-term survival. Finally, given the current rate of listing patients for heart transplantation with the above criteria, and ongoing limitations in the donor supply, cardiac transplantation may not be performed in the near future on outpatients waiting at home for their operation. Rather, it will be available only to the intensive care unit (ICU)-bound patient who may be dependent upon mechanical supports, even though that population may have less than a 50% chance of obtaining a heart.

Recent studies also suggest that patients listed for heart transplantation utilizing the above criteria may be far more stable in their clinical course than previously considered.[42] Recent analysis indicates that there is no incremental survival benefit with cardiac transplantation for patients who have been awaiting transplantation on medical therapy for greater than 6 months. This point is particularly timely, for it suggests that more objective criteria than those enumerated above are necessary in listing patients for cardiac transplantation.

PROPOSED OBJECTIVE CRITERIA FOR CARDIAC TRANSPLANTATION

Recent studies suggest that peak exercise oxygen consumption (VO_2) is the best predictor of mortality in patients awaiting cardiac transplantation.[43] Those individuals with end-stage congestive heart failure and depressed left ventricular ejection fraction with a VO_2 less than 10 ml/kg/min had an annual mortality approaching 70% without cardiac transplantation; those individuals with similar ejection fraction and cardiac index but a peak VO_2 of 20 ml/kg/min having an annual mortality of 5%-10%, a survival that compares favorably to those patients undergoing transplantation. By multivariate analysis, a peak VO_2 is superior to pulmonary capillary wedge pressure, ejection fraction, cardiac index, etiology of congestive heart failure, age, sex, or New York Heart Association Classification in predicting patients' clinical course.[43] Given all these considerations, a recent consensus report has suggested modification to current indications.[44] In addition to the general medical consideration above, this report suggests a 3 group classification as follows:

Group 1: Accepted Indication for Cardiac Transplantation.
1. VO_2 max < 10ml/kg/min with achievement of anaerobic thresholds.
2. Severe ischemia limiting daily activity, not amenable to bypass surgery or angioplasty.
3. Recurrent symptomatic ventricular arrhythmias refractory to all accepted therapeutic modalities.

Group 2: Probable Indication for Cardiac Transplantation.
1. VO_2 max less than 14 ml/kg/min and major limitation of patient's daily activity.
2. Recurrent unstable ischemia not amenable to bypass surgery or angioplasty.
3. Instability in fluid balance and renal function, which is not secondary to compliance issues.

Group 3: Not Adequate Indication for Cardiac Transplantation.
1. Ejection fraction below 20%.
2. History of Class III-IV heart failure.
3. Ventricular arrhythmias.
4. Maximal VO_2 greater than 15 ml/kg/min, without other indications.

One can estimate that perhaps 50% of patients currently listed in the United States fall into category 3. If more objective criteria were utilized in listing patients for cardiac transplantation, the number of recipients might be far less, and the disparity between the number of donors and recipients would be far less acute.

While most clinicians will not become actively involved in the day-to-day decisions on immunosuppressive therapy after cardiac transplantation, their continued involvement is mandatory to optimize long-term survivals. Once a patient is listed at a cardiac transplant center, he or she must be meticulously followed. All patients should receive anticoagulant therapy to reduce the risk of venous and arterial embolization.

While most patients can be satisfactorily managed at home, a small percentage require intermittent inotropic support or prolonged hospitalization. Intra-aortic balloon counter-pulsation may be required, but probably only should be undertaken at the cardiac transplant center, where the patient can be monitored for complications and suitability as a potential recipient can be assessed on a day-to-day basis. Use of a left ventricular assist device or total artificial heart as a bridge to cardiac transplantation has received limited attention; the complications of these devices often preclude cardiac transplantation. The overall results when such bridge devices are used are less impressive than those achieved when the transplant patient is in a more stable condition. This particular dilemma raises many ethical issues about the suitability of using a scarce and limited resource in patients with a hopeless prognosis. Finally, recent experience with medical regimens that are tailored to an individual's needs with invasive monitoring have met with preliminary success and may alleviate the short-term need for transplantation.[45]

Other logistical issues that the clinician should consider include preservation of the right internal jugular vein; thrombosis of this access site may limit options for endomyocardial biopsy. In addition, the potential recipient should receive blood transfusions only when absolutely necessary; frequent transfusions may alter antibody levels, making a suitable match more difficult. Moreover, there is no compelling evidence that repeated transfusions alter rejection episodes for cardiac transplant recipients.

DONOR CRITERIA AND MANAGEMENT OF THE DONOR HEART

The cardiac donor is the other patient essential to the transplant process. Males up to the age of 55 and females to age 60 are generally considered as potential donors once they have fulfilled neurologic criteria for brain death. A suitable cardiac donor is an individual who should have no cardiac disease, no cardiac arrest during their terminal illness, with normal electrocardiogram and normal echocardiogram. A potential donor heart will not be suitable if dependent upon inotropic therapy.

Unfortunately, there has been minimal change in the overall donor supply in the past 5 years. Even if on a national basis we were to achieve maximal donor procurement it would still be far below projected need, being no greater than 8,000-9,000 donors. Given these inevitable limitations to heart transplantation, it is imperative that the potential for all donors be maximized, and involvement of the cardiovascular specialist may be essential to this long-term goal.

The cardiologist should be asked during the early aspects of donor evaluation for expert opinion regarding the adequacy of a potential donor. Electrocardiograms and echocardiograms will need to be reviewed. Cardiac catheterization may be requested by the transplant center if there are either age or risk factor considerations that might predispose the potential donor to subclinical coronary artery disease. Realizing that the donor population is usually defined as a group of patients with catastrophic central nervous system trauma and resultant diabetes insipidus, hypotension in a potential donor should be managed with aggressive volume replacement. Urine output should be matched with intravenous saline, and inotropic support with dobutamine should be avoided until all efforts at volume replacement have failed. Central pulmonary artery lines may be critical to maximize the hemodynamic status of the donor.[46] The cardiovascular subspecialist should learn to work closely with organ procurement organizations in the management of such patients. Efficient donor management benefits the entire population of patients with end stage cardiac disease.

POST-TRANSPLANTATION FOLLOW-UP

Postoperative follow-up is directed toward immunosuppressive requirements, infectious complications, surveillance for the development of malignancy, and the slow evolution of allograft coronary artery disease.

Endomyocardial biopsy continues to be the only reliable means of diagnosing early rejection. Advanced rejection may be diagnosed by hemodynamic compromise or abnormalities in diastolic function as gauged by both echocardiogram and Doppler analysis, but when such findings are present, rejection is often far advanced and may not adequately respond to major changes in immunosuppressive therapy.

Each patient is anticipated to have at least 1 rejection episode as immunosuppressive therapy is titrated to a maintenance regimen. While HLA matching is not done between donor and recipient, there are some general clinical predictors of rejection that are often considered by cardiac transplant centers in individualizing immunosuppressive regimens. Younger patients, multiparous females, those with acute myocarditis, or individuals with a positive cross match characterize patients who will have more intense immunosuppressive requirements. Accordingly, many transplant centers may rapidly taper immunosuppressive regimens in the older male population with coronary artery disease to avoid long-term complications of immunosuppressive therapy.[47]

The general immunosuppressive strategies are summarized in the Table. While Solu-Medrol is used in most patients as induction therapy, monoclonal antibody therapy OKT3 may be considered in patients who have borderline renal dysfunction to avoid the early administration of cyclosporin.

Chronic immunosuppressive regimens almost always include prednisone, azathioprine, and cyclosporine. The prednisone dosage is usually tapered to 0.1 mg/kg over 6 months after cardiac transplantation; and may be withdrawn completely in some patients. Cyclosporine is adjusted to achieve whole blood concentrations of 250-400 ng/ml; and azathioprine is administered at a rate of 1.5-2 mg/kg; the white count should not fall below 4,500. These guidelines are of course arbitrary, for there is a wide variation in the histologic response of patients with cardiac transplantation. Each immunosuppressive regimen must be individualized.

Acute histologic rejection is usually treated with Solu-Medrol (methylprednisolone) therapy; more advanced rejection is treated with either OKT3 monoclonal antibody or antilymphocyte serum.

Patients are often placed upon pneumocystis prophylaxis, usually Bactrim DS (trimethoprim/sulfamethoxazole). Aspirin is often prescribed after cardiac transplantation in an effort to prevent the development of graft atherosclerosis, although the clinical evidence to support this therapy is lacking. Patients are usually maintained on antacids to reduce the possibility of duodenal ulcers. Since cyclosporine therapy is associated with a high renin state, antihypertensive agents are frequently required.

As immunosuppressive regimens are tapered to baseline requirements, potential infectious complications abate. Patients do need to be closely followed for the evolution of post-transplant malignancy;[48] post-transplant lymphoproliferative disorders of primarily B lymphocytes, is a direct result of over immunosuppression, and may resolve as immunosuppression is furthered tapered.[49]

The most ominous complication in the long-term follow-up of patients after cardiac transplantation is the development of allograft coronary artery disease.[50,51] Recent studies suggest that 50%-60% of patients may have tapering of coronary arteries 5 years following transplantation. The clinical presentation of this disease process is particularly unique. Having a denervated heart, these patients rarely have classic anginal discomfort and more often present with symptoms of left or right ventricular heart failure or asymptomatic regional wall motion abnormalities. Coronary arteriography is at times misleading, due to the concentric and diffuse nature of the disease process. Intravascular ultrasound has been recently used as a more reliable means of predicting the extent of pathology. Unfortunately, there are no absolute predictors for the development of coronary artery disease; some studies have suggested the presence of anti-HLA antibodies[52] or activation of intracellular adhesion molecules; other studies have tried to relate this to an active cytomegalovirus infection[53] or to hyperlipidemia.[54] There is insufficient evidence at the present time to justify long-term prophylaxis against cytomegalovirus infection to prevent allograft coronary artery disease. Most recent investigations suggest that allograft coronary artery disease may represent delay type hypersensitivity. Endothelial cells are capable of expressing Class I and Class II HLA antigens. This leads to secretion of cytokines, activation of macrophages, cytokine production, and sustained smooth muscle cell proliferation.[55,56]

Although recent studies suggest that calcium-channel blocking agents may modify the natural history of allograft coronary artery disease,[57] there is no clear current consensus that such therapy is preventive. Isolated case reports indicate success with coronary artery revascularization or angioplasty, although such interventions are at higher risk given the extensive vasculopathy extending to the capillary level.[58] Retransplantation remains the only effective form of therapy for this disease

Table. Immunosuppressive Therapy

Induction Therapy
    Solu-Medrol
    OKT3 Monoclonal Antibody Therapy
    Antilymphocyte Serum

Maintenance Therapy
    Prednisone
    Cyclosporine
    Azathioprine
    Vincristine

Rejection Therapy
    Solu-Medrol
    Oral Prednisone
    OKT3 Monoclonal Therapy
    Antilymphocyte Serum

process.[59] Limited donor supply has reduced enthusiasm for retransplantation within the cardiac transplant community.

After cardiac transplantation, the patient has a denervated heart and the clinician must be aware of certain limitations with this deficit. If allograft coronary artery disease develops, the patient does not have traditional symptoms of angina. Symptoms of transient left ventricular dysfunction or new regional wall motion abnormalities must be aggressively pursued. The patient complaining of paroxysmal exertional dyspnea must be screened for obstructive coronary disease. Yearly coronary arteriography is usually performed.

With a denervated heart, the compensatory response to enhanced physiologic demands may be slower. Hypotension cannot be met with rebound tachycardia. Any heart transplant recipient in whom peripheral vasodilation suddenly develops must be treated with aggressive fluid administration; the most frequent clinical settings are septic shock and general anesthesia for noncardiac surgery. In the latter situation, a liter of volume replacement should be administered before induction of general anesthesia.

REFERENCES

1. Higgins TL, Estafanous FG, Loop FD, et al. Stratification of morbidity and mortality outcome by preoperative risk factors in coronary artery bypass patients. *JAMA.* 1992;267:2344-2348.
2. Cohn LH, Horvath KA. CABG in elderly patients: Risks vs. benefits. *J Myocard Ischemia.* 1991;3(1):13-23.
3. Graver JM, Murphy DA, Jones EL, et al. Concomitant carotid and coronary artery revascularization. *Ann Surg.* 1982;195:712-720.
4. Boldt J, Kling D, Hempetmann G. Right ventricular function and cardiac surgery. *Intensive Care Med.* 1988;14:496-498.
5. Parsons RS, Mohandas K, Riaz N. The effects of an intravenous infusion of isosorbide dinitrate during open heart surgery. *Eur Heart J.* 1988;9(suppl A):195-200.
6. Burman SO. The prophylactic use of digitalis before thoracotomy. *Ann Thorac Surg.* 1972;14:359-368.
7. Selzer A, Walter RM. Adequacy of preoperative digitalis therapy in controlling ventricular rate in postoperative atrial fibrillation. *Circulation.* 1966;34:119-122.
8. Caralps JM, Julet J, Wienhe HR, et al. Results of coronary artery surgery in patients receiving propranolol. *J Thorac Cardiovasc Surg.* 1974;67:526-529.
9. Lauer MS, Eagle KA, Buckley MJ, et al. Atrial fibrillation following coronary artery bypass surgery. *Prog Cardiovas Dis.* 1989;31:367.
10. Ora Y, Frishman W, Becker RN, et al. Clinical Pharmacology of the new beta adrenergic blocking drugs. 10. Beta adrenoceptor blockade and coronary artery surgery. *Am Heart J.* 1980;99:255-269.
11. Muller JE, Gunther S. Nifedipine therapy in Prinzmetal's angina. *Circulation.* 1978;57:137-139.
12. Buring JE, Hennekens CH. Antiplalelet therapy to prevent coronary artery bypass graft occlusion. *Circulation.* 1990;82:1046-1048.
13. Chesebro JH, Clements IP, Fuster V, et al. A platelet inhibitor drug trial in coronary artery bypass operations: Benefit of perioperative dipyridamole and aspirin therapy on early postoperative vein graft patency. *N Engl J Med.* 1982;307:73-78.
14. DiSesa V, Brown E, Mudge GH, et al. Hemodynamic comparison of dopamine and dobutamine in the postoperative volume-loaded, pressure-loaded, and normal ventricle. *J Thorac Cardiovasc Surg.* 1982;83:256-263.
15. Viljoen JF, Estafanous FG, Tarazi RC. Acute hypertension immediately after coronary artery surgery. *J Thorac Cardiovasc Surg.* 1976;71:548-550.
16. Salerno TA, Henderson M, Keith FM, et al. Hypertension after coronary operation. *J Thorac Cardiovasc Surg.* 1981;81:396-399.
17. Cooper TJ, Cluton Brock TH, Jones SN, et al. Factors relating to the development of hypertension after cardiopulmonary bypass. *Br Heart J.* 1985;54:91-95.
18. Niarchos AP, Roberts AJ, Case DB, et al. Hemodynamic characteristics of hypertension after coronary artery bypass surgery and effects of converting enzyme inhibitor. *Am J Cardiol.* 1979;43:586-593.

19. Angelini P, Feldman MI, Lufochanowski R, et al. Cardiac arrhythmias during and after heart surgery: Diagnosis and management. *Prog Cardiovasc Dis.* 1974;16:469-495.
20. Garan H, Ruskin JN, DiMarco JP, et al. Electrophysiologic studies before and after myocardial revascularization in patients with life-threatening ventricular arrhythmias. *Am J Cardiol.* 1983;51:519-524.
21. Douglas P, Hirshfield JW, Edmunds LH. Clinical correlates of postoperative atrial fibrillation. *Circulation.* 1994;70(suppl II):165.
22. Fuller JA, Adams GG, Buxton B. Atrial fibrillation after coronary artery bypass grafting. Is it a disorder of the elderly? *J Thorac Cardiovasc Surg.* 1989;97:821-825.
23. Mohr R, Smolensky A, Goor DA. Prevention of supraventricular tachyarrhythmia with low dose propranolol after coronary bypass. *J Thorac Cardiovasc Surg.* 1981;81:840-845.
24. Waldo AL, MacLean WAN, Karp RB, et al. Continuous rapid atrial pacing to control recurrent or sustained supraventricular tachycardia following open heart surgery. *Circulation.* 1976;54:245-250.
25. London MJ, Hollenberg M, Wong MG, et al. Intraoperative myocardial ischemia: Localization by continuous 12-lead electrocardiography. *Anesthesiology.* 1988;69:232-241.
26. Saour JN, Seck JO, Mamo LA, et al. Trial of different intensities of anticoagulation in patients with prosthetic heart valves. *N Engl J Med.* 1990;322:428-432.
27. Cohn LH, Mudge GH, Pratter F, et al. Five to eight year follow-up of patients undergoing porcine heart-valve replacement. *N Engl J Med.* 1981;304:258-262.
28. Baur HR, Van Tassel RA, Purach CA, et al. Effects of sulfinpyrazone on early graft closure after myocardial revascularization. *Am J Cardiol.* 1982;49:420-424.
29. Fuster V, Cohen M, Halperin J. Aspirin in the prevention of coronary disease. *N Engl J Med.* 1989;321:183-185.
30. Steering Committee of the Physicians' Health Study Research group. Final report on the aspirin component of the ongoing Physicians' Health Study. *N Engl J Med.* 1989;321:129-135.
31. The Consensus Trial Study Group. Effect of enalapril on mortality in severe congestive heart failure. Results of the Cooperative North Scandinavian Enalapril Survival Study (CONSENSUS). *N Engl J Med.* 1987; 316:1429-1435.
32. Young JB, Winters Jr WL, Bourge R, et al. Bethesda Conference on Cardiac Transplantation; Task Force 4: Function of the Heart Transplant Recipient. *J Am Coll Cardiol.* 1993;22:54-64.
33. Evans RW. Executive summary: The National Cooperative Transplantation Study. Report BHARC-100-91-020. Seattle: Battelle Seattle Research Center, June 1991.
34. Olivari MT, Antolick A, Kaye MP, et al. Heart transplantation in elderly patients. *J Heart Transplant.* 1988;7:258-264.
35. Levine TB, Francis GS, Goldsmith SR, et al. Activity of the sympathetic nervous system and renin-angiotensin system assessed by plasma hormone levels and their relationship to hemodynamic abnormalities in congestive heart failure. *Am J Cardiol.* 1982;49:1659-1666.
36. Packer M, Medina N, Yushak M. Relation between serum sodium concentration and the hemodynamic and clinical responses to converting enzyme inhibition with captopril in severe heart failure. *J Am Coll Cardiol.* 1984;3:1035-1043.
37. Engler R, Ray R, Higgins CB, et al. Clinical assessment and follow-up of functional capacity in patients with chronic congestive cardiomyopathy. *Am J Cardiol.* 1982;49:1832-1837.
38. Thompson ME, Kormos RL, Zerke A, et al. Patient selection and results of cardiac transplantation in patients with cardiomyopathy. In: Shaver JA (ed). Cardiomyopathies: Clinical Presentation, Differential Diagnosis and Management. Philadelphia: FA Davis; 1989.
39. Kormos RL, Thompson M, Hardesty RL, et al. Utility of perioperative right heart catheterization data as a predictor of survival after heart transplantation. *J Heart Transplant.* 1986;5:391. Abstract.
40. Costard-Jackle A, Fowler MB. Influence of preoperative pulmonary artery pressure on mortality after heart transplantation: testing of potential reversibility of pulmonary hypertension with nitroprusside is useful in defining a high risk group. *J Am Coll Cardiol.* 1992;19:48-54.
41. Murali S, Uretsky BR, Armitage JM, et al. Utility of prostaglandin E-1 in the pretransplant evaluation of cardiac failure patients with significant pulmonary hypertension. *J Heart Lung Transplant.* 1992;11:716-723.
42. Stevenson LW, Hamilton MA, Tillisch JH, et al. Decreasing survival benefit from cardiac transplantation for outpatients as the waiting list lengthens. *J Am Coll Cardiol.* 1991;18:919-925.
43. Mancini DM, Eisen H, Kussmaul W, et al. Value of peak exercise oxygen consumption for optimal timing of cardiac transplantation in ambulatory patients with heart failure. *Circulation.* 1991;83:778-786.
44. Mudge GH, Goldstein S, Addonizio LJ, et al. Bethesda Conference on Cardiac Transplantation; Task Force 3: Recipient Guidelines; 1993:1-64.
45. Stevenson LW. Tailored therapy before transplantation for treatment of advanced heart failure: effective use of vasodilators and diuretics. *Heart Lung Transplant.* 1991;10:468-476.
46. Baldwin JC, Anderson JL, Boucek MM, et al. Bethesda Conference on Cardiac Transplantation; Task Force 2: Donor Guidelines. 1993:1-64.
47. Miller LW, Schlant RC, Kobashigawa J, et al. Bethesda Conference on Cardiac Transplantation; Task Force 5: Complications. 1993:1-64.
48. Krikorian JG, Anderson JL, Bieber CP, et al. Malignant neoplasms following cardiac transplantation. *JAMA.* 1978;240:639-643.
49. Penn I. Cancer after cyclosporine therapy. *Transplant Proc.* 1988;20:276-279.
50. Hosenpud JD, Shipley GD, Wagner CR. Cardiac allograft vasculopathy: current concepts, recent developments and future directions. *J Heart Lung Transplant.* 1992;11:9-23.
51. Miller LW. Transplant coronary artery disease. *J Heart Lung Transplant.* 1992;11:S1-S4. Editorial.

52. Rose EA, Pepino P, Batt ML, et al. Relation of HLA antibodies and graft atherosclerosis in human cardiac allograft recipients. *J Heart Lung Transplant.* 1992; 11:S120-S123.

53. Grattan MT, Cabral-Moreno CE, Starnes VA, et al. Cytomegalovirus infection is associated with cardiac allograft rejection and atherosclerosis. *JAMA.* 1989;261:3561-3566.

54. Winters GL, Kendall TJ, Radio SJ, et al. Posttransplant obesity and hyperlipidemia: major predictors of severity of coronary arteriopathy in failed human heart allograft. *J Heart Transplant.* 1990;9:364-371.

55. Allen MD, McDonald TO, Carlos T, et al. Endothelial adhesion molecules in heart transplantation. *J Heart Lung Transplant.* 1992;2:S8-S13.

56. Gordon D. Growth factors and cell proliferation in human transplant arteriosclerosis. *J Heart Lung Transplant.* 1992;11:S7. Abstract.

57. Schroeder JS, Gao SZ, Alderman EA, et al. A preliminary study of diltiazem in the prevention of coronary artery disease in heart transplant recipients. *N Engl J Med.* 1993;328:164-170.

58. Halle AA, Wilson RF, Vetrovec GW for the Cardiac Transplant Angioplasty Study Group. Multicenter evaluation of percutaneous transluminal coronary angioplasty in heart transplant recipients. *J Heart Lung Transplant.* 1992;11:S138-S141.

59. Gao SZ, Schroeder JS, Hunt S, et al. Retransplantation for severe accelerated coronary artery disease in heart transplant recipients. *Am J Cardiol.* 1988;62:876-881.

37

Exercise Training and Cardiac Rehabilitation in Patients With Cardiovascular Disease

Joshua M. Hare, MD
Peter H. Stone, MD

Limitation of exercise capability represents a cardinal manifestation of cardiovascular disease, especially coronary artery disease (CAD) and congestive heart failure (CHF). Exercise training, by improving patients' ability to exercise, has the potential, in both of these syndromes, to improve a patient's quality of life. Furthermore, exercise training may actually improve longevity in patents with CAD. In this chapter we will review: (1) normal exercise physiology, (2) the adverse effects of immobilization, (3) the physiologic effects of exercise and (4) the benefits of exercise training and rehabilitation.

MEASUREMENT AND ASSESSMENT OF THE NORMAL PHYSIOLOGIC RESPONSE TO EXERCISE

Peak exercise capacity is defined as "the maximum ability of the cardiovascular system to deliver oxygen to exercising skeletal muscle and of the exercising muscle to extract oxygen from the blood."[1] Normal physiologic function during exercise, therefore, depends on three independent physiologic processes: pulmonary gas exchange, cardiac performance, and skeletal muscle metabolism. From a practical standpoint, exercise capacity may be quantitated through the measurement of oxygen uptake ($\dot{V}O_2$), carbon dioxide production ($\dot{V}CO_2$), and minute ventilation ($\dot{V}E$).[2] These parameters are measured during exercise using rapidly responding gas analyzers capable of breath-by-breath determination of O_2 and CO_2 concentrations. The maximal oxygen uptake ($\dot{V}O_{2max}$) during exercise manifests as a plateau in $\dot{V}O^2$ despite increasing workload (Fig. 1). This parameter reflects maximal exercise capacity as it may be limited by either pulmonary, cardiac or skeletal muscle function.

In addition, $\dot{V}O_{2max}$ has a strong linear correlation with both cardiac output and skeletal muscle blood flow (Fig. 2).[3] The relationship between cardiac output and O_2 consumption forms the basis for the Fick theorem (C.O.=O_2 consumption/arteriovenous O_2 difference). Another index, the anaerobic threshold (AT) is defined as the point at which $\dot{V}E$ increases disproportionately relative to $\dot{V}O_2$, and generally occurs at 60%-70% of $\dot{V}O_2$ (Fig. 1). The AT directly results from the increase in lactic acid production by working muscles. The AT serves as another indicator of exercise capacity and can distinguish between noncardiac pulmonary or musculoskeletal and cardiac causes of exercise limitation. Patients who fatigue prior to reaching AT are likely to have a noncardiac limitation to exercise.[2] Both $\dot{V}O_{2max}$ and AT are useful in assessing severity, progression of, or improvement in exercise capacity. Estimation of exercise capacity can be made by using metabolic equivalent units (METs). One MET is defined as 3.5 milliliters of oxygen uptake per kilogram per minute, and is approximately the oxygen cost of standing quietly.

PHYSIOLOGIC EFFECTS OF IMMOBILIZATION

The traditional concept of placing patients on bed rest following myocardial infarction (MI) derived from the pathologic changes of healing myocardium described by Mallory and colleagues in 1939.[4] Because 6-8 weeks were required for the major portion of the necrotic myocardium to heal and organize, bedrest for 6 weeks post-MI became widely accepted. As early as 1941, however, Tinsley Harrison questioned the wisdom of prolonged bedrest after MI. Controversy surrounded early mobilization after

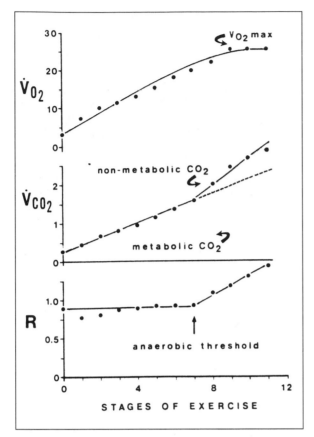

Figure 1. *The response in oxygen uptake ($\dot{V}O_2$), carbon dioxide production($\dot{V}CO_2$) and respiratory gas exchange ratio (R) to incremental treadmill exercise in a normal subject. Maximal oxygen uptake ($\dot{V}O_2$) and onset of anaerobic threshold are identified, as is the metabolic source of carbon dioxide (CO_2) from oxidative metabolism and the nonmetabolic source of carbon dioxide from the buffering of lactate by bicarbonate. Reprinted with permission from Weber KT, Janicki JS. Physiologic Principles and Clinical Applications. W.B. Saunders; 1986:151-167.*

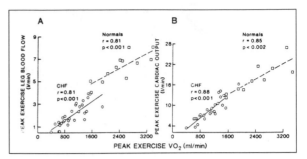

Figure 2. *Plots of relations of peak exercise $\dot{V}O_2$ to single leg blood flow (panel A) and cardiac output (panel B) in patients with chronic heart failure due to systolic LV dysfunction (open circle, solid predicted regression lines) and normal subjects (open box, dashed predicted regression lines); r=correlation coefficient. Reprinted with permission of the American Heart Association, Inc. from Sullivan MJ, et al. Circulation. 1989;80:769-781.*

acute MI until a series of investigations, mainly by Levine and Lown, advocated the "armchair regimen" following MI.[5] This concept was gradually accepted and further advanced to include rapid mobilization, early exercise, and rapid discharge of patients after uncomplicated MI.[6]

Much of the impetus for early mobilization of the post-MI patient came from understanding the deleterious effects of prolonged bedrest. For example, the classic study by Saltin and coworkers showed that physical work capacity decreased strikingly after immobilization. Healthy normal volunteers kept on bedrest for 3 weeks experienced a 20%-25% decrease in $\dot{V}O_{2\ max}$ during exercise,[7] and required 3 weeks of training to restore their pretest physical work capacity. Current studies of the effects of immobilization performed on astronauts preparing for aerospace efforts have confirmed that the most marked alteration after immobilization at bedrest is a decrease in physical work capacity and $\dot{V}O_{2\ max}$.

Immobilization leads to a 700-800 ml decrease in circulating blood volume, causing significant tachycardia and orthostatic hypotension. The plasma volume decreases to a greater extent than does the red blood cell mass; these changes are independent of changes in serum erythropoietin levels, and may predispose to thromboembolism by increasing blood viscosity. A negative nitrogen and protein balance has also been demonstrated. Recent microscopic studies in animal models show that prolonged immobilization is associated with a decrease in cardiac protein synthesis. Structural changes associated with prolonged bedrest include increasing dilation of the sarcoplasmic reticulum and homogenization of mitochondrial cristae. These changes may be significant in the healing phases of MI. Skeletal-muscle strength may diminish by as much as 10%-15% after the first 7-10 days of immobilization. Inefficiently contracting muscle during immobilization demands more oxygen for the same amount of work, imposing a greater cardiac stress in patients with recent MI.

Based on these extensive data about the effects of bedrest, gradually progressive, low-intensity, early ambulation programs were designed to avert or lessen the deleterious effects of prolonged immobilization.[6]

PHYSIOLOGIC RESPONSE TO EXERCISE

The physiologic response to exercise is fundamentally controlled by the autonomic nervous system. The initiation of exercise is associated with both vagal withdrawal, as well as sympathetic discharge. While vagal withdrawal produces a rise in heart rate, sympathetic discharge enhances myocardial contractility and leads to vasoconstriction, which increases venous return. The rise in heart rate, the Frank-Starling mechanism, and the adrenergic-mediated augmentation in myocardial contractility all contribute to increasing cardiac output. Increased sympathetic nerve activity produces vasoconstriction in most circulatory systems, although it leads to vasodilation in the circulations of exercising muscle, brain and the heart.

The significant increases in blood flow to exercising muscle is associated with an increase in oxygen extraction. Total peripheral vascular resistance drops, resulting in an unloading effect on the ventricle, which further facilitates the rise in cardiac output. As a result of the increased cardiac output and decreased systemic vascular resistance, systolic blood pressure increases while diastolic blood pressure changes little or decreases, creating a physiologic situation characteristic of an increased volume load. In terms of the pulmonary circulation, the normal human cardiac output may increase 6-fold without significantly increasing the pulmonary capillary wedge pressure.

Coronary blood flow increases in proportion to myocardial demand during exercise in normal persons. Unlike the peripheral tissues, which can increase their oxygen extraction from the blood in response to exercise, cardiac muscle extracts the maximal amount of oxygen from blood at rest. The resting arteriovenous oxygen difference across the coronary circulation is therefore much greater than that across the peripheral vascular beds. Since the myocardium cannot increase its oxygen extraction during exercise, increased oxygen demand necessitates

an increase in coronary blood flow. In normal persons, coronary blood flow is autoregulated by myocardial oxygen demand, and coronary flow increases in proportion to rises in myocardial oxygen demand or consumption.[8]

Myocardial oxygen demand ($M\dot{V}O_2$) depends on a variety of factors, many of which can be noninvasively measured. The principal determinants of $M\dot{V}O_2$ are heart rate, contractility, and ventricular wall tension, the last being in turn determined by peak ventricular systolic pressure (afterload) and ventricular volume (preload). Measurements of $M\dot{V}O_2$ are helpful in patients with ischemic heart disease because $M\dot{V}O_2$ reflects the limitations of the diseased coronary arteries in providing increased flow during stress. The rate-pressure product (the product of the heart rate and the peak systolic blood pressure) is widely accepted as a useful approximation of the $M\dot{V}O_2$.

THE TRAINING EFFECT

Studies of endurance training in athletes have provided an understanding of the benefits of the "training effect."[9] Conditioned athletes develop higher $\dot{V}O_{2max}$ and AT. Elevation in $\dot{V}O_{2max}$ results from both higher peak cardiac output as well as a widened arteriovenous O_2 content difference. The beneficial effects on the AT result from an increased capacity for aerobic exercise. This contributes significantly to a diminished requirement for ventilation because aerobic exercise requires less oxygen for a given work load and reduces lactate production which stimulates ventilation.[9]

While cardiac output with peak exercise is elevated in conditioned athletes, it is unchanged at rest. Stroke volume, on the other hand, increases at rest. Heart rate is therefore reduced both at rest and at any level of exercise. Conditioning also leads to lower blood pressure during exercise. This may result in part from the dramatic reduction in sympathetic tone that accompanies endurance training.[9]

Exercise conditioning also has significant effects on skeletal muscle which account for the increase in the capacity for aerobic metabolism. Endurance exercise alters the biochemical profile of skeletal muscle such that it becomes more like cardiac muscle, increasing mitochondrial content and capacity to generate ATP from the oxidation of pyruvate and fatty acids. The myoglobin content of skeletal muscle also increases as physical conditioning progresses. In addition to structural changes, O_2 delivery is enhanced by a proliferation of muscle capillaries.[9] Because very little adaptive enhancement of carbohydrate metabolism occurs with exercise training, it appears that physical conditioning shifts the metabolic emphasis toward enhanced utilization of fatty acids, initiating a glycogen-saving effect. The fundamental contractile properties of skeletal muscle, however, are not altered by chronic exercise.

Thus, the training effect raises cardiac functional capacity while lowering O_2 requirements for any given level of work. These benefits arise from alterations in skeletal muscle metabolism and are accompanied by great reductions in sympathetic nervous system activity. Increased work loads are facilitated with lower myocardial O_2 requirements and reductions in pulmonary ventilation.

EFFECT OF EXERCISE IN PATIENTS WITH ISCHEMIC HEART DISEASE

An understanding of these physiologic responses to exercise is particularly germane for management of cardiac patients. These physiologic mechanisms indicate how the patient with ischemic heart disease and/or myocardial dysfunction may be limited in their ability to exercise; equally important, they provide an understanding of the potential role of physical rehabilitation for the cardiac patient.

Figure 3 illustrates the effect of intensive physical training on $\dot{V}O_{2max}$ in patients with ischemic heart disease. After training, there is a dramatic 28% increase in $\dot{V}O_{2max}$[10] although at any given submaximal workload $\dot{V}O_2$ is the same in trained and untrained patients. These benefits of physiologic conditioning are progressively increased with prolonged periods of training

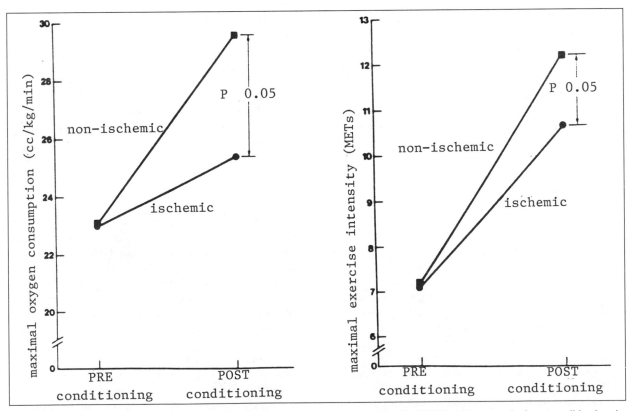

Figure 3. Maximal oxygen consumption and maximal exercise capacity (in METs) before and after conditioning in patients with and without baseline (before conditioning) exercise-induced ischemia. Reprinted with permission from Ades PA, et al.[10]

(Fig. 4).[11] Also, since trained patients have increased their $\dot{V}O_{2max}$, they can exercise for much longer periods (Fig. 5).[12]

The effects of exercise training on the major determinants of myocardial oxygen consumption, $M\dot{V}O_2$, are shown in Figure 6. At submaximal workloads, the heart rate, systolic blood pressure, and rate-pressure product are significantly lower after a period of physical training than they are before conditioning. The $M\dot{V}O_2$ is therefore less at any given workload after training.[13] The physiologic benefits of physical conditioning resemble those of antianginal medications. Physical conditioning leads to a decrease in $M\dot{V}O_2$ by decreasing the determinants of heart rate and blood pressure; antianginal medications decrease $M\dot{V}O_2$ generally by decreasing heart rate, blood pressure, preload, and contractility. Collateral blood flow to the ischemic myocardium is also enhanced by physical training.

Certain investigators have raised concern over the deleterious effects of exercise on infarct remodeling.[14] Jugdutt and colleagues reported that a low-level exercise program starting 15

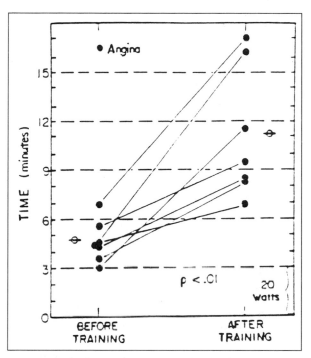

Figure 5. *Effect of training on exercise capacity. Closed circles indicate the time at which angina occurred; barred circles indicate mean values. Dashed lines represent the intervals at which the workload was increased by 20 watts. Reprinted with permission from Redwood DR, et al.[12]*

weeks after a moderate-sized anterior Q-wave MI led to significant exacerbation of left ventricular cavity distortion, an increase in asynergy, and a decrease in ejection fraction compared to the values for a group of nonrandomized control patients who did not exercise after infarction.[14] The authors suggested that exercise training might be deleterious in patients with an extensive transmural infarct that has not healed completely. This concern has been greatly alleviated, however, by the Exercise training in Anterior Myocardial Infarction (EAMI) Trial, a randomized trial of exercise training post-MI in patients with an ejection fraction <40%, which demonstrated that exercise training did not adversely affect the LV remodeling process in patients post-MI.[15]

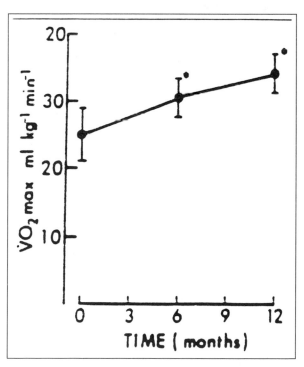

Figure 4. *Progressive increase in response to 12 months of high-intensity exercise training in patients with ischemic heart disease (P < .01) (trained vs untrained state). Reprinted with permission from Ehsani AA.[11]*

EFFECTS OF EXERCISE IN PATIENTS WITH CONGESTIVE HEART FAILURE

Exercise intolerance in patients with congestive heart failure (CHF) results from both central

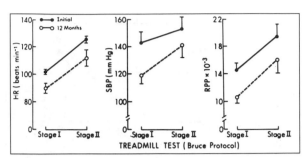

Figure 6. *Effects of endurance training on heart rate (HR), systolic blood pressure (SBP), and rate-pressure product (RPP) at absolute work rate (stages I and II of the Bruce protocol). All the variables after training (open circles) were significantly (P < 0.1) lower than those before training (circles). Reprinted with permission from Ehsani AA, et al.[13]*

hemodynamic and peripheral abnormalities.[3] Hemodynamically, patients with CHF have a reduced cardiac output response. Abnormalities in the autonomic nervous system contribute to this diminished response. Patients with CHF exhibit a reduced contractile and chronotropic response to catecholamines.[16] Thus, the fundamental control mechanisms of heart rate and contractility, which are both important determinants of cardiac output, are hyporesponsive in the failing heart. Augmentation in cardiac output due to the Starling mechanism may also be limited by diastolic dysfunction or pericardial constraint, and mitral regurgitation may additionally contribute to limiting exercise stoke volume in some patients.

As with normal patients, $\dot{V}O_{2max}$ relates in a linear fashion to both peak exercise cardiac output and peak exercise blood flow (Fig. 2). However, the decrease in exercise cardiac output results in decreased perfusion of working skeletal muscles and visceral organs, which in turn results in early anaerobic metabolism and fatigue. Congestive heart failure also leads to increases in pulmonary ventilation.[3] This rise relates to pulmonary hypoperfusion as evidenced by an inverse relationship between ventilation and cardiac output. Gas exchange is likely to be normal as arterial hypoxia does not occur during exercise in patients with CHF. In contrast to normal, patients with CHF demonstrate elevations in the pulmonary wedge pressure during exercise. This is accompanied by equalization with right-atrial pressure and therefore likely reflects pericardial restraint.

Thus, there are pulmonary, cardiac, and muscle metabolism derangements (the 3 determinants of peak exercise capacity) in heart failure.

Exercise training exerts a number of important beneficial effects in patients with heart failure. While training does not improve cardiac function, as evidenced by ejection fraction, baseline cardiac output, or wedge pressure, it does increase *peak* cardiac output and leg-blood flow. $\dot{M}VO_2$ becomes more efficient as similar external work can be performed at lower heart rate and rate-pressure products. Training also leads to decreases in minute ventilation and delayed anaerobic threshold (Fig. 7). Thus, all 3 determinants of peak exercise—pulmonary gas exchange, cardiac efficiency and skeletal muscle metabolism—are improved by exercise training. Finally, in patients with CHF, exercise training produces a reduction in sympathetic tone and an increase in vagal tone at rest, thereby restoring autonomic cardiovascular control towards normal.[17]

ORGANIZATION OF CARDIAC REHABILITATION

With this background of exercise physiology, the organization of the cardiac rehabilitation

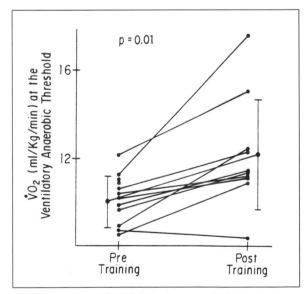

Figure 7. *Plot of individual changes in the ventilatory anaerobic threshold with exercise training in 12 patients with chronic heart failure. Reprinted with permission from Sullivan MJ, et al. Circulation. 1989;79:324-329.*

process can be considered. Cardiac rehabilitation involves all efforts designed to restore and maintain the cardiac patient at an optimal level of function, and attention is therefore directed toward the physiologic, psychosocial, educational, and vocational areas of rehabilitation. Although this review concentrates primarily on the physiologic aspects of cardiac rehabilitation, equally important to the cardiac patient are the nonphysiologic elements of rehabilitation—those elements that help restore the sense of well-being and optimism. Physical therapists, social workers, occupational therapists, and dietitians have a central role in the operation of a complete rehabilitation program.

STRUCTURE OF A FORMAL EXERCISE PROGRAM

The process of cardiac rehabilitation is generally separated into 3 phases. Phase I is the in-hospital phase, which begins during the patient's hospitalization for the acute cardiac event (MI or cardiac surgery). Patients qualify for their rehabilitation program only if they have had an uncomplicated hospital course and do not have recurrent angina, arrhythmias, or CHF. Phase II begins when the patient leaves the hospital, and continues for about 3 months. This is the hospital-based early outpatient rehabilitation phase and involves close medical supervision. Phase III is the maintenance rehabilitation phase that continues indefinitely and generally requires only intermittent supervision and safety checks.[18]

Rehabilitation for the patient with CHF should be reserved for those with chronic CHF once stabilization has been achieved with medical therapy. Full diagnostic evaluation should be considered as patients with certain acute cardiomyopathies such as viral myocarditis should *not* exercise due to their risk of sudden death.

The exercise tolerance test (ETT) provides the objective basis for serial determination of the patient's physical condition, as well as the safety monitor to ensure that a particular degree of activity can be performed safely. If the acute MI is uncomplicated, a low-level ETT is generally performed before hospital discharge. Usually, an arbitrary endpoint of completion of stage I of the modified Bruce protocol (5 METs) or achievement of a target heart rate of 130 beats/min is used to terminate the test. The

patient who tolerates this degree of exercise well is discharged and given an exercise prescription for phase II. After 1 month of phase II training for the post-MI patient, a maximal symptom-limited ETT is performed; if that is safely tolerated, the patient progresses to phase III of rehabilitation. Exercise tolerance tests are then performed at 6- and 12-month intervals to assess safety and the degree of conditioning.

In order for physical conditioning, defined as an increase in $\dot{V}O_{2max}$ or aerobic capacity, to take place, exercise must be of a certain intensity, duration, and frequency. To make the greatest improvement in aerobic capacity with minimal risk, 70%-80% of the maximal heart rate should be reached. The risk of complication from this degree of exercise is negligible. Exercise should generally last for 20-30 min at each workout. Workouts should be performed at least 3 times, and preferably 4 or 5 times, per week.

Sample recommendations for an exercise prescription for cardiac patients are shown in Table 1. During phase I the patient should exercise 2 or 3 times a day, with a target heart rate of about 20 beats/min over the resting rate. Physical activity should be closely supervised, especially during the period of acute hospitalization, to ensure that no untoward effects such as angina, arrhythmias, or congestive failure develop. Activity should last 5-20 min. During phase II the frequency and intensity of the exercise do not change, but the duration increases to 20-40 min. During phase III, in order to maximize conditioning, as noted earlier, exercise should be done 3-5 times/week, at a heart rate of 70% to 85% of the maximal predicted heart rate, for 30-60 min.

VALUE OF CARDIAC REHABILITATION

EFFECT OF CARDIAC REHABILITATION ON MORBIDITY AND MORTALITY

The long-term benefits of cardiac rehabilitation are controversial. It has been difficult to demonstrate mortality benefits for exercise training in individual trials due to small sample size and, often, inadequate compliance. O'Connor and colleagues performed an exhaustive meta-analysis of all randomized trials of cardiac rehabilitation after acute MI examining the effects of

	FREQUENCY	INTENSITY	DURATION (MIN)	MODE

Table 1. Guidelines for Exercise Prescription for Healthy Adults and Cardiac Patients

	FREQUENCY	INTENSITY	DURATION (MIN)	MODE
Healthy adult	3-5 times/wk	60%-80% $\dot{V}O_{2max}$	15-60	Aerobic activities, weights games
Angina	3-5 times/wk	70%-85% anginal threshold	15-60	Walk, jog, bike
MI/CABG				
Phase I	2-3 times/day	$HR_{rest}+20$	5-20	Range of motion, ambulation, stairs
Phase II	3-4 times/wk	$HR_{rest}+20$ or 50%-70% $\dot{V}O_{2max}$	15-60	Range of motion, walk, bike, arm ergometry
Phase III	3-4 times/wk	50%-80% $\dot{V}O_{2max}$	30-60	Range of motion, walk, jog, bike, swim, games, weights
PTCA	Same as phase III			
Transplants				
(outpatient)	3-4 times/wk	RPE 12-14	15-60	Range of motion, walk, bike, arm ergometry
Fixed HR pacemaker	3-4 times/wk	60%-80% systolic BP range	15-60	Walk, jog, bike, swim, games

BP=Blood pressure; CABG=Coronary artery bypass graft; HR=Heart rate; MI=Myocardial infarction; PTCA=Percutaneous transluminal coronary angioplasty; RPE=Relative perceived exertion. From Ward A, et al.[18] Reprinted with permission.

exercise training on recurrence of MI, total death rate, and cardiac death rate. In 4,554 patients, these investigators concluded that exercise significantly reduced the risk of death by 20% and reinfarction by 25% (Fig. 8).[19] The reduced risk of cardiovascular mortality and fatal MI persisted for at least 3 years after the index event, whereas a reduction in sudden death was noted for the first year after MI. No benefit was observed for nonfatal recurrent MI. Another large meta-analysis which used similar trials to those of O'Connor and coworkers reported a similar 24% reduction in total mortality and a 25% reduction for cardiovascular mortality.[20] The benefits of habitual exercise are further supported by the findings of Mittleman and colleagues for the Determinants of Myocardial infarction Onset Study. Interviews were conducted with patients soon after their MI to assess the relationship of heavy exercise with the incidence of MI. Among patients who usually exercised less than once a week, heavy exertion was associated with a relative risk of 107 (95% confidence interval 67-117) of MI. However, patients who exercised 5 or more times per week had a 50-fold less relative risk (2.4, 95% confidence interval 1.5-3.7). Thus, frequent exercise may actually protect against MIs associated with exertion.[21]

While some individual trials favor a program of structured exercise activities, none have demonstrated significant benefits. Perhaps the greatest difficulty has been achieving an adequate sample size. In the United States, the National Exercise and Heart Disease Project[22] was one of the most closely controlled and well-executed randomized studies of the effects of exercise in post-MI patients. The study was a 3-year, multicenter trial that randomized men to a supervised program or to routine post-MI care. In the intervention group, overall mortality was reduced by 37%, cardiovascular deaths by 29%, nonsudden cardiovascular deaths 56%, and all MIs by 24%. Despite enrollment of 651 subjects, none of the differences in the study achieved statistical significance. O'Connor and associates[19] have calculated that a trial would require 4,000 patients to reliably detect a 20% reduction in cardiovascular mortality. Prohibitive costs may prevent the performance of such a study.

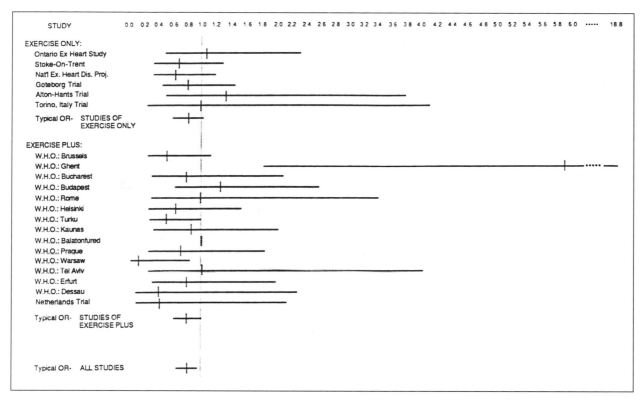

Figure 8. *Chart of effect of pooling from randomized trials of cardiac rehabiliation on the estimate of mortality 3 years after randomization. Short vertical lines indicate the point estimates; horizontal lines depict the 95% confidence intervals. Reprinted with permission from O'Connor GT, et al.[19]*

EFFECT OF CARDIAC REHABILITATION ON RISK FACTORS

The effect of exercise on cardiovascular risk factors represents an additional potential benefit of enhancing cardiorespiratory fitness. Chronic dynamic exercise alters serum lipoprotein levels, which may affect the atherosclerotic process. In patients with normal or elevated cholesterol levels, exercise training has little effect on total cholesterol (-0.5%), but increases high-density lipoprotein (HDL) by 8% and lowers triglyceride levels by 6%. In patients with hypertriglyceridemia, the effects of exercise are more marked: total cholesterol is reduced by about 7%, HDL is increased by about 23%, and triglycerides are reduced by about 37%.[23]

The multicenter Lipid Research Clinics North American Prevalence Study[24] indicated that strenuous exercise may increase protective plasma HDL levels. Although neither treadmill exercise test duration nor heart rate response to submaximal exercise was significantly related to HDL cholesterol levels, participants who report strenuous physical activity at home had higher HDL cholesterol levels than those who reported none. Although triglyceride levels decrease, they often decrease almost equally in the control groups. The significance of decreased triglyceride levels is unknown. The percentage of cigarette smokers is also lower in exercised than in nonexercised groups of post-MI patients, although in some studies more than a third of the exercising patients who continued to smoke claimed to have made substantial reductions in their cigarette consumption. Exercise has beneficial effects on hypertension. Martin and coworkers demonstrated that randomization to an exercise training program led to a significant and meaningful (approximately 10 mm Hg) reduction in diastolic blood pressure in patients with mild essential hypertension.[25] Although exercise itself may contribute relatively little to an improved risk-factor profile in coronary patients, other components of the cardiac rehabilitation program, including dietary modification, stress management, cessation of cigarette smoking, and close control of hypertension and hyperlipidemia may have a major impact on secondary prevention.

EFFECT OF CARDIAC REHABILITATION ON PSYCHOSOCIAL STATUS

The psychologic effects of exercise training are important to explore, since exercise rehabilitation programs may be justified if the patients' sense of well-being and employment activities are improved even if true physiological benefits cannot be documented. The psychological benefits of rehabilitation, however, do not appear to be major. For example, psychological factors seem to play a relatively minor role in whether coronary patients return to work. Most studies that have investigated the typical course of return to vocational functioning among coronary patients suggest that 80% generally resume their pre-illness level of activity. Psychological factors contribute only to a small degree. Oldridge and associates reported that randomization to an 8-week program of exercise conditioning and behavioral counseling failed to increase the percentage of patients returning to work at 1 year.[26] Other investigators estimate that psychological problems after MI are responsible for only 3% to 12% of patients not returning to work. Several investigations suggest that a program of physical exercise leads to a significant reduction in self-reported anxiety and, to a somewhat lesser degree, in depression. In the study of Oldridge and colleagues, a disease-specific, health-related Quality of Life Questionnaire detected statistically significant greater improvement in exercised patients' emotional function, confidence, and self-esteem at 8 weeks.[26] While the magnitude of this increase was very small and was no longer detected at 1-year follow-up, such improvements have the potential to increase motivation for further adherence to rehabilitation regimens and risk factor modification. In perhaps the best study of this type, Ibrahim and associates[27] investigated the effect of group psychotherapy on post-MI patients during the first 18 months after MI. Most patients were eager and faithful

participants in this type of rehabilitation program. The results suggested that patients receiving such therapy experienced less social alienation after MI than patients receiving no therapy. Patients receiving psychotherapy also showed a decrease in levels of competition and in an exaggerated sense of responsibility. However, such effects were short-lived, in that most of the post-MI patients returned to their pre-illness levels of stressful behavior within 6 months after the end of therapy. Many experienced investigators remain skeptical of the psychological benefits of cardiac rehabilitation. While almost all of the participants in training programs say that they feel better as a result of exercising, these changes are difficult to demonstrate objectively by formal psychological testing. In a few randomized controlled studies of psychosocial improvement during cardiac rehabilitation, the effect of exercise on well-being is unimpressive. Shepherd noted that after 12-15 months of rehabilitation, as many as a third of the cohort showed the neurotic triad on the Minnesota Multiphasic Personality Inventory, comprising high scores for hysteria and hypochondriasis and very high depression scores.[28] Over 4 years of rehabilitation, the investigators observed some favorable changes in those who complied with the prescribed exercise regimen. Gains were relatively small, however, even in those who trained themselves to the point of participating in marathon events. On the basis of the most recent studies, expected improvements in psychosocial well-being cannot justify enrollment in cardiac exercise rehabilitation after myocardial infarction.

RECOMMENDATION

Reports from both the Council on Clinical Cardiology of the American Heart Association[29] and the British Working Party on Cardiac Rehabilitation[30] have strongly endorsed efforts to expand cardiac rehabilitation services. Both organizations have concluded that the meta-analyses and studies supporting physiologic risk factor benefits justify exercise rehabilitation and ongoing life-style modification both for patients with cardiovascular disease as well as for healthy people. Exercise is increasingly being recognized for its benefits as primary prevention against CAD.[31]

SUMMARY

A long-term program of intensive physical training enables cardiac patients to perform more work with a decreased physiologic expenditure. Coronary patients can therefore perform their daily activities with fewer symptoms and less disability. Patients with heart failure also appear to derive great symptomatic benefits from exercise training. Recent studies and pooled analyses suggest that exercise may prolong life and decrease reinfarction in patients after MI, but the few controlled clinical trials of long-term exercise training, using relatively small sample sizes, do not support this concept. The effects of exercise itself on coronary risk factors are slight, but a more definitive program of cardiac rehabilitation, including dietary modification and control of hypertension and hyperlipidemia, may have a major impact on secondary prevention.

It is reasonable and appropriate to explain clearly the actual benefits and the limitations of cardiac rehabilitation to cardiac patients and to offer them the appropriate options. Cardiac rehabilitation programs may enable interested patients to live a more active, comfortable, and fruitful life.

ACKNOWLEDGMENT

We are grateful to Mr. John A. Loring for help in the preparation of the manuscript.

REFERENCES

1. Dennis C. Rehabilitation of Patients with Coronary Artery Disease. In: Braunwald E (ed). *Heart Disease, A Textbook of Cardiovascular Medicine*, 4th ed. W.B. Saunders; 1992:1382-1394.

2. McElroy PA, Janicki JS, Weber KT. Cardiopulmonary exercise testing in congestive heart failure. *Am J Cardiol.* 1988;62:35A-40A.

3. Sullivan MJ, Cobb FR. Central hemodynamic response to exercise in patients with chronic heart failure. *Chest.* 1992;101:340S-346S.

4. Mallory GK, White PD, Salcedo-Salgar J. The speed of healing of myocardial infarction: A study of the pathologic anatomy in 72 cases. *Am Heart J.* 1939;18:647-671.

5. Levine SA, Lown B. The "chair" treatment of acute coronary thrombosis. *Trans Assoc Am Physicians.* 1951;64:316-327.

6. Hellerstein HK, Ford AB. Rehabilitation of the cardiac patient. *JAMA.* 1957;164:225-231.

7. Saltin B, Blomqvist G, Mitchell JH, et al. Response to exercise after bed rest and after training. *Circulation.* 1968;38(suppl VII):VII1-VII78.

8. Feigl EO. Coronary Physiology. *Physiol Rev.* 1983; 63:1-205.

9. Casaburi R. Principles of exercise training. *Chest.* 1992;101:263S-267S.

10. Ades PA, Grunvald MH, Weiss RM, et al. Usefulness of myocardial ischemia as predictor of training effect in cardiac rehabilitation after acute myocardial infarction or coronary artery bypass grafting. *Am J Cardiol.* 1989;63:1032-1036.

11. Ehsani AA. Cardiovascular adaptations to endurance exercise training in ischemic heart disease. *Exer Sport Sci Rev.* 1987;15:53-66.

12. Redwood DR, Rosing DR, Epstein SE. Circulatory and symptomatic effects of physical training in patients with coronary artery disease and angina pectoris. *N Engl J Med.* 1972;286:959-965.

13. Ehsani AA, Martin WH, Heath GW, et al. Cardiac effects of prolonged and intense exercise training in patients with coronary artery disease. *Am J Cardiol.* 1982;50:246-254.

14. Jugdutt BI, Michorowski BL, Kappagoda CT. Exercise training after anterior Q-wave myocardial infarction: Importance of regional left ventricular function and topography. *J Am Coll Cardiol.* 1988;12:362-372.

15. Giannuzzi P, Temporelli PL, Tavazzi L, et al. EAMI— Exercise training in anterior myocardial infarction: An ongoing multicenter randomized study. Preliminary results on left ventricular function and remodeling. *Chest.* 1992;101:315S-321S.

16. Colucci WS. In vivo studies of myocardial beta-adrenergic receptor pharmacology in patients with congestive heart failure. *Circulation.* 1990;82(2 suppl):I44-I51.

17. Coats AJS. Exercise rehabilitation in chronic heart failure. *J Am Coll Cardiol.* 1993;22(suppl A):172A-177A.

18. Ward A, Molloy P, Rippe J. Exercise prescription guidelines for normal and cardiac populations. *Cardiol Clin.* 1987;5:197-210.

19. O'Connor GT, Buring JE, Yusuf S, et al. An overview of randomized trials of rehabilitation with exercise after myocardial infarction. *Circulation.* 1989;80:234-244.

20. Oldridge NB, Guyatt GH, Fischer ME, et al. Cardiac rehabilitation after myocardial infarction. Combined experience of randomized clinical trials. *JAMA.* 1988;260:945-950.

21. Mittleman MA, Maclure M, Tofler GH, et al, for the Determinants of Myocardial Infarction Onset Study Investigators. Triggering of acute myocardial infarction by heavy physical exertion. Protection against triggering by regular exertion. *N Engl J Med.* 1993;329:1677-1683.

22. Shaw LW. Effects of a prescribed supervised exercise program on mortality and cardiovascular morbidity in patients after a myocardial infarction. The National Exercise and Heart Disease Project. *Am J Cardiol.* 1980;48:39-46.

23. Superko HR, Hasell WH. The role of exercise training in the therapy of hyperlipoproteins. *Cardiol Clin.* 1987;5:285-310.

24. Goor R, Hosking JD, Dennis BH, et al. Nutrient intake

among selected North American populations in the Lipid Research Clinics Prevalence Study: Comparison of fat intake. *Am J Clin Nutrition.* 1985;41:299-311.

25. Martin JE, Dubbert PM, Cushman WC. Controlled trial of aerobic exercise in hypertension. *Circulation.* 1990;81:1560-1567.

26. Oldridge N, Guyatt G, Jones N, et al. Effects on quality of life with comprehensive rehabilitation after acute myocardial infarction. *Am J Cardiol.* 1991;67:1084-1089.

27. Ibrahim MA, Feldman JG, Sultz HA, et al. Management after myocardial infarction: A controlled trial of the effect of group psychotherapy. *Int J Psychiatric Med.* 1974;5:253-268.

28. Shepard J. Evaluation of earlier studies. In: Cohen LS, Mock MB, Rengqvist I (eds). *Physical Conditioning in Cardiovascular Rehabilitation.* New York: Wiley; 1981:271-288.

29. Fletcher GF, Blair SN, Blumenthal J, et al. Statement on Exercise. Benefits and Recommendations for Physical Activity Programs for All Americans. A Statement for Health Professionals by the Committee on Exercise and Cardiac Rehabilitation of the Council on Clinical Cardiology, American Heart Association. *Circulation.* 1992;86;340-344.

30. Horgan J, Bethell H, Carson P, et al. Working party report on cardiac rehabilitation. *Br Heart J.* 1992; 67:412-418.

31. Berlin JA, Colditz GA. A meta-analysis of physical activity in the prevention of coronary heart disease. *Am J Epidemiol.* 1990;132:612-628.

38 Cardiopulmonary Resuscitation

Richard Wright, MD

Although resuscitation has been attempted for thousands of years, only in the last century has it been performed with any measure of success. Despite reports of external chest compression and artificial ventilation in the late nineteenth century, open-chest cardiac massage was the standard mode of resuscitation until the value of external chest compression was redescribed in 1960.[1] Basic cardiopulmonary resuscitation (CPR) has changed little since then.

Each year more than 500,000 people in the United States suffer sudden cardiac death. Prompt institution of resuscitative efforts could save many of these lives. Reported success rates for CPR vary widely, from less than 2% in those with unwitnessed out of hospital cardiac arrests[2] to 90% in monitored patients with primary ventricular fibrillation. In general, the success rate is low among terminally ill patients and in those in whom the institution of resuscitation is delayed; the success rate is high in patients in whom primary ventricular fibrillation is rapidly identified and treated.

External chest compression and mouth-to-mouth ventilation are temporizing measures, designed to prevent irreversible ischemic deterioration while the patient awaits more definitive therapy. Although no absolute rules predict the outcome of resuscitation, the success rate declines rapidly if basic resuscitation is initiated beyond 4-5 min. If more advanced resuscitative efforts are delayed by 7-8 min, chances of survival are substantially lower. In certain causes of cardiac arrest, particularly hypothermia, these guidelines do not apply and patients may be successfully revived after much longer delays. In general, however, the duration of cardiac arrest is the most important predictor of successful resuscitation.

CAUSES OF CARDIAC ARREST

The most common causes of sudden cardiac death are ventricular tachycardia and ventricular fibrillation. Other tachyarrhythmias, such as atrial fibrillation in the patient with accelerated atrioventricular conduction, may occasionally cause sudden death. Bradyarrhythmias are less common precipitating events; complete heart block or sinus node dysfunction due to ischemia, hypothermia, hypoxia, drug effects, or hyperkalemia are the usual causes.

Other causes of sudden death include primary respiratory arrest; pulseless electrical activity or electromechanical dissociation (absence of effective mechanical systole despite persistent electrical complexes); and acute mechanical lesions, such as extensive acute myocardial infarction, massive pulmonary embolism, acute disruption of the cardiac valves or great vessels, pericardial tamponade, tension pneumothorax, and myocardial rupture. Regardless of the cause of cardiac arrest, the initial approach to the victim is the same.

MECHANISMS OF BLOOD FLOW DURING RESUSCITATION

The success of cardiopulmonary resuscitation depends in large part on achieving adequate blood flow to the heart and brain. External chest compression was initially described as "closed-chest cardiac massage." This term implied that resuscitation-induced blood flow was a result of the heart being squeezed between the sternum and spine, mimicking the action of internal cardiac compression and propelling blood by increasing intracardiac pressure above aortic pressure. Indeed such compression can be directly visualized during CPR in humans.[3]

However, observations and experiments cast doubt on the universal validity of this proposed mechanism and in some victims it is likely that cardiac output during sternal compression is due in part to an increase in intrathoracic pressure during each compression. According to this hypothesis, the heart may act as a conduit for blood flow rather than solely as a pump. When intrathoracic pressure is elevated by chest compression, blood is squeezed out of the thorax. Retrograde flow is prevented by the cardiac and systemic venous valves, and possibly by collapse of the systemic veins as they exit from the thorax. Thus as intrathoracic pressure rises, blood is forced from the lungs through the heart and into the aorta. As pressure on the sternum is released, blood flows back into the pulmonary vascular bed from the systemic veins. Flow from the aorta back into the left ventricle is prevented by the aortic valve.

Evidence for such a flow pattern was originally based on clinical observations. Coughing, which substantially increases intrathoracic pressure, was noted to generate remarkable cardiac output in the absence of cardiac systole;[4] in fact, repetitive coughing can maintain consciousness in humans with ventricular fibrillation. Attempts to duplicate the physiology of the cough, by increasing abdominal pressure (with binding, for example) and by inflating the lungs simultaneously with sternal compression, have resulted in demonstrable increases in forward blood flow during resuscitation. Circumferential chest compression with an inflated vest can successfully revive patients, presumably by cyclical increases in intrathoracic pressure.[5]

Hemodynamic and observational data also support a role for the "chest pump" hypothesis. Measured pressures in the great vessels and the intracardiac chambers can be equal during sternal compression;[6] if forward blood flow were due to direct squeezing of the heart, intracardiac pressures should exceed pressures elsewhere in the thorax. In addition, 2-dimensional and transesophageal echocardiography during sternal compression shows that some patients exhibit flow through open mitral and aortic valves during sternal compression.[7,8] However, with these same techniques there is also evidence

for direct cardiac compression, especially of the right ventricle, during resuscitation in most patients.[3,7,8] It is likely that both mechanisms of flow occur, perhaps related to variations in the victim's anatomy or in the CPR technique.

Supplemental maneuvers, such as abdominal binding and simultaneous lung inflation-chest compression, can further increase intrathoracic pressure and carotid blood flow during sternal compression. However, these techniques have not been shown to improve the success rate of resuscitation and cannot be recommended for general use. Interposed abdominal compression, in which external abdominal pressure is applied between chest compressions, has been shown to improve blood flow and initial, and perhaps long-term, outcome.[9,10] These beneficial effects are presumably related to abdominal aortic compression-counterpulsation and enhanced venous priming of the thorax. This promising technique warrants further study and standardization[11] before it can become recommended therapy.

TECHNIQUE OF CARDIOPULMONARY RESUSCITATION

The figure is a diagram of the process of resuscitation. These techniques have been described in greater detail by the Emergency Care Committee of the American Heart Association.[12]

VENTILATION

The precise need for and timing of the institution of artificial ventilation during CPR is controversial, as some investigators have described initial ventilatory support as being unnecessary.[13] Nevertheless, ventilation is important in longer resuscitative efforts as the amount of air movement during chest compression alone may be low. Once a patient is determined to have stopped breathing, a patent airway must be established. This is accomplished most quickly by placing the patient supine and tilting the head back while simultaneously pulling the jaw forward and opening the mouth slightly. These maneuvers preclude airway

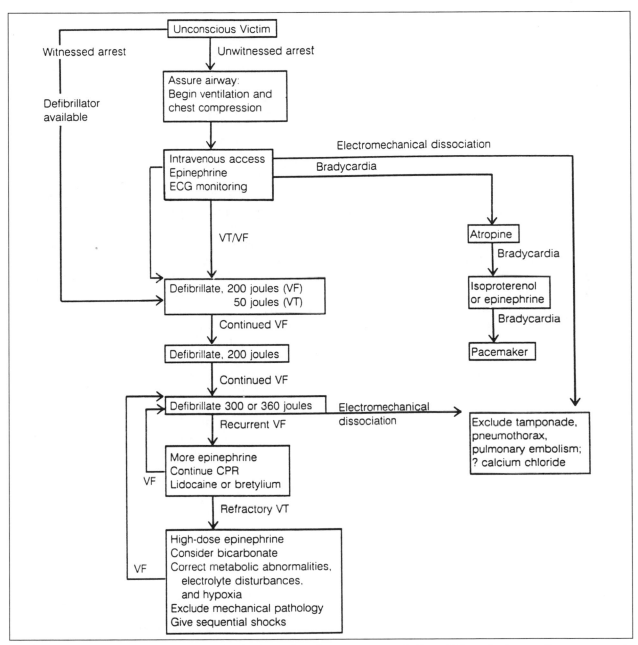

Figure. *The steps instituted during a typical cardiopulmonary resuscitation. If the electrocardiogram reveals ventricular tachycardia, a chest thump may be attempted. See text for further discussion of the use of the chest thump. See text for dosages and dosing intervals.*

obstruction by the tongue and allow inspection of the pharynx if ventilatory difficulties indicate upper airway obstruction. Ventilation at a rate of about 12 to 20 breaths/min can then be instituted. Adequate ventilation can be gauged by the presence of chest expansion and the sounds of the victim's exhalations. Mouth-to-mouth ventilation should be a temporizing measure, as the fractional inspired oxygen so administered is low (approximately 0.17) and hyperventilation is difficult to achieve. Therefore, the use of a respirator bag and a tight-fitting mask, esophageal airway, or endotracheal tube is necessary if initial attempts at restoring spontaneous ventilation are unsuccessful. Endotracheal intubation also provides a route for drug administration if intravenous cannulation is unavailable.

Hyperventilation is frequently necessary to compensate for the metabolic acidosis seen in patients with cardiac arrest. Arterial pH should be maintained at 7.30-7.45. Hypoxia is invariably present because of intrapulmonary shunting; therefore, 100% oxygen should always be administered. Use of high levels of oxygen for brief periods is not dangerous.

Arterial blood gas levels are often poor indicators of tissue acid-base status and oxygenation during resuscitation, but can be useful in assessing the adequacy of ventilation.[14] Mixed venous blood gas levels and end-tidal carbon dioxide levels are better measures of tissue perfusion.[15] This disparity is due to the poor cardiac output achieved during resuscitation. Such low flow leads to poor delivery of carbon dioxide to the lungs, with a resultant striking degree of hypercapnia and acidosis in the tissues and in venous blood. In such situations, arterial blood gases may give insufficient and potentially misleading information regarding the adequacy of tissue perfusion and may fail to indicate the severity of tissue ischemia. On the other hand, measurement of exhaled carbon dioxide is a useful gauge of cardiac output and tissue perfusion, as most carbon dioxide delivered to the lungs is readily transported to the airways.

Upper airway obstruction due to foreign body aspiration, as in the "cafe coronary" syndrome caused by aspiration of food, may be treated successfully by use of the Heimlich maneuver. The rescuer stands behind the victim with the fists clenched beneath the victim's xiphoid and delivers a swift thrust upward and inward. This usually drives the diaphragm up and expels the agent blocking the airway.

CIRCULATION

Adequate blood flow must be achieved simultaneously with or prior to restoration of effective ventilation. In the first minutes following cardiac arrest, artificial ventilation is less important than artificial circulation.[13]

Unfortunately, external chest compression usually produces only 25% or less of the normal cardiac output. This reduced output is directed predominantly cephalad and is often sufficient to perfuse the brain, at least temporarily. Myocardial perfusion is much less optimal. Coronary blood flow during resuscitation may be less than 10% of normal. Insufficient myocardial blood flow is frequently the cause of inability to achieve a stable cardiac rhythm. This suboptimal flow is due to the low diastolic blood pressure (and thus a poor driving force for coronary artery perfusion) attained during resuscitation.[16]

Proper chest compression is important for maximizing blood flow during resuscitation. The rescuer kneels or stands beside the victim and places his interlocked hands, 1 atop the other, on the lower half of the sternum. The exact position is not critical as long as the hands are above the xiphoid process (pressure on the xiphoid may result in ineffective thoracic compression). If sternal placement is impossible, positioning of the hands anywhere on the thorax can be effective; for example, 1 hand can be placed on each hemithorax. Each compression is accomplished by depressing the sternum 4-6 cm. This is most easily done by locking the elbows and leaning over the victim's chest, thereby transmitting the weight of the upper torso to the hands. A force of 70-120 pounds is usually needed. A firm surface beneath the patient makes the job easier and more effective, but successful compressions can be performed with a patient in bed, if necessary.

The optimal rate, force, and velocity of chest compression are controversial. Although early observers noted no significant change in blood flow with rates of 40-120 compressions/min, most reports indicate a rise in output over this range.[17] A rate of 80-120 compressions/min is thus recommended. The duration of compressions may be important: 50% to 60% "downtime" results in improved flow compared to briefer periods of compression during slow rates, but this variable may be less important at faster compression rates. "High impulse" compression, in which the velocity of initial chest compression is increased, may achieve higher blood flow and pressure. Chest compression force is also an important variable: increased force usually results in higher cardiac output.[11] Ventilation should be interposed at least every fourth or fifth compression; if a rescuer is alone, this pattern can be modified so that two ventilations are administered between every 12-15 compressions. In sum, a regimen of 80-120 forceful compressions per minute is recommended.

Recent trials have indicated that different compression techniques might result in more successful resuscitation. One of these methods alternates compression of the chest and abdomen.[9–11] Another employs a device akin to a toilet plunger, alternating sternal compression with thoracic suction, thereby potentially improving cardiac output and resuscitative outcome.[18–21] There is also evidence that use of a rapidly inflated vest to circumferentially compress the thorax may be more effective than standard sternal compression.[5] Widespread uses of these techniques awaits further study.

Open-chest cardiac massage results in demonstrably better cardiac output than sternal compression but is used infrequently. Nevertheless, it is potentially indicated in certain cases of penetrating cardiac trauma; in the postoperative cardiac surgical patient; in some mechanical lesions such as aortic stenosis; in the patient with a grossly unstable chest; and perhaps in some patients with prosthetic valves (external pressure applied over prosthetic valve rings may cause cardiac trauma during chest compression). The technique should be used only if a resuscitatible state was present just before the chest is opened. It is not typically helpful for patients who have failed to respond to prolonged CPR.

The precordial thump has a low success rate and therefore is no longer recommended in the unwitnessed arrest. It may be useful for the patient with witnessed ventricular tachycardia, in which a single thump may convert the patient to sinus rhythm, or with severe bradycardia, in which repetitive thumps may induce cardiac contractions. From a height of 20-30 cm above the victim's chest, the fleshy portion of the fist is used to deliver a swift blow to the midsternum. Conscious patients will not like this maneuver, and alternative modes of therapy, such as intravenous lidocaine for the patient with ventricular tachycardia, should be considered.

ELECTRICAL CARDIOVERSION AND DEFIBRILLATION

Direct current electrical defibrillation is by far the most useful element in successful resuscitation and should be employed as soon as possible. When instituted properly it has a very high success rate in terminating a variety of dysrhythmias. Unfortunately, even early defibrillation is of little help in out of hospital resuscitation if bystander CPR is not promptly instituted.[22] Defibrillators deliver a monophasic depolarization of several thousand volts over a period of about 0.01 seconds. The amount of energy delivered can be varied up to a maximum of 360 joules (watt-seconds).

The optimal power setting for external cardiac defibrillation has been debated. High-energy shocks result in increased electrical injury to the myocardium and a higher incidence of post-shock asystole and atrioventricular block. Current evidence indicates that 200 joules is sufficient for initial attempts at defibrillation; much less energy (10-50 joules) can be used for conversion of ventricular tachycardia.

The technique of defibrillation is straightforward. The machine is set to the desired energy level and the paddles are charged. Exact paddle placement is less critical than ensuring that adequate electrode paste (or saline pads) and firm paddle pressures are used, as these simple maneuvers will maximize the amount of energy delivered to the victim. One paddle is placed just below the right clavicle; the other is placed just lateral to the cardiac apex (or below the left scapula, when a flat posterior paddle is used). When everyone stands clear of the patient and the bed, the shock is delivered. Additional shocks of 200-360 joules are administered if needed, usually in prompt succession.

In the monitored patient with witnessed ventricular tachycardia or ventricular fibrillation, electrical therapy, if immediately available, must not await initiation of chest compression and ventilation. There is no reason to delay the delivery of the definitive treatment for these arrhythmias. In the unwitnessed arrest,

cardiopulmonary resuscitation and pharmacologic intervention are often used for 1-2 min
before countershock is attempted. This may
increase the likelihood of successful conversion;
however, even in an unwitnessed arrest, a
rapidly administered shock may be life-saving
and must be delivered as soon as possible.

Some patients have recovered even after
several hours of ventricular fibrillation and
cardiopulmonary resuscitation; therefore,
attempts at defibrillation should continue until
irreversible cardiac asystole appears. If several
attempts at defibrillation fail, more intensive
pharmacologic therapy, antiarrhythmic agents,
and closer attention to correction of metabolic
abnormalities may improve the likelihood of
subsequent defibrillation. Higher-energy shocks
spaced a few seconds apart occasionally are of
benefit, as the first shock lowers skin impedance
and allows a higher delivery of energy by the
second shock.

Prolonged asystole has the poorest prognosis
of any arrhythmia. Successful shocks have been
reported in cases of asystole, perhaps due to
external "pacing" of the heart via the delivered
energy, or in some cases to unrecognized
ventricular fibrillation. If asystole appears on
the electrocardiographic monitor, the monitor's
gain should be increased and the electrical leads
should be changed to obtain a configuration
perpendicular to the first lead. This ensures that
the tracing is not actually ventricular fibrillation,
which may be isoelectric in a particular lead.

PHARMACOLOGY OF RESUSCITATION

Effective restoration of circulation can often
depend on pharmacologic manipulation
(Table). Rapid placement of an intravenous line
is crucial. Any vein can be used but a vein above
the diaphragm is preferred. Blood flow during
chest compression may be preferentially
directed cephalad; infusion into the saphenous
or femoral veins may therefore result in delayed
entry of instilled medications into the central
circulation. If an arm vein is palpable, it should
be used. Frequently this is not possible due to
the marked venospasm that may accompany
cardiac arrest. In this situation, the external or
internal jugular vein should be cannulated. The

subclavian vein also may be used, but this
approach carries a higher incidence of potentially serious complications and the vein may be
difficult to cannulate while the patient is
undergoing chest compression.

If technical problems preclude rapid
intravenous access, epinephrine, atropine, and
lidocaine can be safely instilled into the
tracheobronchial tree via an endotracheal tube,
in doses equal to initial intravenous doses.
Sodium bicarbonate should not be instilled into
the lungs. Intraosseous infusion is another useful
alternative, especially in pediatric patients.

Except during open-chest massage, intracardiac injection of medications is indicated
only if another route of administration is
unavailable. Potentially serious complications of
this route include coronary artery laceration,
intramyocardial injection, and pericardial
tamponade. Epinephrine is inherently no more
effective when administered by the intracardiac
route. When intracardiac administration is
indicated, the subxiphoid approach is preferable to the parasternal approach.

Volume expansion with 1-2 liters of normal
saline or other volume expander is useful
during resuscitation in the volume-depleted
patient, but is not usually helpful in the
normovolemic patient.

EPINEPHRINE

The most important commonly used drug for
resuscitation is epinephrine. Experimental
evidence clearly shows that administration of
epinephrine enhances survival in cardiac arrest
in animals. The benefits of the drug have been
less apparent in human trials. Since epinephrine
has both α- and ß-adrenergic agonist activity, in
doses given during resuscitation it increases
both peripheral vascular tone (α effect) and
cardiac rate and contractility (ß effect). This
peripheral vasoconstriction results in higher
rates of successful restoration of circulation,
presumably due to augmented myocardial blood
flow resulting from an increase in diastolic
blood pressure. The ß-agonist effect of the drug
may actually be counterproductive, leading
some observers to recommend administration of
a ß-antagonist simultaneously with epinephrine.

DRUG	DOSE	ROUTE	MECHANISM OF ACTION	COMMENTS AND PRECAUTIONS
Epinephrine	≥ 1.0 mg every 5 min or continuous infusion (1 amp=1 mg)	IV, ET, IC	Increases blood pressure and heart rate	Drug of choice for resuscitation; inactivated by sodium bicarbonate
Sodium bicarbonate	After initial 5-10 min, 1 mEq/kg, then 0.5 mEq/kg as needed (1 amp=44.6 or 50 mEq)	IV	May help acidosis	May result in alkalemia, hypernatremia, hyper-osmolar state; inactivates epiniphrine; precipitates with calcium
Calcium chloride	250-1,000 mg (1 amp=1 g)	IV, IC	Increases contractility	Precise role undefined. Intracardiac injection may cause severe bradycardia; precipitates with bicarbonate; contraindicated in digitalis toxicity; may aggravate ischemic cellular injury
Atropine	0.5-1.0 mg every 5 min up to 3 mg	IV, ET, IC	May reverse bradycardia or heart block	Low doses may cause paradoxical bradycardia
Lidocaine	100-300 mg in 50-100 mg boluses; then 1-4 mg/min	IV	May prevent ventricular arrhythmias	High doses may cause central nervous system toxicity; can increase defibrillation threshold
Bretylium	5 mg/kg every 10 min up to 30 mg/kg; then 1-2 mg/min	IV	May prevent or convert ventricular fibrillation; lowers threshold for successful defibrillation	Can cause hypotension

Table. Drugs Frequently Used During Cardiopulmonary Resuscitation

IV=Intravenous; ET=Endotracheal route; IC=Intracardiac; amp=Ampule.

For this reason, purer α-agonists, such as methoxamine, phenylephrine, and norepinephrine, have been used but are less readily available than epinephrine. An α-adrenergic agonist should be administered if initial attempts at cardiac resuscitation are unsuccessful.

Epinephrine, 1 mg or more intravenously at least every 3-5 min throughout the remaining duration of the resuscitation or as a continuous infusion, is the usual choice. The optimal dose is unknown; doses 10-fold higher than this have improved survival rates in some animal studies but not in human trials.[23-25] Frequent administration is necessary due to the rapid metabolism of this drug. If intravenous access is unavailable, epinephrine should be given endotracheally by diluting the desired dose in 10 ml of fluid and instilling this into the endotracheal tube.

SODIUM BICARBONATE

Sodium bicarbonate is frequently used during resuscitation, but its precise role is unclear. Although it is valuable for the temporary correction of metabolic acidosis, premature or excessive use of this drug may result in hypernatremia, the hyperosmolar state, severe alkalemia, or excessive CO_2 production peripherally and centrally, thus potentially worsening intracellular and cerebral acidosis. These conditions can be dangerous and may preclude successful resuscitation. Sodium bicarbonate has not been shown to beneficially affect the outcome of resuscitation,[26] except perhaps in victims undergoing prolonged resuscitative efforts.[27] Therefore, this drug must be administered cautiously. In the witnessed arrest, it usually need not be given for the first 10 min of resuscitation if the patient is being adequately ventilated and metabolic acidosis did not precede the arrest. In the unwitnessed arrest and in the patient with known metabolic acidosis, correction of arterial acidosis may in part be accomplished by hyperventilation-induced hypocarbia. Sodium bicarbonate may still be necessary, usually at an initial dose of 1mEq/kg. Subsequent doses should be gauged by monitoring the bicarbonate concentration or base deficit. If blood gas determinations are unavailable, half of the initial dose can be administered empirically every 10-15 min until spontaneous circulation reappears. Sodium bicarbonate inactivates epinephrine and precipitates with calcium chloride; therefore, these drugs should not be administered concurrently through the same intravenous line.

CALCIUM

Although calcium is necessary for myocardial contraction, no data indicate that calcium salts are therapeutically useful in routine cardiac resuscitation. Studies have failed to demonstrate a beneficial effect of calcium administration for victims of asystole or electromechanical dissociation.[28] Calcium overload may aggravate postischemic cellular injury. Therefore it should not be given during normal CPR. Appropriate indications for calcium administration include hypocalcemia, such as after transfusion with large quantities of citrated blood, and hyperkalemia.

ATROPINE

The parasympatholytic drug atropine is occasionally useful in transiently reversing sinus bradycardia and high-degree atrioventricular block due to excessive vagal tone. It has little role in the initial stages of resuscitation unless bradycardia is identified as the initial rhythm, although in 1 animal model the drug enhanced recovery from electromechanical dissociation.[29] The usual dose is 0.5-1.0 mg every 5 min as needed, to a total of 3 mg. Smaller doses, 0.2 mg or less, should be avoided because they may cause a paradoxical increase in vagal tone.

ISOPROTERENOL

The pure ß-adrenergic agonist isoproterenol is sometimes used to increase the heart rate of patients who remain bradycardic despite atropine and in patients with complete heart block. The usual dose is 1-10 μg/min, titrated to the smallest dose capable of maintaining adequate heart rate. Epinephrine has similar chronotropic efficacy, but neither agent is as effective as artificial pacing for these patients.

ANTIARRHYTHMIC AND OTHER DRUGS

Antiarrhythmic agents can be valuable adjuncts in maintaining sinus rhythm after successful defibrillation. These drugs do not usually directly help to convert ventricular fibrillation to sinus rhythm. Therefore, antiarrhythmics need not be administered during the initial stage of resuscitation of the patient with ventricular fibrillation. If ventricular tachycardia or ventricular fibrillation is persistent or recurrent, the drug of choice is lidocaine (100 mg IV bolus and 50-100 mg IV every 5 min for two more doses to a total of 3 mg/kg, followed by a continuous infusion of 1-4 mg/min). Bretylium (5 mg/kg every 10 min if necessary, to a total dose of 30 mg/kg, followed by a continuous infusion at 1-2 mg/min, if needed) may lower the defibrillation threshold and is recommended in cases of lidocaine failure.

Morphine, ß-blockers, corticosteroids, diuretics, nitrates, and calcium-channel antagonists have no proven role in basic cardiac resuscitation.

MECHANICAL AND ELECTROMECHANICAL SUPPORT

Emergent use of a transcutaneous external pacemaker or placement of a pacing wire is often useful in the symptomatic bradycardic patient, but is unlikely to resuscitate the patient with terminal asystole. Transvenous pacers are preferable to transthoracic wires, as the latter are less often effective and can be associated with serious complications.

Mechanical devices to compress the sternum are effective when properly used and can administer external chest compression more reliably than manual compression. As previously discussed, active compression-decompression of the chest, and circumferential thoracic pneumatic vest inflation, may be more effective than sternal compression alone. Further trials of these devices are pending.

WHEN RESUSCITATION IS FAILING

When initial resuscitative efforts are unsuccessful at restoring spontaneous circulation within 25-30 min, usually little can be done to avert death.[30-32] Rarely, some of these victims can be saved—particularly if ventricular fibrillation persists. Ventilation may be ineffective, perhaps because of improper endotracheal tube placement or tension pneumothorax. Unreliable intravenous access could be a problem; during frenetic resuscitation efforts, subcutaneous

infiltration of an intravenous line may go unnoticed. Severe metabolic abnormalities, such as hyperkalemia, may be present. Volume depletion may be unsuspected and may need empiric treatment if suspicion warrants. Pericardial tamponade may be present; in such instances, pericardiocentesis may result in dramatic hemodynamic improvement. Emergency 2-dimensional or transesophageal echocardiography is extremely useful in these differential diagnoses. Resuscitation should not be abandoned until all potentially reversible causes are investigated, and should be continued until ventricular fibrillation is no longer present.

CEREBRAL PROTECTION AND RESUSCITATION

Despite successful cardiac resuscitation, some patients suffer severe and irreversible ischemic encephalopathy after cardiac arrest. This is due to long periods of cerebral ischemia and to delayed cranial reperfusion after successful restoration of spontaneous circulation. Despite early hopes for effective cerebral protection utilizing high-dose barbiturates, phenytoin, calcium-channel blockers, corticosteroids, anticoagulation, hypothermia, and a variety of other measures, there is little evidence that these interventions are beneficial after resuscitation. Further studies are needed before any regimen can be recommended for routine cerebral protection.

REFERENCES

1. Kouwenhoven WG, Jude JR, Knickerbocker GG. Closed-chest cardiac massage. *JAMA*. 1960;173:1064-1067.
2. Lombardi G, Gallagher EJ, Gennis P. Outcome of out-of-hospital cardiac arrest in New York City. *JAMA*. 1994;271:678-683.
3. Redberg RF, Tucker KJ, Cohen TJ, et al. Physiology of blood flow during cardiopulmonary resuscitation. *Circulation*. 1993;88:534-542.
4. Criley JM, Blaufuss A, Kissel GL. Cough-induced cardiac compression: self-administered form of cardiopulmonary resuscitation. *JAMA*. 1976;236:1246-1250.
5. Halperin HR, Tsitlik JE, Gelfand M, et al. A preliminary study of cardiopulmonary resuscitation by circumferential compression of the chest with use of a pneumatic vest. *N Engl J Med*. 1993;329:762-768.

6. Swenson RD, Weaver WD, Niskanen RA, et al. Hemodynamics in humans during conventional and experimental methods of cardiopulmonary resuscitation. *Circulation*. 1988;78:630-639.

7. Wright RF. Transesophageal echocardiography during cardio-pulmonary resuscitation in humans. *Circulation*. 1990;82(suppl III):III-483.

8. Porter TR, Ornato JP, Guard CS, et al. Transesophageal echocardiography to assess mitral valve function and flow during cardiopulmonary resuscitation. *Am J Cardiol*. 1992;70:1056-1060.

9. Sack JB, Kesselbrenner MB, Bregman D. Survival from in-hospital cardiac arrest with interposed abdominal counterpulsation during cardiopulmonary resuscitation. *JAMA*. 1992;267:379-385.

10. Sack JB, Kesselbrenner MB, Jarrad A. Interposed abdominal compression—cardiopulmonary resuscitation and resuscitation outcome during asystole and electromechanical dissociation. *Circulation*. 1992; 86:1692-1700.

11. Babbs CF. Interposed abdominal compression-cardiopulmonary resuscitation: Are we missing the mark in clinical trials? *Am Heart J*. 1993;126:1035-1041.

12. Emergency Cardiac Care Committee and Subcommittees, American Heart Association. Guidelines for cardiopulmonary resuscitation and emergency cardiac care. *JAMA*. 1992;268:2171-2302.

13. Berg RA, Kern KB, Sanders AB, et al. Bystander cardiopulmonary resuscitation—Is ventilation necessary? *Circulation*. 1993;88:1907-1915.

14. Adrogue HJ, Rashad MN, Gorin AB, et al. Assessing acid-base status in circulatory failure. *N Engl J Med*. 1989;320:1312-1316.

15. Falk JL, Rackow EC, Weil MH. End-tidal carbon dioxide concentration during cardiopulmonary resuscitation. *N Engl J Med*. 1988;318:607-611.

16. Paradis NA, Martin GB, Rivers EP, et al. Coronary perfusion pressure and the return of spontaneous circulation in human cardiopulmonary resuscitation. *JAMA*. 1990;263:1106-1113.

17. Feneley MP, Maier GW, Kern KB, et al. Influence of compression rate on initial success of resuscitation in dogs. *Circulation*. 1988;77:240-250.

18. Cohen TJ, Goldner BG, Maccaro PC, et al. A comparison of active compression-decompression cardiopulmonary resuscitation with standard cardiopulmonary resuscitation for cardiac arrests occurring in the hospital. *N Engl J Med*. 1993;329:1918-1921.

19. Lurie KG, Schultz JJ, Callaham ML, et al. Evaluation of active compression-decompression CPR in victims of out-of-hospital cardiac arrest. *JAMA*. 1994; 271:1405-1411.

20. Lindner KH, Pfenninger EG, Lurie KG, et al. Effects of active compression-decompression resuscitation on myocardial and cerebral blood flow in pigs. *Circulation*. 1993;88:1254-1263.

21. Tucker KJ, Redberg RF, Schiller NB, et al. Active compression-decompression resuscitation: Analysis of transmitral flow and left ventricular volume by transesophageal echocardiography in humans. *J Am Coll Cardiol*. 1993;22:1485-1493.

22. Kellermann AL, Hackman BB, Somes G, et al. Impact of first-responder defibrillation in an urban emergency medical services system. *JAMA*. 1993;270:1708-1713.

23. Stiell IG, Hebert PC, Weitzman BN, et al. High-dose epinephrine in adult cardiac arrest. *N Engl J Med*. 1992;327:1045-1050.

24. Brown CG, Martin DR, Pepe PE, et al. A comparison of standard-dose and high-dose epinephrine in cardiac arrest outside the hospital. *N Engl J Med*. 1992; 327:1051-1055.

25. Callaham M, Madsen CD, Barton CW, et al. A randomized clinical trial of high-dose epinephrine and norepinephrine vs standard-dose epinephrine in prehospital cardiac arrest. *JAMA*. 1992;268:2667-2672.

26. Guerci AD, Chandra N, Johnson E, et al. Failure of sodium bicarbonate to improve resuscitation from ventricular fibrillation in dogs. *Circulation*. 1986;74(suppl IV):IV-75–IV-79.

27. Federiuk CS, Sanders AB, Kern KB, et al. The effect of bicarbonate on resuscitation from cardiac arrest. *Ann Emerg Med*. 1991;20:1173-1177.

28. Thompson BM, Stueven HS, Tonsfeldt DJ, et al. Calcium: Limited indications, some danger. *Circulation*. 1986;74(suppl IV):IV-90–IV-93.

29. Blecic S, Chaskis C, Vincent J, et al. Atropine administration in experimental electromechanical dissociation. *Am J Emerg Med*. 1992;10:515-518.

30. Bonnin MJ, Pepe PE, Kimball KT, et al. Distinct criteria for termination of resuscitation in the out-of-hospital setting. *JAMA*. 1993;270:1457-1462.

31. Kellermann AL, Hackman BB, Somes G. Predicting the outcome of unsuccessful prehospital advanced cardiac life support. *JAMA*. 1993;270:1433-1436.

32. Rosenberg M, Wang C, Hoffman-Wilde S, et al. Results of cardiopulmonary resuscitation. Failure to predict survival in two community hospitals. *Arch Intern Med*. 1993;153:1370-1375.

39 Cardiology in a Changing Managed Care Environment

Richard Caso, MD

The continuing evolution of health care reform will lead to profound changes in the financing, delivery, and payment of health care. This chapter will present a historical overview of managed care, define important terms used in managed care contracts, provide a view of the future practice of cardiology, and discuss a number of strategies to allow cardiologists to position themselves to take advantage of these changes and to develop a successful practice.

HISTORICAL BACKGROUND

The Great Depression of the 1930s led to a number of major changes in the financing of health care. Patients could no longer afford to pay for hospital and medical care directly. This period ushered in the era of private insurance to pay for hospital care in a large and systematic scale. In late 1929, Baylor University Hospital in Dallas, Texas, agreed to provide up to 21 days of hospital coverage to 1,500 public school teachers for a monthly fee of 50 cents per subscriber.[1] Such was the modest beginning of Blue Cross. Strong opposition from organized medicine and state legislatures prohibited providing coverage for physicians' bills. To circumvent this prohibition, Blue Cross was instrumental in aiding the development of the Blue Shield plan to provide payment for physicians' fees. These plans facilitated the development of private employment-based insurance. The growth of workers' unions and their increasing negotiating power in the 1940s resulted in increased enrollment in the private insurance sector.

The 1930s also witnessed the development of pre-paid health care plans. In 1929 two physicians, Dr. Donald Ross and Dr. Clifford Loos, contracted to provide health care to workers and dependents of the Los Angeles Department of Water for a pre-paid fee.[1] This plan ultimately became Ross-Loos, a large regional health maintenance organization (HMO) in southern California (Ross-Loos was subsequently acquired by CIGNA, which was itself a merger of the Insurance Company of North America and Connecticut General Insurance Company).

Dr. Sidney Garfield, a surgeon in southern California, contracted to provide medical care to workers building an aqueduct across the desert to Los Angeles. He later contracted to provide care to Kaiser Steel foundry workers in Fontana, California. The plan was expanded to provide care to the foundry workers' dependents and ultimately led to the formation of the nation's largest HMO, Kaiser-Permanente.

Organized medicine marshaled considerable resources to oppose what it saw as a usurpation of its role in providing health care and formulating policy. Indeed, a number of medical societies expressly prohibited Kaiser physicians from becoming members. A number of hospitals made it nearly impossible for Kaiser physicians to join their medical staffs.

Despite the acrimonious debates in medical society meetings regarding pre-paid health care, the 3 decades between 1940 and 1970 were marked by relatively peaceful co-existence. Kaiser Hospital Foundation built a number of hospitals during this period, and the issue of medical staff privileges became moot. Organized medicine had become complacent and remained reactionary in its policies and outlook. This was the chink in the armor that proved to be its undoing.

FEDERAL HEALTH CARE LAWS

The Medicare and Medicaid (Medi-Cal in California) Act was signed into law by President

Lyndon B. Johnson on July 30, 1965. To appease the various factions, and to counter opposition from the American Medical Association, the debate was framed around the need of the elderly and the poor for adequate health care. These programs established the power and legitimacy of the federal government to fund and regulate healthcare.

Another major landmark in the health care arena was the HMO Act which was signed into law by President Richard M. Nixon in 1973. This act established the legitimacy of pre-paid health care and provided subsidies to health plans to foster their development. California has been in the vanguard of this revolution and today leads the country in the number of subscribers belonging to an HMO.

The implementation of the prospective payment system in 1983 further strengthened the federal government's prerogative to finance health care for Medicare recipients by paying hospitals based on diagnosis-related groups (DRGs). This method of payment provided for 267 diagnostic codes and assigned a specific reimbursement amount. Hospitals were placed at financial risk when providing care to Medicare patients.

These 3 laws signaled a major shift toward increasing federal government regulation and financing of health care and paved the way for the private insurance sector to assume an ever-expanding role in managed care.

MANAGED CARE

Managed care may be broadly defined as a methodologic approach to limit health care costs by controlling access to medical care by a system of gatekeeping, utilization review, and control of specialty referrals while maintaining acceptable standards of quality and patient satisfaction.

The present system of managed health care delivery represents a spectrum of different plans. Traditional indemnity insurance plans added managed care provisions to try to rein in escalating costs. These plans are administered by the large insurance carriers and reimburse or indemnify subscribers for private medical care after they have met a deductible or other co-payment insurance. A number of HMOs provide pre-paid health care to their subscribers through a staff model system in which the physicians are salaried and typically admit patients to HMO-owned or HMO-affiliated hospitals. Other HMOs operate under an Independent Practice Association (IPA) model in which the physicians contract to provide physician services to HMO members under a negotiated discounted fee-for-service or capitation arrangement. Under a' capitation arrangement, the individual IPA physician or IPA group receives a fixed dollar amount monthly based on the number of subscribers in a particular plan and calculated on a per-member per-month basis (PMPM). The IPA is a separate legal entity and may provide care to non-HMO patients. A variant of these HMOs is the group model HMO wherein the HMO contracts with a multispecialty physician group to provide healthcare to the HMO's members under a negotiated fee-for-service or capitated arrangement. In a captive group model HMO, the physicians provide care exclusively to the HMO's subscribers. An example of this model is the Kaiser Foundation Health Plan and its affiliated physician group, the Permanente Medical Group. The Kaiser Foundation Health Plan provides administrative and insurance services and contracts with the Permanente Medical Group physicians to provide medical and surgical care to Kaiser members. Preferred Provider Organizations (PPOs) represent a selected group of participating providers that provide health care services purchased by a large employer benefit plan or by an insurance carrier. Subscribers have a choice of obtaining medical care through the PPO plan or may elect to see non-PPO providers; however, they will have to pay a higher deductible and co-payment if they choose to see a nonparticipating provider. Exclusive Provider Organizations (EPOs) require that members receive all their health care services from the participating provider group. Exclusive Provider Organizations are, therefore, more restrictive than the closely related PPO plan. A relatively recent addition to these plans is the Point-of-Service (POS) plan that allows subscribers to decide at the time of service whether to use a plan provider or a non-plan provider. The POS feature requires subscribers to pay a higher out-of-pocket fee but gives them a choice of providers. Health maintenance organizations added this feature to try to remain competitive with other non-HMO plans. The triple option plan allows subscribers to decide annually whether to obtain their health care through the HMO, PPO, or indemnity plan. Under the triple option plan, the least expensive option with the most benefits and lowest co-payments and deductibles is the HMO option; the most expensive and with fewer benefits is the indemnity plan.

CONSOLIDATION AND MANPOWER

The continued growth of managed care will result in a dwindling number of subscribers in traditional indemnity plans. Indeed, it has been estimated that only 0.7% of the insured population in this country will be enrolled in a traditional nonmanaged indemnity plan by the end of this decade.[2] The indisputable fact is that future health care will be dominated by an ever-decreasing number of payers operating under a tightly managed corporate structure. The continuing consolidation of insurance carriers and health plans will complete the transformation of medical health care delivery from a cottage industry into big business. The traditional doctor-patient relationship will be changed and influenced by corporate guidelines defining access to medical care (gatekeeping), scope of service (benefit design), quality indicators (therapeutic outcomes, length of stay), and economic analysis.

The individual physician, particularly the specialist, will see a continual erosion of his/her patient base as increasing numbers of subscribers and large-employer groups shift to managed-care plans. Prior to the advent of managed care, physicians were selected by patients on the basis of quality, reputation, referral, or hospital affiliation. Physicians entering practice prior to the era of managed care were confident they could build a successful practice by dint of hard work and superior professional and interpersonal skills. This calculus no longer applies in areas with a large managed-care enrollment. The development of a new set of strategies and a willingness to cast aside an obsolete paradigm will be essential elements of a successful practice.

The inexorable move toward consolidation and regionalization of major cardiovascular services will result in a decreased pool of patients requiring interventional procedures in local community hospitals. There is no question that some areas are supersaturated with cardiovascular surgical programs. For example, the entire state of New York has about 27 cardiovascular surgical programs; California, by comparison, has 107 programs.[3] The manpower requirements for specialties will decrease under a fully-evolved managed-care system. The current physician-to-enrollee ratio for cardiology services under an HMO system is 0.6 per 20,000 enrollees; 3.4 per 120,000 enrollees; and 12.8 per 450,000 enrollees. These ratios are approximately 2.5 times less than the national average for non-HMO enrollees.[4]

To be sure, these statistics are based on a number of assumptions which may not be applicable to a non-HMO population. Most HMO enrollees tend to be younger and healthier and, therefore, require fewer services as a group. Moreover, the low HMO physician-to-enrollee ratios lead to decreased access to specialists as a result of the length of time required for an appointment, testing, and treatment. These delays are not as likely to occur in a non-HMO setting. However, these ratios are useful in arriving at a reasonable projection of future manpower requirements and in formulating private-sector policies to achieve a reasonable balance between physician supply and demand within a cost-containment framework.

Manpower issues will dominate health care policy debate because of the direct and inextricable link between the number of specialists and the use of specialty-specific procedures and their attendant costs. However, decreasing the number of trainees in specialty programs is clearly not the answer.

"It is neither feasible nor desirable to implement a public policy that reduces the training of new specialists so that even the best residency programs face extinction. The effects on the evolution of the specialties — the loss of succession and the power for renewal and scientific advancement that the presence of young physicians-in-training provide — would have a severe negative impact on the future of American medicine."[5]

Clearly, the issue of manpower allocation is fraught with philosophic and political dilemmas that will not be easily resolved.

Given these evolutionary and, in some areas, revolutionary changes in health care, several assumptions can be made about the future of cardiology. The most important, and one with the most far-reaching implications, is the continual trend toward consolidation and integration of health care services in the hospital and physician sectors. Of the approximately 5,300 hospitals in the nation, a significant number of them will close or merge. Cardiovascular services will be funneled to large tertiary-care hospitals through their satellite hospitals (spoke and hub concept). These satellite hospitals may offer diagnostic coronary arteriography depending on the expected volume of these procedures at each institution and their proximity to the hub hospital.

As mentioned earlier, the procedural case rates per thousand members will decrease under tight managed-care control. The number of interventional cardiologists that will be required to provide these services will decrease proportionately. A number of cardiologists currently performing interventional procedures will see their volume decrease and may have difficulty maintaining their credentialing to perform these procedures. To illustrate this point, the United States average for percutaneous transluminal coronary angioplasty (PTCA) procedures is 114/100,000 enrollees; the case rate for coronary artery bypass surgery is 105/100,000 enrollees. The respective case rate for Kaiser members is 38/100,000 and 67/100,000 enrollees. One potential strategy to prepare for this possibility is for cardiologists to join large multi-specialty groups or specialty IPAs to maintain a minimum volume of procedures. To be sure, some interventional cardiologists will probably stop performing interventional procedures and limit themselves to diagnostic procedures; some

cardiologists may limit their practice to consultative and noninvasive work. The emphasis on prevention will open new opportunities for these cardiologists. Indeed, a premium will be placed on cognitive as opposed to procedure-oriented services.

Established and newly-minted cardiologists will need to alter a mindset that links the performance of procedures with a tangible financial reward. This linkage will no longer obtain under the new reimbursement paradigm. Cardiologists and cardiovascular surgeons will be reimbursed through a global fee or by capitation. Under global reimbursement, a hospital or medical group will receive a lump sum for a procedure, such as coronary artery bypass surgery. Each specialist involved in the case (cardiologist, anesthesiologist, pulmonologist, cardiovascular surgeon) will be paid from this lump sum according to a pre-determined schedule. Under a capitated system of reimbursement, each specialist or specialty group will receive a fixed amount based on the number of lives (enrollees) in the plan. This latter system of reimbursement accomplishes 2 goals — it decreases the dollar value of procedures and breaks the linkage between the performance of a procedure and its extrinsic "reward." This notion is perhaps the most difficult to accept as it runs counter to the very essence of professionalism. Everyone needs a tangible reward for a job well done or a procedure expertly performed. This reward system is what impels most of us to spend years of rigorous study and training to become professionals. The managed-care philosophy seeks to separate the procedure from the reward to discourage the performance of procedures while encouraging a more conservative approach to health care.

THERAPEUTIC OUTCOMES RESEARCH

A significant component of managed care will address the issue of therapeutic efficacy and relate it to costs. If a particular procedure or test does not add incrementally to the outcome, it will probably be eliminated or modified. For example, an exercise nuclear treadmill stress test may not add any more to the management of a patient than would a regular treadmill stress test in a patient who did not show ischemic changes until at an advanced workload. Another example may be performing a PTCA in a small branch vessel. No one would argue too much with these 2 examples. However, what about the treatment of hypercholesterolemia? The results of large trials will take years before one can be conclusively sure whether patients with hypercholesterolemia and heart disease will derive benefit from aggressive treatment. In the meantime, most physicians will find it prudent to treat hypercholesterolemia.

One potential pitfall of therapeutic outcome analysis is in equating good outcomes with the appropriateness of a particular procedure.

"How well a procedure is performed is not a proxy for whether it needs to be performed. Whether a procedure is needed cannot be known from the characteristics of physicians or patients, but requires a clinical evaluation, and volume will not serve as a proxy for both using a procedure wisely and performing it well. If we do nothing to assess appropriateness, we could end by developing policies that improve the level of quality at which a procedure is performed but that lower population-based measures of health, because the wrong people are receiving the procedure, and thus the net health risk exceeds the benefit."[6]

Fortunately, managed-care plans are increasingly changing their focus from strictly cost to value. These plans are placing greater emphasis on perceived and actual quality of care. A key formula for success may be summarized as follows: **Quality + Cost = Value.**

ETHICAL DILEMMAS

The essence of managed care is based on a methodology of limiting access to specialty care through a system of primary-care gatekeepers who provide the bulk of health care and control access to specialty care. The gatekeeper concept has led to contentious debate on both sides of the issue. Viewed from a managed-care perspective, this system is necessary for the efficient and economic operation of a managed-care plan. Controlling access to specialty care, and the attendant procedures, saves the plan money.

On the other side of the debate are the specialists who view the gatekeepers as interlopers who have a vested interest in not referring patients in a timely fashion. Indeed, they contend that an egregious conflict of interest inheres in the very process of gatekeeping. The fewer the number of specialty referrals, the larger the year-end bonus from the specialty referral pool that will be returned to the primary-care physicians. In a non–managed-care setting, patients can obtain direct access to whichever specialist they deem necessary. Patients with chest pain, for example, can make an appointment with a cardiologist and be promptly seen.

When viewed from a broader perspective, limiting access to health care ensures that care will be appropriate to the condition. This, of course presupposes that the primary-care physician or gatekeeper has the breadth and depth of experience to adequately evaluate a symptom or constellation of symptoms in the broad area of medicine. This may be asking too much of the primary care physicians unless they receive additional training in a particular field. Indeed, specialty training was developed to produce physicians with the requisite skills required for the increasingly more complicated practice of medicine. Requiring primary-care physicians to assume a greater role in the care of patients with cardiovascular conditions carries with it an obligation that they be adequately trained to diagnose and treat a large spectrum of cardiovascular conditions and to promptly refer patients who require more specialized care. Cardiologists will need to work closely and collegially with primary-care physicians to provide quality care to patients with cardiovascular diseases.

A potential quality issue in a managed care system is the very real temptation to delay referring patients or not referring them at all to try to conserve the referral pool funds. No conscientious physician would knowingly do this, but the threshold for referral cannot be but influenced by the managed-care philosophy.

Another ethical issue, and one with profound and far-reaching implications, involves decisions of whether to provide or withhold expensive, experimental, or extensive treatment where the potential outcome may be marginal or futile, or where the patients are of advanced age. Bioethics, a relatively new branch of normative ethics, attempts to analyze the relationship and interdependency of developments in medicine and biologic sciences and provides a philosophic and moral framework for resolving complex issues of medical care. The discipline of bioethics will occupy a central role in articulating issues regarding the provision of expensive, experimental, or extensive treatment where the potential outcome may be marginal or futile, or where patients are of very advanced age. The resolution of these ethical issues will require that allocation of resources and limitation of care for futile cases or very advanced age be viewed from a broader ethical and socioeconomic perspective.

These ethical and moral obligations should likewise apply to health care organizations. They will have to be accountable to patients and physicians and not just to their shareholders. It is immoral and unethical to limit allocation of resources to improve profits while denying needed services.

> "One must be concerned about the potential for confusion between a form of organization that began with an ethic of cost-savings on beneficent grounds and a form of organization that saves money to pay dividends. Insofar as HMOs behave cost-effectively to hold down premiums and reduce the costs in the medical commons, the potential for conflict of interest was a conflict between two salutary moral ends: individual care and social wellbeing. The ethical justification for cost-savings at the margin is harder to sustain if the difference mainly boosts stock prices. As is the case elsewhere in medicine, the profit motive raises issues that no single instututition, HMO or otherwise, can address or solve. However the ethical legitimacy of the entire HMO industry is clearly at stake."[7]

FACING THE FUTURE

Continuing health care reform will forever alter the future practice of cardiology and cardiovascular surgery. Payers will increasingly demand elaborate and extensive practice management and therapeutic outcome data that will require a substantial investment in data acquisition systems and personnel. It will be economically unfeasible for individual or small group practices to develop such systems. One approach is to form large, highly-integrated, and tightly managed specialty groups. Cardiologists will practice in large, widely dispersed groups under a single administration and management structure. The individual cardiologists will be evaluated on the basis of clinical competence, procedural skills, interpersonal relations, and therapeutic and economic outcomes. Statistical models will be used to assess each cardiologist's or cardiovascular surgeon's clinical outcome variance. Physicians consistently falling outside a predetermined optimal variance will be required to obtain additional education and training to try to decrease this variance. Decreasing clinical variance improves outcomes and reduces costs.

It will become increasingly important for cardiovascular specialists to become thoroughly familiar with the concepts and techniques of managed care and to work within the system rather than try to oppose it.

CONCLUDING REMARKS

The ineluctable conclusion is that cardiologists will practice under a new paradigm of health care. The successful group will not cede control of specialty care but will take a strong and decisive role in defining practice parameters and formulating healthcare policy at a local, regional, and national level. These groups will manage change rather than be managed by it.

REFERENCES

1. Starr P. *The Social Transformation of American Medicine.* New York, NY: Basic Books; 1982.
2. The Health Forecasting Group. Cited by: Coile RC Jr, *Revolution.* Knoxville, TN: The Grand Rounds Press, Whittle Books; 1993.

3. *American Hospital Association Guide to the Health Care Field.* Chicago, IL: American Hospital Association; 1991.

4. Kronick R, Goodman DC, Wennberg J, et al. The Marketplace in Health Care Reform. *N Engl J Med.* 1993;328:148-152.

5. Wennberg J, Goodman DC, Nease RF, et al. *Finding Equilibrium in U.S. Phyician Supply.* 1993;Summer:89-103.

6. Brook RH, Park RE, Chassin MR, et al. Predicting the Appropriate Use of Carotid Endarterectomy, Upper Gastrointestinal Endoscopy, and Coronary Angiography. *N Engl J Med.* 1990;323:1173-1177.

7. Povar G, Moreno J. Hippocrates and the Health Maintenance Organization. *Ann Intern Med.* 1988; 109:419-424.

Index